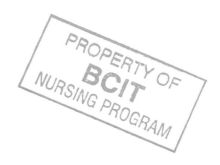

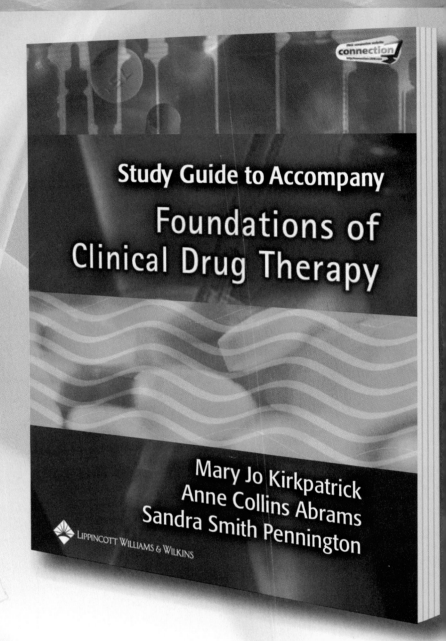
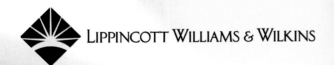

# Foundations of
# Clinical Drug Therapy

**Anne Collins Abrams,** RN, MSN

*Associate Professor, Emeritus*
*Department of Baccalaureate and Graduate Nursing*
*College of Health Sciences*
*Eastern Kentucky University*
*Richmond, Kentucky*


**Sandra Smith Pennington,** RN, PhD

*Associate Professor of Nursing*
*Berea College*
*Berea, Kentucky*

*and*

*Graduate Program Director*
*DSc Program in Nursing*
*Rocky Mountain University of Health Professions*
*Provo, Utah*

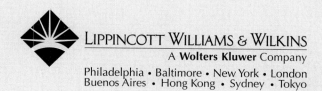

LIPPINCOTT WILLIAMS & WILKINS
A **Wolters Kluwer** Company

Philadelphia • Baltimore • New York • London
Buenos Aires • Hong Kong • Sydney • Tokyo

*Senior Acquisitions Editor:* Margaret Zuccarini
*Developmental Editor:* Megan Klim
*Editorial Assistant:* Carol DeVault
*Production Editor:* Danielle Michaely
*Director of Nursing Production:* Helen Ewan
*Art Director:* Carolyn O'Brien
*Senior Manufacturing Manager:* William Alberti
*Indexer:* Coughlin Indexing Services
*Compositor:* Circle Graphics
*Printer:* R. R. Donnelley-Willard

9 8 7 6 5 4 3 2 1

**Library of Congress Cataloging-in-Publication Data**

Abrams, Anne Collins.
    Foundations of Clinical Drug Therapy / Anne Collins Abrams, Sandra Smith Pennington.
        p. ; cm.
    Includes bibliographical references and index.
    ISBN 0-7817-4921-2 (alk. paper)
    1. Clinical pharmacology—Handbooks, manuals, etc. 2. Therapeutics—Handbooks, manuals, etc. 3. Nursing—Handbooks, manuals, etc. I. Pennington, Sandra Smith. II. Abrams, Anne Collins. Clinical drug therapy. III. Title.
    [DNLM: 1. Pharmaceutical Preparations—Handbooks. 2. Pharmaceutical Preparations—Nurses' Instruction. 3. Drug Therapy—Handbooks. 4. Drug Therapy—Nurses' Instruction. QV 39 A161f 2005]
RM125.A275 2005
615.5'8—dc22
                                                                        2004011367

LWW.com

# Reviewers

Marjorie L. Archer, MS, RNC, WHCNP
Vocational Nursing Coordinator
Health Sciences and Human Services Department
North Central Texas College
Gainesville, Texas

Elizabeth Arnold, RN, MSN, CNS
ADN Faculty of Nursing
Vernon College
Vernon, Texas

Mary C. Bielski
Clinical Education Coordinator, Nursing Faculty
Triton College
River Grove, Illinois

Diane M. Bligh, RN, MS, CNS
Associate Professor of Nursing
Front Range Community College
Westminster, Colorado

Kathy Bode, RN, BS, MS
Chair, Division of Health and Division of Technology
Flint Hills Technical College
Emporia, Kansas

Tori L. Canillas-Dufau, RN, MA, MS, MSEd
Mount St. Mary's College
Los Angeles, California

Donna W. Bohmfalk, MSN, RN
ADN Instructor
School of Nursing
Galveston College
Galveston, Texas

Suzanne H. Carpenter, MSN, RN
Associate Professor of Nursing
Our Lady of the Lake College
Baton Rouge, Louisiana

Gloria Coats, RN, MSN
Nursing Instructor
Modesto Junior College
Modesto, California

Laurel Danes-Webb, RN, MS, FNP, CDE
Professor
School of Nursing and Health
Hocking College
Nelsonville, Ohio

Cheryl Degraw, NP
Florence-Darlington Technical College
Florence, South Carolina

Carrin Dvorak
Assistant Professor of Nursing
Cuyahoga Community College
Cleveland, Ohio

Karen M. Fite, RN, MSN
Level I Coordinator, Professor
Calhoun Community College
Decatur, Alabama

Charlene Beach Gagliardi, RN, BSN, MSN
Instructor, Faculty, BSN Program
Mount Saint Mary's College
Los Angeles, California

Cathy Hansen, RN, MSN
Instructor
Blinn College
Bryan, Texas

Connie S. Heflin, MSN, RN
Professor, Associate Degree Nursing
West Kentucky Community and Technical College
Paducah, Kentucky

Lorraine T. Hester, MSN, RN
Nursing Instructor
Department of Nursing
San Antonio College
San Antonio, Texas

Karen Hill, RN, BS, MN, PhD
Associate Professor of Nursing
Southeastern Louisiana University
Hammond, Louisiana

**Immaculata Igbo, PhD, MSc, BSc**
Assistant Professor
College of Nursing
Prairie View A&M University
Houston, Texas

**Patricia A. Jones, RN, MSN**
Assistant Professor of Nursing
Pensacola Junior College
Pensacola, Florida

**Patricia Meehan Jones, RN, BSN, MSN**
Assistant Professor of Nursing
Pensacola Junior College
Pensacola, Florida

**Elsie Klish, MEd, MS, RN, ARNP-FNP**
Associate Professor of Nursing
Newman University
Wichita, Kansas

**Rose Knapp, RN, MSN, ACNP-C**
Part-time Clinical Associate Professor of Nursing
New York University
New York, New York

**Andrea Knesek, MSN, RN, BC**
Nursing Faculty
Macomb Community College
Clinton Township, Michigan

**Joan W. Kohl, MSN, RNC**
Nursing Instructor
Los Angeles County College of Nursing & Allied Health
Los Angeles, California

**Patricia A. Lange-Otsuka, EdD, MSN, APRN, BC**
Associate Professor of Nursing & Graduate Nursing
    Program Chair
Hawaii Pacific University
Kaneohe, Hawaii

**Patricia E. Lieveld, PharmD, MPH**
Instructor of Nursing
William Carey School of Nursing
New Orleans, Louisiana

**Elizabeth M. Long, RN, MSN, CGNP, CNS**
Nursing Instructor
Lamar University
Beaumont, Texas

**Pamela Y. Mahon, PhD, RN**
Associate Professor
Kingsborough Community College
Brooklyn, New York

**Karen Malloy, MSN, RN**
Department Chair, ADN Mobility Program
San Jacinto College South
Houston, Texas

**Karen S. March, MSN, RN, CCRN, APRN-BC**
Assistant Professor of Nursing
York College of Pennsylvania
York, Pennsylvania

**Darlene Mathis, RN, MSN, APRN-BC, NP-C, CRNP**
Assistant Professor, Family Nurse Practitioner
Samford University
Birmingham, Alabama

**Jeffrey C. McManemy, PhD, RN**
Associate Professor of Nursing & Program Coordinator
St. Louis Community College at Florissant Valley
St. Louis, Missouri

**Tara McMillan-Queen, AA, BSN, MN, ANP-C, GNP-C**
Faculty of Nursing
Mercy School of Nursing
Charlotte, North Carolina

**Lorraine P. McNeil**
Nursing Faculty
School of Nursing
Reading Community College
Reading, Pennsylvania

**Carol L. Moore, PhD, ARNP, BC**
Chairperson & Associate Professor of Nursing
Bethel College
North Newton, Kansas

**Kathleen Pickrell**
Associate Professor & Chair
School of Nursing
Indiana State University
Terre Haute, Indiana

**Laurie Robertson, APRN, BC**
Associate Professor of Nursing
North Harris Montgomery Community College
Conroe, Texas

**Patricia A. Roper, RN, MS**
Professor of Nursing
Columbus State Community College
Columbus, Ohio

**Sally P. Scavone, RN, BSN, MS**
Professor of Nursing
Erie Community College, City Campus
Buffalo, New York

**Barbara Steuble,** RN, MS
Assistant Professor, Nursing
Samuel Merritt College
Oakland, California

**Teryl M. Ward,** RN, MSN
Nursing Instructor
Modesto Junior College
Modesto, California

**Bonnie K. Webster,** RN, MS, BC
Nursing and Informatics Instructor
Health Occupations
Galveston College
Galveston, Texas

**Susan Wilkinson,** PhD, RN, CNS
Assistant Professor & Graduate Advisor
School of Nursing
Angelo State University
San Angelo, Texas

**Linda S. Williams,** MSN, RNBC
Professor of Nursing
Jackson Community College
Jackson, Mississippi

**Thomas Worms,** MSN, RN
Professor of Nursing
Truman College
Chicago, Illinois

# Acknowledgments

I dedicate this book to my family and friends for all their unconditional support.

To my husband, Everett, whose quiet strength, encouragement, humor, and love sustain me.

To my children, Jennifer and Brad, who prove to me on a daily basis that life is richer by being a mom.

To my dad, who has always believed in me; to Gary, Mary Beth, Jason, and Jeremy, for the countless hours of support and encouragement over the years; and to Leah, Matt, Laney, and Maddie and those on Cribbs Hill, who opened their arms and hearts and accepted me as one of them.

To my mother, Helen, and to my mother-in law, Gladys, who, from above, still give me strength and inspiration.

To Anne Abrams, whose energy and commitment to this project was invaluable, and to Margaret Zuccarini, Senior Acquisitions Editor, Megan Klim, Developmental Editor, and Carol DeVault, Editorial Assistant, at Lippincott Williams & Wilkins for their excellent editorial assistance and their encouragement and support when deadlines loomed large.

Sandra Pennington

# Preface

The overall success of *Clinical Drug Therapy: Rationales for Nursing Practice* has led to the development of this foundations text, benefiting students who do not need the extensive detail and scope of the larger book. *Foundations of Clinical Drug Therapy* builds on the same overall purpose as the parent text: promoting safe, effective, and rational drug therapy. In the tradition of *Clinical Drug Therapy: Rationales for Nursing Practice*, this text challenges students to rise to a more advanced level in their knowledge base.

Each chapter delivers current material in a concise, cohesive, and understandable manner. The text uses color highlighting, tables, and boxes to organize and emphasize important information throughout the text. The easy-to-read and easy-to-find format enhances the reader's comprehension of pharmacology. Some material from the parent text has been scaled down, while other information has been placed in appendices, thus presenting students with a manageable amount of content in a streamlined style.

## ORGANIZATIONAL FRAMEWORK

The content of *Foundations of Clinical Drug Therapy* is organized into 11 sections, predominantly by therapeutic drug groups and their effects on particular body systems. This approach supports the student's ability to make logical connections between major drug groups and the conditions for which they are used. The approach also provides a foundation for learning about new drugs, most of which fit into recognized groups.

The first section contains basic information and principles necessary for the learning, understanding, and application of drug knowledge to nursing practice. The chapters in this section present foundational information on drug names, classifications, and prototypes and provide strategies for studying pharmacology. Also included are discussions related to pharmacokinetic and pharmacodynamic processes, systems of weights and measures, methods of dosage calculation, and routes and methods of accurate drug administration. Guidelines for using the nursing process in drug therapy and general principles of drug therapy are also introduced.

The remaining drug sections are designed to facilitate understanding of drug effects on specific body systems, including the central and autonomic nervous systems and the endocrine, reproductive, hematopoietic, immune, respiratory, cardiovascular, and digestive systems. Other drug sections include nutritional support products, drugs used to manage weight control, and drugs used to treat infectious conditions. Chapters within each section emphasize therapeutic and functional classes of drugs, prototypical or commonly used individual drugs, drugs used to treat common disorders, and drugs most frequently encountered in the clinical setting. Herbal and dietary supplements with an emphasis on safety aspects are also included in selected chapters. Content within the chapters is presented in a consistent manner and includes a description of the condition(s) for which the drug group is used; a general description of the drug group (including mechanism[s] of action, indications for use, and contraindications); and descriptions and tables of individual drugs, including recommended dosages for adults and children and routes of administration.

## KEY FEATURES

Some of the most desired features of the seventh edition of *Clinical Drug Therapy: Rationales for Nursing Practice* have been preserved in this text:

- **Nursing Process** sections emphasize the importance of the nursing process in drug therapy. These sections walk students through assessment of the client's clinical condition in relation to the drug group, nursing diagnoses, expected outcomes, necessary interventions, and evaluation of the client's progress toward expected outcomes.
- **Nursing Actions** displays provide specific nursing responsibilities related to drug administration and client observation.
- **Client Teaching Guidelines** emphasize the importance of client teaching and summarize teaching points.
- **Critical Thinking Scenarios** encourage students to explore application of drug therapy in a clinical situation.
- **Drugs at a Glance Tables** provide quick reference to individual drugs and the recommended dosages for adults and children and routes of administration.
- **How Can You Avoid This Medication Error?** features give common drug errors and strategies for avoiding those errors.

*Foundations of Clinical Drug Therapy* retains many recurring features and themes of the parent text, which have prepared nursing students and experienced nurses alike by presenting current drug information and by integrating the nursing process throughout. This text incorporates continuing trends in drug dosage formulations, including a number of fixed-dose combination drug products, long-acting preparations, and nasal or oral inhalation products. In addition, this text includes several unique features:

- **Prototype Profiles** emphasize key features of common prototypes, including the therapeutic considerations, pharmacokinetics, pharmacodynamics, contraindications, precautions, adverse effects, pregnancy considerations, dosages, drug interactions, and herbal supplements and dietary considerations.
- **At the Foundation** boxes facilitate understanding of drug effects by underscoring the essential physiology underlying the clinical conditions.
- **Home Care Considerations** focus on assessing, monitoring, and educating clients in the home setting.
- **Age-related Considerations** emphasize the special drug therapy considerations for children and older adults.

- **Critical Thinking Exercises** at the end of each chapter use **NCLEX-style questions** to promote self-testing of chapter content, challenge critical thinking, and reinforce the chapter objectives.
- **Pregnancy Categories** for all drugs are identified in the drug tables, and an appendix outlining **potential drug interactions with grapefruit juice** is included.

## TEACHING–LEARNING PACKAGE

*Foundations of Clinical Drug Therapy* has an extensive ancillary package, designed with both the student and instructor in mind. A *Study Guide* reinforces key information, allows the student to apply knowledge, and provides a means of self-evaluation. The *Student Resource CD-ROM* included with the book presents additional learning activities, including **dosage calculation exercises** for each chapter. The *Instructor's Resource CD-ROM* provides tools designed to facilitate teaching and learning. The *Connection Web site* contains supplemental information for both instructors and students.

*Anne Collins Abrams, RN, MSN*
*Sandra Smith Pennington, RN, PhD*

# *How to Use*

# Foundations of Clinical Drug Therapy

**Chapter openers** include Objectives and Critical Thinking Scenarios. Objectives guide students by providing the key points and concepts in the chapter. Critical Thinking Scenarios ask students to apply their knowledge in real world situations.

### OBJECTIVES

*After studying this chapter, the student will be able to:*

1 Describe general characteristics of central nervous system (CNS) stimulant drugs.
2 Discuss reasons for decreased use of amphetamines for therapeutic purposes.
3 Give the rationale for treating attention deficit-hyperactivity disorder with CNS stimulant drugs.
4 List effects and sources of caffeine.
5 Identify nursing interventions to prevent, recognize, and treat stimulant overdose.

### CRITICAL THINKING SCENARIO

*M*rs. Williams comes to your office with her 6-year-old son, Tom. She complains that he is a very active child who always seems to be getting into mischief. She likes a clean, orderly house, and he likes to make messes. He seems to be doing okay in school, although she would like to see his grades improve. She was talking to a neighbor, who encouraged her to talk with a health care provider about prescribing Ritalin, because her son may have attention deficit-hyperactivity disorder (ADHD).

✔ What advice would you have for Mrs. Williams?
✔ Identify possible therapeutic effects of prescribing Ritalin if the boy has ADHD.
✔ What are the possible negative effects of giving Tom Ritalin if he does not have ADHD?

**Nursing Process** displays help students think about drug therapy in terms of the nursing process.

### *N*URSING PROCESS

**Assessment**

Assess for muscle spasm and spasticity.
• With muscle spasm, assess for:
  • **Pain.** This is a prominent symptom of muscle spasm and is usually aggravated by movement. Try to determine the location as specifically as possible, as well as the intensity, duration, and precipitating factors (eg, traumatic injury, strenuous exercise).
  • **Accompanying signs and symptoms,** such as bruises (ecchymoses), edema, or signs of inflammation (redness, heat, edema, tenderness to touch)
• With spasticity, assess for pain and impaired functional ability in self-care (eg, eating, dressing). In addition, severe spasticity interferes with ambulation and other movement as well as exercises to maintain joint and muscle mobility.

**Nursing Diagnoses**

• Pain related to muscle spasm
• Impaired Physical Mobility related to spasm and pain
• Bathing/Hygiene Self-Care Deficit related to spasm and pain
• Deficient Knowledge: Nondrug measures to relieve muscle spasm, pain, and spasticity and safe usage of skeletal muscle relaxants
• Risk for Injury: Dizziness, sedation related to CNS depression

**Planning/Goals**

*The client will:*
• Experience relief of pain and spasm
• Experience improved motor function
• Increase self-care abilities in activities of daily living
• Take medications as instructed
• Use nondrug measures appropriately
• Be safeguarded when sedated from drug therapy

**Interventions**

Use adjunctive measures for muscle spasm and spasticity:

• Physical therapy (massage, moist heat, exercises)
• Bed rest for acute muscle spasm
• Relaxation techniques
• Correct posture and lifting techniques (eg, stooping rather than bending to lift objects, holding heavy objects close to the body, *not* lifting excessive amounts of weight)
• Regular exercise and use of warm-up exercises. Strenuous exercise performed on an occasional basis (eg, weekly or monthly) is more likely to cause acute muscle spasm.

**Evaluation**

• Interview and observe for relief of symptoms.
• Interview and observe regarding correct usage of medications and nondrug therapeutic measures.

**Drugs at a Glance** tables present "need to know" information about various drugs. The tables highlight drug routes, dosage ranges, and pregnancy categories.

**DRUG TABLE 6-2**

*Drugs at a Glance*

**Narcotic Antagonists (Antidotes)**

| Generic/Trade Name | Routes and Dosage Ranges | Comments |
|---|---|---|
| **Nalmefene** (Revex) Pregnancy Category B | Reversal of postoperative narcotic depression: (*blue label*, 1-mL ampules containing 100 mcg/L) IV according to body weight (50 kg, 0.125 mL; 60 kg, 0.15 mL; 70 kg, 0.175 mL; 80 kg, 0.2 mL; 90 kg, 0.225 mL; 100 kg, 0.25 mL) Treatment of overdose: (*green label*, 2-mL ampules containing 1 mg/mL) IV 0.5 mg/70 kg as initial dose for clients who are not narcotic dependent, followed by 1 mg/70 kg in 2–5 min if necessary. For known or suspected narcotic-dependent people, give a test dose of 0.1 mg/70 kg. If no signs of opiate withdrawal occur within 2 min, proceed with the above dosage. | Has a longer duration of action than naloxone May be preferred when narcotic depression results from long-acting drugs (eg, methadone) **Warning:** Nalmefene is available in two concentrations: one for postoperative use (*blue label*) and one for treatment of clients with opiate overdoses (*green label*). Health care personnel *must* use the appropriate concentration for the intended purpose. |
| **Naloxone** (Narcan) Pregnancy Category B | *Adults:* Overdose, IV 0.4–2 mg, repeat q2–3min PRN Give IM or Sub-Q, if unable to give IV Postoperative reversal, IV 0.1–0.2 mg q2–3min until desired level of reversal is attained *Children:* IV 0.01 mg/kg initially, repeated q2–3min PRN. Give IM or Sub-Q, if unable to give IV | Usually the drug of choice for treatment of narcotic overdose Therapeutic effects occur in minutes after injection and last 1–2 h Has a shorter duration of action than most narcotics, so repeat injections are usually needed (up to 2–3 d with methadone) Causes few adverse effects, and repeated doses can be given safely |
| **Naltrexone** (ReVia) Pregnancy Category B | PO, 50 mg/day | Clients taking this drug do not respond to narcotic analgesics if pain control is needed Used in the maintenance of opiate-free states in opiate addicts Recommended for use in conjunction with psychological and social counseling |

**Nursing Actions** displays instruct students in drug administration of a particular drug group and include rationales for each step.

## Nursing Actions
### Central Nervous System Stimulants

| Nursing Actions | Rationale/Explanation |
|---|---|
| 1. Administer accurately. | |
| a. Give amphetamines and methylphenidate early in the day, at least 6 hours before bedtime. | To avoid interference with sleep. If insomnia occurs, give the last dose of the day at an earlier time or decrease the dose. |
| b. For children with attention deficit-hyperactivity disorder (ADHD), give amphetamines and methylphenidate about 30 minutes before meals. | To minimize the drugs' appetite-suppressing effects and risks of interference with nutrition and growth. |
| c. Do not crush or open and instruct clients not to bite or chew long-acting forms of methylphenidate (Concerta, Metadate CD, Metadate ER, Ritalin SR). | Breaking the tablets or capsules destroys the extended-release feature and allows the drug to be absorbed faster. An overdose may result. |
| 2. Observe for therapeutic effects. | Therapeutic effects depend on the reason for use. |
| a. Fewer "sleep attacks" with narcolepsy | |
| b. Improved behavior and performance of cognitive and psychomotor tasks with ADHD | |
| c. Increased mental alertness and decreased fatigue | |
| 3. Observe for adverse effects. | Adverse effects may occur with acute or chronic ingestion of any CNS stimulant drugs. |
| a. Excessive central nervous system (CNS) stimulation—hyperactivity, nervousness, insomnia, anxiety, tremors, convulsions, psychotic behavior | These reactions are more likely to occur with large doses. |
| b. Cardiovascular effects—tachycardia, other dysrhythmias, hypertension | These reactions are caused by the sympathomimetic effects of the drugs. |
| c. Gastrointestinal effects—anorexia, gastritis, weight loss, nausea, diarrhea, constipation | |
| 4. Observe for drug interactions. | |
| a. Drugs that *increase* the effects of CNS stimulants: | |
| (1) Other CNS stimulant drugs | Such combinations are potentially dangerous and should be avoided or minimized. |
| (2) Albuterol and related antiasthmatic drugs, pseudoephedrine | These drugs cause CNS and cardiac stimulating effects. |
| b. Drugs that *decrease* effects of CNS stimulants: | |
| (1) CNS depressants | IV diazepam or lorazepam may be used to decrease agitation, hyperactivity, and seizures occurring with stimulant overdose. |
| c. Drugs that *increase* effects of amphetamines: | |
| (1) Alkalinizing agents (eg, antacids) | Drugs that increase the alkalinity of the gastrointestinal tract increase intestinal absorption of amphetamines, and urinary alkalinizers decrease urinary excretion. Increased absorption and decreased excretion serve to potentiate drug effects. |
| (2) Monoamine oxidase (MAO) inhibitors | Potentiate amphetamines by slowing drug metabolism. These drugs thereby increase the risks of headache, subarachnoid hemorrhage, and other signs of a hypertensive crisis. The combination may cause death and should be avoided. |
| d. Drugs that *decrease* effects of amphetamines: | |
| (1) Acidifying agents | Urinary acidifying agents (eg, ammonium chloride) increase urinary excretion and lower blood levels of amphetamines. Decreased absorption and increased excretion serve to decrease drug effects. |

*(continued)*

**How Can You Avoid This Medication Error?** exercises present common mistakes and strategies for avoiding them.

 **How Can You Avoid this Medication Error?**

You are working in a clinic when a patient has a sudden, severe episode of laryngeal edema and hypotension. The physician shouts an order for epinephrine 0.1 mg IV stat. Your stock supply provides epinephrine 1 mg/mL. You draw up 1 mL into a syringe and hand it to the physician for IV administration.

 **How Can You Avoid this Medication Error?**

**Answer:** In this situation, the wrong dose of epinephrine, which could be lethal, is being administered to the patient. IV epinephrine must be diluted to a concentration of 1 : 10,000 (0.1 mg/mL). In an emergency situation, it is easy to pick up the concentration of epinephrine that is intended for intramuscular or subcutaneous use. Labeling on these preparations should include "Not for IV Use" because there is not time to calculate dosage and dilute the solution in an emergency.

**Prototype Profiles** allow students to quickly review important characteristics of a representative drug.

### PROTOTYPE PROFILE 7-1
**P Aspirin** (AS pir in)

**Drug Class**
*Chemical:* Salicylate
*Functional:* Analgesic, anti-inflammatory, antipyretic, platelet aggregation inhibitor

**Trade Names**
Ascriptin, Bayer aspirin, Bufferin, Ecotrin, and others

**Therapeutic Indications**
Treatment of mild to moderate pain, inflammation and fever, prophylaxis of myocardial infarction, stroke and/or transient ischemic episodes, rheumatic fever, management of rheumatoid arthritis (RA), osteoarthritis (OA), and gout

**Pharmacokinetics**
*Absorption*
Well absorbed after oral administration.
*Distribution*
Plasma protein binding: 59%–90%; crosses placenta
*Metabolism*
Hydrolyzed to salicylate, which is metabolized in the liver
*Excretion*
Urine
In alkaline urine (eg, pH of 8), renal excretion of salicylate is greatly increased.

**Pharmacodynamics**
*Onset of Action*
PO: 15–30 minutes; rectal 1–2 hours
*Duration*
4–6 hours

**Contraindications/Precautions**
Hypersensitivity to salicylates, other NSAIDs, inherited or acquired bleeding disorders; third trimester of pregnancy
Should not be used in children <16 years of age owing to association with Reye's disease

**Pregnancy Considerations**
Category: C/D (full dose aspirin in third trimester by expert analysis)
Enters breast milk, use with caution

**Dosage**
*Adults*
Pain, fever: PO, 325–650 mg q4h PRN
Arthritis (OA, RA): PO, 2–6 g/d in divided doses
Prophylaxis of myocardial infarction, transient ischemic attacks (TIAs), and stroke: PO, 81–325 mg/d
TIAs: PO, 1300 mg/d in divided doses
Acute rheumatic fever: PO, 5–8 g/d in divided doses
*Children*
Pain, fever: PO, 10–15 mg/kg mg q4h PRN, up to 60–80 mg/kg/d
Recommended doses for weight: 24–35 lb, 162 mg; 36–47 lb, 243 mg; 48–59 lb, 324 mg; 60–71 lb, 405 mg; 72–95 lb, 486 mg; 96 lb or above, 648 mg
Juvenile rheumatoid arthritis: PO, 60–110 mg/kg/d in divided doses q6–8 h
Acute rheumatic fever: PO, 100 mg/kg/d in divided doses, for 2 weeks, then 75 mg/kg/d for 4 to 6 weeks

**Adverse Effects**
Bleeding, tinnitus; gastric irritation

**Drug Interactions**
*Increased Effects*
Adverse effects with NSAIDs
Risk for bleeding with oral anticoagulants and antiplatelet drugs
Methotrexate and valproic acid levels
*Decreased Effects*
Effect of ACE inhibitors (with high doses of aspirin), beta blockers, thiazide and loop diuretics, probenecid

**Herbal Supplements and Dietary Considerations**
Avoid dong quai, cat's claw, feverfew, garlic, ginger, ginkgo, red clover, green tea, ginseng
Curry powder, licorice, paprika contain 6 mg salicylate in 100 g
Food may decrease the rate but not the extent of absorption
Prunes, raisins, tea, gherkins, and Benedictine liqueur may increase risk for salicylate accumulation

**Client Teaching Guidelines** reinforce the importance of client teaching and summarize key teaching points for a particular drug or drug group.

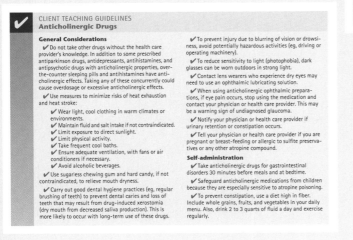

### CLIENT TEACHING GUIDELINES
### Anticholinergic Drugs

**General Considerations**
✔ Do not take other drugs without the health care provider's knowledge. In addition to some prescribed antiparkinson drugs, antidepressants, antihistamines, and antipsychotic drugs with anticholinergic properties, over-the-counter sleeping pills and antihistamines have anticholinergic effects. Taking any of these concurrently could cause overdosage or excessive anticholinergic effects.

✔ Use measures to minimize risks of heat exhaustion and heat stroke:
  ✔ Wear light, cool clothing in warm climates or environments.
  ✔ Maintain fluid and salt intake if not contraindicated.
  ✔ Limit exposure to direct sunlight.
  ✔ Limit physical activity.
  ✔ Take frequent cool baths.
  ✔ Ensure adequate ventilation, with fans or air conditioners if necessary.
  ✔ Avoid alcoholic beverages.

✔ Use sugarless chewing gum and hard candy, if not contraindicated, to relieve mouth dryness.

✔ Carry out good dental hygiene practices (eg, regular brushing of teeth) to prevent dental caries and loss of teeth that may result from drug-induced xerostomia (dry mouth from decreased saliva production). This is more likely to occur with long-term use of these drugs.

✔ To prevent injury due to blurring of vision or drowsiness, avoid potentially hazardous activities (eg, driving or operating machinery).

✔ To reduce sensitivity to light (photophobia), dark glasses can be worn outdoors in strong light.

✔ Contact lens wearers who experience dry eyes may need to use an ophthalmic lubricating solution.

✔ When using anticholinergic ophthalmic preparations, if eye pain occurs, stop using the medication and contact your physician or health care provider. This may be a warning sign of undiagnosed glaucoma.

✔ Notify your physician or health care provider if urinary retention or constipation occurs.

✔ Tell your physician or health care provider if you are pregnant or breast-feeding or allergic to sulfite preservatives or any other atropine compound.

**Self-administration**
✔ Take anticholinergic drugs for gastrointestinal disorders 30 minutes before meals and at bedtime.

✔ Safeguard anticholinergic medications from children because they are especially sensitive to atropine poisoning.

✔ To prevent constipation, use a diet high in fiber. Include whole grains, fruits, and vegetables in your daily menu. Also, drink 2 to 3 quarts of fluid a day and exercise regularly.

**At the Foundation** boxes provide students with the physiological background needed to understand the chapter.

**Age-related Considerations** highlight important aspects of drug therapy in children and older adults.

---

**AT THE FOUNDATION:** *Epilepsy*

Epilepsy is characterized by abnormal and excessive electrical discharges in a group of nerve cells (epileptogenic focus), resulting in alterations in brain function. The neurons experience a paroxysmal shift in depolarization and abrupt changes in the typical membrane potential. The plasma membranes become more permeable and hypersensitive and thus are more easily stimulated by various clinical conditions (hypoxia, hyperthermia, hypoglycemia, hyponatremia, repetitive sensory stimulation, and certain phases of sleep).

The primary abnormality may result in (1) instability in the neuron's resting potential, (2) abnormalities

in potassium conductance or calcium channels, (3) a defect in the GABA inhibitory system, or (4) irregularity in excitatory transmission enhancement.

The involved neurons fire with escalating frequency and amplitude, reach threshold, and spread to adjacent normal neurons through cortical stimulation. If uninhibited at this point, the excitation will spread to other parts of the nervous system. The seizure discharge produces changes typically resulting in altered level of arousal and motor, sensory, autonomic, or psychic clinical manifestations.

---

**Home Care Considerations:**
**Use of Adrenergic Drugs**

***ASSESS:*** the client for compliance with the prescribed regimen and for concurrent use with OTC drugs or herbal drugs containing similar ingredients.

***MONITOR:*** for therapeutic and excessive adverse effects and client's need for additional information, and provide that information.

***EDUCATE:*** on safe use of drugs (especially metered-dose inhalers), on ways to minimize adverse effects, to report excessive CNS or cardiac stimulation to a health care provider, and not to take OTC drugs or herbal preparations with the same or similar ingredients as prescription drugs. Reinforce additional teaching points (see Client Teaching Guidelines: Adrenergic Drugs).

**Home Care Considerations** focus on key considerations for providing drug therapy in this special setting.

---

**Age–Related Considerations:**
**Use of Acetaminophen, Aspirin, and Other NSAIDs**

**USE IN CHILDREN**

Acetaminophen is usually the drug of choice for pain or fever in children. Children seem less susceptible to liver toxicity than adults, apparently because they form less of the toxic metabolite during metabolism of acetaminophen. However, there is a risk for overdose and hepatotoxicity because acetaminophen is a very common ingredient in over-the-counter cold, flu, fever, and pain remedies. An overdose can occur with large doses of one product or smaller amounts of several different products. In addition, toxicity has occurred when parents or caregivers have given the liquid concentration intended for children to infants. The concentrations are different and cannot be given interchangeably. Infants' doses are measured with a dropper; children's doses are measured by a medicine cup. Caution parents and caregivers to ask pediatricians for written instructions on giving acetaminophen to their children, to read the labels of all drug products very carefully, and to avoid giving children acetaminophen from multiple sources.

Ibuprofen also may be given for fever. Aspirin is not recommended because of its association with Reye' syndrome, a life-threatening illness characterized by encephalopathy, hepatic damage, and other serious problems. Reye' syndrome usually occurs after a viral infection, such as influenza or chickenpox, during which aspirin was given for fever. For children with juvenile rheumatoid arthritis, aspirin, ibuprofen, naproxen, or

tolmetin may be given. Pediatric indications for use and dosages have not been established for most of the other drugs.

When an NSAID is given during late pregnancy to prevent premature labor, the fetus' kidneys may be adversely affected. When one is given shortly after birth to close a patent ductus arteriosus, the neonate' kidneys may be adversely affected.

**USE IN OLDER ADULTS**

Acetaminophen is usually safe in recommended doses unless liver damage is present or the person is a chronic alcohol abuser. Aspirin is usually safe in the small doses prescribed for prevention of myocardial infarction and stroke (antiplatelet effects). Aspirin and other NSAIDs are probably safe in therapeutic doses for occasional use as an analgesic or antipyretic. However, older adults have a high incidence of musculoskeletal disorders (eg, osteoarthritis), and an NSAID is often prescribed. Long-term use increases the risk for serious GI bleeding. Small doses, gradual increments, and taking the drug with food or a full glass of water may decrease GI effects. COX-2 inhibitor NSAIDs may be especially beneficial in older adults because they are less likely to cause gastric ulceration and bleeding. Older adults also are more likely than younger adults to acquire nephrotoxicity with NSAIDs, especially with high doses or long-term use, because the drugs may reduce blood flow to the kidneys.

---

**Critical Thinking Exercises**

1. A health care provider prescribes carbamazepine (Tegretol) for tonic-clonic seizures. After 1 month, the client's serum level is 18 mcg/mL. The nurse interprets this level as:

   a. Subtherapeutic
   b. Within normal limits, but in the lower range
   c. Within normal limits, but in the upper range
   d. Toxic

2. A 50 kg client is brought to the emergency department by EMS with seizures. The health care provider orders lorazepam (Ativan), 5 mg IV initially. For which type of seizure is diazepam the drug of choice?

   a. Partial seizure
   b. Tonic-clonic seizure
   c. Absence seizure
   d. Status epilepticus

3. A child is started on phenytoin (Dilantin) after experiencing his first seizure. A teaching plan for the child and family should include strategies to reduce what common side effect?

   a. Hypoglycemia
   b. Photosensitivity
   c. Gingival hyperplasia
   d. Hyponatremia

4. The use of valproate sodium (Depakene) is limited because of which adverse reaction?

   a. Nausea
   b. Sedation
   c. Muscle tremors
   d. Hepatotoxicity

5. A client receiving phenytoin therapy develops nystagmus. The nurse recognizes that the development of this condition is likely:

   a. A sign of toxicity
   b. Unrelated to the phenytoin therapy
   c. An indication that serum levels are subtherapeutic
   d. A normal finding in clients receiving phenytoin

**Critical Thinking Exercises** include NCLEX-style questions that encourage critical thinking and allow self-evaluation.

# Expanded Contents

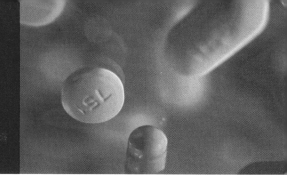

**1**

# Introduction
# to Pharmacology

## OBJECTIVES

*After studying this chapter, the student will be able to:*

1  Differentiate between pharmacology and drug therapy.

2  Distinguish between generic and trade names of drugs.

3  Define a prototypical drug.

4  Select authoritative sources of drug information.

5  Discuss major drug laws and standards.

6  Describe the main categories of controlled substances in relation to therapeutic use and potential for abuse.

7  Discuss nursing responsibilities in handling controlled substances correctly.

8  Explain the role of the U.S. Food and Drug Administration.

9  Analyze the potential impact of drug costs on drug therapy regimens.

10  Develop personal techniques for learning about drugs and using drug knowledge in client care.

## CRITICAL THINKING SCENARIO

*T*his is your first semester of clinical nursing; you will be taking a basic nursing theory course, a skills laboratory, and pharmacology. You anticipate that pharmacology will be challenging. To increase your clinical knowledge and ensure that you will be a safe practitioner, you want to develop a strong foundation in pharmacology.

✔ List successful strategies you have used in the past to learn difficult material. Reflect on which strategies might be helpful this semester.

✔ Assess support for learning at your school (eg, learning center, peer tutors, student study groups) and develop a plan to use them.

✔ Review your course syllabus and pharmacology text. Develop a learning plan (eg, readings, assignments, study times for major tests) and enter this plan into your calendar.

## A MESSAGE TO STUDENTS

The use of medications in Western cultures is common practice. You have probably been taking medications and seeing other people take medications most of your life. Perhaps you have wondered, Why is it usually okay to give children Tylenol but not aspirin? Why do a lot of middle-aged and older people take an aspirin a day? Why do people with high blood pressure, heart failure, or diabetes take ACE inhibitors, and what are ACE inhibitors? When should an antibiotic *not* be prescribed for an infection?

You are embarking on an exciting journey of discovery as you begin or continue your study of pharmacology. Much of what you learn will apply to your personal and family life as well as your professional life as a nurse. The purpose of this book is to help you learn about medicines and the why, what, how, when, and where they are used in daily life. Bon voyage!

## OVERVIEW

*Pharmacology* is the study of drugs (chemicals) that alter functions of living organisms. *Drug therapy*, also called pharmacotherapy, is the use of drugs to prevent, diagnose, or treat signs, symptoms, and disease processes. When prevention or cure is not a reasonable goal, relief of symptoms can greatly improve quality of life and ability to function in activities of daily living. Drugs given for therapeutic purposes are usually called *medications*. Common sources of drugs are outlined in At the Foundation: Sources of Drugs.

Medications may be given for various reasons. In many instances, the goal of drug therapy is to lessen disease processes rather than cure them. To meet this goal, drugs may be given for local or systemic effects. Drugs with local effects, such as sunscreen lotions and local anesthetics, act mainly at the site of application. Those with systemic effects are taken into the body, circulated through the bloodstream to their sites of action in various body tissues, and eventually eliminated from the body. *Most drugs are given for their systemic effects.* Drugs may also be given for relatively immediate effects (eg, in acute problems such as pain or infection) or long-term effects (eg, to relieve signs and symptoms of chronic disorders). Many drugs are given for their long-term effects.

## DRUG CLASSIFICATIONS AND PROTOTYPES

Drugs are classified according to their effects on particular body systems, their therapeutic uses, and their chemical characteristics. For example, morphine can be classified as a central nervous system depressant, a narcotic or opioid analgesic, and an opiate (derived from opium). The names of therapeutic classifications usually reflect the conditions for which the drugs are used (eg, antidepressants, antihypertensives, antidiabetic drugs). However, the names of many drug groups reflect their chemical characteristics rather than therapeutic uses (eg, adrenergics, antiadrenergics, benzodiazepines). Many commonly used drugs fit into multiple groups because they have wide-ranging effects on the human body.

Individual drugs that represent groups of drugs are called *prototypes*. Prototypes, which are often the first drug of a particular group to be developed, are usually the standards with which newer, similar drugs are compared. For example, morphine is the prototype of narcotic analgesics, and penicillin is the prototype of antibacterial drugs.

Drug classifications and prototypes are quite stable, and most new drugs can be assigned to a group and compared with an established prototype. However, some

### AT THE FOUNDATION: *Sources of Drugs*

Historically, drugs were mainly derived from plants (eg, morphine), animals (eg, insulin), and minerals (eg, iron). Now, most drugs are synthetic chemical compounds manufactured in laboratories. Chemists, for example, can often create a useful new drug by altering the chemical structure of an existing drug (eg, by adding, deleting, or altering a side chain). Such techniques and other technologic advances have enabled the production of new drugs as well as synthetic versions of many drugs originally derived from plants and animals. Synthetic drugs are more standardized in their chemical characteristics, more consistent in their effects, and less likely to produce allergic reactions. Semisynthetic drugs (eg, many antibiotics) are naturally occurring substances that have been chemically modified.

Biotechnology is also an important source of drugs. This process involves manipulating deoxyribonucleic acid (DNA) and ribonucleic acid (RNA) and recombining genes into hybrid molecules that can be inserted into living organisms (*Escherichia coli* bacteria are often used) and repeatedly reproduced. Each hybrid molecule produces a genetically identical molecule, called a *clone*. Cloning makes it possible to identify the DNA sequence in a gene and produce the protein product encoded by a gene, including insulin and several other body proteins. Cloning also allows production of adequate amounts of the drug for therapeutic or research purposes.

groups lack a universally accepted prototype, and some prototypes are replaced over time by newer, more commonly used drugs.

## DRUG NAMES

Individual drugs may have several different names, but the two most commonly used are the generic name and the trade name (also called the brand or proprietary name). The *generic name* (eg, amoxicillin) is related to the chemical or official name and is independent of the manufacturer. The generic name often indicates the drug group (eg, drugs with generic names ending in "cillin" are penicillins). The *trade name* is designated and patented by the manufacturer. For example, amoxicillin is manufactured by several pharmaceutical companies, some of which assign a specific trade name (eg, Amoxil, Trimox) and several of which use only the generic name. In drug literature, trade names are capitalized, and generic names are lowercase (unless they appear in a list or at the beginning of a sentence). Drugs may be prescribed and dispensed by generic or trade name.

## DRUG MARKETING

A new drug is protected by patent for 14 years, during which only the pharmaceutical manufacturer that developed it can market it. This is seen as a return on the company's investment in developing a drug, which may require years of work and millions of dollars, and as an incentive for developing other drugs. Other pharmaceutical companies cannot manufacture and market the drug. However, for new drugs that are popular and widely used, other companies often produce similar drugs, with different generic and trade names. For example, the marketing of fluoxetine (Prozac) led to the introduction of similar drugs from different companies, such as citalopram (Celexa), fluvoxamine (Luvox), paroxetine (Paxil), and sertraline (Zoloft). Prozac was approved in 1987 and went off patent in 2001, meaning that any pharmaceutical company could then manufacture and market the generic formulation of fluoxetine. Generic drugs are required to be therapeutically equivalent and are much less expensive than trade name drugs.

## PHARMACOECONOMICS

Pharmacoeconomics involves the costs of drug therapy, including those of purchasing, dispensing (eg, salaries of pharmacists, pharmacy technicians), storage, administration (eg, salaries of nurses, costs of supplies), laboratory and other tests used to monitor client responses, and losses from expiration. Length of illness or hospitalization is also considered.

Costs are increasingly being considered a major factor in choosing medications, and research projects that compare costs have greatly increased in recent years. The goal of most studies is to define drug therapy regimens that provide the desired benefits at the least cost. For drugs or regimens of similar efficacy and toxicity, there is considerable pressure on prescribers (eg, from managed care organizations) to prescribe less costly drugs.

## PRESCRIPTION AND NONPRESCRIPTION DRUGS

Legally, American consumers have two routes of access to therapeutic drugs. One route is by prescription or order from a licensed health care provider, such as a physician, dentist, or nurse practitioner. The other route is by over-the-counter (OTC) purchase of drugs that do not require a prescription. Various drug laws regulate both of these routes. Acquiring and using prescription drugs for nontherapeutic purposes, by persons who are not authorized to have the drugs or for whom they are not prescribed, is illegal.

### American Drug Laws and Standards

Current drug laws and standards have evolved over many years. Their main goal is to protect the public by ensuring that drugs marketed for therapeutic purposes, whether prescription or OTC, are safe and effective. Their main provisions are summarized in Table 1-1.

The Food, Drug, and Cosmetic Act of 1938 was especially important because this law and its amendments regulate the manufacture, distribution, advertising, and labeling of drugs. It also confers official status on drugs listed in *The United States Pharmacopeia*. The letters *USP* may follow the names of these drugs. Official drugs must meet standards of purity and strength as determined by chemical analysis or animal response to specified doses (bioassay). The Durham-Humphrey Amendment designated drugs that must be prescribed by a physician and dispensed by a pharmacist. The U.S. Food and Drug Administration (FDA) is charged with enforcing the law. In addition, the Public Health Service regulates vaccines and other biologic products, and the Federal Trade Commission can suppress misleading advertisements of nonprescription drugs.

Another important law, the Comprehensive Drug Abuse Prevention and Control Act, was passed in 1970. Title II of this law, called the Controlled Substances Act, regulates the manufacture and distribution of narcotics, stimulants, depressants, hallucinogens, and anabolic steroids. These drugs are categorized according to therapeutic usefulness and potential for abuse (Box 1-1) and are labeled as controlled substances (eg, morphine, a Schedule II drug, is labeled C-II).

The Drug Enforcement Administration (DEA) is charged with enforcing the Controlled Substances Act.

## TABLE 1-1  American Drug Laws and Amendments

| Year | Name | Main Provision(s) |
|------|------|-------------------|
| 1906 | Pure Food and Drug Act | Established official standards and requirements for accurate labeling of drug products |
| 1912 | Sherley Amendment | Prohibited fraudulent claims of drug effectiveness |
| 1914 | Harrison Narcotic Act | Restricted the importation, manufacture, sale, and use of opium, cocaine, marijuana, and other drugs that the act defined as narcotics |
| 1938 | Food, Drug, and Cosmetic Act | • Required proof of safety from the manufacturer before a new drug could be marketed<br>• Authorized factory inspections<br>• Established penalties for fraudulent claims and misleading labels |
| 1945 | Amendment | Required governmental certification of biologic products, such as insulin and antibiotics |
| 1952 | Durham-Humphrey Amendment | Designated drugs that must be prescribed by a physician and dispensed by a pharmacist (eg, controlled substances, drugs considered unsafe for use except under supervision by a health care provider, and drugs limited to prescription use under a manufacturer's new drug application) |
| 1962 | Kefauver-Harris Amendment | • Required a manufacturer to provide evidence (from well-controlled research studies) that a drug was effective for claims and conditions identified in the product's labeling<br>• Gave the federal government the authority to standardize drug names |
| 1970 | Comprehensive Drug Abuse Prevention and Control Act; Title II, Controlled Substances Act | • Regulated distribution of narcotics and other drugs of abuse<br>• Categorized these drugs according to therapeutic usefulness and potential for abuse |
| 1978 | Drug Regulation Reform Act | • Established guidelines for research studies and data to be submitted to the FDA by manufacturers<br>• Shortened the time required to develop and market new drugs |
| 1983 | Orphan Drug Act | • Decreased taxes and competition for manufacturers who would produce drugs to treat selected serious disorders affecting relatively few people |
| 1987 | | • Established new regulations designed to speed up the approval process for high-priority medications |
| 1992 | Prescription Drug User Fee Act | • Allowed the FDA to collect user fees from pharmaceutical companies, with each new drug application, to shorten the review time (eg, by hiring more staff)<br>• Specified a review time of 12 months for standard drugs and 6 months for priority drugs |
| 1997 | FDA Modernization Act | • Updated regulation of biologic products<br>• Increased client access to experimental drugs and medical devices<br>• Accelerated review of important new drugs<br>• Allowed drug companies to disseminate information about off-label (non–FDA-approved) uses and costs of drugs<br>• Extended user fees |

FDA, U.S. Food and Drug Administration.

Individuals and companies legally empowered to handle controlled substances must be registered with the DEA, keep accurate records of all transactions, and provide for secure storage. Physicians are assigned a number by the DEA and must include the number on all prescriptions they write for a controlled substance. Prescriptions for Schedule II drugs cannot be refilled; a new prescription is required. Nurses are responsible for storing controlled substances in locked containers, administering them only to people for whom they are prescribed, recording each dose given on agency narcotic sheets and on the client's medication administration record, maintaining an accurate inventory, and reporting discrepancies to the proper authorities.

In addition to federal laws, state laws also regulate the sale and distribution of controlled drugs. These laws may be more stringent than federal laws; if so, the stricter laws usually apply.

## BOX 1-1    Categories of Controlled Substances

**Schedule I**
Drugs that are not approved for medical use and have high abuse potentials: heroin, lysergic acid diethylamide (LSD), peyote, mescaline, tetrahydrocannabinol, marijuana.

**Schedule II**
Drugs that are used medically and have high abuse potentials: narcotic analgesics (eg, codeine, hydromorphone, methadone, meperidine, morphine, oxycodone, oxymorphone), central nervous system (CNS) stimulants (eg, cocaine, methamphetamine, methylphenidate), and barbiturate sedative-hypnotics (amobarbital, pentobarbital, secobarbital).

**Schedule III**
Drugs with less potential for abuse than those in Schedules I and II, but abuse may lead to psychological or physical dependence: androgens and anabolic steroids, some CNS

stimulants (eg, benzphetamine), and mixtures containing small amounts of controlled substances (eg, codeine, barbiturates not listed in other schedules).

**Schedule IV**
Drugs with some potential for abuse: benzodiazepines (eg, diazepam, lorazepam, temazepam), other sedative-hypnotics (eg, phenobarbital, chloral hydrate), and some prescription appetite suppressants (eg, mazindol, phentermine).

**Schedule V**
Products containing moderate amounts of controlled substances. They may be dispensed by the pharmacist without a physician's prescription but with some restrictions regarding amount, record keeping, and other safeguards. Included are antidiarrheal drugs, such as diphenoxylate and atropine (Lomotil).

## Canadian Drug Laws and Standards

Canada and its provinces have laws and standards that parallel those of the United States, particularly those related to controlled substances.

## ■ DRUG APPROVAL PROCESSES

The FDA is responsible for ensuring that new drugs are safe and effective before approving the drugs and allowing them to be marketed. The FDA reviews research studies (usually conducted or sponsored by a pharmaceutical company) about proposed new drugs; the organization does not test the drugs.

Before passage of the Food, Drug, and Cosmetic Act, many drugs were marketed without confirmation of safety or efficacy. Since 1962, however, newly developed drugs have been extensively tested before being marketed for general use. The drugs are carefully evaluated at each step. Testing usually proceeds if there is evidence of safety and effectiveness but may be stopped at any time for inadequate effectiveness or excessive toxicity. Many potential drugs are discarded and never marketed; some drugs are marketed but later withdrawn, usually because of adverse effects that become evident only when the drug is used in a large, diverse population.

## Testing and Clinical Trials

The testing process begins with animal studies to determine potential uses and effects. The next step involves FDA review of the data obtained in the animal studies. The drug then undergoes clinical trials in humans. Most clinical trials use a randomized, controlled experimental design that involves selection of subjects according to

established criteria, random assignment of subjects to experimental groups, and administration of the test drug to one group and a control substance to another group.

In Phase I, a few doses are given to a few healthy volunteers to determine safe dosages, routes of administration, absorption, metabolism, excretion, and toxicity. In Phase II, a few doses are given to a few subjects with the disease or symptom for which the drug is being studied, and responses are compared with those of healthy subjects. In Phase III, the drug is given to a larger and more representative group of subjects. In double-blind, placebo-controlled designs, half the subjects receive the new drug and half receive a placebo, with neither subjects nor researchers knowing who receives which formulation. In crossover studies, subjects serve as their own controls; each subject receives the experimental drug during half the study and a placebo during the other half. Other research methods include control studies, in which some clients receive a known drug rather than a placebo, and subject matching, in which clients are paired with others of similar characteristics. Phase III studies help to determine whether the potential benefits of the drug outweigh the risks.

In Phase IV, the FDA evaluates the data from the first three phases for drug safety and effectiveness, allows the drug to be marketed for general use, and requires manufacturers to continue monitoring the drug's effects. Some adverse drug effects may become evident during the postmarketing phase as the drug is more widely used. Several drugs have been withdrawn in recent years, partly or mainly because of the increased postmarketing surveillance. Critics contend that changes enacted to streamline the approval process have allowed unsafe drugs to be marketed; proponents claim that the faster review process helps clients with serious diseases to gain effective treatment more quickly.

The FDA has increased efforts to monitor marketed drugs more closely in recent years, especially for their adverse effects. One such effort involves contracts with some commercial companies that provide access to databases containing information on the actual use of prescription drugs in adults and children. Examples of information include how long nonhospitalized clients stay on prescribed medications, which combinations of medications are being prescribed to clients, and the use of prescription drugs in hospitalized children. Individual clients are not identified in these databases.

## Food and Drug Administration Approval

The FDA approves many new drugs annually. In 1992, procedures were changed to accelerate the approval process, especially for drugs used to treat acquired immuno-deficiency syndrome (AIDS). Since then, new drugs are categorized according to their review priority and thera-peutic potential: "1P" status indicates a new drug reviewed on a priority basis and with some therapeutic advantages over similar drugs already available; "1S" status indicates standard review and drugs with few, if any, therapeutic advantages (ie, the new drug is similar to one already available). Most newly approved drugs are "1S" prescrip-tion drugs.

The FDA also approves drugs for OTC availability, including the transfer of drugs from prescription to OTC status, and may require additional clinical trials to deter-mine safety and effectiveness of OTC use. Numerous drugs have been transferred from prescription to OTC status in recent years, and the trend is likely to continue. For drugs taken orally, indications for use may be different, and rec-ommended doses are usually lower for the OTC formula-tion. For example, for OTC ibuprofen, which is available under its generic and several trade names (eg, Advil) in 200-mg tablets and is used for pain, fever, and dysmenor-rhea, the recommended dose is usually 200 to 400 mg three or four times daily. With prescription ibuprofen, Motrin is the common trade name, and the dosage may be 400, 600, or 800 mg three or four times daily.

FDA approval of a drug for OTC availability involves evaluation of evidence that the consumer can use the drug safely, using information on the product label, and shifts primary responsibility for safe and effective drug therapy from health care professionals to consumers. With pre-scription drugs, a health care professional diagnoses the condition, often with the help of laboratory and other diagnostic tests, and determines a need for the drug. With OTC drugs, the client must make these decisions, with or without consultation with a health care provider. Ques-tions to be answered include the following:

1. Can consumers accurately self-diagnose the condi-tion for which a drug is indicated?
2. Can consumers read and understand the label well enough to determine the dosage, interpret warnings

and contraindications and determine whether they apply, and recognize drugs already being taken that might interact adversely with the drug being considered?
3. Is the drug effective when used as recommended?
4. Is the drug safe when used as instructed?

Having drugs available OTC has potential advantages and disadvantages for consumers. Advantages include greater autonomy; faster and more convenient access to effective treatment; possibly earlier resumption of usual activities of daily living; fewer visits to a health care provider; and possibly increased efforts by con-sumers to learn about their symptoms, conditions, and recommended treatments. Disadvantages include in-accurate self-diagnoses and potential risk for choosing a wrong or contraindicated drug; delaying treatment by a health care professional; and developing adverse drug reactions and interactions.

When a drug is switched from prescription to OTC sta-tus, pharmaceutical companies' sales and profits increase, and insurance companies' costs decrease. Costs to con-sumers may increase because health insurance policies do not cover OTC drugs. For the year 2000, it was esti-mated that Americans spent more than $19 billion on OTC drugs.

## ■ SOURCES OF DRUG INFORMATION

There are many sources of drug data, including pharma-cology textbooks, drug reference books, journal articles, and Internet sites. For the beginning student of pharma-cology, a textbook is usually the best source of informa-tion because it describes groups of drugs in relation to therapeutic uses. Drug reference books are most helpful in relation to individual drugs. Two authoritative sources are the *American Hospital Formulary Service* and *Drug Facts and Comparisons.* The former is published by the Ameri-can Society of Health-System Pharmacists and updated periodically. The latter is published by the Facts and Comparisons division of Lippincott Williams & Wilkins and updated monthly (loose-leaf edition) or annually (hard-bound edition). A widely available but less author-itative source is the *Physicians' Desk Reference* (PDR). The PDR, published yearly, is a compilation of manufactur-ers' package inserts for selected drugs.

Numerous drug handbooks (eg, Lippincott's *Nursing Drug Guide,* published annually) and pharmacologic, medical, and nursing journals also contain informa-tion about drugs. Journal articles often present infor-mation about drug therapy for clients with specific disease processes and may thereby facilitate application of drug knowledge in clinical practice. Helpful Internet sites include the Food and Drug Administration (http://www.fda.gov), and RxMed (http://www.rxmed.com).

## STRATEGIES FOR STUDYING PHARMACOLOGY

1. *Concentrate on therapeutic classifications and their prototypes.* For example, morphine is the prototype of narcotic analgesics (see Chap. 6). Understanding morphine makes learning about other narcotic analgesics easier because they are compared with morphine.

2. *Compare a newly encountered drug with a prototype when possible.* Relating the unknown to the known aids learning and retention of knowledge.

3. *Try to understand how the drug acts in the body.* This allows you to predict therapeutic effects and to predict, prevent, or minimize adverse effects by early detection and treatment.

4. *Concentrate your study efforts on major characteristics.* These include the main indications for use, common and potentially serious adverse effects, conditions in which the drug is contraindicated or must be used cautiously, and related nursing care needs.

5. *Keep an authoritative, up-to-date drug reference readily available, preferably at work and home.* This is a much more reliable source of drug information than memory, especially for dosage ranges. Use the reference freely whenever you encounter an unfamiliar drug or when a question arises about a familiar one.

6. *Use your own words when taking notes or writing drug information cards.* Also, write notes, answers to review questions, definitions of new terms, and trade names of drugs encountered in clinical practice settings directly into your pharmacology textbook. The mental processing required for these activities helps in both initial learning and later retention of knowledge.

7. *Mentally rehearse applying drug knowledge in nursing care* by asking yourself, "What if I have a client who is receiving this drug? What must I do to administer the drug safely? For what must I assess the client before giving the drug, and for what must I observe the client after drug administration? What if my client is an elderly person or a child?"

## Critical Thinking Exercises

1. The governmental agency responsible for ensuring that new drugs are safe and effective before approving the drugs and allowing them to be marketed is the:
   a. Drug Enforcement Administration
   b. Food and Drug Administration
   c. American Hospital Formulary Service
   d. Federal Trade Commission

2. The drug that is often the first drug of a particular group to be developed, usually the standards, and the one with which newer, similar drugs are compared is called the:
   a. Generic
   b. Therapeutic
   c. Placebo
   d. Prototype

3. When a drug is switched from prescription to OTC status, costs to consumers may:
   a. Increase
   b. Decrease
   c. Remain unchanged
   d. Encourage abuse

4. Five categories of controlled substances exist. The category of drugs that are used medically and have high abuse potentials are classed as:
   a. Schedule I
   b. Schedule II
   c. Schedule III
   d. Schedule IV

## SELECTED REFERENCES

Brass, E. P. (2001). Changing the status of drugs from prescription to over-the-counter availability. *New England Journal of Medicine, 345*(11), 810–816.

Lipsky, M. S., & Sharp, L. K. (2001). From idea to market: The drug approval process. *Journal of the American Board of Family Practice, 14*(5), 362–367.

Schwartz, J. B. (2000). Geriatric clinical pharmacology. In H. D. Humes (Ed.), *Kelley's textbook of internal medicine* (4th ed., pp. 3095–3107). Philadelphia: Lippincott Williams & Wilkins.

U.S. Food and Drug Administration. Frequently asked questions. [On-line.] Available: http://www.fda.gov/opacom/faqs/faqs.html. Accessed 31 March 2000.

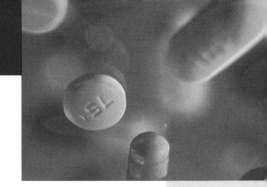

# 2

# Basic Concepts and Processes

## OBJECTIVES

*After studying this chapter, the student will be able to:*

1 Identify the main pathways and mechanisms by which drugs cross biologic membranes and move through the body.

2 Describe each process of pharmacokinetics.

3 Discuss the clinical usefulness of measuring serum drug levels.

4 Give major characteristics of the receptor theory of drug action.

5 Differentiate between agonist drugs and antagonist drugs.

6 Describe drug-related and client-related variables that affect drug actions.

7 Discuss mechanisms and potential effects of drug–drug interactions.

8 Identify signs and symptoms that may occur with adverse drug effects on major body systems.

9 Discuss general management of drug overdose and toxicity.

10 Discuss selected drug antidotes.

## CRITICAL THINKING SCENARIO

*M*rs. Green, an 89-year-old widow, lives alone and has recently started taking many heart medications. She prides herself on being independent and able to manage on her own despite failing memory and failing health. When you visit as a home health nurse, you assess therapeutic and adverse effects of her medications.

✔ Considering Mrs. Green's age, what factors might alter the pharmacokinetics (absorption, distribution, metabolism, excretion) of the drugs she takes? What data will you collect to determine her risk?

✔ What psychosocial factors could affect the therapeutic and adverse effects of Mrs. Green's medications? What data will be important to collect before developing a plan for Mrs. Green?

✔ When clients are taking many medications, the risk for drug interactions and toxicity increases. Describe how you will develop a plan to research possible drug interactions for any client.

## OVERVIEW

All body functions and disease processes and most drug actions occur at the cellular level. Drugs are chemicals that alter basic processes in body cells. They can stimulate or inhibit normal cellular functions and activities; they cannot add functions and activities. To act on body cells, drugs given for systemic effects must reach adequate concentrations in blood and other tissue fluids surrounding the cells. Thus, they must enter the body and be circulated to their sites of action (target cells). After they act on cells, they must be eliminated from the body.

How do systemic drugs reach, interact with, and leave body cells? How do people respond to drug actions? The answers to these questions are derived from cellular physiology, pathways and mechanisms of drug transport, pharmacokinetics, pharmacodynamics, and other basic concepts and processes. These concepts and processes form the foundation of rational drug therapy and the content of this chapter.

## CELLULAR PHYSIOLOGY

Cells (Fig. 2-1) are dynamic, busy "factories." That is, they take in raw materials, manufacture various products required to maintain cellular and bodily functions, and deliver those products to their appropriate destinations in the body. Although cells differ from one tissue to another, their common characteristics include the ability to:

■ Exchange materials with their immediate environment
■ Obtain energy from nutrients
■ Synthesize hormones, neurotransmitters, enzymes, structural proteins, and other complex molecules
■ Duplicate themselves (reproduce)
■ Communicate with each other through various biologic chemicals, such as neurotransmitters and hormones

## DRUG TRANSPORT THROUGH CELL MEMBRANES

Drugs, as well as physiologic substances such as hormones and neurotransmitters, must reach and interact with or cross the cell membrane in order to stimulate or inhibit cellular function. Most drugs are given for effects on body cells that are distant from the sites of administration (ie, systemic effects). To move through the body and reach their sites of action, metabolism, and excretion (Fig. 2-2), drug molecules must cross numerous cell membranes (Fig. 2-3). For example, molecules of most oral drugs must cross the membranes of cells in the gastrointestinal (GI) tract, liver, and capillaries to reach the bloodstream, circulate to their target cells, leave the bloodstream and attach to receptors on cells, perform their action, return to the bloodstream, circulate to the liver, reach drug-metabolizing enzymes in liver cells, reenter the bloodstream (usually as metabolites), circulate to the kidneys, and be excreted in urine. Several transport pathways and mechanisms used to move drug molecules through the body are described in At the Foundation: Drug Transport Pathways and Mechanisms.

## PHARMACOKINETICS

Pharmacokinetics involves drug movement through the body (ie, "what the body does to the drug") to reach sites of action, metabolism, and excretion. Specific processes are absorption, distribution, metabolism (biotransformation), and excretion. Overall, these processes largely

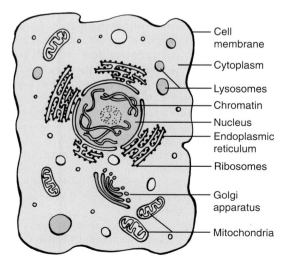

**FIGURE 2–1** Schematic diagram of cell highlighting cytoplasmic organelles.

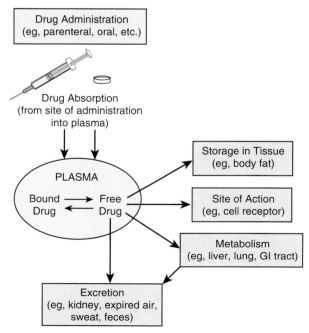

**FIGURE 2–2** Entry and movement of drug molecules through the body to sites of action, metabolism, and excretion.

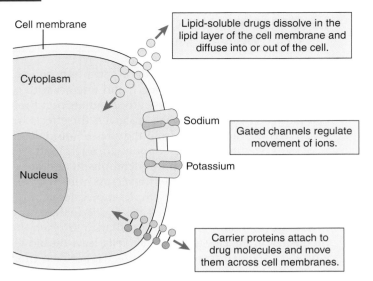

Cell membrane

Lipid-soluble drugs dissolve in the lipid layer of the cell membrane and diffuse into or out of the cell.

Cytoplasm

Sodium

Gated channels regulate movement of ions.

Potassium

Nucleus

Carrier proteins attach to drug molecules and move them across cell membranes.

**FIGURE 2–3** Drug transport pathways. Drug molecules cross cell membranes to move into and out of body cells by directly penetrating the lipid layer, diffusing through open or gated channels, or attaching to carrier proteins.

## AT THE FOUNDATION: *Drug Transport Pathways and Mechanisms*

### Pathways

There are three main pathways of drug movement across cell membranes (see Fig. 2-3). The most common pathway is *direct penetration* of the membrane by lipid-soluble drugs, which are able to dissolve in the lipid layer of the cell membrane. Most systemic drugs are formulated to be lipid soluble so that they can move through cell membranes, even oral tablets and capsules that must be sufficiently water soluble to dissolve in the aqueous fluids of the stomach and small intestine.

A second pathway involves passage through *protein channels* that go all the way through the cell membrane. Only a few drugs are able to use this pathway because most drug molecules are too large to pass through the small channels. Small ions (eg, sodium and potassium) use this pathway, but their movement is regulated by specific channels with a gating mechanism. The gate is a flap of protein, which opens for a few milliseconds to allow ion movement across the cell membrane, and then closes (ie, blocks the channel opening) to prevent additional ion movement. On sodium channels, the gates are located on the outside of the cell membrane; when the gates open, sodium ions ($Na^+$) move from extracellular fluid into the cell. On potassium channels, the gates are located on the inside of the cell membrane; when the gates open, potassium ions ($K^+$) move from the cell into extracellular fluid.

The stimulus for opening and closing the gates may be voltage gating or chemical (also called *ligand*) gating. With voltage gating, the electrical potential across the cell membrane determines whether the gate is open or closed. With chemical gating, a chemical substance (a ligand) binds with the protein forming the channel and changes the shape of the protein to open or close the gate. Chemical gating (eg, by neurotransmitters such as acetylcholine) is very important in the transmission of signals from one nerve cell to another

and from nerve cells to muscle cells to cause muscle contraction.

The third pathway involves *carrier proteins* that transport molecules from one side of the cell membrane to the other. All of the carrier proteins are selective in the substances they transport; a drug's structure determines which carrier will transport it. These transport systems are an important means of moving drug molecules through the body. They are used, for example, to carry oral drugs from the intestine to the bloodstream, to carry hormones to their sites of action inside body cells, and to carry drug molecules from the blood into renal tubules.

### Mechanisms

Once absorbed into the body, drugs are transported to and from target cells by such mechanisms as passive diffusion, facilitated diffusion, and active transport.

*Passive diffusion,* the most common mechanism, involves movement of a drug from an area of higher concentration to one of lower concentration. For example, after oral administration, the initial concentration of a drug is higher in the gastrointestinal tract than in the blood. This promotes movement of the drug into the bloodstream. When the drug is circulated, the concentration is higher in the blood than in body cells, so that the drug moves (from capillaries) into the fluids surrounding the cells or into the cells themselves. Passive diffusion continues until a state of equilibrium is reached between the amount of drug in the tissues and the amount in the blood.

*Facilitated diffusion* is a similar process, except that drug molecules combine with a carrier substance, such as an enzyme or other protein.

In *active transport,* drug molecules are moved from an area of lower concentration to one of higher concentration. This process requires a carrier substance and the release of cellular energy.

determine serum drug levels, onset, peak and duration of drug actions, drug half-life, therapeutic and adverse drug effects, and other important aspects of drug therapy.

## Absorption

*Absorption* is the process that occurs from the time a drug enters the body to the time it enters the bloodstream to be circulated. Onset of drug action is largely determined by the rate of absorption; intensity is determined by the extent of absorption. Numerous factors affect the rate and extent of drug absorption, including dosage form, route of administration, blood flow to the site of administration, GI function, the presence of food or other drugs, and other variables. Dosage form is a major determinant of a drug's bioavailability (the portion of a dose that reaches the systemic circulation and is available to act on body cells). An intravenous (IV) drug is virtually 100% bioavailable; an oral drug is virtually always less than 100% bioavailable because some is not absorbed from the GI tract and some goes to the liver and is partially metabolized before reaching the systemic circulation (first-pass effect).

Most oral drugs must be swallowed, dissolved in gastric fluid, and delivered to the small intestine (which has a large surface area for absorption of nutrients and drugs) before they are absorbed. Liquid medications are absorbed faster than tablets or capsules because they need not be dissolved. Rapid movement through the stomach and small intestine may increase drug absorption by promoting contact with absorptive mucous membrane; it also may decrease absorption because some drugs may move through the small intestine too rapidly to be absorbed. For many drugs, the presence of food in the stomach slows the rate of absorption and may decrease the amount of drug absorbed.

Drugs injected into subcutaneous or intramuscular tissues are usually absorbed more rapidly than oral drugs because they move directly from the injection site to the bloodstream. Absorption is rapid from intramuscular sites because muscle tissue has an abundant blood supply. Drugs injected intravenously do not need to be absorbed because they are placed directly into the bloodstream.

Other absorptive sites include the skin, mucous membranes, and lungs. Most drugs applied to the skin are given for local effects (eg, sunscreens). Systemic absorption is minimal from intact skin but may be considerable when the skin is inflamed or damaged. Also, a number of drugs have been formulated in adhesive skin patches for absorption through the skin (eg, clonidine, estrogen, fentanyl, nitroglycerin, scopolamine). Some drugs applied to mucous membranes also are given for local effects. However, systemic absorption occurs from the mucosa of the oral cavity, nose, eye, vagina, and rectum. Drugs absorbed through mucous membranes pass directly into the bloodstream. The lungs have a large surface area for absorption of anesthetic gases and a few other drugs.

## Distribution

*Distribution* involves the transport of drug molecules within the body. Once a drug is injected or absorbed into the bloodstream, it is carried by the blood and tissue fluids to its sites of pharmacologic action, metabolism, and excretion. Most drug molecules enter and leave the bloodstream at the capillary level, through gaps between the cells that form capillary walls. Distribution depends largely on the adequacy of blood circulation. Drugs are distributed rapidly to organs receiving a large blood supply, such as the heart, liver, and kidneys. Distribution to other internal organs, muscle, fat, and skin is usually slower.

An important factor in drug distribution is *protein binding* (Fig. 2-4). Most drugs form a complex with plasma proteins, mainly albumin, which act as carriers. Drug molecules bound to plasma proteins are pharmacologically inactive because the large size of the complex prevents their leaving the bloodstream through the small openings in capillary walls and reaching their sites of action, metabolism, and excretion. *Only the free or unbound portion of a drug acts on body cells.* As the free drug acts on cells, the decrease in plasma drug levels causes some of the bound drug to be released.

Protein binding allows part of a drug dose to be stored and released as needed. Some drugs also are stored in muscle, fat, or other body tissues and released gradually when plasma drug levels fall. These storage mechanisms maintain lower, more even blood levels and reduce the risk for toxicity. Drugs that are highly bound to plasma proteins or stored extensively in other tissues have a long duration of action.

Drug distribution into the central nervous system (CNS) is limited because the blood–brain barrier, which is composed of capillaries with tight walls, limits move-

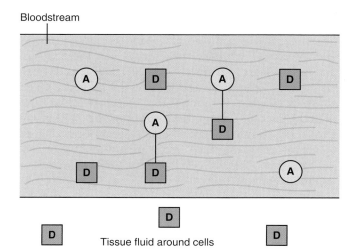

**FIGURE 2-4** Plasma proteins, mainly albumin (A), act as carriers for drug molecules (D). Bound drug (A–D) stays in bloodstream and is pharmacologically inactive. Free drug (D) can leave the bloodstream and act on body cells.

ment of drug molecules into brain tissue. This barrier usually acts as a selectively permeable membrane to protect the CNS. However, it also can make drug therapy of CNS disorders more difficult because drugs must pass *through* cells of the capillary wall rather than *between* cells. As a result, only drugs that are lipid soluble or have a transport system can cross the blood–brain barrier and reach therapeutic concentrations in brain tissue.

Drug distribution during pregnancy and lactation is also unique (see Chap. 23). During pregnancy, most drugs cross the placenta and may affect the fetus. During lactation, many drugs enter breast milk and may affect the nursing infant.

## Metabolism

*Metabolism* is the method by which drugs are inactivated or biotransformed by the body. Most often, an active drug is changed into one or more inactive metabolites, which are then excreted. Some active drugs yield metabolites that are also active and that continue to exert their effects on body cells until they are metabolized further or excreted. Other drugs (called *prodrugs*) are initially inactive and exert no pharmacologic effects until they are metabolized.

Most drugs are lipid soluble, a characteristic that aids their movement across cell membranes. However, the kidneys, which are the primary excretory organs, can excrete only water-soluble substances. Therefore, one function of metabolism is to convert fat-soluble drugs into water-soluble metabolites. Hepatic drug metabolism or clearance is a major mechanism for terminating drug action and eliminating drug molecules from the body.

Most drugs are metabolized by enzymes in the liver (called the *cytochrome P450* [CYP] or the *microsomal enzyme system*); red blood cells, plasma, kidneys, lungs, and GI mucosa also contain drug-metabolizing enzymes. The cytochrome P450 system consists of 12 groups or families, nine of which metabolize endogenous substances and three of which metabolize drugs. The three groups that metabolize drugs are labeled CYP1, CYP2, and CYP3. Of the many drugs metabolized by the liver, the CYP3 group of enzymes is thought to metabolize about 50% of drugs, the CYP2 group about 45%, and the CYP1 group about 5%. Individual members of the groups, each of which metabolizes specific drugs, are further categorized. For example, CYP2D6, CYP2C9, or CYP3A4 enzymes metabolize many drugs.

These enzymes, located within hepatocytes, are complex proteins with binding sites for drug molecules (and endogenous substances). They catalyze the chemical reactions of oxidation, reduction, hydrolysis, and conjugation with endogenous substances, such as glucuronic acid or sulfate. With chronic administration, some drugs stimulate liver cells to produce larger amounts of drug-metabolizing enzymes (a process called *enzyme induction*).

Enzyme induction accelerates drug metabolism because larger amounts of the enzymes (and more binding sites) allow larger amounts of a drug to be metabolized during a given time. As a result, larger doses of the rapidly metabolized drug may be required to produce or maintain therapeutic effects. Rapid metabolism may also increase the production of toxic metabolites with some drugs (eg, acetaminophen). Drugs that induce enzyme production also may increase the rate of metabolism for endogenous steroidal hormones (eg, cortisol, estrogens, testosterone, and vitamin D). However, enzyme induction does not occur for 1 to 3 weeks after an inducing agent is started because new enzyme proteins must be synthesized. Rifampin, an antituberculosis drug, is a strong inducer of CYP1A and CYP3A enzymes.

Metabolism also can be decreased or delayed in a process called *enzyme inhibition*, which most often occurs with concurrent administration of two or more drugs that compete for the same metabolizing enzymes. In this case, smaller doses of the slowly metabolized drug may be needed to avoid adverse reactions and toxicity from drug accumulation. Enzyme inhibition occurs within hours or days of starting an inhibiting agent. Cimetidine, a gastric acid suppressor, inhibits several CYP enzymes (eg, 1A2, 2C, and 3A) and can greatly decrease drug metabolism. The rate of drug metabolism also is reduced in infants (their hepatic enzyme system is immature), in people with impaired blood flow to the liver or severe hepatic or cardiovascular disease, and in people who are malnourished or on low-protein diets.

When drugs are given orally, they are absorbed from the GI tract and carried to the liver through the portal circulation. Some drugs are extensively metabolized in the liver, such as propranolol (Inderal), with only part of the oral drug dose reaching the systemic circulation for distribution to sites of action. This is called the *first-pass effect* or presystemic metabolism.

## Excretion

*Excretion* refers to elimination of a drug from the body. Effective excretion requires adequate functioning of the circulatory system and of the organs of excretion (kidneys, bowel, lungs, and skin). Most drugs are excreted by the kidneys and eliminated unchanged or as metabolites in the urine. Some drugs or metabolites are excreted in bile, and then eliminated in feces; others are excreted in bile, reabsorbed from the small intestine, returned to the liver (called *enterohepatic recirculation*), metabolized, and eventually excreted in urine. Some oral drugs are not absorbed and are excreted in the feces. The lungs mainly remove volatile substances, such as anesthetic gases. The skin has minimal excretory function. Factors impairing excretion, especially severe renal disease, lead to accumulation of numerous drugs and may cause severe adverse effects if dosage is not reduced.

## Serum Drug Levels

A *serum drug level* (Fig. 2-5) is a laboratory measurement of the amount of a drug in the blood at a particular time. It reflects dosage, absorption, bioavailability, half-life, and the rates of metabolism and excretion. A *minimum effective concentration (MEC)* must be present before a drug exerts its pharmacologic action on body cells; this is largely determined by the drug dose and how well it is absorbed into the bloodstream. A *toxic concentration* is an excessive level at which toxicity occurs. Toxic concentrations may stem from a single large dose, repeated small doses, or slow metabolism that allows the drug to accumulate in the body. Between these low and high concentrations is the therapeutic range, which is the goal of drug therapy. That is, enough drug to be beneficial, but not enough to be toxic.

For most drugs, serum levels indicate the onset, peak, and duration of drug action. When a single dose of a drug is given, onset of action occurs when the drug level reaches the MEC. The drug level continues to climb as more of the drug is absorbed, until it reaches its highest concentration and peak drug action occurs. Then, drug levels decline as the drug is eliminated (ie, metabolized and excreted) from the body. Although there may still be numerous drug molecules in the body, drug action stops when drug levels fall below the MEC. The duration of action is the time during which serum drug levels are at or above the MEC. When multiple doses of a drug are given (eg, for chronic, long-lasting conditions), the goal is usually to give sufficient doses often enough to maintain serum drug levels in the therapeutic range and avoid the toxic range.

In clinical practice, measuring serum drug levels is useful in several circumstances:

■ When drugs with a low or narrow therapeutic index are given. These are drugs with a narrow margin of safety because their therapeutic doses are close to their toxic doses (eg, digoxin, aminoglycoside antibiotics, lithium, theophylline)
■ To document the serum drug levels associated with particular drug dosages, therapeutic effects, or possible adverse effects
■ To monitor unexpected responses to a drug dose. This could be either a lack of therapeutic effect or increased adverse effects
■ When a drug overdose is suspected

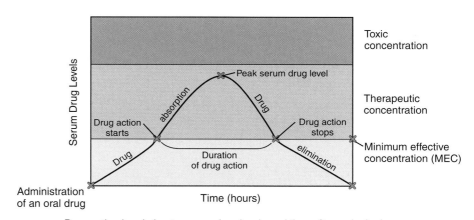

Drug action in relation to serum drug levels and time after a single dose.

**FIGURE 2–5** Serum drug levels with single and multiple oral drug doses. Drug action starts when enough drug is absorbed to reach the minimum effective concentration (MEC), continues as long as the serum level is above the MEC, wanes as drug molecules are metabolized and excreted (if no more doses are given), and stops when the serum level drops below the MEC. The goal of drug therapy is to maintain serum drug levels in the therapeutic range.

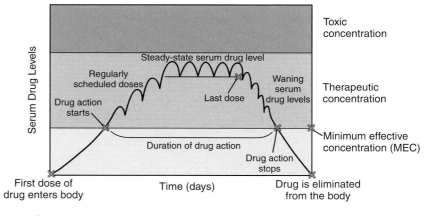

Drug action in relation to serum drug levels with repeated doses.

## Serum Half–Life

*Serum half-life,* also called *elimination half-life,* is the time required for the serum concentration of a drug to decrease by 50%. It is determined primarily by the drug's rates of metabolism and excretion. A drug with a short half-life requires more frequent administration than one with a long half-life.

When a drug is given at a stable dose, four or five half-lives are required to achieve steady-state concentrations and develop equilibrium between tissue and serum concentrations. Because maximal therapeutic effects do not occur until equilibrium is established, some drugs are not fully effective for days or weeks. To maintain steady-state conditions, the amount of drug given must equal the amount eliminated from the body. When a drug dose is changed, an additional four to five half-lives are required to reestablish equilibrium; when a drug is discontinued, it is eliminated gradually over several half-lives.

## ▦ PHARMACODYNAMICS

Pharmacodynamics involves drug actions on target cells and the resulting alterations in cellular biochemical reactions and functions (ie, "what the drug does to the body"). As previously stated, all drug actions occur at the cellular level.

## Receptor Theory of Drug Action

Like the physiologic substances (eg, hormones and neurotransmitters) that normally regulate cell functions, most drugs exert their effects by chemically binding with receptors at the cellular level (Fig. 2-6). Receptors are mainly proteins located on the surfaces of cell membranes or within cells. Specific receptors include *enzymes* involved in essential metabolic or regulatory processes (eg, dihydrofolate reductase, acetylcholinesterase); *proteins* involved in transport (eg, sodium-potassium adenosine triphosphatase) or structural processes (eg, tubulin); and *nucleic acids* (eg, DNA) involved in cellular protein synthesis, reproduction, and other metabolic activities.

When drug molecules bind with receptor molecules, the resulting drug–receptor complex initiates physiochemical reactions that stimulate or inhibit normal cellular functions. One type of reaction involves activation, inactivation, or other alterations of intracellular enzymes. Because enzymes catalyze almost all cellular functions, drug-induced changes can markedly increase or decrease the rate of cellular metabolism. For example, an epinephrine–receptor complex increases the activity of the intracellular enzyme adenyl cyclase, which then causes the formation of cyclic adenosine monophosphate (cAMP). cAMP, in turn, can initiate any one of many different intracellular actions, the exact effect depending on the type of cell.

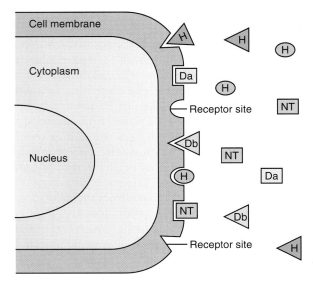

**FIGURE 2–6** Cell membrane contains receptors for physiologic substances such as hormones (H) and neurotransmitters (NT). These substances stimulate or inhibit cellular function. Drug molecules (Da and Db) also interact with receptors to stimulate or inhibit cellular function.

A second type of reaction involves changes in the permeability of cell membranes to one or more ions. The receptor protein is a structural component of the cell membrane, and its binding to a drug molecule may open or close ion channels. In nerve cells, for example, sodium or calcium ion channels may open and allow movement of ions into the cell. This usually causes the cell membrane to depolarize and excite the cell. At other times, potassium channels may open and allow movement of potassium ions out of the cell. This action inhibits neuronal excitability and function. In muscle cells, movement of the ions into the cells may alter intracellular functions, such as the direct effect of calcium ions in stimulating muscle contraction.

A third reaction may modify the synthesis, release, or inactivation of the neurohormones (eg, acetylcholine, norepinephrine, serotonin) that regulate many physiologic processes.

Additional elements and characteristics of the receptor theory include the following:

**1.** The site and extent of drug action on body cells are determined primarily by specific characteristics of receptors and drugs. Receptors vary in type, location, number, and functional capacity. For example, many different types of receptors have been identified. Most types occur in most body tissues, such as receptors for epinephrine and norepinephrine (whether received from stimulation of the sympathetic nervous system or administration of drug formulations) and receptors for hormones, including growth hormone, thyroid hormone, and insulin. Some occur in fewer body tissues, such as receptors for opiates and benzodiazepines in the brain and subgroups of receptors for epinephrine in the heart (beta₁-adrenergic receptors) and lungs (beta₂-adrenergic receptors). Receptor type and location influence drug action. The receptor is often described as a lock into which the drug molecule fits as a key, and only those drugs able to bond chemically to the receptors in a particular body tissue can exert pharmacologic effects on that tissue. Thus, all body cells do not respond to all drugs, even though virtually all cell receptors are exposed to any drug molecules circulating in the bloodstream.

The number of receptor sites available to interact with drug molecules also affects the extent of drug action. Presumably, a minimal number of receptors must be occupied by drug molecules to produce pharmacologic effects. Thus, if many receptors are available, but only a few are occupied by drug molecules, few drug effects occur. In this instance, increasing the drug dosage increases the pharmacologic effects. Conversely, if only a few receptors are available for many drug molecules, receptors may be saturated. In this instance, if most receptor sites are occupied, increasing the drug dosage produces no additional pharmacologic effect.

Drugs vary even more widely than receptors. Because all drugs are chemical substances, chemical characteristics determine drug actions and pharmacologic effects. For example, a drug's chemical structure affects its ability to reach tissue fluids around a cell and bind with its cell receptors. Minor changes in drug structure may produce major changes in pharmacologic effects. Another major factor is the concentration of drug molecules that reach receptor sites in body tissues. Drug- and client-related variables that affect drug actions are further described below.

2. When drug molecules chemically bind with cell receptors, the pharmacologic effects are those due to either agonism or antagonism. *Agonists* are drugs that produce effects similar to those produced by naturally occurring hormones, neurotransmitters, and other substances. Agonists may accelerate or slow normal cellular processes, depending on the type of receptor activated. For example, epinephrine-like drugs act on the heart to increase the heart rate, and acetylcholine-like drugs act on the heart to slow the heart rate; both are agonists. *Antagonists* are drugs that inhibit cell function by occupying receptor sites. This prevents natural body substances or other drugs from occupying the receptor sites and activating cell functions. Once drug action occurs, drug molecules may detach from receptor molecules (ie, the chemical binding is reversible), return to the bloodstream, and circulate to the liver for metabolism and to the kidneys for excretion.

3. Receptors are dynamic cellular components that can be synthesized by body cells and altered by endogenous substances and exogenous drugs. For example, prolonged stimulation of body cells with an excita-

tory agonist usually reduces the number or sensitivity of receptors. As a result, the cell becomes less responsive to the agonist (a process called receptor desensitization, or *down-regulation*). Prolonged inhibition of normal cellular functions with an antagonist may increase receptor number or sensitivity. If the antagonist is suddenly reduced or stopped, the cell becomes excessively responsive to an agonist (a process called receptor *up-regulation*). These changes in receptors may explain why some drugs must be tapered in dosage and discontinued gradually if withdrawal symptoms are to be avoided.

## Nonreceptor Drug Actions

Relatively few drugs act by mechanisms other than combination with receptor sites on cells. These include the following:

- Antacids, which act chemically to neutralize the hydrochloric acid produced by gastric parietal cells and thereby raise the pH of gastric fluid
- Osmotic diuretics (eg, mannitol), which increase the osmolarity of plasma and pull water out of tissues into the bloodstream
- Drugs that are structurally similar to nutrients required by body cells (eg, purines, pyrimidines) and that can be incorporated into cellular constituents, such as nucleic acids. This interferes with normal cell functioning. Several anticancer drugs act by this mechanism
- Metal chelating agents, which combine with toxic metals (eg, lead) to form a complex that can be more readily excreted

## ■ VARIABLES THAT AFFECT DRUG ACTIONS

Expected responses to drugs are largely based on those occurring when a particular drug is given to healthy adult men (18 to 65 years of age) of average weight (150 lb [68 kg]). However, other groups of people (eg, women, children, older adults, different ethnic or racial groups, and clients with diseases or symptoms that the drugs are designed to treat) receive drugs and respond differently than healthy adult men. Therefore, current clinical trials are including more representatives of these groups. In any client, however, responses may be altered by both drug- and client-related variables, some of which are described in the following sections.

## Drug-Related Variables

### Dosage

Although the terms *dose* and *dosage* are often used interchangeably, dose indicates the amount to be given at one time and dosage refers to the frequency, size, and number of doses. Dosage is a major determinant of drug actions and responses, both therapeutic and adverse. If the amount is too small or administered infrequently, no pharmacologic action occurs because the drug does not reach an adequate concentration at target cells. If the amount is too large or administered too often, toxicity (poisoning) may occur. Because dosage includes the amount of the drug and the frequency of administration, overdosage may occur with a single large dose or with chronic ingestion of smaller amounts. Doses that produce signs and symptoms of toxicity are called *toxic doses.* Doses that cause death are called *lethal doses.*

Dosages recommended in drug literature are usually those that produce particular responses in 50% of the people tested. These dosages usually produce a mixture of therapeutic and adverse effects. The dosage of a particular drug depends on many characteristics of the drug (reason for use, potency, pharmacokinetics, route of administration, dosage form, and others) and of the recipient (age, weight, state of health, and function of cardiovascular, renal, and hepatic systems). Thus, the recommended dosages are intended only as guidelines for individualizing dosages.

### Route of Administration

Routes of administration affect drug actions and responses largely by influencing absorption and distribution. For rapid drug action and response, the IV route is most effective because the drug is injected directly into the bloodstream. For some drugs, the intramuscular route also produces drug action within a few minutes because muscles have a large blood supply. The oral route usually produces slower drug action than parenteral routes. Absorption and action of topical drugs vary according to the drug formulation, whether the drug is applied to skin or mucous membranes, and other factors.

### Drug–Diet Interactions

Food may alter the absorption of oral drugs. In many instances, food slows absorption by slowing gastric emptying time and altering GI secretions and motility. When tablets or capsules are taken with or soon after food, they dissolve more slowly; therefore, drug molecules are delivered to absorptive sites in the small intestine more slowly. Food also may decrease absorption by combining with a drug to form an insoluble drug–food complex. In other instances, however, certain drugs or dosage forms are better absorbed with certain types of meals. For example, a fatty meal increases the absorption of some sustained-release forms of theophylline. Interactions that alter drug absorption can be minimized by spacing food and medications.

In addition, some foods contain substances that react with certain drugs. One such interaction occurs between tyramine-containing foods and monoamine oxidase (MAO) inhibitor drugs. Tyramine causes the release of norepinephrine, a strong vasoconstrictive agent, from the adrenal medulla and sympathetic neurons. Normally, norepinephrine is active for only a few milliseconds before it is inactivated by MAO. However, because MAO inhibitor drugs prevent inactivation of norepinephrine, ingesting tyramine-containing foods with an MAO inhibitor may produce severe hypertension or intracranial hemorrhage. MAO inhibitors include the antidepressants isocarboxazid and phenelzine and the antineoplastic procarbazine. These drugs are infrequently used currently, partly because of this potentially serious interaction and partly because other effective drugs are available. Tyramine-rich foods to be avoided by clients taking MAO inhibitors include beer, wine, aged cheeses, yeast products, chicken livers, and pickled herring.

An interaction may occur between warfarin, a frequently used oral anticoagulant, and foods containing vitamin K. Because vitamin K antagonizes the action of warfarin, large amounts of spinach and other green leafy vegetables may offset the anticoagulant effects and predispose the person to thromboembolic disorders.

A third interaction occurs between tetracycline, an antibiotic, and dairy products, such as milk and cheese. The drug combines with the calcium in milk products to form an insoluble, unabsorbable compound that is excreted in the feces.

### *Herbal and Dietary Supplements*

Use of nonprescription herbal and dietary supplements is frequently not reported by the client even though one third of the adults in the United States use these agents. Significant interactions can occur between supplements and prescribed drugs.

### Drug–Drug Interactions

The action of a drug may be increased or decreased by its interaction with another drug in the body. Most interactions occur whenever the interacting drugs are present in the body; some, especially those affecting the absorption of oral drugs, occur when the interacting drugs are given at or near the same time. The basic cause of many drug–drug interactions is altered drug metabolism. For example, drugs metabolized by the same enzymes may compete for enzyme binding sites, and there may not be enough binding sites for two or more drugs. Also, some drugs induce or inhibit the metabolism of other drugs.

---

**?**    **How Can You Avoid**
       **This Medication Error?**

Mrs. Beecher, a 76-year-old nursing home client, has just had a change in her antihypertension medications to felodipine 10 mg qd, a calcium channel blocker. Her blood pressure is 148/70. You give her the tablet with a large glass of grapefruit juice and caution her to swallow the tablet whole. Two days later Mrs. Beecher's blood pressure is 96/60.

Protein binding is also the basis for some important drug–drug interactions. A drug with a strong attraction to protein-binding sites may displace a less tightly bound drug. The displaced drug then becomes pharmacologically active, and the overall effect is the same as taking a larger dose of the displaced drug.

### Increased Drug Effects

Interactions that can increase the therapeutic or adverse effects of drugs are as follows:

1. *Additive effects* occur when two drugs with similar pharmacologic actions are taken.
   *Example:* ethanol + sedative drug → increased sedation
2. *Synergism* or *potentiation* occurs when two drugs with different sites or mechanisms of action produce greater effects when taken together than either does when taken alone.
   *Example:* acetaminophen (non-narcotic analgesic) + codeine (narcotic analgesic) → increased analgesia
3. *Interference* by one drug with the metabolism or elimination of a second drug may result in intensified effects of the second drug
   *Example:* cimetidine inhibits CYP1A, CYP2C, and CYP3A drug-metabolizing enzymes in the liver and therefore interferes with the metabolism of many drugs (eg, benzodiazepine antianxiety and hypnotic drugs, calcium channel blockers, tricyclic antidepressants, some antidysrhythmics, beta blockers and antiseizure drugs, theophylline, and warfarin). When these drugs are given concurrently with cimetidine, they are likely to cause adverse and toxic effects.
4. *Displacement* of one drug from plasma protein-binding sites by a second drug increases the effects of the displaced drug. This increase occurs because the molecules of the displaced drug, freed from their bound form, become pharmacologically active.
   *Example:* aspirin (an anti-inflammatory, analgesic, or antipyretic agent) + warfarin (an anticoagulant) → increased anticoagulant effect

### Decreased Drug Effects

Interactions in which drug effects are decreased are grouped under the term *antagonism*. Examples of such interactions are as follows:

1. In some situations, a drug that is a specific antidote is given to antagonize the toxic effects of another drug.
   *Example:* naloxone (a narcotic antagonist) + morphine (a narcotic or opioid analgesic) → relief of narcotic-induced respiratory depression. Naloxone molecules displace morphine molecules from their receptor sites on nerve cells in the brain, so that the morphine molecules cannot continue to exert their depressant effects.
2. Decreased intestinal absorption of oral drugs occurs when drugs combine to produce nonabsorbable compounds.
   *Example:* aluminum or magnesium hydroxide (antacids) + oral tetracycline (an antibiotic) → binding of tetracycline to aluminum or magnesium, causing decreased absorption and decreased antibiotic effect of tetracycline
3. Activation of drug-metabolizing enzymes in the liver increases the metabolism rate of any drug metabolized primarily by that group of enzymes. Several drugs (eg, phenytoin, rifampin), ethanol, and cigarette smoking are known *enzyme inducers.*
   *Example:* phenobarbital (a barbiturate) + warfarin (an anticoagulant) → decreased effects of warfarin
4. Increased excretion occurs when urinary pH is changed and renal reabsorption is blocked.
   *Example:* sodium bicarbonate + phenobarbital → increased excretion of phenobarbital. The sodium bicarbonate alkalinizes the urine, raising the number of barbiturate ions in the renal filtrate. The ionized particles cannot pass easily through renal tubular membranes. Therefore, less drug is reabsorbed into the blood and more is excreted by the kidneys.

## Client–Related Variables

### Developmental Considerations

#### Neonates and Infants

In children, drug action depends largely on age and developmental stage. Drug distribution, metabolism, and excretion differ markedly in neonates, especially premature infants, because their organ systems are not fully developed. Newborn infants (birth to 1 month) also handle drugs inefficiently. Older infants (1 month to 1 year) reach approximately adult levels of protein binding and kidney function, but liver function and the blood–brain barrier are still immature.

#### Children

Children (1 to 12 years) experience a period of increased activity of drug-metabolizing enzymes, so that some drugs are rapidly metabolized and eliminated. Although the onset and duration of this period are unclear, a few studies have been done with particular drugs. Theophylline, for example, is cleared much faster in a 7-year-old child than in a neonate or adult (18 to 65 years). After approximately 12 years of age, healthy children handle drugs similarly to healthy adults. Specific developmental considerations related to children are identified in subsequent chapters.

#### Pregnancy and Breast-Feeding

During pregnancy, drugs cross the placenta and may harm the fetus. *Teratogenicity* is the ability of a substance to cause abnormal fetal development when taken by pregnant women. Fetuses have no effective mechanisms for metabolizing or eliminating drugs because their liver and kidney functions are immature. Two significant factors to consider when evaluating the teratogenic potential of a medication are the stage of pregnancy at which the exposure occurred and the amount of medication taken. The U.S. Food and Drug Administration (FDA) has established five categories (A, B, C, D, and X) to indicate the potential for a drug to cause birth defects during pregnancy. The categorization is made on the reliability of the reported evidence and the risk-to-benefit ratio with use. The FDA Pregnancy Categories are found in Box 2-1. Pregnancy Categories are reported in individual drug tables in subsequent chapters.

Most drugs that appear in maternal circulation are also secreted in breast milk. During lactation, some medications enter breast milk and may cause potential injury to the infant. Women who breast-feed should be instructed regarding potential adverse reactions and should be referred to a health care provider or pharmacist.

### Older Adults

In older adults (65 years and older), physiologic changes may alter all pharmacokinetic processes. Changes in the GI tract include decreased gastric acidity, decreased blood flow, and decreased motility. Despite these changes, however, there is little difference in absorption. Changes in the cardiovascular system include decreased cardiac output and therefore slower distribution of drug molecules to their sites of action, metabolism, and excretion. In the liver, blood flow and metabolizing enzymes are decreased. Thus, many drugs are metabolized more slowly, have a longer action, and are more likely to accumulate with chronic administration. In the kidneys, there is decreased blood flow, decreased glomerular filtration rate, and decreased tubular secretion of drugs. All of these changes tend to slow excretion and promote accumulation of drugs in the body. *Impaired kidney and liver function greatly increases the risks for adverse drug effects.* In addition, older adults are more likely to have acute and chronic illnesses that require multiple drugs or long-term drug therapy. Thus, possibilities for interactions among drugs and between drugs and diseased organs are greatly multiplied. Specific developmental considerations related to older adults are highlighted in later chapters.

### Body Weight

Body weight affects drug action mainly in relation to dose. The ratio between the amount of drug given and body weight influences drug distribution and concentration at sites of action. In general, people heavier than average need larger doses, provided that their renal, hepatic, and cardiovascular functions are adequate. Recommended doses for many drugs are listed in terms of grams or milligrams per kilogram of body weight.

### Genetic and Ethnic Characteristics

Drugs are given to elicit certain responses that are relatively predictable for most drug recipients. When given the same drug in the same dose, however, some people experience inadequate therapeutic effects, and others experience unusual or exaggerated effects, including increased toxicity. These interindividual variations in drug response are often attributed to genetic or ethnic differences in drug pharmacokinetics or pharmacodynamics. As a result, there is increased awareness that genetic and ethnic characteristics are important factors and that diverse groups must be included in clinical trials.

### Genetics

A person's genetic characteristics may influence drug action in several ways. For example, genes determine the types and amounts of proteins produced in the body. When most drugs enter the body, they interact with proteins (eg, in plasma, tissues, cell membranes, and drug

---

**BOX 2-1    Pregnancy Categories**

**Pregnancy Category A**
Adequate and well-controlled studies have not succeeded in demonstrating a risk to the fetus in the first trimester of pregnancy (and there is no evidence of risk in later trimesters).

**Pregnancy Category B**
Either animal reproduction studies have failed to demonstrate a risk to the fetus with no adequate and well-controlled studies in pregnant women or animal reproduction studies have shown an adverse effect (except for a decrease in fertility) not confirmed in controlled studies in women in the first trimester and no documentation of a risk in later trimesters.

**Pregnancy Category C**
Either animal reproduction studies have revealed an adverse effect on the fetus and there are no adequate and well-controlled studies in humans or studies in women or animals are not available; potential benefits may warrant use of the drug in pregnant women despite potential risks.

**Pregnancy Category D**
There is positive evidence of human fetal risk based on adverse reaction data from investigational or marketing experience or studies in humans, but potential benefits may be acceptable in pregnant women despite potential risks.

**Pregnancy Category X**
Studies in animals or humans have demonstrated fetal abnormalities and/or there is evidence of human fetal risk based on adverse reaction data from investigational or human experience, and the risks involved in use of the drug in pregnant women clearly outweigh potential benefits. The drug is contraindicated in women who are or may become pregnant.

receptor sites) to reach their sites of action, and with other proteins (eg, drug-metabolizing enzymes in the liver and other organs) to be biotransformed and eliminated from the body. Genetic characteristics that alter any of these proteins can alter drug pharmacokinetics or pharmacodynamics.

One of the earliest genetic variations to be identified derived from the observation that some people taking usual doses of isoniazid (an antitubercular drug), hydralazine (an antihypertensive agent), or procainamide (an antidysrhythmic) showed no therapeutic effects, whereas toxicity developed in other people. Research established that these drugs are normally metabolized by acetylation, a chemical conjugation process in which the drug molecule combines with an acetyl group of acetyl coenzyme A. The reaction is catalyzed by a hepatic drug-metabolizing enzyme called *acetyltransferase*. It was further established that humans may acetylate the drug rapidly or slowly, depending largely on genetically controlled differences in acetyltransferase activity. Clinically, rapid acetylators may need larger-than-usual doses to achieve therapeutic effects, and slow acetylators may need smaller-than-usual doses to avoid toxic effects. In addition, several genetic variations of the cytochrome P450 drug-metabolizing system have been identified. Specific variations may influence any of the chemical processes by which drugs are metabolized.

As another example of genetic variation in drug metabolism, some people lack the plasma pseudocholinesterase enzyme that normally inactivates succinylcholine, a potent muscle relaxant used in some surgical procedures. These people may experience prolonged paralysis and apnea if given succinylcholine.

Other people are deficient in glucose-6-phosphate dehydrogenase, an enzyme normally found in red blood cells and other body tissues. These people may have hemolytic anemia when given antimalarial drugs, sulfonamides, analgesics, antipyretics, and other drugs.

### Ethnicity

Most drug information has been derived from clinical drug trials using white men; few subjects of other ethnic groups are included. Interethnic variations became evident when drugs and dosages developed for white people produced unexpected responses, including toxicity, when given to other ethnic groups.

One common interethnic variation is that African Americans are less responsive to some antihypertensive drugs than are white people. For example, angiotensin-converting enzyme (ACE) inhibitors and beta-adrenergic blocking drugs are less effective as single-drug therapy. In general, African-American hypertensive clients respond better to diuretics or calcium channel blockers than to ACE inhibitors and beta blockers. Another interethnic variation is that Asians usually require much smaller doses of some commonly used drugs, including beta blockers and several psychotropic drugs (eg, alprazolam,

an antianxiety agent, and haloperidol, an antipsychotic). Some documented interethnic variations are included in later chapters.

### Gender

Except during pregnancy and lactation, gender has been considered a minor influence on drug action. Most research studies related to drugs have involved men, and clinicians have extrapolated the findings to women. Several reasons have been advanced for excluding women from clinical drug trials, including the risks to a fetus if a woman becomes pregnant and the greater complexity in sample size and data analysis. However, because differences between men and women in responses to drug therapy are being identified, the need to include women in drug studies is evident.

Some gender-related differences in responses to drugs may stem from hormonal fluctuations in women during the menstrual cycle. Although this area has received little attention in research studies and clinical practice, altered responses have been demonstrated in some women taking clonidine, an antihypertensive; lithium, a mood-stabilizing agent; phenytoin, an anticonvulsant; propranolol, a beta-adrenergic blocking drug used in the management of hypertension, angina pectoris, and migraine; and antidepressants. In addition, a significant percentage of women with arthritis, asthma, depression, diabetes mellitus, epilepsy, and migraine experience increased symptoms premenstrually. The increased symptoms may indicate a need for adjustments in their drug therapy regimens. Women with clinical depression, for example, may need higher doses of antidepressant medications premenstrually, if symptoms exacerbate, and lower doses during the rest of the menstrual cycle.

Another example is that women with schizophrenia require lower dosages of antipsychotic medications than men. If given the higher doses required by men, women are likely to have adverse drug reactions.

### Pathologic Conditions

Pathologic conditions may alter pharmacokinetic processes (Table 2-1). In general, all pharmacokinetic processes are decreased in cardiovascular disorders characterized by decreased blood flow to tissues, such as heart failure. In addition, the absorption of oral drugs is decreased with various GI disorders. Distribution is altered in liver or kidney disease and other conditions that alter plasma proteins. Metabolism is decreased in malnutrition (eg, inadequate protein to synthesize drug-metabolizing enzymes) and severe liver disease; it may be increased in conditions that generally increase body metabolism, such as hyperthyroidism and fever. Excretion is decreased in kidney disease.

### Psychological Considerations

Psychological considerations influence individual responses to drug administration, although specific mech-

*(text continues on page 23)*

## TABLE 2-1   Effects of Pathologic Conditions on Drug Pharmacokinetics

| Pathologic Conditions | Pharmacokinetic Consequences |
| --- | --- |
| Cardiovascular disorders that impair the pumping ability of the heart, decrease cardiac output, or impair blood flow to body tissues (eg, acute myocardial infarction, heart failure, hypotension, and shock) | *Absorption* of oral, subcutaneous, intramuscular, and topical drugs is erratic because of decreased blood flow to sites of drug administration. *Distribution* is impaired because of decreased blood flow to body tissues and thus to sites of drug action. *Metabolism* and *excretion* are impaired because of decreased blood flow to the liver and kidneys. |
| Central nervous system (CNS) disorders that alter respiration or circulation (eg, brain trauma or injury, brain ischemia from inadequate cerebral blood flow, drugs that depress or stimulate brain function) | CNS impairment may alter pharmacokinetics indirectly by causing hypo- or hyperventilation and acid–base imbalances. Also, cerebral irritation may occur with head injuries and lead to stimulation of the sympathetic nervous system and increased cardiac output. Increased blood flow may accelerate all pharmacokinetic processes. With faster absorption and distribution, drug action may be more rapid, but faster metabolism and excretion may shorten duration of action. |
| Gastrointestinal (GI) disorders that interfere with GI function or blood flow (eg, trauma or surgery of the GI tract, abdominal infection, paralytic ileus, pancreatitis) | Symptoms of impaired GI function commonly occur with both GI and non-GI disorders. As a result, many patients cannot take oral medications. Those who are able to take oral drugs may experience impaired absorption because of:<br>    Vomiting or diarrhea.<br>    Concurrent administration of drugs that raise the pH of gastric fluids (eg, antacids, histamine-2 blockers, proton pump inhibitors).<br>    Concurrent administration of foods or tube feeding solutions that decrease drug absorption.<br>    Crushing tablets or opening capsules to give a drug through a GI tube. |
| Inflammatory bowel disorders (eg, Crohn's disease, ulcerative colitis) | *Absorption* of oral drugs is variable. It may be increased because GI hypermotility rapidly delivers drug molecules to sites of absorption in the small intestine and the drugs tend to be absorbed more rapidly from inflamed tissue. It may be decreased because hypermotility and diarrhea may move the drug through the GI tract too rapidly to be adequately absorbed. |
| Endocrine disorders that impair function or change hormonal balance<br>    Diabetes-induced cardiovascular disorders | Impaired circulation may decrease all pharmacokinetic processes, as described previously. |
|     Thyroid disorders | The main effect is on metabolism. Hypothyroidism slows metabolism, which prolongs drug action and slows elimination from the body. Hyperthyroidism accelerates metabolism, producing a shorter duration of action and a faster elimination rate. As a thyroid disorder is treated and thyroid function returns to normal, the rate of drug metabolism also returns to normal. Thus, dosages of drugs that are extensively metabolized need adjustments according to the level of thyroid function. |
|     Adrenal disorders resulting from the underlying illness or the stress response that accompanies illness | Increased adrenal function (ie, increased amounts of circulating catecholamines and cortisol) affects drug action by increasing cardiac output, redistributing cardiac output (more blood flow to the heart and brain, less to kidneys, liver, and GI tract), causing fluid retention, and increasing blood volume. Stress also changes plasma protein levels, which can affect the unbound portion of a drug dose. Decreased adrenal function causes hypotension and shock, which impairs all pharmacokinetic processes. |
| Hepatic disorders that impair hepatic function and blood flow (eg, hepatitis, cirrhosis) | Most drugs are eliminated from the body by hepatic metabolism, renal excretion or both. Hepatic metabolism depends on hepatic blood flow, hepatic enzyme activity, and plasma protein binding. Increased hepatic blood flow increases delivery of drug molecules to hepatocytes, where metabolism occurs, and thereby accelerates drug metabolism. Decreased hepatic blood flow slows metabolism. Severe liver disease or cirrhosis may impair all pharmacokinetic processes. |

*(continued)*

## TABLE 2-1   Effects of Pathologic Conditions on Drug Pharmacokinetics (Continued)

| Pathologic Conditions | Pharmacokinetic Consequences |
|---|---|
| | *Absorption* of oral drugs may be decreased in cirrhosis because of edema in the GI tract.<br><br>*Distribution* may be altered by changes in plasma proteins. The impaired liver may be unable to synthesize adequate amounts of plasma proteins, especially albumin. Also, liver impairment leads to inadequate metabolism and accumulation of substances (eg, serum bilirubin) that can displace drugs from protein-binding sites. With decreased protein binding, the serum concentration of active drug is increased and the drug is distributed to sites of action and elimination more rapidly. Thus, onset of drug action may be faster, peak blood levels may be higher and cause adverse effects, and the duration of action may be shorter because the drug is metabolized and excreted more quickly.<br><br>With cirrhosis, oral drugs are distributed directly into the systemic circulation rather than going through the portal circulation and the liver first. This shunting of blood around the liver means that oral drugs that are normally extensively metabolized during their first pass through the liver (eg, propranolol) must be given in reduced doses to prevent high blood levels and toxicity.<br><br>*Metabolism* may be impaired by hepatic and nonhepatic disorders that reduce hepatic blood flow. In addition, an impaired liver may not be able to synthesize adequate amounts of drug-metabolizing enzymes.<br><br>*Excretion* may be increased when protein binding is impaired because larger amounts of free drug are circulating in the bloodstream and being delivered more rapidly to sites of metabolism and excretion. The result is a shorter drug half-life and duration of action. Excretion is decreased when the liver is unable to metabolize lipid-soluble drugs into water-soluble metabolites that can be excreted by the kidneys. |
| Renal impairment—acute renal failure (ARF) and chronic renal failure (CRF) | ARF and CRF can interfere with all pharmacokinetic processes.<br><br>*Absorption* of oral drugs may be decreased indirectly by changes that often occur with renal failure (eg, delayed gastric emptying, changes in gastric pH, GI symptoms such as vomiting and diarrhea). Also, in the presence of generalized edema, edema of the GI tract may impair absorption.<br><br>In CRF, gastric pH may be increased by administration of oral alkalinizing agents (eg, sodium bicarbonate, citrate) and the use of antacids for phosphate-binding effects. This may decrease absorption of oral drugs that require an acidic environment for dissolution and absorption and increase absorption of drugs that are absorbed from a more alkaline environment.<br><br>*Distribution* of many drugs may be altered by changes in extracellular fluid volume (ECF), plasma protein binding, and tissue binding. Water-soluble drugs are distributed throughout the ECF, including edema fluid, which is usually increased in renal impairment because the kidney's ability to eliminate water and sodium is impaired.<br><br>Drug binding with albumin, the main drug-binding plasma protein for acidic drugs, is usually decreased with renal impairment. Protein binding may be decreased because of less albumin or decreased binding capacity of albumin for a drug. Reasons for decreased albumin include hypermetabolic states (eg, stress, trauma, sepsis) in which protein breakdown exceeds protein synthesis, nephrotic states in which albumin is lost in the urine, and liver disease that decreases hepatic synthesis of albumin. Reasons for reduced binding capacity include structural changes in the albumin molecule or uremic toxins that compete with drugs for binding sites. |

*(continued)*

## TABLE 2-1   Effects of Pathologic Conditions on Drug Pharmacokinetics (Continued)

| Pathologic Conditions | Pharmacokinetic Consequences |
|---|---|
| | When less drug is bound to albumin, the higher serum drug levels of unbound or active drug can result in drug toxicity. In addition, more unbound drug is available for distribution into tissues and sites of metabolism and excretion so that faster elimination can decrease drug half-life and therapeutic effects. |
| | For basic drugs (eg, clindamycin, propafenone), alpha$_1$-acid glycoprotein (AAG) is the main binding protein. The amount of AAG increases in some patients, including those with renal transplants and those receiving hemodialysis. If these patients are given a basic drug, a larger amount is bound and a smaller amount is free to exert a pharmacologic effect. |
| | Finally, some conditions that often occur in renal impairment (eg, metabolic acidosis, respiratory alkalosis, others) may alter tissue distribution of some drugs. For example, digoxin can be displaced from tissue-binding sites by metabolic products that cannot be adequately excreted by impaired kidneys. |
| | *Metabolism* can be increased, decreased, or unaffected by renal impairment. |
| | One factor is alteration of drug metabolism in the liver. In uremia, reduction and hydrolysis reactions may be slower, but oxidation by cytochrome P450 enzymes and conjugation with glucuronide or sulfate usually proceed at normal rates. |
| | Another factor is the inability of impaired kidneys to eliminate drugs and pharmacologically active metabolites, which may lead to accumulation and adverse drug reactions with long-term drug therapy. Metabolites may have pharmacologic activity similar to or different from that of the parent drug. |
| | A third factor may be impaired renal metabolism of drugs. Although the role of the kidneys in excretion of drugs and drug metabolites is well known, their role in drug metabolism has received little attention. The kidney itself contains many of the same metabolizing enzymes found in the liver, including renal cytochrome P450 enzymes, which metabolize a variety of chemicals and drugs. |
| | *Excretion* of many drugs and metabolites is reduced by renal impairment. The kidneys normally excrete both the parent drug and metabolites produced by the liver and other tissues. Processes of renal excretion include glomerular filtration, tubular secretion, and tubular reabsorption, all of which may be affected by renal impairment. If the kidneys are unable to excrete drugs and metabolites, some of which may be pharmacologically active, these substances may accumulate and cause adverse or toxic effects. |
| Respiratory impairments | Respiratory impairment may indirectly affect drug metabolism. For example, hypoxemia leads to decreased enzyme production in the liver, decreased efficiency of the enzymes that are produced, and decreased oxygen available for drug biotransformation. Mechanical ventilation leads to decreased blood flow to the liver. |
| Sepsis-induced alterations in cardiovascular function and hepatic blood flow | Sepsis may affect all pharmacokinetic processes. Early sepsis is characterized by hyperdynamic circulation, with increased cardiac output and shunting of blood to vital organs. As a result, absorption, distribution, metabolism, and excretion may be accelerated. Late sepsis is characterized by hypodynamic circulation, with diminished cardiac output and reduced blood flow to major organs. Thus, absorption, distribution, metabolism, and excretion may be impaired. |
| Shock-induced alterations in cardiovascular function and blood flow | Shock may inhibit all pharmacokinetic processes. Absorption is impaired by decreased blood flow to sites of drug administration. Distribution is impaired by decreased blood flow to all body tissues. Metabolism is impaired by decreased blood flow to the liver. Excretion is impaired by decreased blood flow to the kidneys. |

anisms are unknown. An example is the *placebo response.* A placebo is a pharmacologically inactive substance. Placebos are used in clinical drug trials to compare the medication being tested with a "dummy" medication. Interestingly, recipients often report both therapeutic and adverse effects from placebos.

Attitudes and expectations related to drugs in general, a particular drug, or a placebo influence client response. They also influence compliance or the willingness to carry out the prescribed drug regimen, especially with long-term drug therapy.

## ■ TOLERANCE AND CROSS-TOLERANCE

Drug *tolerance* occurs when the body becomes accustomed to a particular drug over time, so that larger doses must be given to produce the same effects. Tolerance may be acquired to the pharmacologic action of many drugs, especially narcotic analgesics, alcohol, and other CNS depressants. Tolerance to pharmacologically related drugs is called *cross-tolerance.* For example, a person who regularly drinks large amounts of alcohol becomes able to ingest even larger amounts before becoming intoxicated—this is tolerance to alcohol. If the person is then given sedative-type drugs or a general anesthetic, larger-than-usual doses are required to produce a pharmacologic effect—this is cross-tolerance.

Tolerance and cross-tolerance are usually attributed to activation of drug-metabolizing enzymes in the liver, which accelerates drug metabolism and excretion. They also are attributed to decreased sensitivity or numbers of receptor sites.

## ■ ADVERSE EFFECTS OF DRUGS

As used in this book, the term *adverse effects* refers to any undesired responses to drug administration, as opposed to *therapeutic effects,* which are desired responses. Most drugs produce a mixture of therapeutic and adverse effects; all drugs can produce adverse effects. Adverse effects may produce essentially any sign, symptom, or disease process and may involve any body system or tissue. They may be common or rare, mild or severe, localized or widespread, depending on the drug and the recipient.

Some adverse effects occur with usual therapeutic doses of drugs (often called *side effects*); others are more likely to occur and to be more severe with high doses. Common or serious adverse effects include the following:

1. *CNS effects* may result from CNS stimulation (eg, agitation, confusion, delirium, disorientation, hallucinations, psychosis, seizures) or CNS depression (dizziness, drowsiness, impaired level of consciousness, sedation, coma, impaired respiration and circulation). CNS effects may occur with many drugs, including most therapeutic groups, substances of abuse, and over-the-counter preparations.

2. *Gastrointestinal effects* (anorexia, nausea, vomiting, constipation, diarrhea) are among the most common adverse reactions to drugs. Nausea and vomiting occur with many drugs from local irritation of the gastrointestinal tract or stimulation of the vomiting center in the brain. Diarrhea occurs with drugs that cause local irritation or increase peristalsis. More serious effects include bleeding or ulceration (most often with aspirin and nonsteroidal anti-inflammatory agents) and severe diarrhea/colitis (most often with antibiotics).

3. *Hematologic effects* (blood coagulation disorders, bleeding disorders, bone marrow depression, anemias, leukopenia, agranulocytosis, thrombocytopenia) are relatively common and potentially life threatening. Excessive bleeding is most often associated with anticoagulants and thrombolytics; bone marrow depression is usually associated with antineoplastic drugs.

4. *Hepatotoxicity* (hepatitis, liver dysfunction or failure, biliary tract inflammation or obstruction) is potentially life threatening. Because most drugs are metabolized by the liver, the liver is especially susceptible to drug-induced injury. Drugs that are hepatotoxic include acetaminophen (Tylenol), isoniazid (INH), methotrexate (Mexate), phenytoin (Dilantin), and aspirin and other salicylates. In the presence of drug- or disease-induced liver damage, the metabolism of many drugs is impaired. Consequently, drugs metabolized by the liver tend to accumulate in the body and cause adverse effects. Besides hepatotoxicity, many drugs produce abnormal values in liver function tests without producing clinical signs of liver dysfunction.

5. *Nephrotoxicity* (nephritis, renal insufficiency or failure) occurs with several antimicrobial agents (eg, gentamicin and other aminoglycosides), nonsteroidal anti-inflammatory agents (eg, ibuprofen and related drugs), and others. It is potentially serious because it may interfere with drug excretion, thereby causing drug accumulation and increased adverse effects.

6. *Hypersensitivity* or *allergy* may occur with almost any drug in susceptible clients. It is largely unpredictable and unrelated to dose. It occurs in those who have previously been exposed to the drug or a similar substance (antigen) and who have developed antibodies. When readministered, the drug reacts with the antibodies to cause cell damage and the release of histamine and other intracellular substances. These substances produce reactions ranging from mild skin rashes to anaphylactic shock. Anaphylactic shock is a life-threatening hypersensitivity reaction characterized by respiratory distress and cardiovascular collapse. It occurs within a few minutes after drug

administration and requires emergency treatment with epinephrine. Some allergic reactions (eg, serum sickness) occur 1 to 2 weeks after the drug is given.

7. *Drug fever* is a fever associated with administration of a medication. Drugs can cause fever by several mechanisms, including allergic reactions, damaging body tissues, increasing body heat or interfering with its dissipation, or acting on the temperature-regulating center in the brain. The most common mechanism is an allergic reaction. Fever may occur alone or with other allergic manifestations (eg, skin rash, hives, joint and muscle pain, enlarged lymph glands, eosinophilia), and its pattern may be low grade and continuous or spiking and intermittent. It may begin within hours after the first dose if the client has taken the drug before, or within approximately 10 days of continued administration if the drug is new to the client. If the causative drug is discontinued, fever usually subsides within 48 to 72 hours unless drug excretion is delayed or significant tissue damage has occurred (eg, hepatitis).

   Many drugs have been implicated as causes of drug fever, including most antimicrobials, several cardiovascular agents (eg, beta blockers, hydralazine, methyldopa, procainamide, quinidine), drugs with anticholinergic properties (eg, atropine, some antihistamines, phenothiazine antipsychotic agents, and tricyclic antidepressants), and some anticonvulsants.

8. *Idiosyncrasy* refers to an unexpected reaction to a drug that occurs the first time it is given. These reactions are usually attributed to genetic characteristics that alter the person's drug-metabolizing enzymes.

9. *Drug dependence* (see Chap. 15) may occur with mind-altering drugs, such as narcotic analgesics, sedative-hypnotic agents, antianxiety agents, and CNS stimulants. Dependence may be physiologic or psychological. Physiologic dependence produces unpleasant physical symptoms when the dose is reduced or the drug is withdrawn. Psychological dependence leads to excessive preoccupation with drugs and drug-seeking behavior.

10. *Carcinogenicity* is the ability of a substance to cause cancer. Several drugs are carcinogens, including some hormones and anticancer drugs. Carcinogenicity apparently results from drug-induced alterations in cellular DNA.

11. *Teratogenicity* is the ability of a substance to cause abnormal fetal development when taken by pregnant women. Drug groups considered teratogenic include analgesics, diuretics, antiepileptic drugs, antihistamines, antibiotics, antiemetics, and others.

## Toxic Effects of Drugs

Drug toxicity (also called poisoning, overdose, or intoxication) results from excessive amounts of a drug and may cause reversible or irreversible damage to body tissues. It is a common problem in both adult and pediatric populations. It may result from a single large dose or from prolonged ingestion of smaller doses. It may involve alcohol or prescription, over-the-counter, or illicit drugs. Poisoned clients may be seen in essentially any setting (eg, inpatient hospital units, clients' homes, long-term care facilities) but are especially likely to be encountered in hospital emergency departments.

In some cases, the client or someone accompanying the client may know the toxic agent (eg, accidental overdose of a therapeutic drug, use of an illicit drug, a suicide attempt). Often, however, multiple drugs have been ingested, the causative drug or drugs are unknown, and the circumstances may involve traumatic injury or impaired mental status that make the client unable to provide useful information. Clinical manifestations are often nonspecific for drug overdoses and may indicate other disease processes. Because of the variable presentation of drug intoxication, health care providers must have a high index of suspicion so that toxicity can be rapidly recognized and treated.

## Drug Overdose: General Management

Most poisoned or overdosed clients are treated in emergency departments and discharged to their homes. A few are admitted to intensive care units (ICUs), often because of unconsciousness and the need for endotracheal intubation and mechanical ventilation. Unconsciousness is a major toxic effect of several commonly ingested substances such as benzodiazepine antianxiety and sedative agents, tricyclic antidepressants, ethanol, and opiates. Serious cardiovascular effects (eg, cardiac arrest, dysrhythmias, circulatory impairment) are also common and warrant admission to an ICU.

The main goals of treatment for a poisoned client are supporting and stabilizing vital functions (ie, airway, breathing, circulation), preventing further damage from the toxic agent by reducing additional absorption or increasing elimination, and administering specific antidotes when available and indicated. General aspects of care are described below; selected antidotes are listed in Table 2-2; and specific aspects of care are described in relevant chapters.

1. For clients who are seriously ill on first contact, enlist help for more rapid assessment and treatment. In general, starting treatment as soon as possible after drug ingestion leads to better client outcomes.

2. The first priority is support of vital functions, as indicated by a rapid assessment of the client's condition (eg, vital signs, level of consciousness). In serious poisonings, an electrocardiogram is indicated, and findings of severe toxicity (eg, dysrhythmias, ischemia) justify more aggressive and invasive care. Standard cardiopulmonary resuscitation (CPR) measures may be needed to maintain breathing and circulation. An

**TABLE 2-2    Antidotes for Overdoses of Selected Therapeutic Drugs**

| Overdosed Drug (Poison) | Antidote | Route and Dosage Ranges | Comments |
|---|---|---|---|
| Acetaminophen (see Chap. 7) | Acetylcysteine (Mucomyst) | PO, 140 mg/kg initially, then 70 mg/kg q4h for 17 doses | Dilute 20% solution to a 5% solution with a cola or other soft drink for oral administration |
| Anticholinergics (atropine; see Chap. 19) | Physostigmine | IV, IM, 2 mg. Give IV slowly, over at least 2 min. | Infrequently used because of its toxicity |
| Benzodiazepines (see Chap. 8) | Flumazenil | IV, 0.2 mg over 30 sec; if no response, may give 0.3 mg. Additional doses of 0.5 mg may be given at 1-min intervals up to a total amount of 3 mg | Should not be given to patients with overdose of unknown drugs or drugs known to cause seizures in overdose (eg, cocaine, lithium) |
| Beta blockers (see Chap. 17) | Glucagon | IV, 50–150 mcg/kg (5–10 mg for adults) over 1 min initially, then 2–5 mg/h by continuous infusion as needed | Glucagon increases myocardial contractility; not FDA-approved for this indication |
| Calcium channel blockers (see Chaps. 41, 43) | Calcium gluconate 10% | IV, 1 g over 5 min; may be repeated | Increases myocardial contractility |
| Cholinergics (see Chap. 18) | Atropine | *Adults:* IV 2 mg, repeated as needed<br>*Children:* IV 0.05 mg/kg, up to 2 mg | If poisoning is due to organophosphates (eg, insecticides), pralidoxime may be given with the atropine |
| Digoxin (see Chap. 39) | Digoxin immune fab (Digibind) | IV, 40 mg (1 vial) for each 0.6 mg of digoxin ingested.<br>Reconstitute each vial with 4 mL Water for Injection, then dilute with sterile isotonic saline to a convenient volume and give over 30 min, through a 0.22-micron filter. If cardiac arrest seems imminent, may give the dose as a bolus injection. | Recommended for severe toxicity; reverses cardiac and extracardiac symptoms in a few minutes<br>*Note:* Serum digoxin levels increase after antidote administration, but the drug is bound and therefore inactive. |
| Heparin (see Chap. 45) | Protamine sulfate | IV, 1 mg/100 units of heparin, slowly, over at least 10 min. A single dose should not exceed 50 mg. | |
| Iron (see Appendix E) | Deferoxamine | IM, 1 g q8h PRN<br>IV, 15 mg/kg/h if hypotensive | Indicated for serum iron levels >500 mg/dL or serum levels >350 mg/dL with GI or cardiovascular symptoms<br>Can bind and remove a portion of an ingested dose; urine becomes red as iron is excreted |

*(continued)*

**TABLE 2-2    Antidotes for Overdoses of Selected Therapeutic Drugs** (Continued)

| Overdosed Drug (Poison) | Antidote | Route and Dosage Ranges | Comments |
|---|---|---|---|
| Isoniazid (see Chap. 32) | Pyridoxine | IV, 1 g per gram of INH ingested, at rate of 1 g q2–3 min. If amount of INH unknown, give 5 g; may be repeated. | Indicated for management of seizures and correction of acidosis |
| Lead | Succimer | *Children:* PO 10 mg/kg q8h for 5 days | |
| Narcotic analgesics (Chap. 6) | Naloxone (Narcan) | *Adults:* IV 0.4–2 mg PRN *Children:* IV 0.1 mg/kg per dose | Can also be given IM, Sub-Q, or by endotracheal tube |
| Phenothiazine antipsychotic agents (see Chap. 9) | Diphenhydramine (Benadryl) | *Adults:* IV 50 mg *Children:* IV 1–2 mg/kg, up to a total of 50 mg | Given to relieve extrapyramidal symptoms (movement disorders) |
| Thrombolytics (see Chap. 45) | Aminocaproic acid (Amicar) | PO, IV infusion, 5 g initially, then 1–1.25 g/h for 8 h or until bleeding is controlled. Maximum dose, 30 g/24h | |
| Tricyclic antidepressants (see Chap. 10) | Sodium bicarbonate | IV, 1–2 mEq/kg initially, then continuous IV drip to maintain serum pH of 7.5 | To treat cardiac dysrhythmias, conduction disturbances, and hypotension |
| Warfarin (see Chap. 45) | Vitamin K₁ | PO, 5–10 mg daily IV (severe overdose), continuous infusion at rate no faster than 1 mg/min | |

IV line is usually needed to administer fluids and drugs and invasive treatment or monitoring devices may be inserted.

Endotracheal intubation and mechanical ventilation are often required to maintain breathing (in unconscious clients), correct hypoxemia, and protect the airway. Hypoxemia must be corrected quickly to avoid brain injury, myocardial ischemia, and cardiac dysrhythmias. Ventilation with positive end-expiratory pressure (PEEP) should be used cautiously in hypotensive clients because it decreases venous return to the heart and worsens hypotension. Serious cardiovascular manifestations often require pharmacologic treatment. Hypotension and hypoperfusion may be treated with inotropic and vasopressor drugs. Dysrhythmias are treated according to Advanced Cardiac Life Support (ACLS) protocols. Recurring seizures or status epilepticus requires treatment with anticonvulsant drugs.

3. For unconscious clients, as soon as an IV line is established, some authorities recommend a dose of naloxone (2 mg IV) for possible narcotic overdose and thiamine (100 mg IV) for possible brain dysfunction due to thiamine deficiency. In addition, a finger-stick blood glucose test should be done and, if hypoglycemia is indicated, 50% dextrose (50 mL IV) should be given.

4. Once the client is out of immediate danger, a thorough physical examination and efforts to determine the drugs, the amounts, and the time lapse since exposure are needed. If the client is unable to supply needed information, interview anyone else who may be able to do so. Ask about the use of prescription, over-the-counter, alcohol, and illicit substances.

5. There are no standard laboratory tests for poisoned clients. The client's condition and the clinician's judgment determine which laboratory tests are needed, although baseline tests of liver and kidney function are usually indicated. Specimens of blood, urine, or gastric fluids may be obtained for laboratory analysis.

Screening tests for toxic substances are not very helpful because test results may be delayed, many substances are not detected, and the results rarely affect initial treatment. Initial treatment should never be delayed to obtain results of a toxicology screen.

Identification of an unknown drug or poison is often based on the client's history and signs and symptoms, with specific tests as confirmation.

To assist with treatment, serum drug levels are needed when acetaminophen, alcohol, digoxin, lithium, aspirin, or theophylline is known to be an ingested drug.

6. For orally ingested drugs, GI decontamination has become a controversial topic. For many years, standard techniques for removing drugs from the GI tract included ipecac syrup for alert clients, to induce emesis; gastric lavage for clients with decreased levels of consciousness; activated charcoal to adsorb the ingested drug in the GI tract; and a cathartic (usually 70% sorbitol) to accelerate elimination of the adsorbed drug. More recently, whole bowel irrigation (WBI) was introduced as an additional technique.

Now, there are differences of opinion regarding whether and when these techniques are indicated. These differences led to the convening of a consensus group of toxicologists from the American Academy of Clinical Toxicology (AACT) and the European Association of Poison Centres and Clinical Toxicologists (EAPCCT). This group issued treatment guidelines that have also been endorsed by other toxicology organizations. Generally, the recommendations state that none of the aforementioned techniques should be used routinely and that adequate data to support or exclude their use are often lacking. Opinions expressed by the consensus group and others are described below:

■ *Ipecac.* Use in hospital settings has declined. Its use may delay administration or reduce effectiveness of activated charcoal, oral antidotes, and WBI. Because of the risk for aspiration, ipecac is contraindicated in clients who are less than fully alert. Ipecac is also used to treat mild poisonings in the home, especially in children. Parents should call a poison control center or a health care provider before giving ipecac. If instructed to use, it is most beneficial if administered within an hour after ingestion of a toxic drug dose.

■ *Gastric lavage.* Its usefulness is being increasingly questioned. It is contraindicated in less than alert clients unless the client has an endotracheal tube in place (to prevent aspiration). It may be beneficial in serious overdoses if performed within an hour of drug ingestion. If the ingested agent delays gastric emptying (eg, tricyclic antidepressants and other drugs with anticholinergic effects), the time limit may be extended. When used after ingestion of pills or capsules, the tube lumen should be large enough to allow removal of pill fragments.

■ *Activated charcoal.* Sometimes called the universal antidote, it is useful in many poisoning situations. It is being used alone for mild or moderate overdoses and with gastric lavage in serious poisonings. It effec-

tively adsorbs many toxins and rarely causes complications. It is most beneficial when given within an hour of ingestion of a potentially toxic amount of a drug known to bind to charcoal. Its effectiveness decreases with time, and there are inadequate data to support or exclude its use later than one hour after ingestion. Activated charcoal is usually mixed in water (about 50 g or 10 heaping tablespoons in 8 oz water) to make a slurry, which is gritty and unpleasant to swallow. It is often given by GI tube. The charcoal blackens later bowel movements. Adverse effects include pulmonary aspiration and impaction of the charcoal–drug complex. If used with WBI, activated charcoal should be given before the WBI solution is started. If given during WBI, the binding capacity of the charcoal is decreased.

■ *Cathartic.* It is not recommended alone, and its use with activated charcoal has produced conflicting data. If used, it should be limited to a single dose to minimize adverse effects.

■ *Whole bowel irrigation.* This technique is most useful for removing toxic ingestions of long-acting, sustained-release drugs (eg, many beta blockers, calcium channel blockers, and theophylline preparations); enteric coated drugs; and toxins that do not bind well with activated charcoal (eg, iron, lithium, lead). It may also be helpful in removing packets of illicit drugs, such as cocaine or heroin. When given, polyethylene glycol solution (eg, Colyte), 1 to 2 L/hour to a total of 10 L, is recommended. WBI is contraindicated in clients with serious bowel disorders (eg, obstruction, perforation, ileus), hemodynamic instability, or respiratory impairment (unless intubated).

7. Urinary elimination of some drugs and toxic metabolites can be accelerated by changing the pH of urine (eg, acidifying with amphetamine overdose; alkalinizing with salicylate overdose), diuresis, or hemodialysis. Hemodialysis is the treatment of choice in severe lithium and aspirin (salicylate) poisoning.

8. Administer specific antidotes when available and indicated by the client's clinical condition. Available antidotes vary widely in effectiveness. Some are very effective and rapidly reverse toxic manifestations (eg, naloxone for opiates, flumazenil for benzodiazepines, specific Fab fragments for digoxin). Others are less effective (eg, deferoxamine for acute iron ingestion) or potentially toxic themselves (eg, physostigmine for tricyclic antidepressant overdose).

When an antidote is used, its half-life relative to the toxin's half-life must be considered. For example, the half-life of naloxone, a narcotic antagonist, is relatively short compared with the half-life of the longer-acting opiates such as methadone. Similarly, flumazenil has a shorter half-life than most benzodiazepines. Thus, repeated doses of these agents may be needed to prevent recurrence of the toxic state.

**Answer:** Grapefruit juice interacts with many medications, including felodipine. The drug level of felodipine increases because the grapefruit juice inhibits the isozyme of cytochrome P450, which is important in the metabolism of felodipine. As the blood level increases, serious toxic effects can occur. Other juices do not impact cytochrome P450 so it would be safe to have Mrs. Beecher take her medication with another type of juice or water. Notify the physician regarding Mrs. Beecher's hypotension and the drug–food interaction. If Mrs. Beecher remains on felodipine, she must be cautioned to eliminate grapefruit juice from her diet.

## Critical Thinking Exercises

1. A client comes to the emergency department with a fractured wrist and is experiencing moderate pain. The health care provider prescribes Tylenol #3 (acetaminophen and codeine). Adding acetaminophen with codeine produces which type of effect?
   a. Cumulative
   b. Addictive
   c. Synergistic
   d. Paradoxical

2. Protein binding allows part of a drug to be stored and released as needed, reducing the risk for toxicity. Drugs that are highly bound to plasma proteins have a:
   a. Long duration of action
   b. Limited bioavailability
   c. First-pass effect
   d. Cross-tolerance response

3. A client with alcohol abuse is scheduled for surgery. The anesthesiologist anticipates that the client will need a larger than usual dose to produce a pharmacologic effect. This effect is called:
   a. Synergistic
   b. Paradoxical
   c. Cross-tolerance
   d. Addictive

4. Drugs that produce effects similar to those produced by naturally occurring hormones, neurotransmitters, and other substances are called:
   a. Receptors
   b. Antagonists
   c. Agonists
   d. Addictive

5. A client receives a second round of amoxicillin for a chronic wound infection. After taking a dose, the client begins to complain of itching, a skin rash, flank pain, and shortness of breath. This is likely a:
   a. Hypersensitivity reaction
   b. Synergistic effect
   c. Drug interference effect
   d. Cumulative effect

## SELECTED REFERENCES

Barone, J. A., & Hermes-DeSantis, E. R. (2000). Adverse drug reactions and drug-induced diseases. In E. T. Herfindal & D. R. Gourley (Eds.), *Textbook of therapeutics: Drug and disease management* (7th ed., pp. 21–34). Philadelphia: Lippincott Williams & Wilkins.

Brater, D. C. (2000). Principles of clinical pharmacology. In H. D. Humes (Ed.), *Kelley's textbook of internal medicine* (4th ed., pp. 311–319). Philadelphia: Lippincott Williams & Wilkins.

*Drug facts and comparisons.* (Updated monthly). St. Louis: Facts and Comparisons.

Ensom, M. H. H. (2000). Gender-based differences and menstrual cycle-related changes in specific diseases: Implications for pharmacotherapy. *Pharmacotherapy, 20*(5), 523–539.

Guyton, A. C., & Hall, J. E. (2000). *Textbook of medical physiology* (10th ed.). Philadelphia: W. B. Saunders.

Klein-Schwartz, W., & Oderda, G. M. (2000). Clinical toxicology. In E. T. Herfindal & D. R. Gourley (Eds.), *Textbook of therapeutics: Drug and disease management* (7th ed., pp. 51–68). Philadelphia: Lippincott Williams & Wilkins.

Matthews, H. W., & Johnson, J. (2000). Racial, ethnic, and gender differences in response to drugs. In E. T. Herfindal & D. R. Gourley (Eds.), *Textbook of therapeutics: Drug and disease management* (7th ed., pp. 93–103). Philadelphia: Lippincott Williams & Wilkins.

Lacy, C. F., Armstrong, L. L., Goldman, M. P., & Lance, L. L. (2003). *Lexi-Comp's drug information handbook* (11th ed.). Hudson, OH: American Pharmaceutical Association.

Tatro, D. S. (2000). Drug interactions. In E. T. Herfindal & D. R. Gourley (Eds.), *Textbook of therapeutics: Drug and disease management* (7th ed., pp. 35–49). Philadelphia: Lippincott Williams & Wilkins.

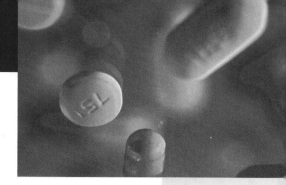

# 3

# Dosage Calculations

## OBJECTIVES

*After studying this chapter, the student will be able to:*

1 Identify common systems of measurement and their equivalents.

2 Convert measurements among the metric, apothecary, and household systems.

3 Compute medication calculations using the metric system.

## CRITICAL THINKING SCENARIO

*M*rs. Morgan, an 82-year-old housewife, has started taking some of her medications in liquid form because of difficulty swallowing following a cerebral vascular accident (CVA). During a home visit, you find that Mrs. Morgan has symptoms of an adverse drug reaction related to her medications. Further questioning reveals that she has been using household spoons to measure her medications.

✔ What changes in expected results, side effects, and adverse reactions may occur when clients do not use standardized measurement instruments?

✔ What strategies and resources will you use to get Mrs. Morgan to take her medication with standard measurement instruments?

## OVERVIEW

Dosage calculation involves the use of mathematical processes to determine the correct amount of medication to be given to a client. Accuracy in calculation is essential to ensure client safety. Three established systems of measurement are used to calculate and administer medications. These systems are the metric, apothecary, and household systems. This chapter focuses primarily on the metric system because nearly all medication orders are written using this system. However, because the apothecary and household measurement systems also may be used, nurses need to be familiar with these systems, which are briefly outlined in this chapter.

## SYSTEMS OF WEIGHTS AND MEASUREMENT

The metric, apothecary, and household systems of measurement are most commonly involved with medication administration. The metric system is used in all drug labels and most prescriptions in the United States. However, the apothecary and household systems may be used for liquid doses. Additionally, medicine cups used for liquid medications commonly are marked in metric, apothecary, and household units. Therefore, the nurse must be familiar with each system and be able to convert from one system to another. For example, when measuring liquid doses, the nurse must be knowledgeable about the apothecary and household systems and their equivalents to ensure that the proper amount of medication is prepared and administered. Nurses also need to keep in mind that equivalents are approximate. Table 3-1 lists equivalent measurements within and among these three systems.

Occasionally, a certain drug is ordered and measured in terms of units or milliequivalents (mEq). *Units* express biologic activity in animal tests (ie, the amount of drug required to produce a particular response). For example, concentrations of insulin and heparin are expressed in units. These drugs are usually ordered in the number of units per dose (eg, NPH insulin, 30 units subcutaneously every morning; or heparin, 5000 units subcutaneously every 12 hours). However, the units for each drug are unique and unrelated. In other words, there is no relationship between a unit of insulin and a unit of heparin. For example, although labels for both drugs state the number of units per milliliter, the number of units varies. Insulin labeled U 100 contains 100 units/mL, whereas heparin may have 1000, 5000, or 10,000 units/mL.

*Milliequivalents* express the ionic activity of a drug. Drugs such as potassium chloride are ordered and labeled in the number of milliequivalents per dose, tablet, or milliliter.

## Metric System

As previously noted, the most commonly used system of measurement is the *metric system,* in which the meter is used for linear measure, the gram for weight, and the liter for volume. One milliliter (mL) equals 1 cubic centimeter (cc), and both equal 1 gram (g) of water. The metric system is a decimal system, based on multiples of 10; all units are derived by multiplying or dividing by 10, 100, or 1000. Metric prefixes indicate the portion of the unit being considered. For instance, a milliliter is 1/1000 of a liter; a centimeter is 1/100 of a meter, and a microgram is 1/1,000,000 of a gram. Table 3-2 outlines common metric abbreviations and equivalents.

## Apothecary System

The *apothecary system,* now rarely used, involves measurements called grains, minims, drams, ounces, pounds, pints, and quarts. The notations are rather unusual and

### TABLE 3-1   Equivalents

| Metric | Apothecary | Household |
|---|---|---|
| 1 mL = 1 cc | = 15 or 16 minims | = 15 or 16 drops |
| 4 or 5 mL | = 1 fluid dram | = 1 tsp |
| 60 or 65 mg | = 1 gr | |
| 30 or 32 mg | = ½ gr | |
| 30 g = 30 mL | = 1 oz | = 2 tbsp |
| 250 mL | = 8 oz | = 1 cup |
| 454 g | = 1 lb | |
| 500 mL = 500 cc | = 16 oz | = 1 pint |
| 1 L = 1000 mL | = 32 oz | = 1 quart |
| 1000 mcg = 1 mg | | |
| 1000 mg | = 1 g | |
| 1000 g = 1 kg | = 2.2 lb | = 2.2 lb |
| 0.6 g = 600 mg or 650 mg | = 10 gr | |

mcg, microgram.

## TABLE 3-2  Metric Units and Equivalents

| | Units (Abbreviations) | Equivalents |
|---|---|---|
| **Weight** | gram (g) | 1 g = 1000 mg |
| | milligram (mg) | 1 mg = 1000 mcg or 0.001 g |
| | microgram (mcg) | 1 mcg = 0.001 mg or 0.000001 g |
| | kilogram (kg) | 1 kg = 1000 g |
| **Volume** | liter (L) | 1 L = 1000 mL |
| | milliliter (mL) | 1 mL = 0.001 L or 1 cc |
| | cubic centimeter (cc) | 1 cc = 0.0001 L or 1 mL |
| **Length** | meter (m) | 1 m = 100 cm or 1000 mm |
| | centimeter (cm) | 1 cm = 0.01 m or 10 mm |
| | millimeter (mm) | 1 mm = 0.002 m or 0.1 cm |

differ from notations in the other systems. Several rules govern the use of notations in this system:

- The only solid unit of measure in this system is the grain (gr)
- The dram (ʒ), the ounce (ℨ), and the drop (gt) are liquid measures
- The unit precedes the amount (gr x, ℨ iii)
- Lower-case Roman numerals are used to express the whole numbers of 1 through 10, 20, and 30 (gr xx); Arabic numbers are used for all other amounts (ℨ 12)
- Amounts less than 1 are designated as fractions (gr 1/3); the fraction 1/2 is designated by the symbol śś (ℨ vśś)

Conversions for apothecary weights and volumes are listed in Table 3-3. However, whenever possible, the metric system should be used.

## Household System

The *household system*, with measurements of drops, teaspoons, tablespoons, and cups, is infrequently used in health care agencies but may be used by clients in their home. Because of the lack of standardization of measurements (ie, drops, spoons, and cups), this is the least accurate of the three major measurement systems. Often, on discharge from the hospital or while the home health nurse is visiting in the home, clients request assistance in converting metric to household measurements. It is recommended that the client be encouraged to use stan-

dardized measurements, instead of household spoons and cups, to ensure safe and accurate medication administration. Conversions in the household system are listed in Box 3-1.

## ■ METHODS OF CALCULATION

Most drug orders and labels are expressed in metric units of measurement. If the amount specified in the order is the same as that on the drug label, no calculations are required, and preparing the right dose is a simple matter. For example, if the order reads "ibuprofen, 400 mg PO" and the drug label reads "ibuprofen, 400 mg per tablet," it is clear that one tablet is to be given. However, what happens if the order calls for a 400-mg dose, and 200-mg tablets are available? The question is, "How many 200-mg tablets are needed to give a dose of 400 mg?" In this case, the answer can be readily calculated mentally to indicate 2 tablets.

Although a relatively simple calculation, this example also can be used to illustrate mathematical calculations that may be required in other situations. This problem can be solved by several acceptable methods: (1) basic equations; (2) ratio proportion equations; or (3) fractional dose equations. A nurse should be familiar with one of these methods and use it consistently. The following sections outline calculation formulas using each method and use the above question example to illustrate application of the formula. In addition, calculations involving

## TABLE 3-3  Apothecary Weights and Volumes

| Apothecary Weight | Apothecary Volume |
|---|---|
| 60 grains = 1 dram | 60 minims = 1 fluidram |
| 8 drams (or 480 grains) = 1 ounce | 8 fluid drams (or 480 minims) = 1 fluidounce |
| 12 ounces = 1 pound | 16 fluidounces = 1 pint |
| | 2 pints = 1 quart |
| | 4 quarts = 1 gallon |

> ## BOX 3-1   Household Equivalents
>
> 1 drop (gt) = 1 minim
> 1 teaspoon (tsp) = 60 drops (gtt)
> 1 tablespoon (tbsp) = 3 teaspoons (tsp)
> 1 ounce (oz) = 2 tablespoons (tbsp)
> 1 measuring cup = 8 ounces (oz)

body weight and body surface area, methods commonly used to determine doses for infants and small children, are provided.

## Basic Equations

The basic equation is commonly used and is represented by the formula:

$$\frac{D}{H} \times V = A$$

Where:
D is the desired dose
H is the amount on hand
V is the vehicle
A is the amount to be administered to the client

Using the example, the basic equation would look like this:

$$\frac{400}{200} \times 1 \text{ tablet} = 2 \text{ tablets}$$

Therefore, the nurse would administer 2 tablets.

## Ratio and Proportion Equations

One of the oldest methods of calculation is the ratio and proportion equation and can be expressed by the formula:

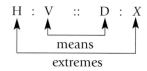

$$H : V :: D : X$$
means
extremes

Where:
D is the desired dose
H is the amount on hand
V is the vehicle (or form in which the drug comes)
A is the amount to be administered to the client (commonly designated as X or x)

Using fractions, proportions are set up so that similar units are across from each other.

The first fraction is the known equivalent, and the second fraction is the unknown and desired amount. All measurements need to be in the same system and in the same unit or size. Using the example, the ratio and proportion would look like this:

$$\frac{V}{H} = \frac{A (\text{or } X)}{D}$$

$$\frac{1 \text{ tablet}}{200} = \frac{X \text{ tablets}}{400}$$

With this equation, you would cross-multiply and solve for $X$

$$\frac{1 \text{ tablet}}{200} \times \frac{X \text{ tablets}}{400}$$

1 tablet × 400 = X tablets × 200
400 = 200X
2 = X

Therefore, the nurse would administer 2 tablets.

## Fractional Dose Equations

The fractional dose equation is similar to the ratio and proportion equation. The formula can be expressed as the following:

$$\frac{H}{V} = \frac{D}{X}$$

Where:
D is the desired dose
H is the amount on hand
V is the vehicle
A is the amount to be administered to the client (commonly designated as X or x)

With this equation, you would cross-multiply and solve for X, or A.

Using the example:

$$\frac{200}{1 \text{ tablet}} \times \frac{400}{X \text{ tablets}}$$

Therefore, the nurse would administer 2 tablets.

What happens if the order and the label are written in different units? For example, the order may read "ibuprofen, 0.4 g," and the label may read "ibuprofen, 200 mg/tablet." To calculate the number of tablets needed for the dose, the first step is to convert 0.4 g to the equivalent number of milligrams, or convert 400 mg to the equivalent number of grams. The desired or ordered dose and the available or label dose *must* be in the same units of measurement. Using the equivalents (ie, 1 g = 1000 mg) listed in Table 3-2, an equation can be set up as follows:

$$0.4 \text{ g} = 400 \text{ mg}$$

The next step is to use the new information in the formula, which then becomes:

1 tablet × 400 = X tablets × 200
400 = 200X
2 = X

Therefore, the nurse would administer 2 tablets.

# Dosages Based on Body Weight and Body Surface Area

Some dosages are based on body weight or body surface area (BSA). Commonly, dosages for infants and children are ordered in this fashion owing to wide variations in age, growth and development, and weight in this group. Often, the amount needed for a specific dose must be calculated as a fraction of the adult dose. The following two methods are used for these calculations.

Clark's rule is based on weight and is used for children at least 2 years of age. The following is the mathematical formula representing Clark's rule:

$$\frac{\text{weight (in pounds)}}{150} \times \text{adult dose} = \text{child's dose}$$

Calculating dosage based on body surface area (BSA) is considered a more accurate method for dosage calcu-

**? How Can You Avoid This Medication Error?**

Jane Johnson, a 9-year-old child with a congenital heart defect, is started on digoxin for her heart failure. A digitalizing dose of 0.02 mg/kg PO in 4 divided doses over 24 hours is ordered. The child weighs 77 pounds. A nurse, who was pulled from an adult medical-surgical floor, transcribes the order and schedules the doses to be administered at 9 AM, 3 PM, 9 PM, and 3 AM the following morning. The nurse administers 0.385 mg PO to the child. After two doses, the child develops nausea, vomiting, photophobia, and confusion.

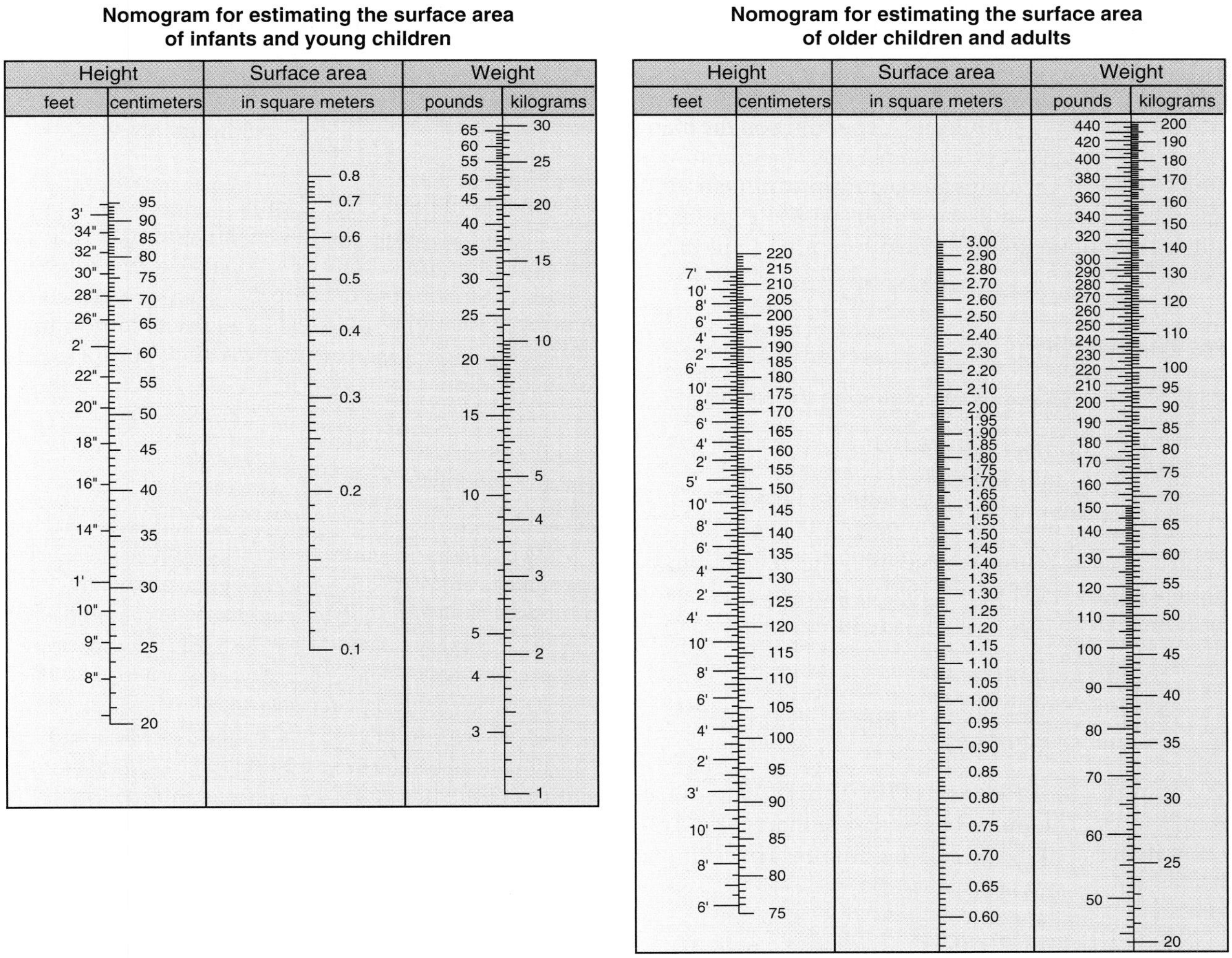

lation. Body surface area, based on height and weight, is estimated using a nomogram (Fig. 3-1). To calculate the child's dose using the estimated body surface area, use the following formula:

**Nomogram for estimating the surface area of infants and young children**

| Height | | Surface area | Weight | |
|---|---|---|---|---|
| feet | centimeters | in square meters | pounds | kilograms |

**Nomogram for estimating the surface area of older children and adults**

| Height | | Surface area | Weight | |
|---|---|---|---|---|
| feet | centimeters | in square meters | pounds | kilograms |

**FIGURE 3-1** Body surface nomograms. To determine the surface area of the client, draw a straight line between the point representing his or her height on the left vertical scale to the point representing weight on the right vertical scale. The point at which this line intersects the middle vertical scale represents the client's surface area in square meters (Courtesy of Abbott Laboratories).

$$\frac{\text{body surface area (in square meters)}}{1.73 \text{ square meters } (m^2)} \times \text{adult dose} = \text{child's dose}$$

Administering a safe dose is crucial for all clients, but especially for infants and children, because many pediatric dosages are minute. Thus, even a slight miscalculation or error can cause harm. A review of the literature should indicate the safe dose range. The calculated dose should fall within the stated low and high safe ranges.

## ■ CALCULATION OF INTRAVENOUS FLOW RATES

Intravenous (IV) fluids are administered using infusion sets that are set to the proper flow rate. IV flow rates are usually calculated in milliliters per hours and drops (gtts) per minute. To calculate the flow rate, specific information is required, including the amount of solution or medication to be infused, the time or duration of the infusion, and the number of drops per milliliter (drop factor) that the intravenous administration set delivers. For example, the drop factor of macrodrip administration sets may be 10, 15, or 20 drops per milliliter, depending on the manufacturer. Most agencies use mainly one manufacturer's product. The drop factor for all microdrip administration sets is 60 drops/mL. Infusion pumps typically are set in milliliters per hour, so the calculations are in milliliters per hour (mL/hour).

### Rate of Infusions

The rate of the infusion is calculated by the formula:

$$\frac{\text{total number of milliliters (mL) ordered}}{\text{number of hours to run}} = \text{number of mL/h}$$

If an infusion pump is available, the calculation is complete. If the drop factor varies, as it does with macrodrip tubing, an additional step is required.

$$\frac{\text{number of milliliters per hour} \times \text{drop factor}}{\text{number of minutes}} = \text{drops per minute}$$

For example, the order reads "1000 mL D5W to run at 100 mL/hour." The nurse has available macrodrip tubing that delivers 20 drops/mL per minute. The formula looks like this:

$$\frac{100 \text{ mL} \times 20}{60} = \frac{2000}{60} = 33.3 \text{ drops/minute}$$

Therefore, the nurse would set the infusion to run at 33 drops/minute.

If microdrip tubing was used in the above example, the calculation is as follows:

$$\frac{100 \text{ mL} \times 60}{60} = 100 \text{ drops/minute}$$

The nurse would set the infusion to run at 100 drops/minute.

### Length of Infusion

In many cases, it is useful to calculate how long an IV infusion will take. The calculation formula is simply stated as:

$$\frac{\text{number of milliliters ordered}}{\text{number of milliliters per hour}} = \text{number of hours to infuse}$$

Consider this example. The order reads "1000 mL 0.9% saline to run at 125 mL/hour." Setting up the formula to determine the infusion time would look like this:

$$\frac{1000 \text{ mL}}{125 \text{ mL/h}} = 8 \text{ hours}$$

The IV will infuse for 8 hours.

Calculating drug dosages is an essential skill for a nurse because inaccurate dosage calculations can harm a client. A nurse must develop proficiency in calculating among measurement systems and use common mathematical calculations to determine the appropriate dose of medication.

---

**?** **How Can You Avoid This Medication Error?**

**Answer:** Dosage calculations, particularly in children, require rigorous attention to detail. In calculating the dosage based on weight, the nurse failed to convert pounds to kilograms and ultimately administered more than twice the desired dose. Additionally, the dose given is above the recommended safe dose for children. Literature indicates that children 2 to 10 years of age should receive an oral digitalizing dose of 0.02 to 0.04 mg/kg in 4 divided doses over 24 hours. Moreover, the symptoms exhibited in the child are signs of an adverse reaction. Nurses administering medication to any client must be knowledgeable about specific drug actions and effects so they can readily assess for signs of an adverse reaction. Nurses unfamiliar with working with children and common pediatric dosages may be at greater risk for making a medication error. Using unit dose systems and having another nurse review your calculations before administering the medication aid in error prevention.

## Critical Thinking Exercises

1. The most commonly used system of measurement in calculating and administering medications is the:
   a. Metric system
   b. Apothecary system
   c. Household system
   d. Calculation system

2. Body surface area, based on height and weight, is estimated using a:
   a. Calculator
   b. Nomogram
   c. Growth chart
   d. Hemodynamic monitor

3. A client weighs 110 pounds. His weight in kilograms is:
   a. 50
   b. 55
   c. 60
   d. 65

4. Using the metric system, one milliliter (mL) equals:
   a. 2 cubic centimeter (cc)
   b. 2 grams of water
   c. 1 cubic centimeter (cc)
   d. 0.5 gram of water

## SELECTED REFERENCES

Buchholz, S., & Henke, S. G. (2003). *Henke's med-math dosage calculation, preparation and administration* (4th ed.). Philadelphia: Lippincott Williams & Wilkins.

Craven, R. F., & Hirnle, C. J. (2003). *Fundamentals of nursing: Human health and function* (4th ed.). Philadelphia: Lippincott Williams & Wilkins.

Pickar, G. D. (1999). *Dosage calculations* (6th ed.). Albany, NY: Delmar.

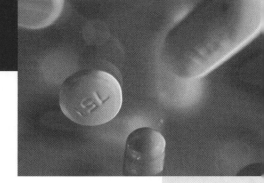

# 4

# Administering Medications

## OBJECTIVES

*After studying this chapter, the student will be able to:*

1 Give the seven rights of drug administration.

2 Discuss knowledge and skills needed to implement the seven rights.

3 List requirements of a complete drug order or prescription.

4 Accurately interpret drug orders containing common abbreviations.

5 Differentiate drug dosage forms for various routes and purposes of administration.

6 Discuss advantages and disadvantages of oral, parenteral, and topical routes of drug administration.

7 Identify supplies, techniques, and observations needed for safe and accurate administration by different routes.

## CRITICAL THINKING SCENARIO

*M*s. Mabel Zack is transferred to your rehabilitation facility after a cerebral vascular accident (stroke) 2 weeks ago. When you review her chart, it indicates she has right-sided hemiparesis, memory deficits, and dysphagia (difficulty swallowing).

✔ Outline appropriate assessments to determine whether it is safe to give Ms. Zack oral medications.

✔ If a swallowing evaluation indicates that Ms. Zack can take medications orally, what precautions can you take to help ensure her safety?

✔ How might you individualize your teaching plan, considering Ms. Zack's memory deficits?

# OVERVIEW

Drugs given for therapeutic purposes are called *medications*. Giving medications to clients is an important nursing responsibility in many health care settings, including ambulatory care, hospitals, long-term care facilities, and clients' homes. The basic requirements for accurate drug administration were traditionally called the "five rights": giving the right *drug*, in the right *dose*, to the right *client*, by the right *route*, at the right *time*. Two additional rights, the right *documentation* and the client's right *to refuse* medication, place priority on the rights of the client to possess sufficient basic knowledge to make an educated decision (informed consent). These current "seven rights" include that the nurse provide to the client complete information regarding the medication, the therapeutic basis for administering, potential side effects, any diet modifications or lifestyle adjustments required of the client, and additional management requirements. Additionally, appropriate and timely documentation of administration of the medication and the client's response must be noted in the hospital record. This requires knowledge of the drugs to be given

and the clients who are to receive them as well as specific nursing skills and interventions. When one of these rights is violated, medication errors can occur. Nurses need to recognize circumstances in which errors are likely to occur and intervene to prevent errors and protect clients. This chapter is concerned with safe and accurate medication administration. Universal principles of accurate drug administration are found in At the Foundation: General Principles of Accurate Drug Administration.

# LEGAL RESPONSIBILITIES

Registered and licensed practical nurses are legally empowered, under state nurse practice acts, to give medications ordered by licensed physicians and dentists. In some states, nurse practitioners may prescribe medications.

*When giving medications, the nurse is legally responsible for safe and accurate administration.* This means the nurse may be held liable for not giving a drug or for giving a wrong drug or a wrong dose. In addition, *the nurse is expected to possess sufficient drug knowledge to recognize and question*

## AT THE FOUNDATION: *General Principles of Accurate Drug Administration*

Follow the "seven rights" of medication administration consistently.

Identify essential information about each drug to be given (eg, indications for use, contraindications, therapeutic effects, adverse effects, and any specific instructions about administration).

Interpret the prescriber's order accurately (ie, drug name, dose, frequency of administration). Question the prescriber if any information is unclear or if the drug seems inappropriate for the client's condition.

Examine the labels of drug containers for the drug name and concentration (usually in milligrams per tablet, capsule, or milliliter of solution).

Minimize the use of abbreviations for drug names, doses, routes of administration, and times of administration. This promotes safer administration and reduces errors.

Calculate doses accurately. Current nursing practice requires few dosage calculations (most are done by pharmacists). However, when they are needed, accuracy is essential (see Chapter 3). For medications with a narrow safety margin or potentially serious adverse effects, ask a pharmacist or a colleague to do the calculation also and compare the results. This is especially important when calculating children's dosages.

Measure doses accurately. Ask a colleague to double-check measurements of insulin and heparin, unusual doses (ie, large or small), and any drugs to be given intravenously.

Use the correct procedures and techniques for all routes of administration.

Seek information about the client's medical diagnoses and condition in relation to drug administration (eg, ability to swallow oral medications; allergies or contraindications to prescription drugs; new signs or symptoms that may indicate adverse effects of administered drugs; heart, liver, or kidney disorders that may interfere with the client's ability to eliminate drugs).

Verify the identity of all clients before administering medications; check identification bands on clients who have them (eg, in hospitals or long-term facilities).

Omit or delay doses as indicated by the client's condition; report or record omissions appropriately.

Be especially vigilant when giving medications to children because there is a high risk for medication errors. One reason is their great diversity in age from birth to 18 years and in weight from 2 to 3 kilograms (kg) to 100 kg or more. Another reason is that most drugs have not been tested in children. A third reason is that many drugs are marketed in dosage forms and concentrations suitable for adults. This requires dilution, calculation, preparation, and administration of very small doses. A fourth reason is that children have limited sites for administration of IV drugs, and several may be given through the same site. In many cases, the need for small volumes of fluid limits flushing between drugs (which may produce undesirable interactions with other drugs and IV solutions).

**?** **How Can You Avoid This Medication Error?**

It is 6 AM and you are administering morning medications to a client on a medical unit. You enter Mr. Gonzales' room, gently shake him awake, and call him by name. He slowly awakens and appears groggy. You explain that you have his medications, which he takes and quickly falls back to sleep. On exiting the room, you look at the room number and realize that you just gave medications to Mr. Sanchez.

*erroneous orders.* If, after questioning the prescriber and seeking information from other authoritative sources, the nurse considers that giving a drug is unsafe, the nurse must refuse to give the drug. The fact that a health care provider wrote an erroneous order does not excuse the nurse from legal liability if he or she carries out that order.

The nurse also is legally responsible for actions delegated to people who are inadequately prepared for or legally barred from administering medications (such as nursing assistants). However, certified medical assistants (CMAs) administer medications in physicians' offices, and certified medication aides (nursing assistants with a short course of training, also called CMAs,) often administer medications in long-term care facilities.

The nurse who consistently follows safe practices in giving medications does not need to be excessively concerned about legal liability. The basic techniques and guidelines described in this chapter are aimed at safe and accurate preparation and administration; most errors result when these practices are not followed.

Legal responsibilities in other aspects of drug therapy are less tangible and clearcut. However, in general, nurses are expected to monitor clients' responses to drug therapy (eg, therapeutic and adverse effects) and to teach clients safe and effective self-administration of drugs when indicated. These aspects are described more fully in Chap. 5.

## MEDICATION ERRORS

Increasing attention is being paid to the number and consequences of medication errors. Studies suggest that medication errors account for about one third of adverse drug events and are thus preventable. In one study of 1116 hospitals, medication errors (a total of 430,586) were reported in approximately 5% of admitted clients. In 913 of those hospitals, more than 17,000 errors (0.25% of admitted clients) reportedly caused adverse client outcomes (usually described as serious illness, conditions that prolong hospitalization or require additional treatment, or death). Other studies have reported that common errors include giving an incorrect dose, not giving an ordered drug, and giving an unordered drug. Specific drugs often associated with errors include insulin, heparin, and warfarin.

In addition to the actual harm to clients, medication-related errors are costly in relation to health care costs. One study at two prestigious teaching hospitals reported that in 2 of every 100 admissions, a preventable adverse drug event resulted in an average increased hospital cost of $4700. If these findings can be generalized, increased hospital costs from preventable inpatient adverse drug events for the nation as a whole are estimated at $2 billion. This estimate does not include costs from other populations at risk, including providers' offices, clinics, nursing homes, outpatient surgical centers, and home care.

Not all costs can be measured directly. Medication errors can significantly diminish the loss of trust in a hospital or health care system by clients and families and significantly reduce satisfaction for both clients and health care providers.

There are several steps and numerous people involved in getting each dose of a medication to the intended client. Each step or person has a potential for contributing to a medication error (Box 4-1). All health care providers involved in drug therapy must be extremely vigilant in all phases of drug administration.

## MEDICATION SYSTEMS

Each agency has a system for distributing drugs. The unit-dose system, in which most drugs are dispensed in single-dose containers for individual clients, is widely used. Drug orders are checked by a pharmacist or pharmacy technician, who then places the indicated number of doses in the client's medication drawer at scheduled intervals. When a dose is due, the nurse removes the medication and takes it to the client. *Unit-dose wrappings of oral drugs should be left in place until the nurse is in the presence of the client and ready to give the medication.* Each dose of a drug must be recorded on the client's medication administration record (MAR) as soon as possible after administration.

Increasingly, agencies are using automated, computerized, locked cabinets for which each nurse on a unit has a password or code for accessing the cabinet and obtaining a drug dose. These automated systems maintain an inventory, and drugs are restocked as needed.

Controlled drugs, such as narcotic analgesics, are usually kept as a stock supply in a locked drawer or automated cabinet and replaced as needed. Each dose is signed for and recorded on the client's MAR. Each nurse must comply with legal regulations and agency policies for dispensing and recording controlled drugs.

## MEDICATION ORDERS

Medication orders should include the full name of the client; the generic or trade name of the drug; the dose, route, and frequency of administration; and the date, time, and signature of the prescriber.

Most orders in a health care agency are handwritten on an order sheet in the client's medical record or typed into a computer. Occasionally, verbal or telephone orders are

## BOX 4-1    Sources of Medication Errors

Medication errors may occur during any phase of drug therapy, including prescribing, dispensing, and administration. The main purpose of including potential sources of errors here is to increase the ability of health care providers to recognize risky situations and to prevent errors when possible.

### Health Care Providers

**Prescribers** may write orders illegibly; order a drug that is not indicated by the client's condition; fail to order a drug that is indicated; fail to consider the client's age, size, kidney function, liver function, and disease process when selecting a drug or dosage; fail to consider other medications the client is taking, including prescription and over-the-counter drugs; lack sufficient knowledge about the drug; fail to monitor for, or instruct others to monitor for, effects of administered drugs; and fail to discontinue drugs appropriately. **Pharmacists** may not know the client's condition or recognize an inappropriate or erroneous physician's order. They may dispense incorrect medications, mislabel containers, or fail to ask outpatients about other drugs being taken. **Nurses** may have inadequate knowledge about a drug or about the client receiving the drug; not follow the "seven rights"; fail to question the medication order when indicated.

### Clients/Consumers

People may take drugs from several prescribers; fail to inform one physician about drugs prescribed by another; get prescriptions filled at more than one pharmacy; fail to get prescriptions filled or refilled; underuse or overuse an appropriately prescribed drug; take drugs left over from a previous illness or prescribed for someone else; fail to follow instructions for drug administration or storage; fail to keep appointments for follow-up care; and fail to ask for information about prescription and nonprescription drugs when needed.

### Drugs

Drugs may have similar names that can lead to erroneous prescribing, dispensing, or administration. For example, the antiseizure drug Lamictal (generic name, lamotrigine) has been confused with Lamisil, an antifungal drug, lamivudine, an antiviral drug, and others. As a result, the FDA-proposed labeling changes to make the differences more noticeable. The Institution of Safe Medication Practices has urged the use of "tall-man-lettering" by generic manufacturers currently recommended by the FDA. By combining large and small letters with bolding (ie, predni**SONE** and predniso**LONE**) it is anticipated that errors caused by confusing name look-alikes will be reduced. The FDA is also looking at proposed trade names of new drugs prior to marketing, to see if they are likely to be confused with older drugs, and increasing surveillance of medication errors attributed to drug name confusion.

In addition to similar names, many drugs, especially those produced by the same manufacturer, have similar packaging. This can lead to errors if container labels are not read carefully, especially if the products are shelved or stored next to each other.

Long-acting oral dosage forms with various, sometimes unclear indicators (eg, LA, XL, XR), may be crushed, chewed, or otherwise broken so that the long-acting feature is destroyed. This can cause an overdose.

### Health Care System

Much attention has been given to the environment or system in which health care providers work to help understand and respond to medication errors. Prescribers, pharmacists, and nurses may have a heavy workload with resultant rushing of prescribing, dispensing, or administering medications. They may also experience distractions by interruptions, noise, and other events in the work environment that make it difficult to pay needed attention to the medication-related task. Attributes of a safe medication system, wherever the health care provider practices, include (1) preventing errors, (2) making errors visible, and (3) mitigating the effects of errors that reach the client.

---

acceptable by institutional policy. These are written on the client's order sheet, signed by the person taking the order, and later countersigned by the prescriber. Once the order is written, a copy is sent to the pharmacy, where the order is recorded and the drug is dispensed to the appropriate client care unit. In many agencies, pharmacy staff prepare a computer-generated MAR for each 24-hour period.

For clients in ambulatory care settings, the procedure is essentially the same for drugs to be given immediately. For drugs to be taken at home, written prescriptions are given. In addition to the previous information, a prescription should include instructions for taking the drug (eg, dose and frequency) and whether the prescription can be refilled. Prescriptions for Schedule II controlled drugs cannot be refilled. In 1998, the Food and Drug Administration published a requirement that new drugs likely to be important or frequently used in the treatment of children should be labeled with instructions for safe pediatric use.

To interpret medication orders accurately, the nurse must know commonly used abbreviations for routes, dosages, and times of drug administration (Table 4-1). If the nurse cannot read the health care provider's order, or if the order seems erroneous, the nurse must question the order before giving the drug.

## DRUG PREPARATIONS AND DOSAGE FORMS

Drug preparations and dosage forms vary according to the drug's chemical characteristics, reason for use, and route of administration. Some drugs are available in only one dosage form; others are available in several forms. Characteristics of various dosage forms are described below and in Table 4-2.

Dosage forms of systemic drugs include liquids, tablets, capsules, suppositories, and transdermal and pump deliv-

## TABLE 4-1   Common Abbreviations

### Routes of Drug Administration

| | |
|---|---|
| IM | intramuscular |
| IV | intravenous |
| OD | right eye* |
| OS | left eye* |
| OU | both eyes* |
| PO | by mouth, oral |
| Sub-Q** | subcutaneous |
| SL | sublingual |

### Drug Dosages

| | |
|---|---|
| cc | cubic centimeter |
| g | gram |
| gr | grain |
| gt | drop† |
| mcg | microgram |
| mg | milligram |
| mL | milliliter |
| oz | ounce |
| tbsp | tablespoon |
| tsp | teaspoon |

### Times of Drug Administration

| | |
|---|---|
| ac | before meals |
| ad lib | as desired |
| bid | twice daily |
| hs | bedtime |
| pc | after meals |
| PRN | when needed |
| qd | every day, daily |
| q4h | every four hours |
| qid | four times daily |
| qod | every other day |
| stat | immediately |
| tid | three times daily |

*Because of errors made with the abbreviations, some authorities recommend spelling out the site (eg, right eye).

**The Joint Commission on Accreditation of Healthcare Organizations (JCAHO) recommends using "Sub-Q" instead of "SC" to avoid misinterpretation; the Institute for Safe Medication Practices (ISMP) recommends using "subcut." or spelling out "subcutaneous".

†drops = gtt.

ery systems. Systemic liquids are given orally (PO) or by injection. Those given by injection must be sterile.

Tablets and capsules are given PO. Tablets contain active-drug plus binders, colorants, preservatives, and other substances. Capsules contain active drug enclosed in a gelatin capsule. Most tablets and capsules dissolve in the acid fluids of the stomach and are absorbed in the alkaline fluids of the upper small intestine. Enteric-coated tablets and capsules are coated with a substance that is insoluble in stomach acids. This delays dissolution until the medication reaches the intestine, usually to avoid gastric irritation or to keep the drug from being destroyed by gastric acid. Tablets for sublingual or buccal administration must be specifically formulated for such use.

Several controlled-release dosage forms and drug delivery systems are available, and more continue to be developed. These formulations maintain more consistent serum drug levels and allow less frequent administration, which is more convenient for clients. Oral tablets and capsules are called by a variety of names (eg, timed release, sustained release, extended release), and their names usually include SR, XL, or other indications that they are long-acting formulations. Most of these formulations are given once or twice daily. Some drugs (eg, alendronate for osteoporosis and fluoxetine for major depression) are available in formulations that deliver a full week's dosage in one oral tablet. *Because controlled-release tablets and capsules contain high amounts of drug intended to be absorbed slowly and act over a prolonged period of time, they should never be broken, opened, crushed, or chewed. Such an action allows the full dose to be absorbed immediately and constitutes an overdose, with potential organ damage or death.* Transdermal (skin patch) formulations include systemically absorbed clonidine, estrogen, fentanyl, nitroglycerin, and scopolamine. These medications are slowly absorbed from the skin patches over varying periods of time (eg, 1 week for clonidine and estrogen). Pump delivery systems may be external or implanted under the skin and refillable or long acting without refills. Pumps are used to administer insulin, narcotic analgesics, antineoplastic agents, and other drugs.

Solutions, ointments, creams, and suppositories are applied topically to skin or mucous membranes. They are formulated for the intended route of administration. For example, several drugs are available in solutions for nasal or oral inhalation; they are usually self-administered as a spray into the nose or mouth.

Many combination products containing fixed doses of two or more drugs are also available. Commonly used combinations include analgesics, antihypertensive drugs, and cold remedies. Most are oral tablets, capsules, or solutions.

## ■ CALCULATING DRUG DOSAGES

When calculating drug doses, the importance of accuracy cannot be overemphasized. Accuracy requires basic skills in mathematics, knowledge of common units of measurement, and methods of using data in performing calculations. Chapter 3 outlines the concepts and processes of each measurement system used in dosage calculations.

## ■ ROUTES OF ADMINISTRATION

Routes of administration depend on drug characteristics, client characteristics, and desired responses. The major routes are oral, parenteral, and topical. Each has advantages, disadvantages, indications for use, and specific

## TABLE 4-2    Drug Dosage Forms

| Dosage Forms and Their Routes of Administration | Characteristics | Considerations/Precautions |
|---|---|---|
| *Tablets* | | |
| *Regular:* PO, GI tube (crushed and mixed with water) | • Contain active drug plus binders, dyes, preservatives<br>• Dissolve in gastric fluids | 8 oz of water recommended when taken orally, to promote dissolution and absorption |
| *Chewable:* PO | • Colorful and flavored, mainly for young children who are unable to swallow or who refuse regular tablets | Colors and flavors appeal to children; keep out of reach to avoid accidental overdose. |
| *Enteric coated:* PO | • Dissolve in small intestine rather than stomach; mainly used for medications that cause gastric irritation | *Do not crush;* instruct clients not to chew or crush. |
| *Extended release* (XL): PO | • Also called sustained release (SR), long acting (LA), and others<br>• Formulated for slow absorption and prolonged action<br>• Effects of most last 12–24 hours<br>• Contain relatively large doses of active drug | **Warning:** Crushing to give orally or through a GI tube administers an overdose, with potentially serious adverse effects or death!!<br>*Never* crush; instruct clients not to chew or crush. |
| *Sublingual:* Under the tongue | • Dissolve quickly and exerts rapid systemic effect | Few medications formulated for administration by these routes |
| *Buccal:* Held in cheek | • Medication absorbed directly into the bloodstream and exerts rapid systemic effects | Few medications formulated for administration by these routes |
| *Capsules* | | |
| *Regular:* PO | • Contain active drug, fillers, and preservatives in a gelatin capsule<br>• Gelatin capsules dissolve in gastric fluid and release medication | As with oral tablets, 8 oz of fluid recommended to promote dissolution of capsule and absorption of medication |
| *Extended release* (XL): PO | • Also called sustained release (SR), long acting (LA), and others<br>• Formulated for slow absorption and prolonged action<br>• Effects of most last 12–24 hours<br>• Contain relatively large doses of active drug | **Warning:** Emptying a capsule to give the medication orally or through a GI tube administers an overdose, with potentially serious adverse effects or death!!<br>Instruct clients not to bite, chew, or empty these capsules. |
| *Solutions* | | |
| *Oral:* PO, GI tube | • Absorbed rapidly because they do not need to be dissolved | Use of appropriate measuring devices and accurate measurement are extremely important. |
| *Parenteral:* IV, IM Sub-Q, intradermal | • Medications and all administration devices must be sterile<br>• IV produces rapid effects; Sub-Q is used mainly for insulin and heparin; IM is used for only a few drugs; intradermal is used mainly to inject skin test material rather than therapeutic drugs. | Use of appropriate equipment (eg, needles, syringes, IV administration sets) and accurate measurement are extremely important. Insulin syringes should always be used for insulin and tuberculin syringes are recommended for measuring small amounts of other drugs. |
| *Suspensions* | | |
| PO, Sub-Q (NPH and Lente insulins) | • These are particles of active drug suspended in a liquid; the liquid must be rotated or shaken before measuring a dose. | Drug particles settle to the bottom on standing. If not remixed, the liquid vehicle is given rather than the drug dose. |

*(continued)*

**TABLE 4-2    Drug Dosage Forms** (Continued)

| Dosage Forms and Their Routes of Administration | Characteristics | Considerations/Precautions |
|---|---|---|
| **Dermatologic Creams, Lotions, Ointments**<br><br>Topically to skin | • Most are formulated for minimal absorption through skin and local effects at the site of application; medications in skin patch formulations are absorbed and exert systemic effects. | Formulations vary with intended uses and are not interchangeable.<br>When removed from the client, skin patches must be disposed of properly to prevent someone else from being exposed to the active drug remaining in the patch. |
| **Solutions and Powders for Oral or Nasal Inhalation, Including Metered Dose Inhalers (MDIs)** | • Oral inhalations are used mainly for asthma; nasal sprays for nasal allergies (allergic rhinitis)<br>• Effective with less systemic effect than oral drugs<br>• Deliver a specified dose per inhalation | Several research studies indicate that patients often do not use MDIs correctly and sometimes are incorrectly taught by health care providers. Correct use is essential to obtaining therapeutic effects and avoiding adverse effects. |
| **Eye Solutions and Ointments** | • Should be sterile<br>• Most are packaged in small amounts, to be used by a single patient | Can be systemically absorbed and cause systemic adverse effects |
| **Throat Lozenges** | • Used for cough and sore throat | |
| **Ear Solutions** | • Used mainly for ear infections | |
| **Vaginal Creams and Suppositories** | • Formulated for insertion into the vagina<br>• Commonly used to treat vaginal infections | |
| **Rectal Suppositories and Enemas** | • Formulated for insertion into the rectum<br>• Suppositories may be used to administer sedatives, analgesics, laxatives<br>• Medicated enemas are used to treat inflammatory bowel diseases (eg, ulcerative colitis) | Effects somewhat unpredictable because absorption is erratic |

PO, oral; GI, gastrointestinal; IV, intravenous; IM, intramuscular; Sub-Q, subcutaneous.

techniques of administration (Table 4-3). The term *parenteral* refers to any route other than gastrointestinal (enteral) but is commonly used to indicate subcutaneous (Sub-Q), intramuscular (IM), and intravenous (IV) injections. Injections require special drug preparations, equipment, and techniques. General characteristics are described later; specific considerations for the intravenous route are described in Box 4-2.

## Drugs for Injection

Parenteral drugs must be prepared, packaged, and administered in ways to maintain sterility. Vials are closed glass or plastic containers with rubber stoppers through which a sterile needle can be inserted for withdrawing medication. Single-dose vials usually do not contain a preservative and must be discarded after a dose is withdrawn; multiple-dose vials contain a preservative and may be reused if aseptic technique is maintained.

Ampules are sealed glass containers, the tops of which must be broken off to allow insertion of a needle and withdrawal of the medication. Broken ampules and any remaining medication are discarded; they are no longer sterile and cannot be reused. When vials or ampules contain a powder form of the drug, a sterile solution of water or 0.9% sodium chloride must be added and the drug dissolved before withdrawal. Use a filter needle to withdraw the medication from an ampule or vial because broken glass or rubber fragments may need to be removed from the drug solution. Replace the filter needle with a regular needle before injecting the client.

Many injectable drugs (eg, morphine, heparin) are available in prefilled syringes with attached needles. These *(text continues on page 46)*

## TABLE 4-3 Routes of Drug Administration

| Route and Description | Advantages | Disadvantages | Comments |
|---|---|---|---|
| Oral | • Simple and can be used by most people<br>• Convenient; does not require complex equipment<br>• Relatively inexpensive | • Amount of drug acting on body cells is unknown because varying portions of a dose are absorbed and some drug is metabolized in the liver before reaching the bloodstream for circulation<br>• Slow drug action<br>• Irritation of gastrointestinal mucosa by some drugs | The oral route should generally be used when possible, considering the client's condition and ability to take or tolerate oral drugs. |
| GI tubes (eg, nasogastric, gastrostomy) | • Allows use of GI tract in clients who cannot take oral drugs<br>• Can be used over long periods of time, if necessary<br>• May avoid or decrease injections | • With nasogastric tubes, medications may be aspirated into the lungs<br>• Small-bore tubes often become clogged<br>• Requires special precautions to give correctly and avoid complications | • Liquid preparations are preferred over crushed tablets and emptied capsules, when available.<br>• Tube should be rinsed before and after instilling medication. |
| Subcutaneous (Sub-Q) injection—injection of drugs under the skin, into the underlying fatty tissue | • Relatively painless<br>• Very small needles can be used<br>• Insulin and heparin, commonly used medications that often require multiple daily injections, can be given Sub-Q | • Only a small amount of drug (up to 1 mL) can be given<br>• Drug absorption is relatively slow<br>• Only a few drugs can be given Sub-Q | The Sub-Q route is commonly used for only a few drugs because many drugs are irritating to Sub-Q tissues. Such drugs may cause pain, necrosis, and abscess formation if injected Sub-Q. |
| Intramuscular (IM) injection—injection of drugs into selected muscles | • May be used for several drugs<br>• Drug absorption is rapid because muscle tissue has an abundant blood supply | • A relatively small amount of drug (up to 3 mL) can be given<br>• Risks of damage to blood vessels or nerves if needle is not positioned correctly | It is very important to use anatomic landmarks when selecting IM injection sites. |
| Intravenous (IV) injection—injection of a drug into the bloodstream | • Allows medications to be given to a patient who cannot take fluids or drugs by GI tract<br>• Bypasses barriers to drug absorption that occur with other routes<br>• Rapid drug action<br>• Larger amounts can be given than by Sub-Q and IM routes<br>• Allows slow administration when indicated | • Time and skill required for venipuncture and maintaining an IV line<br>• Once injected, drug cannot be retrieved if adverse effects or overdoses occur<br>• High potential for adverse reactions from rapid drug action and possible complications of IV therapy (ie, bleeding, infection, fluid overload, extravasation)<br>• Phlebitis commonly occurs and increases risks of thrombosis<br>• Phlebitis and thrombosis cause discomfort or pain, may take days or weeks to subside, and limit the veins available for future therapy | • The nurse should wear latex gloves to start IV infusions, for protection against exposure to blood-borne pathogens.<br>• Phlebitis and thrombosis result from injury to the endothelial cells that form the inner lining (intima) of veins and may be caused by repeated venipunctures, the IV catheter, hypertonic IV fluid, or irritating drugs. |

*(continued)*

## TABLE 4-3   Routes of Drug Administration (Continued)

| Route and Description | Advantages | Disadvantages | Comments |
|---|---|---|---|
| Topical administration— application to skin or mucous membranes. Application to mucous membranes includes drugs given by nasal or oral inhalation; by instillation into the lungs, eyes, or nose; and by insertion under the tongue (sublingual), into the cheek (buccal), and into the vagina or rectum. | • With application to intact skin, most medications act at the site of application, with little systemic absorption or systemic adverse effects.<br>• Some drugs are given topically for systemic effects (eg, medicated skin patches). Effects may last several days and the patches are usually convenient for clients.<br>• With application to mucous membranes, most drugs are well and rapidly absorbed | • Some drugs irritate skin or mucous membranes and cause itching, rash, or discomfort<br>• With inflamed, abraded, or damaged skin, drug absorption is increased and systemic adverse effects may occur<br>• Application to mucous membranes may cause systemic adverse effects (eg, beta blocker eye drops, used to treat glaucoma, can cause bradycardia just as oral beta blockers can)<br>• Specific drug preparations must be used for the various routes (ie, dermatologics for skin; ophthalmics for eyes; sublingual, buccal, vaginal, and rectal preparations for those sites). | When available and effective, topical drugs are often preferred over oral or injected drugs, because of fewer and/or less severe systemic adverse effects. |

## BOX 4-2   Principles and Techniques With IV Drug Therapy

### Methods

**IV injection** or **IV push** is the direct injection of a medication into the vein. The drug may be injected through an injection site on IV tubing or an intermittent infusion device. Most IV push medications should be injected slowly. The time depends on the particular drug, but is often 2 minutes or longer for a dose. Rapid injection should generally be avoided because the drug produces high blood levels and is quickly circulated to the heart and brain, where it may cause adverse or toxic effects. Although IV push may be useful with a few drugs or in emergency situations, slower infusion of more dilute drugs is usually preferred.

**Intermittent infusion** is administration of intermittent doses, often diluted in 50 to 100 mL of fluid and infused over 30–60 minutes. The drug dose is usually prepared in a pharmacy and connected to an IV administration set that controls the amount and flow rate. Intermittent infusions are often connected to an injection port on a primary IV line, through which IV fluids are infusing continuously. The purpose of the primary IV line may be to provide fluids to the client or to keep the vein open for periodic administration of medications. The IV fluids are usually stopped for the medication infusion, then restarted. Drug doses may also be infused through an intermittent infusion device (eg, a heparin lock) to conserve veins and allow freedom of motion between drug doses. The devices decrease the amount of IV fluids given to patients who do not need them (ie, who are able to ingest adequate amounts of oral fluids) and those who are at risk of fluid overload, especially children and older adults.

An intermittent infusion device may be part of an initial IV line or used to adapt a continuous IV for intermittent use. The devices include a heparin lock or a resealable adapter added to a peripheral or central IV catheter. These devices must be flushed routinely to maintain patency. If the IV catheter has more than one lumen, all must be flushed, whether being used or not. Saline is probably the most commonly used flushing solution; heparin may also be used if recommended by the device's manufacturer or required by institutional policy. For example, heparin (3 to 5 mL of 100 units/mL, after each use or monthly if not in use) is recommended for implanted catheters.

**Continuous infusion** indicates medications mixed in a large volume of IV fluid and infused continuously, over several hours. For example, vitamins and minerals (eg, potassium chloride) are usually added to liters of IV fluids. Greater

*(continued)*

BOX
4-2    Principles and Techniques With IV Drug Therapy (Continued)

dilution of the drug and administration over a longer time decrease risks of accumulation and toxicity, as well as venous irritation and thrombophlebitis.

## Equipment

Equipment varies considerably from one health care agency to another. Nurses must become familiar with the equipment available in their work setting, including IV catheters, types of IV tubing, needles and needleless systems, types of volume control devices, and electronic infusion devices (IV pumps).

**Catheters** vary in size (both gauge and length), design and composition (eg, polyvinyl chloride, polyurethane, silicone). The most common design type is over the needle; the needle is used to start the IV, then it is removed. When choosing a catheter to start an IV, one that is much smaller than the lumen of the vein is recommended. This allows good blood flow and rapidly dilutes drug solutions as they enter the vein. This, in turn, prevents high drug concentrations and risks of toxicity. Also, once a catheter is inserted, it is very important to tape it securely so that it does not move around. Movement of the catheter increases venous irritation and risks of thrombophlebitis and infection. If signs of venous irritation and inflammation develop, the catheter should be removed and a new one inserted at another site. Additional recommendations include application of a topical antibiotic or antiseptic ointment at the IV site after catheter insertion, a sterile occlusive dressing over the site, and limiting the duration of placement to a few days.

Many medications are administered through peripherally inserted central catheters (PICC lines) or central venous catheters, in which the catheter tips are inserted into the superior vena cava, next to the right atrium of the heart. Central venous catheters may have single, double, or triple lumens. Other products, which are especially useful for long-term IV drug therapy, include a variety of implanted ports, pumps, and reservoirs.

*If a catheter becomes clogged, do not irrigate it. Doing so may push a clot into the circulation and result in a pulmonary embolus, myocardial infarction, or stroke. It may also cause septicemia, if the clot is infected.*

**Needleless systems** are one of the most important advances in IV therapy. Most products have a blunt-tipped plastic insertion device and an injection port that opens. These systems greatly decrease needle-stick injuries and exposure to blood-borne pathogens.

**Electronic infusion devices** allow amounts and flow rates of IV drug solutions to be set and controlled by a computer. Although the devices save nursing time, because the nurse does not need to count drops and continually adjust flow rates, probably the biggest advantage is the steady rate of drug administration. The devices are used in most settings where IV drugs and IV fluids are administered, but they are especially valuable in pediatrics, where very small amounts of medication and IV fluid are needed, and in intensive care units, where strong drugs and varying amounts

of IV fluid are usually required. Several types of pumps are available, even within the same health care agency. It is extremely important that nurses become familiar with the devices used in their work setting, so they can program them accurately and determine whether or not they are functioning properly (ie, delivering medications as ordered).

## Site Selection

IV needles are usually inserted into a vein on the hand or forearm; IV catheters may be inserted in a peripheral site or centrally (the catheter tip ends in the superior vena cava, near the right atrium of the heart, and medications and fluids are rapidly diluted and flow directly into the heart). In general, recommendations are:

- Start at the most distal location. This conserves more proximal veins for later use, if needed. Veins on the back of the hand and on the forearm are often used. These sites usually provide more comfort and freedom of movement for clients than other sites.
- Use veins with a large blood volume flowing through them when possible. Many drugs cause irritation and phlebitis in small veins.
- When possible, avoid the antecubital vein on the inner surface of the elbow, veins over or close to joints, and veins on the inner aspect of the wrists. Reasons include the difficulty of stabilizing and maintaining an IV line at these sites. In addition, the antecubital vein is often used to draw blood samples for laboratory analysis and inner wrist venipunctures are very painful. *Do not perform venipuncture in foot or leg veins.* The risks of serious or fatal complications are too high.
- Rotate sites when long-term use (more than a few days) of IV fluid or drug therapy is required. Venous irritation occurs with longer duration of site use and with the administration of irritating drugs or fluids. When it is necessary to change an IV site, use the opposite arm if possible.

## Drug Preparation

Most IV drugs are prepared for administration in pharmacies and this is the safest practice. When a nurse must prepare a medication, considerations include the following.

- Only drug formulations manufactured for IV use should be given IV. Other formulations contain various substances that are not sterile, pure enough, or soluble enough to be injected into the bloodstream. *In recent years, there have been numerous reports of medication errors resulting from IV administration of drug preparations intended for oral use!!* Such errors can and should be prevented. For example, when liquid medications intended for oral use are measured or dispensed in a syringe (as they often are for children, adults with difficulty in swallowing tablets and capsules, or for administration through a gastrointestinal [GI] tube), the syringe should have a blunt tip that will not connect to or penetrate IV tubing injection sites.

*(continued)*

BOX
4-2    **Principles and Techniques With IV Drug Therapy** (Continued)

- Use sterile technique during all phases of IV drug preparation.
- Follow the manufacturer's instructions for mixing and diluting IV medications. Some liquid IV medications need to be diluted prior to IV administration and powdered medications must be reconstituted appropriately (eg, the correct amount of the recommended diluent added). The diluent recommended by the drug's manufacturer should be used because different drugs require different diluents. In addition, be sure any reconstituted drug is completely dissolved to avoid particles that may be injected into the systemic circulation and lead to thrombus formation or embolism. A filtered aspiration needle should be used when withdrawing medication from a vial or ampule, to remove any particles in the solution. The filter needle should then be discarded, to prevent filtered particles from being injected when the medication is added to the IV fluid. Filters added to IV tubing also help to remove particles.
- Check the expiration date on all IV medications. Many drugs have a limited period of stability after they are reconstituted or diluted for IV administration.
- IV medications should be compatible with the infusing IV fluids. Most are compatible with 5% dextrose in water or saline solutions.
- If adding a medication to a container of IV fluid, invert the container to be sure the additive is well mixed with the solution.
- For any IV medication that is prepared or added to an IV bag, label the medication vial or IV bag with the name of the patient, drug, dosage, date, time of mixing, expiration date, and the preparer's signature.

**Drug Administration**
- Most IV medications are injected into a self-sealing site in any of several IV set-ups, including a scalp–vein needle and tubing, a plastic catheter connected to a heparin lock or other intermittent infusion device, or IV tubing and a plastic bag containing IV fluid.
- Before injecting any IV medication, be sure the IV line is open and functioning properly (eg, catheter not clotted, IV fluid not leaking into surrounding tissues, phlebitis not present). If leakage occurs, some drugs are very irritating to subcutaneous tissues and may cause tissue necrosis.
- Maintain sterility of all IV fluids, tubings, injection sites, drug solutions, and equipment coming into contact with the IV system. Because medications and fluids are injected directly into the bloodstream, breaks in sterile technique can lead to serious systemic infections (septicemia) and death.
- When two or more medications are to be given one after the other, flush the IV tubing and catheter (with the infusing IV fluid or with sterile 0.9% sodium chloride injection) so that the drugs do not come into contact with each other.
- If a medication is to be injected or infused through an intermittent infusion device containing heparin, the drug should be compatible with heparin or the device should be irrigated with sterile saline before and after medication administration. After irrigation, heparin then needs to be reinstilled. This is not a common event, because most heparin locks and other intermittent infusion devices are now filled with saline rather than heparin.
- In general, administer slowly to allow greater dilution of the drug in the bloodstream. Most drugs given by IV push (direct injection) can be given over 2–5 minutes and most drugs diluted in 50–100 mL of IV fluid can be infused in 30–60 minutes.
- When injecting or infusing medications into IV solutions that contain other additives (eg, vitamins, insulin, minerals such as potassium or magnesium), be sure the medications are compatible with the other substances. Consult compatibility charts (usually available on nursing units) or pharmacists when indicated.
- IV flow rates are usually calculated in mL/hour and drops per minute. Required information includes the amount of solution or medication to be infused, the time or duration of the infusion, and the drop factor of the IV administration set to be used. The drop factor of macrodrip sets may be 10, 15, or 20 drops per milliliter, depending on the manufacturer. Most agencies use mainly one manufacturer's product. The drop factor of all microdrip sets is 60 drops per mL.

units are inserted into specially designed holders and used like other needle and syringe units.

## Equipment for Injections

Sterile needles and syringes are used to measure and administer parenteral medications; they may be packaged together or separately. Needles are available in various gauges and lengths. The term *gauge* refers to lumen size, with larger numbers indicating smaller lumen sizes. For example, a 25-gauge needle is smaller than an 18-gauge needle. Choice of needle gauge and length depends on the route of administration, the viscosity (thickness) of the solution to be given, and the size of the client. Usually, a 25-gauge, $5/_8$-inch needle is used for Sub-Q injections and a 22- or 20-gauge, $1^1/_2$-inch needle for IM injections. Other needle sizes are available for special uses, such as insulin or intradermal injections. When needles are used, avoid recapping them, and dispose of them in appropriate containers. Such containers are designed to prevent accidental needle-stick injuries to health care and housekeeping personnel.

In many settings, needleless systems are being used. These involve a plastic tip on the syringe that can be used to enter vials and injection sites on IV tubing. Openings created by the tip reseal themselves. Needleless systems were developed to reduce the risk for injury and spread of blood-borne pathogens, such as the viruses that cause acquired immunodeficiency syndrome (AIDS) and hepatitis B.

Syringes also are available in various sizes. The 3-mL size is probably used most often. It is usually plastic and is available with or without an attached needle. Syringes are calibrated so that drug doses can be measured accurately. However, the calibrations vary according to the size and type of syringe.

Insulin and tuberculin syringes are used for specific purposes. Insulin syringes are calibrated to measure up to 100 units of insulin. Safe practice requires that *only* insulin syringes be used to measure insulin and that they be used for no other drugs. Tuberculin syringes have a capacity of 1 mL. They should be used for small doses of any drug because measurements are more accurate than with larger syringes.

## Sites for Injections

Sites for subcutaneous injections are the upper arms, abdomen, back, and thighs. Locations for intramuscular injections are the deltoid, dorsogluteal, ventrogluteal, and vastus lateralis muscles. Common sites for intravenous injections are the veins on the back of the hands and on the forearms; other sites (eg, subclavian and jugular veins) are also used, mainly in critically ill clients. Additional parenteral routes include injection into layers of the skin (intradermal), arteries (intraarterial), joints (intraarticular), and cerebrospinal fluid (intrathecal). Nurses may administer drugs intradermally or, rarely, intraarterially (if an established arterial line is present); physicians administer intraarticular and intrathecal medications.

## *Nursing Actions*
## Drug Administration

| *Nursing Actions* | *Rationale/Explanation* |
|---|---|
| 1. Follow general rules for administering medications safety and effectively. | |
| a. Prepare and give drugs in well-lighted areas, as free of interruptions and distractions as possible. | To prevent errors in selecting ordered drugs, calculating dosages, and identifying clients |
| b. Wash hands before preparing medications and, if needed, during administration. | To prevent infection and cross-contamination |
| c. Use sterile technique in preparing and administering injections. | To prevent infection. Sterile technique involves using sterile needles and syringes, using sterile drug solutions, not touching sterile objects to any unsterile objects, and cleansing injection sites with an antiseptic. |
| d. Read the medication administration record (MAR) carefully. Read the label on the drug container, and compare with the MAR in terms of drug, dosage or concentration, and route of administration. | For accurate drug administration. Most nursing texts instruct the nurse to read a drug label three times: when removing the container, while measuring the dose, and before returning the container. |
| e. Do not leave medications unattended. | To prevent accidental or deliberate ingestion by anyone other than the intended person. Also, to prevent contamination or spilling of medications. |
| f. Identify the client, preferably by comparing the identification wristband to the medication sheet. | This is the best way to verify identity. Calling by name, relying on the name on a door or bed, and asking someone else are unreliable methods, although they must be used occasionally when the client lacks a name band. |
| g. Identify yourself, if indicated, and state your reason for approaching the client. For example, "I'm . . . I have your medication for you." | Explaining actions helps to decrease client anxiety and increase cooperation in taking prescribed medication. |
| h. Position the client appropriately for the intended route of administration. | To prevent complications, such as aspiration of oral drugs into the lungs |
| i. Provide water or other supplies as needed. | To promote comfort of the client and to ensure drug administration |
| j. Do not leave medications at the bedside as a general rule. Common exceptions are antacids, nitroglycerin, and eye medications. | To prevent omitting or losing the drug or hoarding of the drug by the client |
| k. Do not give a drug when signs and symptoms of toxicity are present. Notify the health care provider, and record that the drug was omitted and why. | Additional doses of a drug increase toxicity. However, drugs are not omitted without a careful assessment of the client's condition and a valid reason. |
| l. Record drug administration (or omission) as soon as possible and according to agency policies. | To maintain an accurate record of drugs received by the client |

*(continued)*

## Nursing Actions
### Drug Administration (Continued)

| Nursing Actions | Rationale/Explanation |
|---|---|
| m. If it is necessary to omit a scheduled dose for some reason, the decision to give the dose later or omit it depends largely on the drug and frequency of administration. Generally, give drugs ordered once or twice daily at a later time. For others, omit the one dose, and give the drug at the next scheduled time. | Clients may be unable to take the drug at the scheduled time because of diagnostic tests or many other reasons. A temporary change in the time of administration—usually for one dose only—may be necessary to maintain therapeutic effects. |
| n. For medications ordered as needed (PRN), assess the client's condition; check the physician's orders or MAR for the name, dose, and frequency of administration; and determine the time of the most recently administered dose. | Administration of PRN medications requires nursing assessment and decision making. Analgesics, antiemetics, and antipyretics are often ordered PRN. |
| o. For narcotics and other controlled substances, sign drugs out on separate narcotic records according to agency policies. | To meet legal requirements for dispensing controlled substances |
| p. If, at any time during drug preparation or administration, any question arises regarding the drug, the dose, or whether the client is supposed to receive it, check the original health care provider's order. If the order is not clear, call the health care provider for clarification before giving the drug. | To promote safety and prevent errors. The same procedure applies when the client questions drug orders at the bedside. For example, the client may state he has been receiving different drugs or different doses. |
| 2. **For oral medications:** | |
| a. With adults | |
| (1) To give tablets or capsules, open the unit-dose wrapper, place medication in a medicine cup, and give the cup to the client. For solutions, hold the cup at eye level, and measure the dosage at the bottom of the meniscus. For suspensions, shake or invert containers to mix the medication before measuring the dose. | To maintain clean technique and measure doses accurately. Suspensions settle on standing, and if not mixed, diluent may be given rather than the active drug. |
| (2) Have the client in a sitting position when not contraindicated. | To decrease risks of aspirating medication into lungs. Aspiration may lead to difficulty in breathing and aspiration pneumonia. |
| (3) Give before, with, or after meals as indicated by the specific drug. | Food in the stomach usually delays drug absorption and action. It also decreases gastric irritation, a common side effect of oral drugs. Giving drugs at appropriate times in relation to food intake can increase therapeutic effects and decrease adverse effects. |
| (4) Give most oral drugs with a full glass (8 oz) of water or other fluid. | To promote dissolution and absorption of tablets and capsules. Also, to decrease gastric irritation by diluting drug concentration. |
| b. With children, liquids or chewable tablets are usually given. | Children under 5 years of age are often unable to swallow tablets or capsules. |
| (1) Measure and give liquids to infants with a dropper or syringe, placing medication on the tongue or buccal mucosa and giving slowly. | For accurate measurement and administration. Giving slowly decreases risks of aspiration. |
| (2) Medications are often mixed with juice, applesauce, or other vehicle. | To increase the child's ability and willingness to take the medication. If this is done, use a small amount, and be sure the child takes all of it; otherwise, less than the ordered dose is given. |
| c. Do not give oral drugs if the client is: | |
| (1) NPO (receiving nothing by mouth) | Oral drugs and fluids may interfere with diagnostic tests or be otherwise contraindicated. Most drugs can be given after diagnostic tests are completed. If the client is having surgery, preoperative drug orders are cancelled. New orders are written postoperatively. |

*(continued)*

## Nursing Actions
### Drug Administration (Continued)

| Nursing Actions | Rationale/Explanation |
|---|---|
| (2) Vomiting | Oral drugs and fluids increase vomiting. Thus, no benefit results from the drug. Also, fluid and electrolyte problems may result from loss of gastric acid. |
| (3) Excessively sedated or unconscious | To avoid aspiration of drugs into the lungs owing to impaired ability to swallow |
| 3. For medications given by nasogastric tube: | |
| a. Use a liquid preparation when possible. If necessary, crush a tablet or empty a capsule into about 30 mL of water and mix well. **Do not crush enteric-coated or sustained-release products, and do not empty sustained-release capsules.** | Particles of tablets or powders from capsules may obstruct the tube lumen. Altering sustained-release products increases risks of overdosage and adverse effects. |
| b. Use a clean bulb syringe or other catheter-tipped syringe. | The syringe allows aspiration and serves as a funnel for instillation of medication and fluids into the stomach. |
| c. Before instilling medication, aspirate gastric fluid or use another method to check tube placement. | To be sure the tube is in the stomach |
| d. Instill medication by gravity flow, and follow it with at least 50 mL of water. Do not allow the syringe to empty completely between additions. | Gravity flow is safer than applying pressure. Water "pushes" the drug into the stomach and rinses the tube, thereby maintaining tube patency. Additional water or other fluids may be given according to fluid needs of the client. Add fluids to avoid instilling air into the stomach unnecessarily, with possible client discomfort. |
| e. Clamp off the tube from suction or drainage for at least 30 minutes. | To avoid removing the medication from the stomach |
| 4. For subcutaneous (Sub-Q) injections: | |
| a. Use only sterile drug preparations labeled or commonly used for Sub-Q injections. | Many parenteral drugs are too irritating to subcutaneous tissue for use by this route. |
| b. Use a 25-gauge, $\frac{5}{8}$-inch needle for most Sub-Q injections. | This size needle is effective for most clients and drugs. |
| c. Select an appropriate injection site, based on client preferences, drug characteristics, and visual inspection of possible sites. In long-term therapy, such as with insulin, rotate injection sites. Avoid areas with lumps, bruises, or other lesions. | These techniques allow the client to participate in his or her care; avoid tissue damage and unpredictable absorption, which occur with repeated injections in the same location; and increase client comfort and cooperation |
| d. Cleanse the site with an alcohol sponge. | To prevent infection |
| e. Tighten the skin or pinch a fold of skin and tissue between thumb and fingers. | Either is acceptable for most clients. If the client is obese, tightening the skin may be easier. If the client is very thin, the tissue fold may keep the needle from hitting bone. |
| f. Hold the syringe like a pencil, and insert the needle quickly at a 45-degree angle. Use enough force to penetrate the skin and subcutaneous tissue in one smooth movement. | To give the drug correctly with minimal client discomfort. |
| g. Release the skin so that both hands are free to manipulate the syringe. Pull back gently on the plunger (aspirate). If no blood enters the syringe, inject the drug. If blood is aspirated into the syringe, remove the needle, and reprepare the medication. | To prevent accidental injection into the bloodstream. Blood return in the syringe is an uncommon occurrence. |
| h. Remove the needle quickly and apply gentle pressure for a few seconds. | To prevent bleeding |
| 5. For intramuscular (IM) injections: | |
| a. Use only drug preparations labeled or commonly used for IM injections. Check label instructions for mixing drugs in powder form. | Some parenteral drug preparations cannot be given safely by the IM route. |

*(continued)*

## Nursing Actions

## Drug Administration (Continued)

| Nursing Actions | Rationale/Explanation |
|---|---|
| b. Use a 1½-inch needle for most adults and a ⅝- to 1½-inch needle for children, depending on the size of the client. | A long needle is necessary to reach muscle tissue, which underlies subcutaneous fat. |
| c. Use the smallest-gauge needle that will accommodate the medication. A 22-gauge is satisfactory for most drugs; a 20-gauge may be used for viscous medications. | To decrease tissue damage and client discomfort |
| d. Select an appropriate injection site, based on client preferences, drug characteristics, anatomic landmarks, and visual inspection of possible sites. Rotate sites if frequent injections are being given, and avoid areas with lumps, bruises, or other lesions. | To increase client comfort and participation and to avoid tissue damage. Identification of anatomic landmarks is mandatory for safe administration of IM drugs. |
| e. Cleanse the site with an alcohol sponge. | To prevent infection |
| f. Tighten the skin, hold the syringe like a pencil, and insert the needle quickly at a 90-degree angle. Use enough force to penetrate the skin and subcutaneous tissue into the muscle in one smooth motion. | To give the drug correctly with minimal client discomfort |
| g. Aspirate (see 4g, Sub-Q injections). | |
| h. Remove the needle quickly and apply pressure for several seconds. | To prevent bleeding |
| 6. **For intravenous (IV) injections:** | |
| a. Use only drug preparations that are labeled for IV use. | Others are not pure enough for safe injection into the bloodstream or are not compatible with the normal blood pH (7.35–7.45). |
| b. Check label instructions for the type and amount of fluid to use for dissolving or diluting the drug. | Some drugs require special preparation techniques to maintain solubility or pharmacologic activity. Most drugs in powder form can be dissolved in sterile water or sodium chloride for injection. Most drug solutions can be given with dextrose or dextrose and sodium chloride IV solutions. |
| c. Prepare drugs just before use, as a general rule. Also, add drugs to IV fluids just before use. | Some drugs are unstable in solution. In some agencies, drugs are mixed and added to IV fluids in the pharmacy. This is the preferred method because sterility can be better maintained. |
| d. For venipuncture and direct injection into a vein, apply a tourniquet, select a site in the arm, cleanse the skin with an antiseptic (eg, povidone-iodine or alcohol), insert the needle, and aspirate a small amount of blood into the syringe to be sure that the needle is in the vein. Remove the tourniquet, and inject the drug slowly. Remove the needle and apply pressure until there is no evidence of bleeding. | For safe and accurate drug administration with minimal risk to the client. The length of time required to give the drug depends on the specific drug and the amount. Slow administration, over several minutes, allows immediate discontinuation if adverse effects occur. |
| e. For administration by an established IV line: | |
| (1) Check the infusion for patency and flow rate. Check the venipuncture site for signs of infiltration and phlebitis before each drug dose. | The solution must be flowing freely for accurate drug administration. If infiltration or phlebitis is present, do not give the drug until a new IV line is begun. |
| (2) For direct injection, cleanse an injection site on the IV tubing, insert the needle, and inject the drug slowly. | Most tubings have injection sites to facilitate drug administration. |
| (3) To use a volume-control set, fill it with 50–100 mL of IV fluid, and clamp it so that no further fluid enters the chamber and dilutes the drug. Inject the drug into an injection site after cleansing the site with an alcohol sponge and infuse, usually in 1 hour or less. Once the drug is infused, add solution to maintain the infusion. | This method is used for administration of antibiotics on an intermittent schedule. Dilution of the drug decreases adverse effects. |

(continued)

## *Nursing Actions*

## Drug Administration (Continued)

| *Nursing Actions* | *Rationale/Explanation* |
|---|---|
| (4) To use a "piggyback" method, add the drug to 50–100 mL of IV solution in a separate container. Attach the IV tubing and a needle. Insert the needle in an injection site on the main IV tubing after cleansing the site. Infuse the drug over 15–60 minutes, depending on the drug. | This method is also used for intermittent administration of antibiotics and other drugs. Whether a volume-control or piggyback apparatus is used depends on agency policy and equipment available. |
| f. When more than one drug is to be given, flush the line between drugs. Do not mix drugs in syringes or in IV fluids unless the drug literature states that the drugs are compatible. | Physical and chemical interactions between the drugs may occur and cause precipitation, inactivation, or increased toxicity. Most nursing units have charts depicting drug compatibility, or information may be obtained from the pharmacy. |
| **7. For application to skin:**<br>a. Use drug preparations labeled for dermatologic use. Cleanse the skin, remove any previously applied medication, and apply the drug in a thin layer. For broken skin or open lesions, use sterile gloves, tongue blade, or cotton-tipped applicator to apply the drug. | To promote therapeutic effects and minimize adverse effects |
| **8. For instillation of eye drops:**<br>a. Use drug preparations labeled for ophthalmic use. Wash your hands, open the eye to expose the conjunctival sac, and drop the medication into the sac, not on the eyeball, without touching the dropper tip to anything. Provide a tissue for blotting any excess drug. If two or more eye drops are scheduled at the same time, wait 1–5 minutes between instillations. | Ophthalmic preparations must be sterile to avoid infection. Blot any excess drug from the inner canthus near the nose to decrease systemic absorption of the drug. |
| With children, prepare the medication, place the child in a head-lowered position, steady the hand holding the medication on the child's head, gently retract the lower lid, and instill the medication into the conjunctival sac. | Careful positioning and restraint to avoid sudden movements are necessary to decrease risks of injury to the eye. |
| **9. For instillation of nose drops and nasal sprays:**<br>a. Have the client hold his or her head back, and drop the medication into the nostrils. Give only as ordered<br>With children, place in a supine position with the head lowered, instill the medication, and maintain the position for 2–3 minutes. Then, place the child in a prone position. | When nose drops are used for rhinitis and nasal congestion accompanying the common cold, overuse results in a rebound congestion that may be worse than the original symptom. |
| **10. For instillation of ear medications:**<br>a. Open the ear canal by pulling the ear up and back for adults, down and back for children, and drop the medication on the side of the canal. | To straighten the canal and promote maximal contact between medication and tissue |
| **11. For rectal suppositories:**<br>a. Lubricate the end with a water-soluble lubricant, wear a glove or finger cot, and insert into the rectum the length of the finger. Place the suppository next to the mucosal wall. If the client prefers and is able, provide supplies for self-administration. | To promote absorption. Allowing self-administration may prevent embarrassment to the client. Be sure the client knows the correct procedure. |
| **12. For vaginal medications:**<br>a. Use gloves or an applicator for insertion. If an applicator is used, wash thoroughly with soap and water after each use. If the client prefers and is able, provide supplies for self-administration. | Some women may be embarrassed and prefer self-administration. Be sure the client knows the correct procedure. |

## ❓ How Can You Avoid This Medication Error?

**Answer:** This medication error occurred because the medication was given to the wrong client. The nurse did not check the client's name band and relied on the client to respond to her calling his name. In this situation, the client had been asleep and may have been responding simply to being awakened. Also, language and culture may have been a factor. Accurate identification of the client is imperative, especially when the client may be confused or unable to respond appropriately.

## Critical Thinking Exercises

1. The drop factor for all intravenous microdrip sets is:
   a. 10 gtts/mL
   b. 20 gtts/mL
   c. 30 gtts/mL
   d. 60 gtts/mL

2. The nurse is administering an oral suspension of a drug to a client. Failure to shake or invert the container before measuring the dose may:
   a. Increase amount available for absorption
   b. Decrease amount available for absorption
   c. Inactivate the suspension
   d. Likely have little effect on the dosage

3. If, after questioning the prescriber and seeking information from other authoritative sources, the nurse considers that giving a drug is unsafe, the nurse should:
   a. Refuse to give the drug
   b. Administer the drug
   c. Wait to ask the nurse on the next shift what she or he would do
   d. Substitute a safer drug and administer

4. After a thorough explanation, a client makes an informed decision and refuses to take his morning dose of furosemide (Lasix), stating, "I'm not going to take that water pill anymore." The nurse should:
   a. Document the reason for the refusal and notify the prescriber
   b. See if another nurse can convince the client to take the medicine
   c. Bring the medicine back later and tell the client it is a vitamin pill
   d. Crush the pill and mix the medication with the applesauce on his breakfast tray

5. It is particularly important that a nurse be especially vigilant when giving medications to children because:
   a. There is a high risk for medication errors in this population
   b. Many drugs are marketed in dosage forms and concentrations suitable for adults
   c. Most drugs have not been tested in children
   d. All of the above

## SELECTED REFERENCES

Argo, A. L., Cox, K. K., & Kelley, W. N. (2000). The ten most common lethal medication errors in hospital patients. *Hospital Pharmacy, 35*(5), 470–474.

Craven, R. F., & Hirnle, C. J. (2000). *Fundamentals of nursing: Human health and function* (3rd ed.). Philadelphia: Lippincott Williams & Wilkins.

*Drug facts and comparisons.* (Updated monthly). St. Louis: Facts and Comparisons.

Institute for Safe Medication Practices. (September 19, 2001). New tall-man lettering will reduce mix-ups due to generic drug name confusion. *ISMP Medication Safety Alert.* [On-line.] Available: http://www.ismp.org. Accessed July 2003.

Lacy, C. F., Armstrong, L. L., Goldman, M. P., & Lance, L. L. (2003). *Lexi-Comp's drug information handbook* (11th ed.). Hudson, OH: American Pharmaceutical Association.

Togger, D. A., & Brenner, P. S. (2001). Metered dose inhalers. *American Journal of Nursing, 101*(10), 26–32.

Weinstein, S. M. (2001). *Plumer's principles and practice of intravenous therapy* (7th ed.). Philadelphia: Lippincott Williams & Wilkins.

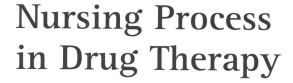

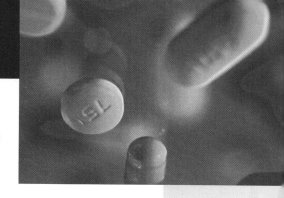

# 5

# Nursing Process in Drug Therapy

## OBJECTIVES

*After studying this chapter, the student will be able to:*

1 Assess the client's condition in relation to age, weight, health status, and lifestyle habits likely to influence drug effects.

2 Obtain a medication history about the client's use of prescription, over-the-counter, and social drugs as well as herbal and dietary supplements.

3 Identify nonpharmacologic interventions to prevent or decrease the need for drug therapy.

4 Discuss interventions to increase benefits and decrease hazards of drug therapy.

5 Explain guidelines for rational choices of drugs, dosages, routes, and times of administration.

6 Observe clients for therapeutic and adverse responses to drug therapy.

7 Teach clients and family members how to use prescription and over-the-counter drugs safely and effectively.

8 When indicated, teach clients about the potential effects of herbal and dietary supplements.

9 For clients who use herbal and dietary supplements, provide or assist them in obtaining reliable information.

10 Describe major considerations in drug therapy for clients with impaired renal or hepatic function.

11 Discuss application of the nursing process in home care settings.

## CRITICAL THINKING SCENARIO

*Y*ou are making the first home visit to Paul Robinson, an elderly client. He has arthritis and hypertension and is taking the following medications:

Ibuprofen, 800 mg PO every 4 hours

Prednisone, 5 mg PO daily

Lasix, 20 mg PO twice a day

Captopril, 25 mg PO twice a day

Pepcid, 20 mg PO at bedtime

✔ Look up each of these medications. Note the drug class and why you think this client is taking them.

✔ Are these acceptable doses for elderly clients?

✔ What criteria will you use to determine therapeutic effects for each drug?

✔ Note any side effects that are likely for each drug and what assessment data will be important to collect.

## OVERVIEW

Drug therapy involves the use of drugs to prevent or treat disease processes and manifestations. It may save lives, improve the quality of life, and otherwise benefit recipients. It also may cause adverse effects. Adverse effects and failure to achieve therapeutic effects may occur with correct use, but they are more likely to occur with incorrect use. Physicians, pharmacists, clients, and nurses all have important roles to play in the safe and effective use of drugs.

For the nurse, drug therapy is one of many responsibilities in client care. To fulfill this responsibility, the nurse must be knowledgeable about pharmacology (drugs and their effects on the body), physiology (normal body functions), and pathophysiology (alterations in physical and mental functions due to disease processes) and must be adept at using all steps of the nursing process. The nurse should also recognize sources in the literature that synthesize known data about drug therapy and apply the nursing process using evidenced-based practice.

Chapter 1 includes general information about drugs and suggested strategies for studying pharmacology. Chapter 2 describes cellular physiology and concepts and processes essential to understanding drug effects in humans. Chapter 3 includes general information regarding the metric, apothecary, and household systems and common methods used in calculating medication problems. Chapter 4 emphasizes drug preparation and administration. Although the importance of safe and accurate administration cannot be overemphasized, this is only one aspect of the nursing process in drug therapy. The nurse also must monitor responses to drug therapy, both therapeutic and adverse, and teach clients about drugs, both prescribed and over the counter. To help the nurse continue to acquire knowledge and skills related to drug therapy, this chapter includes nursing process guidelines, general principles of drug therapy, and general nursing actions. Guidelines and actions related to specific drug groups and individual drugs are included in appropriate chapters throughout this text.

## NURSING PROCESS IN DRUG THERAPY

The nursing process is a systematic way of gathering and using information to plan and provide individualized client care and to evaluate the outcomes of care. It involves both cognitive and psychomotor skills. Knowledge and skill in the nursing process are required for drug therapy, as in other aspects of client care. The five steps of the nursing process are assessment, nursing diagnosis, planning and establishing goals for nursing care, interventions, and evaluation. One might say that assessment and interventions are the "action" phases, whereas analysis of assessment data and establishing nursing diagnoses and goals are "thinking" phases. However, knowledge and informed, rational thinking should underlie all data collection, decision making, and interventions.

### Assessment

Assessment involves collecting data about client characteristics known to affect drug therapy. This can be done by observing and interviewing the client, interviewing family members or others involved in client care, completing a physical assessment, reviewing medical records for pertinent laboratory and diagnostic test reports, and other methods. Although listed as the important first step in the nursing process, assessment is actually a component of all steps and occurs with every contact with the client. For example, the initial assessment needs to be especially thorough because the information gained may guide the care provided by oneself, other nurses, and other health care providers (eg, dietitians, pharmacists). All available sources of assessment data should be used (eg, client, family members, medical records). Later assessments of a client's condition and response to treatment are ongoing; they provide a basis for decisions about continuing or revising nursing care. Some guidelines for obtaining needed assessment data are described as follows:

On initial contact with a client, before drug therapy is started, assess age, weight, health status, pathologic conditions, and ability to function in usual activities of daily living. The effects of these client-related factors on drug therapy are discussed in Chapter 2.

Assess for previous and current use of prescription, nonprescription, and nontherapeutic (eg, alcohol, caffeine, nicotine, cocaine, marijuana) drugs. A medication history (see Box 5-1) is useful, or the information can be incorporated into any data collection tool.

Specific questions and areas of assessment include:

■ What are current drug orders?
■ What does the client know about current drugs? Is teaching needed?
■ What drugs has the client taken before? Include any drugs taken regularly, such as those taken for chronic illnesses (eg, hypertension, diabetes mellitus, arthritis). It also may be helpful to ask about nonprescription drugs for headache, colds, indigestion, or constipation because some people do not think of these preparations as drugs.
■ Has the client ever had an allergic reaction to a drug? If so, what signs and symptoms occurred? This information is necessary because many people describe minor nausea and other symptoms as allergic reactions. Unless the reaction is further explored, the client may have therapy withheld inappropriately.
■ What are the client's attitudes about drugs? Try to obtain information to help assess whether the client takes drugs freely or reluctantly, is likely to comply with a prescribed drug regimen, or is likely to abuse drugs.
■ If long-term drug therapy is likely, can the client afford to buy medications? Is transportation available for

## BOX 5-1 Medication History

Name_____ Age_____
Health problems, acute and chronic
Are you allergic to any medications?
If yes, describe specific effects or symptoms.

### Part 1: Prescription Medications

1. Do you take any prescription medications on a regular basis?
2. If yes, ask the following about each medication.

| | |
|---|---|
| Name | Dose |
| Frequency | Specific times |
| How long taken | Reason for use          Perceived effectiveness |

3. Do you have any difficulty in taking your medicines? If yes, ask to specify problem areas.
4. Have you had any symptoms or problems that you think are caused by your medicines? If yes, ask to specify.
5. Do you need help from another person to take your medicines?
6. Do you take any prescription medications on an irregular basis? If yes, ask the following about each medication.

| | |
|---|---|
| Name | Dose |
| Frequency | Reason |
| How long taken | |

### Part 2: Nonprescription Medications

Do you take over-the-counter medications?

| | | Medication | | | |
|---|---|---|---|---|---|
| Problem | Yes/No | Name | Amount | Frequency | Perceived Effectiveness |
| Pain | | | | | |
| Headache | | | | | |
| Sleep | | | | | |
| Cold | | | | | |
| Indigestion | | | | | |
| Heartburn | | | | | |
| Diarrhea | | | | | |
| Constipation | | | | | |
| Other | | | | | |

### Part 3: Social Drugs

| | Yes/No | Amount/day | Perceived Effect |
|---|---|---|---|
| Coffee | | | |
| Tea | | | |
| Cola drinks | | | |
| Alcohol | | | |
| Tobacco | | | |
| Other substances | | | |

### Part 4: Herbal or Dietary Supplements

Do you take any herbal or dietary supplements (eg, ginkgo, glucosamine/chondroitin, kava)? If so, ask for names, how much and how often taken, reason for use, perceived effectiveness, any adverse effects.

obtaining medications or seeing a health care provider for monitoring and follow-up care?
■ Can the client communicate his or her needs, such as requesting medication? Can he or she swallow oral medications?
■ Are any other conditions present that influence drug therapy? For example, all seriously ill clients should be assessed for risk factors and manifestations of impaired function of vital organs. Early recognition and treatment may prevent or decrease organ impairment.

■ Assess for previous or current use of herbal or dietary supplements (eg, echinacea, ginkgo, glucosamine, chondroitin). If used, ask for names, how much and how often taken, for how long, their reason for use, and perceived benefits or adverse effects.
■ In addition to nursing assessment data, use progress notes, laboratory reports, and other sources as available and relevant. As part of the initial assessment, obtain baseline data on measurements to be used in monitoring therapeutic or adverse effects. Specific data to be

acquired depend on the medication and the client's condition. Laboratory tests of liver, kidney, and bone marrow function are often helpful because some drugs may damage these organs. Also, if liver or kidney damage exists, drug metabolism or excretion may be altered. Some specific laboratory tests include serum potassium levels before diuretic therapy, culture and susceptibility studies before antimicrobial therapy, and blood clotting tests before anticoagulant therapy. Other data that may be relevant include physical assessment data, vital signs, weight, and urine output.

■ Seek information about ordered drugs, if needed.

Once assessment data are obtained, they need to be analyzed for their relevance to the client's current condition and nursing care needs. In general, nurses must provide care based on available information while knowing that assessment data are always relatively incomplete. As a result, continued assessment is needed. With later contacts and after drug therapy is begun, assess the client's response in relation to therapeutic and adverse effects, ability and willingness to take the drugs as prescribed, and other aspects of safe and effective drug therapy.

## Nursing Diagnoses

These statements, as developed by the North American Nursing Diagnosis Association, describe client problems or needs and are based on assessment data. They should be individualized according to the client's condition and the drugs prescribed. Thus, the nursing diagnoses needed to reflect adequately the client's condition vary considerably. Because almost any nursing diagnosis may apply in specific circumstances, this text emphasizes those diagnoses that generally apply to any course of drug therapy.

■ Deficient Knowledge: Drug therapy regimen (eg, drug ordered, reason for use, expected effects, and monitoring of response by health care providers, including diagnostic tests and office visits)
■ Deficient Knowledge: Safe and effective self-administration (when appropriate)
■ Risk for Injury related to adverse drug effects
■ Noncompliance: Overuse
■ Noncompliance: Underuse

## Planning and Goals

This step involves stating the expected outcomes of the prescribed drug therapy. As a general rule, goals should be stated in terms of client behavior, not nurse behavior. For example, the client will:

■ Receive or take drugs as prescribed
■ Experience relief of signs and symptoms
■ Avoid preventable adverse drug effects
■ Avoid unnecessary drug ingestion
■ Self-administer drugs safely and accurately
■ Verbalize essential drug information

■ Keep appointments for monitoring and follow-up
■ Use any herbal and dietary supplements with caution
■ Report the use of herbal and dietary supplements to health care providers

## Interventions

This step involves implementing planned activities and actually includes any task performed on a client's behalf. Areas of nursing intervention may include assessment, drug administration, teaching about medications, solving problems related to drug therapy, promoting compliance with the prescribed drug therapy regimen, identifying barriers to compliance, identifying resources (eg, financial assistance for obtaining medications), and others. Interventions should be based on best practice and consistent with evidence.

*General interventions* include promoting health, preventing or decreasing the need for drug therapy, and using nonpharmacologic measures to enhance therapeutic effects or to decrease adverse effects. Some examples include:

■ Promoting healthful lifestyles in terms of nutrition, fluids, exercise, rest, and sleep
■ Hand washing and other measures to prevent infection
■ Positioning
■ Assisting to cough and deep breathe
■ Ambulating
■ Applying heat or cold
■ Increasing or decreasing sensory stimulation
■ Scheduling activities to allow periods of rest or sleep
■ Recording vital signs, fluid intake, urine output, and other assessment data
■ Implementing specific interventions indicated by a particular drug or the client's condition. For example, weighing seriously ill clients helps in calculating dosages of several drugs and in assessing changes in the client's fluid balance or nutritional status; ensuring that blood samples for serum drug levels are drawn at correct times in relation to drug administration helps to increase the usefulness and accuracy of these tests in monitoring the client's condition; and, in clients at risk for developing acute renal failure (ARF), ensuring adequate fluid intake and blood pressure and avoiding or following safety precautions with nephrotoxic drugs (eg, aminoglycoside antibiotics) helps to prevent ARF.

Client teaching as a nursing intervention is presented separately to emphasize its importance. Teaching about drug therapy is essential because most medications are self-administered and clients need information and assistance to use therapeutic drugs safely and effectively. When medications are given by another caregiver, rather than self-administered, the caregiver needs to understand about the medications. Adequate knowledge and preparation are required to fulfill teaching responsibilities. Teaching aids to assist the nurse in this endeavor include Box 5-2: Preparing to Teach a Client or Caregiver; Client Teaching

BOX
5-2      Preparing to Teach a Client or Caregiver

- Assess learning needs, especially when new drugs are added or new conditions are being treated. This includes finding out what the person already knows about a particular drug. If the client has been taking a drug for awhile, verify by questions and observations that he or she already knows essential drug information and takes the drug correctly. Do not assume that teaching is unneeded.
- Assess ability to manage a drug therapy regimen (ie, read printed instructions and drug labels, remember dosage schedules, self-administer medications by ordered routes). A medication history (see Box 5–1) helps to assess the client's knowledge and attitudes about drug therapy.
- From assessment data, develop an individualized teaching plan. This saves time for both nurse and client by avoiding repetition of known material. It also promotes compliance with prescribed drug therapy.
- Clients and caregivers may feel overwhelmed by complicated medication regimens and are more likely to make errors with large numbers of medications or changes in the medication regimen. Try to decrease their anxiety and provide positive reinforcement for effort.
- Choose an appropriate time (eg, when the client is mentally alert and not in acute distress [eg, from pain, difficulty in breathing, or other symptoms]) and a place with minimal noise and distractions.
- Proceed slowly, in small steps; emphasize essential information; and provide ample opportunities to express concerns or ask questions.
- Usually, a combination of verbal and written instructions is more effective than either alone. Minimize medical jargon and be aware that clients may have difficulty understanding and retaining the material being taught because of the stress of the illness.
- When explaining a drug therapy regimen to a hospitalized client, describe the name, purpose, expected effects, and so on. In many instances, the drug is familiar and can be described from personal knowledge. If the drug is unfamiliar, use available resources (eg, drug reference books, pharmacists) to learn about the drug and provide accurate information to the client.

   The client should know the name, preferably both the generic and a trade name, of any drugs being taken. Such knowledge is a safety measure, especially if an allergic or other potentially serious adverse reaction or overdose occurs. It also decreases the risk of mistaking one drug for another and promotes a greater sense of control and responsibility regarding drug therapy. The client should also know the purpose of prescribed drugs. Although people vary in the amount of drug information they want and need, the purpose can usually be simply stated in terms of symptoms to be relieved or other expected benefits.

- When teaching a client about medications to be taken at home, provide specific instructions about taking the medications. Also teach the client and caregiver to observe for beneficial and adverse effects. If side effects occur, teach them how to manage minor ones and which ones to report to a health care provider. In addition, discuss specific ways to take medications so that usual activities of daily living are minimally disrupted. Planning with a client to develop a convenient routine, within the limitations imposed by individual drugs, may help increase compliance with the prescribed regimen. Allow time for questions and try to ensure that the client understands how, when, and why to take the medications.
- When teaching a client about potential adverse drug effects, the goal is to provide needed information without causing unnecessary anxiety. Most drugs produce undesirable effects; some are minor, some are potentially serious. Many people stop taking a drug rather than report adverse reactions. If reactions are reported, it may be possible to continue drug therapy by reducing dosage, changing the time of administration, or other measures. The occurrence of severe reactions indicates that the drug should be stopped and the prescribing health care provider should be notified.
- Throughout the teaching session and perhaps at other contacts, emphasize the importance of taking medications as prescribed. Common client errors include taking incorrect doses, taking doses at the wrong times, forgetting to take doses, and stopping a medication too soon. Treatment failure can often be directly traced to these errors. For example, missed doses of glaucoma medication can lead to optic nerve damage and blindness.
- Reassess learning needs when medication orders are changed (eg, when medications are added because of a new illness or stopped).

Guidelines: Safe and Effective Use of Prescription Medications; and Client Teaching Guidelines: Safe and Effective Use of Over-the-Counter (OTC) Medications. Later, drug-related chapters contain client teaching guidelines for the drugs discussed in particular chapters.

Other nursing interventions presented in a separate section of most chapters are the actions needed once a drug is ordered (ie, accurate administration, assessing for therapeutic and adverse effects, observing for drug interactions). These are presented under the heading of "Nursing Actions," and rationales for the interventions are included.

In addition, nursing interventions are integrated into the text with background information and client characteristics to assist in individualizing care. General principles or guidelines are included in this chapter; those related to particular drug groups are included in later chapters.

## Evaluation

This step involves evaluating the client's status in relation to stated goals and expected outcomes. Some outcomes can be evaluated within a few minutes of drug

(text continues on page 60)

CLIENT TEACHING GUIDELINES
## Safe and Effective Use of Prescription Medications

### General Considerations

✔ Use drugs cautiously and only when necessary because all drugs affect body functions and may cause adverse effects.

✔ Use non-pharmacological measures, when possible, to prevent the need for drug therapy or to enhance beneficial effects and decrease adverse effects of drugs.

✔ Do not take drugs left over from a previous illness or prescribed for someone else and do not share prescription drugs with anyone else. The likelihood of having the right drug in the right dose is remote and the risk of adverse effects is high in such circumstances.

✔ Keep all health care providers informed about all the drugs being taken, including over-the-counter (OTC) products and herbal or dietary supplements. One way to do this is to keep a written record of all current medicines, including their names and doses and how they are taken. It is a good idea to carry a copy of this list at all times. This information can help avoid new prescriptions or OTC drugs that have similar effects or cancel each other's effects.

✔ Take drugs as prescribed and for the length of time prescribed; notify a health care provider if unable to obtain or take a medication. Therapeutic effects greatly depend on taking medications correctly. Altering the dose or time may cause underdosage or overdosage. Stopping a medication may cause a recurrence of the problem for which it was given or withdrawal symptoms. Some medications need to be tapered in dosage and gradually discontinued. If problems occur with taking the drug, report them to the prescribing physician rather than stopping the drug. Often, an adjustment in dosage or other aspect of administration may solve the problem.

✔ Follow instructions for follow-up care (eg, office visits, laboratory or other diagnostic tests that monitor therapeutic or adverse effects of drugs). Some drugs require more frequent monitoring than others. However, safety requires periodic checks with essentially all medications. With long-term use of a medication, responses may change over time with aging, changes in kidney function, and so on.

✔ Take drugs in current use when seeing a health care provider for any health-related problem. It may be helpful to remind the health care provider periodically of the medications being taken and ask if any can be discontinued or reduced in dosage.

✔ Get all prescriptions filled at the same pharmacy, when possible. This is an important safety factor in helping to avoid several prescriptions of the same or similar drugs and to minimize undesirable interactions of newly prescribed drugs with those already in use.

✔ Report any drug allergies to all health care providers and wear a medical identification emblem that lists allergens.

✔ Ask questions (and write down the answers) about newly prescribed medications, such as:
What is the medicine's name?
What is it supposed to do (ie, what symptoms or problems will it relieve)?
How and when do I take it, and for how long?
Should it be taken with food or on an empty stomach?
While taking this medicine, should I avoid certain foods, beverages, other medications, certain activities? (For example, alcoholic beverages and driving a car should be avoided with medications that cause drowsiness or decrease alertness.)
Will this medication work safely with the others I'm already taking?
What side effects are likely and what do I do if they occur?
Will the medication affect my ability to sleep or work?
What should I do if I miss a dose?
Is there a drug information sheet I can have?

✔ Store medications out of reach of children and never refer to medications as "candy", to prevent accidental ingestion.

✔ Develop a plan for renewing or refilling prescriptions so that the medication supply does not run out when the prescribing health care provider is unavailable or the pharmacy is closed.

✔ When taking prescription medications, talk to a doctor, pharmacist, or nurse before starting an OTC medication or herbal or dietary supplement. This is a safety factor to avoid undesirable drug interactions.

✔ Inform health care providers if you have diabetes or kidney or liver disease. These conditions require special precautions with drug therapy.

✔ If pregnant, consult your obstetrician before taking any medications prescribed by another health care provider.

✔ If breast-feeding, consult your obstetrician or pediatrician before taking any medications prescribed by another health care provider.

### Self-administration

✔ Develop a routine for taking medications (eg, at the same time and place each day). A schedule that minimally disrupts usual household activities is more convenient and more likely to be followed accurately.

✔ Take medications in a well-lighted area and read labels of containers to ensure taking the intended drug. Do not take medications if you are not alert or cannot see clearly.

✔ Most tablets and capsules should be taken whole. If unable to take them whole, ask a health care provider before splitting, chewing, or crushing tablets or taking the medication out of capsules. Some long-acting preparations are dangerous if altered so that the entire dose is absorbed at the same time.

*(continued)*

CLIENT TEACHING GUIDELINES
## Safe and Effective Use of Prescription Medications (Continued)

✔ As a general rule, take oral medications with 6–8 oz of water, in a sitting or standing position. The water helps tablets and capsules dissolve in the stomach, "dilutes" the drug so that it is less likely to upset the stomach, and promotes absorption of the drug into the bloodstream. The upright position helps the drug reach the stomach rather than getting stuck in the throat or esophagus.

✔ Take most oral drugs at evenly spaced intervals around the clock. For example, if ordered once daily, take about the same time every day. If ordered twice daily or morning and evening, take about 12 hours apart.

✔ Follow instructions about taking a medication with food or on an empty stomach, about taking with other medications, or taking with fluids other than water. Prescription medications often include instructions to take on an empty stomach or with food. If taking several medications, ask a health care provider whether they may be taken together or at different times. For example, an antacid usually should not be taken at the same time as other oral medications because the antacid decreases absorption of many other drugs.

✔ If a dose is missed, most authorities recommend taking the dose if remembered soon after the scheduled time and omitting the dose if it is not remembered for several hours. If a dose is omitted, the next dose should be taken at the next scheduled time. Do not double the dose.

✔ If taking a liquid medication (or giving one to a child), measure with a calibrated medication cup or measuring spoon. A dose cannot be measured accurately with household teaspoons or tablespoons because they are different sizes and deliver varying amounts of medication. If the liquid medication is packaged with a measuring cup that shows teaspoons or tablespoons, that should be used to measure doses, for adults or children. This is especially important for young children because most of their medications are given in liquid form.

✔ Use other types of medications according to instructions. If not clear how a medication is to be used, be sure to ask a health care provider. Correct use of oral or nasal inhalers, eye drops, and skin medications is essential for therapeutic effects.

✔ Report problems or new symptoms to a health care provider.

✔ Store medications safely, in a cool, dry place. Do not store them in a bathroom; heat, light, and moisture may cause them to decompose. Do not store them near a dangerous substance, which could be taken by mistake. Keep medications in the container in which they were dispensed by the pharmacy, where the label identifies it and gives directions. Do not put several different tablets or capsules in one container. Although this may be more convenient, especially when away from home for work or travel, it is never a safe practice because it increases the likelihood of taking the wrong drug.

✔ Discard outdated medications; do not keep drugs for long periods. Drugs are chemicals that may deteriorate over time, especially if exposed to heat and moisture. In addition, having many containers increases the risks of medication errors and adverse drug interactions.

CLIENT TEACHING GUIDELINES
## Safe and Effective Use of Over-the-Counter (OTC) Medications

✔ Read product labels carefully. The labels contain essential information about the name, ingredients, indications for use, usual dosage, when to stop using the medication or when to see a health care provider, possible side effects, and expiration dates.

✔ Use a magnifying glass, if necessary, to read the fine print.

✔ If you do not understand the information on labels, ask a physician, pharmacist, or nurse.

✔ Do not take OTC medications longer or in higher doses than recommended.

✔ Note that all OTC medications are not safe for everyone. Many OTC medications warn against use with certain illnesses (eg, hypertension, thyroid disorders). Consult a health care provider before taking the product if you have one of the contraindicated conditions.

✔ If taking any prescription medications, consult a health care provider before taking any nonprescription drugs to avoid undesirable drug interactions and adverse effects. Some specific precautions include the following:

Avoid alcohol if taking antihistamines, cough or cold remedies containing dextromethorphan, or sleeping pills. Because all these drugs cause drowsiness, combining any of them with alcohol may result in excessive, potentially dangerous, sedation.

Avoid OTC sleeping aids if you are taking a prescription sedative-type drug (eg, for nervousness or depression).

Ask a health care provider before taking products containing aspirin if you are taking an anticoagulant (eg, Coumadin).

Ask a health care provider before taking other products containing aspirin if you are already taking a regular dose of aspirin to prevent blood clots, heart attack, or stroke. Aspirin is commonly used for this purpose, often in doses of 81 mg or 325 mg.

*(continued)*

Do not take a laxative if you have stomach pain, nausea, or vomiting, to avoid worsening the problem.

Do not take a nasal decongestant (eg, Sudafed), a multisymptom cold remedy containing pseudo-ephedrine (eg, Actifed, Sinutab), an antihistamine-decongestant combination (eg, Claritin D), or the herbal medicine ephedra (Ma Huang) if you are taking a prescription medication for high blood pressure. Such products can raise blood pressure and decrease or cancel the blood pressure–lowering effect of the prescription drug. This could lead to severe hypertension and stroke.

✔ Store OTC drugs in a cool, dry place, in their original containers; check expiration dates periodically and discard those that have expired.

✔ If pregnant, consult your obstetrician before taking any OTC medications.

✔ If breast-feeding, consult your pediatrician or family doctor before taking any OTC medications.

✔ For children, follow any age limits on the label.

✔ Measure liquid OTC medications with the measuring device that is supplied with the product (some have a dropper or plastic cup calibrated in milliliters, teaspoons, or tablespoons). If such a device is not available, use a measuring spoon. It is not safe to use household teaspoons or tablespoons because they are different sizes and deliver varying amounts of medication. Accurate measurement of doses is especially important for young children because most of their medications are given in liquid form.

✔ Do not assume continued safety of an OTC medication you have taken for years. Older people are more likely to have adverse drug reactions and interactions because of changes in heart, kidneys, and other organs that occur with aging and various disease processes.

✔ Note tamper-resistant features and do not buy products with damaged packages.

---

administration (eg, relief of acute pain after administration of an analgesic). Most, however, require much longer periods of time, often extending from hospitalization and direct observation by the nurse to self-care at home and occasional contact with a health care provider.

With the current emphasis on outpatient treatment and short hospitalizations, the client is likely to experience brief contacts with many health care providers rather than extensive contacts with a few health care providers. These factors, plus a client's usual reluctance to admit noncompliance, contribute to difficulties in evaluating outcomes of drug therapy. These difficulties can be managed by using appropriate techniques and criteria of evaluation.

■ Techniques include directly observing the client's status; interviewing the client or others about the client's response to drug therapy; and checking appropriate medical records, including medication records and laboratory and other diagnostic test reports. With outpatients, "pill counts" may be done to compare doses remaining with the number prescribed during a designated time. These techniques may be used at every contact with a client, if appropriate.

■ General criteria include progress toward stated outcomes, such as relief of symptoms, accurate administration, avoidance of preventable adverse effects, compliance with instructions, and others. Specific criteria indicate the parameters that must be measured to evaluate responses to particular drugs (eg, blood sugar with antidiabetic drugs, blood pressure with antihypertensive drugs).

## INTEGRATING NURSING PROCESS, CLINICAL PRACTICE GUIDELINES, AND DRUG THERAPY

In many agencies, nursing responsibilities related to drug therapy are designated in clinical practice guidelines (CPGs) that support informed clinical decisions for the care of clients with particular conditions. These CPGs may assume a variety of forms, including *care standards*, *clinical pathways*, *care maps*, *protocols*, and *algorithms*. Research evidence is interpreted and blended with other sources of knowledge, including theoretical guidelines and clinical expertise to direct informed clinical decisions.

Depending on the clinical condition, many CPGs have specific guidelines related to drug therapy. These guidelines may affect any step of the nursing process. With assessment, for example, the critical path may state, "Assess for bleeding if on anticoagulant."

## HERBAL AND DIETARY SUPPLEMENTS

In recent years, an additional nursing concern has emerged in the form of herbal and dietary supplements. These supplements are increasingly being used, and clients who take them are likely to be encountered in any clinical practice setting. Herbal medicines, also called *botanicals*, *phytochemicals*, and *nutriceuticals*, are derived from plants; other dietary supplements may be derived from a variety of sources. The 1994 Dietary Supplement Health and Education Act (DSHEA) defined a dietary supplement as "a vitamin, a mineral, an herb or other botanical used to supplement the diet." Under this law, herbs can be labeled according to their possible effects on the human body, but the products cannot claim to diagnose, prevent, relieve, or cure specific human diseases unless approved by the U.S. Food and Drug Administration (FDA). Most products have not been studied sufficiently to evaluate their safety or effectiveness; most available information involves self-reports of a few people. Overall, the effects of these products in particular consumers, in combination with other herbal and dietary supplements, and in combination with pharmaceutical drugs, are essentially unknown.

What is the nursing role in relation to these products and safe and effective drug therapy? Two major concerns are that use of supplements may keep the client from seeking treatment from a health care provider when indicated and that the products may interact with prescription drugs to decrease therapeutic effects or increase adverse effects. In general, nurses need to have an ade-quate knowledge base and to incorporate their knowledge in all steps of the nursing process (see later). Nurses should seek information from authoritative, objective sources rather than product labels, advertisements, or personal testimonials from family members, friends, or celebrities. With the continued caution that limited reliable information is available about these products, several resources are provided in this text, including the following:

■ Table 5-1 describes some commonly used herbal and dietary supplements. In later chapters, when information is available and deemed clinically relevant, selected herbal and dietary supplements with some scientific support for their use are described in more detail. For example, in Chapter 7, some products reported to be useful in relieving pain, fever, inflammation, or migraine are described.

■ *Client teaching guidelines.* In this chapter, general information is provided (see Client Teaching Guidelines: General Information About Herbal and Dietary Supplements). In later chapters, guidelines may emphasize

(text continues on page 66)

## TABLE 5-1    Herbal and Dietary Supplements

| Name | Characteristics | Uses | Remarks |
|---|---|---|---|
| Black cohosh | • Thought to relieve menopausal symptoms by suppressing the release of luteinizing hormone (LH) from the pituitary gland and dysmenorrhea by relaxing uterine muscle<br>• Well tolerated; may cause occasional stomach upset. In overdose may cause nausea, vomiting, dizziness, visual disturbances, and reduced pulse rate<br>• Most clinical trials done with Remefemin, in small numbers of women; other trade names include Estroven and Femtrol | • Most often used to relieve symptoms of menopause (eg, flushes, vaginal dryness, irritability)<br>• May also relieve premenstrual syndrome (PMS) and dysmenorrhea | • No apparent advantage over traditional estrogen replacement therapy (ERT)<br>• May be useful when ERT is contraindicated for a client or the client refuses ERT<br>• Recommended dose is 1 tab standardized to contain 20 mg of herbal drug, twice daily<br>• Not recommended for use for longer than 6 months because long-term effects are unknown<br>• Apparently has no effect on endometrium, so progesterone not needed in women with an intact uterus |
| Capsaicin (see Chap. 6) | • Derived from cayenne pepper<br>• Pain with first application<br>• Adverse effects include skin irritation, itching, redness, and stinging | • Capsaicin is a topical analgesic that may inhibit the synthesis, transport, and release of substance P, a peripheral neurotransmitter of pain.<br>• Used to treat pain associated with neuralgia, neuropathy, and osteoarthritis.<br>• Self-defense as the active ingredient in "pepper spray" | Applied topically |

*(continued)*

**TABLE 5-1** **Herbal and Dietary Supplements** (Continued)

| Name | Characteristics | Uses | Remarks |
|------|----------------|------|---------|
| Chamomile | • Usually ingested as a tea<br>• May cause contact dermatitis<br>• May cause severe hypersensitivity reactions, including anaphylaxis, in people allergic to ragweed, asters, and chrysanthemums<br>• May delay absorption of oral medications<br>• May increase risks of bleeding (contains coumarins, the substances from which warfarin, an oral anticoagulant, is derived) | Used mainly for antispasmodic effects in the gastrointestinal (GI) tract; may relieve abdominal cramping | Few studies and little data to support use and effectiveness in GI disorders |
| Chondroitin (see Chap. 7) | • Derived from the trachea cartilage of cattle slaughtered for food<br>• Usually taken with glucosamine<br>• Adverse effects minor, may include GI upset, nausea, and headache | Arthritis | Several studies support use |
| Creatine | • An amino acid produced in liver and kidneys and stored in muscles<br>• Causes weight gain, usually within 2 weeks of starting use<br>• Legal and available in health food stores as a powder to be mixed with water or juice, a liquid, as tablets and capsules | Athletes take creatine supplements to gain extra energy, to train longer and harder, and improve performance | • Not recommended for use by children because studies have not been done and effects in children are unknown<br>• Nurses and parents need to actively discourage children and adolescents from using creatine supplements |
| Echinacea | • Many species but *E. purpurea* most often used medicinally<br>• Effects on immune system include stimulation of phagocytes and monocytes<br>• Contraindicated in persons with immune system disorders because stimulation of the immune system may aggravate autoimmune disorders<br>• Hepatotoxic with long-term use | Most often used for the common cold, but also advertised for many other uses (immune system stimulant, anti-infective) | • Hard to interpret validity of medicinal claims because various combinations of species and preparations used in reported studies<br>• A few studies support use in common cold, with reports of shorter durations and possibly decreased severity of symptoms |
| Ephedra (Ma Huang) | • Acts the same as the adrenergic drugs ephedrine and pseudoephedrine, which are cardiac and central nervous system (CNS) stimulants as well as decongestants and bronchodilators (see Chap. 18)<br>• Commonly found in herbal weight-loss products | Anorexiant for weight loss, decongestant, bronchodilator, stimulant | • The Food and Drug Administration (FDA) has issued warnings against use of ephedra because of potentially severe adverse effects, including death and has taken it off the market.<br>• Ephedra is considered especially hazardous for people with conditions that might |

*(continued)*

## TABLE 5-1    Herbal and Dietary Supplements (Continued)

| Name | Characteristics | Uses | Remarks |
|------|-----------------|------|---------|
| | • May cause or aggravate hypertension, cardiac dysrhythmias, nervousness, nausea, vomiting, tremor, headache, seizures, strokes, myocardial infarctions<br>• May increase effects of other cardiac and CNS stimulants and cause potentially life-threatening illnesses<br>• May decrease effects of antihypertensive medications | | be aggravated (eg, hypertension, seizures, cardiac palpitations) or who take medications associated with significant drug interactions (eg, decreased therapeutic effects or increased adverse effects). |
| Feverfew (see Chap. 7) | • May increase clotting time and risk of bleeding<br>• May cause hypersensitivity reactions in people allergic to ragweed, asters, chrysanthemums, or daisies<br>• May cause withdrawal syndrome if use is stopped abruptly | Migraines, menstrual irregularities, arthritis | Some studies support use in migraine |
| Garlic | • Active ingredient is thought to be allicin<br>• Has antiplatelet activity and may increase risk of bleeding; should not be used with anticoagulants<br>• May decrease blood sugar and cholesterol<br>• Adverse effects include allergic reactions (asthma, dermatitis), dizziness, irritation of GI tract, nausea, vomiting | • Used mainly to lower serum cholesterol levels, although a recent study did not support its effectiveness for this purpose<br>• Also used for antihypertensive and antibiotic effects, but there is little reliable evidence for such use | Medicinal effects probably exaggerated, especially those of deodorized supplements |
| Ginger | • Inhibits platelet aggregation; may increase clotting time<br>• Gastroprotective effects in animal studies | Used mainly to treat nausea, including motion sickness and postoperative nausea | Should not be used for morning sickness associated with pregnancy—may increase risk of miscarriage |
| Ginkgo biloba | • Reportedly increases blood flow to the brain; improves memory and decreases dizziness and ringing in the ears (tinnitus)<br>• Improves blood flow to legs and decreases intermittent claudication associated with peripheral arterial insufficiency<br>• Antioxidant<br>• Inhibits platelet aggregation<br>• Adverse effects include GI upset, headache, bleeding, allergic skin reaction<br>• May increase risks of bleeding with any drug that has antiplatelet effects (eg, aspirin and other nonsteroidal anti-inflammatory drugs [NSAIDs], warfarin, heparin, clopidogrel) | Used mainly to improve memory and cognitive function in people with Alzheimer's disease; may be useful in treating peripheral arterial disease | • Some studies indicate slight improvement in Alzheimer's disease. Whether this shows clinically significant benefits is still unclear. A disadvantage is a delayed response, up to 6 or 8 weeks, and a recommendation to use no longer than 3 months.<br>• In European studies, patients with intermittent claudication showed significant improvement. |

*(continued)*

**TABLE 5-1 Herbal and Dietary Supplements** (Continued)

| Name | Characteristics | Uses | Remarks |
|---|---|---|---|
| Ginseng | • Active ingredients called ginsenosides or panaxosides<br>• Has a variety of pharmacologic effects that vary with dose and duration of use (eg, inhibits platelet aggregation; may depress or stimulate central nervous system [CNS], thus possible mood elevating, antistress, antidepression, and sedative effects; decreases blood glucose and cholesterol)<br>• Adverse effects include hypertension, diarrhea, nervousness, depression, headache, amenorrhea, insomnia, skin rashes, chest pain, epistaxis, headache, impotence, nausea, palpitations, pruritus, vaginal bleeding, and vomiting<br>• May increase risks of bleeding with any drug that has antiplatelet effects (eg, aspirin and other NSAIDs, warfarin, heparin, clopidogrel)<br>• Increases risk of hypoglycemic reactions if taken concurrently with insulin or oral antidiabetic agents<br>• Should not be taken concurrently with other herbs or drugs that inhibit monoamine oxidase (eg, St. John's wort, phenelzine, selegiline, tranylcypromine); headache, mania, and tremors may occur | Used to increase stamina, strength, endurance, and mental acuity. Also to promote sleep and relieve depression | • A few small studies in humans support benefits of ginseng in improving psychomotor and cognitive functioning and sleep. However, additional well-controlled studies are needed before the herb can be recommended for these uses.<br>• A ginseng abuse syndrome, with symptoms of insomnia, hypotonia, and edema, has been reported. Caution clients to avoid ingesting excessive amounts.<br>• Diabetics should use ginseng very cautiously, if at all, because of its hypoglycemic effect alone and apparent ability to increase the hypoglycemic effects of insulin and oral antidiabetic drugs. If a client insists on using, urge him or her to check blood glucose frequently until ginseng's effects on blood sugar are known.<br>• Instruct clients with cardiovascular disease, diabetes mellitus, or hypertension to check with their primary health care provider before taking ginseng.<br>• Instruct any client taking ginseng to avoid long-term use. Siberian ginseng should not be used longer than 3 weeks. |
| Glucosamine (see Chap. 7) | • Usually used with chondroitin<br>• Has beneficial effects on cartilage<br>• Adverse effects mild, may include GI upset, drowsiness | Arthritis | Several studies support use |
| Kava kava (see Chap. 8) | • Produces mild euphoria and sedation; may have antiseizure effects<br>• May act similarly to benzodiazepines, by enhancing effects of GABA (an inhibitory neurotransmitter in the CNS)<br>• Adverse effects include impaired coordination, gait, and judgment; pupil dilation | Most studied and used to treat anxiety, stress, emotional excitability and restlessness; additional claims include treatment of depression, insomnia, asthma, pain, rheumatism, muscle spasms, and promotion of wound healing | • Use as a calming agent is supported by limited evidence from a few small clinical trials; other therapeutic claims are poorly documented<br>• Should be used cautiously by people with renal disease, thrombocytopenia, or neutropenia |

*(continued)*

## TABLE 5-1  Herbal and Dietary Supplements (Continued)

| Name | Characteristics | Uses | Remarks |
|---|---|---|---|
| | • Chronic heavy use may cause hematologic abnormalities (eg, decreased platelets, lymphocytes, plasma proteins, bilirubin and urea), weight loss, and hepatotoxicity<br>• May increase effects of alcohol and other CNS depressants (any herb or drug that causes drowsiness and sedation); such combinations should be avoided | | • Should be avoided by people with hepatic disease, during pregnancy and lactation, and in children under 12 years old |
| Melatonin (Chap. 8) | • Several studies of effects on sleep, energy level, fatigue, mental alertness, and mood indicate some improvement, compared with placebo<br>• Contraindicated in persons with hepatic insufficiency (especially cirrhosis, because of slowed melatonin clearance), a history of cerebrovascular disease, depression, or neurologic disorders<br>• Adverse effects include altered sleep patterns, confusion, headache, itching, sedation, tachycardia | Used mainly for treatment of insomnia and prevention and treatment of jet lag | Patients with renal impairment should use cautiously |
| St. John's wort (Chap. 10) | • Active component thought to be hypericin, but at least 10 potentially active components have been identified<br>• Thought to act similarly to fluoxetine (Prozac), which increases serotonin in the brain<br>• Studies (most lasting 6 months or less) indicate improvement in mild to moderate depression<br>• Apparently not effective in major or serious depression<br>• Adverse effects include photosensitivity (especially in fair-skinned persons), dizziness, GI upset, fatigue, and confusion<br>• May interact with numerous drugs to increase their effects, probably by inhibiting their metabolism. These include antidepressants, adrenergics and others | Used mainly for treatment of depression | • Should not be combined with monoamine oxidase inhibitor (MAOI) or selective serotonin reuptake inhibitor (SSRI) antidepressants; unsafe when combined with ephedra<br>• Can decrease effectiveness of birth control pills, antineoplastic drugs, antivirals used to treat acquired immunodeficiency syndrome (AIDS), and organ transplant drugs (immunosuppressants) |

(continued)

**TABLE 5-1  Herbal and Dietary Supplements** (Continued)

| Name | Characteristics | Uses | Remarks |
|------|-----------------|------|---------|
| Saw palmetto | • Action unknown; may have antiandrogenic effects<br>• Generally well tolerated; adverse effects usually minor but may include GI upset, headache. Diarrhea may occur with high doses | Used mainly to relieve urinary symptoms in men with benign prostatic hyperplasia (BPH) | • Reportedly effective in doses of 320 mg/d for 1–3 months<br>• Men should have a prostate specific antigen (PSA) test (a blood test for prostate cancer) before starting saw palmetto, because the herb can reduce levels of PSA and produce a false-negative result. |
| Valerian (Chap. 8) | • Sedative effects may be due to increasing GABA in the brain<br>• Adverse effects with acute overdose or chronic use include blurred vision, drowsiness, dizziness, excitability, headache, hypersensitivity reactions, insomnia, nausea. Also, risk of liver damage from combination products containing valerian and from overdoses averaging 2.5 g<br>• May cause additive sedation if combined with other CNS depressants; these combinations should be avoided | Used mainly to promote sleep and allay anxiety and nervousness. Also has muscle relaxant effects | • Should not be combined with sedative drugs and should not be used regularly<br>• Many extract products contain 40%–60% alcohol and may not be appropriate for all patients<br>• Most studies flawed—experts do not believe there is sufficient evidence to support the use of valerian for treatment of insomnia |

avoidance or caution in using supplements thought to interact adversely with prescribed drugs or particular client conditions.

■ *Assessment guidelines.* In this chapter, general information about the use or nonuse of supplements is assessed. In later chapters, the nurse can ask about the use of specific supplements that may interact with the drug groups discussed in that chapter. For example, some supplements are known to increase blood pressure (see Chap. 42) or risk for excessive bleeding (see Chap. 44).

One of the best sources of information is the National Center for Complementary and Alternative Medicine (NCCAM) at the National Institutes of Health. Contact:

NCCAM Clearinghouse
PO Box 8218
Silver Spring, MD 20907-8218
Tel: 1-888-644-6226
Web site: www.nccam.nih.gov

Nurses should provide information about herbal supplements and assess use. Ask clients whether they use herbal medicines or other dietary supplements. If so, try to determine the name, dose, and frequency and duration of use. Teach clients about these products and their possible interactions with each other and with their prescription drugs (when such information is available).

## GENERAL PRINCIPLES OF DRUG THERAPY

General guiding principles of drug therapy include universal aims and strategies, found in At the Foundation: General Goals and Guidelines of Drug Therapy. In addition, drug selection and dosage considerations must be considered individually for each client. Developmental, clinical, and environmental considerations also play important roles in safe drug delivery.

### General Drug Selection and Dosage Considerations

Numerous factors must be considered when choosing a drug and dosage range for a particular client, including the following:

1. For the most part, use as few drugs in as few doses as possible. Minimizing the number of drugs and the frequency of administration increases client compliance with the prescribed drug regimen and decreases risks for serious adverse effects, including hazardous drug–drug interactions. There are notable exceptions to this basic rule. For example, multiple drugs are

## CLIENT TEACHING GUIDELINES
### General Information About Herbal and Dietary Supplements

✔ Herbal and dietary products are chemicals that have drug-like effects in people. Unfortunately, their effects are largely unknown and may be dangerous for some people because there is little reliable information about them. For most products, little research has been done to determine either their benefits or their adverse effects.

✔ The safety and effectiveness of these products are not documented or regulated by laws designed to protect consumers, as are pharmaceutical drugs. As a result, the types and amounts of ingredients may not be standardized or even identified on the product label. In fact, most products contain several active ingredients and it is often not known which ingredient has the desired pharmacologic effect. In addition, components and active ingredients of plants can vary considerably, depending on the soil, water, and climate where the plants are grown.

✔ These products can be used more safely if they are manufactured by a reputable company that states the ingredients are standardized (meaning that the dose of medicine in each tablet or capsule is the same).

✔ The product label should also state specific percentages, amounts, and strengths of active ingredients. With herbal medicines especially, different brands of the same herb vary in the amounts of active ingredients per recommended dose. Dosing is also difficult because a particular herb may be available in several different dosage forms (eg, tablet, capsule, tea, extract) with different amounts of active ingredients.

✔ These products are often advertised as "natural." Many people interpret this to mean the products are safe and better than synthetic or man-made products. This is not true; "natural" does not mean safe, especially when taken concurrently with other herbals, dietary supplements, or drugs.

✔ When taking herbal or dietary supplements, follow the instructions on the product label. Inappropriate use or taking excessive amounts may cause dangerous side effects.

✔ Inform health care providers when taking any kind of herbal or dietary supplement, to reduce risks of severe adverse effects or drug–supplement interactions.

✔ Most herbal and dietary supplements should be avoided during pregnancy or lactation and in young children.

✔ The American Society of Anesthesiologists recommends that all herbal products be discontinued 2–3 weeks before any surgical procedure. Some products (eg, echinacea, ephedra, feverfew, garlic, ginkgo, ginseng, kava kava, valerian, and St. John's wort) can interfere with or increase the effects of some drugs, affect blood pressure or heart rhythm, or increase risks of bleeding; some have unknown effects when combined with anesthetics, other perioperative medications, and surgical procedures.

✔ Store herbal and dietary supplements out of the reach of children.

---

commonly used to treat severe hypertension or serious infections.

2. Although individual drugs allow greater flexibility of dosage than fixed-dose combinations, fixed-dose combinations are increasingly available and commonly used, mainly because clients are more likely to take them. Also, many of the combination products are formulated to be long acting, which also promotes compliance.

3. The least amount of the least potent drug that yields therapeutic benefit should be given to decrease adverse reactions. For example, if a mild non-narcotic and a strong narcotic analgesic are both ordered, give the non-narcotic drug if it is effective in relieving pain.

4. In drug literature, recommended dosages are listed in amounts likely to be effective for most people. However, they are only guidelines to be interpreted according to the client's condition. For example, clients with serious illnesses may require larger doses of some drugs than clients with milder illnesses; clients with severe kidney disease often need much smaller doses of renally excreted drugs.

---

## AT THE FOUNDATION: *General Goals and Guidelines of Drug Therapy*

1. *The goal of drug therapy should be to maximize beneficial effects and minimize adverse effects.*

2. *Expected benefits should outweigh potential adverse effects.* Thus, drugs usually should not be prescribed for trivial problems or problems for which nonpharmacologic measures are effective.

3. *Drug therapy should be individualized.* Many variables influence a drug's effects on the human body. Failure to consider these variables may decrease therapeutic effects or increase risks for adverse effects to an unacceptable level.

4. *Drug effects on quality of life should be considered in designing a drug therapy regimen.* Quality-of-life issues are also being emphasized in research studies, with expectations of measurable improvement as a result of drug therapy.

5. A drug can be started rapidly or slowly. If it has a long half-life and optimal therapeutic effects do not usually occur for several days or weeks, the health care provider may order a limited number of relatively large (loading) doses followed by a regular schedule of smaller (maintenance) doses. When drug actions are not urgent, therapy may be initiated with a maintenance dose.

6. In general, different salts of the same drug rarely differ pharmacologically. Hydrochloride, sulfate, and sodium salts are often used. Pharmacists and chemists choose salts on the basis of cost, convenience, solubility, and stability. For example, solubility is especially important with parenteral drugs; taste is a factor with oral drugs. Dermatologic drugs are often formulated in different salts and dosage forms, however, according to their intended uses (eg, application to intact skin or the mucous membranes of the eye, nose, mouth, vagina, or rectum).

# Developmental Considerations in Drug Therapy

In any population, general nursing process guidelines and principles of drug therapy apply. In addition, drug therapy in children requires special consideration because adverse effects are likely due to the child's changing size, developmental level, and organ function. Particular consideration is also given to older adults who frequently require adjustment in drug therapy because of changes associated with aging or disease. In older adults, organ function, particularly hepatic and renal function, is a key consideration.

## Drug Therapy in Children

Drug therapy in neonates (birth to 1 month), infants (1 month to 1 year), and children (approximately 1 to 12 years) demonstrates physiologic differences that alter drug pharmacokinetics (Table 5-2), and drug therapy is less predictable than in adults. Neonates are especially

---

**TABLE 5-2   Neonates, Infants, and Children: Physiologic Characteristics and Pharmacokinetic Consequences**

| Physiologic Characteristics | Pharmacokinetic Consequences |
|---|---|
| Increased thinness and permeability of skin in neonates and infants | Increased absorption of topical drugs (eg, corticosteroids may be absorbed sufficiently to suppress adrenocortical function) |
| Immature blood–brain barrier in neonates and infants | Increased distribution of drugs into the central nervous system because myelinization (which creates the blood–brain barrier to the passage of drugs) is not mature until approximately 2 years of age |
| Increased percentage of body water (70% to 80% in neonates and infants, compared with 50% to 60% in children older than 2 years of age and adults) | Usually increased volume of distribution in infants and young children, compared with adults. This would seem to indicate a need for larger doses. However, prolonged drug half-life and decreased rate of drug clearance may offset. The net effect is often a need for decreased dosage. |
| Altered protein binding until approximately 1 year of age, when it reaches adult levels | The amount and binding capacity of plasma proteins may be reduced. This may result in a greater proportion of unbound or pharmacologically active drug and greater risks of adverse drug effects. Dosage requirements may be decreased or modified by other factors. Drugs with decreased protein binding in neonates, compared with older children and adults, include ampicillin (Omnipen, others), diazepam (Valium), digoxin (Lanoxin), lidocaine (Xylocaine), nafcillin (Unipen), phenobarbital, phenytoin (Dilantin), salicylates (eg, aspirin), and theophylline (Theolair). |
| Decreased glomerular filtration rate in neonates and infants, compared with older children and adults. Kidney function develops progressively during the first few months of life and is fairly mature by 1 year of age. | In neonates and infants, slowed excretion of drugs eliminated by the kidneys. Dosage of these drugs may need to be decreased, depending on the infant's age and level of growth and development. |
| Decreased activity of liver drug-metabolizing enzyme systems in neonates and infants | Decreased capacity for biotransformation of drugs. This results in slowed metabolism and elimination, with increased risks of drug accumulation and adverse effects. |
| Increased activity of liver drug-metabolizing enzyme systems in children | Increased capacity for biotransformation of some drugs. This results in a rapid rate of metabolism and elimination. For example, theophylline is cleared about 30% faster in a 7-year-old child than in an adult and approximately four times faster than in a neonate. |

vulnerable to adverse drug effects because of their immature liver and kidney function; neonatal therapeutics are discussed further in Chapter 23.

Most drug use in children is empiric in nature because few studies have been done in that population. For many drugs, manufacturers' literature states "safety and effectiveness for use in children have not been established." Most drugs given to adults also are given to children, and general principles, techniques of drug administration, and nursing process guidelines apply. Additional principles and guidelines include the following:

1. All aspects of pediatric drug therapy must be guided by the child's age, weight, and level of growth and development.

2. Choice of drug is often restricted because many drugs commonly used in adult drug therapy have not been sufficiently investigated to ensure safety and effectiveness in children.

3. Safe therapeutic dosage ranges are less well defined for children than for adults. Some drugs are not recommended for use in children, and therefore dosages have not been established. For many drugs, doses for children are extrapolated from those established for adults. When pediatric dosage ranges are listed in drug literature, these should be used. Often, however, they are expressed in the amount of drug to be given per kilogram of body weight or square meter of body surface area, and the amount needed for a specific dose must be calculated as a fraction of the adult dose. The methods used for these calculations are found in Chapter 3. Dosages obtained from these calculations are approximate and must be individualized. These doses can be used initially and then increased or decreased according to the child's response.

4. Use the oral route of drug administration when possible. Try to obtain the child's cooperation; never force oral medications because forcing may lead to aspiration.

5. If intramuscular injections are required in infants, use the thigh muscles (vastus lateralis) because the deltoid muscles are quite small and the gluteal muscles (gluteus maximus and minimus) do not develop until the child is walking.

6. For safety, keep all medications in childproof containers, out of reach of children, and do not refer to medications as "candy."

### Drug Therapy in Older Adults

Aging is a continuum; precisely when a person becomes an "older adult" is not clearly established, but in this book, people 65 years of age and older are so categorized. In this population, general nursing process guidelines and principles of drug therapy apply. In addition, adverse effects are likely because of physiologic changes associated with aging (Table 5-3), pathologic changes due to disease processes, multiple drug therapy for acute

> **? How Can You Avoid This Medication Error?**
>
> Amoxicillin is prescribed for Jamie to treat an ear infection. The order is for 300 mg daily, to be administered q8h in equally divided doses. Jamie weighs 10 kg and the recommendations for infants are 20–40 mg/kg/day. The amoxicillin is supplied in syrup containing 100 mg/10 mL. The nurse gives Jamie 30 mL of amoxicillin for his morning dose.

and chronic disorders, impaired memory and cognition, and difficulty in complying with drug orders. Overall, the goal of drug therapy may be "care" rather than "cure," with efforts to prevent or control symptoms and maintain the client's ability to function in usual activities of daily living.

Additional principles include the following:

1. Although age in years is an important factor, older adults are quite heterogeneous in their responses to drug therapy, and responses differ widely within the same age group. Responses also differ in the same person over time. Physiologic age (ie, organ function) is more important than chronologic age.

2. It may be difficult to separate the effects of aging from the effects of disease processes or drug therapy, particularly long-term drug therapy. Symptoms attributed to aging or disease may be caused by medications. This occurs because older adults are usually less able to metabolize and excrete drugs efficiently. As a result, drugs are more likely to accumulate.

3. Both prescription and nonprescription drugs should be taken only when necessary.

4. Any prescriber should review current medications, including nonprescription drugs, before prescribing new drugs. In addition, unnecessary drugs should be discontinued. Some drugs, especially with long-term use, need to be tapered in dosage and discontinued gradually to avoid withdrawal symptoms.

5. When drug therapy is required, the choice of drug should be based on available drug information regarding effects in older adults.

6. The basic principle of giving the smallest effective number of drugs applies especially to older adults. A regimen of several drugs increases the incidence of adverse reactions and potentially hazardous drug interactions. In addition, many older adults are unable to self-administer more than three or four drugs correctly.

7. All drugs should be given for the shortest effective time. This interval is not established for most drugs, and many drugs are continued for years. Health care providers must reassess drug regimens periodically to see whether drugs, dosages, or other aspects need to be revised. This is especially important when a

**TABLE 5-3  Older Adults: Physiologic Characteristics and Pharmacokinetic Consequences**

| Physiologic Characteristics | Pharmacokinetic Consequences |
| --- | --- |
| Decreased gastrointestinal secretions and motility | Minimal effects on absorption of most oral drugs; effects on extended-release formulations are unknown |
| Decreased cardiac output | Slower absorption from some sites of administration (eg, gastro-intestinal tract, subcutaneous or muscle tissue); effects on absorption from skin and mucous membranes are unknown<br>Decreased distribution to sites of action in tissues, with potential for delaying the onset and reducing the extent of therapeutic effects |
| Decreased blood flow to the liver and kidneys | Delayed metabolism and excretion, which may lead to drug accumu-lation and increased risks of adverse or toxic effects |
| Decreased total body water and lean body mass per kg of weight; increased body fat | Water-soluble drugs (eg, ethanol, lithium) are distributed into a smaller area, with resultant higher plasma concentrations and higher risks of toxicity with a given dose. Fat-soluble drugs (eg, diazepam) are distributed to a larger area, accumulate in fat, and have a longer duration of action in the body. |
| Decreased serum albumin | Decreased availability of protein for binding and transporting drug molecules. This increases serum concentration of free, pharmaco-logically active drug, especially for those that are normally highly protein bound (eg, aspirin, warfarin). This may increase risks of adverse effects. However, the drug also may be metabolized and excreted more rapidly, thereby offsetting at least some of the risks.<br>In addition, drug interactions occur with co-administration of multiple drugs that are highly protein bound. The drugs compete for protein-binding sites and are more likely to cause adverse effects with decreased levels of serum albumin. As above, the result is larger concentrations of free drug. |
| Decreased blood flow to the liver; decreased size of the liver; decreased number and activity of the cytochrome P450 (CYP) oxidative drug-metabolizing enzymes | Slowed metabolism and detoxification of many drugs, with increased risks of drug accumulation and toxic effects. (Numerous drugs metabolized by the CYP enzymes are often prescribed for older adults, including beta blockers, calcium channel blockers, anti-microbials, the statin cholesterol-lowering drugs, and antiulcer drugs. Metabolism of drugs metabolized by conjugative reactions [eg, acetaminophen, diazepam, morphine, steroids] does not change significantly with aging.) |
| Decreased blood flow to the kidneys, decreased number of functioning nephrons, decreased glomerular filtration rate, and decreased tubular secretion | Impaired drug excretion, prolonged half-life, and increased risks of toxicity<br>Age-related alterations in renal function are consistent and well described. When renal blood flow is decreased, less drug is deliv-ered to the kidney for elimination. Renal mass is also decreased and older adults may be more sensitive to drugs that further impair renal function (eg, nonsteroidal anti-inflammatory drugs such as ibuprofen, which older adults often take for pain or arthritis). |

serious illness or significant changes in health status have occurred.

8. The smallest number of effective doses should be prescribed. This allows less disruption of usual activities and promotes compliance with the prescribed regimen.

9. When any drug is started, the dosage should usually be smaller than for younger adults. The dosage can then be increased or decreased according to response.

If an increased dosage is indicated, increments should be smaller and made at longer intervals in older adults. This conservative, safe approach is sometimes called "start low, go slow."

10. Use nonpharmacologic measures to decrease the need for drugs and to increase their effectiveness or decrease their adverse effects. For example, insomnia is a common complaint among older adults. Preventing it (eg, by avoiding caffeine-containing

beverages and excessive napping) is much safer than taking sedative-hypnotic drugs.

11. For people receiving long-term drug therapy at home, use measures to help them take drugs safely and effectively.

   a. If vision is impaired, label drug containers with large lettering for easier readability. A magnifying glass also may be useful.

   b. Be sure the client can open drug containers. For example, avoid childproof containers for an older adult with arthritic hands who does not have young children in the home.

   c. Several devices may be used to schedule drug doses and decrease risks for omitting or repeating doses. These include written schedules, calendars, and charts. Also available are drug containers with doses prepared and clearly labeled as to the day and time each dose is to be taken. With the latter system, the client can tell at a glance whether a dose has been taken.

   d. Enlist family members or friends when necessary.

12. When a client acquires new symptoms or becomes less capable of functioning in usual activities of daily living, consider the possibility of adverse drug effects. Often, new signs and symptoms are attributed to aging or disease. They may then be ignored or treated by prescribing a new drug, when stopping or reducing the dose of an old drug is the indicated intervention.

## Clinical Considerations in Drug Therapy

Many clients have or are at risk for impaired renal or hepatic function. Drug therapy must be especially cautious in clients with renal and hepatic impairment because of the risks for drug accumulation and adverse effects.

Clients with disease processes such as diabetes, hypertension, or heart failure may have renal insufficiency on first contact, and this may be worsened by illness, major surgery or trauma, or administration of nephrotoxic drugs. In clients with normal renal function, renal failure may develop from depletion of intravascular fluid volume, shock due to sepsis or blood loss, seriously impaired cardiovascular function, major surgery, nephrotoxic drugs, or other conditions.

Most drugs are eliminated from the body by hepatic metabolism, renal excretion, or both. Hepatic metabolism depends mainly on blood flow and enzyme activity in the liver and protein binding in the plasma. Clients at risk for impaired liver function include those with primary liver disease (eg, hepatitis, cirrhosis) and those with disease processes that impair blood flow to the liver (eg, heart failure, shock, major surgery or trauma) or hepatic enzyme production. An additional factor is hepatotoxic drugs. Fortunately, although the liver is often damaged, it has a great capacity for cell repair and may be able to function with as little as 10% of undamaged hepatic cells.

## Drug Therapy in Renal Impairment

Acute renal failure (ARF) may occur in any illness in which renal blood flow or function is impaired. Chronic renal failure (CRF) usually results from disease processes that destroy renal tissue.

With ARF, renal function may recover if the impairment is recognized promptly, contributing factors are eliminated or treated effectively, and medication dosages are adjusted according to the extent of renal impairment. With CRF, effective treatment can help to conserve functioning nephrons and delay progression to end-stage renal disease (ESRD). If ESRD develops, dialysis or transplantation is required.

In relation to drug therapy, the major concern with renal impairment is the high risk for drug accumulation and adverse effects because the kidneys are unable to excrete drugs and drug metabolites. Guidelines have been established for the use of many drugs; health care providers need to know and use these recommendations to maximize the safety and effectiveness of drug therapy. Some general guidelines are listed here; specific guidelines for particular drug groups are included in appropriate chapters.

1. When possible, nephrologists should design drug therapy regimens. However, all health care providers need to be knowledgeable about risk factors for development of renal impairment, illnesses and their physiologic changes (eg, hemodynamic, renal, hepatic, and metabolic alterations) that affect renal function, and the effects of various drugs on renal function.

2. Renal status should be monitored in any client with renal insufficiency or risk factors for development of renal insufficiency. Signs and symptoms of ARF include decreased urine output (<600 mL per 24 hours), increased blood urea nitrogen or increased serum creatinine (>2 mg/dL or an increase of ≥0.5 mg/dL over a baseline value of <3.0 mg/dL). In addition, an adequate fluid intake is required to excrete drugs by the kidneys. Any factors that deplete extracellular fluid volume (eg, inadequate fluid intake, diuretic drugs, loss of body fluids with blood loss, vomiting, or diarrhea) increase the risk for worsening renal impairment in clients who already have impairment or of causing impairment in those who previously had normal function.

3. Clients with renal impairment may respond to a drug dose or serum concentration differently than clients with normal renal function because of the physiologic and biochemical changes. Thus, drug therapy must be individualized according to the extent of renal impairment. This is usually determined by measuring serum creatinine, which is then used to calculate creatinine clearance as a measure of the glomerular filtration rate (GFR). Because serum creatinine is determined by muscle mass as well as the GFR, the serum creatinine measurement cannot be used as the sole indicator of renal function unless the client is a young,

relatively healthy, well-nourished person with a sudden acute illness. Estimations of creatinine clearance are more accurate for clients with stable renal function (ie, stable serum creatinine) and average muscle mass (for their age, weight, and height). Estimations are less accurate for emaciated and obese clients and for those with changing renal function, as often occurs in acute illness. If a fluctuating serum creatinine is used to calculate the GFR, an erroneous value will be obtained. If a client is oliguric (<400 mL urine per 24 hours), for example, the creatinine clearance should be estimated to be less than 10 mL/minute, regardless of the serum creatinine concentration.

Serum creatinine is also a relatively unreliable indicator of renal function in elderly or malnourished clients. Because these clients usually have diminished muscle mass, they may have a normal serum level of creatinine even if their renal function and GFR are markedly reduced.

Some medications can increase serum creatinine levels and create a false impression of renal failure. These drugs, which include cimetidine and trimethoprim, interfere with secretion of creatinine into kidney tubules. As a result, serum creatinine levels are increased without an associated decrease in renal function.

4. **Drug selection** should be guided by baseline renal function and the known effects of drugs on renal function, when possible. Many commonly used drugs may adversely affect renal function, including nonsteroidal anti-inflammatory drugs such as prescription or over-the-counter ibuprofen (Motrin, Advil). Some drugs are excreted exclusively (eg, aminoglycoside antibiotics, lithium) and most are excreted primarily or to some extent by the kidneys. Some drugs are contraindicated in renal impairment (eg, tetracyclines except doxycycline); others can be used if safety guidelines are followed (eg, reducing dosage, monitoring serum drug levels and renal function tests, avoiding dehydration). Drugs known to be nephrotoxic should be avoided when possible. In some instances, however, there are no effective substitutes, and nephrotoxic drugs must be given. Some commonly used nephrotoxic drugs include aminoglycoside antibiotics, amphotericin B, and cisplatin.

5. **Dosage** of many drugs needs to be decreased in renal failure, including aminoglycoside antibiotics, most cephalosporin antibiotics, fluoroquinolones, and digoxin. For some drugs, a smaller dose or a longer interval between doses is recommended for clients with moderate (creatinine clearance 10 to 50 mL/minute) or severe (creatinine clearance <10 mL/minute) renal insufficiency. However, for many commonly used drugs, the most effective dosage adjustments are based on the client's clinical responses and serum drug levels.

For clients receiving renal replacement therapy (eg, hemodialysis or some type of filtration), the treatment removes variable amounts of drugs that are usually excreted through the kidneys. With some drugs, such as many antimicrobials, a supplemental dose may be needed to maintain therapeutic blood levels of drug.

## Drug Therapy in Hepatic Impairment

In relation to drug therapy, acute liver impairment may interfere with drug metabolism and elimination, whereas chronic cirrhosis or severe liver impairment may affect all pharmacokinetic processes. It is difficult to predict the effects of drug therapy because of wide variations in liver function and few helpful diagnostic tests. In addition, with severe hepatic impairment, extrahepatic sites of drug metabolism (eg, intestine, kidneys, lungs) may become more important in eliminating drugs from the body. Thus, guidelines for drug selection, dosage, and duration of use are not well established. Some general guidelines for increasing drug safety and effectiveness are listed here; known guidelines for particular drug groups are included in appropriate chapters.

1. During drug therapy, clients with impaired liver function require close monitoring for signs and symptoms (eg, nausea, vomiting, jaundice, liver enlargement) and abnormal results of laboratory tests of liver function (see 4, below).

2. **Drug selection** should be based on knowledge of drug effects on hepatic function. Hepatotoxic drugs should be avoided when possible. If they cannot be avoided, they should be used in the smallest effective doses, for the shortest effective time. Commonly used hepatotoxic drugs include acetaminophen, isoniazid, and cholesterol-lowering statins. Alcohol is toxic to the liver by itself and increases the risks for hepatotoxicity with other drugs.

   In addition to hepatotoxic drugs, many other drugs can cause or aggravate liver impairment by decreasing hepatic blood flow and drug-metabolizing capacity. For example, epinephrine and related drugs may cause vasoconstriction in the hepatic artery and portal vein, the two main sources of the liver's blood supply. Beta-adrenergic blocking agents decrease hepatic blood flow by decreasing cardiac output. Several drugs (eg, cimetidine, fluoxetine, ketoconazole) inhibit hepatic metabolism of many coadministered drugs. The consequence may be toxicity from the inhibited drugs if the dose is not decreased.

3. **Dosage** should be reduced for drugs that are extensively metabolized in the liver because, if doses are not reduced, serum drug levels are higher, elimination is slower, and toxicity is more likely to occur in a client with hepatic disease. For example, lidocaine is normally rapidly deactivated by hepatic metabolism. If blood flow is impaired so that lidocaine molecules in the blood are unable to reach drug-metabolizing liver cells, more drug stays in the bloodstream longer. Also, some oral drugs are normally extensively metabolized during their "first pass" through the liver, so that a rel-

atively small portion of an oral dose reaches the systemic circulation. With cirrhosis, the blood carrying the drug molecules is shunted around the liver so that oral drugs go directly into the systemic circulation. Some drugs whose dosages should be decreased in hepatic failure include cefoperazone, cimetidine, clindamycin, diazepam, labetalol, lorazepam, meperidine, morphine, phenytoin, propranolol, quinidine, ranitidine, theophylline, and verapamil.

4. Liver function tests should be monitored in clients with or at risk for liver impairment, especially when clients are receiving potentially hepatotoxic drugs. Indicators of hepatic impairment include serum bilirubin levels above 4 to 5 mg/dL, a prothrombin time greater than 1.5 times control, a serum albumin level below 2.0 g/dL, and elevated serum alanine (ALT) and aspartate (AST) aminotransferases. In some clients, abnormal liver function test results may occur without indicating severe liver damage and are often reversible.

## Environmental Considerations in Drug Therapy

Whether the client is hospitalized or at home, the environment plays a key role in aspects of drug therapy. Clients are hospitalized during critical illness most often in critical care environments, such as an intensive care unit (ICU). However, nurses in numerous other settings also care for critically ill clients. For example, nurses in emergency departments often initiate and maintain treatment for several hours; nurses on other hospital units care for clients who are transferred to or from ICUs; and, increasingly, clients formerly cared for in an ICU are on medical-surgical hospital units, in long-term care facilities, or even at home. Moreover, increasing numbers of nursing students are introduced to critical care during their educational programs, many new graduates seek employment in critical care settings, and experienced nurses may transfer to an ICU. Thus, all nurses need to know about drug therapy in critically ill clients.

Home care is an expanding area of health care evolving from efforts to reduce health care costs, especially the costs of hospitalization. The consequences of this trend include increased outpatient care and brief hospitalizations for severe illness or major surgery. In both instances, clients of all age groups are often discharged to their homes for follow-up care and recovery. Skilled nursing care, such as managing medication regimens, is essential for clients during periods of critical illness and as follow-up in the home after any health condition.

### Drug Therapy in Critical Illness

The term *critical illness*, as used here, denotes the care of clients who are experiencing acute, serious, or life-threatening illness. Critically ill clients are at risk for multiple organ failure, including cardiovascular, renal, and hepatic impairments that influence all aspects of drug therapy. Overall, critically ill clients exhibit varying degrees of organ dysfunction, and their conditions tend to change rapidly, so that drug pharmacokinetics and pharmacodynamics vary widely. Although blood volume is often decreased, drug distribution is usually increased because of less protein binding and increased extracellular fluid. Drug elimination is usually impaired because of decreased blood flow and decreased function of the liver and kidneys.

Some general guidelines to increase safety and effectiveness of drug therapy in critical illness are listed here:

1. Drug therapy in clients who are critically ill is often more complex, more problematic, and less predictable than in most other populations. One reason is that clients often have multiple organ impairments that alter drug effects and increase the risks for adverse drug reactions. Another reason is that critically ill clients often require aggressive treatment with large numbers, large doses, and combinations of highly potent medications. Overall, therapeutic effects may be decreased, and risks for adverse reactions and interactions may be increased because the client's body may be unable to process or respond to drugs effectively.

   In this at-risk population, safe and effective drug therapy requires that all involved health care providers be knowledgeable about common critical illnesses, the physiologic changes (eg, hemodynamic, renal, hepatic, and metabolic alterations) that can be caused by the illnesses, and the drugs used to treat the illnesses. Nurses need to be especially diligent in administering drugs and vigilant in observing client responses.

2. Drugs used in critical illness represent most drug classifications and are also discussed in other chapters. Commonly used drugs include analgesics, antimicrobials, cardiovascular agents, gastric acid suppressants, neuromuscular blocking agents, and sedatives.

3. In many instances, the goal of drug therapy is to support vital functions and relieve life-threatening symptoms until healing can occur or definitive treatment can be instituted.

4. **Drug selection** should be guided by the client's clinical status (eg, symptoms, severity of illness) and organ function, especially cardiovascular, renal, and hepatic functions.

5. **Route of administration** should also be guided by the client's clinical status. Most drugs are given by the intravenous (IV) route because critically ill clients are often unable to take oral medications and require many drugs, rapid drug action, and relatively large doses. In addition, the IV route achieves more reliable and measurable blood levels.

   When a drug is given by IV route, it reaches the heart and brain quickly because the sympathetic nervous system and other homeostatic mechanisms attempt to maintain blood flow to the heart and brain at the expense of blood flow to other organs such as the kidneys, gastrointestinal (GI) tract, liver, and skin. As a result, cardiovascular and CNS effects may be faster, more pronounced, and longer lasting than usual. If the drug is a sedative, effects may include excessive sedation and cardiac depression.

If the client is able to take oral medications, this is probably the preferred route. However, many factors may interfere with drug effects (eg, impaired function of the GI tract, heart, kidneys, or liver), and drug–drug and drug–food interactions may occur if precautions are not taken. For example, antiulcer drugs, which are often given to prevent stress ulcers and GI bleeding, may decrease absorption of other drugs.

For clients who receive oral medications or nutritional solutions through a nasogastric, gastrostomy, or jejunostomy tube, there may be drug–food interactions that impair drug absorption. In addition, crushing tablets or opening capsules to give a drug by a GI tube may alter the absorption and chemical stability of the drug.

Sublingual, oral inhalation, and transdermal medications may be used effectively in some critically ill clients. However, few drugs are available in these formulations.

For clients with hypotension and shock, drugs usually should not be given orally, subcutaneously, intramuscularly, or by skin patch because shock impairs absorption from these sites of administration, distribution to body cells is unpredictable, the liver cannot metabolize drugs effectively, and the kidneys cannot excrete drugs effectively.

6. **Dosage** requirements may vary considerably among clients and within the same client at different times during an illness. A standard dose may be effective, subtherapeutic, or toxic. Thus, it is especially important that initial dosages are individualized according to the severity of the condition being treated and client characteristics such as age and organ function, and that maintenance dosages are titrated according to client responses and changes in organ function (eg, as indicated by symptoms or laboratory tests).

7. With many drugs, the timing of administration may be important in increasing therapeutic effects and decreasing adverse effects. Once-daily drug doses should be given at approximately the same time each day; multiple daily doses should be given at approximately even intervals around the clock.

8. Weigh clients when possible, initially and periodically, because dosage of many drugs is based on weight. In addition, periodic weights help to assess clients for loss of body mass or gain in body water, both of which affect the pharmacokinetics of the drugs administered.

9. Laboratory tests are often needed before and during drug therapy of critical illnesses to assess the client's condition (eg, cardiovascular, renal and hepatic functions, fluid and electrolyte balance) and response to treatment. Other tests may include measurement of serum drug levels. The results of these tests may indicate that changes are needed in drug therapy.

10. Serum protein levels should be monitored in critically ill clients because drug binding may be significantly altered. Serum albumin, which binds acidic drugs such as phenytoin and diazepam, is usually decreased during critical illness for a variety of reasons, including inadequate production by the liver. If there is not enough albumin to bind a drug, blood levels are higher and may cause adverse effects. Also, unbound molecules are metabolized and excreted more readily so that therapeutic effects may be decreased.

Alpha$_1$-acid glycoprotein binds basic drugs, and its synthesis may increase during critical illness. As a result, the bound portion of a dose increases for some drugs (eg, meperidine, propranolol, imipramine, lidocaine) and therapeutic blood levels may not be achieved unless higher doses are given. In addition, these drugs are eliminated more slowly than usual.

## Drug Therapy in Home Care

Most general principles and nursing responsibilities related to drug therapy apply in home care as in other health care settings. Some additional principles and factors include the following:

1. Clients may require short- or long-term drug therapy. In most instances, the role of the nurse is to teach the client or caregiver to administer medications and monitor their effects.

2. In a client's home, the nurse is a guest and must work within the environment to establish rapport, elicit cooperation, and provide nursing care. The initial contact is usually by telephone, and one purpose is to schedule a home visit, preferably at a convenient time for the client and caregiver. In addition, state the main purpose of the visit and approximately how long the visit will be. Establish a method for contact in case the appointment must be canceled by either party.

3. Assess the client's attitude toward the prescribed medication regimen and his or her ability to provide self-care. If the client is unable, who will be the primary caregiver for medication administration and observing for medication effects? What are the learning needs of the client or caregiver in relation to the medication regimen?

4. Ask to see all prescribed and over-the-counter medications the client takes, and ask how and when the client takes each one. With this information, the

nurse may be able to reinforce the client's compliance or identify potential problem areas (eg, differences between instructions and client usage of medications, drugs with opposing or duplicate effects, continued use of medications that were supposed to be discontinued, drugs discontinued because of adverse effects).

5. Ask if the client takes any herbal medicines or dietary supplements. If so, try to determine the amount, frequency, duration of use, reasons for use, and perceived beneficial or adverse effects. Explain that the nurse needs this information because some herbals and dietary supplements may cause various health problems or react adversely with prescription or over-the-counter medications.

6. Assess the environment for potential safety hazards (eg, risk for infection with corticosteroids and other immunosuppressants, risk for falls and other injuries with narcotic analgesics and other drugs with sedating effects). In addition, assess the client's ability to obtain medications and keep appointments for follow-up visits to health care providers.

7. Provide whatever information and assistance are needed for home management of the drug therapy regimen. Most people are accustomed to taking oral drugs, but they may need information about timing in relation to food intake, whether a tablet can be crushed, when to omit the drug, and other aspects. With other routes, the nurse may initially need to demonstrate administration or coach the client or caregiver through each step. Demonstrating and having the client or caregiver do a return demonstration is a good way to teach psychomotor skills such as giving a medication through a GI tube, preparing and administering an injection, or manipulating an intravenous infusion pump.

8. In addition to safe and accurate administration, teach the client and caregiver to observe for beneficial and adverse effects. If side effects occur, teach them how to manage minor ones and which ones to report to a health care provider.

9. Between home visits, the home care nurse can maintain contact with clients and caregivers to monitor progress, answer questions, identify problems, and provide reassurance. Clients and caregivers should be given a telephone number to call with questions about medications, side effects, and so forth. The nurse may wish to schedule a daily time for receiving and making nonemergency calls. For clients and nurses with computers and Internet access, electronic mail may be a convenient and efficient method of communication.

## Nursing Actions
### Monitoring Drug Therapy

| Nursing Actions | Rationale/Explanation |
|---|---|
| 1. Prepare medications for administration. | If giving medications to a group of clients, start preparing about 30 minutes before the scheduled administration time when possible, to avoid rushing and increasing the risk of errors. |
| a. Assemble appropriate supplies and equipment. | Medications and supplies are usually kept on a medication cart in a hospital or long-term care facility. |
| b. Calculate doses when indicated. | Except for very simple calculations, use pencil and paper to decrease the risk of errors. If unsure about the results, ask a colleague or a pharmacist to do the calculation. Compare results. Accuracy is vital. |
| c. Check vital signs when indicated. | Check blood pressure (recent recordings) before giving antihypertensive drugs. Check temperature before giving an antipyretic. |
| d. Check laboratory reports when indicated. | Commonly needed reports include serum potassium levels before giving diuretics; prothrombin time or international normalized ratio (INR) before giving Coumadin; culture and susceptibility reports before giving an antibiotic. |
| e. Check drug references when indicated. | This is often needed to look up new or unfamiliar drugs; other uses include assessing a drug in relation to a particular client (eg, Is it contraindicated? Is it likely to interact with other drugs the client is taking? Does the client's ordered dose fit within the dosage range listed in the drug reference? Can a tablet be crushed or a capsule opened without decreasing therapeutic effects or increasing adverse effects?) |

*(continued)*

## Nursing Actions

## Monitoring Drug Therapy (Continued)

| Nursing Actions | Rationale/Explanation |
|---|---|
| **2. Administer drugs accurately (see Chap. 4).**<br>a. Practice the seven rights of drug administration (right *drug,* right *client,* right *dose,* right *route,* and right *time,* right *documentation,* and *client's right to refuse*). | These rights are ensured if the techniques described in Chapter 4 are consistently followed. The time may vary by approximately 30 minutes. For example, a drug ordered for 9 AM can be usually given between 8:30 AM and 9:30 AM. No variation is allowed in the other rights. |
| b. Use correct techniques for different routes of administration.<br>c. Follow label instructions regarding mixing or other aspects of giving specific drugs.<br>d. In general, do not give antacids with any other oral drugs. When both are ordered, administer at least 2 hours apart. | For example, sterile equipment and techniques are required for injection of any drug.<br>Some drugs require specific techniques of preparation and administration.<br>Antacids decrease absorption of many oral drugs. |
| **2. Observe for therapeutic effects.**<br>a. Look for improvement in signs and symptoms, laboratory or other diagnostic test reports, or ability to function.<br>b. Ask questions to determine whether the client is feeling better. | In general, the nurse should know the expected effects and when they are likely to occur.<br><br>Specific observations depend on the specific drug or drugs being given. |
| **3. Observe for adverse effects.**<br>a. Look for signs and symptoms of new problems or worsening of previous disorders. If noted, compare the client's symptoms with your knowledge base about adverse effects associated with the drugs or consult a drug reference.<br>b. Check laboratory (eg, complete blood count [CBC], electrolytes, blood urea nitrogen and serum creatinine, liver function tests) and other diagnostic test reports for abnormal values.<br>c. Assess for decreasing ability to function at previous levels.<br>d. Ask questions to determine how the client is feeling and whether he or she is having difficulties that may be associated with drug therapy. | All drugs are potentially harmful, although the incidence and severity of adverse reactions vary among drugs and clients. People most likely to have adverse reactions are those with severe liver or kidney disease, those who are very young or very old, those taking several drugs, and those receiving large doses of any drug. Specific adverse effects for which to observe depend on the drugs being given. |
| **4. Observe for drug interactions.**<br>a. Consider a possible interaction when a client does not experience expected therapeutic effects or develops adverse effects.<br>b. Look for signs and symptoms of new problems or worsening of previous ones. If noted, compare the client's symptoms with your knowledge base about interactions associated with the drugs or consult a drug reference to validate your observations. | Interactions may occur whenever the client is receiving two or more drugs concurrently and the number of possible interactions is very large. Although no one can be expected to know or recognize all potential or actual interactions, it is helpful to build a knowledge base about important interactions with commonly used drugs (eg, warfarin, sedatives, cardiovascular drugs). |

## ? How Can You Avoid This Medication Error?

**Answer:** The nurse administered the wrong dose of medication to Jamie. Thirty milliliters would provide the entire daily dose of amoxicillin, rather than 100 mg, which should be administered every 8 hours. Carefully reread the order and recalculate the dosage ordered. Unit dosing can help double-check calculations and avoid errors.

## Critical Thinking Exercises

1. The primary reason that the nurse should never force oral medications on a child is that:
   a. Forcing may lead to aspiration
   b. Aggression threatens the therapeutic relationship
   c. Forcing may cause gastric upset in the child
   d. The child may refuse to take the medicine at home

**2.** The nurse recognizes that intramuscular injections in infants should be administered in the:

a. Thigh muscles

b. Deltoid muscles

c. Gluteus maximus muscle

d. Gluteus minimus muscle

**3.** Several measures are used to decrease the risk for omitting or repeating administration of a medication in an older adult. A client can tell at a glance whether a dose has been taken by using:

a. Schedules

b. Calendars

c. Charts

d. Drug containers with doses prepared and clearly labeled as to the day and time each dose is to be taken

**4.** The nurse recognizes that clients in renal failure may not need dosage reduction in which of the following drugs?

a. Aminoglycoside antibiotics

b. Cephalosporin antibiotics

c. Fluoroquinolones

d. Acetaminophen

**5.** Clients at risk for impaired liver function include those:

a. With primary liver disease

b. With disease processes that impair blood flow to the liver

c. Receiving hepatotoxic drugs

d. All the above

## SELECTED REFERENCES

Boullata, J. I., & Nace, A. M. (2000). Safety issues with herbal medicine. *Pharmacotherapy, 20*(3), 257–269.

DerMarderosian, A. (Ed.) (2001). *The review of natural products.* St. Louis: Facts and Comparisons.

Fetrow, C. W., & Avila, J. R. (1999). *Professional's handbook of complementary & alternative medicines.* Springhouse, PA: Springhouse Corp.

Hardy, M. L. (2000). Women's Health series: Herbs of special interest to women. *Journal of the American Pharmaceutical Association, 40*(2), 234–242.

Hatcher, T. (2001). The proverbial herb. *American Journal of Nursing, 101*(2), 36–43.

Metzl, J., Small, E., & Levine, S. R. (2001). Creatine use among young athletes. *Pediatrics, 108*(2), 421–425.

Miller, L. G., Hume, A., Harris, I. M., Jackson, E. A., Kanmaz, T. J., Cauffield, J. S., et al. (2000). White paper on herbal products. *Pharmacotherapy, 20*(7), 877–891.

Multach, M. (2000). Alternative medicine: Prevalence, cost, and usefulness. In H. D. Humes (Ed.), *Kelley's textbook of internal medicine* (4th ed., pp. 319–323). Philadelphia: Lippincott Williams & Wilkins.

Murch, S. J., KrishnaRaj, S., & Saxena, P. K. (2000). Phytopharmaceuticals: Problems, limitations, and solutions. *Scientific Review of Alternative Medicines, 4*(2), 33–37. [On-line.] Available: http://www.medscape.com/prometheus/SRAM/2000/v04.n02/sram0402.02. murc/sram0402.02.murc-01.html. Accessed July 2003.

Schwartz, J. B. (2000). Geriatric clinical pharmacology. In H. D. Humes (Ed.), *Kelley's textbook of internal medicine* (4th ed., pp. 3095–3107). Philadelphia: Lippincott Williams & Wilkins.

Tyler, V. E. (2000). Product definition deficiencies in clinical studies of herbal medicines. *Scientific Review of Alternative Medicines, 4*(2), 17–21. [On-line.] Available: http://www.medscape.com/prometheus/SRAM/2000/v04.n02/sram0402.01.tyle/sram0402.01.tyle.html. Accessed July 2003.

Waddell, D. L., Hummel, M. E., & Sumners, A. D. (2001). Three herbs you should get to know. *American Journal of Nursing, 101*(4), 48–53.

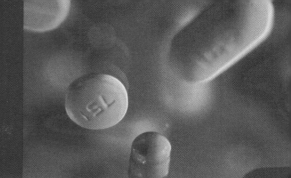

## 6

# Narcotic Analgesics and Narcotic Antagonists

### OBJECTIVES

*After studying this chapter, the student will be able to:*

1 Describe characteristics of pain.

2 Discuss the nurse's role in assessing and managing clients' pain.

3 List characteristics of narcotic analgesics in terms of mechanism of action, indications for use, and major adverse effects.

4 Use morphine sulfate as the prototype to discuss characteristics of narcotic analgesics.

5 Contrast the use of narcotic analgesics in opiate-naive and opiate-tolerant clients.

6 Discuss the nursing process for using narcotic analgesics in specific populations.

7 Identify signs and symptoms of narcotic overdose and withdrawal and the treatment of each.

8 Teach clients about safe, effective use of narcotic analgesics.

9 Discuss the clinical use of narcotic antagonists.

### CRITICAL THINKING SCENARIO

*J*ohn Shone, 65 years of age, has terminal cancer that was diagnosed 9 months ago. One month ago, he was prescribed morphine sulfate (MS Contin, 30 mg twice daily) for pain. When you assess him, you note that he is very quiet and seems reluctant to move. His vital signs are as follows: blood pressure, 152/88 mm Hg; pulse, 88 beats/minute; and respirations, 20 breaths/minute. He rates his pain as 9 on a 1-to-10 scale, saying that during the past week, his pain seemed to be getting much worse. Previously, Mr. Shone and his wife expressed their concern regarding "having to take so much medication and not wanting to become addicted to pain medication."

✔ Based on the data collected, assess Mr. Shone's pain.

✔ Reflect on teaching what Mr. Shone and his wife may need regarding chronic pain and its treatment. What suggestions do you have for Mr. Shone's pain management plan?

### PROTOTYPE PROFILE

morphine sulfate, p. 91

# OVERVIEW

Pain is the most common symptom prompting people to seek health care. It is an unpleasant sensation that usually indicates tissue damage and impels the person to remove the cause of the damage or seek relief from the pain. Narcotic (opioid) analgesics are drugs that relieve moderate to severe pain. To aid understanding of drug actions, selected characteristics of pain are described in At the Foundation: Pain. A description of endogenous (within the body) pain-relieving substances is also detailed.

# ENDOGENOUS ANALGESIA SYSTEM

The central nervous system (CNS) has its own system for suppressing the transmission of pain signals from peripheral nerves. The system can be activated by nervous signals entering the periaqueductal gray area of the brain or by morphine-like drugs. Important elements include opiate receptors and endogenous peptides with actions similar to those of morphine sulfate. Narcotic opiate receptors are highly concentrated in some regions of the CNS, including the ascending and descending pain pathways and portions of the brain essential to the endogenous analgesia system. The opioid peptides (ie, the enkephalins, dynorphins, and beta-endorphins) interact with opiate receptors to inhibit pain transmission. All are important in the endogenous opiate system, but the three types of peptides differ in precursors and anatomic locations. Enkephalins are believed to interrupt the transmission of pain signals at the spinal cord level by inhibiting the release of substance P from C nerve fibers. The endogenous analgesia system may also inhibit pain signals at other points in the pain pathway.

# NARCOTIC ANALGESICS

Narcotic analgesics are drugs that relieve moderate to severe pain by inhibiting the release of substance P in both central and peripheral nerves (which inhibits transmission of pain signals from peripheral tissues to the brain), reducing the perception of pain sensation in the brain, producing sedation, and decreasing the emotional

---

**AT THE FOUNDATION:** *Pain*

Pain occurs when tissue damage activates the free nerve endings (pain receptors or nociceptors) of peripheral nerves. Pain receptors are abundant in the skin and underlying soft tissue, muscle fascia, joint surfaces, arterial walls, and periosteum; most internal organs, such as lung and uterine tissue, contain few pain receptors.

Bradykinin, one of the strongest pain-producing substances, is quickly metabolized during tissue damage and therefore may be involved in acute pain. Prostaglandins increase bradykinin's pain-provoking effects by increasing the sensitivity of pain receptors. Several other substances are also thought to produce pain, including acetylcholine, adenosine triphosphate, histamine, leukotrienes, potassium, serotonin, and substance P. Overall, these chemical mediators produce pain by activating and sensitizing peripheral pain receptors or stimulating the release of pain-producing substances.

For a person to feel pain, the signal must be transmitted to the spinal cord, then to the hypothalamus and cerebral cortex in the brain. The signal is carried to the spinal cord by two types of peripheral nerve cells: A-delta fibers, which transmit fast, sharp, well-localized pain signals, and C fibers, which conduct the pain signal slowly and produce a poorly localized, dull, or burning type of pain. Tissue damage from an acute injury often produces an initial sharp pain transmitted by A-delta fibers, followed by a dull ache or burning sensation transmitted by C fibers. C fibers release somatostatin and substance P at synapses in the spinal cord. Glutamate, aspartate, substance P, and perhaps other chemical mediators are thought to enhance transmission of the pain signal.

The dorsal horn of the spinal cord is the control center or relay station for information from the A-delta and C nerve fibers, for local modulation of the pain impulse, and for descending influences from higher centers in the CNS (eg, attention, emotion, memory). Here, nociceptive nerve fibers synapse with non-nociceptive nerve fibers (neurons that carry information other than pain signals). Another major inhibitory pathway is noradrenergic and originates in the pons. Thus, increasing the concentration of norepinephrine and serotonin in the synapse interrupts or inhibits transmission of nerve impulses that carry pain signals to the brain and spinal cord. (This is thought to account for the pain-relieving effects of the tricyclic antidepressants, drugs that increase the amounts of serotonin and norepinephrine in the synapse by inhibiting their reuptake by presynaptic nerve endings.)

In the brain, the thalamus is a relay station for incoming sensory stimuli, including pain. Perception of pain is a primitive awareness in the thalamus, and sensation is not well localized or specific. From the thalamus, pain messages are relayed to the cerebral cortex, where they are perceived more specifically and analyzed to determine actions needed.

upsets often associated with pain. They also inhibit the production of pain and inflammation by prostaglandins in peripheral tissues. Most of these analgesics are Schedule II drugs under federal narcotic laws and may lead to drug abuse and dependence. These exogenous analgesics are called *opioids* because they act like 🅟 **morphine sulfate** in the body.

Narcotic analgesics are well absorbed with oral, intramuscular, or subcutaneous administration. Oral preparations undergo significant first-pass metabolism in the liver, so that oral doses must be larger than parenteral doses for equivalent therapeutic effects. The drugs are extensively metabolized in the liver, and metabolites are excreted in urine. Morphine sulfate and meperidine form pharmacologically active metabolites. Thus, liver impairment can interfere with metabolism, and kidney impairment can interfere with excretion. Drug accumulation and increased adverse effects may occur if dosage is not reduced. In clients with renal impairment, the drugs should be given in minimal doses, for the shortest effective time, because usual doses may produce profound sedation and a prolonged duration of action.

Narcotics exert widespread pharmacologic effects, especially in the CNS and the gastrointestinal (GI) system. These effects occur with usual doses and may be therapeutic or adverse, depending on the reason for use. CNS effects include analgesia, CNS depression ranging from drowsiness to sleep to unconsciousness, decreased mental and physical activity, respiratory depression, nausea and vomiting, and pupil constriction. Sedation and respiratory depression are major adverse effects and are potentially life threatening. Most new narcotic analgesics have been developed in an effort to find drugs as effective as morphine sulfate in relieving pain while causing less sedation, respiratory depression, and dependence. However, this effort has not been successful: *equianalgesic doses of these drugs produce sedative and respiratory depressant effects comparable with those of morphine sulfate.* Equianalgesic comparisons of narcotics are found in Table 6-1. In the GI tract, narcotic analgesics slow motility and may cause constipation and smooth muscle spasms in the bowel and biliary tract.

## Mechanism of Action

Narcotics relieve pain mainly by binding to opioid receptors in the brain and spinal cord; some receptors have been found in the periphery as well. They also activate the endogenous analgesia system. The major types of receptors are mu, kappa, and delta. Most opioid effects (analgesia, CNS depression with respiratory depression and sedation, euphoria, decreased GI motility, and physical dependence) are attributed to activation of the mu receptors. Analgesia, sedation, and decreased GI motility also occur with activation of kappa receptors. Delta receptors are important in the endogenous analgesia system,

| TABLE 6-1 | Equianalgesic Comparisons of Common Narcotics | |
|---|---|---|
| | **Approximate Equianalgesic Doses Based on Morphine 10 mg IM or Sub-Q** | |
| **Drug** | *Oral (mg)* | *Parenteral (mg)* |
| Codeine | 180–200 | IM: 120–130 Sub-Q: 120 |
| Hydrocodone | 30 | No data available |
| Hydromorphone (Dilaudid) | 7.5 | IM: 1.3–1.5 Sub-Q: 1–1.5 |
| Levorphanol (Levo-Dromoran) | 4 | IM: 2 Sub-Q: 2 |
| Meperidine (Demerol) | 300 | IM: 75 Sub-Q: 75–100 |
| Methadone (Dolophine) | 10–20 | IM: 10 Sub-Q: 8–10 |
| **Morphine** | 30–60 | IM: 10 Sub-Q: 10 |
| Oxycodone (Roxicodone, others) | 30 | IM: 10–15 Sub-Q: 10–15 |
| Oxymorphone (Numorphan) | No data available on oral dosing (rectal, 5 or 10) | IM: 1 Sub-Q: 1–1.5 |
| Propoxyphene (Darvon) | 130 | Not available |

but it is not clear whether they bind with opioid drugs. Narcotic analgesics and narcotic antagonists bind to different receptors to varying degrees, and their pharmacologic actions can be differentiated and classified on this basis.

## Indications for Use

The main indication for the use of narcotics is to prevent or relieve acute or chronic pain. Specific conditions in which narcotics are used for analgesic effects include acute myocardial infarction, biliary colic, renal colic, burns and other traumatic injuries, postoperative states, and cancer. These drugs are usually given for chronic pain only when other measures and milder drugs are ineffective, as in terminal malignancy. Other clinical uses include the following:

1. Before and during surgery to promote sedation, decrease anxiety, facilitate induction of anesthesia, and decrease the amount of anesthesia required
2. Before and during invasive diagnostic procedures, such as angiograms and endoscopic examinations
3. During labor and delivery (obstetric analgesia)
4. In treating GI disorders, such as abdominal cramping and diarrhea
5. In treating acute pulmonary edema (morphine sulfate is used)
6. In treating severe, unproductive cough (codeine is often used)

## Contraindications to Use

These drugs are contraindicated or must be used very cautiously in people with respiratory depression, chronic lung disease, liver or kidney disease, prostatic hypertrophy, increased intracranial pressure, or hypersensitivity reactions to narcotics and related drugs.

## ◼ NEED FOR EFFECTIVE PAIN MANAGEMENT

Numerous studies have indicated ineffective management of clients' pain, especially moderate to severe pain associated with surgery or cancer. Much of the difficulty has been attributed to inadequate or improper use of narcotic analgesics, including administering the wrong drug, prescribing inadequate dosage, or leaving long intervals between doses. Even when ordered appropriately, nurses or clients and family members may not administer the drugs effectively. Traditionally, concerns about respiratory depression, excessive sedation, drug dependence, and other adverse effects have contributed to reluctance and delay in administering narcotic analgesics. Inadequate management of pain often leads to anxiety, depression, and other emotional upsets from anticipation of pain recurrence.

In recent years, a more humane approach to pain management has evolved. Basic assumptions of this approach are that no one should suffer pain needlessly; that pain occurs when the client says it does and should be relieved by whatever means are required, including pharmacologic and nonpharmacologic treatments; that doses of narcotics should be titrated to achieve maximal effectiveness and minimal toxicity; and that dependence rarely results from drugs taken for physical pain. Proponents of this view emphasize the need to assess and monitor all clients receiving narcotic analgesics.

## Management Considerations

Several factors govern the type of narcotic ordered for a client. The type of drug ordered, route selection, and dosage and administration schedule may vary with clinical condition and goals of therapy.

Narcotic analgesics are widely used in the home for both acute and chronic pain. With acute pain, such as postoperative recovery, the use of a narcotic analgesic is often limited to a short period, and clients self-administer their medications. The need for strong pain medication recedes as healing occurs. Home care may be an essential component in the management of individuals taking narcotics for various health conditions. Guidelines for ongoing evaluation and intervention are addressed in Home Care Considerations.

In addition, age-specific considerations are important in the management of individuals taking narcotics. In general, there is little understanding of the physiology, pathology, assessment, and management of pain in children. Many authorities indicate that children's pain is often ignored or undertreated, including children having surgical and other painful procedures for which adults routinely receive an anesthetic, a strong analgesic, or both. This is especially true in preterm and full-term neonates.

Narcotic analgesics should be used cautiously in older adults, especially if they are debilitated; have hepatic,

### Home Care Considerations: Use of Narcotics

***ASSESS:*** the frequency and severity of the pain and how successfully the pain is managed, including alternative methods of relieving discomfort.

***MONITOR:*** the response to narcotics, modification of risk factors, and quality of life.

***EDUCATE:*** on safe use of the drugs (eg, that the drugs decrease mental alertness and physical agility, so that potentially hazardous activities should be avoided), nonpharmacologic methods of managing pain, and ways to prevent adverse effects of narcotics (eg, excessive sedation, constipation). Reinforce additional teaching points (see Client Teaching Guidelines: Opioid [Narcotic] Analgesics).

renal, or respiratory impairment; or are receiving other drugs that depress the CNS. Despite these factors, the older adult should receive adequate analgesia and attentive observation. Discussion of specific management considerations in children and older adults is found in Age-related Considerations.

## Drug Selection

1. Morphine sulfate is often the drug of first choice for severe pain. It is effective, available in various dosage strengths and forms, and useful on a short- or long-term basis, and its adverse effects are well known. In addition, it is a "nonceiling" drug because there is no upper limit to the dosage that can be given to clients who have developed tolerance to previous dosages. This characteristic is especially valuable in clients with severe cancer-related pain because the drug dosage can be increased and titrated to relieve pain when pain increases or tolerance develops. Thus, some clients have safely received extremely large doses. Hydromorphone, levorphanol, and methadone are other nonceiling drugs.

2. When more than one analgesic drug is ordered, use the least potent drug that is effective in relieving pain. For example, use a non-narcotic analgesic, such as acetaminophen, rather than a narcotic analgesic when feasible.

3. Non-narcotic analgesics may be alternated or given concurrently with narcotic analgesics, especially in chronic pain. This increases client comfort, reduces the likelihood of drug abuse and dependence, and decreases tolerance to the pain-relieving effects of the narcotic analgesics.

4. In many instances, the drug preparation of choice may be one that combines a narcotic and a non-narcotic such as acetaminophen (see Table 6-2). The drugs act by different mechanisms and therefore produce greater analgesic effects.

## Route Selection

Narcotic analgesics can be given by several routes, either noninvasively (orally, rectally, or transdermally) or invasively (subcutaneously, intravenously, or by spinal infusion). *When the route is changed (eg, from oral to injection or vice versa), the dose must also be changed to prevent overdosage or underdosage.*

1. Oral drugs are preferred when feasible, and most clients achieve relief with a short-acting or sustained-release oral preparation.

2. IV injection is usually preferred for rapid relief of acute, severe pain. Small, frequent intravenous (IV) doses are often effective in relieving pain with minimal risk for serious adverse effects. This is especially advantageous during a serious illness or after surgery.

   A technique called *patient-controlled analgesia* (PCA) allows self-administration. One device consists of a syringe of diluted drug connected to an IV line and infusion pump; another device uses a specially designed IV bag and special tubing. These devices deliver a dose when the client pushes a button. Some PCA pumps can also deliver a basic amount of analgesic by continuous infusion, with the client injecting additional doses when needed. The amount of drug delivered with each dose and the intervals between doses are preset and limited. PCA requires an alert, cooperative client who can press a button when pain occurs. Studies indicate that analgesia is more effective, client satisfaction is high, and smaller amounts of drug are used than with conventional as-needed (PRN) administration. PCA is especially useful for clients with postoperative pain or high narcotic requirements and provides a more uniform narcotic serum concentration than intermittent dosing methods.

3. Continuous IV infusion may be used to treat severe pain.

4. Two other routes of administration are used to manage acute pain. One route involves injection of narcotic analgesics directly into the CNS through a catheter placed into the epidural or intrathecal space by an anesthesiologist or other health care provider. This method provides effective analgesia while minimizing depressant effects. This type of pain control was developed after opioid receptors were found on neurons in the spinal cord. The other route involves the injection of local anesthetics to provide local or regional analgesia. Both of these methods interrupt the transmission of pain signals and are effective in relieving pain, but they also require special techniques and monitoring procedures for safe use.

   PCA can be administered by the epidural route, and less narcotic analgesic is required for pain relief. Morphine sulfate or fentanyl may be used alone or combined with the local anesthetic bupivacaine.

5. For clients with chronic pain and contraindications to oral or injected medications, some narcotics are available in rectal suppositories or skin patches. Morphine sulfate, oxymorphone, and hydromorphone can be given rectally with similar potencies and half-lives as when given orally. For clients who cannot take oral medications and whose narcotic requirement is too large for rectal administration, the transdermal route is preferred over the IV and subcutaneous routes. A fentanyl skin patch (Duragesic) is effective and commonly used. When first applied, pain relief is delayed approximately 12 hours (as the drug is gradually absorbed). Because of the delayed effects, doses of a short-acting narcotic should be ordered and given as needed during the first 48 hours after the patch is applied. With continued use, the old patch is removed, and a new one is applied approximately every 72 hours. Narcotic overdose can occur with fentanyl patches if the client has fever (hastens drug absorption) or liver impairment (slows drug metabolism).

## Age-related Considerations: Use of Narcotics

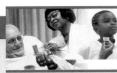

### USE IN CHILDREN

One reason for inadequate prevention and management of pain in newborns has been a common belief that they did not experience pain because of immature nervous systems. However, research indicates that neonates have abundant C fibers and that A-delta fibers are developing during the first few months of life. These are the nerve fibers that carry pain signals from peripheral tissues to the spinal cord. In addition, brain pain centers and the endogenous analgesia system seem to be developed and functional. Endogenous narcotics are released at birth and in response to fetal and neonatal distress such as asphyxia or other difficulty associated with the birth process.

Older infants and children may experience pain even when analgesics have been ordered and are readily available. For example, children may fear injections or may be unable to communicate their discomfort. Health care providers or parents may fear adverse effects of narcotic analgesics, including excessive sedation, respiratory depression, and addiction.

Other than reduced dosage, there have been few guidelines about the use of narcotic analgesics in children. With increased knowledge about pain mechanisms and the recommendations prepared by the Acute Pain Management Guideline Panel in 1992, every nurse who works with children should be able to manage pain effectively. Some specific considerations include the following:

1. Narcotic analgesics administered during labor and delivery may depress fetal and neonatal respiration. The drugs cross the blood–brain barrier of the infant more readily than that of the mother. Therefore, doses that do not depress maternal respiration may profoundly depress the infant's respiration. Respiration should be monitored closely in neonates, and the narcotic antagonist naloxone should be readily available.

2. Expressions of pain may differ according to age and developmental level. Infants may cry and have muscular rigidity and thrashing behavior. Preschoolers may behave aggressively or complain verbally of discomfort. Young school-aged children may express pain verbally or behaviorally, often with regression to behaviors used at younger ages. Adolescents may be reluctant to admit they are uncomfortable or need help. With chronic pain, children of all ages tend to withdraw and regress to an earlier stage of development.

3. The Acute Pain Management Guideline Panel recommends that narcotic analgesics be given by routes (eg, PO, IV, epidurally) other than IM injections because IM injections are painful and frightening for children. For any child receiving parenteral narcotics, vital signs and level of consciousness must be assessed regularly.

4. Narcotic formulations specifically for children are not generally available. When children's doses are calculated from adult doses, the fractions and decimals that often result greatly increase the risk for a dosage error.

5. Narcotic rectal suppositories may be used more often in children than in adults. Although they may be useful when oral or parenteral routes are not indicated, the dose of medication actually received by the child is unknown because drug absorption is erratic and because adult suppositories are sometimes cut in half or otherwise altered.

6. Narcotic effects in children may differ from those expected in adults because of physiologic and pharmacokinetic differences. Assess regularly and be alert for unusual signs and symptoms.

7. Hydromorphone, methadone, oxycodone, and oxymorphone are not recommended for use in children because safety, efficacy, or dosages have not been established.

8. Like adults, children seem more able to cope with pain when they are informed about what is happening to them and are assisted in developing coping strategies. Age-appropriate doll play, a favorite videotape, diversionary activities, and other techniques can be used effectively. However, such techniques should be used in conjunction with adequate analgesia, not as a substitute for pain medication.

### USE IN OLDER ADULTS

Older adults are especially sensitive to respiratory depression, excessive sedation, confusion, and other adverse effects. However, they should receive adequate analgesia, along with vigilant monitoring. Specific recommendations include the following:

1. Use nondrug measures (eg, heat or cold applications, exercise) and non-narcotic analgesics to relieve pain, when effective.

2. When narcotic analgesics are needed, use those with short half-lives (eg, oxycodone or hydromorphone) because they are less likely to accumulate.

3. Start with low doses and increase doses gradually, if necessary.

4. Give the drugs less often than for younger adults because the duration of action may be longer.

5. Monitor carefully for sedation or confusion. Also, monitor voiding and urine output because acute urinary retention is more likely to occur in older adults.

6. Assess older adults for ability to self-administer narcotic analgesics safely. Those with short-term memory loss (common in this population) may require assistance and supervision.

## TABLE 6-2 Selected Combination Narcotic-Acetaminophen Products

| Trade Name/ Dosage Forms | Narcotic Component | Amount of Acetaminophen | Average Adult Dosage Ranges |
|---|---|---|---|
| *Schedule II* | | | |
| **Percocet** | Oxycodone 5 mg | 325 mg | 1 tab q6h |
| **Roxicet** tablets | Oxycodone 5 mg | 325 mg | 1 tab q6h |
| **Roxicet oral solution** | Oxycodone 5 mg | 325 mg | 5 mL q6h |
| **Roxicet 5/500** caplets | Oxycodone 5 mg | 500 mg | 1 cap q6h |
| **Tylox** capsules | Oxycodone 5 mg | 500 mg | 1 cap q6h |
| *Schedule III* | | | |
| **Hydrocet** capsules | Hydrocodone 5 mg | 500 mg | 1–2 tabs q4–6h, up to 8 tabs/d |
| **Lorcet HD** tablets | Hydrocodone 5 mg | 500 mg | 1–2 tabs q4–6h, up to 8 tabs/d |
| **Lorcet Plus** tablets | Hydrocodone 7.5 mg | 650 mg | 1 tab q4–6h |
| **Lorcet 10/650** tablets | Hydrocodone 10 mg | 650 mg | 1 tab q4–6h |
| **Lortab** elixir | Hydrocodone 2.5 mg | 167 mg | 15 mL q4–6h, up to 6 doses/d |
| **Lortab 2.5/500** tablets | Hydrocodone 2.5 mg | 500 mg | 1–2 tabs q4–6h, up to 8 tabs/d |
| **Lortab 5/500** tablets | Hydrocodone 5 mg | 500 mg | 1–2 tabs q4–6h, up to 8 tabs/d |
| **Lortab 7.5/L500** tablets | Hydrocodone 7.5 mg | 500 mg | 1 tab q4–6h |
| **Lortab 10/500** tablets | Hydrocodone 10 mg | 500 mg | 1 tab q4–6h up to 6/d |
| **Tylenol with codeine #2** tablets | Codeine 15 mg | 300 mg | 1–4 tabs q4h |
| **Tylenol with codeine #3** tablets | Codeine 30 mg | 300 mg | 0.5–2 tabs q4h |
| **Tylenol with codeine #4** tablets | Codeine 60 mg | 300 mg | 1 tab q4h |
| **Vicodin** tablets | Hydrocodone 5 g | 500 mg | 1–2 tabs q4–6h, up to 8 tabs/d |
| **Vicodin ES** tablets | Hydrocodone 7.5 mg | 750 mg | 1 tab q4–6h, up to 5 tabs/d |
| **Vicodin HP** tablets | Hydrocodone 10 mg | 660 mg | 1 tab q4–6h |
| *Schedule V* | | | |
| **Tylenol with codeine** elixir | Codeine 12 mg | 120 mg | 15 mL q4h |
| *Non-narcotic* | | | |
| **Ultracet** tablets | Tramadol 37.5 mg | 325 mg | 2 tabs q4–6h, up to 8 tabs/d for 5 days |

## Dosage

Dosages of narcotic analgesics should be sufficient to relieve pain without causing unacceptable adverse effects. Thus, dosages should be individualized according to the type and severity of pain; the client's age, size, and health status; whether the client is opiate naive (has not received sufficient narcotics for development of tolerance) or opiate tolerant (has previously taken narcotics and drug tolerance has developed, so that larger-than-usual doses are needed to relieve pain); whether the client has progressive or worsening disease; and other characteristics that influence responses to pain. Guidelines include the following:

1. Small to moderate doses relieve constant, dull pain; moderate to large doses relieve intermittent, sharp pain caused by trauma or conditions affecting the viscera.
2. When a narcotic analgesic is ordered in variable amounts (eg, 8 to 10 mg of morphine sulfate), give the smaller amount as long as it is effective in relieving pain.
3. Dosages of narcotic analgesics should be reduced for clients who also are receiving other CNS depressants, such as sedating antianxiety, antidepressant, antihistaminic, antipsychotic, or other sedative-type drugs.

4. Dosages often differ according to the route of administration. Oral doses undergo extensive metabolism on their first pass through the liver so that oral doses are usually much larger than injected doses.

## Scheduling

Narcotic analgesics may be given as needed, within designated time limits, or on a regular schedule. Traditionally, the drugs have often been scheduled every 4 to 6 hours PRN. Numerous studies have indicated that such a schedule is often ineffective in managing clients' pain. Because these analgesics are used for moderate to severe pain, they should in general be scheduled to provide effective and consistent pain relief. Some guidelines for scheduling drugs include the following:

1. When analgesics are ordered PRN, have a clearcut system by which the client reports pain or requests medication. The client should know that analgesic drugs have been ordered and will be given promptly when needed. If a drug cannot be given or if administration must be delayed, explain this to the client. In addition, offer or give the drug when indicated by the client's condition rather than waiting for the client to request medication.

2. In acute pain, narcotic analgesics are most effective when given parenterally and at the onset of pain. In chronic, severe pain, narcotic analgesics are most effective when given on a regular schedule, around the clock. To prevent pain recurrence, sleeping clients may need to be awakened to take their medication.

3. When needed, analgesics should be given before coughing and deep-breathing exercises, dressing changes, and other therapeutic and diagnostic procedures.

4. Narcotics are not recommended for prolonged periods except for advanced malignant disease. Health care agencies usually have an automatic "stop order" for narcotics after 48 to 72 hours; this means that the drug is discontinued when the time limit expires if the health care provider does not reorder it.

## ▨ INDIVIDUAL DRUGS

The two main subgroups of narcotic analgesics are agonists and agonists/antagonists. Agonists include morphine sulfate and morphine sulfate–like drugs. These agents have activity at mu and kappa opioid receptors and thus produce prototypical opioid effects. The agonists/antagonists have agonist activity at some receptors and antagonist activity at other receptors. Because of their agonist activity, they are strong analgesics with a lower abuse potential than pure agonists; because of their antagonist activity, they may produce withdrawal symptoms in people with opiate dependence. In addition, numerous combinations of a narcotic and acetaminophen, a non-narcotic analgesic (see Chap. 7), are available and commonly used in both inpatient and outpatient health care settings. Narcotic antagonists are antidote drugs that reverse the effects of narcotic agonists. Individual drugs are described later; trade names and dosages are listed in Drugs at a Glance 6-1: Narcotic Analgesics, and Drugs at a Glance 6-2: Narcotic Antagonists (Antidotes).

## Agonists

Morphine sulfate, the prototype, is a naturally occurring opium alkaloid used mainly to relieve severe acute or chronic pain. However, many health care providers do not use it in clients with pain from pancreatic or biliary tract disease because of its spasm-producing effects. It is a Schedule II narcotic that is given orally and parenterally. Client response depends on route and dosage. Specific characteristics of the drug are found in Prototype Profile 6-1: Morphine Sulfate. The drug and its active metabolite accumulate in clients with impaired liver or kidney function and may cause prolonged sedation if dosage is not reduced. Older adults may also need small doses.

Oral administration of morphine sulfate is common for chronic pain associated with cancer. When given orally, relatively high doses are required because part of each dose is metabolized in the liver and never reaches the systemic circulation. Concentrated solutions (eg, Roxanol, which contains 20 mg morphine sulfate/mL) and controlled-release tablets (eg, MS Contin, which contains 30 mg/tablet) have been developed for oral administration of these high doses.

In some cases of severe pain that cannot be controlled by other methods, morphine sulfate is administered as a continuous IV infusion. Other routes of administration include epidural, in which the drug is instilled through a catheter placed in the epidural space and slowly diffuses into the spinal cord, and intrathecal, in which the drug is injected directly into the spinal cord. Epidural and intrathecal morphine sulfate provide pain relief with very small doses, once or twice daily. When clients cannot take oral medications and injections are undesirable, rectal suppositories are often given.

**Alfentanil** (Alfenta), **fentanyl** (Sublimaze), **remifentanil** (Ultiva), and **sufentanil** (Sufenta) are potent drugs with a short duration of action. They are most often used in anesthesia (see Appendix D) as analgesic adjuncts or primary anesthetic agents in open-heart surgery or complicated neurologic and orthopedic procedures.

Fentanyl also is used for preanesthetic medication, postoperative analgesia, and chronic pain that requires a narcotic analgesic. A transmucosal formulation (Fentanyl Oralet, also called a lozenge or "lollipop") is available for conscious sedation or anesthesia premedication in children and adults. Because of a high risk for respiratory depression, recommended dosages must not be exceeded, and the drug should be given only in an area with staff and equipment for emergency care (eg, intensive care

**DRUG TABLE 6-1**

*Drugs at a Glance*

**Narcotic Analgesics**

| Generic/Trade Name | Routes and Dosage Ranges | Comments |
|---|---|---|
| **Agonists**<br>**Alfentanil** (Alfenta)<br>Pregnancy Category C | *Adults:* Analgesic adjunct in general anesthesia; IV initial dose, 8–50 mcg/kg; maintenance injection, 3–5 mcg/kg; maintenance infusion, 0.5–1 mcg/kg/min<br>Anesthesia induction; IV injection, 130–245 mcg/kg over 3 min or IV infusion 50–75 mcg/kg<br>Anesthesia maintenance; IV infusion, 0.5–3 mcg/kg/min | Therapeutic serum reference range 100–340 ng/mL<br>Drug is titrated to desired response within a wide range of doses; reflects degree of desired analgesia and anesthesia |
| **Codeine**<br>Pregnancy Category C; D with prolonged use or at term | *Adults:* Pain: PO, Sub-Q, IM, 15–60 mg q4–6h PRN; usual dose 30 mg; maximum, 360 mg/24 h<br>Cough: PO 10–20 mg q4h PRN; maximum, 120 mg/24 h<br>*Children:* 1 y or older, Pain: PO, Sub-Q, IM 0.5 mg/kg q4–6h PRN<br>6–12 y, Cough: PO, 5–10 mg q4–6h; maximum, 60 mg/24 h<br>2–6 y, Cough: PO, 2.5–5 mg q4–6h; maximum, 30 mg/24 h | Therapeutic reference range not established; toxicity occurs at greater than 1.1 mcg/mL |
| **Fentanyl** (Actiq, Duragesic, Sublimaze)<br>Pregnancy Category C; D with prolonged use or at term | *Adults:* Preanesthetic sedation; IM, 0.05–0.1 mg 30–60 min before surgery; oral lozenge, 200–400 mcg, 20–40 min before a procedure, with instructions to suck, not chew, the medication. Maximum dose of oral lozenge, 400 mcg<br>Analgesic adjunct to general anesthesia; IV, total dose of 0.002–0.05 mg/kg, depending on the surgical procedure<br>Adjunct to regional anesthesia; IM or slow IV (over 1–2 min), 0.05–0.1 mg PRN<br>Postoperative analgesia; IM, 0.05–0.1 mg, repeat in 1–2 h if needed<br>General anesthesia; IV, 0.05–0.1 mg/kg with oxygen and a muscle relaxant (maximum dose, 0.15 mg/kg with open-heart surgery, other major surgeries, and complicated neurologic or orthopedic procedures)<br>Chronic pain, transdermal system, 2.5–10 mg every 72 h<br>*Children:* Weight at least 10 kg: Conscious sedation or preanesthetic sedation, 5–15 mcg/kg of body weight (100–400 mcg), depending on weight, type of procedure, and other factors. Maximum dose, 400 mcg, regardless of age and weight<br>2–12 y: General anesthesia induction and maintenance, IV 2–3 mcg/kg | Oral lozenge (Actiq) has 2 g of sugar per unit, so that serum glucose level may be affected<br>Clinical effects of transdermal patch can continue 12 hours or more after discontinuing product; caregiver should wear gloves and avoid touching while applying patch; if accidental contact occurs, do not use alcohol or soap because this increases absorption; keep all preparations out of the hands of children |

*(continued)*

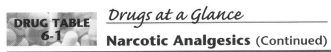

**DRUG TABLE
6-1**

## *Drugs at a Glance*

## Narcotic Analgesics (Continued)

| Generic/Trade Name | Routes and Dosage Ranges | Comments |
|---|---|---|
| **Hydromorphone** (Dilaudid)<br>Pregnancy Category B; D with prolonged use or high doses at term | *Adults:* PO, 2–4 mg q4–6h PRN<br>IM, Sub-Q, IV 1–2 mg q4–6h PRN (may be increased to 4 mg for severe pain)<br>Rectal suppository 3 mg q6–8h<br>*Children:* Dosage not established | As with all narcotics, monitor for pain relief, respiratory status, level of consciousness, and blood pressure |
| **Levorphanol** (Levo-Dromoran)<br>Pregnancy Category B; D with prolonged use or high doses at term | *Adults:* PO or Sub-Q, 2–3 mg q4–6h PRN<br>*Children:* Dosage not established | Dosage reduction is necessary in clients with liver disease |
| **Meperidine** (Demerol)<br>Pregnancy Category B; D with prolonged use or high doses at term | *Adults:* IM, IV, Sub-Q, PO 50–100 mg q2–4h<br>Obstetric analgesia, IM, Sub-Q, 50–100 mg q2–4h for three or four doses<br>*Children:* IM, Sub-Q, PO 1.1–1.75 mg/kg, up to adult dose, q3–4h | Should not be used in clients with renal impairment because a toxic metabolite, normeperidine, may accumulate. Normeperidine is pharmacologically active and is a CNS stimulant that may cause muscle spasms, seizures, and psychosis. Narcotic antagonists such as naloxone do not reverse these effects. |
| **Methadone** (Dolophine)<br>Pregnancy Category B; D with prolonged use or high doses at term | *Adults:* IM, Sub-Q, PO 2.5–10 mg q3–4h PRN<br>*Children:* Not recommended, lack of data | Therapeutic reference range: 100 to 400 ng/mL; toxicity: >2 mcg/mL<br>Oral tablets must not be used for injection |
| **Morphine sulfate** (MSIR, MS Contin, Roxanol others) | See Prototype Profile 6-1: Morphine Sulfate | |
| **Oxycodone** (OxyContin, Roxicodone, others)<br>Pregnancy Category B; D with prolonged use or high doses at term | *Adults:* PO, immediate release, 5 mg q6h PRN (OxyIR, Oxydose, OxyFAST); 10–30 mg q4h PRN for other formulations PO, controlled release, 10 mg q12h, increased if necessary<br>*Children:* Not recommended for children <12 y | Do not crush controlled-release tablets |
| **Oxymorphone** (Numorphan)<br>Pregnancy Category B; D with prolonged use or high doses at term | *Adults:* IM, Sub-Q, 1–1.5 mg q4–6h PRN IV, 0.5 mg q4–6h PRN<br>Rectal, 5 mg q4–6h PRN<br>Obstetric analgesia, IM 0.5–1 mg<br>*Children:* Dosage not established | Refrigerate suppository |
| **Propoxyphene** (Darvon)<br>Pregnancy Category C; D with prolonged use | Propoxyphene hydrochloride<br>*Adults:* PO, 65 mg q4h PRN (maximal daily dose, 390 mg)<br>*Children:* Not recommended<br>Propoxyphene napsylate<br>*Adults:* PO, 100 mg q4h PRN (maximal daily dose, 600 mg)<br>*Children:* Not recommended for use | Therapeutic reference range: 0.1–0.4 mcg/mL; toxicity: >0.5 mcg/mL<br>Recognized as a primary cause of drug-related deaths<br>Causes a false-positive test for methadone |
| **Remifentanil** (Ultiva)<br>Pregnancy Category C | *Adults:* Anesthesia induction, IV infusion, 0.5–1.0 mcg/kg/min<br>*Children:* ≥ 2y: Same as adults | Short duration of action; not appropriate as the sole agent for induction of anesthesia |

*(continued)*

**DRUG TABLE 6-1**

## *Drugs at a Glance*

### Narcotic Analgesics (Continued)

| Generic/Trade Name | Routes and Dosage Ranges | Comments |
|---|---|---|
| **Sufentanil** (Sufenta)<br>Pregnancy Category C | *Adults:* Analgesic adjunct to general anesthesia, IV initial dose, 1–8 mcg/kg; maintenance, 10–25 mcg PRN<br>General anesthesia, IV induction, 8–30 mcg/kg; maintenance, 10–25 mcg PRN<br>*Children:* <12 y: Anesthesia, 10–20 mcg/kg (total dosage) for induction and maintenance | Clients may manifest rebound postoperative respiratory depression |
| **Tramadol** (Ultram)<br>Pregnancy Category C | *Adults:* PO 50–100 mg q4–6h PRN (maximum, 400 mg/day)<br>Renal impairment (creatinine clearance, <30 mL/min): PO 50–100 mg q12h (maximum dose, 200 mg/day)<br>Hepatic impairment (cirrhosis): PO 50 mg q12h<br>*Older adults* (65–75 y): Same as adults, unless they also have renal or hepatic impairment<br>*Older adults* (>75 y): <300 mg daily, in divided doses<br>*Children:* Dosage not established | Serum level monitoring is not necessary though reference range is 100–300 ng/mL<br>Observe ranges for hepatic and renal impairment |
| *Agonists/Antagonists* | | |
| **Buprenorphine** (Buprenex, Subutex)<br>Pregnancy Category C | *Adults:* IM or slow IV (over 2 min) 0.3 mg q6h PRN<br>*Children:* Dosage not established | Withdrawal has been observed in infants of mothers who received drug during pregnancy |
| **Butorphanol** (Stadol)<br>Pregnancy Category C; D with prolonged use or high doses at term | *Adults:* IM, IV, 1–4 mg q3–4h PRN<br>Nasal spray, 1 mg (one spray in one nostril) q3–4h PRN<br>*Older adults:* IM, 1–2 mg q6–8h PRN<br>Renal or hepatic impairment IM 1–2 mg q6–8h<br>*Children:* Not recommended for children younger than 18 years of age | Therapeutic reference range: 0.7–1.5 ng/mL<br>Nasal spray can be used for severe pain associated with migraines; concomitant use of other migraine nasal sprays should be avoided or administration should be separated by 30 min |
| **Nalbuphine** (Nubain)<br>Pregnancy Category B; D with prolonged use or high doses at term | *Adults:* IM, IV, Sub-Q, 10 mg/70 kg q3–6h PRN<br>*Children:* Not recommended | Should reduce dosage in hepatic failure |
| **Pentazocine** (Talwin, Talwin NX)<br>Pregnancy Category B; D with prolonged use or high doses at term | PO, 50–100 mg q3–4h (maximum, 600 mg/day)<br>IM, Sub-Q, IV 30–60 mg q3–4h (maximum, 360 mg/day)<br>*Children:* Not recommended for children <12 y | Talwin NX contains naloxone to prevent abuse by using dissolved drug as injection |

unit, operating room, emergency room). As with other routes of administration, dosage of the oral lozenge should be individualized according to age, weight, illness, other medications, type of procedure and anesthesia, and other factors. A transdermal formulation (Duragesic) is used in the treatment of chronic pain. The active drug is deposited in the skin and slowly absorbed systemically. Thus, the skin patches have a slow onset of action (12 to 24 hours), but they last 3 days. When a patch is removed, the drug continues to be absorbed from the skin deposits for 24 hours or longer.

**Codeine** is a naturally occurring opium alkaloid, Schedule II drug used for analgesic and antitussive effects. Codeine produces weaker analgesic and antitussive effects and milder adverse effects than morphine sulfate. Compared with other narcotic analgesics, codeine is more

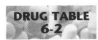

**DRUG TABLE 6-2**

*Drugs at a Glance*

## Narcotic Antagonists (Antidotes)

| Generic/Trade Name | Routes and Dosage Ranges | Comments |
|---|---|---|
| **Nalmefene** (Revex)<br>Pregnancy Category B | Reversal of postoperative narcotic depression: (*blue label*, 1-mL ampules containing 100 mcg) IV according to body weight (50 kg, 0.125 mL; 60 kg, 0.15 mL; 70 kg, 0.175 mL; 80 kg, 0.2 mL; 90 kg, 0.225 mL; 100 kg, 0.25 mL)<br>Treatment of overdose: (*green label*, 2-mL ampules containing 1 mg) IV 0.5 mg/70 kg as initial dose for clients who are not narcotic dependent, followed by 1 mg/70 kg in 2–5 min if necessary. For known or suspected narcotic-dependent people, give a test dose of 0.1 mg/70 kg. If no signs of opiate withdrawal occur within 2 min, proceed with the above dosage. | Has a longer duration of action than naloxone<br>May be preferred when narcotic depression results from long-acting drugs (eg, methadone)<br>**Warning:** Nalmefene is available in two concentrations: one for postoperative use (*blue label*) and one for treatment of clients with opiate overdoses (*green label*). Health care personnel *must* use the appropriate concentration for the intended purpose. |
| **Naloxone** (Narcan)<br>Pregnancy Category B | *Adults:* Overdose, IV 0.4–2 mg, repeat q2–3min PRN<br>Give IM or Sub-Q, if unable to give IV<br>Postoperative reversal, IV 0.1–0.2 mg q2–3min until desired level of reversal is attained<br>*Children:* IV 0.01 mg/kg initially, repeated q2–3min PRN. Give IM or Sub-Q, if unable to give IV | Usually the drug of choice for treatment of narcotic overdose<br>Therapeutic effects occur in minutes after injection and last 1–2 h<br>Has a shorter duration of action than most narcotics, so repeat injections are usually needed (up to 2–3 d with methadone)<br>Causes few adverse effects, and repeated doses can be given safely |
| **Naltrexone** (ReVia)<br>Pregnancy Category B | PO, 50 mg/day | Clients taking this drug do not respond to narcotic analgesics if pain control is needed<br>Used in the maintenance of opiate-free states in opiate addicts<br>Recommended for use in conjunction with psychological and social counseling |

effective when given orally and is less likely to lead to abuse and dependence. Injected drug is more effective than oral drug in relieving pain, but onset (15 to 30 minutes), peak (30 to 60 minutes), and duration of action (4 to 6 hours) are about the same. Half-life is about 3 hours. Larger doses are required for analgesic than for antitussive effects. Codeine is often given with acetaminophen for additive analgesic effects.

Codeine is metabolized to morphine sulfate, which is responsible for its analgesic effects, by the cytochrome P450 2D6 family of enzymes. Up to 10% of whites, Asians, and African Americans have inadequate amounts or activity of the 2D6 enzymes and may therefore receive less pain relief with usual therapeutic doses.

**Hydrocodone,** which is similar to codeine in its analgesic and antitussive effects, is a Schedule III drug. It is available in oral combination products for cough and with acetaminophen or ibuprofen for pain. Its half-life is about 4 hours, and its duration of action is 4 to 6 hours. Hydrocodone is metabolized to hydromorphone by the cytochrome P450 2D6 enzymes.

**Hydromorphone** (Dilaudid) is a semisynthetic derivative of morphine sulfate that has the same actions, uses, contraindications, and adverse effects as morphine sulfate. It is more potent on a milligram basis and relatively more effective orally than morphine sulfate. Effects occur in 15 to 30 minutes, peak in 30 to 90 minutes, and last 4 to 5 hours. It produces less euphoria, nausea, and pruri-

## PROTOTYPE PROFILE 6-1

### P Morphine Sulfate (MOR feen SUL fate)

**Drug Class**
*Chemical:* opioid
*Functional:* analgesic; narcotic

**Trade Names**
Astramorph PF, Duramorph, MS Contin, Oramorph SR, Roxanol, and others

**Therapeutic Indications**
Relief of moderate to severe acute and chronic pain; relief of pain associated with myocardial infarction; relief of dyspnea in pulmonary edema

**Pharmacokinetics**
Oral and parenteral effectiveness varies with chronic use

*Absorption*
variable

*Distribution*
binds to opioid receptors in the CNS and periphery; plasma protein binding: 30%.

*Metabolism*
hepatic; significant first-pass effects limit bioavailability orally

*Excretion*
active metabolites that are excreted by the kidneys

**Pharmacodynamics**
*Onset of Action (maximal analgesia and respiratory depression):*
IV, 10–20 min
IM, 30 minutes
Sub-Q, 60–90 minutes
PO, 60 minutes

*Duration*
5–7 h

**Contraindications**
Hypersensitivity to morphine sulfate, increased intracranial pressure

**Pregnancy Considerations**
Category: B/D (with high doses at term or with prolonged use)
Enters breast milk, use with caution

**Dosage**
Titrated to pain relief and prevention
*Adults:* PO immediate-release, 5–30 mg q4h PRN
PO controlled-release, 30 mg q8–12h
IM, Sub-Q, 5–20 mg/70 kg q4h PRN
IV injection, 2–10 mg/70 kg, diluted in 5 mL water for injection and injected slowly, over 5 min, PRN
IV continuous infusion, 0.1–1 mg/mL in 5% dextrose in water, by controlled infusion pump
Epidurally, 2–5 mg/24 h; Intrathecally, 0.2–1 mg/24 h
Rectal, 10–20 mg q4h
*Children:* IM, Sub-Q, 0.05–0.2 mg/kg (up to 15 mg) q4h

**Adverse Effects**
Respiratory depression, physical and psychological dependence, antidiuretic hormone (ADH) release, pruritus, constipation, flushing

**Drug Interactions**
*Increased Effects*
Effect/toxicity with CNS depressants and ethanol
Analgesic effect with dextroamphetamine
Adverse effects with concurrent use of monoamine oxidase (MAO) inhibitors and meperidine

*Decreased Effects*
Diuretic effects (due to ADH release)

**Herbal Supplements and Dietary Considerations**
Avoid St. John's wort, valerian, kava kava, gotu cola
May irritate stomach; oral administration with food (except Oramorph SR) may increase bioavailability, so be consistent in taking with or without food

---

tus than morphine sulfate when given epidurally. Hydromorphone is metabolized in the liver to inactive metabolites that are excreted through the kidneys.

**Levorphanol** (Levo-Dromoran) is a synthetic drug with the same uses and adverse effects as morphine sulfate, although some reports indicate less nausea and vomiting. The average dose is probably equianalgesic with 10 mg of morphine sulfate. Maximal analgesia occurs 60 to 90 minutes after subcutaneous injection. Effects last 4 to 8 hours.

**Meperidine** (Demerol) is a synthetic drug that is similar to morphine sulfate in pharmacologic actions. An injection of 80 to 100 mg is equivalent to 10 mg of morphine sulfate. After injection, analgesia occurs in 10 to 20 minutes, peaks in 1 hour, and lasts 2 to 4 hours. Oral

meperidine is only half as effective as a parenteral dose because approximately half is metabolized in the liver and never reaches the systemic circulation. Compared with morphine sulfate, meperidine produces similar sedation and respiratory depression but has a shorter duration of action, requires more frequent administration, has little antitussive effect, causes less respiratory depression in newborns when used for obstetric analgesia, causes less smooth muscle spasm, and is preferred in renal and biliary colic.

A unique feature of meperidine is that a neurotoxic metabolite (normeperidine) accumulates with chronic use, large doses, or renal failure. Normeperidine also accumulates more rapidly in patients who have taken drugs that induce hepatic drug-metabolizing enzymes (eg, phenytoin, isoniazid, rifampin) because faster metabolism of meperidine produces more normeperidine. Accumulation produces CNS stimulation characterized by agitation, convulsions, hallucinations, and tremors. The half-life of normeperidine is 15 to 30 hours, depending on renal function, and the effects of normeperidine are not reversible with narcotic antagonist drugs.

As a result of these factors, the use of this once popular drug has greatly declined in recent years. Now, meperidine is recommended for short-term use in healthy individuals and is contraindicated for treatment of cancer pain, which often requires progressively higher doses over a long period of time. It is also contraindicated in patients who have taken amphetamines or monoamine oxidase inhibitor drugs (eg, phenelzine) within the past 21 days because this can precipitate a fatal syndrome (called *serotonin syndrome*) of excitation, high fever, and seizures.

**Methadone** (Dolophine) is a synthetic drug similar to morphine sulfate. Compared with morphine sulfate, methadone has a longer duration of action and is relatively more effective when given orally. It is usually given orally, with which onset and peak of action occur in 30 to 60 minutes. Effects last 4 to 6 hours initially and longer with repeated use. Half-life is 15 to 30 hours, which also lengthens with repeated use. Methadone is used for severe pain and in the detoxification and maintenance treatment of opiate addicts.

**Oxycodone** (Roxicodone, others) is a semisynthetic derivative of codeine used to relieve moderate pain. It is less potent and less likely to produce dependence than morphine sulfate but is more potent and more likely to produce dependence than codeine. It is a Schedule II drug of abuse. Pharmacologic actions are similar to those of other narcotic analgesics. Action starts in 15 to 30 minutes, peaks in 60 minutes, and lasts 4 to 6 hours. Its half-life is unknown. It is metabolized by the cytochrome P450 2D6 enzymes and excreted through the kidneys.

Oxycodone has been widely used for many years, often in combination with aspirin or acetaminophen. It is also available alone in oral, immediate-release tablets and solutions. A few years ago, controlled-release tablets (OxyContin) in 10-, 20-, 40-, 80-, and 160-mg sizes were marketed for extended treatment of moderate to severe pain (the 80- and 160-mg tablets should be used only by patients who have developed drug tolerance through long-term use of lesser doses). When given every 12 hours, the tablets could relieve pain around the clock. These effects are very advantageous to patients with terminal cancer or other chronically painful conditions. However, OxyContin soon became a popular drug of abuse, leading to dozens of deaths and much criminal activity. Most deaths have resulted from inappropriate use (ie, not legally prescribed for the user) and by crushing and snorting or injecting the drug. Crushing destroys the long-acting feature and constitutes an overdose. Subsequently, the manufacturer and the U.S. Food and Drug Adminis-

tration (FDA) have issued precautions for prescribing OxyContin and warnings not to crush the product. Some people have proposed taking the drug off the market.

**Oxymorphone** (Numorphan) is a semisynthetic derivative of morphine sulfate. Its actions, uses, and adverse effects are similar to those of morphine sulfate, except that it has little antitussive effect. It is available as a solution for injection and as a rectal suppository. With injection, action starts in 5 to 10 minutes, peaks in 30 to 60 minutes, and lasts 3 to 6 hours.

**Propoxyphene** (Darvon) is a synthetic, Schedule IV drug that is chemically related to methadone. It is used for mild to moderate pain but is considered no more effective than 650 mg of aspirin or acetaminophen, with which it is usually given. Propoxyphene is abused (alone and with alcohol or other CNS depressant drugs), and deaths have occurred from overdoses. In addition, its metabolism produces an active metabolite, norpropoxyphene, which is eliminated in urine. Norpropoxyphene is not a narcotic but it has a long half-life and accumulates with repeated administration of propoxyphene. Accumulation is associated with dysrhythmias and pulmonary edema; there have also been reports of apnea, cardiac arrest, and death. Norpropoxyphene cannot be effectively removed by hemodialysis, and naloxone, a narcotic antagonist, does not reverse its effects.

As a result of these characteristics, propoxyphene is not recommended for use in children, clients at risk for suicide or addiction, or older adults, or for long-term use. Despite these characteristics, dangers, and warnings from authoritative clinicians, the drug continues to be prescribed.

**Tramadol** (Ultram) is an oral, synthetic, centrally active analgesic for moderate to severe pain. It is effective and well tolerated in older adults and people with acute or chronic pain, back pain, fibromyalgia, osteoarthritis, and neuropathic pain. Because it has a low potential for producing tolerance and abuse, it may be used for the long-term management of chronic pain. It is not chemically related to opioids and is not a controlled drug. Its mechanism of action is unclear but includes binding to mu opioid receptors and inhibiting reuptake of norepinephrine and serotonin in the brain, actions that interfere with pain transmission. Analgesia occurs within 1 hour after administration and peaks in 2 to 3 hours. Tramadol causes significantly less respiratory depression than morphine sulfate but may cause other morphine sulfate–like adverse effects (eg, drowsiness, nausea, constipation, pruritus, orthostatic hypotension).

Tramadol is well absorbed after oral administration, even if taken with food. It is minimally bound (20%) to plasma proteins, and its half-life is 6 to 7 hours. It is metabolized by the cytochrome P450 3A4 and 2D6 enzymes and forms an active metabolite. Approximately 30% of a dose is excreted unchanged in the urine, and 60% is excreted as metabolites. Dosage should be reduced in people with renal or hepatic impairment. Tramadol is available in oral tablets alone and in combination with acetaminophen.

## Agonists/Antagonists

These agents have agonist activity at some receptors and antagonist activity at others. Because of their agonist activity, they are potent analgesics with a lower abuse potential than pure agonists; because of their antagonist activity, they may produce withdrawal symptoms in people with opiate dependence.

**Buprenorphine** (Buprenex) is a semisynthetic, Schedule V narcotic with a long duration of action and a low incidence of causing physical dependence. These characteristics are attributed to its high affinity for and slow dissociation from mu receptors. With intramuscular administration, analgesia occurs in 15 minutes, peaks in 60 minutes, and lasts approximately 6 hours. Buprenorphine may also be given intravenously. It is highly protein bound (96%) and has an elimination half-life of 2 to 3 hours. It is metabolized in the liver, and clearance is related to hepatic blood flow. It is excreted mainly in feces. Adverse effects include dizziness, sedation, hypoventilation, hypotension, and nausea and vomiting. Symptoms of narcotic withdrawal occur infrequently with coadministered narcotics.

**Butorphanol** (Stadol) is a synthetic, Schedule IV agonist similar to morphine sulfate and meperidine in analgesic effects and ability to cause respiratory depression. It is used in moderate to severe pain and is given parenterally or topically to nasal mucosa by a metered spray (Stadol NS). After IM or IV administration, analgesia peaks in 30 to 60 minutes. After nasal application, analgesia peaks within 1 to 2 hours. Butorphanol also has antagonist activity and therefore should not be given to people who have been receiving narcotic analgesics or who have narcotic dependence. Other adverse effects include drowsiness and nausea and vomiting. Butorphanol is not recommended for use in children younger than 18 years of age.

**Nalbuphine** (Nubain) is a synthetic analgesic used for moderate to severe pain. It is not a controlled drug. It is given intravenously, intramuscularly, or subcutaneously. After IV injection, action starts in 2 to 3 minutes, peaks in 15 to 20 minutes, and lasts 3 to 6 hours. After intramuscular or subcutaneous injection, action begins in less than 15 minutes, peaks in 30 to 60 minutes, and lasts 3 to 6 hours. Half-life is 5 hours. The most common adverse effect is sedation. Others include dizziness, sweating, headache, and psychotic symptoms, but these are reportedly minimal at doses of 10 mg or less.

**Pentazocine** (Talwin) is a synthetic, Schedule IV analgesic drug of abuse and may produce physical and psychological dependence. It is used for the same clinical indications as other strong analgesics and causes similar adverse effects. Recommended doses for analgesia are less effective than usual doses of morphine sulfate or meperidine, but some people may tolerate pentazocine better than morphine sulfate or meperidine. Parenteral pentazocine usually produces analgesia within 10 to 30 minutes and lasts 2 to 3 hours. Adverse effects include hallucinations, bizarre dreams or nightmares, depression, nervousness, feelings of depersonalization, extreme euphoria, tissue damage with ulceration and necrosis or fibrosis at injection sites with long-term use, and respiratory depression.

Oral pentazocine tablets contain naloxone 0.5 mg, a narcotic antagonist that prevents the effects of pentazocine if the oral tablet is injected. It has no pharmacologic action if taken orally. Naloxone was added to prevent a method of abuse in which oral tablets of pentazocine and tripelennamine, an antihistamine, were dissolved and injected intravenously. The mixture caused pulmonary emboli and stroke (from obstruction of blood vessels by talc and other insoluble ingredients in the tablets). Pentazocine is not recommended for use.

## Narcotic Antagonists

Narcotic antagonists reverse or block analgesia, CNS and respiratory depression, and other physiologic effects of narcotic agonists. They compete with opioids for opioid receptor sites in the brain and thereby prevent opioid binding with receptors or displace opioids already occupying receptor sites. When a narcotic cannot bind to receptor sites, it is "neutralized" and cannot exert its effects on body cells. Narcotic antagonists do not relieve the depressant effects of other drugs, such as sedative-hypnotic, antianxiety, and antipsychotic agents. The chief clinical use of these drugs is to relieve CNS and respiratory depression induced by therapeutic doses or overdoses of narcotics. The drugs are also used to reverse postoperative narcotic depression, and naltrexone is approved for the treatment of narcotic and alcohol dependence. These drugs produce withdrawal symptoms when given to narcotic-dependent people.

**Naloxone** (Narcan), **nalmefene** (Revex), and **naltrexone** (ReVia) are structurally and pharmacologically similar. Naloxone is the oldest and has long been the drug of choice in respiratory depression known or thought to be caused by a narcotic drug. Therapeutic effects occur within minutes after IV, intramuscular, or subcutaneous injection and last 1 to 2 hours. Naloxone has a shorter duration of action than narcotics, and repeated injections are usually needed. For a long-acting drug such as methadone, injections may be needed for 2 to 3 days. Naloxone produces few adverse effects, and repeated injections can be given safely. This drug should be readily available in all health care settings where narcotics are given. Nalmefene is a newer agent whose main difference from naloxone is a longer duration of action. It may be preferred when narcotic depression results from long-acting drugs such as methadone. Nalmefene is available in two concentrations: one for postoperative use and one for treatment of clients with narcotic overdoses. Health care personnel must use the appropriate concentration for the intended purpose. Naltrexone is used in the maintenance of opiate-free states in opiate addicts. It is apparently effective in highly motivated, detoxified people. If given before the client is detoxified, acute withdrawal symptoms occur. Clients receiving naltrexone do not respond to analgesics if pain control is needed. The drug is recommended for use in conjunction with psychological and social counseling.

## Dietary and Herbal Supplements

**Capsaicin** (Zostrix), a product derived from cayenne chili peppers, is applied topically to the skin to relieve pain associated with osteoarthritis, rheumatoid arthritis, postherpetic neuralgia after a herpes zoster infection (shingles), diabetic neuropathy, postsurgical pain (including pain after mastectomy and amputation), and other neuropathic pain and complex pain syndromes. Its analgesic effects are attributed to depletion in nerve endings of substance P, which is thought to be a mediator in the transmission of painful stimuli from peripheral tissues to the spinal cord. An additional analgesic effect may result from interference with production of prostaglandins and leukotrienes.

Capsaicin is available in a gel, creams, and lotions in concentrations ranging from 0.025% to 0.25%, for topical application to the skin. It is most effective when applied 3 or 4 times daily; effects last about 4 to 5 hours. Less frequent application produces less effective analgesia. The main adverse effects are itching and stinging, which decrease with continued use.

Capsaicin also is the active ingredient in a popular nonlethal self-defense spray (pepper spray).

## ■ DRUG USE IN SPECIFIC SITUATIONS

## Cancer

When narcotic analgesics are required in chronic pain associated with malignancy, the main consideration is client comfort, not preventing drug addiction. Effective treatment requires that pain be relieved and prevented from recurring. With disease progression and the development of drug tolerance, extremely large doses and frequent administration may be required. The nurse also must be proficient in using and teaching various routes of drug administration and in arranging regimens with potentially very large doses and various combinations of drugs. Additional guidelines include the following:

1. Analgesics should be given on a regular schedule, around the clock. Clients should be awakened, if necessary, to prevent pain recurrence.

2. Oral, rectal, and transdermal routes of administration are generally preferred over injections.

3. A non-narcotic analgesic (see Chap. 7) may be used alone for mild pain.

4. Oxycodone or codeine can be used for moderate pain, often with a non-narcotic analgesic. A combination of the two types of drugs produces additive analgesic effects and may allow smaller doses of the narcotic.

5. Morphine sulfate or another strong narcotic is given for severe pain. Although the dose of morphine sulfate can be titrated upward for adequate analgesia, unacceptable adverse effects (eg, excessive sedation, respiratory depression, nausea and vomiting) may limit the dose. The oral route of administration is preferred; the initial oral dosage of morphine sulfate is usually 10 to 20 mg every 3 to 4 hours.

6. When long-acting forms of narcotic analgesics are being given on a regular schedule (eg, sustained-release forms of morphine sulfate or fentanyl skin patches), fast-acting forms also need to be ordered and available for "breakthrough" pain. If additional doses are needed frequently, the baseline dose of long-acting medication may need to be increased.

7. In addition to narcotic analgesics, other drugs may be used to increase client comfort. For example, tricyclic antidepressants (TCAs) have analgesic effects, especially in neuropathic pain. Lower doses of TCAs are required for analgesia than for depression, but analgesic effects may not occur for 2 to 3 weeks. Antiemetics may be given for nausea and vomiting; laxatives or stool softeners should be used along with a bowel program to prevent or relieve constipation because tolerance does not develop to the constipating effects of narcotics.

## Biliary, Renal, or Ureteral Colic

When narcotic analgesics are used to relieve the acute, severe pain associated with various types of colic, an antispasmodic drug such as atropine may be needed as well. Narcotic analgesics may increase smooth muscle tone and cause spasm. Atropine does not have strong antispasmodic properties of its own in usual doses, but it reduces the spasm-producing effects of narcotic analgesics.

### Postoperative Use

When analgesics are used postoperatively, the goal is to relieve pain without excessive sedation so that clients can do deep-breathing exercises, cough, ambulate, and implement other measures to promote recovery.

### Burns

In severely burned clients, narcotic analgesics should be used cautiously. A common cause of respiratory arrest in burned clients is excessive administration of analgesics. Agitation in a burned person usually should be interpreted as hypoxia or hypovolemia rather than pain, until proved otherwise. When narcotic analgesics are necessary,

## ᴺURSING PROCESS

### Assessment

Pain is a subjective experience (whatever the person says it is), and humans display a wide variety of responses. Although pain thresholds (the point at which a tissue-damaging stimulus produces a sensation of pain) are similar, people differ in their perceptions, behaviors, and tolerance of pain. Differences in pain perception may result from psychological components. Stressors such as anxiety, depression, fatigue, anger, and fear tend to increase pain; rest, mood elevation, and diversionary activities tend to decrease pain. Differences in behaviors may or may not indicate pain to observers, and overt signs and symptoms are not reliable indicators of the presence or extent of pain. Especially with chronic pain, overt signs and symptoms may be absent. Differences in tolerance of pain (the amount or duration of pain a person is willing to suffer before seeking relief) often reflect the person's concern about the meaning of the pain and the type or intensity of the painful stimulus. Thus, pain is a complex physiologic, psychological, and sociocultural phenomenon that must be thoroughly assessed if it is to be managed effectively.

The nurse must assess every client in relation to pain, initially to determine appropriate interventions and later to determine whether the interventions were effective in preventing or relieving pain. Although the client is usually the best source of data, other people may be questioned about the client's words and behaviors that indicate pain. This is especially important with young children. During assessment, keep in mind that acute pain may coexist with or be superimposed on chronic pain. Specific assessment data usually include:

- **Location.** Determining the location may assist in relieving the pain or identifying its underlying cause. Ask the client to show you where it hurts, if possible, and whether the pain stays in one place or radiates to other parts of the body. The term referred pain is used when pain arising from tissue damage in one area of the body is felt in another area. Patterns of referred pain may be helpful in diagnosis. For example, pain of cardiac origin may radiate to the neck, shoulders, chest muscles, and down the arms, often on the left side. This form of pain usually results from myocardial ischemia due to atherosclerosis of coronary arteries. Stomach pain is usually referred to the epigastrium and may indicate gastritis or peptic ulcer. Gallbladder and bile duct pain is often localized in the right upper quadrant of the abdomen. Uterine pain is usually felt as abdominal cramping or low back pain. Deep or chronic pain is usually more difficult to localize than superficial or acute pain.
- **Intensity or severity.** Because pain is a subjective experience and cannot be objectively measured, assessment of severity is based on the client's description and the nurse's observations. Various scales have been developed to measure and quantify pain. These include verbal descriptor scales in which the client is asked to rate pain as mild, moderate, or severe; numeric scales, with 0 representing no pain and 10 representing severe, intense pain; and visual analog scales, in which the client chooses the location indicating the level of pain on a continuum. Scales have also been created specifically for use with children. The scale FACES

illustrates this type of scale. It combines words, numbers, and faces for use with children as young as 3 years.

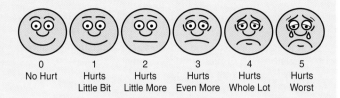

| 0 | 1 | 2 | 3 | 4 | 5 |
|---|---|---|---|---|---|
| No Hurt | Hurts Little Bit | Hurts Little More | Hurts Even More | Hurts Whole Lot | Hurts Worst |

- **Relation to time, activities, and other signs and symptoms.** Specific questions include:
  - When did the pain start?
  - What activities were occurring when the pain started?
  - Does the pain occur with exercise or when at rest?
  - Do other signs and symptoms occur before, during, or after the pain?
  - Is this the first episode or a recurrent pain?
  - How long does the pain last?
  - What, if anything, decreases or relieves the pain?
  - What, if anything, aggravates the pain?
- **Other data.** For example, do not assume that postoperative pain is incisional and requires narcotic analgesics for relief. A person who has had abdominal surgery may have headache, musculoskeletal discomfort, or "gas pains." Also, restlessness may be caused by hypoxia or anxiety rather than pain.

### Nursing Diagnoses

- Acute Pain
- Chronic Pain
- Impaired Gas Exchange related to sedation and decreased mobility
- Risk for Injury related to sedation and decreased mobility
- Constipation related to slowed peristalsis
- Deficient Knowledge: Effects and appropriate use of opioid analgesics
- Noncompliance: Drug dependence related to overuse

### Planning/Goals

*The client will:*

- Avoid or be relieved of pain
- Use opioid analgesics appropriately
- Avoid preventable adverse effects
- Avoid excessive sedation and respiratory depression
- Be able to communicate and perform other activities of daily living when feasible

### Interventions

Use measures to prevent, relieve, or decrease pain when possible. General measures include those that promote optimal body functioning and those that prevent trauma, inflammation, infection, and other sources of painful stimuli. Specific measures include:

- Encourage pulmonary hygiene techniques (eg, coughing, deep breathing, ambulation) to promote respiration and

*(continued)*

## NURSING PROCESS (Continued)

prevent pulmonary complications, such as pneumonia and atelectasis.
- Use sterile technique when caring for wounds, urinary catheters, or intravenous (IV) lines.
- Use exercises, ambulation, and position changes to promote circulation and musculoskeletal function.
- Handle any injured tissue very gently to avoid further trauma.
- Prevent bowel or bladder distention.
- Apply heat or cold.
- Use relaxation or distraction techniques.
- If a client is in pain on initial contact, try to relieve the pain as soon as possible. Once pain is controlled, plan with the client to avoid or manage future episodes.
- If a client is not in pain initially but anticipates surgery or an uncomfortable diagnostic procedure, plan with the client ways to minimize and manage discomfort.
- If using PCA, instruct the client and significant other as to the purpose, pump features, including safety considerations, and importance of adequate pain control. The nurse

should evaluate the pattern of use by the client to indicate the degree of understanding of method used and the degree of pain control (ie, multiple attempts within lock-out interval may indicate inadequate pain control). The nurse should assess and the client should be instructed to report side effects or adverse reactions of the narcotic being infused. Naloxone (Narcan) should be readily available should reversal of the narcotic be necessary.

### Evaluation
- Ask clients about their levels of comfort or relief from pain.
- Observe behaviors that indicate the presence or absence of pain.
- Observe participation and ability to function in usual activities of daily living.
- Observe for presence or absence of sedation and respiratory depression.
- Observe for drug-seeking behavior (possibly indicating dependence).

---

they are usually given intravenously in small doses. Drugs given by other routes are absorbed erratically in the presence of shock and hypovolemia and may not relieve pain. In addition, unabsorbed drugs may be rapidly absorbed when circulation improves, with the potential for excessive dosage and toxic effects.

## ◼ TOXICITY: RECOGNITION AND MANAGEMENT OF OVERDOSE

Acute toxicity or narcotic overdose can occur from therapeutic use or from abuse by drug-dependent people. Overdose may produce severe respiratory depression and coma. The main goal of treatment is to restore and maintain adequate respiratory function. This can be accomplished by inserting an endotracheal tube and starting mechanical ventilation, or by giving a narcotic antagonist, such as naloxone or nalmefene. Thus, emergency supplies should be readily available in any setting where narcotic analgesics are used, including ambulatory settings and clients' homes.

## ◼ PREVENTION AND MANAGEMENT OF WITHDRAWAL SYMPTOMS

Abstinence from opiates after chronic use produces a withdrawal syndrome characterized by anxiety; aggressiveness; restlessness; generalized body aches; insomnia; lacrimation; rhinorrhea; perspiration; pupil dilation; piloerection (goose flesh); anorexia, nausea, and vomiting; diarrhea; elevation of body temperature, respiratory rate, and systolic blood pressure; abdominal and other muscle cramps; dehydration; and weight loss. Although

all narcotics produce similar withdrawal syndromes, the onset, severity, and duration vary. With morphine sulfate, symptoms begin within a few hours of the last dose, reach peak intensity in 36 to 72 hours, and subside over approximately 10 days. With methadone, symptoms begin in 1 to 2 days, peak in approximately 3 days, and subside over several weeks. Heroin, meperidine, methadone, morphine sulfate, oxycodone, and oxymorphone are associated with more severe withdrawal symptoms than other narcotics. If a narcotic antagonist such as naloxone (Narcan) is given, withdrawal symptoms occur rapidly and are more intense but of shorter duration. Despite the discomfort that occurs, withdrawal from narcotics is rarely life threatening unless other problems are present. An exception is narcotic withdrawal in neonates, which has a high mortality rate if not treated effectively. Signs and symptoms in neonates include tremor, jitteriness, increased muscle tone, screaming, fever, sweating, tachycardia, vomiting, diarrhea, respiratory distress, and possibly seizures.

Recognition and treatment of early, mild symptoms of withdrawal can prevent progression to severe symptoms. Both narcotics and non-narcotics are used for treatment. Narcotics may be used in two ways to provide a safe, comfortable, and therapeutic withdrawal. One technique is to give the narcotic from which the person is withdrawing, which immediately reverses the signs and symptoms of withdrawal. Then, dosage is gradually reduced over several days. Another technique is to substitute a long-acting narcotic (eg, methadone) for a short-acting narcotic of abuse. Methadone is usually given in an adequate dose to control symptoms, once or twice daily, then gradually tapered over 5 to 10 days. In neonates undergoing narcotic withdrawal, methadone or paregoric may be used.

## CLIENT TEACHING GUIDELINES
### Narcotic (Opioid) Analgesics

**General Considerations**

✔ Use nonpharmacologic treatments of pain (eg, exercise, heat and cold applications) instead of or along with analgesics, when effective.

✔ For pain that is not relieved by nondrug treatments, a non-narcotic analgesic (eg, acetaminophen or ibuprofen) may be taken.

✔ For pain that is not relieved by a non-narcotic analgesic, a narcotic may be alternated with a non-narcotic analgesic or a combination product containing a narcotic and non-narcotic may be effective. Use of a narcotic analgesic for acute pain is acceptable and unlikely to lead to addiction.

✔ Most combination products (eg, Lorcet, Lortab, Percocet, Vicodin, Tylenol No. 3) contain acetaminophen and there is a risk of liver failure from high doses of acetaminophen or from lower doses in people who already have liver damage (eg, alcohol abusers). The maximum recommended daily dose, whether taken alone or in a combination product, is 4000 milligrams (eg, 8 tablets or capsules containing 500 mg each or 12 tablets containing 325 mg each). If unsure whether a combination product contains acetaminophen, ask a health care provider.

✔ For acute episodes of pain, most opioids may be taken as needed; for chronic pain, the drugs should be taken on a regular schedule, around the clock.

✔ When a choice of analgesics is available, use the least amount of the mildest drug that is likely to be effective in a particular situation.

✔ Take only as prescribed. If desired effects are not achieved, report to the physician. Do not increase the dose and do not take medication more often than prescribed. Although these principles apply to all medications, they are especially important with opioid analgesics because of potentially serious adverse reactions, including drug dependence, and because analgesics may mask pain for which medical attention is needed.

✔ Do not drink alcohol or take other drugs that cause drowsiness (eg, some antihistamines, sedative-type drugs for nervousness or anxiety, sleeping pills) while taking opioid analgesics. Combining drugs with similar effects may lead to excessive sedation, even coma, and difficulty in breathing.

✔ Do not smoke, cook, drive a car, or operate machinery when drowsy or dizzy or when vision is blurred from medication.

✔ Stay in bed at least 30–60 minutes after receiving an opioid analgesic by injection. Injected drugs may cause dizziness, drowsiness, and falls when walking around. If it is necessary to get out of bed, ask someone for assistance.

✔ When hospitalized, ask the physician or nurse about potential methods of pain management. For example, if anticipating surgery, ask how postoperative pain will be handled, how you need to report pain and request pain medication, and so on. It is better to take adequate medication and be able to cough, deep breathe, and ambulate than to avoid or minimize pain medication and be unable to perform activities that promote recovery and healing. Do not object to having bedrails up and asking for assistance to ambulate when receiving a strong narcotic analgesic. These are safety measures to prevent falls or other injuries because these analgesics may cause drowsiness, weakness, unsteady gait, and blurred vision.

✔ Constipation is a common adverse effect of opioid analgesics. It may be prevented or managed by eating high-fiber foods, such as whole-grain cereals, fruits, and vegetables; drinking 2–3 quarts of fluid daily; and being as active as tolerated. For someone unable to take these preventive measures, Metamucil daily or a mild laxative every other day may be needed.

**Self-administration**

✔ Take oral narcotics with 6–8 oz of water, with or after food to reduce nausea.

✔ Do not crush or chew long-acting tablets (eg, MS Contin, Oxycontin). The tablets are formulated to release the active drug slowly, over several hours. Crushing or chewing causes immediate release of the drug, with a high risk of overdose and adverse effects, and shortens the duration of action.

✔ Omit one or more doses if severe adverse effects occur (eg, excessive drowsiness, difficulty in breathing, severe nausea, vomiting, or constipation) and report to a health care provider.

---

Clonidine, an antihypertensive drug, is a non-narcotic that may be used to treat narcotic withdrawal. Clonidine reduces the release of norepinephrine in the brain and thus reduces symptoms associated with excessive stimulation of the sympathetic nervous system (eg, anxiety, restlessness, insomnia). Blood pressure must be closely monitored during clonidine therapy. Other medications (non-narcotic analgesics, antiemetics, antidiarrheals) are often required to treat other symptoms.

## USE IN OPIATE-TOLERANT PEOPLE

Whether opiate tolerance results from the use of prescribed, therapeutic drugs or the abuse of street drugs, there are two main considerations in using narcotic analgesics in this population. First, larger-than-usual doses are required to treat pain. Second, signs and symptoms of withdrawal occur if adequate dosage is not maintained or if narcotic antagonists are given.

## *Nursing Actions*
## Narcotic Analgesics

| *Nursing Actions* | *Rationale/Explanation* |
|---|---|
| 1. Administer accurately. | Respiratory depression is a major adverse effect of strong analgesics. Assessing respirations before each dose can help prevent or minimize potentially life-threatening respiratory depression. |
| a. Check the rate, depth, and rhythm of respirations before each dose. If the rate is below 12 per minute, delay or omit the dose and report to the physician. | |
| b. Have the client lie down to receive injections of opioid analgesics and for at least a few minutes afterward. | To prevent or minimize hypotension, nausea, and vomiting. These effects are more likely to occur in ambulatory clients. Also, clients may be sedated enough to increase risk of falls or other injuries if they try to ambulate. |
| c. When injecting opioid analgesics intravenously, give small doses; inject slowly over several minutes; and have opioid antagonist drugs, artificial airways, and equipment for artificial ventilation readily available. | Large doses or rapid intravenous injection may cause severe respiratory depression and hypotension. |
| d. Put siderails up; instruct the client not to smoke or try to ambulate without help. Keep the call light within reach. | To prevent falls or other injuries |
| e. *When giving controlled-release tablets, do NOT crush them, and instruct the client not to chew them.* | Crushing or chewing causes immediate release of drug, with a high risk of overdose and toxicity. |
| f. To apply transdermal fentanyl: | Correct preparation of the site and application of the medicated adhesive patch are necessary for drug absorption and effectiveness. |
| (1) Clip (do not shave) hair, if needed, on a flat surface of the upper trunk. | |
| (2) If it is necessary to cleanse the site, use plain water; do not use soaps, oils, lotions, alcohol, or other substances. Let the skin dry. | |
| (3) Apply the skin patch and press it in place for a few seconds. | |
| (4) Leave in place for 72 hours. | |
| (5) When a new patch is to be applied, remove the old one, fold it so that the medication is on the inside, and flush the patch down the toilet. Apply the new patch to a different skin site. | |
| 2. Observe for drug interactions. | |
| a. Drugs that *increase* effects of opioid analgesics: | |
| (1) CNS depressants—alcohol, general anesthetics, benzodiazepine antianxiety and hypnotic agents, tricyclic antidepressants, sedating antihistamines, antipsychotic agents, barbiturates, and other drugs that cause sedation | All these drugs alone, as well as the opioid analgesics, produce CNS depression. When combined, additive CNS depression results. If dosage of one or more interacting drugs is high, severe respiratory depression, coma, and death may ensue. |
| (2) Anticholinergics—atropine and other drugs with anticholinergic effects (eg, antihistamines, tricyclic antidepressants, phenothiazine antipsychotic drugs) | Increased constipation and urinary retention |
| (3) Antihypertensive drugs | Orthostatic hypotension, an adverse effect of both strong analgesics and antihypertensive drugs, may be increased if the two drug groups are given concurrently. |
| (4) Monoamine oxidase (MAO) inhibitors | These drugs interfere with detoxification of some opioid analgesics, especially meperidine. They may cause additive CNS depression with hypotension and respiratory depression or CNS stimulation with hyperexcitability and convulsions. If an MAO inhibitor is necessary, dosage should be reduced because the combination is potentially life threatening. |

*(continued)*

## Nursing Actions

### Narcotic Analgesics (Continued)

| Nursing Actions | Rationale/Explanation |
|---|---|
| (5) Protease inhibitors—ritonavir, saquinavir, others | May increase CNS and respiratory depression |
| (6) Cimetidine | May increase CNS and respiratory depression, probably by inhibiting the cytochrome P450 enzymes that normally metabolize opioids |
| b. Drugs that *decrease* effects of opioid analgesics:<br>(1) Narcotic antagonists | These drugs reverse respiratory depression produced by opioid analgesics. This is their only clinical use, and they should not be given unless severe respiratory depression is present. They do not reverse respiratory depression caused by other CNS depressants. |
| (2) Butorphanol, nalbuphine | These analgesics are weak antagonists of opioid analgesics, and they may cause withdrawal symptoms in people who have been receiving opiates or who are physically dependent on opioid analgesics. |

## Critical Thinking Exercises

1. A narcotic is considered a "nonceiling" drug when:
   a. There is no upper limit to the dosage that can be given to clients who have developed tolerance to previous dosages
   b. The dosage must be increased on a consistent basis to maintain pain control
   c. The drug is ineffective for high levels of pain
   d. It is the most effective pain control measure for a client

2. When narcotic analgesics are required in chronic pain associated with malignancy, the main consideration is:
   a. Client comfort
   b. Preventing drug addiction
   c. Drug tolerance
   d. Minimizing side effects

3. Why do oral pentazocine (Talwin) tablets contain naloxone (Narcan) 0.5 mg?
   a. To reverse respiratory depression caused by non-narcotic CNS depressants
   b. The combination increases the drug's effectiveness as an agonist
   c. To decrease the need for around-the-clock dosing of pentazocine when used individually
   d. To prevent the complications of IV injection if combined with tripelennamine as a method of substance abuse

4. Why should short-acting narcotics be ordered and given as needed during the first 48 hours after applying a fentanyl skin patch (Duragesic)?
   a. To counteract the rapid absorption when using the skin patch
   b. To prevent the adverse effects associated with dermal application of the patch
   c. When first applied, pain relief is delayed because the patch has delayed effects from gradual absorption
   d. To minimize narcotic withdrawal following an acute episode of pain

5. Up to 10% of whites, Asians, and African Americans have inadequate amounts or activity of the 2D6 enzymes necessary for codeine to metabolize to morphine sulfate. What result has been reported in this group because of this deficiency?
   a. Increased analgesic effect
   b. Increased risk for adverse effects
   c. Extended respiratory depression
   d. Less pain relief with usual therapeutic doses

## SELECTED REFERENCES

Abrahm, J. L. (2000). Cancer pain management. In H. D. Humes (Ed.), *Kelley's textbook of internal medicine* (4th ed., pp. 1875–1880). Philadelphia: Lippincott Williams & Wilkins.

Acute Pain Management Guideline Panel. (1992). *Acute pain management: Operative or medical procedures and trauma. Clinical practice guideline.* AHCPR Pub. No. 92-0032. Rockville, MD: Agency for Health Care Policy and Research, Public Health Service, U.S. Department of Health and Human Services for Health Care Policy and Research.

Barkin, R. L., & Barkin, D. (2001). Pharmacologic management of acute and chronic pain. *Southern Medical Journal, 94*(8), 756–812.

Devine, E. C. (2002). Somatosensory function and pain. In C. M. Porth (Ed.), *Pathophysiology: Concepts of altered health states* (6th ed., pp. 1091–1122). Philadelphia: Lippincott Williams & Wilkins.

*Drug facts and comparisons.* (Updated monthly). St. Louis: Facts and Comparisons.

Guyton, A. C., & Hall, J. E. (2000). *Textbook of medical physiology* (10th ed.). Philadelphia: W. B. Saunders.

Hadbavny, A. M., & Hoyt, J. W. (2000). Sedatives and analgesics in critical care. In A. Grevnik, S. M. Ayres, P. R. Holbrook, & W. C. Shoemaker (Eds.), *Textbook of critical care* (4th ed., pp. 961–971). Philadelphia: W. B. Saunders.

Kim, R. B. (Ed.) (2001). *The medical letter handbook of adverse drug interactions.* New Rochelle, NY: The Medical Letter, Inc.

Lacy, C. F., Armstrong, L. L., Goldman, M. P., & Lance, L. L. (2003). *Lexi-Comp's drug information handbook* (11th ed.). Hudson, OH: American Pharmaceutical Association.

Reisner, L. A. (2000). Pain management. In E. T. Herfindal & D. R. Gourley (Eds.), *Textbook of therapeutics: Drug and disease management* (pp. 1157–1183). Philadelphia: Lippincott Williams & Wilkins.

Wilkie, D. (2000). Pain perception and management. In R. F. Craven & C. J. Hirnle (Eds.), *Fundamentals of nursing: Human health and function* (3rd ed., pp. 1141–1172). Philadelphia: Lippincott Williams & Wilkins.

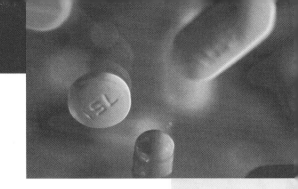

# 7

# Analgesic–Antipyretic–
# Anti-inflammatory
# and Related Drugs

## OBJECTIVES

*After studying this chapter, the student will be able to:*

1  Describe the role of prostaglandins in the etiology of pain, fever, and inflammation.

2  Discuss aspirin and other nonsteroidal anti-inflammatory drugs (NSAIDs) in terms of mechanism of action, indications for use, contraindications to use, and the nursing process.

3  Compare and contrast aspirin, other NSAIDs, and acetaminophen in terms of indications for use and adverse effects.

4  Differentiate among antiplatelet, analgesic, and anti-inflammatory doses of aspirin.

5  Distinguish between traditional NSAIDs and cyclooxygenase-2 inhibitors.

6  Teach clients interventions to prevent or decrease adverse effects of aspirin, other NSAIDs, and acetaminophen.

7  Identify age-related considerations influencing the use of aspirin, NSAIDs, and acetaminophen.

8  Discuss recognition and management of acetaminophen toxicity.

9  Discuss the use of NSAIDs and antigout drugs.

10  Discuss the use of NSAIDs, triptans, and ergot antimigraine drugs.

## CRITICAL THINKING SCENARIO

*Y*ou are working in an emergency room when parents bring in their 2-year-old son, Miguel. He has just ingested half a bottle of acetaminophen (Tylenol). His parents have recently come to this country from Mexico and speak very little English. The child does not appear acutely ill, and the parents become very upset when the health care provider wants to admit the child.

✔ Why is Tylenol overdose potentially so serious for this young child?

✔ What would emergency and follow-up treatment for Tylenol overdose be?

✔ How has this child's developmental stage increased the likelihood of accidental poisoning?

✔ Develop a teaching plan for this family to prevent recurrence.

## PROTOTYPE PROFILE

aspirin, p. 113

## OVERVIEW

The analgesic–antipyretic–anti-inflammatory drug group includes chemically and pharmacologically diverse drugs that share the ability to relieve pain, fever, and inflammation, symptoms associated with many injuries and illnesses. Drugs discussed in this chapter include ⓟ aspirin (acetylsalicylic acid, or ASA), the prototype, aspirin-related drugs that are often called nonsteroidal anti-inflammatory drugs (NSAIDs, such as ibuprofen), acetaminophen, and drugs used to prevent or treat gout and migraine.

Aspirin, NSAIDs, and acetaminophen can also be called antiprostaglandin drugs because they inhibit the synthesis of prostaglandins. Prostaglandins are chemical mediators found in most body tissues; they help regulate many cell functions and participate in the inflammatory response. They are formed when cellular injury occurs and phospholipids in cell membranes release arachidonic acid. Arachidonic acid is then metabolized by cyclooxygenase enzymes to produce prostaglandins, which act briefly in the area where they are produced and are then inactivated. Prostaglandins exert various and opposing effects in different body tissues (Table 7-1). To aid understanding of prostaglandins, their functions in pain, fever, and inflammation are described in At the Foundation: Prostaglandins' Roles in Pain, Fever, and Inflammation.

## ANALGESIC, ANTIPYRETIC, AND ANTI-INFLAMMATORY DRUGS

### Mechanism of Action

Aspirin, NSAIDs, and acetaminophen inactivate cyclooxygenases, the enzymes required for prostaglandin formation (Fig. 7-1). Two forms of cyclooxygenase, called COX-1 and COX-2, have been identified. Aspirin and traditional NSAIDs inhibit both COX-1 and COX-2 enzymes.

COX-1 is normally synthesized continuously and is present in all tissues and cell types, especially platelets, endothelial cells, the gastrointestinal (GI) tract, and the kidneys. Prostaglandins produced by COX-1 are important in numerous homeostatic functions and are associated with protective effects on the stomach and kidneys. In the stomach, they decrease gastric acid secretion, increase mucus secretion, and regulate blood circulation. In the kidneys, these prostaglandins help to maintain adequate blood flow and function. In the cardiovascular system, the prostaglandins help regulate vascular tone (ie, vasoconstriction and vasodilation) and platelet function. Drug-induced inhibition of these prostaglandins results in the adverse effects associated with aspirin and related drugs, especially gastric irritation, ulceration, and bleeding. Inhibition of COX-1 activity in platelets may be more responsible for GI bleeding than inhibition in gastric mucosa.

COX-2 is also normally present in several tissues (eg, brain, bone, kidneys, GI tract, and the female reproductive system). However, it is thought to occur in small amounts or to be inactive until stimulated by pain and inflammation. In inflamed tissues, COX-2 is induced by inflammatory chemical mediators such as interleukin-1 (IL-1) and tumor necrosis factor–alpha (TNF-alpha). In the GI tract, COX-2 is also induced by trauma and *Helicobacter pylori* infection, a common cause of peptic ulcer disease. Overall, prostaglandins produced by COX-2 are associated with pain and other signs of inflammation. Inhibition of COX-2 results in the therapeutic

| TABLE 7-1 | Prostaglandins | |
|---|---|---|
| **Prostaglandin** | **Locations** | **Effects** |
| D$_2$ | Airways, brain, mast cells | • Bronchoconstriction |
| E$_2$ | Brain, kidneys, vascular smooth muscle cells, platelets | • Bronchodilation<br>• Gastroprotection<br>• Increased activity of GI smooth muscle<br>• Increased sensitivity to pain<br>• Increased body temperature<br>• Vasodilation |
| F$_2$ | Airways, eyes, uterus, vascular smooth muscle | • Bronchoconstriction<br>• Increased activity of GI smooth muscle<br>• Increased uterine contraction (eg, menstrual cramps) |
| I$_2$ (Prostacyclin) | Brain, endothelium, kidneys, platelets | • Decreased platelet aggregation<br>• Gastroprotection<br>• Vasodilation |
| Thromboxane A$_2$ | Kidneys, macrophages, platelets, vascular smooth muscle | • Increased platelet aggregation<br>• Vasoconstriction |

**AT THE FOUNDATION:** *Prostaglandins' Roles in Pain, Fever, and Inflammation*

### Pain

Pain is the sensation of discomfort, hurt, or distress. It is a common human ailment and may occur with tissue injury and inflammation. Prostaglandins sensitize pain receptors and increase the pain associated with other chemical mediators such as bradykinin and histamine (see Box 7-1).

### Fever

Fever is an elevation of body temperature above the normal range. Body temperature is controlled by a regulating center in the hypothalamus. Normally, there is a balance between heat production and heat loss so that a constant body temperature is maintained. When there is excessive heat production, mechanisms to increase heat loss are activated. As a result, blood vessels dilate, more blood flows through the skin, sweating occurs, and body temperature usually stays within normal range. When fever occurs, the heat-regulating center in the hypothalamus is reset so that it tolerates a higher body temperature. Dehydration, inflammation, infectious processes, some drugs, brain injury, or diseases involving the hypothalamus may produce fever. Prostaglandin formation is stimulated by such circumstances, and along with bacterial toxins and other substances, prostaglandins act as pyrogens (fever-producing agents).

### Inflammation

Inflammation is the normal body response to tissue damage from any source, and it may occur in any tissue or organ. It is an attempt by the body to remove the damaging agent and repair the damaged tissue. Local manifestations are redness, heat, edema, and pain. Redness and heat result from vasodilation and increased blood supply; edema results from leakage of blood plasma into the area; and pain occurs when pain receptors on nerve endings are stimulated by heat, edema, pressure, chemicals released by the damaged cells, and prostaglandins. Systemic manifestations include leukocytosis, increased erythrocyte sedimentation rate, fever, headache, loss of appetite, lethargy or malaise, and weakness. Both local and systemic manifestations vary according to the cause and extent of tissue damage. In addition, inflammation may be acute or chronic.

effects of analgesia and anti-inflammatory activity. The COX-2 inhibitor drugs are NSAIDs designed to inhibit COX-2 selectively and to relieve pain and inflammation with fewer adverse effects, especially stomach damage.

To relieve pain, aspirin acts to block the transmission of pain impulses both centrally and peripherally. Related drugs act peripherally to prevent sensitization of pain receptors to various chemical substances released by damaged cells. To relieve fever, the drugs act on the hypothalamus to decrease its response to pyrogens and reset the "thermostat" at a lower level. For inflammation, the drugs prevent prostaglandins from increasing the pain and edema produced by other substances released by damaged cells. Although these drugs relieve symptoms and contribute greatly to the client's comfort and quality of life, they do not cure the underlying disorders that cause the symptoms.

Aspirin and traditional NSAIDs also have antiplatelet effects that differ in mechanism and extent. When aspirin is absorbed into the bloodstream, the acetyl portion dissociates, then binds irreversibly to platelet COX-1. This action prevents synthesis of thromboxane $A_2$, a prostaglandin derivative, and thereby inhibits platelet aggregation. A small single dose (325 mg) irreversibly acetylates circulating platelets within a few minutes, and its effects last for the lifespan of the platelets (7 to 10 days). Most other NSAIDs bind reversibly with platelet COX-1 so that antiplatelet effects occur only while the drug is present in the blood. Thus, aspirin has greater effects, but all the drugs except acetaminophen and the COX-2 inhibitors inhibit platelet aggregation, interfere with blood coagulation, and increase the risk for bleeding.

## Indications for Use

These drugs are widely used to prevent and treat mild to moderate pain or inflammation associated with musculoskeletal disorders (eg, osteoarthritis [OA], tendonitis, gout), headache, dysmenorrhea, minor trauma (eg, athletic injuries such as sprains), minor surgery (eg, dental extraction, episiotomy), and other acute and chronic conditions. Despite many similarities, however, aspirin and other NSAIDs differ in their approved uses. Although aspirin is effective in many disorders, its use has declined for most indications, largely because of adverse effects on the GI tract and the advent of newer drugs. At the same time, low-dose aspirin is increasingly prescribed for clients at risk for myocardial infarction or stroke from thrombosis. This indication stems from its antiplatelet activity and resultant effects on blood coagulation (ie, decreased clot formation). Some NSAIDs, such as ibuprofen (Motrin) and related drugs, are widely used as anti-inflammatory agents and analgesics; ketorolac (Toradol), which can be given orally and parenterally, is used only as an analgesic. Most of the other NSAIDs are too toxic to use as analgesics and antipyretics.

BOX
7-1    **Chemical Mediators of Inflammation and Immunity**

*Bradykinin* is a kinin in body fluids that becomes physiologically active with tissue injury. When tissue cells are damaged, white blood cells (WBCs) increase in the area and ingest damaged cells to remove them from the area. When the WBCs die, they release enzymes that activate kinins. The activated kinins increase and prolong the vasodilation and increased vascular permeability caused by histamine. They also cause pain by stimulating nerve endings for pain in the area. Thus, bradykinin may aggravate and prolong the erythema, heat, and pain of local inflammatory reactions. It also increases mucous gland secretion.

*Complement* is a group of plasma proteins essential to normal inflammatory and immunologic processes. More specifically, complement destroys cell membranes of body cells (eg, red blood cells, lymphocytes, platelets) and pathogenic microorganisms (eg, bacteria, viruses). The system is initiated by an antigen–antibody reaction or by tissue injury. Components of the system (called C1 through C9) are activated in a cascade type of reaction in which each component becomes a proteolytic enzyme that splits the next component in the series. Activation yields products with profound inflammatory effects. C3a and C5a, also called anaphylatoxins, act mainly by liberating histamine from mast cells and platelets, and their effects are therefore similar to those of histamine. C3a causes or increases smooth muscle contraction, vasodilation, vascular permeability, degranulation of mast cells and basophils, and secretion of lysosomal enzymes by leukocytes. C5a performs the same functions as C3a and also promotes movement of WBCs into the injured area (chemotaxis). In addition, it activates the lipoxygenase pathway of arachidonic acid metabolism in neutrophils and macrophages, thereby inducing formation of leukotrienes and other substances that increase vascular permeability and chemotaxis.

In the immune response, the complement system breaks down antigen–antibody complexes, especially those in which the antigen is a microbial agent. It enables the body to produce inflammation and localize an infective agent. More specific reactions include increased vascular permeability, chemotaxis, and opsonization (coating a microbe or other antigen so it can be more readily phagocytized).

*Cytokines* may act on the cells that produce them, on surrounding cells, or on distant cells if sufficient amounts reach the bloodstream. Thus, cytokines act locally and systemically to produce inflammatory and immune responses, including increased vascular permeability and chemotaxis of macrophages, neutrophils, and basophils. Two major types of cytokines are interleukins (produced by leukocytes) and interferons (produced by T lymphocytes or fibroblasts). Interleukin-1 (IL-1) mediates several inflammatory responses, including fever, and IL-2 (also called T-cell growth factor) is required for the growth and function of T lymphocytes. Interferons are cytokines that protect nearby cells from invasion by intracellular microorganisms, such as viruses and rickettsiae. They also limit the growth of some cancer cells.

*Histamine* is formed (from the amino acid histidine) and stored in most body tissue, with high concentrations in mast cells, basophils, and platelets. Mast cells, which are abundant in skin and connective tissue, release histamine into the vascular system in response to stimuli (eg, antigen–antibody reaction, tissue injury, and some drugs). Once released, histamine is highly vasoactive, causing vasodilation (increasing blood flow to the area and producing hypotension) and increasing permeability of capillaries and venules (producing edema). Other effects include contracting smooth muscles in the bronchi (producing bronchoconstriction and respiratory distress), gastrointestinal (GI) tract, and uterus; stimulating salivary, gastric, bronchial, and intestinal secretions; stimulating sensory nerve endings to cause pain and itching; and stimulating movement of eosinophils into injured tissue. Histamine is the first chemical mediator released in the inflammatory response and immediate hypersensitivity reactions (anaphylaxis).

When histamine is released from mast cells and basophils, it diffuses rapidly into other tissues. It then acts on target tissues through both histamine-1 ($H_1$) and histamine-2 ($H_2$) receptors. $H_1$ receptors are located mainly on smooth muscle cells in blood vessels and the respiratory and GI tracts. When histamine binds with these receptors, resulting events include contraction of smooth muscle, increased vascular permeability, production of nasal mucus, stimulation of sensory nerves, pruritus, and dilation of capillaries in the skin. H2 receptors are also located in the airways, GI tract, and other tissues. When histamine binds to these receptors, there is increased secretion of gastric acid by parietal cells in the stomach mucosal lining, increased mucus secretion and bronchodilation in the airways, contraction of esophageal muscles, tachycardia, inhibition of lymphocyte function, and degranulation of basophils (with additional release of histamine and other mediators) in the bloodstream. In allergic reactions, both types of receptors mediate hypotension (in anaphylaxis), skin flushing, and headache. The peak effects of histamine occur within 1 to 2 minutes of its release and may last as long as 10 minutes, after which it is inactivated by histaminase (produced by eosinophils) or N-methyltransferase.

*Platelet-activating factor (PAF),* like prostaglandins and leukotrienes, is derived from arachidonic acid metabolism and has multiple inflammatory activities. It is produced by mast cells, neutrophils, monocytes, and platelets. Because these cells are widely distributed, PAF effects can occur in virtually every organ and tissue. Besides causing platelet aggregation, PAF activates neutrophils, attracts eosinophils, increases vascular permeability, causes vasodilation, and causes IL-1 and tumor necrosis factor–alpha (TNF-alpha) to be released. PAF, IL-1, and TNF-alpha can induce each other's release.

They are used primarily in rheumatoid arthritis (RA) and other musculoskeletal disorders that do not respond to safer drugs. Celecoxib (Celebrex) is also used to treat familial adenomatous polyposis, in which the drug reduces the number of polyps and may decrease the risk for colon cancer. Several NSAIDs are formulated as eye drops for use in treating eye disorders (see Appendix G).

**Acetaminophen,** which differs chemically from aspirin and other NSAIDs, is commonly used as an aspirin sub-

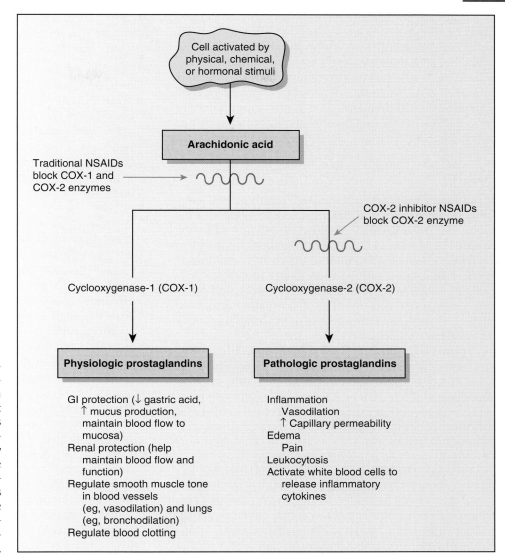

**FIGURE 7–1** Physiologic and pathologic (ie, inflammatory) prostaglandins: Actions of antiprostaglandin drugs. Prostaglandins play important roles in normal body functions as well as inflammatory processes. Inhibition of both COX-1 and COX-2 by traditional NSAIDs produces adverse effects on the stomach (eg, irritation, ulceration, bleeding) as well as anti-inflammatory effects. Selective inhibition of COX-2 produces anti-inflammatory effects while maintaining protective effects on the stomach.

stitute for pain and fever, but it lacks anti-inflammatory and antiplatelet effects.

## Contraindications to Use

Contraindications to aspirin and nonselective NSAIDs include peptic ulcer disease, GI or other bleeding disorders, history of hypersensitivity reactions, and impaired renal function. In people who are allergic to aspirin, nonaspirin NSAIDs also are contraindicated because hypersensitivity reactions may occur with any drugs that inhibit prostaglandin synthesis. In children and adolescents, aspirin is contraindicated in the presence of viral infections such as influenza or chickenpox because of its association with Reye's syndrome. Selective COX-2 inhibitors are contraindicated for clients with a history of peptic ulcers, GI bleeding, asthma, an allergic reaction to other NSAIDs, or severe renal impairment. In addition, **celecoxib** is contraindicated in clients who are allergic to sulfonamides, and **ketorolac** is contraindicated in clients at risk for excessive bleeding. Thus, ketorolac should not be adminis-

tered during labor and delivery; before or during any major surgery; with suspected or confirmed cerebrovascular bleeding; or to clients who are currently taking aspirin or other NSAIDs.

Over-the-counter (OTC) products containing these drugs are contraindicated for chronic alcohol abusers because of possible liver damage (with acetaminophen) or stomach bleeding (with aspirin, ibuprofen, ketoprofen, or naproxen). The U.S. Food and Drug Administration (FDA) requires an alcohol warning on the labels of all OTC pain relievers and fever reducers. This warning states that people who drink three or more alcoholic drinks daily should ask their doctors before taking the products.

## Subgroups and Individual Drugs

Subgroups and selected individual drugs are described below; indications for use, trade names, and dosage ranges of individual drugs are listed in Drugs at a Glance 7-1: Analgesic, Antipyretic, Anti-inflammatory Drugs.

Home care is an essential component in the management of clients taking these drugs. Guidelines for ongoing evaluation and intervention are addressed in Home Care Considerations. Age-specific considerations are also important in clients taking acetaminophen, aspirin, and other NSAIDs. Discussion of specific management considerations in children and older adults is found in Age-related Considerations: Use of Acetaminophen, Aspirin, and Other NSAIDs.

## Aspirin

Aspirin is the prototype of the analgesic–antipyretic–anti-inflammatory drugs and the most commonly used salicylate. Information can be found in Prototype Profile 7-1: Aspirin. Because it is a nonprescription drug and is widely available, people tend to underestimate its usefulness. It is effective in pain of low to moderate intensity, especially that involving the skin, muscles, joints, and other connective tissue. It is useful in inflammatory disorders, such as arthritis, but many people prefer drugs that cause less gastric irritation.

Aspirin is a home remedy for headaches, colds, influenza and other respiratory infections, muscular aches, and fever. It can be purchased in plain, chewable, enteric-coated, and effervescent tablets and rectal suppositories. It is not marketed in liquid form because it is unstable in solution. Aspirin is nephrotoxic in high doses, and protein binding of aspirin is reduced in renal failure so that blood levels of active drug are higher.

**Diflunisal** (Dolobid) is a salicylic acid derivative that differs chemically from aspirin. It is reportedly equal or superior to aspirin in mild to moderate pain, RA, and OA. Compared with aspirin, it has less antipyretic effect, causes less gastric irritation, and has a longer duration of action.

Aspirin and other NSAIDs can decrease blood flow in the kidneys by inhibiting synthesis of prostaglandins that dilate renal blood vessels. When renal blood flow is normal, these prostaglandins have limited activity. When renal blood flow is decreased, however, their synthesis is increased, and they protect the kidneys from ischemia and hypoxia by antagonizing the vasoconstrictive effects of angiotensin II, norepinephrine, and other substances. Thus, in clients who depend on prostaglandins to maintain an adequate renal blood flow, the prostaglandin-blocking effects of aspirin and NSAIDs result in constriction of renal arteries and arterioles, decreased renal blood flow, decreased glomerular filtration rate, and retention of salt and water. NSAIDs can also cause kidney damage by other mechanisms, including a hypersensitivity reaction that leads to acute renal failure, manifested by proteinuria, hematuria, or pyuria. Biopsy reports usually indicate inflammatory reactions such as glomerulonephritis or interstitial nephritis.

### Guidelines for Therapy With Aspirin

When pain, fever, or inflammation is present, aspirin is effective across a wide range of clinical conditions. Like any other drug, aspirin must be used appropriately to maximize therapeutic benefits and minimize adverse reactions. Some guidelines include the following:

1. For *pain,* aspirin is useful alone when the discomfort is of low to moderate intensity. For more severe pain, aspirin may be combined with an oral narcotic (eg, codeine) or given between narcotic doses. Aspirin and narcotic analgesics act by different mechanisms; hence, such use is rational. For acute pain, aspirin is taken when the pain occurs and is often effective within a few minutes. For chronic pain, a regular schedule of administration, such as every 4 to 6 hours, is more effective.
2. For *fever,* aspirin is effective if drug therapy is indicated. In children, however, aspirin is contraindicated because of its association with Reye's syndrome.
3. For *inflammation,* aspirin is useful in both short- and long-term therapy of conditions characterized by pain and inflammation, such as RA or OA. Although effective, the high doses and frequent administration required for anti-inflammatory effects increase the risks for GI upset, ulceration, and bleeding.
4. For acute pain or fever, plain aspirin tablets are preferred. For chronic pain, long-term use in arthritis, and daily use for antiplatelet effects, enteric-coated tablets may be better tolerated. Rectal suppositories are sometimes used when oral administration is contraindicated.
5. Aspirin dosage depends mainly on the condition being treated. Low doses are used for antiplatelet effects in preventing arterial thrombotic disorders such as myocardial infarction or stroke. Lower-than-average doses are needed for clients with low serum albumin levels because a larger proportion of each dose is free to exert pharmacologic activity. Larger doses are needed for anti-inflammatory effects than for analgesic and antipyretic effects.
6. In general, clients taking low-dose aspirin to prevent myocardial infarction or stroke should continue the aspirin if prescribed a COX-2 inhibitor NSAID. The COX-2 inhibitors have little effect on platelet function.

### Toxicology: Salicylate Poisoning

Salicylate intoxication (salicylism) may occur with an acute overdose or chronic use of therapeutic doses, especially the higher doses taken for anti-inflammatory effects. Chronic ingestion of large doses saturates a major metabolic pathway, thereby slowing drug elimination, prolonging the serum half-life, and causing drug accumulation.

### *Prevention*

To decrease the risk for toxicity, plasma salicylate levels should be measured when an acute overdose is suspected and periodically when large doses of aspirin are taken

*(text continues on page 111)*

## DRUG TABLE 7-1

*Drugs at a Glance*

### Analgesic, Antipyretic, Anti-inflammatory Drugs

| Generic/ Trade Name | Indications for Use | Routes and Dosage Ranges | Comments |
|---|---|---|---|
| **Acetaminophen** (Tylenol, others) Pregnancy Category B | Pain Fever | *Adults:* PO 325–650 mg q4–6h, or 1000 mg three or four times per day; maximum 4 g/d<br>*Children:* PO 10 mg/kg or according to age as follows: 0–3 mo, 40 mg; 4–11 mo, 80 mg; 1–2 y, 120 mg; 2–3 y, 160 mg; 4–5 y, 240 mg; 6–8 y, 320 mg; 9–10 y, 400 mg; 11 y, 480 mg. Doses may be given q4–6h to a maximum of 5 doses in 24 h.<br>*Adults:* Rectal suppository 650 mg q4–6h, maximum of 6 in 24 h<br>*Children:* Rectal suppository: age under 3 y, consult physician; age 3–6 y, 120 mg q4–6h, maximum, 720 mg in 24 h; age 6–12 y, 325 mg q4–6h, maximum 2.6 g in 24 h | **Warning:** Overdoses may cause fatal liver damage. Maximum recommended dose for adults is 4 g/d, from all sources. Parents and caregivers should ask pediatricians about the amounts of acetaminophen children may take safely. |
| **Aspirin** | See Prototype Profile 7-1: Aspirin | | |
| **Celecoxib** (Celebrex) Pregnancy Category C; D after 34 weeks gestation | Osteoarthritis (OA) Rheumatoid arthritis (RA) Familial adenomatous polyposis (FAP) | *Adults: OA,* PO 100 mg twice daily or 200 mg once daily<br>*RA:* PO 100–200 mg twice daily<br>*FAP:* PO 200 mg twice daily<br>*Children:* Dosage not established | 200-mg doses should be taken with food |
| **Diclofenac potassium** (Cataflam) **Diclofenac sodium** (Voltaren, Voltaren XR) Pregnancy Category B; D (3rd trimester) | Osteoarthritis Rheumatoid arthritis | *Adults: OA,* PO 100–150 mg/d in divided doses (eg, 50 mg two or three times or 75 mg twice or 100 mg once daily)<br>*RA:* PO 150–200 mg/d in two, three, or four divided doses<br>*Children:* Dosage not established | Diclofenac potassium is available only in 50-mg, immediate-release tablets. It may be used for all indications. This drug has a more rapid onset of action than diclofenac sodium because it is absorbed in the stomach instead of the duodenum. |
| | Ankylosing spondylitis (AS) Pain, dysmenorrhea | *Adults: AS:* PO 100–125 mg/d in four or five divided doses (eg, 25 mg four or five times daily)<br>Pain, dysmenorrhea: (diclofenac potassium only) PO 50 mg three times daily | Diclofenac sodium is available in 25-, 50-, and 75-mg delayed-release tablets and a 100-mg extended-release (XR) tablet. It is not recommended for acute pain or dysmenorrhea. |

*(continued)*

**DRUG TABLE 7-1** _Drugs at a Glance_

## Analgesic, Antipyretic, Anti-inflammatory Drugs (Continued)

| Generic/ Trade Name | Indications for Use | Routes and Dosage Ranges | Comments |
|---|---|---|---|
| **Diflunisal** (Dolobid) Pregnancy Category C, D 3rd trimester | Osteoarthritis Rheumatoid arthritis Pain | _Adults: OA, RA:_ PO 500–1000 mg/d, in two divided doses, increased to a maximum of 1500 mg/d if necessary<br>_Pain:_ PO 500–1000 mg initially, then 250–500 mg q8–12h<br>_Children:_ Not recommended for use in children <12 years of age | Swallow tablet whole; do not chew or crush |
| **Etodolac** (Lodine, Lodine XL) Pregnancy Category C; D 3rd trimester | Osteoarthritis Rheumatoid arthritis Pain | _Adults: OA, RA:_ PO 600–1200 mg/d in two to four divided doses<br>_Pain:_ PO 200–400 mg q6–8h Maximum according to weight: 1200 mg/d for 60 kg (132 lbs) or more; 20 mg/kg/d for <60 kg<br>_Children:_ Dosage not established | Available in immediate-release and extended-release (XL) tablets of various strengths. The immediate-release forms should be used to treat acute pain.<br>Swallow tablets whole; do not chew or crush |
| **Fenoprofen** (Nalfon) Pregnancy Category C; D 3rd trimester or near delivery | Osteoarthritis Rheumatoid arthritis Pain | _Adults: OA, RA:_ PO 300–600 mg three or four times per day<br>_Pain:_ PO 200 mg q4–6h PRN Maximum, 3200 mg/d<br>_Children:_ Dosage not established | Do not chew or crush tablet; take with food, water, or milk |
| **Flurbiprofen** (Ansaid) Pregnancy Category C; D 3rd trimester | Osteoarthritis Rheumatoid arthritis | _Adults: OA, RA:_ PO 200–300 mg/d in two, three, or four divided doses<br>_Children:_ Dosage not established | Take oral form with food |
| **Ibuprofen** (Advil, Motrin, PediaCare) Pregnancy Category B; D 3rd trimester | Osteoarthritis Rheumatoid arthritis Pain, dysmenorrhea Fever | _Adults: OA, RA:_ PO 300–600 mg 3 or 4 times per day; maximum, 2400 mg/d<br>Pain, dysmenorrhea: PO 400 mg q4–6h PRN Maximum, 3200 mg/d<br>_Children: 1–12 y:_ Fever, initial temperature 39.2°C (102.5°F) or less, PO 5 mg/kg q6–8h; initial temperature above 39.2°C (102.5°F), PO 10 mg/kg q6–8h; maximum dose, 40 mg/kg/d<br>Juvenile arthritis, PO 20–40 mg/kg/d, in three or four divided doses | Available in numerous dosage forms and concentrations, including regular tablets; chewable tablets; capsules; oral suspensions (of 100 mg/5 mL); and oral drops (of 40 mg/mL, for infants) |

_(continued)_

**DRUG TABLE 7-1**

## *Drugs at a Glance*

### Analgesic, Antipyretic, Anti-inflammatory Drugs (Continued)

| Generic/Trade Name | Indications for Use | Routes and Dosage Ranges | Comments |
|---|---|---|---|
| **Indomethacin** (Indocin, Indocin SR) Pregnancy Category B; D if taken after 34 weeks gestation or for longer than 48 hours | Osteoarthritis Rheumatoid arthritis Ankylosing spondylitis Tendinitis Bursitis Acute painful shoulder Acute gout Closure of patent ductus arteriosus (IV only) | *Adults:* PO, rectal suppository, 75 mg/d initially, increased by 25 mg/d at weekly intervals to a maximum of 150–200 mg/d, if necessary Acute gouty arthritis, acute painful shoulder, PO 75–150 mg/d in three or four divided doses until pain and inflammation are controlled (eg, 3–5 d for gout; 7–14 d for painful shoulder), then discontinued *Children:* Premature infants with patent ductus arteriosus, IV 0.2–0.3 mg/kg q12h for a total of three doses | The sustained-release form is not recommended for acute gouty arthritis and must be swallowed intact. |
| **Ketoprofen** (Orudis, Oruvail) Pregnancy Category B; D 3rd trimester | Pain Dysmenorrhea Osteoarthritis Rheumatoid arthritis | *Adults: Pain, dysmenorrhea:* PO 25–50 mg q6–8h PRN *OA, RA:* PO 150–300 mg/d in three or four divided doses Sustained-release (Oruvail SR), 200 mg once daily Maximum, 300 mg/d for regular formulation; 200 mg/d for extended release; 100–150 mg/d for clients with impaired renal function *Children:* Do not give to children <16 years unless directed by a physician. | Extended-release capsules are available as generic ketoprofen and Oruvail. Note that the names do not contain any letters (eg, SR, XL) that indicate long-acting dosage forms. May cause drowsiness or dizziness |
| **Ketorolac** (Toradol) Pregnancy Category B; D 3rd trimester | Moderately severe, acute pain, for short term (up to 5 days) treatment | *Adults:* IV, IM 30 mg q6h PRN to a maximum of 120 mg/d PO 10 mg q4–6h to a maximum of 40 mg/d Older adults (>65 y), those with renal impairment, those with weight < 50 kg (110 lbs), IV, IM 15 mg q6h to a maximum of 60 mg/d *Children:* Dosage not established | Treatment is started with one or more injected doses, followed by oral doses when the client is able to take them. Maximum duration of both injected and oral doses, 5 days. May cause drowsiness or dizziness |
| **Meloxicam** (Mobic) Pregnancy Category C; D 3rd trimester | Osteoarthritis | *Adults:* PO 7.5 once daily; increased to 15 mg once daily if necessary *Children:* Dosage not established | May be taken without regard to meals |
| **Nabumetone** (Relafen) Pregnancy Category C; D 3rd trimester | Osteoarthritis Rheumatoid arthritis | *Adults:* PO 1000–2000 mg/day in one or two doses *Children:* Dosage not established | Available in 500-mg and 750-mg tablets Avoid GI irritants with use |

*(continued)*

**DRUG TABLE 7-1**

*Drugs at a Glance*

## Analgesic, Antipyretic, Anti-inflammatory Drugs (Continued)

| Generic/ Trade Name | Indications for Use | Routes and Dosage Ranges | Comments |
|---|---|---|---|
| **Naproxen** (Naprosyn) **Naproxen sodium** (Aleve, Anaprox, Naprelan) Pregnancy Category B; D 3rd trimester or near delivery | Osteoarthritis Rheumatoid arthritis Juvenile arthritis Ankylosing spondylitis Pain Dysmenorrhea Bursitis Tendinitis Acute gout | *Adults: Naproxen:* PO 250–500 mg twice daily Gout: PO 750 mg initially, then 250 mg q8h until symptoms subside Maximum, 1250 mg/d *Naproxen sodium: Pain, dysmenorrhea, acute tendinitis, bursitis:* PO 550 mg q12h or 275 mg q6–8h Maximum, 1375 mg/d OA, RA, AS: PO 275–550 mg twice a day *Acute gout:* PO 825 mg initially, then 275 mg q8h until symptoms subside Controlled-release (Naprelan), 750–1000 mg once daily *Children:* Juvenile arthritis (naproxen only): PO 10 mg/kg/d in two divided doses. Oral suspension (125 mg/5 mL) twice daily according to weight: 13 kg (29 lb), 2.5 mL; 25 kg (55 lb), 5 mL; 39 kg (84 lb), 7.5 mL OTC preparation not recommended for children < 12 y | Available in several dosage strength tablets, in a suspension, and in immediate- and delayed-release formulations |
| **Oxaprozin** (Daypro) Pregnancy Category C; D 3rd trimester | Osteoarthritis Rheumatoid arthritis | *Adults:* PO 600–1200 mg once daily Maximum, 1800 mg/d or 26 mg/kg/d, whichever is lower, in divided doses *Children:* Dosage not established | Lower doses recommended for patients with low body weight or milder disease Monitor ocular, renal, and hepatic function |
| **Piroxicam** (Feldene) Pregnancy Category B; D 3rd trimester | Osteoarthritis Rheumatoid arthritis | *Adults:* PO 20 mg/d or 10 mg twice daily *Children:* Dosage not established | Monitor ocular, renal, and hepatic function |
| **Rofecoxib** (Vioxx) Pregnancy Category C; D 3rd trimester or near delivery | Osteoarthritis Pain Dysmenorrhea | *Adults: OA,* PO 12.5–25 mg once daily *Acute pain, dysmenorrhea:* PO 50 mg once daily as needed *Children:* Dosage not established | Available in tablets of 12.5, 25, and 50 mg and a suspension containing 12.5 mg/5 mL or 25 mg/5 mL May be taken with or without food |
| **Sulindac** (Clinoril) Pregnancy Category B; D at term | Osteoarthritis Rheumatoid arthritis Ankylosing spondylitis Bursitis Tendinitis Acute painful shoulder Acute gout | *Adults:* PO 150–200 mg twice a day; maximum, 400 mg/d *Acute gout, acute painful shoulder:* PO 200 mg twice a day until pain and inflammation subside (eg, 7–14 d), then reduce dosage or discontinue *Children:* Dosage not established | Inform surgeon or dentist of risk of prolonged bleeding time; may cause drowsiness, dizziness, or impaired judgment |

*(continued)*

**DRUG TABLE 7-1**

## *Drugs at a Glance*
### Analgesic, Antipyretic, Anti-inflammatory Drugs (Continued)

| Generic/ Trade Name | Indications for Use | Routes and Dosage Ranges | Comments |
|---|---|---|---|
| **Tolmetin** (Tolectin) Pregnancy Category C; D at term | Osteoarthritis Rheumatoid arthritis Juvenile rheumatoid arthritis | *Adults:* PO 400 mg three times daily initially, increased to 1800 mg/d if necessary *Children:* Juvenile *RA:* PO 20 mg/kg/d in three or four divided doses | Take with food, water or milk; may cause drowsiness or impaired judgment |
| **Valdecoxib** (Bextra) Pregnancy Category C; D 3rd trimester | Osteoarthritis Rheumatoid arthritis Dysmenorrhea | *Adults:* OA, RA: PO 10 mg once daily Dysmenorrhea: PO 20 mg twice daily as needed *Children:* Dosage not established | |

long-term. Therapeutic levels are 150 to 300 mcg/mL. Signs of salicylate toxicity occur at serum levels greater than 200 mcg/mL; severe toxic effects may occur at levels greater than 400 mcg/mL.

### Recognition: Signs and Symptoms
Manifestations of salicylism include nausea, vomiting, fever, fluid and electrolyte deficiencies, tinnitus, decreased hearing, visual changes, drowsiness, confusion, hyperventilation, and others. Severe central nervous system dysfunction (eg, delirium, stupor, coma, seizures) indicates life-threatening toxicity.

### Treatment
In mild salicylism, stopping the drug or reducing the dose is usually sufficient. In severe salicylate overdose,

## Home Care Considerations: Use of Analgesic, Antipyretic, and Anti-inflammatory Drugs

**ASSESS:** the adverse drug effects that should be reviewed with clients; clients for characteristics (eg, older age group, renal impairment, overuse of the drugs) that increase the risks for adverse effects.

**MONITOR:** the therapeutic and adverse effects of the drugs and the client's need for additional information and provide that information.

**EDUCATE:** regarding the importance of reading and following instructions on labels of OTC analgesics, not exceeding recommended dosages without consulting a health care provider, avoiding multiple sources of acetaminophen or NSAIDs (eg, multiple OTC NSAIDs or an OTC and a prescription NSAID); reinforce additional teaching points (see Client Teaching Guidelines: Acetaminophen, Aspirin, and Other NSAIDs)

treatment is symptomatic and aimed at preventing further absorption from the GI tract; increasing urinary excretion; and correcting fluid, electrolyte, and acid–base imbalances. When the drug may still be in the GI tract, gastric lavage and activated charcoal help reduce absorption. Intravenous (IV) sodium bicarbonate produces an alkaline urine in which salicylates are more rapidly excreted, and hemodialysis effectively removes salicylates from the blood. IV fluids are indicated when high fever or dehydration is present. The specific content of IV fluids depends on the serum electrolyte and acid–base status.

## Nonsteroidal Anti–inflammatory Drugs

**Propionic acid derivatives** include fenoprofen (Nalfon), flurbiprofen (Ansaid), ibuprofen (Motrin, Advil), ketoprofen (Orudis), naproxen (Naprosyn), and oxaprozin (Daypro). In addition to their use as anti-inflammatory agents, some are used as analgesics and antipyretics. Ibuprofen, ketoprofen, and naproxen are available OTC, with recommended doses smaller and durations of use shorter than those for prescription formulations. Although these drugs are usually better tolerated than aspirin, they are much more expensive and may cause all the adverse effects associated with aspirin and other prostaglandin inhibitors.

**Ibuprofen,** a commonly used drug, is well absorbed with oral administration. Its action starts in about 30 minutes, peaks in 1 to 2 hours, and lasts 4 to 6 hours. The drug is highly bound (about 99%) to plasma proteins and has a half-life of about 2 hours. It is metabolized in the liver and excreted through the kidneys. It is available by prescription and OTC, in tablets, chewable tablets, capsules, oral suspension, and oral drops, for use by adults and children.

**Acetic acid derivatives** include indomethacin (Indocin), sulindac (Clinoril), and tolmetin (Tolectin).

## Age-related Considerations:
## Use of Acetaminophen, Aspirin, and Other NSAIDs

### USE IN CHILDREN

Acetaminophen is usually the drug of choice for pain or fever in children. Children seem less susceptible to liver toxicity than adults, apparently because they form less of the toxic metabolite during metabolism of acetaminophen. However, there is a risk for overdose and hepatotoxicity because acetaminophen is a very common ingredient in over-the-counter cold, flu, fever, and pain remedies. An overdose can occur with large doses of one product or smaller amounts of several different products. In addition, toxicity has occurred when parents or caregivers have given the liquid concentration intended for children to infants. The concentrations are different and cannot be given interchangeably. Infants' doses are measured with a dropper; children's doses are measured by a medicine cup. Caution parents and caregivers to ask pediatricians for written instructions on giving acetaminophen to their children, to read the labels of all drug products very carefully, and to avoid giving children acetaminophen from multiple sources.

Ibuprofen also may be given for fever. Aspirin is not recommended because of its association with Reye's syndrome, a life-threatening illness characterized by encephalopathy, hepatic damage, and other serious problems. Reye's syndrome usually occurs after a viral infection, such as influenza or chickenpox, during which aspirin was given for fever. For children with juvenile rheumatoid arthritis, aspirin, ibuprofen, naproxen, or tolmetin may be given. Pediatric indications for use and dosages have not been established for most of the other drugs.

When an NSAID is given during late pregnancy to prevent premature labor, the fetus' kidneys may be adversely affected. When one is given shortly after birth to close a patent ductus arteriosus, the neonate's kidneys may be adversely affected.

### USE IN OLDER ADULTS

Acetaminophen is usually safe in recommended doses unless liver damage is present or the person is a chronic alcohol abuser. Aspirin is usually safe in the small doses prescribed for prevention of myocardial infarction and stroke (antiplatelet effects). Aspirin and other NSAIDs are probably safe in therapeutic doses for occasional use as an analgesic or antipyretic. However, older adults have a high incidence of musculoskeletal disorders (eg, osteoarthritis), and an NSAID is often prescribed. Long-term use increases the risk for serious GI bleeding. Small doses, gradual increments, and taking the drug with food or a full glass of water may decrease GI effects. COX-2 inhibitor NSAIDs may be especially beneficial in older adults because they are less likely to cause gastric ulceration and bleeding. Older adults also are more likely than younger adults to acquire nephrotoxicity with NSAIDs, especially with high doses or long-term use, because the drugs may reduce blood flow to the kidneys.

---

These drugs have strong anti-inflammatory effects and more severe adverse effects than the propionic acid derivatives. Potentially serious adverse effects include GI ulceration, bone marrow depression, hemolytic anemia, mental confusion, depression, and psychosis. These effects are especially associated with indomethacin; the other drugs were developed in an effort to find equally effective but less toxic derivatives of indomethacin. Although adverse reactions occur less often with sulindac and tolmetin, they are still common.

In addition to other uses, IV indomethacin is approved for treatment of patent ductus arteriosus in premature infants. (The ductus arteriosus joins the pulmonary artery to the aorta in the fetal circulation. When it fails to close, blood is shunted from the aorta to the pulmonary artery, causing severe cardiopulmonary problems.)

Other drugs related to this group are etodolac (Lodine), ketorolac (Toradol), and nabumetone (Relafen). Etodolac reportedly causes less gastric irritation, especially in older adults at high risk for GI bleeding. Ketorolac is used only for pain, and although it can be given orally, its unique characteristic is that it can be given by injection. Parenteral ketorolac reportedly compares with morphine sulfate and other narcotics in analgesic effectiveness for moderate or severe pain. However, its use is limited to 5 days because it increases the risk for bleeding. Hematomas and wound bleeding have been reported with postoperative use.

**Oxicam** drugs include meloxicam (Mobic) and piroxicam (Feldene). Meloxicam has a serum half-life of 15 to 20 hours and is excreted about equally through urine and feces. Piroxicam has a half-life of about 50 hours. The long half-lives allow the drugs to be given once daily, but optimal efficacy may not occur for 1 to 2 weeks.

**Diclofenac** sodium (Voltaren) is chemically different but pharmacologically similar to other NSAIDs. Formulations are delayed or extended release, and onset of action is therefore delayed. Peak action occurs in about 2 hours, and effects last 12 to 15 hours. The formulation of diclofenac potassium (Cataflam) is immediate release; action starts quickly, peaks in about 20 minutes to 2 hours, and also lasts 12 to 15 hours. As a result, the potassium salt may be given for rapid relief of pain and primary dysmenorrhea. Diclofenac has a serum half-life of about 2 hours and is excreted mainly in the urine.

**Cyclooxygenase-2 inhibitors** block production of prostaglandins associated with pain and inflammation without blocking those associated with protective effects

## PROTOTYPE PROFILE 7-1
## P Aspirin (AS pir in)

### Drug Class
**Chemical:** Salicylate
**Functional:** Analgesic, anti-inflammatory, antipyretic, platelet aggregation inhibitor

### Trade Names
Ascriptin, Bayer aspirin, Bufferin, Ecotrin, and others

### Therapeutic Indications
Treatment of mild to moderate pain, inflammation and fever, prophylaxis of myocardial infarction, stroke and/or transient ischemic episodes, rheumatic fever, management of rheumatoid arthritis (RA), osteoarthritis (OA), and gout

### Pharmacokinetics
*Absorption*
Well absorbed after oral administration.

*Distribution*
Plasma protein binding: 59%–90%; crosses placenta

*Metabolism*
Hydrolyzed to salicylate, which is metabolized in the liver

*Excretion*
Urine
In alkaline urine (eg, pH of 8), renal excretion of salicylate is greatly increased.

### Pharmacodynamics
*Onset of Action*
PO: 15–30 minutes; rectal 1–2 hours

*Duration*
4–6 hours

### Contraindications/Precautions
Hypersensitivity to salicylates, other NSAIDs, inherited or acquired bleeding disorders; third trimester of pregnancy
Should not be used in children <16 years of age owing to association with Reye's disease

### Pregnancy Considerations
Category: C/D (full dose aspirin in third trimester by expert analysis)
Enters breast milk, use with caution

### Dosage
*Adults*
Pain, fever: PO, 325–650 mg q4h PRN
Arthritis (OA, RA): PO, 2–6 g/d in divided doses
Prophylaxis of myocardial infarction, transient ischemic attacks (TIAs), and stroke: PO, 81–325 mg/d
TIAs: PO, 1300 mg/d in divided doses
Acute rheumatic fever: PO, 5–8 g/d in divided doses

*Children*
Pain, fever: PO, 10–15 mg/kg mg q4h
PRN, up to 60–80 mg/kg/d
Recommended doses for weight: 24–35 lb, 162 mg; 36–47 lb, 243 mg; 48–59 lb, 324 mg; 60–71 lb, 405 mg; 72–95 lb, 486 mg; 96 lb or above, 648 mg
Juvenile rheumatoid arthritis: PO, 60–110 mg/kg/d in divided doses q6–8 h
Acute rheumatic fever: PO, 100 mg/kg/d in divided doses, for 2 weeks, then 75 mg/kg/d for 4 to 6 weeks

### Adverse Effects
Bleeding, tinnitus; gastric irritation

### Drug Interactions
*Increased Effects*
Adverse effects with NSAIDs
Risk for bleeding with oral anticoagulants and antiplatelet drugs
Methotrexate and valproic acid levels

*Decreased Effects*
Effect of ACE inhibitors (with high doses of aspirin), beta blockers, thiazide and loop diuretics, probenecid

### Herbal Supplements and Dietary Considerations
Avoid dong quai, cat's claw, feverfew, garlic, ginger, ginkgo, red clover, green tea, ginseng
Curry powder, licorice, paprika contain 6 mg salicylate in 100 g
Food may decrease the rate but not the extent of absorption
Prunes, raisins, tea, gherkins, and Benedictine liqueur may increase risk for salicylate accumulation

---

on gastric mucosa. Thus, they produce less gastric irritation than aspirin and other NSAIDs. In addition, they are not associated with increased risk for bleeding because they do not have the antiplatelet effects of aspirin and other NSAIDs. Despite the relative safety of these drugs, there have been a few cases reported in which hypertension was acutely worsened by the drugs (blood pressure returned to previous levels when the drugs were discontinued; the drugs do not raise blood pressure in normotensive clients), and some clients receiving a COX-2 inhibitor had a small increase in the incidence of myocardial infarc-

tion and stroke due to thrombosis, compared with clients receiving a nonselective NSAID (naproxen) or placebo. These concerns are being investigated.

The role of COX-2 inhibitor NSAIDs in renal impairment is not clear. Although it was hoped that these drugs would have protective effects on the kidneys as they do on the stomach, studies indicate that their effects on the kidneys are similar to those of the older NSAIDs.

**Celecoxib** (Celebrex) is well absorbed with oral administration; peak plasma levels and peak action occur approximately 3 hours after an oral dose. It is highly protein bound (97%), and its serum half-life is about 11 hours. It is metabolized by the cytochrome P450 enzymes in the liver to inactive metabolites that are then excreted in the urine. A small amount is excreted unchanged in the urine. **Rofecoxib** (Vioxx) acts within 45 minutes and peaks in 2 to 3 hours. It is 87% protein bound and has a half-life of 17 hours. It is metabolized in the liver and excreted in urine and feces. **Valdecoxib** (Bextra) is a newer COX-2 inhibitor; others are being developed.

### Guidelines for Therapy With Nonsteroidal Anti-inflammatory Drugs

Nonaspirin NSAIDs are widely used and preferred by many people because of less gastric irritation and GI upset, compared with aspirin. Many NSAIDs are prescription drugs used primarily for analgesia and anti-inflammatory effects in arthritis and other musculoskeletal disorders. However, several are approved for more general use as an analgesic or antipyretic. Ibuprofen, ketoprofen, and naproxen are available by prescription and OTC. Clients must be instructed to avoid combined use of prescription and nonprescription NSAIDs because of the high risk for adverse effects. NSAIDs commonly cause gastric mucosal damage, and their prolonged use may lead to gastric ulceration and bleeding. Because NSAIDs lead to renal impairment in some clients, blood urea nitrogen and serum creatinine should be checked approximately 2 weeks after starting any of the agents.

NSAIDs inhibit platelet activity only while drug molecules are in the bloodstream, not for the life of the platelet (approximately 1 week) as aspirin does. Thus, they are not prescribed therapeutically for antiplatelet effects.

The effects of NSAIDs on liver function and the effects of hepatic impairment on most NSAIDs are largely unknown. Because the drugs are metabolized in the liver, they should be used with caution and in lower doses in people with impaired hepatic function or a history of liver disease.

In cirrhotic liver disease, naproxen and sulindac may be metabolized more slowly and aggravate hepatic impairment if dosage is not reduced. Thus, the drugs should be used cautiously, possibly in reduced dosage.

### Effects of Nonsteroidal Anti-inflammatory Drugs on Other Drugs

NSAIDs decrease effects of angiotensin-converting enzyme (ACE) inhibitors, beta blockers, and diuretics. With **ACE inhibitors,** there are decreased antihypertensive effects, probably because of sodium and water retention. With **beta blockers,** decreased antihypertensive effects are attributed to NSAID inhibition of renal prostaglandin synthesis, which allows unopposed pressor systems to produce hypertension. With **diuretics,** decreased effects on hypertension and edema are attributed to retention of sodium and water.

NSAIDs increase effects of a variety of drugs. With anticoagulants, prothrombin time may be prolonged, and NSAID-induced gastric irritation and antiplatelet effects increase the risk for bleeding. With cyclosporine, nephro-

toxicity associated with both drugs may be increased. With digoxin, ibuprofen and indomethacin may increase serum levels. With phenytoin, serum drug levels and pharmacologic effects, including adverse or toxic effects, may be increased. With lithium, serum drug levels and risk for toxicity may be increased (except with sulindac, which has no effect or may decrease serum lithium levels). With methotrexate, risk for toxicity (eg, stomatitis, bone marrow suppression, nephrotoxicity) may be increased. Celecoxib and meloxicam apparently do *not* increase methotrexate toxicity.

## Acetaminophen

Acetaminophen (also called APAP, an abbreviation for *N*-acetyl-p-aminophenol) is a nonprescription drug commonly used as an aspirin substitute because it does not cause nausea, vomiting, or GI bleeding and does not interfere with blood clotting. It is equal to aspirin in analgesic and antipyretic effects, but it lacks anti-inflammatory activity.

Acetaminophen is well absorbed with oral administration, and peak plasma concentrations are reached within 30 to 120 minutes. Duration of action is 3 to 4 hours.

Acetaminophen is metabolized in the liver; approximately 94% is excreted in the urine as inactive glucuronate and sulfate conjugates. Approximately 4% is metabolized to a toxic metabolite, which is normally inactivated by conjugation with glutathione and excreted in urine. With usual therapeutic doses, a sufficient amount of glutathione is available in the liver to detoxify acetaminophen. In acute or chronic overdose situations, however, the supply of glutathione may become depleted. In the absence of glutathione, the toxic metabolite combines with liver cells and causes damage or fatal liver necrosis.

In people who abuse alcohol, usual therapeutic doses may cause or increase liver damage. The probable mechanism for increased risk for hepatotoxicity in this population is that ethanol induces drug-metabolizing enzymes in the liver. The resulting rapid metabolism of acetaminophen produces enough toxic metabolite to exceed the available glutathione. Additionally, these metabolites may accumulate in clients with renal failure. In addition, acetaminophen is nephrotoxic in overdose because it forms a metabolite that attacks kidney cells and may cause necrosis.

Acetaminophen is available in tablet, liquid, and rectal suppository forms and is in numerous combination products marketed as analgesics and cold remedies. It is often prescribed with codeine, hydrocodone, or oxycodone for added analgesic effects.

### Guidelines for Therapy With Acetaminophen

Acetaminophen is effective and widely used for the treatment of pain and fever. Two major advantages over aspirin are that acetaminophen does not cause gastric irritation and it does not increase the risk for bleeding. It is the drug of choice for children with febrile illness (because of the association of aspirin with Reye's syndrome), elderly adults with impaired renal function (because aspirin and NSAIDs may cause further impairment), and pregnant women (because aspirin is associated with several maternal and fetal disorders, including bleeding).

As previously mentioned, despite its high degree of safety when used appropriately, acetaminophen is probably not the drug of choice for people with hepatitis or other liver disorders or those who drink substantial amounts of alcoholic beverages. The major drawback to acetaminophen use is potentially fatal liver damage with overdose because the drug forms a metabolite that can destroy liver cells, causing necrosis. The hepatotoxic metabolite is formed more rapidly when drug-metabolizing enzymes in the liver have been stimulated by ingestion of alcohol, cigarette smoking, and drugs such as anticonvulsants and others. Thus, alcoholics are at high risk for hepatotoxicity with usual therapeutic doses. The kidneys and myocardium may also be damaged.

## Toxicology: Acetaminophen Poisoning

Poisoning may occur with a single large dose (possibly as little as 6 g, but usually 10 to 15 g), or chronic ingestion of excessive doses (5 to 8 g/day for several weeks or 3 to 4 g/day for 1 year). Potentially fatal hepatotoxicity is the main concern and is most likely to occur with doses of 20 g or more. Metabolism of acetaminophen produces a toxic metabolite that is normally inactivated by combining with glutathione. In overdose situations, the supply of glutathione is depleted, and the toxic metabolite accumulates and directly damages liver cells. Acute renal failure may also occur.

### Prevention

The recommended maximum daily dose is 4 g for adults; additional amounts constitute an overdose. Ingestion of an overdose may be accidental or intentional. A contributing factor may be that some people think the drug is so safe that they can take any amount without harm. Another may be that people take the drug in several formulations without calculating or realizing that they are taking potentially harmful amounts. For example, numerous brand names of acetaminophen are available OTC, and acetaminophen is an ingredient in many prescription and OTC combination products (eg, Percocet, and OTC cold, flu, headache, and sinus remedies). For chronic alcohol abusers, short-term ingestion of usual therapeutic doses may cause hepatotoxicity, and it is recommended that they ingest no more than 2 g daily. If they ingest three or more alcoholic drinks daily, they should avoid acetaminophen or ask a health care provider before using even small doses. Another recommendation is to limit duration of use (5 days or less in children, 10 days or less in adults, and 3 days in both adults and children when used to reduce fever) unless directed by a health care provider.

Because of multiple reports of liver damage from acetaminophen poisoning, the FDA may strengthen the warning on products containing acetaminophen and emphasize that the maximum dose of 4 g daily, from all sources, should not be exceeded.

### Recognition: Signs and Symptoms

Early symptoms (12 to 24 hours after ingestion) are non-specific (eg, anorexia, nausea, vomiting, diaphoresis) and may not be considered serious or important enough to report or seek treatment. After 24 to 48 hours, symptoms may subside. but tests of liver function (eg, aspartate transaminase [AST], alanine transaminase [ALT], bilirubin, prothrombin time) begin to increase. Later manifestations may include jaundice, vomiting, and central nervous system stimulation with excitement and delirium, followed by vascular collapse, coma, and death. Peak hepatotoxicity occurs in 3 to 4 days; recovery in nonfatal overdoses occurs in 7 to 8 days.

Plasma acetaminophen levels should be obtained when an overdose is known or suspected, preferably within 4 hours after ingestion and every 24 hours for several days. Minimal hepatotoxicity is associated with plasma levels of less than 120 mcg/mL at 4 hours after ingestion or less than 30 mcg/mL at 12 hours after ingestion. With blood levels greater than 300 mcg/mL at 4 hours after ingestion, about 90% of clients develop liver damage.

### Treatment

Gastric lavage is recommended if overdose is detected within 4 hours after ingestion and activated charcoal can be given to inhibit absorption. In addition, the specific antidote is acetylcysteine (Mucomyst), a mucolytic agent given by inhalation in respiratory disorders. For acetaminophen poisoning, it is usually given orally (dosage is listed with other antidotes in Chap. 2). The drug provides cysteine, a precursor substance required for the synthesis of glutathione. Glutathione combines with a toxic metabolite and decreases hepatotoxicity if acetylcysteine is given. Acetylcysteine is most beneficial if given within 8 to 10 hours of acetaminophen ingestion, but it may be helpful up to 36 hours. It does not reverse damage that has already occurred.

## Herbal and Dietary Supplements

In addition to the drugs described previously, many herbal medicines are used to relieve pain and inflammation. For most of these (eg, comfrey, marigold, peppermint, primrose), such usage is anecdotal and unsupported by clinical studies. For a few supplements, there is some evidence of effectiveness with few adverse effects; these are described below.

**Chondroitin sulfate** (CS), a supplement extracted from animal cartilage or manufactured synthetically and used to treat arthritis, is thought to delay the breakdown of joint cartilage (by inhibiting elastase, a proteolytic enzyme found in synovial membranes), to stimulate synthesis of new cartilage (by stimulating chondrocytes to produce collagen and proteoglycan), and to promote the "shock-absorbing" quality of cartilage (by retaining water).

Chondroitin is a normal component of joint cartilage, which contains water (65% to 80%), collagen, proteoglycans, and chondrocytes that produce new collagen and proteoglycans. CS was first used as a dietary supplement because studies suggested that it would promote healing of cartilage damaged by inflammation or injury. The daily dose is based on the client's weight: less than 120 lb, 800 mg CS; 120 to 200 lb, 1200 mg CS; more than 200 lb, 1600 mg CS. CS is usually taken with food, in two to four divided doses.

Proponents of CS cite clinical trials that indicate beneficial effects. Proponents also tout the safety of CS in comparison with the adverse effects of NSAIDs. The main adverse effect is reportedly minor stomach upset. In addition, there is a theoretical risk for bleeding because of the drug's structural similarity to heparin, but there have been no reports of bleeding from the use of CS.

Opponents question the quality of the studies, whether CS is absorbed systemically, because of its large molecule size, and whether it is able to reach cartilage cells. They also state that little is known about long-term toxicity of the compound.

**Feverfew** is an herbal medicine with some evidence of effectiveness in migraine, especially in reducing the incidence and severity. Its main active ingredient is thought to be parthenolide. Feverfew is thought to inhibit platelet aggregation, prostaglandin synthesis, and the release of inflammatory mediators such as histamine, but its exact mechanism in migraine prophylaxis is unknown. It is contraindicated in pregnant and lactating women.

In general, clients should be encouraged to try standard methods of preventing and treating migraine before taking products with uncertain benefits and risks. For example, commercial preparations are not standardized and may contain different amounts of parthenolide. The usual recommended dose is 25 to 50 mg daily with food, but more studies are needed.

Adverse effects include hypersensitivity reactions in people who are allergic to ragweed, asters, chrysanthemums, or daisies, and stopping the preparation abruptly can result in withdrawal symptoms of pain and stiffness. No interactions with OTC or prescription drugs have been reported, but there is a potential for increasing the risk for bleeding in clients taking an antiplatelet drug (eg, aspirin) or an anticoagulant (eg, warfarin).

**Glucosamine,** a synthetic supplement, is also taken for arthritis. Glucosamine is an essential structural component of joint connective tissue. With OA, glucosamine production is decreased, synovial fluid becomes thin and less effective in lubricating the joint, and joint cartilage deteriorates. The rationale for taking supplementary glucosamine is to reduce cartilage breakdown and improve cartilage production and repair.

Some studies indicate that glucosamine may decrease mild to moderate OA pain in some clients, possibly as well as NSAIDs; other studies indicate little or no benefit when glucosamine is compared with placebo. There is controversy about glucosamine's ability to affect cartilage structure and delay joint deterioration. Most studies are criticized as being too small and of too short duration, and of having flawed designs. A study of 212 clients with knee OA indicated that long-term use of glucosamine improves symptoms and prevents changes in joint structure. These clients took 1500 mg of glucosamine sulfate or placebo once a day for 3 years; radiographs of the knees were taken before starting glucosamine and after 1 and 3 years of treatment. The researchers concluded that significant improvement of symptoms and less joint deterioration occurred in clients receiving glucosamine. Some reviewers of this study said the pain relief was minor and the radiographic changes were insignificant and did not indicate improvement in disease progression.

Glucosamine is available as a hydrochloride salt and as a sulfate salt. Most studies have been done with glucosamine sulfate (GS), and this is the preferred form. Dosage is based on the client's weight: less than 120 lb, 1000 mg GS; 120 to 200 lb, 1500 mg GS; more than 200 lb, 2000 mg GS. The total daily dosage is usually taken with food in two to four divided doses.

There are no known contraindications to the use of glucosamine, but it should be avoided during pregnancy and lactation and in children because effects are unknown. Adverse effects include GI upset (eg, epigastric pain, heartburn, nausea, constipation, diarrhea), drowsiness, headache, and skin rash. No interactions with OTC or prescription drugs have been reported.

**Glucosamine and chondroitin** can each be used alone but are more often taken in combination, with the same dosages as listed previously. Use of this combination greatly increased after it was highly praised in *The Arthritis Cure*, by J. Theodosakis.

As with studies of the individual components, many of the studies involving glucosamine and chondroitin are flawed. The American College of Rheumatology and the Arthritis Foundation do not recommend the use of these supplements because they do not believe reported research studies adequately demonstrate significant relief of symptoms or slowing of the disease process. These organizations say longer clinical trials with larger groups of people are needed. When questioned by clients, some health care providers suggest taking the supplement for 3 months (glucosamine, 500 mg, and chondroitin, 400 mg, 3 times a day) and decide for themselves whether their symptoms improve (eg, less pain, improved ability to walk) and whether they want to continue.

## ▨ DRUG USE IN SPECIAL SITUATIONS

### Drugs Used in Gout and Hyperuricemia

Individual drugs are described below; dosages are listed in Drugs at a Glance 7-2: Drugs for Gout.

**Allopurinol** (Zyloprim) is used to prevent or treat hyperuricemia, which occurs with gout and with antineoplastic drug therapy. Uric acid is formed by purine metabolism and an enzyme called xanthine oxidase. Allopurinol

## _Drugs at a Glance_
## Drugs for Gout

| Generic/Trade Name | Routes and Dosage Ranges | Comments |
|---|---|---|
| **Allopurinol** (Zyloprim)<br>Pregnancy Category C | _Adults:_ Mild gout, PO, 200–400 mg/d; severe gout, PO, 400–600 mg/d; hyperuricemia in clients with renal insufficiency, PO, 100–200 mg/d; secondary hyperuricemia from anticancer drugs, PO, 100–200 mg/d, maximum 800 mg/d<br>_Children:_ Secondary hyperuricemia from anticancer drugs: <6 y, PO, 150 mg/d; 6–10 y, PO, 300 mg/d | Alcohol decreases effectiveness<br>Administer oral forms after meals with plenty of water |
| **Colchicine**<br>Pregnancy Category C (oral), D (parenteral) | _Adults:_ Acute attacks, PO, 0.5 mg q1h until pain is relieved or toxicity (nausea, vomiting, diarrhea) occurs; 3-d interval between courses of therapy<br>IV, 1–2 mg initially, then 0.5 mg q3–6h until response is obtained; maximum total dose 4 mg<br>Prophylaxis, PO, 0.5–1 mg/d<br>_Children:_ Dosage not established | $B_{12}$ absorption may decrease, so supplementation may be necessary; extravasation of tissue with IV infiltration; do not administer IM or Sub-Q |
| **Probenecid** (Benemid)<br>Pregnancy Category B | _Adults:_ PO, 250 mg twice a day for 1 wk, then 500 mg twice a day<br>_Children:_ >2 years: PO, 40 mg/kg/d in divided doses | Give with food if GI distress occurs; instruct clients to drink plenty of fluids to reduce risk for uric acid stones |
| **Sulfinpyrazone** (Anturane)<br>Pregnancy Category C/D (near term by expert analysis) | _Adults:_ PO, 100–200 mg twice a day, gradually increased over 1 wk to a maximum of 400–800 mg/d<br>_Children:_ Dosage not established | Monitor serum and urine uric acid levels |

prevents formation of uric acid by inhibiting xanthine oxidase. It is especially useful in chronic gout characterized by tophi (deposits of uric acid crystals in the joints, kidneys, and soft tissues) and impaired renal function.

The drug promotes resorption of urate deposits and prevents their further development. Acute attacks of gout may result when urate deposits are mobilized. These may be prevented by concomitant administration of colchicine until serum uric acid levels are lowered.

**Colchicine** is an anti-inflammatory drug used to prevent or treat acute attacks of gout. In acute attacks, it is the drug of choice for relieving joint pain and edema. Colchicine decreases inflammation by decreasing the movement of leukocytes into body tissues containing urate crystals. It has no analgesic or antipyretic effects.

**Probenecid** (Benemid) increases the urinary excretion of uric acid. This uricosuric action is used therapeutically to treat hyperuricemia and gout. It is not effective in acute attacks of gouty arthritis but prevents hyperuricemia and tophi associated with chronic gout. Probenecid may precipitate acute gout until serum uric acid levels are within the normal range; concomitant administration of colchicine prevents this effect. (Probenecid also is used

with penicillin, most often in treating sexually transmitted diseases. It increases blood levels and prolongs the action of penicillin by decreasing the rate of urinary excretion.)

**Sulfinpyrazone** (Anturane) is a uricosuric agent similar to probenecid. It is not effective in acute gout but prevents or decreases tissue changes of chronic gout. Colchicine is usually given during initial sulfinpyrazone therapy to prevent acute gout.

### Guidelines for Treating Hyperuricemia and Gout

Opinions differ regarding treatment of asymptomatic hyperuricemia. Some authorities do not think drug therapy is indicated; others think that lowering serum uric acid levels may prevent joint inflammation and renal calculi. Allopurinol, probenecid, or sulfinpyrazone may be given for this purpose. Colchicine also should be given for several weeks to prevent acute attacks of gout while serum uric acid levels are being lowered. During initial administration of these drugs, a high fluid intake (to produce approximately 2000 mL of urine per day) and alkaline urine are recommended to prevent renal calculi. Urate crystals are more likely to precipitate in acid urine.

## CLIENT TEACHING GUIDELINES
### Acetaminophen, Aspirin, and Other NSAIDs

### General Considerations

✔ Aspirin and other nonsteroidal anti-inflammatory drugs (NSAIDs) such as ibuprofen (Advil, Motrin) are used to relieve pain, fever, and inflammation. Aspirin is as effective as the more costly NSAIDs, but is more likely to cause stomach irritation and bleeding problems. This advantage of NSAIDs may be minimal if high doses are taken.

Because these drugs are so widely used and available, there is a high risk of overdosing on different products containing the same drug or products containing similar drugs. Knowing drug names, reading product labels, and using the following precautions can increase safety in using these drugs:

1. If you are taking aspirin or an NSAID regularly for pain or inflammation, generally avoid taking additional aspirin in over-the-counter (OTC) aspirin or products containing aspirin (eg, Alka-Seltzer, Anacin, Arthritis Pain Formula, Ascriptin, Bufferin, Doan's Pills/Caplets, Ecotrin, Excedrin, Midol, Vanquish). There are two exceptions if you are taking a small dose of aspirin daily (usually 81–325 mg), to prevent heart attack and stroke. First, you should continue taking the aspirin if Celebrex, Vioxx, or Bextra is prescribed. Second, it is generally safe to take occasional doses of aspirin or an NSAID for pain or fever.

2. If you are taking any prescription NSAID regularly, avoid OTC products containing ibuprofen (eg, Advil, Dristan Sinus, Midol IB, Motrin IB, Sine-Aid IB), ketoprofen (Actron, Orudis KT), or naproxen (Aleve). Also, do not combine the OTC products with each other or with aspirin. These drugs are available as both prescription and OTC products. OTC ibuprofen is the same medication as prescription Motrin; OTC naproxen is the same as prescription Naprosyn; OTC ketoprofen is the same as prescription Orudis. Recommended doses are smaller for OTC products than for prescription drugs. However, any combination of these drugs could constitute an overdose.

✔ With NSAIDs, if one is not effective, another one may work because people vary in responses to the drugs. Improvement of symptoms depends on the reason for use. When taken for pain, the drugs usually act within 30 to 60 minutes; when taken for inflammatory disorders, such as arthritis, improvement may occur within 24 to 48 hours with aspirin and 1 to 2 weeks with other NSAIDs.

✔ Taking a medication for fever is not usually recommended unless the fever is high or is accompanied by other symptoms. Fever is one way the body fights infection.

✔ Do not take OTC ibuprofen more than 3 days for fever or 10 days for pain. If these symptoms persist or worsen, or if new symptoms develop, contact a health care provider.

✔ Avoid aspirin for approximately 2 weeks before and after major surgery or dental work to decrease the risk of excessive bleeding. If pregnant, do not take aspirin for approximately 2 weeks before the estimated delivery date.

✔ Inform any health care provider if taking aspirin, ibuprofen, or any other NSAID regularly.

✔ Inform health care providers if you have ever had an allergic reaction (eg, asthma, difficulty in breathing, hives) or severe GI symptoms (eg, ulcer, bleeding) after taking aspirin, ibuprofen, or similar drugs.

✔ Avoid or minimize alcoholic beverages because alcohol increases gastric irritation and risks of bleeding. The Food and Drug Administration requires an alcohol warning on the labels of OTC pain and fever relievers and urges people who drink three or more alcoholic drinks every day to ask their doctors before using the products.

✔ To avoid accidental ingestion and aspirin poisoning, store aspirin in a closed childproof container and keep out of children's reach.

### Self-administration

✔ Take aspirin, ibuprofen, and other NSAIDs with a full glass of liquid and food to decrease stomach irritation. Rofecoxib (Vioxx) and meloxicam (Mobic) may be taken without regard to food.

✔ Swallow enteric-coated aspirin (eg, Ecotrin) whole; do not chew or crush. The coating is applied to decrease stomach irritation by making the tablet dissolve in the intestine. Also, do not take with an antacid, which can cause the tablet to dissolve in the stomach.

✔ Swallow any long-acting pills or capsules whole; do not chew or crush. These include diclofenac sodium (Voltaren or Voltaren XR); diflunisal (Dolobid); etodolac (Lodine XL); ketoprofen or Oruvail extended-release capsules; naproxen delayed-release (EC-Naprosyn) or controlled-release (Naprelan) tablets.

*Note:* These are prescription drugs and most are also available in short-acting products; if unsure whether the medicine you are taking is long-acting, ask a health care provider.

✔ Drink 2–3 quarts of fluid daily when taking an NSAID regularly. This decreases gastric irritation and helps to maintain good kidney function.

✔ Report signs of bleeding (eg, nose bleed, vomiting blood, bruising, blood in urine or stools), difficulty breathing, skin rash or hives, ringing in ears, dizziness, severe stomach upset, or swelling and weight gain.

### Acetaminophen

✔ Acetaminophen is often the initial drug of choice for relieving mild-to-moderate pain and fever because it is effective and does not cause gastric irritation or bleeding. It may be taken on an empty stomach.

*(continued)*

## CLIENT TEACHING GUIDELINES
### Acetaminophen, Aspirin, and Other NSAIDs (Continued)

✔ Acetaminophen is an effective aspirin substitute for pain or fever but not for inflammation or preventing heart attack or stroke.

✔ Acetaminophen is available in its generic form and with many OTC brand names (eg, Tylenol). Most preparations contain 500 mg of drug per tablet or capsule. In addition, almost all OTC pain relievers (often labeled "nonaspirin") and cold, flu, and sinus remedies contain acetaminophen. Thus, all consumers should read product labels carefully to avoid taking the drug in several products, with potential overdoses.

✔ Do not exceed recommended doses. For occasional pain or fever, 650–1000 mg may be taken three or four times daily. For daily, long-term use (eg, in osteoarthritis), do not take more than 4000 mg (eg, eight 500 mg or extra-strength tablets or capsules) daily. Larger doses may cause life-threatening liver damage. People who have hepatitis or other liver disorders and those who ingest alcoholic beverages frequently should take no more than 2000 mg daily.

✔ Do not exceed recommended duration of use (longer than 5 days in children, 10 days in adults, or 3 days for fever in adults and children) without consulting a physician.

✔ Avoid or minimize alcoholic beverages because alcohol increases risk of liver damage. The Food and Drug Administration requires an alcohol warning on the labels of OTC pain and fever relievers and urges people who drink three or more alcoholic drinks every day to ask their doctors before taking products containing acetaminophen.

#### Antigout Drugs

✔ When colchicine is taken for acute gout, pain is usually relieved in 4–12 hours with IV administration and 24–48 hours with oral administration. Inflammation and edema may not decrease for several days.

✔ With colchicine for chronic gout, carry the drug and start taking it as directed (usually one pill every hour for several hours until relief is obtained or nausea, vomiting, and diarrhea occur) when joint pain starts. This prevents or minimizes acute attacks of gout.

✔ Drink 2–3 quarts of fluid daily with antigout drugs. An adequate fluid intake helps prevent formation of uric acid kidney stones. Fluid intake is especially important initially, when uric acid levels in the blood are high and large amounts of uric acid are being excreted in the urine.

✔ When allopurinol is taken, blood levels of uric acid usually decrease to normal range within 1–3 weeks.

## Drugs Used for Migraines

Individual drugs are described below; dosages are listed in Drugs at a Glance 7-3: Drugs for Migraine.

**Almotriptan** (Axert), **frovatriptan** (Frova), **naratriptan** (Amerge), **rizatriptan** (Maxalt), **sumatriptan** (Imitrex), and **zolmitriptan** (Zomig), called *triptans*, were developed specifically for the treatment of moderate or severe migraines. They are called selective serotonin 5-HT$_1$ receptor agonists because they act on a specific subtype of serotonin receptor to increase serotonin (5-hydroxytryptamine, or 5-HT) in the brain. They relieve migraine by constricting blood vessels. Because of their vasoconstrictive properties, the drugs are contraindicated in clients with a history of angina pectoris, myocardial infarction, or uncontrolled hypertension. The drugs vary in onset of action, with subcutaneous sumatriptan acting the most rapidly and starting to relieve migraine headache within 10 minutes. Most clients get relief within 1 to 2 hours with all of the oral drugs. The drugs are metabolized in the liver by monoamine oxidase or cytochrome P450 enzymes; metabolism of rizatriptan and zolmitriptan produces active metabolites. Subcutaneous sumatriptan produces more adverse effects than the oral drugs, which have similar adverse effects (eg, pain, paresthesias, nausea, dizziness, and drowsiness). These drugs are considered safer than ergot alkaloids.

**Ergotamine tartrate** (Ergomar) is an ergot alkaloid used only in the treatment of migraine. Ergot preparations relieve migraine by constricting blood vessels. Ergotamine is most effective when given sublingually or by inhalation at the onset of headache. When given orally, ergotamine is erratically absorbed, and therapeutic effects may be delayed for 20 to 30 minutes. Ergotamine is contraindicated during pregnancy and in the presence of severe hypertension, peripheral vascular disease, coronary artery disease, renal or hepatic disease, and severe infections.

**Ergotamine tartrate and caffeine** (Cafergot) is a commonly used antimigraine preparation. Caffeine reportedly increases the absorption and vasoconstrictive effects of ergotamine. **Dihydroergotamine mesylate** (DHE 45) is a semisynthetic derivative of ergotamine that is less toxic and less effective than the parent drug.

### Guidelines for Treating Migraine

For infrequent or mild migraine attacks, acetaminophen, aspirin, or other NSAIDs may be effective. For example, NSAIDs are often effective in migraines associated with menstruation. For moderate to severe migraine attacks, sumatriptan and related drugs are effective, and they cause fewer adverse effects than ergot preparations. They are usually well tolerated; adverse effects are relatively minor and usually brief. However, because they are strong vasoconstrictors, people with coronary artery disease or hypertension should not take them. They are also expensive compared with other antimigraine drugs. If an

## DRUG TABLE 7-3

### *Drugs at a Glance*
### Drugs for Migraines

| Generic/Trade Name | Routes and Dosage Ranges | Comments |
|---|---|---|
| *Serotonin agonists (Triptans)* | | |
| **Almotriptan** (Axert)<br>Pregnancy Category C | PO, 6.25 mg, repeat after 2 h if necessary. Maximum, 12.5 mg/24 h (2 doses) | Used to reduce migraine; does not prevent or reduce number of attacks; cardiac events have been reported with use |
| **Naratriptan** (Amerge)<br>Pregnancy Category C | PO, 1–2.5 mg as a single dose; repeat in 4 h if necessary. Maximum, 5 mg/d | Do not crush or chew tablets.<br>Used to reduce migraine, not to prevent or reduce number of attacks; cardiac events have been reported with use. |
| **Rizatriptan** (Maxalt)<br>Pregnancy Category C | PO, 5–10 mg as a single dose; repeat after 2 h if necessary. Maximum dose, 30 mg/d (15 mg/d maximum if taking propranolol) | Maxalt-MLT (orally disintegrating tablets) contain phenylalanine; store in blister packs until administering; open with dry hands |
| **Sumatriptan** (Imitrex)<br>Pregnancy Category C | PO, 25–100 mg as a single dose. Maximum dose, 200 mg/d<br>Sub-Q, 6 mg as a single dose. Maximum, 12 mg/d<br>Nasal spray 5, 10, or 20 mg by unit-dose spray device. Maximum, 40 mg/d | PO dose in older adults not recommended due to prevalence of heart disease in that group<br>Significant hepatic first-pass metabolism with oral route |
| **Zolmitriptan** (Zomig)<br>Pregnancy Category C | PO, 1.25–2.5 mg as a single dose; may repeat after 2 h if necessary. Maximum dose, 10 mg/d | Used to reduce migraine; does not prevent or reduce number of attacks; cardiac events have been reported with use |
| *Ergot Preparations* | | |
| **Ergotamine tartrate** (Ergomar)<br>Pregnancy Category X | PO, sublingually, 1–2 mg at onset of migraine, then 2 mg q30min, if necessary, to a maximum of 6 mg/24 h or 10 mg/wk<br>Inhalation, 0.36 mg (one inhalation) at onset of migraine, repeat in 5 min, if necessary, to a maximum of 6 inhalations/24 h | Do not take with pregnancy because drug crosses placenta and may cause reduced placental blood flow<br>Do not crush sublingual products<br>Avoid caffeinated beverages because they may increase gastric absorption of drug; grapefruit juice may increase drug levels, leading to toxicity |
| **Ergotamine tartrate and caffeine** (Cafergot)<br>Pregnancy Category X | *Adults:* PO, 2 tablets at onset of migraine, then 1 tablet q30min, if necessary, up to 6 tablets per attack or 10 tablets/wk<br>Rectal suppository, 0.5–1 suppository at onset of migraine, repeat in 1 h, if necessary, up to two suppositories per attack or five suppositories/wk<br>*Children:* PO, 0.5–1 tablet initially, then 0.5 tablet q30min, if necessary, to a maximum of three tablets | Do not take with pregnancy because ergotamine and caffeine cross placenta and may cause reduced placental blood flow<br>Avoid caffeinated beverages because they may increase gastric absorption of drug; grapefruit juice may increase drug levels, leading to toxicity |
| **Dihydroergotamine mesylate** (DHE 45, Migranal)<br>Pregnancy Category X | IM, Sub-Q, 1 mg at onset of migraine, may be repeated hourly, if necessary, to a total of 3 mg<br>*Nasal spray,* 1 spray (0.5 mg) into each nostril, may be repeated after 15 min up to 4 sprays. Maximum, 3 mg/d. Do not exceed 8 sprays (4 mg)/wk<br>IV, 1 mg, repeated, if necessary, after 1 h; maximum dose 2 mg. Do not exceed 6 mg/wk | Should not be taken in pregnancy, with heart disease, high blood pressure, or liver disease<br>Do not tilt head back or inhale when using nasal dosing |

ergot preparation is used, it should be given at the onset of headache, and the client should lie down in a quiet, darkened room.

For frequent (two or more per month) or severe migraine attacks, prophylactic therapy is needed. Those for whom the triptans and ergot preparations are contraindicated for acute attacks and those whose attacks are predictable (eg, perimenstrual) may also need drug therapy to reduce the incidence and severity of acute attacks. Numerous medications have been used for prophylaxis, including aspirin (650 mg twice daily) and NSAIDs (ibuprofen 300 to 600 mg three times daily; ketoprofen (50 to 75 mg twice or three times daily); and naproxen (250 to 750 mg daily or 250 mg three times daily). When used to prevent migraine associated with menses, they should be started approximately 1 week before and continued through the menstrual period. Although these drugs are usually well tolerated, long-term use is not recommended because of GI and renal toxicity associated with chronic inhibition of prostaglandin production. Other prophylactic drugs include propranolol and other beta-adrenergic blocking agents (see Chap. 19).

# Drugs Used for Arthritis

Individual drugs have been previously described or are identified in subsequent chapters. Goals of drug therapy for OA and RA are described below.

## Guidelines for Treating Arthritis

The primary goals of treatment are to control pain and inflammation and to minimize immobilization and disability. Rest, exercise, physical therapy, and drugs are used to attain these goals. Few of these measures prevent or slow joint destruction.

### Osteoarthritis

The main goal of drug therapy is relief of pain. Acetaminophen is probably the initial drug of choice. For clients whose pain is inadequately relieved by acetaminophen, an NSAID is usually given. Ibuprofen and other propionic acid derivatives are often used, although available NSAIDs have comparable effectiveness. A drug may be given for 2 or 3 weeks on a trial basis. If therapeutic benefits occur, the drug may be continued; if

---

## CLIENT TEACHING GUIDELINES
## Drugs for Migraines

### General Considerations

✔ Try to identify and avoid situations known to precipitate acute attacks of migraine.

✔ For mild or infrequent migraine attacks, acetaminophen, aspirin, or another nonsteroidal anti-inflammatory drug may be effective.

✔ For moderate to severe migraine attacks, the drug of first choice is probably sumatriptan (Imitrex) or a related drug, if not contraindicated (eg, by heart disease or hypertension). However, one of these drugs should not be taken if an ergot preparation has been taken within the previous 24 hours.

✔ If you have frequent or severe migraine attacks, consult a physician about medications to prevent or reduce the frequency of acute attacks.

✔ Never take an antimigraine medication prescribed for someone else or allow someone else to take yours. The medications used to relieve acute migraine can constrict blood vessels, raise blood pressure, and cause serious adverse effects.

### Self-administration

✔ Take medication at onset of pain, when possible, to prevent development of more severe symptoms.

✔ With triptans, take oral drugs (except for rizatriptan orally disintegrating tablets) with fluids. If symptoms recur, a second dose may be taken. However, do not take a second dose of sumatriptan or zolmitriptan sooner than 2 hours after the first dose, or a second dose of naratriptan sooner than 4 hours after the first dose. Do not take

more than 12.5 mg of almotriptan, 7.5 mg of frovatriptan, 5 mg of naratriptan, or 10 mg of zolmitriptan in any 24-hour period.

✔ Rizatriptan is available in a regular tablet, which can be taken with fluids, and in an orally disintegrating tablet, which can be dissolved on the tongue and swallowed without fluids. The tablet should be removed from its package with dry hands and placed on the tongue immediately.

✔ Sumatriptan can be taken by mouth, injection, or nasal spray. Instructions should be strictly followed for the prescribed method of administration. For the nasal spray, the usual dose is one spray into one nostril. If symptoms return, a second spray may be taken 2 hours or longer after the first spray. Do not take more than 40 mg of nasal spray or 200 mg orally or by injection in any 24-hour period. If self-administering injectable sumatriptan, be sure to give in fatty tissue under the skin. This drug must not be taken intravenously; serious, potentially fatal reactions may occur.

✔ If symptoms of an allergic reaction (eg, shortness of breath, wheezing, heart pounding, swelling of eyelids, face or lips, skin rash, or hives) occur after taking a triptan drug, tell your prescribing physician immediately and do not take any additional doses without specific instructions to do so.

✔ With ergot preparations, report signs of poor blood circulation, such as tingling sensations or coldness, numbness, or weakness of the arms and legs. These are symptoms of ergot toxicity. To avoid potentially serious adverse effects, do not exceed recommended doses.

no benefits seem evident or toxicity occurs, another drug may be tried. A COX-2 inhibitor may be preferred for clients at high risk for GI ulceration and bleeding. NSAIDs are usually given in analgesic doses for OA, rather than the larger anti-inflammatory doses given for RA.

Additional treatments for knee OA include topical capsaicin; oral chondroitin and glucosamine; intraarticular injections of corticosteroids (see Chap. 35); or hyaluronic acid (eg, Synvisc, a product that helps restore the shock-absorbing ability of joint structures). Clients who continue to have severe pain and functional impairment despite medical treatment may need knee replacement surgery.

*Rheumatoid Arthritis*
Acetaminophen may relieve pain; aspirin or another NSAID may relieve pain and inflammation. Aspirin is effective, but many people are unable to tolerate the adverse effects associated with anti-inflammatory doses. When aspirin is used, dosage usually ranges between 2 and 6 g daily but should be individualized to relieve symptoms, maintain therapeutic salicylate blood levels, and minimize adverse effects. For people who cannot take aspirin, another NSAID may be given. For those who cannot take aspirin or a nonselective NSAID because of gastric irritation, peptic ulcer disease, bleeding disorders, or other contraindications, a selective COX-2 inhibitor NSAID may be preferred. NSAIDs are usually given in larger, anti-inflammatory doses for RA, rather than the smaller, analgesic doses given for OA.

Second-line drugs, for moderate or severe RA, include corticosteroids and immunosuppressants (see Chap. 35). The goal of treatment with corticosteroids is to relieve symptoms; the goal with immunosuppressants is to relieve symptoms and also slow tissue damage (so-called disease-modifying effects). Both groups of drugs may cause serious adverse effects, including greatly increased susceptibility to infection. Methotrexate (MTX), which is also used in cancer chemotherapy, is given in smaller doses for RA. It is unknown whether MTX has disease-modifying effects or just improves symptoms and quality of life. About 75% of clients have a beneficial response, with improvement usually evident within 4 to 8 weeks (ie, less morning stiffness, pain, joint edema, and fatigue).

Three newer immunosuppressants used to treat RA are etanercept (Enbrel), infliximab (Remicade), and leflunomide (Arava). Clinical improvement usually occurs within a few weeks. One of these drugs may be used alone or given along with MTX in clients whose symptoms are inadequately controlled by MTX alone.

## Perioperative Use of Aspirin and Other Nonsteroidal Anti-inflammatory Drugs

Aspirin should generally be avoided for 1 to 2 weeks before and after surgery because it increases the risk for bleeding. Most other NSAIDs should be discontinued approximately 3 days before surgery; nabumetone and piroxicam have long half-lives and must be discontinued approximately 1 week before surgery. After surgery, especially after relatively minor procedures, such as dental extractions and episiotomies, several of the drugs are used to relieve pain. Caution is needed because of increased risk for bleeding, and the drugs should not be given if there are other risk factors for bleeding. In addition, ketorolac, the only injectable NSAID, has been used in more extensive surgeries. Although the drug has several advantages over narcotic analgesics, bleeding and hematomas may occur.

## Use of Acetaminophen, Aspirin, and Other Nonsteroidal Anti-inflammatory Drugs for Cancer Pain

Cancer often produces chronic pain from tumor invasion of tissues or complications of treatment (chemotherapy, surgery, or radiation). As with acute pain, these drugs prevent sensitization of peripheral pain receptors by inhibiting prostaglandin formation. They are especially effective for pain associated with bone metastases. For mild pain, acetaminophen or an NSAID may be used alone; for moderate to severe pain, these drugs may be continued and a narcotic analgesic added. Non-narcotic and narcotic analgesics can be given together or alternated; a combination of analgesics is often needed to provide optimal pain relief. Aspirin is contraindicated for the client receiving chemotherapy that depresses the bone marrow, because of the high risk for thrombocytopenia and bleeding.

## Nursing Process

### Assessment
- Assess for signs and symptoms of pain, such as location, severity, duration, and factors that cause or relieve the pain (see Chap. 6).
- Assess for fever (thermometer readings above 99.6°F [37.3°C] are usually considered fever). Hot, dry skin; flushed face; reduced urine output; and concentrated urine may accompany fever if the person also is dehydrated.
- Assess for inflammation. Local signs are redness, heat, edema, and pain or tenderness; systemic signs include fever, elevated white blood cell count (leukocytosis), and weakness.

*(continued)*

## NURSING PROCESS (Continued)

- With arthritis or other musculoskeletal disorders, assess for pain and limitations in activity and mobility.
- Ask about use of OTC analgesic, antipyretic, or anti-inflammatory drugs and herbal or dietary supplements.
- Ask about allergic reactions to aspirin or NSAIDs.
- Assess for history of peptic ulcer disease, GI bleeding, or kidney disorders.
- With migraine, assess severity and patterns of occurrences.

### Nursing Diagnoses

- Acute Pain
- Chronic Pain
- Activity Intolerance related to pain
- Risk for Poisoning: Acetaminophen overdose
- Risk for Injury related to adverse drug effects (GI bleeding, renal insufficiency)
- Deficient Knowledge: Therapeutic and adverse effects of commonly used drugs
- Deficient Knowledge: Correct use of OTC drugs for pain, fever, and inflammation

### Planning/Goals

*The client will:*

- Experience relief of discomfort with minimal adverse drug effects
- Experience increased mobility and activity tolerance
- Inform health care providers if taking aspirin or an NSAID regularly
- Self-administer the drugs safely
- Avoid overuse of the drugs
- Use measures to prevent accidental ingestion or overdose, especially in children
- Experience fewer and less severe attacks of migraine

### Interventions

Implement measures to prevent or minimize pain, fever, and inflammation:

- Treat the disease processes (eg, infection, arthritis) or circumstances (eg, impaired blood supply, lack of physical activity, poor positioning or body alignment) thought to be causing pain, fever, or inflammation
- Treat pain as soon as possible; early treatment may prevent severe pain and anxiety and allow the use of milder analgesic drugs. Use distraction, relaxation techniques, other nonpharmacologic techniques along with drug therapy, when appropriate.
- With acute musculoskeletal injuries (eg, sprains), cold applications can decrease pain, swelling, and inflammation. Apply for approximately 20 minutes, then remove.
- Assist clients with migraine to identify and avoid "triggers."

Assist clients to drink 2 to 3 L of fluid daily when taking an NSAID regularly. This decreases gastric irritation and helps to maintain good kidney function. With long-term use of aspirin, fluids help to prevent precipitation of salicylate crystals in the urinary tract. With antigout drugs, fluids help to prevent precipitation of urate crystals and formation of urate kidney stones. Fluid intake is especially important initially when serum uric acid levels are high and large amounts of uric acid are being excreted.

### Evaluation

- Interview and observe regarding relief of symptoms.
- Interview and observe regarding mobility and activity levels.
- Interview and observe regarding safe, effective use of the drugs.
- Select drugs appropriately.

---

## *Nursing Actions*

## Analgesic–Antipyretic–Anti-inflammatory and Related Drugs

| Nursing Actions | Rationale/Explanation |
|---|---|
| 1. Administer accurately. <br>   a. Give aspirin and other nonsteroidal anti-inflammatory drugs (NSAIDs) with a full glass of water or other fluid and with or just after food. <br>   b. Do not crush tablets or open capsules of long-acting dosage forms and instruct patients not to crush or chew the products. Examples include: <br>     (1) Enteric-coated aspirin (eg, Ecotrin) <br>     (2) Diclofenac *sodium* (Voltaren or Voltaren XR). <br>     (3) Diflunisal (Dolobid) <br>     (4) Etodolac (Lodine XL) <br>     (5) Indomethacin or Indocin SR <br>     (6) Ketoprofen or Oruvail extended-release capsules <br>     (7) Naproxen delayed-release (EC-Naprosyn) or naproxen sodium controlled-release (Naprelan) | To decrease gastric irritation. Even though food delays absorption and decreases peak plasma levels of some of the drugs, it is probably safer to give them with food. Rofecoxib and meloxicam may be given without regard to food. Breaking the tablets or capsules allows faster absorption, destroys the long-acting feature, and increases risks of adverse effects and toxicity from overdose. |

*(continued)*

## Nursing Actions

## Analgesic–Antipyretic–Anti-inflammatory and Related Drugs (Continued)

| Nursing Actions | Rationale/Explanation |
|---|---|
| c. Give antimigraine preparations at the onset of headache. | To prevent development of more severe symptoms. |
| **2. Observe for therapeutic effects.** | |
| a. When drugs are given for pain, observe for decreased or absent manifestations of pain. | Pain relief is usually evident within 30–60 minutes. |
| b. When drugs are given for fever, record temperature every 2 to 4 hours, and observe for a decrease. | |
| c. When drugs are given for arthritis and other inflammatory disorders, observe for decreased pain, edema, redness, heat, and stiffness of joints. Also observe for increased joint mobility and exercise tolerance. | With aspirin, improvement is usually noted within 24–48 hours. With most of the NSAIDs, 1–2 weeks may be required before beneficial effects become evident. |
| d. When colchicine is given for acute gouty arthritis, observe for decreased pain and inflammation in involved joints. | Therapeutic effects occur within 4–12 hours after intravenous colchicine administration and 24–48 hours after oral administration. Edema may not decrease for several days. |
| e. When allopurinol, probenecid, or sulfinpyrazone is given for hyperuricemia, observe for normal serum uric acid level (approximately 2–8 mg/100 mL). | Serum uric acid levels usually decrease to normal range within 1–3 weeks. |
| f. When the above drugs are given for chronic gout, observe for decreased size of tophi, absence of new tophi, decreased joint pain and increased joint mobility, and normal serum uric acid levels. | |
| g. When triptans or ergot preparations are given in migraine headache, observe for relief of symptoms. | Therapeutic effects are usually evident within 15–30 minutes. |
| **3. Observe for adverse effects.** | |
| a. With analgesic–antipyretic–anti-inflammatory and antigout agents, observe for: | |
| (1) Gastrointestinal problems—anorexia, nausea, vomiting, diarrhea, bleeding, ulceration | These are common reactions, more likely with aspirin, indomethacin, piroxicam, sulindac, tolmetin, colchicine, and sulfinpyrazone and less likely with acetaminophen, celecoxib, diflunisal, etodolac, fenoprofen, ibuprofen, naproxen, rofecoxib, and valdecoxib. |
| (2) Hematologic problems—petechiae, bruises, hematuria, melena, epistaxis, and bone marrow depression (leukopenia, thrombocytopenia, anemia) | Bone marrow depression is more likely to occur with colchicine. |
| (3) Central nervous system effects—headache, dizziness, fainting, ataxia, insomnia, confusion, drowsiness | These effects are relatively common with indomethacin and may occur with most of the other drugs, especially with high dosages. |
| (4) Skin rashes, dermatitis | |
| (5) Hypersensitivity reactions with dyspnea, bronchospasm, skin rashes | These effects may simulate asthma in people who are allergic to aspirin and aspirin-like drugs. Most likely to occur in patients with a history of nasal polyps, asthma, or rhinitis. May result in severe symptoms, including potentially fatal bronchospasm. |
| (6) Tinnitus, blurred vision | Tinnitus (ringing or roaring in the ears) is a classic sign of aspirin overdose (salicylate intoxication). It occurs with NSAIDs as well, especially with overdosage. |
| (7) Nephrotoxicity—decreased urine output, increased blood urea nitrogen (BUN), increased serum creatinine, hyperkalemia, retention of sodium and water with resultant edema | More likely to occur in people with preexisting renal impairment, especially when fluid intake is decreased or fluid loss is increased. Older adults are at greater risk because of decreased renal blood flow and increased incidence of congestive heart failure and diuretic therapy. Renal damage is usually reversible when the drug is discontinued. |

*(continued)*

## *Nursing Actions*

### Analgesic–Antipyretic–Anti-inflammatory and Related Drugs (Continued)

| Nursing Actions | Rationale/Explanation |
|---|---|
| (8) Cardiovascular effects—increased hypertension | Long known to occur with older NSAIDs, probably due to retention of sodium and water. A few cases have been reported with COX-2 inhibitors, mechanism unknown. |
| (9) Hepatotoxicity—liver damage or failure | Occurs mainly with acetaminophen, in overdose or in people with underlying liver disease |
| b. With triptan antimigraine drugs, observe for: | Most adverse effects are mild and transient. However, because of their vasoconstrictive effects, they may cause or aggravate angina pectoris and hypertension. |
|   (1) Chest tightness or pain, hypertension, drowsiness, dizziness, nausea, fatigue, paresthesias | |
| c. With ergot antimigraine drugs, observe for: | |
|   (1) Nausea, vomiting, diarrhea | These drugs have a direct effect on the vomiting center of the brain and stimulate contraction of gastrointestinal smooth muscle. |
|   (2) Symptoms of ergot poisoning (ergotism)— coolness, numbness, and tingling of the extremities, headache, vomiting, dizziness, thirst, convulsions, weak pulse, confusion, angina-like chest pain, transient tachycardia or bradycardia, muscle weakness and pain, cyanosis, gangrene of the extremities | The ergot alkaloids are highly toxic; poisoning may be acute or chronic. Acute poisoning is rare; chronic poisoning is usually a result of overdosage. Circulatory impairments may result from vasoconstriction and vascular insufficiency. Large doses also damage capillary endothelium and may cause thrombosis and occlusion. Gangrene of extremities rarely occurs with usual doses unless peripheral vascular disease or other contraindications are also present. |
|   (3) Hypertension | Blood pressure may rise as a result of generalized vasoconstriction induced by the ergot preparation. |
|   (4) Hypersensitivity reactions—local edema and pruritus, anaphylactic shock | Allergic reactions are relatively uncommon. |
| **4. Observe for drug interactions.** | |
|   a. Drugs that *increase* effects of aspirin and other NSAIDs: | |
|     (1) Acidifying agents (eg, ascorbic acid) | Acidify urine and thereby decrease the urinary excretion rate of salicylates |
|     (2) Alcohol | Increases gastric irritation and occult blood loss |
|     (3) Anticoagulants, oral | Increase risk of bleeding substantially. People taking anticoagulants should avoid aspirin and aspirin-containing products. |
|     (4) Codeine, hydrocodone, oxycodone | Additive analgesic effects because of different mechanisms of action. Aspirin or an NSAID can often be used with these drugs to provide adequate pain relief without excessive doses and sedation. |
|     (5) Corticosteroids (eg, prednisone) | Additive gastric irritation and possible ulcerogenic effects |
|   b. Drug that *increases* effects of celecoxib: | |
|     (1) Fluconazole (and possibly other azole antifungal drugs) | Inhibits liver enzymes that normally metabolize celecoxib; increases serum celecoxib levels |
|   c. Drugs that *decrease* effects of aspirin and other NSAIDs: | |
|     (1) Alkalinizing agents (eg, sodium bicarbonate) | Increase rate of renal excretion |
|     (2) Misoprostol (Cytotec) | This drug, a prostaglandin, was developed specifically to prevent aspirin and NSAID-induced gastric ulcers. |
|   d. Drug that *decreases* effects of fenoprofen: | |
|     (1) Phenobarbital | Induces drug-metabolizing enzymes in the liver and decreases blood levels of fenoprofen. Dosage of fenoprofen may need to be increased if phenobarbital is started or decreased if phenobarbital is discontinued. |

*(continued)*

## *Nursing Actions*

## Analgesic–Antipyretic–Anti-inflammatory and Related Drugs (Continued)

| *Nursing Actions* | *Rationale/Explanation* |
|---|---|
| e. Drug that *decreases* effects of rofecoxib | |
| (1) Rifampin | Induces drug-metabolizing enzymes in the liver and decreases blood levels of rofecoxib |
| f. Drugs that *increase* effects of indomethacin: | |
| (1) Anticoagulants, oral | Increase risk of gastrointestinal bleeding. Indomethacin causes gastric irritation and is considered an ulcerogenic drug. |
| (2) Corticosteroids | Increase ulcerogenic effect |
| (3) Salicylates | Increase ulcerogenic effect |
| (4) Heparin | Increases risk of bleeding. These drugs should not be used concurrently. |
| g. Drugs that *decrease* effects of indomethacin: | |
| (1) Antacids | Delay absorption from the gastrointestinal tract |
| h. Drugs that *decrease* effects of allopurinol, probenecid, and sulfinpyrazone: | |
| (1) Alkalinizing agents (eg, sodium bicarbonate) | Decrease risks of renal calculi from precipitation of uric acid crystals. Alkalinizing agents are recommended until serum uric acid levels return to normal. |
| (2) Colchicine | Decreases attacks of acute gout. Recommended for concurrent use until serum uric acid levels return to normal. |
| (3) Diuretics | Decrease uricosuric effects |
| (4) Salicylates | Mainly at salicylate doses of less than 2 g/day, decrease uricosuric effects of probenecid and sulfinpyrazone but do not interfere with the action of allopurinol. Salicylates are uricosuric at doses greater than 5 g/day. |
| i. Drugs that *increase* effects of ergot preparations: | |
| (1) Vasoconstrictors (eg, ephedrine, epinephrine, phenylephrine) | Additive vasoconstriction with risks of severe, persistent hypertension and intracranial hemorrhage |
| j. Drugs that *increase* the effects of triptan antimigraine drugs: | |
| (1) Monoamine oxidase inhibitors (MAOIs) | Increase serum levels of triptans and may cause serious adverse effects, including cardiac arrhythmias and myocardial infarction. **Triptans and MAOIs must not be taken concurrently; a triptan should not be taken for at least 2 weeks after an MAOI is discontinued.** |
| (2) Ergot preparations | **Triptans and ergot preparations should not be taken concurrently or within 24 hours of each other, because severe hypertension and stroke may occur.** |

## Critical Thinking Exercises

**1.** Cyclooxygenase-2 inhibitors block production of prostaglandins associated with pain and inflammation but differ from aspirin in that COX-2 inhibitors:

a. Block prostaglandins associated with protective effects on gastric mucosa
b. Produce more gastric irritation
c. Have greater antiplatelet effects
d. Are not associated with increased risk for bleeding

**2.** When an NSAID is given during late pregnancy to prevent premature labor, what fetal organ may be adversely affected?

a. Brain
b. Spleen
c. Kidneys
d. Lungs

**3.** For a 50-year-old client with RA and peptic ulcer disease, what drug would typically be prescribed to manage the condition?

a. Aspirin
b. Nonselective NSAID
c. Acetaminophen
d. Selective COX-2 inhibitor NSAID

**4.** In an individual who is allergic to aspirin, which drug may be an acceptable alternative for mild pain relief?

a. Meperidine (Demerol)
b. Acetaminophen
c. Morphine sulfate
d. Nonaspirin NSAID

**5.** An OTC product pain reliever and fever reducer that is contraindicated for chronic alcohol abusers because of possible liver damage is:

a. Acetaminophen
b. Aspirin
c. Ibuprofen
d. Naproxen

## SELECTED REFERENCES

Barkin, R. L., & Barkin, D. (2001). Pharmacologic management of acute and chronic pain. *Southern Medical Journal, 94*(8), 756–812.

*Drug facts and comparisons.* (Updated monthly.) St. Louis: Facts and Comparisons.

Fetrow, C. W., & Avila, J. R. (1999). *Professional's handbook of complementary and alternative medicines.* Springhouse, PA: Springhouse Corporation.

Fitzgerald, G. A., & Patrono, C. (2001). The coxibs, selective inhibitors of cyclooxygenase-2. *New England Journal of Medicine, 345*(6), 433–442.

Graves, J. W., & Hunder, I. A. (2000). Worsening of hypertension by cyclooxygenase-2 inhibitors. *Journal of Clinical Hypertension, 2*(6), 396–398.

Hughes, R. A., & Carr, A. J. (2000). A randomized, double-blind, placebo-controlled trial of glucosamine to control pain in osteoarthritis of the knee. Program and abstracts from the 64th Annual Scientific Meeting of the American College of Rheumatology; October 29—November 2, 2000; Philadelphia. Abstract 1903.

Lacy, C. F., Armstrong, L. L., Goldman, M. P., & Lance, L. L. (2003). *Lexi-Comp's drug information handbook* (11th ed.). Hudson, OH: American Pharmaceutical Association.

Lance, J. W. (2000). Approach to the patient with headache. In H. D. Humes (Ed.), *Kelley's textbook of internal medicine* (4th ed., pp. 2836–2844). Philadelphia: Lippincott Williams & Wilkins.

McAlindon, T. E., LaValley, M. P., Gulin, J. P., & Felson, D. T. (2000). Glucosamine and chondroitin for treatment of osteoarthritis. *Journal of the American Medical Association, 283,* 1469–1475.

Whitaker, A. L., & Small, R. E. (2000). Osteoarthritis. In E. T. Herfindal & D. R. Gourley (Eds.), *Textbook of therapeutics: Drug and disease management* (7th ed., pp. 667–678).

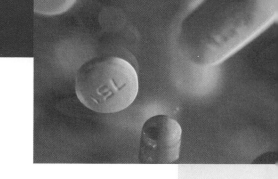

# 8

# Antianxiety and Sedative–Hypnotic Drugs

## OBJECTIVES

*After studying this chapter, the student will be able to:*

1 Identify characteristics, sources, and signs and symptoms of anxiety.

2 Discuss functions of sleep and consequences of sleep deprivation.

3 Describe nonpharmacologic interventions to decrease anxiety and insomnia.

4 List characteristics of benzodiazepine antianxiety and hypnotic drugs in terms of mechanism of action, indications for use, nursing process implications, and potential for abuse and dependence.

5 Describe strategies for preventing, recognizing, and treating benzodiazepine withdrawal reactions.

6 Contrast characteristics of selected nonbenzodiazepines and benzodiazepines.

7 Teach clients guidelines for rational, safe use of antianxiety and sedative-hypnotic drugs

8 Discuss the use of flumazenil and other treatment measures for overdose of benzodiazepines.

## CRITICAL THINKING SCENARIO

*J*ane Morgan, 37 years of age and recently divorced, presents to her primary care provider complaining of anxiety and inability to sleep at night. Her doctor prescribes diazepam (Valium), 5 mg PO three times daily, and triazolam (Halcion), 0.25 mg PO half-strength PRN. You are the nurse responsible for developing a teaching plan for Ms. Morgan.

✔ How would you establish a therapeutic rapport while obtaining additional important information?

✔ Describe nonpharmacologic methods to reduce anxiety and improve sleep.

✔ Identify essential information about these new medications that can be taught in 5 minutes.

✔ Discuss teaching and evaluation strategies that might be helpful in this situation.

## PROTOTYPE PROFILE

**diazepam** (Valium), p. 129

## OVERVIEW

Antianxiety and sedative-hypnotic agents are central nervous system (CNS) depressants with similar effects. Antianxiety drugs and sedatives promote relaxation; hypnotics produce sleep. The difference between the effects depends largely on dosage: large doses of antianxiety and sedative agents produce sleep, and small doses of hypnotics produce antianxiety or sedative effects. In addition, therapeutic doses of hypnotics given at bedtime may have residual sedative effects ("morning hangover") the following day. Because these drugs produce varying degrees of CNS depression, some are also used as anticonvulsant and anesthetic agents.

Antianxiety and sedative-hypnotic drugs are often used in critically ill clients to relieve stress, anxiety, and agitation. By their calming effects, they may also decrease cardiac workload (eg, heart rate, blood pressure, force of myocardial contraction, myocardial oxygen consumption) and respiratory effort. Additional benefits include improving tolerance of treatment measures (eg, mechanical ventilation); keeping confused clients from harming themselves by pulling out intravenous (IV) catheters, feeding or drainage tubes, wound drains, and other treatment devices; and allowing clients to rest or sleep more. In addition to sedation, the drugs often induce amnesia, which may be a desirable effect in critically ill clients.

The drugs most often used to treat both anxiety and insomnia belong to a chemical group called *benzodiazepines*. **ⓟ Diazepam** (Valium) is the prototype benzodiazepine and is highlighted in Prototype Profile 8-1: Diazepam, although alprazolam (Xanax) and lorazepam (Ativan) may be more commonly prescribed. Several

---

### PROTOTYPE PROFILE 8-1
### ⓟ Diazepam (dye AZ e pam)

**Drug Class**
*Chemical:* Benzodiazepine
*Functional:* Antianxiety agent; sedative; anticonvulsant

**Trade Name**
Valium

**Therapeutic Indications**
Used for anxiety, seizure disorders, acute alcohol withdrawal, muscle spasm, and preoperative sedation

**Pharmacokinetics**
*Absorption*
PO: 85% to 100%, more reliable than IM

*Distribution*
Plasma protein binding: 98%; crosses the blood–brain barrier and placenta

*Metabolism*
Hepatic; some metabolites are active CNS depressants

*Excretion*
Hepatic

**Pharmacodynamics**
*Onset of Action*
PO: 30–60 min; IV: 1–5 min; IM: within 20 min

*Duration*
PO: up to 24h; IV: 30–100 min; IM: unknown

**Contraindications/Precautions**
Severe respiratory disorders, severe liver or kidney disease, hypersensitivity reactions, and a history of alcohol or other drug abuse

**Pregnancy Considerations**
Category D
Enters breast milk, contraindicated

**Dosage**
*Adults:* PO, 2–10 mg 2–4 times daily IM, IV, 5–10 mg, repeated in 3–4 hours if necessary. Give IV slowly, no faster than 5 mg (1 mL) per minute
*Older or debilitated adults:* PO, 2–5 mg once or twice daily, increased gradually if needed and tolerated
*Children:* PO, 1–2.5 mg 3–4 times daily, increased gradually if needed and tolerated
>30 days and < 5 y: Seizures IM, IV, 0.2–0.5 mg/2–5 min to a maximum of 5 mg
5 yr or older: Seizures, IM, IV, 1 mg/2–5 min to a maximum of 10 mg

**Adverse Effects**
Hypotension, drowsiness, dizziness, ataxia, headache, anxiety, depression, confusion

**Drug Interactions**
*Increased Effects*
Potentiates the CNS depressant effects of narcotic analgesics, antihistamines, barbiturates, alcohol, phenothiazines, and MAO inhibitors
Diazepam toxicity with concurrent drugs that inhibit

*Decreased Effects*
Decreased therapeutic effect of diazepam with concurrent use with carbamazepine, rifabutin, and rifampin
Decreased efficacy of levodopa with concurrent use
Sedative effect may be decreased with theophylline

**Herbal Supplements and Dietary Considerations**
Avoid valerian, St. John's wort, kava kava, chamomile, and hops because they may increase CNS depression
Avoid ethanol

other drugs are also used, including some miscellaneous drugs and antidepressants (see Chap. 10). The main focus of this chapter is the benzodiazepines; the other drugs are discussed in relation to their use in treating anxiety or insomnia.

Anxiety is a common disorder that may be referred to as nervousness, tension, worry, or other terms that denote an unpleasant feeling state. It occurs when a person perceives a situation as threatening to physical, emotional, social, or economic well-being. Many causes occur with everyday events associated with home, work, school, social activities, and chronic illness. Others occur episodically, such as an acute illness, death, divorce, loss of a job, starting a new job, or taking a test. Situational anxiety is a normal response to a stressful situation. It may be beneficial when it motivates the person toward constructive, problem-solving, coping activities. Symptoms may be quite severe, but they usually last only 2 to 3 weeks.

Although there is no clear boundary between normal and abnormal anxiety, it is called an *anxiety disorder* when it is severe or prolonged and impairs the ability to function in usual activities of daily living. The American Psychiatric Association delineates anxiety disorders as medical diagnoses in the *Diagnostic and Statistical Manual of Mental Disorders*, 4th edition (revised). This classification includes several types of anxiety disorders (Box 8-1). *Generalized anxiety disorder* is emphasized in this chapter.

To aid understanding of the uses and effects of these drugs, anxiety and insomnia are described in At the Foundation: Anxiety and Sleep. The clinical manifestations of these disorders are similar and overlapping; that is, daytime anxiety may be manifested as nighttime difficulty in sleeping because the person cannot "turn off" worries, and difficulty in sleeping may be manifested as anxiety, fatigue, and decreased ability to function during usual waking hours.

As stated above, the main drugs used to treat anxiety and insomnia are the benzodiazepines; a few nonbenzodiazepines are also used. In addition, antidepressants are increasingly being used to treat some types of anxiety. The barbiturates, a historically important group of CNS depressants, are obsolete for most uses, including treatment of anxiety and insomnia. A few may be used as intravenous general anesthetics (see Appendix D), phenobarbital may be used to treat seizure disorders (see Chap. 11), and some are abused (see Chap. 14). The benzodiazepines are described below; pharmacokinetic profiles are listed in Table 8-1; trade names, indications for use, and dosage ranges of individual drugs are listed in Drugs at a Glance 8-1: Benzodiazepines. Miscellaneous nonbenzodiazepines are described later and listed in Drugs at a Glance 8-2: Miscellaneous Antianxiety and Sedative-Hypnotic Agents.

## ▨ BENZODIAZEPINES

Benzodiazepines are widely used for anxiety and insomnia and are also used for several other indications. They have a wide margin of safety between therapeutic and toxic doses and are rarely fatal, even in overdose, unless combined with other CNS depressant drugs, such as alcohol. They are Schedule IV drugs under the Controlled Substances Act. They do not induce drug-metabolizing enzymes or suppress rapid-eye-movement (REM) sleep. Because they are drugs of abuse and may cause physiologic dependence, withdrawal symptoms occur if the drugs are stopped abruptly. To avoid withdrawal symptoms, the drugs should be gradually tapered and discontinued.

In addition to abuse and dependence, benzodiazepines may cause characteristic effects of CNS depression, including excessive sedation, impairment of physical and mental activities, and respiratory depression. They are not recommended for long-term use.

Benzodiazepines differ mainly in their plasma half-lives, production of active metabolites, and clinical uses. Drugs with half-lives longer than 24 hours (eg, chlordiazepoxide, diazepam, clorazepate, flurazepam, and quazepam) form active metabolites that also have long half-lives and tend to accumulate, especially in older adults and people with impaired liver function. These drugs require 5 to 7 days to reach steady-state serum levels. Therapeutic effects (eg, decreased anxiety or insomnia) and adverse effects (eg, sedation, ataxia) are more likely to occur after 2 or 3 days of therapy than initially. Such effects accumulate with chronic usage and persist for several days after the drugs are discontinued. Drugs with half-lives shorter than 24 hours (eg, alprazolam, lorazepam, midazolam, oxazepam, temazepam, and triazolam) do not have active metabolites and do not accumulate. Although the drugs produce similar effects, they differ in clinical uses mainly because their manufacturers developed and promoted them for particular purposes.

## Mechanism of Action and Pharmacokinetics

Benzodiazepines bind with benzodiazepine receptors in nerve cells of the brain; this receptor complex also has binding sites for gamma-aminobutyric acid (GABA), an inhibitory neurotransmitter. This GABA–benzodiazepine receptor complex regulates the entry of chloride ions into the cell. When GABA binds to the receptor complex, chloride ions enter the cell and stabilize (hyperpolarize) the cell membrane so that it is less responsive to excitatory neurotransmitters, such as norepinephrine. Benzodiazepines bind at a different site on the receptor complex and enhance the inhibitory effect of GABA to relieve anxiety, tension, and nervousness and to produce sleep. The decreased neuronal excitability also accounts for the usefulness of benzodiazepines as muscle relaxants, hypnotics, and anticonvulsants.

At least two benzodiazepine receptors, called BZ1 and BZ2, have been identified in the brain. BZ1 is thought to be concerned with sleep mechanisms; BZ2 is associated with memory, motor, sensory, and cognitive functions.

Benzodiazepines are well absorbed with oral administration, and most are given orally; a few (eg, diazepam, lorazepam) are given both orally and parenterally. They

BOX
8-1    **Anxiety Disorders**

### Generalized Anxiety Disorder (GAD)

Major diagnostic criteria for GAD include worry about two or more circumstances and multiple symptoms for 6 months or longer, and elimination of disease processes or drugs as possible causes. The frequency, duration, or intensity of the worry is exaggerated or out of proportion to the actual situation. Symptoms are related to motor tension (eg, muscle tension, restlessness, trembling, fatigue), overactivity of the autonomic nervous system (eg, dyspnea, palpitations, tachycardia, sweating, dry mouth, dizziness, nausea, diarrhea), and increased vigilance (feeling fearful, nervous, or keyed up; difficulty concentrating, irritability, insomnia).

Symptoms of anxiety occur with numerous disease processes, including medical disorders (eg, hyperthyroidism, cardiovascular disease, cancer) and psychiatric disorders (eg, mood disorders, schizophrenia, substance use disorders). They also frequently occur with drugs that affect the CNS. With CNS stimulants (eg, nasal decongestants, antiasthma drugs, nicotine, caffeine), symptoms occur with drug administration; with CNS depressants (eg, alcohol, benzodiazepines), symptoms are more likely to occur when the drug is stopped, especially if stopped abruptly.

When the symptoms are secondary to medical illness, they may decrease as the illness improves. However, most persons with GAD experience little relief when one stressful situation or problem is resolved. Instead, they quickly move on to another worry. Additional characteristics of GAD include its chronicity, although the severity of symptoms fluctuates over time; its frequent association with somatic symptoms (eg, headache, gastrointestinal complaints, including irritable bowel syndrome); and its frequent coexistence with depression, other anxiety disorders, and substance abuse or dependence.

### Obsessive-Compulsive Disorder (OCD)

An obsession involves an uncontrollable desire to dwell on a thought or a feeling; a compulsion involves repeated performance of some act to relieve the fear and anxiety associated with an obsession. OCD is characterized by obsessions or compulsions that are severe enough to be time consuming (eg, take more than an hour per day), cause marked distress, or impair the person's ability to function in usual activities or relationships. The compulsive behavior provides some relief from anxiety but is not pleasurable. The person recognizes that the obsessions or compulsions are excessive or unreasonable and attempts to resist them. When patients resist or are prevented from performing the compulsive behavior, they experience increasing anxiety and often abuse alcohol or antianxiety, sedative type drugs in the attempt to relieve anxiety.

### Panic Disorder

Panic disorder involves acute, sudden, recurrent attacks of anxiety, with feelings of intense fear, terror, or impending doom. It may be accompanied by such symptoms as palpita-tions, sweating, trembling, shortness of breath or smothering, chest pain, nausea, or dizziness. Symptoms usually build to a peak over about 10 minutes and may require medication to be relieved. Afterward, the person is usually preoccupied and worried about future attacks.

A significant number (50%–65%) of patients with panic disorder are thought to also have major depression. In addition, some patients with panic disorder also develop agoraphobia, a fear of having a panic attack in a place or situation where one cannot escape or get help. Combined panic disorder and agoraphobia often involves a chronic, relapsing pattern of significant functional impairment and may require lifetime treatment.

### Post-Traumatic Stress Disorder (PTSD)

PTSD develops after seeing or being involved in highly stressful events that involve actual or threatened death or serious injury (eg, natural disasters, military combat, violent acts such as rape or murder, explosions or bombings, serious automobile accidents). The person responds to such an event with thoughts and feelings of intense fear, helplessness, or horror and develops symptoms such as hyperarousal, irritability, outbursts of anger, difficulty sleeping, difficulty concentrating, and an exaggerated startle response. These thoughts, feelings, and symptoms persist as the traumatic event is relived through recurring thoughts, images, nightmares, or flashbacks in which the actual event seems to be occurring. The intense psychic discomfort leads people to avoid situations that remind them of the event, become detached from other people, have less interest in activities they formerly enjoyed, and develop other disorders (eg, anxiety disorders, major depression, alcohol or other substance abuse).

The response to stress is highly individualized and the same event or type of event might precipitate PTSD in one person and have little effect in another. Thus, most people experience major stresses and traumatic events during their lifetimes, but many do not develop PTSD. This point needs emphasis because many people seem to assume that PTSD is the normal response to a tragic event and that intensive counseling is needed. For example, counselors converge upon schools in response to events that are perceived to be tragic or stressful. Some authorities take the opposing view, however, that talking about and reliving a traumatic event may increase anxiety in some people and thereby increase the likelihood that PTSD will occur.

### Social Phobia

This disorder involves excessive concern about scrutiny by others, which may start in childhood and last lifelong. Affected persons are afraid they will say or do something that will embarrass or humiliate them. As a result, they try to avoid certain situations (eg, public speaking) or experience considerable distress if they cannot avoid them. They are often uncomfortable around other people or experience anxiety in many social situations.

## AT THE FOUNDATION: *Anxiety and Sleep*

### Anxiety

The pathophysiology of anxiety disorders is unknown, but there is evidence of a biologic basis and possible imbalances among several neurotransmission systems. A simplistic view involves an excess of excitatory neurotransmitters (eg, norepinephrine) or a deficiency of inhibitory neurotransmitters (eg, gamma-aminobutyric acid [GABA]). Although other neurotransmission systems may be involved, the noradrenergic and GABA-ergic systems are relevant to anxiety and its pharmacologic treatment.

The noradrenergic system is associated with the hyperarousal state experienced by clients with anxiety (ie, feelings of panic, restlessness, tremulousness, palpitations, hyperventilation), which are attributed to excessive norepinephrine. Norepinephrine is released from the locus ceruleus (LC) in response to an actual or a perceived threat. The LC is a brain-stem nucleus that contains many noradrenergic neurons and has extensive projections to the limbic system, cerebral cortex, and cerebellum. The involvement of the noradrenergic system in anxiety is supported by the observations that drugs that stimulate activity in the LC (eg, caffeine) may cause symptoms of anxiety and drugs used to treat anxiety (eg, benzodiazepines) decrease neuronal firing and norepinephrine release in the LC.

Neuroendocrine factors also play a role in anxiety disorders. Perceived threat or stress activates the hypothalamic-pituitary-adrenal (HPA) axis and corticotropin-releasing factor (CRF), one of its components. CRF activates the LC, which then releases norepinephrine and generates anxiety. Overall, CRF is considered important in integrating the endocrine, autonomic, and behavioral responses to stress.

GABA is the major inhibitory neurotransmitter in the brain and spinal cord. GABA-A receptors are attached to chloride channels in nerve cell membranes. When GABA interacts with GABA-A receptors, chloride channels open, chloride ions move into the neuron, and the nerve cell is less able to be excited (ie, generate an electrical impulse).

Additional causes of anxiety disorders include medical conditions (anxiety disorder due to a general medical condition according to the DSM-IV), psychiatric disorders, and substance abuse. Almost all major psychiatric illnesses may be associated with symptoms of anxiety (eg, dementia, major depression, mania, schizophrenia). Anxiety related to substance abuse is categorized in the DSM-IV as substance-induced anxiety disorder.

### Sleep and Insomnia

Sleep is a recurrent period of decreased mental and physical activity during which the person is relatively unresponsive to sensory and environmental stimuli. Normal sleep allows rest, renewal of energy for performing activities of daily living, and alertness on awakening. When a person retires for sleep, there is an initial period of drowsiness or sleep latency, which lasts about 30 minutes. Once the person is asleep, cycles occur approximately every 90 minutes during the sleep period. During each cycle, the sleeper progresses from drowsiness (stage I) to deep sleep (stages III and IV). These stages are characterized by depressed body functions, non–rapid eye movements (non-REM), and nondreaming, and are thought to be physically restorative. Activities that occur during these stages include *increased* tissue repair, synthesis of skeletal muscle protein, and secretion of growth hormone. At the same time, there is *decreased* body temperature, metabolic rate, glucose consumption, and production of catabolic hormones. Stage IV is followed by a period of 5 to 20 minutes of REM, dreaming, and increased physiologic activity. REM sleep is thought to be mentally and emotionally restorative; REM deprivation can lead to serious psychological problems, including psychosis.

It is estimated that a person spends about 75% of sleeping hours in non-REM sleep and about 25% in REM sleep. Older adults, however, often have a different pattern, with less deep sleep, more light sleep, more frequent awakenings, and generally more disruptions.

Insomnia, prolonged difficulty in going to sleep or staying asleep long enough to feel rested, is the most common sleep disorder. Insomnia has many causes, including such stressors as pain, anxiety, illness, changes in lifestyle or environment, and various drugs. Occasional sleeplessness is a normal response to many stimuli and is not usually harmful. As in anxiety, several neurotransmission systems are apparently involved in regulating sleep–wake cycles and producing insomnia.

---

are widely distributed in body tissues, and their high lipid solubility allows them to enter the CNS easily and perform their actions. The drugs are then redistributed to peripheral tissues, from which they are slowly eliminated. Thus, the pharmacodynamic effects (eg, sedation) do not correlate with plasma drug levels because the drugs move in and out of the CNS rapidly. This redistribution allows a client to awaken even though the drug may remain in the blood and other peripheral tissues for days or weeks before it is completely eliminated.

The drugs are mainly metabolized in the liver by the cytochrome P450 enzymes (3A4 subgroup) and glucuronide conjugation. Some (eg, midazolam) are also metabolized by CYP3A4 enzymes in the intestine. Most benzodiazepines are oxidized by the enzymes to metabolites that are then conjugated. For example, diazepam is converted to N-desmethyldiazepam (N-DMDZ), an active metabolite with a long elimination half-life (up to 200 hours). N-DMDZ is further oxidized to oxazepam,

*(text continues on page 136)*

## TABLE 8-1  Benzodiazepine Pharmacokinetics

| Generic Name | Protein Binding (%) | Half-life (h) | Metabolite(s) | Action | | |
|---|---|---|---|---|---|---|
| | | | | Onset | Peak | Duration |
| Alprazolam | 80 | 7–15 | Active | 30 min | 1–2 h | 4–6 h |
| Chlordiazepoxide | 96 | 5–30 | Active | 10–15 min | 1–4 h | 2–3 d |
| Clonazepam | 97 | 20–50 | Inactive | varies | 1–4 h | weeks |
| Clorazepate | 97 | 40–50 | Active | rapid | 1–2 h | days |
| Diazepam | 98 | 20–80 | Active | PO 30–60 min | 1–2 h | 3 h |
| | | | | IV 1–5 min | 30 min | 15–60 min |
| Estazolam | 93 | 8–28 | Inactive | 30–60 min | 2 h | 24 h |
| Flurazepam | 97 | 2–3 | Active | 15–45 min | 30–60 min | 6–8 h |
| Lorazepam | 85 | 10–20 | Inactive | PO 1–30 min | 2–4 h | 12–24 h |
| | | | | IM 15–30 min | 60–90 min | 12–24 h |
| | | | | IV 5–20 min | 30 min | 4 h |
| Midazolam | | 1–2 | Active | 15 min | | 30–60 min |
| Oxazepam | 87 | 5–20 | Inactive | slow | 2–4 h | 2–4 h |
| Quazepam | >95 | 41 | Active | 30 min | 2 h | 12–24 h |
| Temazepam | 96 | 9–12 | Inactive | 30–60 min | 2–3 h | 6–8 h |
| Triazolam | 78–89 | 2–5 | Inactive | 15–30 min | 1–2 h | 4–6 h |

### DRUG TABLE 8-1

## *Drugs at a Glance*
## Benzodiazepines

| Generic/Trade Name | Routes and Dosage Ranges | Comments |
|---|---|---|
| **Alprazolam** (Xanax) Pregnancy Category D | *Adults:* Anxiety: PO, 0.25–0.5 mg 3 times daily; maximum, 4 mg daily in divided doses *Older or debilitated adults:* PO, 0.25 mg 2–3 times daily, increased gradually if necessary *Panic disorder:* PO, 0.5 mg 3 times daily initially, gradually increase to 4–10 mg daily *Children:* Dosage not established | Indicated for anxiety and panic disorder; abrupt discontinuation after long-term use may cause withdrawal symptoms |
| **Chlordiazepoxide** (Librium) Pregnancy Category D | *Adults:* PO, 15–100 mg daily, once at bedtime or in 3–4 divided doses. IM, IV 50–100 mg, maximum, 300 mg daily *Older or debilitated adults:* PO, 5 mg 2–4 times daily; IM, IV, 25–50 mg *Children:* <6 y: Not recommended >6 y: PO, 5–10 mg 2–4 times daily | Indicated for anxiety and acute alcohol withdrawal; avoid use with hepatic impairment |
| **Clonazepam** (Klonopin) Pregnancy Category D | *Adults:* PO, 0.5 mg 3 times daily, increased by 0.5–1 mg every 3 days until seizures are controlled or adverse effects occur. Maximum, 20 mg daily *Children:* Up to 10 y or 30 kg: 0.01–0.03 mg/kg/d initially, not to exceed 0.05 mg/kg/d, in 2 or 3 divided doses. Increase by 0.25 to 0.5 mg every third day until a daily dose of 0.1 to 0.2 mg/kg is reached | Used for seizure disorders; relationship between serum level of drug and seizure control is not well established |

*(continued)*

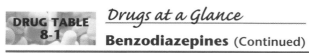

**DRUG TABLE 8-1**

*Drugs at a Glance*

**Benzodiazepines** (Continued)

| Generic/Trade Name | Routes and Dosage Ranges | Comments |
|---|---|---|
| **Clorazepate** (Tranxene)<br>Pregnancy Category D | *Adults:* PO, 7.5 mg 3 times daily, increased by no more than 7.5 mg/wk. Maximum, 90 mg daily<br>*Children:*<br>&lt;9 y: Not recommended<br>9–12 y: PO, 7.5 mg 2 times daily, increased by no more than 7.5 mg/wk. Maximum, 60 mg daily | Indicated for anxiety and seizure disorders; monitor clients for excessive sedation or respiratory depression |
| **Diazepam** (Valium) | See Prototype Profile 8-1: Diazepam | |
| **Estazolam** (ProSom)<br>Pregnancy Category X | *Adults:* PO, 1–2 mg<br>*Children:* Not for use in children &lt;18 y | Short-term management of insomnia |
| **Flurazepam** (Dalmane)<br>Pregnancy Category X | *Adults:* PO, 15–30 mg<br>*Children:* Not for use in children &lt;15 y | Indicated for insomnia; avoid alcohol and other CNS depressants |
| **Lorazepam** (Ativan)<br>Pregnancy Category D | *Adults:* PO, 2–6 mg/d in 2–3 divided doses<br>IM, 0.05 mg/kg to a maximum of 4 mg<br>IV, 2 mg, diluted with 2 mL of sterile water, sodium chloride, or 5% dextrose injection. Do not exceed 2 mg/min.<br>*Older or debilitated adults:* PO, 1–2 mg/d in divided doses | Used for anxiety and preoperative sedation; inadvertent intraarterial injection may cause arteriospasm that could lead to amputation |
| **Midazolam** (Versed)<br>Pregnancy Category D | *Adults:* Preoperative sedation, IM, 0.05–0.08 mg/kg approximately 1 h before surgery<br>Prediagnostic test sedation: IV 0.1–0.15 mg/kg or up to 0.2 mg/kg initially; maintenance dose, approximately 25% of initial dose. Reduce dose by 25% to 30% if an opioid analgesic is also given.<br>Induction of anesthesia: IV 0.3–0.35 mg/kg initially, then reduce dose as above for maintenance. Reduce initial dose to 0.15–0.3 mg/kg if a narcotic is also given.<br>*Children:* Preoperative or preprocedure sedation, induction of anesthesia: PO, syrup 0.25–1 mg/kg (maximum dose, 20 mg) as a single dose | Indicated for preoperative sedation; sedation before short diagnostic tests and endoscopic examinations; induction of general anesthesia; supplementation of nitrous oxide and oxygen anesthesia for short surgical procedures<br>Emergency respiratory resuscitation equipment should be available with use |
| **Oxazepam** (Serax)<br>Pregnancy Category D | *Adults:* PO, 10–30 mg 3–4 times daily<br>*Older or debilitated adults:* PO, 10 mg 3 times daily, gradually increased to 15 mg 3 times daily if necessary | Used for short-term anxiety and acute alcohol withdrawal |
| **Quazepam** (Doral)<br>Pregnancy Category X | *Adults:* PO, 7.5–15 mg<br>*Children:* Not for use in children &lt;18 y | Indicated for insomnia |
| **Temazepam** (Restoril)<br>Pregnancy Category X | *Adults:* PO, 15–30 mg<br>*Children:* Not for use in children &lt;18 y | Indicated for insomnia |
| **Triazolam** (Halcion)<br>Pregnancy Category X | *Adults:* PO, 0.125–0.25 mg<br>*Children:* Not for use in children &lt;18 y | Indicated for insomnia; short acting with less tendency to cause morning drowsiness |

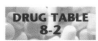

**DRUG TABLE 8-2**

*Drugs at a Glance*

## Miscellaneous Antianxiety and Sedative-Hypnotic Agents

| Generic/Trade Name | Routes and Dosage Ranges | Comments |
|---|---|---|
| ***Antianxiety Agents*** | | |
| **Buspirone** (BuSpar)<br>Pregnancy Category B | *Adults:* PO, 5 mg 3 times daily, increased by 5 mg/d at 2- to 3-day intervals if necessary. Usual mainte-nance dose 20–30 mg/d in divided doses; maximum dose 60 mg/d<br>*Children:* Not recommended | Used for treatment of anxiety; contra-indicated in clients with severe renal impairment; metabolized in the liver and should not be used in clients with severe hepatic impairment |
| **Clomipramine** (Anafranil)<br>Pregnancy Category C | *Adults:* PO, 25 mg/d initially; increase to 100 mg/d during the first 2 wk and to a maximum dose of 250 mg/d over several weeks if necessary<br>*Children:* PO, 25 mg/d initially, gradu-ally increased over 2 wk to a maxi-mum of 3 mg/kg/d or 100 mg, whichever is smaller. Then increase to 3 mg/kg/d or 200 mg per day if necessary | Management of OCD |
| **Hydroxyzine** (Vistaril)<br>Pregnancy Category C | *Adults:* PO, 75–400 mg/d in 3 or 4 divided doses. Pre- and postoperative and pre- and postpartum sedation, IM 25–100 mg in a single dose<br>*Children:* PO, 2 mg/kg per day in 4 divided doses. Pre- and postoperative sedation, IM 1 mg/kg in a single dose | Used for anxiety, sedation, pruritus |
| **Sertraline** (Zoloft)<br>Pregnancy Category C | *Adults:* OCD, PO, 50 mg once daily Panic disorder and PTSD, PO 25 mg once daily initially, increased after 1 wk to 50 mg once daily<br>*Children:* OCD, 6–12 y: PO, 25 mg once daily; 13–17 y, PO, 50 mg once daily | Indicated in OCD, panic disorder, and PTSD |
| **Venlafaxine** extended release (Effexor XR)<br>Pregnancy Category C | *Adults:* PO, 37.5–75 mg once daily ini-tially, increased up to 225 mg daily if necessary<br>*Children:* Dosage not established | Indicated in generalized anxiety disorder |
| ***Sedative-Hypnotic Agents*** | | |
| **Chloral hydrate**<br>Pregnancy Category C | *Adults:* Sedative: PO, rectal suppository 250 mg 3 times per day<br>Hypnotic: PO, rectal suppository 500–1000 mg at bedtime; maximum dose, 2 g/d<br>*Children:* Sedative: PO, rectal supposi-tory 25 mg/kg per day, in 3 or 4 divided doses.<br>Hypnotic: PO, rectal suppository 50 mg/kg at bedtime; maximum single dose, 1 g | Used as sedative, hypnotic |
| **Dexmedetomidine** (Precedex)<br>Pregnancy Category B | *Adults:* IV infusion, 1 mcg/kg over 10 min initially, then 0.2–0.7 mcg/kg/h to maintain the desired level of sedation<br>*Children:* not recommended for chil-dren <18 y | Indicated for sedation of intubated, mechanically ventilated clients in intensive care units |

*(continued)*

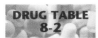

**DRUG TABLE 8-2**

## Drugs at a Glance

### Miscellaneous Antianxiety and Sedative-Hypnotic Agents (Continued)

| Generic/Trade Name | Routes and Dosage Ranges | Comments |
|---|---|---|
| **Zaleplon** (Sonata)<br>Pregnancy Category C | *Adults:* PO, 10 mg at bedtime; 5 mg for adults who are elderly, of low weight, or have mild to moderate hepatic impairment<br>*Children:* Dosage not established | Used as hypnotic; may be used in renal impairment and does not require dosage reduction; not recommended for clients with severe liver impairment |
| **Zolpidem** (Ambien)<br>Pregnancy Category B | *Adults:* PO, 10 mg at bedtime; 5 mg for older adults and those with hepatic impairment<br>*Children:* Not recommended | Used as hypnotic; may be used in renal impairment and does not require dosage reduction |

OCD, obsessive-compulsive disorder; PTSD, post-traumatic stress disorder.

then conjugated and excreted. With repeated drug doses, N-DMDZ accumulates and may contribute to both long-lasting antianxiety effects and adverse effects. If oxidation is impaired (eg, in older adults, in liver disease, or with concurrent use of drugs that inhibit oxidation), higher blood levels of both the parent drugs and metabolites increase the risk for adverse drug effects. In contrast, lorazepam, oxazepam, and temazepam are conjugated only; thus, their elimination is not impaired by the previously described factors. Drug metabolites are excreted through the kidneys.

## Indications for Use

Major clinical uses of the benzodiazepines are as antianxiety, hypnotic, and anticonvulsant agents. They also are given for preoperative sedation, prevention of agitation and delirium tremens in acute alcohol withdrawal, and treatment of anxiety symptoms associated with depression, acute psychosis, or mania. Thus, they are often given concurrently with antidepressants, antipsychotics, and mood stabilizers. Not all benzodiazepines are approved for all uses; see Drugs at a Glance 8-1: Benzodiazepines for indications for the use of individual benzodiazepines. Diazepam has been extensively studied and has more approved uses than others.

Clinical indications for the use of sedative-hypnotics include short-term treatment of insomnia and sedation before surgery or invasive diagnostic tests (eg, angiograms, endoscopies).

Although antianxiety and sedative-hypnotic drugs are not recommended for long-term use, they are often used at home. Guidelines for strategies for ongoing evaluation and intervention in the home are addressed in Home Care Considerations. In addition, age-specific considerations are important in the treatment of these conditions. Discussion of specific management factors in children and older adults is found in Age-related Considerations.

## Management Considerations

### Duration of Therapy

Benzodiazepines should be given for the shortest effective period to decrease the likelihood of drug abuse and physiologic and psychological dependence. Few problems develop with short-term use unless an overdose is taken or other CNS depressant drugs (eg, alcohol) are taken concurrently. Most problems occur with long-term use, especially of larger-than-usual doses. In general, an antianxiety benzodiazepine should not be taken for longer than 4 months, and a hypnotic benzodiazepine should

### Home Care Considerations: Use of Antianxiety and Sedative–Hypnotic Drugs

***ASSESS:*** for signs and symptoms of overuse, withdrawal, and use of other sedating drugs, including alcohol, sedating antihistamines, and other prescription drugs.

***MONITOR:*** for adverse effects that may increase the risks for injuries if mental and physical responses are slowed by the drugs.

***EDUCATE:*** on taking the drug exactly as prescribed; avoiding OTC drugs that contain CNS depressants, such as alcohol or antihistamines; the use of nonpharmacologic methods of reducing anxiety and insomnia; and not giving any prescribed drugs to family or friends. Reinforce additional teaching points (see Client Teaching Guidelines: Antianxiety and Sedative-Hypnotic Drugs).

# Age-related Considerations:
# Use of Antianxiety and Sedative-Hypnotic Drugs

## USE IN CHILDREN

Anxiety is a common disorder among children and adolescents. When given antianxiety and sedative-hypnotic drugs, children may have unanticipated or variable responses, including paradoxical CNS stimulation and excitement rather than CNS depression and calming. Few studies have been done in children. Thus, much clinical usage of these drugs is empiric, not approved by the FDA, and not supported by data. Some considerations include the following:

1. Drug pharmacodynamics and pharmacokinetics are likely to be different in children than in adults. Pharmacodynamic differences may stem from changes in neurotransmission systems in the brain as the child grows. Pharmacokinetic differences may stem from changes in distribution or metabolism of drugs; absorption seems similar to that in adults. In relation to distribution, children usually have a smaller percentage of body fat than adults. Thus, antianxiety and sedative-hypnotic drugs, which are usually highly lipid soluble, cannot be as readily stored in fat as they are in adults. This often leads to shorter half-lives and the need for more frequent administration. In relation to metabolism, young children (eg, preschoolers) usually have a faster rate than adults and may therefore require relatively high doses for their size and weight. In relation to excretion, renal function is usually similar to that of adults, and most of the drugs are largely inactive. Thus, with normal renal function, excretion probably has little effect on blood levels of active drug or the child's response to the drug.

2. Oral and parenteral diazepam has been used extensively in children, in all age groups older than 6 months. Other benzodiazepines are not recommended for particular age groups (eg, oral lorazepam in children younger than 12 years of age; alprazolam and injectable lorazepam in children younger than 18 years of age).

3. As with other populations, benzodiazepines should be given to children only when clearly indicated, in the lowest effective dose, for the shortest effective time.

4. Effects of buspirone, zaleplon, and zolpidem in children are unknown, and these drugs are not recommended for use in children.

## USE IN OLDER ADULTS

Most antianxiety and sedative-hypnotic drugs are metabolized and excreted more slowly in older adults; hence the effects of a given dose last longer. Also, several of the benzodiazepines produce pharmacologically active metabolites, which prolong drug actions. Thus, the drugs may accumulate and increase adverse effects if dosages are not reduced. The initial dose of any antianxiety or sedative-hypnotic drug should be small, and any increments should be made gradually to decrease the risks for adverse effects. Adverse effects include oversedation, dizziness, confusion, hypotension, and impaired mobility, which may contribute to falls and other injuries unless clients are carefully monitored and safeguarded.

Benzodiazepines should be tapered rather than discontinued abruptly in older adults, as in other populations. Withdrawal symptoms may occur within 24 hours after abruptly stopping a short-acting drug but may not occur for several days after stopping a long-acting agent.

For anxiety, short-acting benzodiazepines, such as alprazolam or lorazepam, are preferred over long-acting agents, such as diazepam. Buspirone may be preferred over a benzodiazepine because it does not cause sedation, psychomotor impairment, or increased risk for falls. However, it must be taken on a regular schedule and is not effective for PRN use.

For insomnia, sedative-hypnotic drugs should usually be avoided or their use minimized in older adults. Finding and treating the causes and using nondrug measures to aid sleep are much safer. If a sedative-hypnotic is used, shorter-acting benzodiazepines are preferred because they are eliminated more rapidly and are therefore less likely to accumulate and cause adverse effects. In addition, dosages should be smaller than for younger adults, the drugs should not be used every night or for longer than a few days, and older adults should be monitored closely for adverse effects. If zaleplon or zolpidem is used, the recommended dose for older adults is half that of younger adults (5 mg).

---

not be taken more than 3 or 4 nights a week for approximately 3 weeks.

For buspirone, recommendations for duration of therapy have not been established. For zaleplon and zolpidem, the recommended duration is no longer than 10 days.

### Dosage

With benzodiazepines, dosage must be individualized and carefully titrated because requirements vary widely among clients. With antianxiety agents, the goal is to find the lowest effective dose that does not cause excessive daytime drowsiness or impaired mobility. In general, start with the smallest dose likely to be effective (eg, diazepam, 2 mg three times daily, or equivalent doses of others). Then, according to client response, doses can be titrated upward to relieve symptoms of anxiety and avoid adverse drug effects. The maximum daily dose with diazepam is 40 mg/day, or equivalent doses of other agents. With hypnotics, the lowest effective doses should be taken on an intermittent basis, not every night. All benzodiazepines undergo hepatic metabolism and then elimination in urine. Several of the drugs produce active metabolites that are normally excreted by the kidney. In the presence of liver disease (eg, cirrhosis, hepatitis), the metabolism of most benzodiazepines is slowed, with resultant accumulation and increased risk for adverse effects. If renal excretion is impaired, the active metabolites may accumulate and cause excessive sedation and respiratory depression. If a benzodiazepine is needed, lorazepam and oxazepam are preferred antianxiety agents, and temazepam is the preferred hypnotic. Additional guidelines include the following:

1. Smaller-than-usual doses may be indicated in clients receiving cimetidine or other drugs that decrease the hepatic metabolism of benzodiazepines, in older adults, and in debilitated clients. With alprazolam, the most commonly prescribed benzodiazepine, the dose should be reduced by 50% if given concurrently with the antidepressant fluvoxamine.

   In older adults, most benzodiazepines are metabolized more slowly, and half-lives are longer than in younger adults. Exceptions are lorazepam and oxazepam, whose half-lives and dosages are the same for older adults as for younger ones. The recommended initial dose of zaleplon and zolpidem is 5 mg, one half of that recommended for younger adults.

2. Larger-than-usual doses may be needed for clients who are severely anxious or agitated. Also, large doses are usually required to relax skeletal muscle, control muscle spasm, control seizures, and provide sedation before surgery, cardioversion, endoscopy, and angiography.

3. When benzodiazepines are used with opioid analgesics, the analgesic dose should be reduced initially and increased gradually to avoid excessive CNS depression.

## Scheduling

The antianxiety benzodiazepines are often given in three or four daily doses. This is necessary for the short-acting agents, but there is no pharmacologic basis for multiple daily doses of the long-acting drugs. Because of their prolonged actions, all or most of the daily dose can be given at bedtime. This schedule promotes sleep, and there is usually enough residual sedation to maintain antianxiety effects throughout the next day. If necessary, one or two small supplemental doses may be given during the day. Although the hypnotic benzodiazepines vary in their onset of action, they should be taken at bedtime because it is safer for clients to be recumbent when drowsiness occurs. Zaleplon and zolpidem also should be taken at bedtime because of their rapid onset of action.

## Contraindications to Use

Contraindications to benzodiazepines include severe respiratory disorders, severe liver or kidney disease, hypersensitivity reactions, and a history of alcohol or other drug abuse. The drugs must be used very cautiously when taken concurrently with any other CNS depressant drugs.

## ■ MISCELLANEOUS DRUGS

Several nonbenzodiazepine drugs of varied characteristics are also used as antianxiety and sedative-hypnotic agents. These include buspirone, clomipramine, and hydroxyzine as antianxiety agents and chloral hydrate, dexmedetomidine, zaleplon, and zolpidem as sedative-hypnotics.

**Buspirone** (BuSpar) differs chemically and pharmacologically from other antianxiety drugs. Its mechanism of action is unclear, but it apparently interacts with serotonin and dopamine receptors in the brain. Compared with the benzodiazepines, buspirone lacks muscle relaxant and anticonvulsant effects, does not cause sedation or physical or psychological dependence, does not increase the CNS depression of alcohol and other drugs, and is not a controlled substance. Adverse effects include nervousness and excitement. Thus, clients wanting and accustomed to sedative effects may not like the drug or comply with instructions for its use. Its only clinical indication for use is the short-term treatment of anxiety. Although some beneficial effects may occur within 7 to 10 days, optimal effects may require 3 to 4 weeks. Because therapeutic effects may be delayed, buspirone is not considered beneficial for immediate effects or occasional (PRN) use. Buspirone is rapidly absorbed after oral administration. Peak plasma levels occur within 45 to 90 minutes. It is metabolized by the liver to inactive metabolites, which are then excreted in the urine and feces. Its elimination half-life is 2 to 3 hours.

**Chloral hydrate,** the oldest sedative-hypnotic drug, is relatively safe, effective, and inexpensive in usual therapeutic doses. It reportedly does not suppress REM sleep. Tolerance develops after approximately 2 weeks of continual use. It is a drug of abuse and may cause physical dependence.

**Clomipramine** (Anafranil), **fluoxetine** (Prozac, Sarafem), **fluvoxamine** (Luvox), **paroxetine** (Paxil), **sertraline** (Zoloft), and **venlafaxine** (Effexor, extended release only) are antidepressants (see Chap. 10) used for the treatment of one or more anxiety disorders.

**Dexmedetomidine** (Precedex) is a sedative that is approved only for short-term sedation (less than 24 hours) of clients in critical care settings who are being mechanically ventilated. It is given by continuous IV infusion and has a half-life of 2 hours. Dosage should be reduced in older adults, clients with impaired liver function, and clients who are receiving other CNS depressant drugs. Common adverse effects include bradycardia and hypotension.

**Hydroxyzine** (Vistaril) is an antihistamine with sedative and antiemetic properties. Clinical indications for use include anxiety, preoperative sedation, nausea and vomiting associated with surgery or motion sickness, and pruritus and urticaria associated with allergic dermatoses.

**Zaleplon** (Sonata) is an oral, nonbenzodiazepine hypnotic approved for the short-term treatment (7 to 10 days) of insomnia. It binds to the benzodiazepine BZ1 receptor and apparently enhances the inhibitory effects of GABA, as do the benzodiazepines. It is a Schedule IV controlled substance; a few studies indicate abuse potential similar to that associated with benzodiazepines.

Zaleplon is well absorbed, but bioavailability is only about 30% because of extensive presystemic or "first-pass" hepatic metabolism. Action onset is rapid and peaks in 1 hour. A high-fat, heavy meal slows absorption and may reduce the drug's effectiveness in inducing sleep. It is 60% bound to plasma proteins, and its half-life is 1 hour. The drug is metabolized mainly by aldehyde oxidase and slightly by the cytochrome P450 3A4 enzymes to inactive metabolites. The metabolites and a small amount of unchanged drug are excreted in urine.

Zaleplon is contraindicated in clients with hypersensitivity reactions and during lactation; it should be used cautiously during pregnancy and in people who are depressed or have impaired hepatic or respiratory function. Adverse effects include depression, drowsiness, nausea, dizziness, headache, hypersensitivity, impaired coordination, and short-term memory impairment. To decrease the risk for adverse effects, the dosage should be reduced in clients with mild to moderate hepatic impairment, and the drug should be avoided in those with severe hepatic impairment. No dosage adjustment is needed with mild to moderate renal impairment; drug effects with severe renal impairment have not been studied. Dosage should also be reduced in older adults; drug safety and effectiveness in children have not been established. Japanese clients may be at higher-than-average risk for adverse effects because these subjects had higher peak plasma levels and longer durations of action in clinical trials. These effects were attributed to differences in body weight or drug metabolizing enzymes resulting from dietary, environmental, or other factors.

Zaleplon should not be taken concurrently with alcohol or other CNS depressant drugs because of the increased risk for excessive sedation and respiratory depression. There is also a risk for increased serum zaleplon levels if the drug is taken concurrently with cimetidine (see Chap. 46). Cimetidine inhibits both the aldehyde oxidase and cytochrome P450 3A4 enzymes that metabolize zaleplon. If cimetidine is taken, zaleplon dosage should be reduced to 5 mg. It is very important that clients taking zaleplon be taught about this interaction because cimetidine is available without prescription and the client may not inform the health care provider who prescribes zaleplon about taking cimetidine.

Overall, zaleplon is effective in helping a person get to sleep and has several advantages as a hypnotic, including its rapid onset of action, absence of active metabolites, absence of clinically significant cytochrome P450 drug interactions, rapid clearance from the body, and absence of major memory impairments. However, it may not increase total sleep time or decrease the number of awakenings during sleeping hours.

**Zolpidem** (Ambien) is a hypnotic that differs structurally from the benzodiazepines but produces similar effects. It is also similar to zaleplon. It is a Schedule IV drug approved for short-term treatment (7 to 10 days) of insomnia. Zolpidem should be given with caution to clients with signs and symptoms of major depression because of increased risk for intentional overdose.

Zolpidem is well absorbed with oral administration and has a rapid onset of action, usually within 20 to 30 minutes. Its half-life is 2.5 hours, and its hypnotic effects last 6 to 8 hours. It is 90% bound to plasma proteins. Bioavailability, peak plasma concentration, and half-life are increased in older adults and clients with impaired hepatic function. Dosage should be reduced for these groups. Zolpidem is metabolized to inactive metabolites that are then eliminated by renal excretion. Dosage reductions are not required for clients with renal impairment, but they should be closely monitored.

Adverse effects are usually few and mild (eg, daytime drowsiness, dizziness, nausea, diarrhea), but rebound insomnia may occur for a night or two after stopping the drug, and withdrawal symptoms may occur if it is stopped abruptly after approximately a week of regular use. Zolpidem should not be taken concurrently with alcohol or other CNS depressant drugs because of the increased risk for excessive sedation and respiratory depression.

## Herbal and Dietary Supplements

Numerous preparations have been used to relieve anxiety and insomnia; none has been adequately studied regarding dosage, effects, or interactions with prescribed drugs, over-the-counter drugs, or other supplements. Three commonly used products are kava kava, melatonin, and valerian.

### Kava Kava

Kava kava is derived from a shrub found in many South Pacific islands. It is claimed to be useful in numerous disorders, including anxiety, depression, insomnia, asthma, pain, rheumatism, muscle spasms, and seizures. It suppresses emotional excitability and may produce a mild euphoria. Effects include analgesia, sedation, diminished reflexes, impaired gait, and pupil dilation. Kava kava has been used or studied most often for treatment of anxiety, stress, and restlessness. It is thought to act similarly to the benzodiazepines by interacting with GABA receptors on nerve cell membranes. This action and limited evidence from a few small clinical trials may support the herb's use in treating anxiety, insomnia, and seizure disorders. However, additional studies are needed to delineate therapeutic and adverse effects, dosing recommendations, and drug interactions when used for these conditions.

Adverse effects include impaired thinking, judgment, motor reflexes, and vision. Serious adverse effects may occur with long-term, heavy use, including decreased plasma proteins, decreased platelet and lymphocyte counts, dyspnea, and pulmonary hypertension. Kava kava should not be taken concurrently with any other CNS depressant drugs (eg, benzodiazepines, ethanol), anti-platelet drugs, or levodopa (increases parkinsonian symptoms). It should not be taken by women who are pregnant or lactating or by children younger than 12 years of age; it should be used cautiously by clients with renal disease, thrombocytopenia, or neutropenia.

In December 2001, the U.S. Food and Drug Administration (FDA) issued a warning that products containing kava kava have been implicated in at least 25 cases of severe liver toxicity (hepatitis, cirrhosis, liver failure).

## Melatonin

Melatonin is a hormone produced by the pineal gland, an endocrine gland in the brain. Endogenous melatonin is derived from the amino acid tryptophan, which is converted to serotonin; serotonin is then enzymatically converted to melatonin in the pineal gland. Exogenous preparations are produced synthetically and may contain other ingredients.

Melatonin influences sleep–wake cycles; it is released during sleep, and serum levels are very low during waking hours. Prolonged intake of exogenous melatonin can reset the sleep–wake cycle. As a result, it is widely promoted for prevention and treatment of jet lag (considered a circadian rhythm disorder) and treatment of insomnia. It is thought to act similarly to the benzodiazepines in inducing sleep. In several studies of clients with sleep disturbances, those taking melatonin experienced modest improvement compared with those taking a placebo. Other studies suggest that a melatonin supplement improves sleep in older adults with melatonin deficiency and decreases weight loss in clients with cancer.

Melatonin supplements are contraindicated in clients with hepatic insufficiency, because of reduced clearance. They are also contraindicated in people with a history of cerebrovascular disease, depression, or neurologic disorders. Individuals with renal impairment and those taking benzodiazepines or other CNS depressant drugs should use them cautiously. Adverse effects include altered sleep patterns, confusion, headache, hypothermia, pruritus, sedation, and tachycardia.

Melatonin products are widely available. Recommended doses on product labels usually range from 0.3 to 5 mg. Large, controlled studies are needed to determine the most effective regimen when used for jet lag and the effects of long-term use.

## Valerian

Valerian is an herb used mainly as a sedative-hypnotic. It apparently increases the amount of GABA in the brain, probably by inhibiting the transaminase enzyme that normally metabolizes GABA. Increasing GABA, an inhibitory neurotransmitter, results in calming, sedative effects.

There are differences of opinion about the clinical usefulness of valerian, with some saying studies indicate the herb's effectiveness as a sleep aid and mild antianxiety agent and others saying studies were flawed by small samples, short durations, and poor definitions of client populations. An expert panel convened by the U.S. Pharmacopeia advised that there is insufficient evidence to support the use of valerian for treating insomnia.

Adverse effects with acute overdose or chronic use include blurred vision, cardiac disturbance, excitability, headache, hypersensitivity reactions, insomnia, and nausea. There is a risk for hepatotoxicity from overdosage and from combination herbal products containing valerian. Valerian should not be taken by people with hepatic impairment (risk for increased liver damage) or by pregnant or breast-feeding women (effects are unknown). The herb should not be taken concurrently with any other sedatives, hypnotics, alcohol, or CNS depressants, because of the potential for additive CNS depression.

---

# NURSING PROCESS

### Assessment

Assess the client's need for antianxiety or sedative-hypnotic drugs, including intensity and duration of symptoms. Manifestations are more obvious with moderate to severe anxiety or insomnia. Some guidelines for assessment include the following:

- What is the client's statement of the problem? Does the problem interfere with usual activities of daily living? If so, how much and for how long?
- Try to identify factors that precipitate anxiety or insomnia in the client. Some common ones are physical symptoms; feeling worried, tense, or nervous; factors such as illness, death of a friend or family member, divorce, or job stress; and excessive CNS stimulation from caffeine-containing beverages or drugs such as bronchodilators and nasal decongestants. In addition, excessive daytime sleep and too little exercise and activity may cause insomnia, especially in older clients.
- Observe for behavioral manifestations of anxiety, such as psychomotor agitation, facial grimaces, tense posture, and others.
- Observe for physiologic manifestations of anxiety. These may include increased blood pressure and pulse rate, increased rate and depth of respiration, increased muscle tension, and pale, cool skin.
- If behavioral or physiologic manifestations seem to indicate anxiety, try to determine whether this is actually the case. Because similar manifestations may indicate pain or other problems rather than anxiety, the observer's perceptions must be validated by the client before appropriate action can be taken.

(continued)

## 𝑁URSING PROCESS (Continued)

- If insomnia is reported, observe for signs of sleep deprivation such as drowsiness, slow movements or speech, and difficulty concentrating or focusing attention.
- Obtain a careful drug history, including the use of alcohol and sedative-hypnotic drugs, and assess the likelihood of drug abuse and dependence. People who abuse other drugs, including alcohol, are likely to abuse antianxiety and sedative-hypnotic drugs. Also assess for use of CNS stimulant drugs (eg, appetite suppressants, bronchodilators, nasal decongestants, caffeine, cocaine) and herbs (eg, ephedra).
- Identify coping mechanisms used in managing previous situations of stress, anxiety, and insomnia. These are very individualized. Reading, watching television, listening to music, or talking to a friend are examples. Some people are quiet and inactive; others participate in strenuous activity. Some prefer to be alone; others prefer being with a friend or family member or a group.
- Once drug therapy for anxiety or insomnia is begun, assess the client's level of consciousness and functional ability before each dose so that excessive sedation can be avoided.

### Nursing Diagnoses

- Ineffective Individual Coping related to need for antianxiety or sedative-hypnotic drug
- Deficient Knowledge: Appropriate uses and effects of antianxiety or sedative-hypnotic drugs
- Deficient Knowledge: Nondrug measures for relieving anxiety and insomnia
- Noncompliance: Overuse
- Risk for Injury related to sedation, respiratory depression, impaired mobility, and other adverse effects
- Sleep Pattern Disturbance: Insomnia related to one or more causes (eg, anxiety, daytime sleep)

### Planning/Goals

*The client will:*

- Feel more calm, relaxed, and comfortable with anxiety; experience improved quantity and quality of sleep with insomnia
- Be monitored for excessive sedation and impaired mobility to prevent falls or other injuries (in health care settings)
- Verbalize and demonstrate nondrug activities to reduce or manage anxiety or insomnia
- Demonstrate safe, accurate drug usage
- Notify a health care provider if he or she wants to stop taking a benzodiazepine; will not stop taking a benzodiazepine abruptly
- Avoid preventable adverse effects, including abuse and dependence

### Interventions

Use nondrug measures to relieve anxiety or to enhance the effectiveness of antianxiety drugs.

- Assist clients to identify and avoid or decrease situations that cause anxiety and insomnia, when possible. In addi-

tion, help them to understand that medications do not solve underlying problems.

- Support the client's usual coping mechanisms when feasible. Provide the opportunity for reading, exercising, listening to music, or watching television; promote contact with significant others, or simply allow the client to be alone and uninterrupted for a while.
- Use interpersonal and communication techniques to help the client manage anxiety. The degree of anxiety and the clinical situation largely determine which techniques are appropriate. For example, staying with the client, showing interest, listening, and allowing him or her to verbalize concerns may be beneficial.
- Providing information may be a therapeutic technique when anxiety is related to medical conditions. People vary in the amount and kind of information they want, but usually the following topics should be included:
  - The overall treatment plan, including medical or surgical treatment, choice of outpatient care or hospitalization, expected length of treatment, and expected outcomes in terms of health and ability to function in activities of daily living
  - Specific diagnostic tests, including preparation, after-effects if any, and how the client will be informed of results
  - Specific medication and treatment measures, including expected therapeutic results
  - What the client must do to carry out the plan of treatment
- When offering information and explanations, keep in mind that anxiety interferes with intellectual functioning. Thus, communication should be brief, clear, and repeated as necessary because clients may misunderstand or forget what is said.
- Modify the environment to decrease anxiety-provoking stimuli. Modifications may involve altering temperature, light, and noise levels.
- Use measures to increase physical comfort. These may include a wide variety of activities, such as positioning, helping the client bathe or ambulate, giving back rubs, or providing fluids of the client's choice.
- Consult with other services and departments on the client's behalf. For example, if financial problems were identified as a cause of anxiety, social services may be able to help.
- When a benzodiazepine is used with diagnostic tests or minor surgery, provide instructions for postprocedure care to the client or to family members, preferably in written form.

Implement measures to decrease the need for or increase the effectiveness of sedative-hypnotic drugs, such as the following:

- Modify the environment to promote rest and sleep (eg, reduce noise and light).
- Plan care to allow uninterrupted periods of rest and sleep when possible.
- Relieve symptoms that interfere with rest and sleep. Drugs such as analgesics for pain or antitussives for cough are

*(continued)*

## NURSING PROCESS (Continued)

usually safer and more effective than sedative-hypnotic drugs. Nondrug measures, such as positioning, exercise, and back rubs, may be helpful in relieving muscle tension and other discomforts. Allowing the client to verbalize concerns, providing information so that he or she knows what to expect, or consulting other personnel (eg, social worker, chaplain) may be useful in decreasing anxiety.

- Help the client modify lifestyle habits to promote rest and sleep (eg, limiting intake of caffeine-containing beverages, limiting intake of fluids during evening hours if nocturia interferes with sleep, avoiding daytime naps,

having a regular schedule of rest and sleep periods, increasing physical activity, and not trying to sleep unless tired or drowsy).

### Evaluation

- Decreased symptoms of anxiety or insomnia and increased rest and sleep are reported or observed.
- Excessive sedation and motor impairment are not observed.
- The client reports no serious adverse effects.
- Monitoring of prescriptions (eg, "pill counts") does not indicate excessive use.

---

## CLIENT TEACHING GUIDELINES
## Antianxiety and Sedative-Hypnotic Drugs

### General Considerations

✔ "Nerve pills" and "sleeping pills" can relieve symptoms temporarily but they do not cure or solve the underlying problems. With rare exceptions, these drugs are recommended only for short-term use. For long-term relief, counseling or psychotherapy may be more beneficial because it can help you learn other ways to decrease your nervousness and difficulty in sleeping.

✔ Use nondrug measures to promote relaxation, rest, and sleep when possible. Physical exercise, reading, craft work, stress management, and relaxation techniques are safer than any drug.

✔ Try to identify and avoid factors that cause nervousness or insomnia, such as caffeine-containing beverages and stimulant drugs. This may prevent or decrease the severity of nervousness or insomnia so that sedative-type drugs are not needed. If the drugs are used, these factors can cancel or decrease the drugs' effects. Stimulant drugs include asthma and cold remedies and appetite suppressants.

✔ Most "nerve pills" and "sleeping pills" belong to the same chemical group and have similar effects, including the ability to decrease nervousness, cause drowsiness, and cause dependence. Thus, there is no logical reason to take a combination of the drugs for anxiety, or to take one drug for daytime sedation and another for sleep. Ativan, Xanax, Valium, and Restoril are commonly used examples of this group, but there are several others as well.

✔ Inform all health care providers when taking a sedative-type medication, preferably by the generic and trade names. This helps avoid multiple prescriptions of drugs with similar effects and reduces the risk of serious adverse effects from overdose.

✔ Do not perform tasks that require alertness if drowsy from medication. The drugs often impair mental and physical functioning, especially during the first several days of use, and thereby make routine activities poten-

tially hazardous. Avoid smoking, ambulating without help, driving a car, operating machinery, and other potentially hazardous tasks. These activities may lead to falls or other injuries if undertaken while alertness is impaired.

✔ Avoid alcohol and other depressant drugs (eg, over-the-counter [OTC] antihistamines and sleeping pills, narcotic analgesics, sedating herbs such as kava kava and valerian, and the dietary supplement melatonin) while taking any antianxiety or sedative-hypnotic drugs (except buspirone). An antihistamine that causes drowsiness is the active ingredient in OTC sleep aids (eg, Compoz, Nytol, Sominex, Unisom) and many pain reliever products with "PM" as part of their names (eg, Tylenol PM). Because these drugs depress brain functioning when taken alone, combining them produces additive depression and may lead to excessive drowsiness, difficulty breathing, traumatic injuries, and other potentially serious adverse drug effects.

✔ Store drugs safely, out of reach of children and adults who are confused or less than alert. Accidental or intentional ingestion may lead to serious adverse effects. Also, do not keep the drug container at the bedside, because a person sedated by a previous dose may take additional doses.

✔ Do not share these drugs with anyone else. These mind-altering, brain-depressant drugs should be taken only by those people for whom they are prescribed.

✔ Do not stop taking a Valium-related drug abruptly. Withdrawal symptoms can occur. When being discontinued, dosage should be gradually reduced, as directed and with the supervision of a health care provider.

✔ Do not take "sleeping pills" every night. These drugs lose their effectiveness in 2–4 weeks if taken nightly, and cause sleep disturbances when stopped.

✔ Alprazolam (Xanax), is sometimes confused with ranitidine (Zantac), a drug for heartburn and peptic ulcers.

*(continued)*

**CLIENT TEACHING GUIDELINES**
## Antianxiety and Sedative-Hypnotic Drugs (Continued)

**Self-administration**

✔ Follow instructions carefully about how much, how often, and how long to take the drugs. These drugs produce more beneficial effects and fewer adverse reactions when used in the smallest effective doses and for the shortest duration feasible in particular circumstances. All of the Valium-related drugs, zaleplon (Sonata), and zolpidem (Ambien) can cause physical dependence, which may eventually cause worse problems than the original anxiety or insomnia.

✔ Take sleeping pills just before going to bed so that you are lying down when the expected drowsiness occurs.

✔ Omit one or more doses if excessive drowsiness occurs to avoid difficulty breathing, falls, and other adverse drug effects.

✔ Take oral benzodiazepines with a glass of water; they may be taken with food if stomach upset occurs.

✔ Take buspirone on a daily schedule. It is not fully effective until after 3–4 weeks of regular use; it is ineffective for occasional use.

✔ Take zolpidem on an empty stomach, at bedtime, because the drug acts quickly to cause drowsiness.

## ▨ DRUG USE IN SPECIFIC SITUATIONS

### Use in Anxiety Disorders

Antianxiety drugs are not recommended for treating everyday stress and anxiety. Some authorities believe such use promotes reliance on drugs and decreases development of healthier coping mechanisms. For severe anxiety associated with a temporary stressful situation, an anxiolytic drug may be beneficial for short-term, "as-needed" use; prolonged drug therapy is not recommended. These drugs are most clearly indicated when anxiety causes disability and interferes with job performance, interpersonal relationships, and other activities of daily living. The drugs are not recommended for long-term use. Because anxiety often accompanies pain, antianxiety agents are sometimes used to manage pain. In the management of chronic pain, however, antianxiety drugs have not demonstrated a definite benefit. Anxiety about recurrence of pain is probably better controlled by adequate analgesia than by antianxiety drugs.

The antianxiety benzodiazepines are often the drugs of choice for treating anxiety. Because they are equally effective in relieving anxiety, other factors may assist the prescriber in choosing a particular drug for a particular client. For example, alprazolam, clorazepate, and diazepam decrease anxiety within 30 to 60 minutes. Thus, one of these drugs may be preferred when rapid onset of drug action is desired. Lorazepam, oxazepam, and prazepam have a slower onset of action and thus are not recommended for acute symptoms of anxiety. Because they have short half-lives and their elimination does not depend on the cytochrome P450 oxidizing enzymes in the liver, lorazepam and oxazepam are the drugs of choice for clients who are elderly, have liver disease, or are taking drugs that interfere with hepatic drug-metabolizing enzymes.

When benzodiazepines are used to treat generalized anxiety disorder (GAD), clients often experience relief of symptoms within a few days. In addition, these clients rarely develop tolerance to anxiety-relieving effects or abuse the drugs. Persons most likely to abuse the drugs are those who have a history of drug abuse.

Buspirone is also an effective antianxiety agent, especially for clients with conditions that may be aggravated by the sedative and respiratory depressant effects of benzodiazepines (eg, chronic obstructive lung disease). However, anxiety-relieving effects may be delayed for 2 to 4 weeks. Thus, buspirone is not useful for acute episodes of anxiety, and it may be difficult to persuade some clients to take the drug long enough to be effective. Adverse effects are usually mild and can include nausea and dizziness. Buspirone should not be taken in combination with monoamine oxidase inhibitors; otherwise, buspirone has few drug–drug interactions. When used to treat generalized anxiety disorder, some clinicians recommend relatively high doses of 30 to 60 mg daily (in two or three divided doses).

Antidepressant medications are increasingly being used as a first-line treatment for several anxiety disorders, including GAD. Although several other agents have been used, paroxetine and extended release venlafaxine are approved by the FDA for treatment of GAD. In studies comparing the effects of antidepressants and benzodiazepines for treating GAD, it was concluded that benzodiazepines work faster (within a few days), but that antidepressants are more effective after 4 to 6 weeks. Some clinicians prescribe a combination of a benzodiazepine and an antidepressant. The benzodiazepine provides relief during the 2 to 3 weeks required for antidepressant effects, and then it is tapered and discontinued while the antidepressant is continued. Antidepressants do not cause cognitive impairment or dependence, as benzodiazepines do. In addition, clients with GAD often have depression as well. Thus, an antidepressant can relieve both anxiety and depression, but a benzodiazepine is not effective for treating depression.

One factor to consider in the use of antidepressants is that these drugs can increase the agitation and hyperarousal already present in the client with GAD. To minimize stimulation, initial doses of antidepressants should be about 50% less than the doses for depression. Then, the dose can be increased over 1 to 2 weeks. The optimal maintenance dose of an antidepressant for GAD is usually the same as the antidepressant dose. Another factor is that clients may not be willing to take antidepressants long-term, because of the sexual dysfunction and weight gain associated with the drugs.

Overall, a combination of drug therapy and psychotherapy may be the most effective treatment for GAD. Benzodiazepines, buspirone, and antidepressants are the drugs of choice; cognitive behavioral therapy (CBT) is probably the nonpharmacologic treatment of choice. Drug therapy can relieve the symptoms; CBT can help clients learn to manage their anxiety and decrease their negative thinking. Once anxiety is under control, some clinicians recommend continuing drug therapy for at least a year.

## Use in Insomnia

In general, sedative-hypnotic drugs should be used only when insomnia causes significant distress and resists management by nonpharmacologic means; they should not be used for occasional sleeplessness. When drug therapy is required, guidelines for effective use include the following:

1. The goal of treatment is to relieve anxiety or sleeplessness without permitting sensory perception, responsiveness to the environment, or alertness to drop below safe levels.
2. The drugs of choice for most clients are the benzodiazepines and the BZ1 receptor–specific drugs zaleplon and zolpidem. However, for clients with insomnia associated with major depression, antidepressants are preferred.
3. Do not give sedative-hypnotic drugs every night unless necessary. Intermittent administration helps maintain drug effectiveness and decreases the risks for drug abuse and dependence. It also decreases disturbances of normal sleep patterns.
4. When sedative-hypnotic drugs are prescribed for outpatients, the prescription should limit the number of doses dispensed and the number of refills. This is one way of decreasing the risks for abuse and suicide.
5. In chronic insomnia, no hypnotic drug is recommended for long-term treatment. Most benzodiazepine hypnotics lose their effectiveness in producing sleep after 4 weeks of daily use; triazolam loses effectiveness in 2 weeks. It is not helpful to switch from one drug to another because cross-tolerance develops. To restore the sleep-producing effect, administration of the hypnotic drug must be interrupted for 1 to 2 weeks.
6. As with the antianxiety benzodiazepines, most hypnotic benzodiazepines are oxidized in the liver by the cytochrome P450 enzymes to metabolites that

are then conjugated and excreted through the kidneys. An exception is temazepam (Restoril), which is eliminated only by conjugation with glucuronide. Thus, temazepam is the drug of choice for clients who are elderly, have liver disease, or are taking drugs that interfere with hepatic drug-metabolizing enzymes.

## Prevention and Management of Benzodiazepine Withdrawal

Physical dependence on benzodiazepines, which is associated with longer use and higher doses, is indicated by withdrawal symptoms when the drugs are stopped. Mild symptoms occur in approximately half the clients taking therapeutic doses for 6 to 12 weeks; severe symptoms are most likely to occur when high doses are taken regularly for more than 4 months and then abruptly discontinued. Although the drugs have not been proved effective for more than 4 months of regular use, this period is probably exceeded quite often in clinical practice.

Withdrawal symptoms may be caused by the abrupt separation of benzodiazepine molecules from their receptor sites and the acute decrease in GABA neurotransmission that results. Because GABA is an inhibitory neurotransmitter, less GABA may produce a less inhibited CNS and symptoms of hyperarousal or CNS stimulation. Thus, common manifestations include increased anxiety, psychomotor agitation, insomnia, irritability, headache, tremor, and palpitations. Less common but more serious manifestations include confusion, abnormal perception of movement, depersonalization, psychosis, and seizures.

Severe symptoms are most likely to occur with short-acting drugs (eg, alprazolam, lorazepam, and triazolam) unless they are discontinued very gradually. Symptoms may occur within 24 hours of stopping a short-acting drug but usually occur 4 to 5 days after stopping a long-acting drug such as diazepam. Symptoms can be relieved by administration of a benzodiazepine.

To prevent withdrawal symptoms, the drug should be tapered in dose and gradually discontinued. Reducing the dose by 10% to 25% every 1 or 2 weeks over 4 to 16 weeks usually is effective. However, the rate may need to be even slower with high doses or long-term use. After the drug is discontinued, the client should be monitored for a few weeks for symptoms of withdrawal or recurrence of symptoms for which the drug was originally prescribed.

## Toxicity of Benzodiazepines: Recognition and Management

Toxic effects of benzodiazepines include excessive sedation, respiratory depression, and coma. Flumazenil (Romazicon) is a specific antidote that competes with benzodiazepines for benzodiazepine receptors and reverses toxicity. Clinical indications for use include benzodiazepine overdose and reversal of sedation after diagnostic or therapeutic procedures. The degree of sedation reversal depends on the plasma concentration of the ingested benzodiazepine and the flumazenil dose and frequency of administration. The drug acts rapidly, with onset within 2 minutes and peak effects within 6 to 10 minutes. However, the duration of action is short (serum half-life of 60 to 90 minutes) compared with that of most benzodiazepines; thus, repeated doses are usually required. Adverse effects include precipitation of acute benzodiazepine withdrawal symptoms, agitation, confusion, seizures, and cardiac arrest. Resedation and hypoventilation may occur if flumazenil is not given long enough to coincide with the duration of action of the benzodiazepine. Although the risk for adverse effects with a benzodiazepine is high in critically ill clients, routine use of the benzodiazepine antidote, flumazenil, is generally not recommended because the drug may cause seizures.

The drug should be injected into a freely flowing IV line in a large vein. Dosage recommendations vary with use. For reversal of conscious sedation or general anesthesia, the initial dose is 0.2 mg over 15 seconds, then 0.2 mg every 60 seconds, if necessary, to a maximum of 1.0 mg (total of five doses). For overdose, the initial dose is 0.2 mg over 30 seconds, wait 30 seconds, then 0.3 mg over 30 seconds, then 0.5 mg every 60 seconds up to a total dose of 3 mg, if necessary, for the client to reach the desired level of consciousness. Slow administration and repeated doses are recommended to awaken the client gradually and decrease the risk for causing acute withdrawal symptoms. A client who does not respond within 5 minutes of administering the total recommended dose should be reassessed for other causes of sedation.

## Use in Hypoalbuminemia

Clients with hypoalbuminemia (eg, from malnutrition or liver disease) are at risk for adverse effects with drugs that are highly bound to plasma proteins, such as the benzodiazepines, buspirone, and zolpidem. If a benzodiazepine is given to clients with low serum albumin levels, alprazolam or lorazepam is preferred because these drugs are less extensively bound to plasma proteins and less likely to cause adverse effects. If buspirone or zolpidem is given, dosage may need to be reduced.

## Nursing Actions

### Antianxiety and Sedative-Hypnotic Drugs

| Nursing Actions | Rationale/Explanation |
|---|---|
| 1. Administer accurately. | |
| a. If a client appears excessively sedated when a dose of an antianxiety or sedative-hypnotic drug is due, omit the dose and record the reason. | To avoid excessive sedation and other adverse effects |
| b. For oral sedative-hypnotics: | |
| (1) Prepare the client for sleep before giving hypnotic doses of any drug. | Most of the drugs cause drowsiness within 15–30 minutes. The client should be in bed when he or she becomes drowsy to increase the therapeutic effectiveness of the drug and to decrease the likelihood of falls or other injuries. |
| (2) Give with a glass of water or other fluid. | The fluid enhances dissolution and absorption of the drug for a quicker onset of action. |
| (3) Raise bedrails and instruct the client to stay in bed or ask for help if necessary to get out of bed. | To avoid falls and other injuries related to sedation and impaired mobility |
| c. For benzodiazepines: | |
| (1) Give orally, when feasible. | These drugs are well absorbed from the gastrointestinal (GI) tract, and onset of action occurs within a few minutes. Diazepam is better absorbed orally than IM. When given IM, the drug crystallizes in tissue and is absorbed very slowly. |
| (2) Do not mix injectable diazepam with any other drug in a syringe or add to intravenous (IV) fluids. | Diazepam is physically incompatible with other drugs and solutions. |
| (3) Give intramuscular (IM) benzodiazepines undiluted, deeply, into large muscle masses, such as the gluteus muscle of the hip. | These drugs are irritating to tissues and may cause pain at injection sites. |
| (4) With intravenous benzodiazepines, be very careful to avoid intra-arterial injection or extravasation into surrounding tissues. Have equipment available for respiratory assistance. | These drugs are very irritating to tissues and may cause venous thrombosis, phlebitis, local irritation, edema, and vascular impairment. They may also cause respiratory depression and apnea. |

*(continued)*

## Nursing Actions

## Antianxiety and Sedative-Hypnotic Drugs (Continued)

| Nursing Actions | Rationale/Explanation |
|---|---|
| (5) Give IV **diazepam** slowly, over at least 1 minute for 5 mg (1 mL); into large veins (not hand or wrist veins); by direct injection into the vein or into IV infusion tubing as close as possible to the venipuncture site. | To avoid apnea and tissue irritation |
| (6) Give IV **lorazepam** slowly, over at least 1 minute for 2 mg, by direct injection into the vein or into IV infusion tubing. Immediately before injection, dilute with an equal volume of sterile water for injection, sodium chloride injection, or 5% dextrose injection. | To avoid apnea, hypotension, and tissue irritation |
| (7) Give IV **midazolam** slowly, over approximately 2 minutes, after diluting the dose with 0.9% sodium chloride injection or 5% dextrose in water. | Rapid IV injection may cause severe respiratory depression and apnea; dilution facilitates slow injection. |
| (8) Midazolam may be mixed in the same syringe with morphine sulfate, and atropine sulfate. | No apparent chemical or physical incompatibilities occur with these substances. |
| d. Give **hydroxyzine** orally or deep IM only. When given IM for preoperative sedation, it can be mixed in the same syringe with atropine, and most opioid analgesics likely to be ordered at the same time. | IM hydroxyzine is very irritating to tissues. |
| e. Give **clomipramine** in divided doses, with meals, initially; after titration to a stable dose, give the total daily dose at bedtime. | Giving with meals decreases adverse effects on the GI tract; giving the total dose once daily at bedtime decreases daytime sedation. |
| 2. **Observe for therapeutic effects.** | Therapeutic effects depend largely on the reason for use. |
| a. When a drug is given for antianxiety effects, observe for: | |
| (1) An appearance of being relaxed, perhaps drowsy, but easily aroused | With benzodiazepines, decreased anxiety and drowsiness may appear within a few minutes. |
| (2) Verbal statements such as "less worried," "more relaxed," "resting better" | With buspirone, antianxiety effects may occur within 7–10 days of regular use, with optimal effects in 3–4 weeks. |
| (3) Decrease in or absence of manifestations of anxiety, such as rigid posture, facial grimaces, crying, elevated blood pressure and heart rate | |
| (4) Less time spent in worrying or compulsive behaviors | |
| b. When a drug is given for hypnotic effects, drowsiness should be evident within approximately 30 minutes, and the client usually sleeps for several hours. | |
| c. When diazepam or lorazepam is given IV for control of acute convulsive disorders, seizure activity should decrease or stop almost immediately. When a drug is given for chronic anticonvulsant effects, lack of seizure activity is a therapeutic effect. | |
| d. When hydroxyzine is given for nausea and vomiting, absence of vomiting and verbal statements of relief indicate therapeutic effects. | |
| e. When hydroxyzine is given for antihistaminic effects in skin disorders, observe for decreased itching and fewer statements of discomfort. | |

(continued)

## *Nursing Actions*

## Antianxiety and Sedative-Hypnotic Drugs (Continued)

| *Nursing Actions* | *Rationale/Explanation* |
|---|---|
| 3. Observe for adverse effects. | Most adverse effects are caused by central nervous system (CNS) depression. |
| a. Excessive sedation—drowsiness, stupor, difficult to arouse, impaired mental processes, impaired mobility, respiratory depression, confusion | These effects are more likely to occur with large doses or if the recipient is elderly, debilitated, or has liver disease that slows drug metabolism. Respiratory depression and apnea stem from depression of the respiratory center in the medulla oblongata; they are most likely to occur with large doses or rapid IV administration of diazepam, lorazepam, or midazolam. Excessive drowsiness is more likely to occur when drug therapy is begun, and it usually decreases within a week. |
| b. Hypotension | Hypotension probably results from depression of the vasomotor center in the brain and is more likely to occur with large doses or rapid IV administration of diazepam, lorazepam, or midazolam. |
| c. Pain and induration at injection sites | Parenteral solutions are irritating to tissues. |
| d. Paradoxical excitement, anger, aggression, and hallucinations | |
| e. Chronic intoxication—sedation, confusion, emotional lability, muscular incoordination, impaired mental processes, mental depression, GI problems, weight loss | These signs and symptoms may occur with benzodiazepines and are similar to those occurring with chronic alcohol abuse (see Chap. 14). |
| f. Withdrawal or abstinence syndrome—anxiety, insomnia, restlessness, irritability, tremors, postural hypotension, seizures | These signs and symptoms may occur when benzodiazepines are discontinued abruptly, especially after high doses or long-term use. |
| g. With buspirone, the most common adverse effects are headache, dizziness, nausea, nervousness, fatigue, and excitement. Less frequent effects include dry mouth, chest pain, tachycardia, palpitations, drowsiness, confusion, and depression | |
| h. With zaleplon and zolpidem, common adverse effects include daytime drowsiness, dizziness, headache, nausea, and diarrhea. Less frequent effects include ataxia, confusion, paradoxical excitation. | |
| 4. Observe for drug interactions. | |
| a. Drugs that *increase* effects of antianxiety and sedative-hypnotic drugs: | |
| (1) CNS depressants—alcohol, opioid analgesics, tricyclic antidepressants, sedating antihistamines, phenothiazine and other antipsychotic agents | All these drugs produce CNS depression when given alone. Any combination increases CNS depression, sedation, and respiratory depression. Combinations of these drugs are hazardous and should be avoided. Ingesting alcohol with antianxiety or sedative-hypnotic drugs may cause respiratory depression, coma, and convulsions. Although buspirone does not appear to cause additive CNS depression, concurrent use with other CNS depressants is best avoided. |
| (2) Amprenavir, clarithromycin, cimetidine, diltiazem, erythromycin, fluoxetine, fluvoxamine, itraconazole, ketoconazole, metoprolol, omeprazole, oral contraceptives, propranolol, ritonavir, valproic acid | These drugs inhibit cytochrome P450 3A4 enzymes that metabolize most benzodiazepines. Midazolam should be avoided in patients receiving a CYP3A4 inhibitor drug; lorazepam or propofol may be used for sedation. These drugs do not affect elimination of lorazepam or temazepam. |

*(continued)*

## Nursing Actions
### Antianxiety and Sedative-Hypnotic Drugs (Continued)

| Nursing Actions | Rationale/Explanation |
|---|---|
| b. Drugs that *decrease* effects of antianxiety and sedative-hypnotic agents:<br>(1) CNS stimulants—antiasthma drugs, appetite suppressants, bronchodilators (eg, albuterol, theophylline), nasal decongestants (eg, phenylephrine, pseudoephedrine), and lifestyle drugs (eg, caffeine, nicotine) | Phenylephrine and pseudoephedrine are available alone or in multisymptom cold remedies. |
| (2) Enzyme inducers (eg, carbamazepine, isoniazid, phenytoin, rifampin) | With chronic use, these drugs antagonize their own actions and the actions of other drugs metabolized by the same enzymes in the liver. They increase the rate of drug metabolism and elimination from the body. |
| c. Drug that increases effects of zaleplon:<br>(1) Cimetidine | Inhibits both aldehyde oxidase and CYP3A4 enzymes that metabolize zaleplon, thereby greatly increasing serum levels and risks of toxicity |
| d. Drug that increases effects of zolpidem:<br>(1) Ritonavir | Inhibits hepatic metabolism of zolpidem and may cause severe sedation and respiratory depression. **These drugs should not be given concurrently.** |

## Critical Thinking Exercises

1. Benzodiazepines bind with benzodiazepine receptors in the brain; they also have binding sites for gamma-aminobutyric acid (GABA), an inhibitory neurotransmitter. This GABA–benzodiazepine receptor complex regulates the entry of what ions into the cell?
   a. Sodium
   b. Potassium
   c. Chloride
   d. Magnesium

2. There is also a risk for increased serum zaleplon levels if the drug is taken concurrently with which of the following?
   a. Cimetidine
   b. Alcohol
   c. Coffee
   d. Chocolate

3. Which of the following drugs may be preferred when rapid onset of drug action is desired to decrease acute symptoms of anxiety?
   a. Lorazepam
   b. Oxazepam
   c. Prazepam
   d. Alprazolam

4. Drugs such as the benzodiazepines are highly bound to plasma proteins. When administering the drug in a client with a low serum albumin level, the drug:
   a. Dosage may need to be increased
   b. Should not be administered
   c. Dosage may need to be decreased
   d. Can be administered without concern for adverse effects

5. Buspirone differs from other antianxiety agents, particularly the benzodiazepines, in that:
   a. The drug can be taken in combination with monoamine oxidase inhibitors
   b. Anxiety-relieving effects may be delayed for 2 to 4 weeks
   c. The drug is useful for acute episodes of anxiety
   d. The sedative and respiratory depressant effects are significant

## SELECTED REFERENCES

American Psychiatric Association (2000). *Diagnostic and statistical manual of mental disorders* (4th ed., revised). Washington, DC: Author.

Canales, P. L., Cates, M., & Wells, B. G. (2000). Anxiety disorders. In E. T. Herfindal & D. R. Gourley (Eds.), *Textbook of therapeutics: Drug and disease management* (7th ed., pp. 1185–1202). Philadelphia: Lippincott Williams & Wilkins.

Dresser, G. K., Spence, J. D., & Bailey, D. G. (2000). Pharmaco-kinetic-pharmacodynamic consequences and clinical relevance of cytochrome P450 3A4 inhibition. *Clinical Pharmacokinetics, 38*(1), 41–57.

*Drug facts and comparisons.* (Updated monthly). St. Louis: Facts and Comparisons.

Fetrow, C. W., & Avila, J. R. (2000). *Professional's handbook of complementary and alternative medicines.* Springhouse, PA: Springhouse Corporation.

Hadbavny, A. M., & Hoyt, J. W. (2000). Sedatives and analgesics in critical care. In A. Grenvik, S. M. Ayres, P. R. Holbrook, & W. C. Shoemaker (Eds.), *Textbook of critical care* (4th ed., pp. 961–971). Philadelphia: W.B. Saunders.

Hembree, E. A., & Foa, E. B. (2000). Posttraumatic stress disorder: Psychological factors and psychosocial interventions. *Journal of Clinical Psychiatry, 61*(Suppl. 7), 33–99.

Lacy, C. F., Armstrong, L. L., Goldman, M. P., & Lance, L. L. (2003). *Lexi-Comp's drug information handbook* (11th ed.). Hudson, OH: American Pharmaceutical Association.

Rickels, K., Pollack, M. H., Sheehan, D. V., & Haskins, J. T. (2000). Efficacy of extended-release venlafaxine in non-depressed outpatients with generalized anxiety disorder. *American Journal of Psychiatry, 157,* 968–974.

Waddell, D. L., Hummel, M. E., & Sumners, A. D. (2001). Three herbs you should get to know. *American Journal of Nursing 101*(4), 48–53.

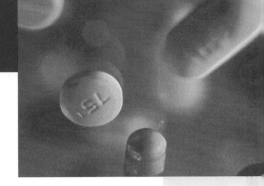

# 9

# Antipsychotic Drugs

## CRITICAL THINKING SCENARIO

*A*s a nurse in an acute psychiatric facility, you attend the family conference for a young man, Jeff Smith, who has recently been diagnosed as schizophrenic and started on antipsychotic medications. It is apparent that the family members are in shock, still not believing that a member of their family could be mentally ill. They also have just experienced a very stressful week in which Mr. Smith was psychotic, experiencing delusions and severe agitation, and threatening the family.

✔ How would you feel if someone you love were diagnosed with a serious, chronic mental health condition? How are these feelings similar to or different from when a loved one is diagnosed with a chronic physical condition?

✔ What questions do you think these family members might ask about schizophrenia or the medications prescribed to control it?

✔ What factors might influence compliance with antipsychotic medications?

## PROTOTYPE PROFILE

clozapine (Clozaril), p. 162

# PSYCHOSIS

Antipsychotic drugs are used mainly for the treatment of *psychosis,* a severe mental disorder characterized by disordered thought processes (disorganized and often bizarre thinking); blunted or inappropriate emotional responses; bizarre behavior ranging from hypoactivity to hyperactivity with agitation, aggressiveness, hostility, and combativeness; social withdrawal in which a person pays less than usual attention to the environment and other people; deterioration from previous levels of occupational and social functioning (poor self-care and interpersonal skills); hallucinations; and paranoid delusions. *Hallucinations* are sensory perceptions of people or objects that are not present in the external environment. More specifically, people see, hear, or feel stimuli that are not visible to external observers and cannot distinguish between these false perceptions and reality. Hallucinations occur with delirium, dementias, schizophrenia, and other psychotic states. Those occurring in schizophrenia or bipolar affective disorder are usually auditory, those in delirium are usually visual or tactile, and those in dementias are usually visual. *Delusions* are false beliefs that persist in the absence of reason or evidence. Deluded people often believe that other people control their thoughts, feelings, and behaviors or seek to harm them (paranoia). Delusions indicate severe mental illness. Although they are commonly associated with schizophrenia, delusions also occur with delirium, dementias, and other psychotic disorders.

Psychosis may be acute or chronic. Acute episodes, also called confusion or delirium, have a sudden onset over hours to days and may be precipitated by physical disorders (eg, brain damage related to cerebrovascular disease or head injury, metabolic disorders, infections); drug intoxication with adrenergics, antidepressants, some anticonvulsants, amphetamines, cocaine, and others; and drug withdrawal after chronic use (eg, alcohol, benzodiazepine antianxiety or sedative-hypnotic agents). In addition, acute psychotic episodes may be superimposed on chronic dementias and psychoses, such as schizophrenia. This chapter focuses primarily on schizophrenia as a chronic psychosis.

# SCHIZOPHRENIA

Although schizophrenia is often referred to as a single disease, it includes a variety of related disorders. Risk factors include a genetic predisposition and environmental stresses. Symptoms may begin gradually or suddenly, usually during adolescence or early adulthood. According to the American Psychiatric Association's *Diagnostic and Statistical Manual of Mental Disorders,* 4th edition, Text Revision (DSM-IV-TR, 2000), overt psychotic symptoms must be present for 6 months before schizophrenia can be diagnosed.

Behavioral manifestations of schizophrenia are categorized as positive and negative symptoms. Positive symptoms are characterized by central nervous system (CNS) stimulation and include agitation, behavioral disturbances, delusions, disorganized speech, hallucinations, insomnia, and paranoia. Negative symptoms are characterized by a lack of pleasure (anhedonia), a lack of motivation, a blunted affect, poor grooming and hygiene, poor social skills, poverty of speech, and social withdrawal. However, all of these symptoms may occur with other disorders.

## Etiology

The etiology of schizophrenia is unclear. However, there is evidence that it results from abnormal neurotransmission systems in the brain, especially in the dopaminergic, serotonergic, and glutamatergic systems. There is also evidence of extensive interactions among neurotransmission systems. For example, the serotonergic and glutamatergic systems can alter dopaminergic activity, and drugs that may cause psychosis affect several systems (eg, adrenergics increase norepinephrine and antidepressants increase norepinephrine, serotonin, or both). Thus, schizophrenia probably results from imbalances and abnormal integration among several neurotransmission systems. In addition, illnesses or drugs that alter neurotransmission in one system are likely to alter neurotransmission in other systems. The most-studied systems are the dopaminergic, serotonin, and glutamatergic; these are discussed in At the Foundation: Neurotransmission Systems.

# ANTIPSYCHOTIC DRUGS

Antipsychotic drugs are derived from several chemical groups and broadly categorized as "typical," conventional, or first-generation agents (phenothiazines and older nonphenothiazines with similar pharmacologic actions) and the "atypical" or second-generation agents, which can also be called newer nonphenothiazines.

## Phenothiazines

These drugs are historically important because **chlorpromazine** (Thorazine), the first drug to treat psychotic disorders effectively, belongs to this group. These drugs have been used since the 1950s, but their use and clinical importance have waned in recent years.

The phenothiazines are well absorbed after oral and parenteral administration. They are distributed to most body tissues and reach high concentrations in the brain. They are metabolized in the liver by the cytochrome P450 enzyme system; several produce pharmacologically active metabolites. Metabolites are excreted in urine. These drugs do not cause psychological dependence, but they may cause physical dependence manifested by withdrawal

## AT THE FOUNDATION: *Neurotransmission Systems*

### Dopaminergic System

This system has been more extensively studied than other systems because schizophrenia has long been attributed to increased dopamine activity in the brain. Stimulation of dopamine can initiate psychotic symptoms or exacerbate an existing psychotic disorder. The importance of dopamine is further supported by the findings that antipsychotic drugs exert their therapeutic effects by decreasing dopamine activity (ie, blocking dopamine receptors) and that drugs that increase dopamine levels in the brain (eg, bromocriptine, cocaine, levodopa) can cause signs and symptoms of psychosis.

In addition to the increased amount of dopamine, dopamine receptors are also involved. Two groups of dopamine receptors have been differentiated, mainly by the effects of the dopamine–receptor complex on intracellular functions. One group stimulates cellular functions, whereas the other group decreases cellular functions and alters the movement of calcium and potassium ions across neuronal cell membranes. The second group ($D_2$ receptors) is considered important in the pathophysiology of schizophrenia. Thus, at the cellular level, dopamine activity is determined by its interaction with various receptors and the simultaneous actions of other neurotransmitters at the same target neurons. In general, overactivity of dopamine in some parts of the brain is thought to account for the positive symptoms of schizophrenia, and underactivity in another part of the brain is thought to account for the negative symptoms.

### Serotonergic System

The serotonergic system, which is widespread in the brain, is mainly inhibitory in nature. In schizophrenia, serotonin apparently decreases dopamine activity in the part of the brain associated with negative symptoms and causes or aggravates these symptoms.

### Glutamatergic System

This neurotransmission system involves glutamate, the major excitatory neurotransmitter in the CNS. Glutamate receptors are widespread and possibly located on every neuron in the brain. They are also diverse, and their functions may vary according to subtypes and their locations in particular parts of the brain. When glutamate binds to its receptors, the resulting neuronal depolarization activates signaling molecules (eg, calcium, nitric oxide) within and between brain cells. Thus, glutamatergic transmission may affect every CNS neuron and is considered essential for all mental, sensory, motor, and affective functions. Dysfunction of glutamatergic neurotransmission has been implicated in the development of psychosis.

In addition, the glutamatergic system interacts with the dopaminergic, GABAergic, and possibly other neurotransmission systems. In schizophrenia, evidence indicates abnormalities in the number, density, composition, and function of glutamate receptors. In addition, glutamate receptors are genetically encoded and can interact with environmental factors (eg, stress, alcohol and other drugs) during brain development. Thus, glutamatergic dysfunction may account for the roles of genetic and environmental risk factors in the development of schizophrenia as well as the cognitive impairments and negative symptoms associated with the disorder.

---

symptoms (eg, lethargy and difficulty sleeping) if abruptly discontinued.

Phenothiazines exert many effects in the body, including CNS depression, autonomic nervous system depression (antiadrenergic and anticholinergic effects), antiemetic effects, lowering of body temperature, hypersensitivity reactions, and others. They differ mainly in potency and adverse effects. Differences in potency are demonstrated by the fact that some phenothiazines are as effective in doses of a few milligrams as others are in doses of several hundred milligrams. All phenothiazines produce the same kinds of adverse effects, but individual drugs differ in the incidence and severity of particular adverse effects. Jaundice has been associated with phenothiazines, usually after 2 to 4 weeks of therapy. It is considered a hypersensitivity reaction, and clients should not be reexposed to a phenothiazine. Selected adverse effects, dosages, and pharmacokinetic characteristics of individual drugs are listed in Drugs at a Glance 9-1: Phenothiazine Antipsychotic Drugs and in Table 9-1.

## Nonphenothiazines

The older nonphenothiazines (eg, haloperidol [Haldol]) are similar to phenothiazines in their pharmacologic actions, clinical uses, and adverse effects. The atypical, or newer, nonphenothiazines have become the drugs of first choice in recent years and have virtually replaced phenothiazines and related drugs, except for clients doing well on older drugs and for treatment of acute psychotic episodes.

The atypical drugs (eg, risperidone [Risperdal]) have both similarities and differences compared with other antipsychotic drugs and with each other. The main similarity is their effectiveness in treating the positive symptoms of psychosis; the main differences are greater effectiveness in relieving negative symptoms of schizophrenia and fewer movement disorders (ie, extrapyramidal symptoms such as acute dystonia, parkinsonism, akathisia, and tardive dyskinesia). Although adverse effects are generally milder and more tolerable than with older

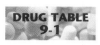

**DRUG TABLE 9-1**

## Drugs at a Glance

## Phenothiazine Antipsychotic Drugs

| Generic/ Trade Name | Routes of Administration and Dosage Ranges | Major Side Effects (Incidence) | | |
|---|---|---|---|---|
| | | Sedation | Extrapyramidal Reactions | Hypotension |
| **Chlorpromazine** (Thorazine) Pregnancy Category C | *Adults:* PO, 200–600 mg daily in divided doses. Dose may be increased by 100 mg daily q2–3 days until symptoms are controlled, adverse effects occur, or a maximum daily dose of 2 g is reached. IM, 25–100 mg initially for acute psychotic symptoms, repeated in 1–4 hours PRN until control is achieved. *Elderly or debilitated adults:* PO, one third to one half usual adult dose, increased by 25 mg daily q2–3 days if necessary. IM, 10 mg q6–8h until acute symptoms are controlled *Children:* PO, IM, 0.5 mg/kg q4–8h. Maximum IM dose, 40 mg daily in children under 5 y of age and 75 mg for older children | High | Moderate | Moderate to high |
| **Fluphenazine decanoate and enanthate** (Prolixin Decanoate; Prolixin Enanthate) Pregnancy Category C | *Adults < 50 y:* IM, Sub-Q, 12.5 mg initially followed by 25 mg every 2 weeks. Dosage requirements rarely exceed 100 mg q2–6 wk. *Adults > 50 y, debilitated clients, or clients with a history of extrapyramidal reactions:* 2.5 mg initially followed by 2.5–5 mg q10–14 days *Children:* No dosage established | Low to moderate | High | Low |
| **Fluphenazine hydrochloride** (Prolixin, Permitil) Pregnancy Category C | *Adults:* PO, 2.5–10 mg initially, gradually reduced to maintenance dose of 1–5 mg (doses above 3 mg are rarely necessary). Acute psychosis: 1.25 mg initially, increased gradually to 2.5–10 mg daily in 3–4 divided doses *Elderly or debilitated adults:* PO, 1–2.5 mg daily; IM one third to one half the usual adult dose *Children:* PO, 0.75–10 mg daily in children 5 to 12 y. IM, no dosage established | Low to moderate | High | Low |
| **Mesoridazine** (Serentil) Pregnancy Category C | *Adults and children > 12 y:* PO, 150 mg daily in divided doses initially, increased gradually in 50-mg increments until symptoms are controlled. Usual dose range, 100–400 mg. IM, 25–175 mg daily in divided doses *Elderly and debilitated adults:* one third to one half usual adult dose *Children < 12 y:* no dosage established | High | Low | Moderate |

*(continued)*

**DRUG TABLE 9-1**

## *Drugs at a Glance*

## Phenothiazine Antipsychotic Drugs (Continued)

| Generic/ Trade Name | Routes of Administration and Dosage Ranges | Major Side Effects (Incidence) | | |
|---|---|---|---|---|
| | | Sedation | Extrapyramidal Reactions | Hypotension |
| **Perphenazine** (Trilafon) Pregnancy Category C | *Adults:* PO, 16–64 mg daily in divided doses. Acute psychoses: IM, 5–10 mg initially, then 5 mg q6h if necessary. Maximum daily dose, 15 mg for ambulatory clients and 30 mg for hospitalized clients *Elderly or debilitated adults:* PO, IM, one-third to one-half usual adult dose *Children:* PO dosages not established, but the following amounts have been given in divided doses: ages 1–6 y, 4–6 mg daily; 6–12 y, 6 mg daily; over 12 y, 6–12 mg daily | Low to moderate | High | Low |
| **Prochlorperazine** (Compazine) Pregnancy Category C | *Adults:* PO, 10 mg 3–4 times daily, increased gradually (usual daily dose, 100–150 mg). IM 10–20 mg; may be repeated in 2–4 h. Switch to oral form as soon as possible. *Children > 2 y:* PO, rectal 2.5 mg 2–3 times daily; IM 0.06 mg/lb | Moderate | High | Low |
| **Promazine** (Sparine) Pregnancy Category C | *Adults:* Initially, 50–150 mg IM; mainte-nance, PO, IM, 10–200 mg q4–6h *Children > 12 y:* 10–25 mg q4–6h | Moderate | Moderate | Moderate |
| **Trifluoperazine** (Stelazine) Pregnancy Category C | *Adults:* Outpatients; PO, 2–4 mg daily in divided doses. Hospitalized clients: PO, 4–10 mg daily in divided doses. Acute psychoses: IM, 1–2 mg q4–5h, maximum of 10 mg daily *Elderly or debilitated adults:* PO, IM, one third to one half usual adult dose. If given IM, give at less frequent inter-vals than above. *Children ≥ 6 y:* PO, IM, 1–2 mg daily, maximum daily dose 15 mg *Children < 6 y:* no dosage established | Moderate | High | Low |

drugs, clozapine may cause life-threatening agranulocy-tosis, and some have been associated with weight gain, hyperglycemia, and diabetes.

The drugs' ability to decrease adverse effects is seen as a significant advantage because clients are more likely to take the drugs. Better compliance with drug therapy helps to prevent acute episodes of psychosis and repeated hos-pitalizations. Although these drugs are more expensive than the older ones, studies indicate that they reduce the overall cost of care by reducing acute psychotic episodes and hospitalizations.

Because typical and atypical nonphenothiazines vary in their characteristics, individual drugs are described in later sections, in Table 9-1, and in Drugs at a Glance 9-2: Nonphenothiazine Antipsychotic Drugs.

## Mechanism of Action

Most antipsychotic drugs bind to $D_2$ dopamine receptors and block the action of dopamine (Fig. 9-1). However, drug binding to the receptors does not explain antipsy-chotic effects because binding occurs within a few hours after a drug dose, and antipsychotic effects may not occur until the drugs have been given for a few weeks. Manifes-tations of hyperarousal (eg, anxiety, agitation, hyper-activity, insomnia, aggressive or combative behavior) are

## TABLE 9-1 Pharmacokinetics of Antipsychotic Drugs

| Generic Name | Route | Action | | | Half-life (h) |
| | | Onset | Peak | Duration | |
|---|---|---|---|---|---|
| Chlorpromazine | PO | 30–60 min | 2–4 h | 4–6 h (10–12 h for extended release) | 3–40 |
| | IM | 15–30 min | 2–3 h | 4–8 h | 3–40 |
| Clozapine | PO | Unknown | 1–6 h | 4–12 h | 9–17 |
| Fluphenazine hydrochloride | PO | 60 min | 3–5 h | 6–8 h | 5–15 |
| Fluphenazine decanoate | IM | 24–72 h | 24 h | 1–3 wks | 7–10 days |
| Fluphenazine enanthate | IM | 24–72 h | 48 h | >4 wks | 4 days |
| Haloperidol | PO | 2 h | 2–6 h | 8–12 h | 21–24 |
| | IM | 20–30 min | 30–45 min | 4–8 h | |
| Haloperidol decanoate | IM | 3–9 days | Unknown | 1 month | 3 wk |
| Loxapine | PO | 30 min | 1.5–3 h | 12 h | 3–4 |
| Mesoridazine | PO | Varies | 2–4 h | 4–6 h | 24–48 |
| | IM | Rapid | 30 min | 6–8 h | |
| Molindone | PO | Varies | 30–90 min | 24–36 h | 1.5–6 |
| Olanzapine | PO | Varies | 4–5 h | weeks | 20–27 |
| Perphenazine | PO | Varies | Unknown | Unknown | Unknown |
| | IM/IV | 5–10 min | 1–2 h | 6 h | |
| Promazine | PO | 30 min | unknown | 4–6 h | Unknown |
| Quetiapine | PO | Varies | 2–4 h | 8–10 h | 6 |
| Risperidone | PO | 1–2 h | 3–17 h | weeks | 20–30 |
| Thiothixene | PO | Slow | 1–3 h | 12 h | 3–4 |
| Trifluoperazine | PO | Varies | 2–4 h | <12 h | 3–40 |
| | IM | Rapid | 1–2 h | <12 h | 3–40 |
| Ziprasidone | PO | Varies | 1 h | 6–8 h | 3 |

relieved more quickly than hallucinations, delusions, and thought disorders. One view of the delayed effects is that the blockade of dopamine receptors leads to changes in the receptors and postreceptor effects on cell metabolism and function. With chronic drug administration (ie, chronic blockade of dopamine receptors), there is an increased number of dopamine receptors on postsynaptic and possibly presynaptic nerve cell membranes (up-regulation). Clozapine (Clozaril) and other atypical agents interact with dopamine, serotonin, and glutamate receptors. Overall, the drugs re-regulate the abnormal neurotransmission systems associated with psychosis.

## Indications for Use

The major clinical indication for use of antipsychotic drugs is schizophrenia. The drugs also are used to treat psychotic symptoms associated with brain impairment induced by head injury, tumor, stroke, alcohol withdrawal, overdoses of CNS stimulant drugs, and other disorders. They may be useful in the manic phase of bipolar affective disorder to control manic behavior until lithium, the drug of choice, becomes effective.

The phenothiazines are also used for clinical indications not associated with psychiatric illness. These include treatment of nausea, vomiting, and intractable hiccups. The drugs relieve nausea and vomiting by blocking dopamine receptors in the chemoreceptor trigger zone, a group of neurons in the medulla oblongata that causes nausea and vomiting when activated by physical or psychological stimuli. **Promethazine** (Phenergan) is not used for antipsychotic effects but is often used for antiemetic, sedative, and antihistaminic effects. The mechanism by which the drugs relieve hiccups is unclear.

Childhood schizophrenia is often characterized by more severe symptoms and a more chronic course than adult schizophrenia. Drug therapy is largely empiric because few studies have been done in children and adolescents. Antipsychotic drugs should be used cautiously in older adults. Before they are started, a thorough assessment is needed because psychiatric symptoms are often caused by organic disease or other drugs. If this is the case, treating the disease or stopping the offending drug may cancel the need for an antipsychotic drug. Additional developmental factors are highlighted in Age-related Considerations.

## Contraindications to Use

Because of their wide-ranging adverse effects, antipsychotic drugs may cause or aggravate a number of condi-

(text continues on page 158)

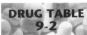

*Drugs at a Glance*

**DRUG TABLE 9-2**

## Nonphenothiazine Antipsychotic Drugs

| Generic/Trade Name | Routes and Dosage Ranges | Comments |
|---|---|---|
| ***First-Generation "Typical" Drugs*** | | |
| **Haloperidol** (Haldol) Pregnancy Category C | *Adults:* Acute psychosis: PO, 1–15 mg/d initially in divided doses, gradually increased to 100 mg/d, if necessary; usual maintenance dose, 2–8 mg daily; IM, 2–10 mg q1–8h until symptoms are controlled (usually within 72 h) | May cause anticholinergic effects (blurred vision, urinary retention, constipation, dry mouth, confusion) |
| | Chronic schizophrenia: PO, 6–15 mg/d; maximum 100 mg/d; dosage is reduced for maintenance, usually 15–20 mg/d. Haloperidol decanoate IM, initial dose up to 100 mg, depending on the previous dose of oral drug, then titrated according to response. Usually given every 4 weeks | Avoid alcohol and other CNS depressants |
| | | Skin contact with oral suspension may cause contact dermatitis |
| | | Solution may be administered if slightly yellow in color; should be discarded if markedly discolored because potency may be decreased |
| | Tourette's syndrome: PO, 6–15 mg/d; maximum 100 mg/d; usual maintenance dose, 9 mg/d | |
| | Mental retardation with hyperkinesia: PO, 80–120 mg/d, gradually reduced to a maintenance dose of approximately 60 mg/d; IM, 20 mg/d in divided doses, gradually increased to 60 mg/d if necessary | |
| | Oral administration should be substituted after symptoms are controlled | |
| | *Elderly or debilitated adults:* Same as for children <12 y | |
| | *Children > 12 y:* Acute psychosis, chronic refractory schizophrenia, Tourette's syndrome, mental retardation with hyperkinesia: same as for adults | |
| | *<12 y:* Acute psychosis: PO, 0.5–1.5 mg/d initially, gradually increased in increments of 0.5 mg; usual maintenance dose, 2–4 mg/d | |
| | IM dosage not established | |
| | Chronic refractory schizophrenia, dosage not established | |
| | Tourette's syndrome: PO, 1.5–6 mg/d initially in divided doses; usual maintenance dose, 1.5 mg/d | |
| | Mental retardation with hyperkinesia: PO, 1.5 mg/d initially, in divided doses, gradually increased to a maximum of 15 mg/d, if necessary. When symptoms are controlled, dosage is gradually reduced to the minimum effective level. IM dosage not established | |

*(continued)*

**DRUG TABLE 9-2**

*Drugs at a Glance*

## Nonphenothiazine Antipsychotic Drugs (Continued)

| Generic/Trade Name | Routes and Dosage Ranges | Comments |
|---|---|---|
| **Loxapine** (Loxitane) Pregnancy Category C | *Adults:* PO, 10 mg twice a day initially, may be increased to 50 mg/d in severe psychoses; usual maintenance dose 20–60 mg/d; maximum dose 250 mg/d | May cause extrapyramidal reactions and anticholinergic effects |
| | IM, 12.5–50 mg q4–6h or longer, depending on response. Change to oral drug when symptoms controlled | Observe for hypotension when administering IM; should not be administered IV |
| | *Elderly or debilitated adults:* One third to one half the usual adult dosage *Children ≥ 16 y:* Same as adults *<16 y:* Not recommended | |
| **Molindone** (Moban) Pregnancy Category C | *Adults:* PO, 50–75 mg/d, increased gradually if necessary up to 225 mg/d, then reduced for maintenance; usual maintenance dose, 15–40 mg/d | Observe for signs of tardive dyskinesia and neuroleptic malignant syndrome May increase appetite and craving for sweets |
| | *Elderly or debilitated adults:* One third to one half the usual adult dosage *Children <12 y:* Dosage not established | |
| **Pimozide** (Orap) Pregnancy Category C | *Adults:* PO, 1–2 mg/d in divided doses initially, increased if necessary; usual maintenance dose approximately 10 mg/d; maximum dose 20 mg/d (doses greater than 10 mg/d generally not recommended) | Suppresses severe motor and phonic tics in clients with Tourette's disorder who have failed other standard treatment |
| **Thiothixene** (Navane) Pregnancy Category C | *Adults:* PO, 6–10 mg/d in divided doses; maximum 60 mg/d | Phenothiazines cause anticholinergic effects |
| | Acute psychosis: IM, 8–16 mg/d in divided doses; maximum 30 mg/d | Monitor for extrapyramidal symptoms |
| | *Elderly or debilitated adults:* PO, IM, one third to one half the usual adult dosage *Children ≥ 12 y:* Same as adults *<12 y:* Dosage not established | |

### Second-Generation "Atypical" Drugs

| Generic/Trade Name | Routes and Dosage Ranges | Comments |
|---|---|---|
| **Clozapine** (Clozaril) | See Prototype Profile 9-1: Clozapine | |
| **Olanzapine** (Zyprexa) Pregnancy Category C | *Adults:* PO, 5–10 mg/d initially; given once daily at bedtime; increased over several weeks to 20 mg/d, if necessary *Children:* Dosage not established | May cause anticholinergic effects and extrapyramidal reactions Orally disintegrating tablets contain phenylalanine; do not push through foil packet but peel back foil and place in mouth immediately |
| **Quetiapine** (Seroquel) Pregnancy Category C | *Adults:* PO, 25 mg bid initially; increased by 25–50 mg two or three times daily on second and third days, as tolerated, to 300–400 mg, in two or three divided doses on the fourth day. Additional increments or decrements can be made at 2-day intervals; maximum dose 800 mg/d | May cause orthostatic hypotension May increase the risk for cataracts; eye examinations should occur on onset of administration and at 6-mo intervals |

*(continued)*

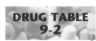

*Drugs at a Glance*

## Nonphenothiazine Antipsychotic Drugs (Continued)

| Generic/Trade Name | Routes and Dosage Ranges | Comments |
|---|---|---|
| | *Elderly or debilitated adults:* Use lower initial doses and increase more gradually, to a lower target dose than for other adults<br>*Hepatic impairment:* PO, same as for elderly or debilitated adults<br>*Children:* Dosage not established | |
| **Risperidone** (Risperdal)<br>Pregnancy Category C | *Adults:* PO, initially 1 mg twice daily (2 mg/d); increase to 2 mg twice daily on the second day (4 mg/d); increase to 3 mg twice daily on the third day (6 mg/d), if necessary. Usual maintenance dose, 4 to 8 mg/d. After initial titration, dosage increases or decreases should be made at a rate of 1 mg/wk<br>*Elderly or debilitated adults:* PO, initially 0.5 mg twice daily (1 mg/d); increase in 0.5 mg increments to 1.5 mg twice daily (3 mg/d)<br>*Children < 12 y:* Dosage not established | May cause anticholinergic effects and extrapyramidal reactions<br>Risperidone may antagonize the effects of levodopa<br>Because risperidone is metabolized to an active metabolite, recommended dosage reductions and titrations for clients with renal impairment are the same as those for older adults |
| **Ziprasidone** (Geodon)<br>Pregnancy Category C | *Adults:* PO, 20 mg twice daily with food, initially, gradually increased up to 80 mg twice daily, if necessary | May cause dose-related ECG changes (prolonged QT interval associated with torsades de pointes) |

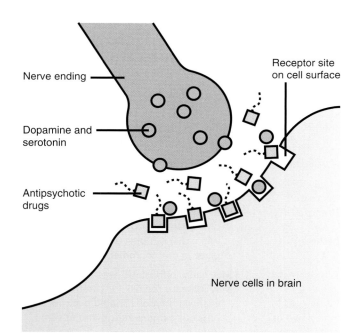

**FIGURE 9–1** Antipsychotic drugs prevent dopamine and serotonin from occupying receptor sites on neuronal cell membranes and exerting their effects on cellular functions. This action leads to changes in receptors and cell functions that account for therapeutic effects (ie, relief of psychotic symptoms). Other neurotransmitters and receptors may also be involved.

tions. Thus, they are contraindicated in clients with liver damage, coronary artery disease, cerebrovascular disease, parkinsonism, bone marrow depression, severe hypotension or hypertension, coma, or severely depressed states. They should be used cautiously in seizure disorders, diabetes mellitus, glaucoma, prostatic hypertrophy, peptic ulcer disease, and chronic respiratory disorders.

## Management Considerations

### Goals of Treatment

Overall, the goal of treatment is to relieve symptoms with minimal or tolerable adverse drug effects. For acute psychosis, the goal during the first week is to decrease symptoms (eg, aggression, agitation, combativeness, hostility) and normalize patterns of sleeping and eating. The next goals may be increased ability for self-care and increased socialization. Therapeutic effects usually occur gradually, over 1 to 2 months. Long-term goals include increasing the client's ability to cope with the environment, promoting optimal functioning in self-care and activities of daily living, and preventing acute episodes and hospitalizations. With drug therapy, clients often can participate in psychotherapy, group therapy, or other treatment modalities; return to community settings; and return to their pre-illness level of functioning.

# Age-related Considerations: Use of Antipsychotic Drugs

## USE IN CHILDREN

Guidelines for the use of antipsychotic drugs in children were published by the American Academy of Child and Adolescent Psychiatry (AACAP) in its *Practice Parameter for the Assessment and Treatment of Children and Adolescents with Schizophrenia.* Major recommendations are as follows:

- A thorough psychiatric and physical examination before starting drug therapy
- Choosing a medication based on potency, adverse effects, and the client's medication response history, if available. A newer, atypical drug is probably the drug of first choice.
- Giving the chosen drug at least 4 to 6 weeks before evaluating its effectiveness. If an inadequate response is then evident, a new antipsychotic should be tried.
- Once an adequate response is obtained, drug therapy should be continued at least for several months. For newly diagnosed children who are symptom free for 6 to 12 months, it may be feasible to stop the drug for a trial period to reassess condition and drug dosage. In general, the lowest effective dose is recommended.
- Using psychosocial and psychotherapeutic interventions along with antipsychotic drugs
- Having a health care provider maintain contact with the child and parents or guardian and monitor responses to the medication. For example, weight charts and calculations of the body mass index should be maintained with the atypical drugs because most are associated with weight gain and some are associated with the development of diabetes.
- More controlled studies of drug effects in children and adolescents

Drug pharmacodynamics and pharmacokinetics are likely to be different in children, compared with adults. Pharmacodynamic differences may stem from changes in neurotransmission systems in the brain as the child grows. Pharmacokinetic differences may stem from changes in distribution or metabolism of drugs; absorption seems similar to that in adults. In relation to distribution, children usually have a lesser percentage of body fat than adults. Thus, antipsychotic drugs, which are highly lipid soluble, cannot be as readily stored in fat as they are in adults. This often leads to shorter half-lives and the need for more frequent administration. In relation to metabolism, children usually have a faster rate than adults and may therefore require relatively high doses for their size and weight. In relation to excretion, renal function is usually similar to that of adults, and most of the drugs are largely inactivated by liver metabolism. Thus, with normal renal function, excretion probably has little effect on blood levels of active drug or the child's response to the drug.

It is not clear which antipsychotics are safest and most effective in children and adolescents. Although the newer drugs are being used, children's dosages have not been established, and long-term effects are unknown. Traditional drugs are not usually recommended for children younger than 12 years of age. However, prochlorperazine (Compazine), trifluoperazine (Stelazine), and haloperidol (Haldol) may be used in children aged 2 to 12 years.

Dosage regulation is difficult because children may require lower plasma levels for therapeutic effects, but they also metabolize antipsychotic drugs more rapidly than adults. A conservative approach is to begin with a low dose and increase it gradually (no more than once or twice a week), if necessary. Divided doses may be useful initially, with later conversion to once-daily doses at bedtime. Older adolescents may require doses comparable with those of adults.

Adverse effects may be different in children. For example, extrapyramidal symptoms with conventional drugs are more likely to occur in children than adults. If they do occur, dosage reduction is more effective in alleviating them than the anticholinergic antiparkinson drugs commonly used in adults. In addition, hypotension is more likely to develop in children. Blood pressure should be closely monitored during initial dosage titration.

## USE IN OLDER ADULTS

Older adults are more likely to have problems in which the antipsychotic drugs are contraindicated (eg, severe cardiovascular disease, liver damage, Parkinson's disease) or must be used very cautiously (eg, diabetes mellitus, glaucoma, prostatic hypertrophy, peptic ulcer disease, chronic respiratory disorders).

If antipsychotic drugs are used to control acute agitation in older adults, they should be used in the lowest effective dose for the shortest effective duration. If the drugs are used to treat dementias, they may relieve some symptoms (eg, agitation, hallucinations, hostility, suspiciousness, and uncooperativeness), but they do not improve memory loss and may further impair cognitive functioning.

For older adults in long-term care facilities, there is concern that antipsychotic drugs may be overused to control agitated or disruptive behavior that is caused by nonpsychotic disorders and for which other treatments are preferable. For example, clients with dementias may become agitated from environmental or medical problems. Alleviating such causes, when possible, is safer and more effective than administering antipsychotic drugs. Inappropriate use of the drugs exposes clients to adverse drug effects and does not resolve underlying problems. Because of the many implications for client safety and welfare, federal regulations were established for the use of antipsychotics in facilities receiving Medicare and Medicaid funds. These regulations include indications that are appropriate (eg, psychotic disorders, delusions, schizophrenia, and dementia and delirium that meet certain criteria) and inappropriate (eg, agitation not thought to indicate potential harm to the resident or others, anxiety, depression, uncooperativeness, wandering). When the drugs are required in older adults, considerations include the following:

- *Drug selection.* With traditional antipsychotic drugs, haloperidol and fluphenazine may be better tolerated, but

*(continued)*

## Age-related Considerations: Use of Antipsychotic Drugs (Continued)

they cause a high incidence of extrapyramidal symptoms. With atypical drugs, clozapine is a second-line agent because it produces many adverse effects. Olanzapine, quetiapine, risperidone, or ziprasidone may be useful, but little information is available about their use in older adults. Ziprasidone should not be used in older adults with cardiac dysrhythmias or severe cardiovascular disease.

• *Dosage.* When the drugs are required, the recommended starting dosage is 25% to 33% of the dosage recommended for younger adults. Dosage should also be increased more gradually, if necessary, and according to clinical response. The basic principle of "start low, go slow" is especially applicable. Once symptoms are controlled, dosage should be reduced to the lowest effective level. Some specific drugs and dosage ranges include haloperidol, 0.25 to 1.5 mg qd to qid; clozapine, 6.25 mg qd, initially; risperidone, 0.5 mg qd, initially; quetiapine, a lower initial dose, slower dose titration, and a lower target dose in older adults.

• As in other populations, antipsychotic drugs should be tapered in dosage and discontinued gradually rather than discontinued abruptly.

• *Adverse effects.* Older adults are at high risk for adverse effects because metabolism and excretion are usually slower or more likely to be impaired than in younger adults. With traditional antipsychotic drugs, anticholinergic effects (eg, confusion, memory impairment, hallucinations, urinary retention, constipation, heat stroke) may be especially problematic. In addition, cardiovascular (hypotension, dysrhythmias) effects may be especially dangerous in older adults, who often have underlying cardiovascular diseases. Tardive dyskinesia, which may occur with long-term use of the typical antipsychotic drugs, may develop more rapidly and at lower drug doses in older adults than in younger clients. There is also a risk for neuroleptic malignant syndrome, a rare but serious disorder characterized by confusion, dizziness, fever, and rigidity. Other adverse effects include oversedation, dizziness, confusion, and impaired mobility, which may contribute to falls and other injuries unless clients are carefully monitored and safeguarded. With atypical drugs, many of these adverse effects are less likely to occur, especially at the reduced doses recommended for older adults.

### Drug Selection

The health care provider caring for a client with psychosis has a greater choice of drugs than ever before. Some general factors to consider include the client's age and physical condition, the severity and duration of illness, the frequency and severity of adverse effects produced by each drug, the use of and response to antipsychotic drugs in the past, the supervision available, and the health care provider's experience with a particular drug. Some specific factors include the following:

1. The atypical drugs (eg, risperidone) are the drugs of choice, especially for newly diagnosed schizophrenic clients, because they may be more effective in relieving some symptoms, they usually produce milder adverse effects, and clients seem to take them more consistently. A major drawback is their high cost, which may preclude their use in some clients.

   An additional drawback and concern is weight gain and abnormal glucose metabolism. Most of the drugs in this group have been associated with weight gain, especially with the chronic use required for treatment of schizophrenia. Recent reports also associate clozapine, olanzapine, and quetiapine with changes in blood glucose, including hyperglycemia and diabetes mellitus. A causal relationship between use of these drugs and onset of diabetes has not been established. However, before starting one of the drugs, clients should be assessed for diabetes or risk factors related to the development of diabetes (eg, obesity, personal or family history of diabetes, symptoms of diabetes

such as polyuria, polydipsia, and polyphagia). If symptoms or risk factors are identified, blood glucose levels should be checked before starting the drug and periodically during treatment.

2. The traditional or typical antipsychotic drugs are apparently equally effective, but some clients who do not respond well to one may respond to another. Because the drugs are similarly effective, some health care providers base their choice on a drug's adverse effects. In addition, some health care providers use a phenothiazine first and prescribe a nonphenothiazine as a second-line agent for clients with chronic schizophrenia whose symptoms have not been controlled by the phenothiazines and for clients with hypersensitivity reactions to the phenothiazines. Thioridazine (Mellaril), formerly a commonly used drug, is now indicated only when other drugs are ineffective, because of its association with serious cardiac dysrhythmias.

3. Clients who are unable or unwilling to take daily doses of a maintenance antipsychotic drug may be given periodic injections of a long-acting form of fluphenazine or haloperidol.

4. Any person who has had an allergic or hypersensitivity reaction to an antipsychotic drug usually should not be given that drug again or any drug in the same chemical group. Cross-sensitivity occurs, and the likelihood of another allergic reaction is high.

5. There is no logical basis for giving more than one antipsychotic agent at a time. There is no therapeutic advantage, and the risk for serious adverse reactions is increased.

### Dosage and Administration

Dosage and route of administration must be individualized according to the client's condition and response. Oral drugs undergo extensive first-pass metabolism in the liver so that a significant portion of a dose does not reach the systemic circulation and low serum drug levels are produced. In contrast, intramuscular doses avoid first-pass metabolism and produce serum drug levels approximately double those of oral doses. Thus, usual intramuscular doses are approximately half the oral doses.

Initial drug therapy for acute psychotic episodes may require intramuscular administration and hospitalization; symptoms are usually controlled within 48 to 72 hours, after which oral drugs can be given. When treatment is initiated with oral drugs, divided daily doses are recommended. For maintenance therapy, once-daily dosing is usually preferred. A single bedtime dose is effective for most clients. This schedule increases compliance with prescribed drug therapy, allows better nighttime sleep, and decreases hypotension and daytime sedation. Effective maintenance therapy requires close supervision and contact with the client and family members.

### Duration of Therapy

In schizophrenia, antipsychotic drugs are usually given for years because there is a high rate of relapse (acute psychotic episodes) when drug therapy is discontinued, most often by clients who become unwilling or unable to continue their medication regimen. Drug therapy usually is indicated for at least 1 year after an initial psychotic episode and for at least 5 years, perhaps for life, after multiple episodes. Several studies indicate that low-dose, continuous maintenance therapy is effective in long-term prevention of recurrent psychosis. With wider use of maintenance therapy and the newer, better-tolerated antipsychotic drugs, clients may experience fewer psychotic episodes and hospitalizations.

Chronically mentally ill clients, such as individuals with schizophrenia, are among the most challenging in a home care nurse's caseload. Major recurring problems include failure to take antipsychotic medications as prescribed and the concurrent use of alcohol and other drugs of abuse. Either problem is likely to lead to acute psychotic episodes and hospitalizations. Guidelines for ongoing evaluation and intervention are addressed in Home Care Considerations.

## Individual Phenothiazine–similar Drugs

**Haloperidol** (Haldol) is a butyrophenone used in psychiatric disorders; a related drug, droperidol, is used in anesthesia and as an antiemetic. Haloperidol is a frequently used, potent, long-acting drug. It is well absorbed after oral or intramuscular administration, metabolized in the liver, and excreted in urine and bile. It may cause adverse effects

**Home Care Considerations: Use of Antipsychotic Drugs**

***ASSESS:*** the caregivers' efforts to maintain medications and manage adverse drug effects, other aspects of daily care, follow-up psychiatric care, and quality of life.

***MONITOR:*** for therapeutic and adverse effects; the presence or absence of psychotic symptoms such as agitation, hyperactivity, combativeness, and bizarre behavior; coordination of the collaborative efforts of multiple health and social service agencies or providers.

***EDUCATE:*** on safe use of the drugs (eg, that the drugs decrease mental alertness and physical agility, so potentially hazardous activities should be avoided) and about the importance of tapering dosage and discontinuing gradually. Reinforce additional teaching points (see Client Teaching Guidelines: Antipsychotic Drugs).

similar to those of the phenothiazines. Usually, it produces a relatively low incidence of hypotension and sedation and a high incidence of extrapyramidal effects.

Haloperidol may be used as the initial drug for treating psychotic disorders or as a substitute in clients who are hypersensitive or refractory to the phenothiazines. It also is used for some conditions in which other antipsychotic drugs are not used, including mental retardation with hyperkinesia (abnormally increased motor activity), Tourette's syndrome (a rare disorder characterized by involuntary movements and vocalizations), and Huntington's disease (a rare genetic disorder that involves progressive psychiatric symptoms and involuntary movements). For clients who are unable or unwilling to take the oral drug as prescribed, a slowly absorbed, long-acting formulation (haloperidol decanoate) may be given intramuscularly, once a month.

**Loxapine** (Loxitane) is similar to phenothiazines and related drugs. It is recommended for use only in the treatment of schizophrenia.

**Molindone** (Moban) differs chemically from other agents but has similar pharmacologic actions.

**Pimozide** (Orap) is approved only for the treatment of Tourette's syndrome in clients who fail to respond to haloperidol. Potentially serious adverse effects include tardive dyskinesia, major motor seizures, and sudden death.

**Thiothixene** (Navane) is used only for antipsychotic effects, although it produces other effects similar to those of the phenothiazines.

## Atypical Antipsychotic Drugs

**Clozapine** (Clozaril), the prototype of the atypical agents, is chemically different from the older antipsychotic drugs. It blocks both dopamine and serotonin receptors in the brain. It is recommended only for clients with schizophrenia, for whom it may improve negative symptoms and does not cause the extrapyramidal effects associated with older antipsychotic drugs. Despite these advantages, however, it is a second-line drug, recommended only for clients who have not responded to treatment with at least two other antipsychotic drugs or who have disabling tardive dyskinesia. The reason for clozapine's second-line status is its association with agranulocytosis, a life-threatening decrease in white blood cells (WBCs), which usually occurs during the first 3 months of therapy. Weekly WBC counts are required. In addition, clozapine is reportedly more likely to cause constipation, dizziness, drowsiness, hypotension, seizures, and weight gain than other atypical agents. An overview of the drug is found in Prototype Profile 9-1: Clozapine.

**Olanzapine** (Zyprexa) has therapeutic effects similar to those of clozapine, but adverse effects may differ. Compared with clozapine, olanzapine is more likely to cause extrapyramidal effects and less likely to cause agranulocytosis. Compared with typical antipsychotics, olanzapine reportedly causes less sedation, extrapyramidal symptoms, anticholinergic effects, and orthostatic

hypotension. However, it has been associated with weight gain, hyperglycemia, and initiation or aggravation of diabetes mellitus.

The drug is well absorbed after oral administration; its absorption is not affected by food. A steady-state concentration is reached in approximately 1 week of once-daily administration. It is metabolized in the liver and excreted in urine and feces.

**Quetiapine** (Seroquel), like the other atypical agents, blocks both dopamine and serotonin receptors and relieves both positive and negative symptoms of psychosis. After oral administration, quetiapine is well absorbed and may be taken without regard for meals. It is extensively metabolized in the liver by the cytochrome P450 enzyme system. Clinically significant drug interactions may occur with drugs that induce or inhibit the liver enzymes; dosage of quetiapine may need to be increased with enzyme inducers (eg, carbamazepine, phenytoin, rifampin) or decreased with enzyme inhibitors (eg, cimetidine, erythromycin). Common adverse effects include drowsiness, headache, orthostatic hypotension, and weight gain.

**Risperidone** (Risperdal), like other atypical antipsychotic agents, blocks both dopamine and serotonin recep-

---

### PROTOTYPE PROFILE 9-1
### *P* Clozapine (KLOZ za peen)

**Drug Class**
*Chemical:* Dibenzodiazepine
*Functional:* Atypical Antipsychotic Agent

**Trade Name**
Clozaril

**Therapeutic Indications**
Treatment of refractory schizophrenia

**Pharmacokinetics**
*Absorption*
Variable

*Distribution*
Plasma protein binding: 95%

*Metabolism*
Hepatic

*Excretion*
Urine and feces

**Pharmacodynamics**
*Onset of Action*
Unknown

*Duration*
4–12h

**Contraindications/Precautions**
Avoid abrupt withdrawal; may lead to psychosis and cholinergic rebound (headache, nausea, vomiting, and diarrhea)

**Pregnancy Considerations**
Category B
Enters breast milk; contraindicated

**Dosage**
Available on through a distribution system
*Adult:* PO, 25 mg once or twice daily initially, increased by 25–50 mg/d, if tolerated, to 300–450 mg/d by the end of 2nd wk
*Children:* Dosage not established

**Adverse Effects**
Agranulocytosis, seizures, orthostasis, tachycardia, drowsiness, dizziness, constipation, urinary incontinence, weight gain

**Drug Interactions**
*Increased Effects*
Anticholinergic and hypotensive effects of other drugs
Respiratory depression and hypotension with benzodiazepines, especially in early weeks of therapy
Risk for extrapyramidal symptoms with metoclopramide
Serum levels by a large number of drugs, such as amiodarone, cimetidine, diltiazem, isoniazid, and erythromycin

*Decreased Effects*
Serum levels with phenytoin, carbamazepine, primidone, and valproic acid

**Herbal Supplements and Dietary Considerations**
St. John's wort may decrease clozapine levels
Kava kava, gotu kola, St. John's wort, and valerian may increase CNS depression
May be taken without regard to food

tors and relieves both positive and negative symptoms of psychosis. It is a frequently prescribed, first-choice agent that is usually well tolerated. In a study that compared risperidone and olanzapine, researchers concluded that both drugs were well tolerated and effective in treating schizophrenia, but risperidone relieved positive symptoms, anxiety, and depression to a greater degree and caused less weight gain than olanzapine.

Risperidone is well absorbed with oral administration. Peak blood levels occur in 1 to 2 hours, but therapeutic effects are delayed for 1 to 2 weeks. It is metabolized mainly in the liver by the cytochrome P450 2D6 enzymes and produces an active metabolite. Effects are attributed approximately equally to risperidone and the metabolite. Most (70%) is excreted in urine; some (14%) is excreted in feces. Adverse effects include agitation, anxiety, headache, insomnia, dizziness, and hypotension. It may also cause parkinsonism and other movement disorders, especially at higher doses, but is less likely to do so than the typical antipsychotic drugs.

**Ziprasidone** (Geodon) is a newer atypical agent used to treat schizophrenia. It is effective in suppressing many of the negative symptoms such as blunted affect, lack of motivation, and social withdrawal. It is contraindicated in people who are allergic to the drug, who are pregnant or lactating, who have a prolonged QT/QTc interval on electrocardiogram, or who have a history of severe heart disease. It must be used cautiously in people with impaired renal or hepatic function and cardiovascular disease. Because it may prolong the QT/QTc interval and cause torsades de pointes, a potentially fatal type of ventricular tachycardia, ziprasidone is probably not a drug of first choice.

Ziprasidone is metabolized in the liver and excreted in urine. Adverse effects include cardiac dysrhythmias, drowsiness, headache, and nausea; weight gain is less likely than with other antipsychotic drugs.

## ■ DRUG USE IN SPECIFIC SITUATIONS

### Management of Drug Withdrawal

Antipsychotic drugs can cause symptoms of withdrawal when suddenly or rapidly discontinued. Specific symptoms are related to a drug's potency, extent of dopaminergic blockade, and its anticholinergic effects. Low-potency drugs (eg, chlorpromazine), for example, have strong anticholinergic effects, and sudden withdrawal can cause cholinergic effects such as diarrhea, drooling, and insomnia. To prevent withdrawal symptoms, drugs should be tapered in dosage and gradually discontinued over several weeks.

### Management of Extrapyramidal Symptoms

Extrapyramidal effects (eg, abnormal movements) are more likely to occur with older antipsychotic drugs than with the newer atypical agents. If they do occur, an anticholinergic antiparkinson drug (see Chap. 12) can be given. Such neuromuscular symptoms appear in fewer than half the clients taking traditional antipsychotic drugs and are better handled by reducing dosage, if this does not cause recurrence of psychotic symptoms. If antiparkinson drugs are given, they should be gradually discontinued in about 3 months. Extrapyramidal symptoms do not usually recur despite continued administration of the same antipsychotic drug at the same dosage.

## Genetic or Ethnic Considerations With Drug Therapy

Antipsychotic drug therapy for nonwhite populations in the United States is based primarily on dosage recommendations, pharmacokinetic data, adverse effects, and other characteristics of antipsychotic drugs derived from white recipients. However, some groups respond differently. Most of the differences are attributed to variations in hepatic drug-metabolizing enzymes. Those with strong enzyme activity are known as extensive or fast metabolizers, whereas those with slower rates of enzyme activity are poor or slow metabolizers. Fast metabolizers eliminate drugs rapidly and may need a larger-than-usual dose to achieve therapeutic effects; poor metabolizers eliminate drugs slowly and therefore are at risk for drug accumulation and adverse effects. For example, risperidone has a half-life of 3 hours, and its active metabolite has a half-life of 21 hours in extensive metabolizers. In slow metabolizers, risperidone has a half-life of 20 hours, and the metabolite has a half-life of 30 hours. About 6% to 8% of white people are thought to be slow metabolizers. Although little research has been done, especially with the atypical drugs, and other factors may be involved, several studies document differences in antipsychotic drug effects in nonwhite populations, including the following:

1. *African Americans* tend to respond more rapidly, experience a higher incidence of adverse effects, including tardive dyskinesia, and metabolize antipsychotic drugs more slowly than whites.

   In addition, compared with whites with psychotic disorders, African Americans may be given higher doses and more frequent injections of long-acting antipsychotic drugs, both of which may increase the incidence and severity of adverse effects.

2. *Asians* generally metabolize antipsychotic drugs slowly and therefore have higher plasma drug levels for a given dose than whites. Most studies have been done with haloperidol and in a limited number of Asian subgroups. Thus, it cannot be assumed that all antipsychotic drugs and all people of Asian heritage respond in the same way. To avoid drug toxicity, initial doses should be approximately half the usual doses given to whites, and later doses should be titrated according to clinical response and serum drug levels.

3. *Hispanics'* responses to antipsychotic drugs are largely unknown. Some are extremely fast metabolizers who may have low plasma drug levels in relation to a given dose.

## NURSING PROCESS

### Assessment

Assess the client's mental health status, need for anti-psychotic drugs, and response to drug therapy. There is a wide variation in response to drug therapy. Close observation of physical and behavioral reactions is necessary to evaluate effectiveness and to individualize dosage schedules. Accurate assessment is especially important when starting drug therapy and when increasing or decreasing dosage. Some assessment factors include the following:

- Interview the client and family members. Attempts to interview an acutely psychotic person yield little useful information because of the client's distorted perception of reality. The nurse may be able to assess the client's level of orientation and delusional and hallucinatory activity. If possible, try to determine from family members or others what the client was doing or experiencing when the acute episode began (ie, predisposing factors, such as increased environmental stress or alcohol or drug ingestion); whether this is a first or a repeated episode of psychotic behavior; whether the person has physical illnesses, takes any drugs, or uses alcohol; whether the client seems to be a hazard to self or others; and some description of pre-illness personality traits, level of social interaction, and ability to function in usual activities of daily living.
- Observe the client for the presence or absence of psychotic symptoms such as agitation, hyperactivity, combativeness, and bizarre behavior.
- Obtain baseline data to help monitor the client's response to drug therapy. Some authorities advocate initial and periodic laboratory tests of liver, kidney, and blood functions, as well as electrocardiograms. Such tests may assist in early detection and treatment of adverse drug effects. Baseline blood pressure readings also may be helpful.
- Continue assessing the client's response to drug therapy and his or her ability to function in activities of daily living, whether the client is hospitalized or receiving outpatient treatment.

### Nursing Diagnoses

- Altered Thought Processes related to psychosis
- Self-Care Deficit related to the disease process or drug-induced sedation
- Impaired Physical Mobility related to sedation
- Altered Tissue Perfusion related to hypotension
- Risk for Injury related to excessive sedation and movement disorders (extrapyramidal effects)
- Risk for Violence: Self-Directed or Directed at Others
- Noncompliance related to underuse of prescribed drugs

### Planning/Goals

*The client will:*

- Become less agitated within a few hours after drug therapy is started and less psychotic within 1–3 weeks
- Be safe while sedated from drug therapy
- Meet care needs in areas of nutrition, hygiene, exercise, and social interactions even when unable to provide self-care
- Improve in ability to participate in self-care activities

- Avoid preventable adverse drug effects, especially those that impair safety
- Take medications as prescribed and return for follow-up appointments with health care providers

### Interventions

Use nondrug measures when appropriate to increase the effectiveness of drug therapy and to decrease adverse reactions.

- Drug therapy is ineffective if the client does not receive sufficient medication and many people are unable or unwilling to take medications as prescribed. Any nursing action aimed toward more accurate drug administration increases the effectiveness of drug therapy.

  Specific nursing actions must be individualized to the client and/or caregiver. Some general nursing actions that may be helpful include emphasizing the therapeutic benefits expected from drug therapy, answering questions or providing information about drug therapy and other aspects of the treatment plan, devising a schedule of administration times that is as convenient as possible for the client, and assisting the client or caregiver in preventing or managing adverse drug effects. Most adverse effects are less likely to occur or be severe with the newer atypical drugs than with phenothiazines and other older drugs.
- Supervise ambulation to prevent falls or other injuries if the client is drowsy or elderly or has postural hypotension.
- Several measures can help prevent or minimize hypotension, such as having the client lie down for approximately an hour after a large oral dose or an injection of antipsychotic medication; applying elastic stockings; and instructing the client to change positions gradually, elevate legs when sitting, avoid standing for prolonged periods, and avoid hot baths (hot baths cause vasodilation and increase the incidence of hypotension). In addition, the daily dose can be decreased or divided into smaller amounts.
- Dry mouth and oral infections can be decreased by frequent brushing of the teeth, rinsing the mouth with water, chewing sugarless gum or candy, and ensuring an adequate fluid intake. Excessive water intake should be discouraged because it may lead to serum electrolyte deficiencies.
- The usual measures of increasing fluid intake, dietary fiber, and exercise can help prevent constipation.
- Support caregivers in efforts to maintain contact with inpatients and provide care for outpatients. One way is to provide caregivers with telephone numbers of health care providers and to make periodic telephone calls to caregivers.

### Evaluation

- Interview the client to determine the presence and extent of hallucinations and delusions.
- Observe the client for decreased signs and symptoms.
- Document abilities and limitations in self-care.
- Note whether any injuries have occurred during drug therapy.
- Interview the caregiver about the client's behavior and medication response (ie, during a home visit or telephone call).

## CLIENT TEACHING GUIDELINES
### Antipsychotic Drugs

Antipsychotic drugs are given to clients with schizophrenia, a chronic mental illness. Because of the nature of the disease, a responsible adult caregiver is needed to prompt a client about taking particular doses and to manage other aspects of the drug therapy regimen, as follows.

### General Considerations

✔ Ask about the planned drug therapy regimen, including the desired results, when results can be expected, and the tentative length of drug therapy.

✔ Maintain an adequate supply of medication to ensure regular administration. Consistent blood levels are necessary to control symptoms and prevent recurring episodes of acute illness and hospitalization.

✔ Do not allow the client to drive a car, operate machinery, or perform activities that require alertness when drowsy from medication. Drowsiness, slowed thinking, and impaired muscle coordination are especially likely during the first 2 weeks of drug therapy but tend to decrease with time.

✔ Report unusual side effects and all physical illnesses, because changes in drug therapy may be indicated.

✔ Try to prevent the client from taking unprescribed medications, including those available without prescription or those prescribed for another person, to prevent undesirable drug interactions. Alcohol and sleeping pills should be avoided because they may cause excessive drowsiness and decreased awareness of safety hazards in the environment.

✔ Keep all health care providers informed about all the medications being taken by the client, to decrease risks of undesirable drug interactions.

✔ These drugs should be tapered in dosage and discontinued gradually; they should not be stopped abruptly.

### Medication Administration

Assist or prompt the client to:

✔ Take medications in the correct doses and at the correct times, to maintain blood levels and beneficial effects.

✔ Avoid taking these medications with antacids. If an antacid is needed (eg, for heartburn), it should be taken 1 hour before or 2 hours after the antipsychotic drug. Antacids decrease absorption of these drugs from the intestine.

✔ Lie down for approximately an hour after receiving medication, if dizziness and faintness occur.

✔ Take the medication at bedtime, if able, so that drowsiness aids sleep and is minimized during waking hours.

✔ Practice good oral hygiene, including dental checkups, thorough and frequent toothbrushing, drinking fluids, and frequent mouth rinsing. Mouth dryness is a common side effect of the drugs. Although it is usually not serious, dry mouth can lead to mouth infections and dental cavities.

✔ Minimize exposure to sunlight, wear protective clothing, and use sunscreen lotions. Sensitivity to sunlight occurs with some of the drugs and may produce a sunburn-type of skin reaction.

✔ Avoid exposure to excessive heat. Some of these medications may cause fever and heat prostration with high environmental temperatures. In hot weather or climates, keep the client indoors and use air conditioning or fans during the hours of highest heat levels.

## Use in Perioperative Periods

A major concern about giving traditional antipsychotic drugs perioperatively is their potential for adverse interactions with other drugs. For example, the drugs potentiate the effects of general anesthetics and other CNS depressants that are often used before, during, and after surgery. As a result, risks for hypotension and excessive sedation are increased unless doses of other agents are reduced. If hypotension occurs and requires vasopressor drugs, phenylephrine or norepinephrine should be used rather than epinephrine because antipsychotic drugs inhibit the vasoconstrictive (blood pressure–raising) effects of epinephrine. Guidelines for perioperative use of the newer, atypical agents have not been developed. Cautious use is indicated because they may also cause hypotension, sedation, and other adverse effects.

*(text continues on page 170)*

## Nursing Actions
### Antipsychotic Drugs

| Nursing Actions | Rationale/Explanation |
| --- | --- |
| 1. Administer accurately.<br>a. Check doses carefully, especially when starting or stopping an antipsychotic drug, or substituting one for another. | Doses are often changed. When a drug is started, initial doses are usually titrated upward over days or weeks, then reduced for maintenance; when the drug is stopped, doses are gradually reduced; when substituting, dosage of one may be increased while dosage of the other is decreased. |

*(continued)*

## Nursing Actions

### Antipsychotic Drugs (Continued)

| Nursing Actions | Rationale/Explanation |
|---|---|
| b. With older, typical drugs: | |
| (1) Give once daily, 1–2 hours before bedtime, when feasible. | Peak sedation occurs in about 2 hours and aids sleep. Also, adverse effects such as dry mouth and hypotension are less bothersome. |
| (2) When preparing solutions, try to avoid skin contact. If contact is made, wash the area immediately. | These solutions are irritating to the skin and many cause contact dermatitis. |
| (3) Mix liquid concentrates with at least 60 mL of fruit juice or water just before administration. | To mask the taste. If the client does not like juice or water, check the package insert for other diluents. Some of the drugs may be mixed with coffee, tea, milk, or carbonated beverages. |
| (4) For intramuscular injections, give only those preparations labeled for IM use; do not mix with any other drugs in a syringe; change the needle after filling the syringe; inject slowly and deeply into gluteal muscles; and have the client lie down for 30–60 minutes after the injection. | These drugs are physically incompatible with many other drugs, and a precipitate may occur; parenteral solutions are irritating to body tissues and changing needles helps protect the tissues of the injection tract from unnecessary contact with the drug; injecting into a large muscle mass decreases tissue irritation; lying down helps to prevent orthostatic hypotension. |
| (5) With parenteral fluphenazine, give the hydrochloride salt IM only; give the decanoate and enanthate salts IM or Sub-Q. | To decrease tissue irritation |
| c. With newer, atypical drugs: | |
| (1) Give olanzapine once daily, without regard to meals; with oral disintegrating tablets, peel back foil covering, transfer tablet to dry cup or fingers, and place the tablet into the mouth. | Manufacturer's recommendations. The disintegrating tablet does not require fluid. |
| (2) Give quetiapine in 2 or 3 daily doses. | |
| (3) Give risperidone twice daily; mix the oral solution with 3–4 oz of water, coffee, orange juice, or low-fat milk; do not mix with cola drinks or tea. | Manufacturer's recommendations |
| (4) Give ziprasidone twice daily with food. | Manufacturer's recommendation |
| 2. Observe for therapeutic effects. | |
| a. When the drug is given for acute psychotic episodes, observe for decreased agitation, combativeness, and psychomotor activity. | The sedative effects of antipsychotic drugs are exerted within 48–72 hours. Sedation that occurs with treatment of acute psychotic episodes is a therapeutic effect. Sedation that occurs with treatment of nonacute psychotic disorders, or excessive sedation at any time, is an adverse reaction. |
| b. When the drug is given for acute or chronic psychosis, observe for decreased psychotic behavior, such as: | These therapeutic effects may not be evident for 3–6 weeks after drug therapy is begun. |
| (1) Decreased auditory and visual hallucinations | |
| (2) Decreased delusions | |
| (3) Continued decrease in or absence of agitation, hostility, hyperactivity, and other behavior associated with acute psychosis | |
| (4) Increased socialization | |
| (5) Increased ability in self-care activities | |
| (6) Increased ability to participate in other therapeutic modalities along with drug therapy. | |
| c. When the drug is given for antiemetic effects, observe for decreased or absent nausea or vomiting. | |

(continued)

## Nursing Actions

## Antipsychotic Drugs (Continued)

| Nursing Actions | Rationale/Explanation |
|---|---|
| 3. Observe for adverse effects. | |
| a. With phenothiazines and related drugs, observe for: | |
| (1) Excessive sedation—drowsiness, lethargy, fatigue, slurred speech, impaired mobility, and impaired mental processes | Excessive sedation is most likely to occur during the first few days of treatment of an acute psychotic episode, when large doses are usually given. Psychotic clients also seem sedated because the drug lets them catch up on psychosis-induced sleep deprivation. Sedation is more likely to occur in elderly or debilitated people. Tolerance to the drugs' sedative effects develops, and sedation tends to decrease with continued drug therapy. |
| (2) Extrapyramidal reactions *Akathisia*—compulsive, involuntary restlessness and body movements | Akathisia is the most common extrapyramidal reaction, and it may occur about 5–60 days after the start of antipsychotic drug therapy. The motor restlessness may be erroneously interpreted as psychotic agitation necessitating increased drug dosage. This condition can sometimes be controlled by substituting an antipsychotic drug that is less likely to cause extrapyramidal effects or by giving an anticholinergic antiparkinson drug. |
| *Parkinsonism*—loss of muscle movement (akinesia), muscular rigidity and tremors, shuffling gait, postural abnormalities, mask-like facial expression, hypersalivation, and drooling | These symptoms are the same as those occurring with idiopathic Parkinson's disease. They can be controlled with anticholinergic antiparkinson drugs, given along with the antipsychotic drug for about 3 months, then discontinued. This reaction may occur about 5–30 days after antipsychotic drug therapy is begun. |
| *Dyskinesias* (involuntary, rhythmic body movements) and *dystonias* (uncoordinated, bizarre movements of the neck, face, eyes, tongue, trunk, or extremities) | These are less common extrapyramidal reactions, but they may occur suddenly, approximately 1–5 days after drug therapy is started, and be very frightening to the client and health care personnel. The movements are caused by muscle spasms and result in exaggerated posture and facial distortions. These symptoms are sometimes misinterpreted as seizures, hysteria, or other disorders. Antiparkinson drugs are given parenterally during acute dystonic reactions, but continued administration is not usually required. These reactions occur most often in younger people. |
| *Tardive dyskinesia*—hyperkinetic movements of the face (sucking and smacking of lips, tongue protrusion, and facial grimaces) and choreiform movements of the trunk and limbs | This syndrome occurs after months or years of high-dose antipsychotic drug therapy. The drugs may mask the symptoms so that the syndrome is more likely to be diagnosed when dosage is decreased or the drug is discontinued for a few days. It occurs gradually and at any age but is more common in older people, women, and people with organic brain disorders. The condition is usually irreversible, and there is no effective treatment. Symptoms are not controlled and may be worsened by antiparkinson drugs. Low dosage and short-term use of antipsychotic drugs help prevent tardive dyskinesia; drug-free periods may aid early detection. |
| (3) Antiadrenergic effects—hypotension, tachycardia, dizziness, faintness, and fatigue. | Hypotension is potentially one of the most serious adverse reactions to the antipsychotic drugs. It is most likely to occur when the client assumes an upright position after sitting or lying down (orthostatic or postural hypotension) but it does occur in the recumbent position. It is caused by peripheral vasodilation. Orthostatic hypotension can be assessed by comparing blood pressure readings taken with the client in supine and standing positions. Tachycardia occurs as a compensatory mechanism in response to hypotension and as an anticholinergic effect in which the normal vagus nerve action of slowing the heart rate is blocked. |

*(continued)*

## Nursing Actions
### Antipsychotic Drugs (Continued)

| Nursing Actions | Rationale/Explanation |
|---|---|
| (4) Anticholinergic effects—dry mouth, dental caries, blurred vision, constipation, paralytic ileus, urinary retention | These atropine-like effects are common with therapeutic doses and are increased with large doses of phenothiazines. |
| (5) Respiratory depression—slow, shallow breathing and decreased ability to breathe deeply, cough, and remove secretions from the respiratory tract | This stems from general central nervous system (CNS) depression, which causes drowsiness and decreased movement. It may cause pneumonia or other respiratory problems, especially in people with hypercarbia and chronic lung disease. |
| (6) Endocrine effects—menstrual irregularities, possibly impotence and decreased libido in the male client, weight gain | These apparently result from drug-induced changes in pituitary and hypothalamic functions. |
| (7) Hypothermia or hyperthermia | Antipsychotic drugs may impair the temperature-regulating center in the hypothalamus. Hypothermia is more likely to occur. Hyperthermia occurs with high doses and warm environmental temperatures. |
| (8) Hypersensitivity reactions:<br>*Cholestatic hepatitis*—may begin with fever and influenza-like symptoms followed in approximately 1 week by jaundice | Cholestatic hepatitis results from drug-induced edema of the bile ducts and obstruction of the bile flow. It occurs most often in women and after 2–4 weeks of receiving the drug. It is usually reversible if the drug is discontinued. |
| *Blood dyscrasias*—leukopenia, agranulocytosis (fever, sore throat, weakness) | Some degree of leukopenia occurs rather often and does not seem to be serious. Agranulocytosis, on the other hand, occurs rarely but is life threatening. Agranulocytosis is most likely to occur during the first 4–10 weeks of drug therapy, in women, and in older people. |
| *Skin reactions*—photosensitivity, dermatoses | Skin pigmentation and discoloration may occur with exposure to sunlight. |
| (9) Electrocardiogram (ECG) changes, cardiac dysrhythmias | ECG changes may portend dysrhythmias, especially in people with underlying heart disease. Ziprasidone may prolong the QT/QTc interval, an ECG change associated with torsades de pointes, a life-threatening dysrhythmia. |
| (10) Neuroleptic malignant syndrome—fever (may be confused with heat stroke), muscle rigidity, agitation, confusion, delirium, dyspnea, tachycardia, respiratory failure, acute renal failure | A rare but potentially fatal reaction that may occur hours to months after initial drug use. Symptoms usually develop rapidly over 24–72 hours. Treatment includes stopping the antipsychotic drug, giving supportive care related to fever and other symptoms, and drug therapy (dantrolene, a skeletal muscle relaxant, and amantadine or bromocriptine, dopamine-stimulating drugs). |
| b. With clozapine, observe for:<br>(1) CNS effects—drowsiness, dizziness, headache, seizures<br>(2) Gastrointestinal (GI) effects—nausea, vomiting, constipation<br>(3) Cardiovascular effects—hypotension, tachycardia<br>(4) Hematologic effects—agranulocytosis | This is the most life-threatening adverse effect of clozapine. Clients' white blood cell counts must be checked before starting clozapine, every week during therapy, and for 4 weeks after the drug is discontinued. |
| c. With olanzapine, observe for:<br>(1) CNS effects—drowsiness, dizziness, akathisia, tardive dyskinesia, neuroleptic malignant syndrome<br>(2) GI effects—constipation<br>(3) Cardiovascular effects—hypotension, tachycardia<br>(4) Other—weight gain, hyperglycemia, diabetes mellitus | |

*(continued)*

## Nursing Actions

### Antipsychotic Drugs (Continued)

| Nursing Actions | Rationale/Explanation |
|---|---|
| d. With quetiapine, observe for: | |
|    (1) CNS effects—drowsiness, dizziness, headache, tardive dyskinesia, neuroleptic malignant syndrome | |
|    (2) GI effects—anorexia, nausea, vomiting | |
|    (3) Cardiovascular effects—orthostatic hypotension, tachycardia | |
|    (4) Other—weight gain, hyperglycemia, diabetes mellitus | |
| e. With risperidone, observe for: | |
|    (1) CNS effects—agitation, anxiety, drowsiness, dizziness, headache, insomnia, tardive dyskinesia, neuroleptic malignant syndrome | |
|    (2) GI effects—nausea, vomiting, constipation | |
|    (3) Cardiovascular effects—orthostatic hypotension, arrhythmias | |
|    (4) Other—photosensitivity | |
| f. With ziprasidone, observe for: | |
|    (1) CNS effects—drowsiness, headache, extrapyramidal reactions | |
|    (2) GI effects—nausea, constipation | |
|    (3) Cardiovascular effects—dysrhythmias, hypotension, ECG changes | |
|    (4) Other—fever | |
| **4. Observe for drug interactions.** | |
| a. Drugs that *increase* effects of antipsychotic drugs: | |
|    (1) Anticholinergics (eg, atropine) | Additive anticholinergic effects |
|    (2) Antidepressants, tricyclic | Potentiation of sedative and anticholinergic effects. Additive CNS depression, sedation, orthostatic hypotension, urinary retention, and glaucoma may occur unless dosages are decreased. Apparently these two drug groups inhibit the metabolism of each other, thus prolonging the actions of both groups if they are given concurrently. |
|    (3) Antihistamines | Additive CNS depression and sedation |
|    (4) CNS depressants—alcohol, opioid analgesics, antianxiety agents, sedative-hypnotics | Additive CNS depression. Also, severe hypotension, urinary retention, seizures, severe atropine-like reactions, and others may occur, depending on which group of CNS depressant drugs is given. |
|    (5) Propranolol | Additive hypotensive and ECG effects |
|    (6) Thiazide diuretics, such as hydrochlorothiazide | Additive hypotension |
|    (7) Lithium | Acute encephalopathy, including irreversible brain damage and dyskinesias, has been reported. |
| b. Drugs that *decrease* effects of antipsychotic drugs: | |
|    (1) Antacids | Oral antacids, especially aluminum hydroxide and magnesium trisilicate, may inhibit gastrointestinal absorption of antipsychotic drugs. |
|    (2) Carbamazepine, phenytoin, rifampin | By induction of drug-metabolizing enzymes in the liver |
|    (3) Norepinephrine, phenylephrine | Antagonize the hypotensive effects of antipsychotic drugs |
| c. Drugs that alter effects of quetiapine: | |
|    (1) Cimetidine, erythromycin, itraconazole, and ketoconazole *increase* effects. | These drugs *inhibit* cytochrome P450 3A4 enzymes and slow the metabolism of quetiapine. |
|    (2) Carbamazepine, phenytoin, and rifampin *decrease* effects. | These drugs *induce* cytochrome P450 3A4 enzymes and speed up the metabolism of quetiapine. |

## Critical Thinking Exercises

1. The atypical antipsychotic drugs, such as risperidone, are the drugs of choice, especially for newly diagnosed schizophrenics. A major drawback that may preclude their use in some clients is the drug's:
   a. High cost
   b. Severe side effects
   c. Lack of effectiveness in relieving some symptoms
   d. Availability

2. Olanzapine (Zyprexa) is started in your client with schizophrenia. Which condition warrants close monitoring during olanzapine therapy?
   a. Thyroid disease
   b. Diabetes mellitus
   c. Asthma
   d. Peripheral vascular disease

3. A client taking chlorpromazine abruptly stops taking the drug and develops diarrhea, drooling, and insomnia. Which drug effect is responsible for this adverse reaction?
   a. Anticholinergic
   b. Adrenergic
   c. Extrapyramidal
   d. Cholinergic

4. A client with dementia receiving haloperidol becomes agitated. While drawing up the solution, the nurse notices a slight yellow color to the medication. The nurse should:
   a. Call the health care provider and ask about the action to take
   b. Administer the medication; a slight yellow color is acceptable
   c. Discard the medication; the potency has decreased
   d. Administer the medication; the normal color of the solution is yellow

5. A client on maintenance therapy with antipsychotic drugs tells the nurse that she takes a single bedtime dose while at home. The nurse recognizes that this dosing schedule is effective for most clients for all of the following reasons, except that the once-daily dosing:
   a. Prevents adverse reactions
   b. Allows for better nighttime sleep
   c. Decreases daytime hypotension
   d. Decreases daytime sedation

## SELECTED REFERENCES

American Psychiatric Association. (2000). *Diagnostic and statistical manual of mental disorders* (4th ed.). Text Revision (DSM-IV-TR). Washington, DC: Author.

Conley, R. R., & Mahmoud, R. (2001). A randomized double-blind study of risperidone and olanzapine in the treatment of schizophrenia or schizoaffective disorder. *American Journal of Psychiatry, 158,* 765–774.

*Drug facts and comparisons.* (Updated monthly). St. Louis: Facts and Comparisons.

Glassman, A. H., & Bigger, J. T., Jr. (2001). Antipsychotic drugs: Prolonged QT interval, torsades de pointes, and sudden death. *American Journal of Psychiatry, 158*(11), 1774–1782.

Goff, D. C., & Coyle, J. T. (2001). The emerging role of glutamate in the pathophysiology and treatment of schizophrenia. *American Journal of Psychiatry, 158*(9), 1367–1375.

Hadbavny, A. M., & Hoyt, J. W. (2000). Sedatives and analgesics in critical care. In A. Grenvik, S. M. Ayres, P. R. Holbrook, & W. C. Shoemaker (Eds.), *Textbook of critical care* (4th ed., pp. 961–971). Philadelphia: W. B. Saunders.

Lacy, C. F., Armstrong, L. L., Goldman, M. P., & Lance, L. L. (2003). *Lexi-Comp's drug information handbook* (11th ed.). Hudson, OH: American Pharmaceutical Association.

The Practice Parameter for the Assessment and Treatment of Children and Adolescents with Schizophrenia (2001). *Journal of the American Academy of Child & Adolescent Psychiatry, 40*(7), 4S–23S.

Silva, R. R. (2000). Psycholopharmacology news. *Journal of Child and Adolescent Development, 10*(3), 155.

Silva, R. R. (2001). Psycholopharmacology news. *Journal of Child and Adolescent Development, 11*(3), 215.

Stimmel, G. L. (2000). Schizophrenia. In E. T. Herfindal & D. R. Gourley (Eds.), *Textbook of therapeutics: Drug and disease management* (7th ed., pp. 1217–1227). Philadelphia: Lippincott Williams & Wilkins.

Tamminga, C. A., & Frost, D. O. (2001). Changing concepts in the neurochemistry of schizophrenia (Editorial). *American Journal of Psychiatry, 158*(9), 1365–1366.

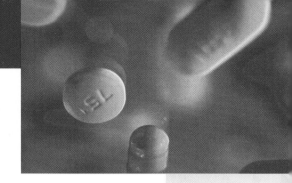

# 10

# Drugs for Mood Disorders: Antidepressants and Mood Stabilizers

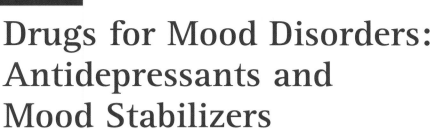

## OBJECTIVES

*After studying this chapter, the student will be able to:*

1 Give major features of depression and bipolar disorder.

2 Identify characteristics of antidepressants in terms of mechanism of action, indications for use, adverse effects, principles of therapy, and nursing process implications.

3 Compare and contrast selective serotonin reuptake inhibitors with tricyclic antidepressants.

4 List selected characteristics of bupropion, mirtazapine, nefazodone, and venlafaxine.

5 Describe the use of lithium in bipolar disorder.

6 Discuss interventions to increase safety of lithium therapy.

7 Describe the nursing role in preventing, recognizing, and treating overdoses of antidepressant drugs and lithium.

## CRITICAL THINKING SCENARIO

*B*etty McGrath, 73 years of age, was recently widowed. She depended on her husband to handle their finances, maintain their home, and make major decisions. She enjoyed the role of homemaker and never worked outside the home. Her children live out of state, but they write and call often. Mrs. McGrath's daughter calls you because she is concerned about her mother. Mrs. McGrath seems to be losing weight, stays home most of the time, complains she feels very tired, and sleeps much more than usual. She is also reluctant to go out with friends or visit her children.

✔ List factors that might increase Mrs. McGrath's risk for depression.

✔ What symptoms does Mrs. McGrath have that may indicate she is depressed?

✔ What additional data would support a diagnosis of depression?

✔ At this point, what suggestions would you have for Mrs. McGrath and her daughter?

## PROTOTYPE PROFILES

amitriptyline (Elavil), p. 181

fluoxetine (Prozac), p. 182

lithium carbonate (Eskalith, Lithobid), p. 184

# MOOD DISORDERS

Mood disorders include depression, dysthymia, bipolar disorder, and cyclothymia (Box 10-1).

## Depression

Depression is estimated to affect 5% to 10% of adults in the United States and to be increasing in children and adolescents. It is associated with impaired ability to function in usual activities and relationships. The average depressive episode lasts about 5 months, and having one episode is a risk factor for developing another episode. Depression and antidepressant drug therapy are emphasized in this chapter; bipolar disorder and mood-stabilizing drugs are also discussed. Despite extensive study and identification of numerous potential contributory factors, the etiology of depression is unclear. It is likely that depression results from interactions among several complex factors. Two of the major theories of depression pathogenesis are described in At the Foundation: Biochemistry and Depression.

Additional factors thought to play a role in the etiology of depression include the immune system, genetic factors, and environmental factors.

Immune cells (eg, T lymphocytes and B lymphocytes) produce cytokines (eg, interleukins, interferons, and tumor necrosis factor) that affect neurotransmission. Possible mechanisms of cytokine-induced depression include increased corticotropin-releasing factor (CRF) and activation of the hypothalamic-pituitary-adrenal (HPA) axis, alteration of monoamine neurotransmitters in several areas of the brain, or cytokines functioning as neurotransmitters and exerting direct effects on brain function.

Genetic factors are considered important mainly because close relatives of a depressed person are more likely to experience depression.

Environmental factors include stressful life events, which apparently change brain structure and function and contribute to the development of depression in some people. Changes have been identified in CRF, the HPA axis, and the noradrenergic neurotransmission system, all of which are activated as part of the stress response. These changes are thought to cause a hypersensitive or exaggerated response to later stressful events, including mild stress or daily life events. Most studies have involved early life trauma such as physical or sexual abuse in childhood.

## Bipolar Disorder

Like depression, mania and hypomania may result from abnormal functioning of neurotransmitters or recep-

---

## BOX 10-1    Types of Mood Disorders

### Depression
Depression, often described as the most common mental illness, is characterized by depressed mood, feelings of sadness, or emotional upset, and it occurs in all age groups. Mild depression occurs in everyone as a normal response to life stresses and losses and usually does not require treatment; severe or major depression is a psychiatric illness and requires treatment. Major depression also is categorized as unipolar, in which people of usually normal moods experience recurrent episodes of depression.

### Major Depression
The American Psychiatric Association's *Diagnostic and Statistical Manual of Mental Disorders,* 4th edition (Text Revision), lists criteria for a major depressive episode as a depressed mood plus at least five of the following symptoms for at least 2 weeks:

- Loss of energy, fatigue
- Indecisiveness
- Difficulty thinking and concentrating
- Loss of interest in appearance, work, and leisure and sexual activities
- Inappropriate feelings of guilt and worthlessness
- Loss of appetite and weight loss, or excessive eating and weight gain
- Sleep disorders (hypersomnia or insomnia)
- Somatic symptoms (eg, constipation, headache, atypical pain)
- Obsession with death, thoughts of suicide
- Psychotic symptoms, such as hallucinations and delusions

### Dysthymia
Dysthymia involves a chronically depressed mood and at least two other symptoms (eg, anorexia, overeating, insomnia, hypersomnia, low energy, low self-esteem, poor concentration, feelings of hopelessness) for two years. Although the symptoms may cause significant social and work-related impairments, they are not severe enough to meet the criteria for major depression.

### Bipolar Disorder
Bipolar disorder involves episodes of depression alternating with episodes of mania. *Mania* is characterized by excessive central nervous system (CNS) stimulation with physical and mental hyperactivity (eg, agitation, constant talking, constant movement, grandiose ideas, impulsiveness, inflated self-esteem, little need for sleep, poor concentration, racing thoughts, short attention span) for at least one week. Symptoms are similar to those of acute psychosis or schizophrenia. *Hypomania* involves the same symptoms, but they are less severe, indicate less CNS stimulation and hyperactivity, and last 3 or 4 days.

### Cyclothymia
Cyclothymia is a mild type of bipolar disorder which involves periods of hypomania and depression that do not meet the criteria for mania and major depression. Symptoms must be present for at least two years. It does not usually require drug therapy.

**AT THE FOUNDATION:** *Biochemistry and Depression*

### Monoamine Neurotransmitter Dysfunction

Depression is thought to result from a deficiency of nor-epinephrine and/or serotonin. This hypothesis stemmed from studies demonstrating that antidepressant drugs increase the amounts of one or both of these neuro-transmitters in the CNS synapse by inhibiting their reuptake into the presynaptic neuron. Serotonin received increased attention after the SSRI antidepres-sants were marketed. Serotonin helps regulate several behaviors that are disturbed in depression, such as mood, sleep, appetite, energy level, and cognitive and psychomotor functions.

Emphasis shifted toward receptors because the neuro-transmitter view did not explain why the amounts of neurotransmitter increased within hours after single doses of a drug, but relief of depression occurred only after weeks of drug therapy. Researchers identified changes in norepinephrine and serotonin receptors with chronic antidepressant drug therapy. Studies demonstrated that chronic drug administration (ie, increased neurotransmitter in the synapse for several weeks) results in fewer receptors on the post-synaptic membrane. This down-regulation of receptors, first noted with beta-adrenergic receptors, corresponds with therapeutic drug effects. All known treatments for depression lead to the down-regulation of beta recep-tors and occur in the same period as the behavioral changes associated with antidepressant drug therapy.

Alpha$_2$-adrenergic receptors (called *autoreceptors*), located on presynaptic nerve terminals, may also play a role. When these receptors are stimulated, they inhibit the release of norepinephrine. There is evidence that alpha$_2$ receptors are also down-regulated by antidepres-sant drugs, thus allowing increased norepinephrine release. With serotonin receptors, available antidepres-sants may increase the sensitivity of postsynaptic recep-tors and decrease the sensitivity of presynaptic receptors.

Physiologically, presynaptic receptors regulate the release and reuptake of neurotransmitters; postsynaptic receptors participate in the transmission of nerve impulses to target tissues. It seems apparent that long-term administration of antidepressant drugs produces complex changes in the sensitivities of both presynaptic and postsynaptic receptor sites.

Overall, there is increasing awareness that balance, integration, and interactions among norepinephrine, serotonin, and possibly other neurotransmission sys-tems (eg, dopamine, acetylcholine) are probably more important etiologic factors than single neurotransmitter or receptor alterations. For example, animal studies indicate that serotonin is required for optimal function-ing of the neurons that produce norepinephrine. Changes in neurons may also play a major role.

### Neuroendocrine Factors

In addition to monoamine neurotransmission systems, researchers have identified nonmonoamine systems that influence neurotransmission and are significantly altered in depression. A major nonmonoamine is corticotropin-releasing factor, or hormone (CRF, or CRH), whose secretion is increased in depression. CRF-secreting neurons are widespread in the CNS, and CRF appar-ently functions as a neurotransmitter and mediator of the endocrine, autonomic, immune, and behavioral responses to stress as well as a releasing factor for corti-cotropin. Hypothalamic CRF is part of the HPA axis, which becomes hyperactive in depression. As a result, there is increased secretion of CRF by the hypothala-mus, adrenocorticotropic hormone (ACTH) by the ante-rior pituitary, and cortisol by the adrenal cortex. The increased cortisol (part of the normal physiologic response to stress) is thought to decrease the numbers or sensitivity of cortisol receptors (down-regulation) and lead to depression. This view is supported by ani-mal studies indicating that antidepressant drugs restore the ability of cortisol receptors to bind with cortisol. This alteration of cortisol receptors takes about 2 weeks, the approximate time interval required for the drugs to improve symptoms of depression. Extrahypothalamic CRF is also increased in depression. Secretion of both hypothalamic and extrahypothalamic CRF apparently returns to normal with recovery from depression.

Other neuroendocrine factors in depression are thought to include abnormalities in the secretion and function of thyroid and growth hormones.

---

tors, such as a relative excess of excitatory neurotrans-mitters (eg, norepinephrine) or a relative deficiency of inhibitory neurotransmitters (eg, gamma-aminobutyric acid [GABA]). Drugs that stimulate the central nervous system (CNS) can cause manic and hypomanic behaviors that are easily confused with schizophreniform psychoses.

## ANTIDEPRESSANT DRUGS

Drugs used in the pharmacologic management of depressive disorders are derived from several chemical groups. Older antidepressants include the tricyclic antidepressants (TCAs) and the monoamine oxidase inhibitors (MAOIs). Newer drugs include the selective serotonin reuptake inhibitors (SSRIs) and several indi-vidual drugs that differ from TCAs, MAOIs, and SSRIs. General characteristics of antidepressants include the following:

■ All are effective in relieving depression, but they differ in their adverse effects.
■ All must be taken for 2 to 4 weeks before depressive symptoms improve.

■ They are given orally, absorbed from the small bowel, enter the portal circulation, and circulate through the liver, where they undergo extensive first-pass metabolism before reaching the systemic circulation.

■ They are metabolized by the cytochrome P450 enzymes in the liver. Many antidepressants and other drugs are metabolized by the 2D6 or 3A4 subgroup of the enzymes.

Thus, antidepressants may interact with each other and with a wide variety of drugs that are normally metabolized by the same subgroups of enzymes.

## Mechanisms of Action

Although their actions are still being studied in relation to newer information about brain function and the etiology of mood disorders, antidepressant drugs apparently normalize abnormal neurotransmission systems in the brain by altering the amounts of neurotransmitters and the number or sensitivity of receptors. They may also modify interactions among neurotransmission systems and affect endocrine function (eg, the HPA axis and cortisol activity).

After neurotransmitters are released from presynaptic nerve endings, the molecules that are not bound to receptors are normally inactivated by reuptake into the presynaptic nerve fibers that released them or metabolized by MAO. Most antidepressants prevent the reuptake of multiple neurotransmitters; SSRIs selectively inhibit the reuptake of serotonin. MAOIs prevent the metabolism of neurotransmitter molecules. These mechanisms thereby increase the amount of neurotransmitter available to bind to receptors.

With chronic drug administration, receptors adapt to the presence of increased neurotransmitter by decreasing their number or sensitivity to the neurotransmitter. More specifically, norepinephrine receptors, especially postsynaptic beta receptors and presynaptic alpha$_2$ receptors, are down-regulated. The serotonin-$_2$ receptor, a postsynaptic receptor, and cortisol (glucocorticoid) receptors may also be down-regulated.

Thus, antidepressant effects are attributed to changes in receptors rather than changes in neurotransmitters. Although some of the drugs act more selectively on one neurotransmission system than another initially, this selectivity seems to be lost with chronic administration.

With lithium, the exact mechanism of action is unknown. However, it is known to affect the synthesis, release, and reuptake of several neurotransmitters in the brain, including acetylcholine, dopamine, GABA, and norepinephrine. For example, the drug may increase the activity of GABA, an inhibitory neurotransmitter. It also stabilizes postsynaptic receptor sensitivity to neurotransmitters, probably by competing with calcium, magnesium, potassium, and sodium ions for binding sites.

## Indications for Use

Antidepressant drug therapy may be indicated if depressive symptoms persist at least 2 weeks, impair social relationships or work performance, and occur independently of life events. In addition, antidepressants are increasingly being used for treatment of anxiety disorders. TCAs may be used in children and adolescents in the management of enuresis (bed-wetting or involuntary urination resulting from a physical or psychological disorder). In this setting, a TCA may be given after physical causes (eg, urethral irritation, excessive intake of fluids) have been ruled out. TCAs are also commonly used in the treatment of neuropathic pain. MAOIs are considered third-line drugs, largely because of their potential for serious interactions with certain foods and other drugs.

Depression commonly occurs in children and adolescents, and antidepressant drugs are widely prescribed. However, drug therapy is largely empiric and of unproven effectiveness. Although some antidepressants are approved for other uses in children (eg, two SSRIs, fluvoxamine and sertraline, are approved for treatment of obsessive-compulsive disorder, and some TCAs are approved for treatment of enuresis), none is approved for treatment of depression. Moreover, the long-term effects of antidepressant drugs on the developing brain are unknown. Overall, there are few reliable data or guidelines for the use of antidepressants in children and adolescents; considerations for this age group and older adults are found in Age-related Considerations.

## Contraindications to Use

Antidepressant drugs are contraindicated or must be used with caution in clients with acute schizophrenia; mixed mania and depression; suicidal tendencies; severe renal, hepatic, or cardiovascular disease; narrow-angle glaucoma; and seizure disorders. Hepatic impairment leads to reduced first-pass metabolism of most antidepressant drugs, with resultant higher plasma levels. The drugs should be used cautiously in clients with severe liver impairment. Cautious use means lower doses, longer intervals between doses, and slower dose increases than usual.

## Management Considerations

### Drug Selection

Because the available drugs seem similarly effective, the choice of an antidepressant depends on the client's age, medical conditions, previous history of drug response, if any, and a specific drug's adverse effects. Cost also needs to be considered. The newer drugs are much more expensive than the TCAs. However, they may be more cost effective overall because TCAs are more likely to cause serious adverse effects, they require monitoring of plasma drug levels and electrocardiograms (ECGs), and clients are more likely to stop taking them. Additional guidelines for choosing a drug include the following:

## Age-related Considerations: Use of Antidepressants

### USE IN CHILDREN

Considerations for use in children include the following:

1. For most children and adolescents, it is probably best to reserve drug therapy for those who do not respond to nonpharmacologic treatment and for those whose depression is persistent or severe enough to impair function in usual activities of daily living.

2. For adolescents, it may be important to discuss sexual effects because the SSRIs and venlafaxine cause a high incidence of sexual dysfunction (eg, anorgasmia, decreased libido, erectile dysfunction). Bupropion, mirtazapine, and nefazodone are unlikely to cause sexual dysfunction.

3. SSRIs are not approved in children (<18 years of age), and their safety and effectiveness have not been established. However, for children, as for other groups, these drugs are considered first-line antidepressants and safer than TCAs and MAOIs. Common adverse effects include sedation and activation; it is often difficult to distinguish therapeutic effects (improvement of mood, increased energy and motivation) from the adverse effects of behavioral activation (agitation, hypomania, restlessness).

4. TCAs are not recommended for use in children younger than 12 years of age except for short-term treatment of enuresis in children older than 6 years of age. However, they are used to treat depression, mainly amitriptyline, desipramine, imipramine, and nortriptyline. Because of potentially serious adverse effects, blood pressure, ECGs, and plasma drug levels should be monitored. There is evidence that children metabolize TCAs faster than adults, and withdrawal symptoms (eg, increased GI motility, malaise, headache) are more common in children than in adults.

   Divided doses may be better tolerated and minimize withdrawal symptoms. When a TCA is used for enuresis, effectiveness may decrease over time, and no residual benefits continue once the drug is stopped. Common adverse effects include sedation, fatigue, nervousness, and sleep disorders. A TCA probably is not a drug of first choice for adolescents because TCAs are more toxic in overdose than other antidepressants, and suicide is a leading cause of death in adolescents.

5. Safety and effectiveness have not been established for amoxapine and MAOIs in children younger than 16 years of age or for bupropion, mirtazapine, nefazodone, and venlafaxine in children younger than 18 years of age.

6. Lithium is not approved for use in children younger than 12 years of age, but it has been used to treat bipolar disorder and aggressiveness. Children normally excrete lithium more rapidly than adults. As for adults, initial doses should be relatively low and gradually increased according to regular measurements of serum drug levels.

### USE IN OLDER ADULTS

SSRIs are the drugs of choice in older adults as in younger ones because they produce fewer sedative, anticholinergic, cardiotoxic, and psychomotor adverse effects than the TCAs and related antidepressants. These drugs produce similar adverse effects in older adults as in younger adults. Although their effects in older adults are not well delineated, SSRIs may be eliminated more slowly, and smaller or less frequent doses may be prudent. The weight loss often associated with SSRIs may be undesirable in older adults. Venlafaxine may also be used in older adults, with smaller initial doses and increments recommended.

TCAs may cause or aggravate conditions that are common in older adults (eg, cardiac conduction abnormalities, urinary retention, narrow-angle glaucoma). In addition, impaired compensatory mechanisms make older adults more likely to experience anticholinergic effects, confusion, hypotension, and sedation. If a TCA is chosen for an older adult, nortriptyline or desipramine is preferred. In addition, any TCA should be given in small doses initially and gradually increased over several weeks, if necessary, to achieve therapeutic effects. Initial and maintenance doses should be small because the drugs are metabolized and excreted more slowly than in younger adults. Initial dosage should be decreased by 30% to 50% to avoid serious adverse reactions; increments should be small. Vital signs, serum drug levels, and ECGs should be monitored regularly.

MAOIs may be more likely to cause hypertensive crises in older adults because cardiovascular, renal, and hepatic functions are often diminished.

With lithium, initial doses should be low and increased gradually, according to regular measurements of serum drug levels.

---

1. The SSRIs are the drugs of first choice. These drugs are effective and usually produce fewer and milder adverse effects than other drugs. Guidelines for choosing one SSRI over another have not been established.

2. With TCAs, initial selection may be based on the client's previous response or susceptibility to adverse effects. For example, if a client (or a close family member) responded well to a particular drug in the past, that is probably the drug of choice for repeated episodes of depression. The response of family members to individual drugs may be significant because there is a strong genetic component to depression and drug response. If therapeutic effects do not occur within 4 weeks, the TCA probably should be discontinued or changed because some clients tolerate or respond better to one TCA than to another. For a

potentially suicidal client, an SSRI or another newer drug is preferred over a TCA because the TCAs are much more toxic in overdoses.

3. MAOIs are third-line drugs for the treatment of depression because of their potential interactions with other drugs and certain foods. An MAOI is most likely to be prescribed when the client does not respond to other antidepressant drugs or when electroconvulsive therapy is refused or contraindicated.

4. Criteria for choosing bupropion, mirtazapine, nefazodone, and venlafaxine are not clearly defined. Bupropion does not cause orthostatic hypotension or sexual dysfunction. Mirtazapine decreases anxiety, agitation, migraines, and insomnia as well as depression. In addition, it does not cause sexual dysfunction or clinically significant drug–drug interactions. Nefazodone has sedating and anxiolytic properties that may be useful for clients with severe insomnia, anxiety, and agitation. However, it has been associated with liver failure and probably should not be given to clients with significant liver impairment. In addition, serum nefazodone levels are increased in clients with cirrhosis and the drug inhibits cytochrome P450 3A4 enzymes that metabolize many drugs. Venlafaxine has stimulant effects, increases blood pressure, and causes sexual dysfunction, but does not cause significant drug–drug interactions.

5. For clients with cardiovascular disorders, most antidepressants can cause hypotension, but the SSRIs, bupropion, nefazodone, and venlafaxine are rarely associated with cardiac dysrhythmias. Venlafaxine and MAOIs can increase blood pressure.

6. For clients with seizure disorders, bupropion, clomipramine, and maprotiline should be avoided; SSRIs, MAOIs, and desipramine are less likely to cause seizures.

7. For clients with diabetes mellitus, SSRIs may have a hypoglycemic effect, and bupropion and venlafaxine have little effect on blood sugar levels.

8. Lithium is the drug of choice for clients with bipolar disorder. When used therapeutically, lithium is effective in controlling mania in 65% to 80% of clients. When used prophylactically, the drug decreases the frequency and intensity of manic cycles. Carbamazepine (Tegretol), an anticonvulsant, may be as effective as lithium as a mood-stabilizing agent. It is often used in clients who do not respond to lithium, although it has not been approved by the U.S. Food and Drug Administration (FDA) for that purpose.

## Dosage and Administration

Dosage of antidepressant drugs should be individualized according to clinical response. Antidepressant drug therapy is usually initiated with small, divided doses that are gradually increased until therapeutic or adverse effects occur. Specific guidelines for dosage include the following:

1. With SSRIs, nefazodone, and venlafaxine, therapy is begun with once-daily oral administration of the manufacturer's recommended dosage. Dosage may be increased after 3 or 4 weeks if depression is not relieved. With nefazodone, an optimal response may require 300 to 500 mg daily. As with most other drugs, smaller doses may be indicated in older adults and clients taking multiple medications.

2. With TCAs, therapy is begun with small doses, which are increased to the desired dose over 1 to 2 weeks. TCAs can be administered once or twice daily because they have long elimination half-lives. Once dosage is established, TCAs are often given once daily at bedtime. This regimen is effective and well tolerated by most clients. Elderly clients may experience fewer adverse reactions if divided doses are continued. With TCAs, plasma levels are helpful in adjusting dosages.

3. With bupropion, seizures are more likely to occur with large single doses, large total doses, and large or abrupt increases in dosage. Recommendations to avoid these risk factors are:
   a. Give the drug in equally divided doses, three times daily (at least 6 hours apart), for immediate-release tablets, twice daily for sustained-release tablets.
   b. The maximal single dose of immediate-release tablets is 150 mg (sustained-release, 200 mg).
   c. The recommended initial dose is 200 mg, gradually increased to 300 mg. If no clinical improvement occurs after several weeks of 300 mg/day, dosage may be increased to 450 mg, the maximal daily dose for immediate-release tablets (sustained-release maximum, 400 mg).
   d. The recommended maintenance dose is the lowest amount that maintains remission.

4. With lithium, dosage should be based on serum lithium levels, control of symptoms, and occurrence of adverse effects. Serum levels are required because therapeutic doses are only slightly lower than toxic doses and because clients vary widely in rates of lithium absorption and excretion. Thus, a dose that is therapeutic in one client may be toxic in another. Lower doses are indicated for older adults and for clients with conditions that impair lithium excretion (eg, diuretic drug therapy, dehydration, low-salt diet, renal impairment, decreased cardiac output).

   When lithium therapy is being initiated, the serum drug concentration should be measured two or three times weekly in the morning, 12 hours after the last dose of lithium. For most clients, the therapeutic range of serum levels is 0.6 to 1.2 mEq/L (SI units, 0. to 1.2 mmol/L). Serum lithium levels should not exceed 1.5 mEq/L because the risk for serious toxicity is increased at higher levels.

   Once symptoms of mania are controlled, lithium doses should be lowered. Serum lithium levels should be measured at least every 3 months during long-term maintenance therapy.

## Duration of Drug Therapy

Guidelines for the duration of antidepressant drug therapy are not well established, and there are differences of opinion. Some authorities recommend 9 months of treatment after symptoms subside for a first episode of depression, 5 years after symptoms subside for a second episode, and long-term therapy after a third episode. One argument for long-term maintenance therapy is that depression tends to relapse or recur, and successive episodes often are more severe and more difficult to treat.

Maintenance therapy for depression requires close supervision and periodic reassessment of the client's condition and response. With the use of TCAs for acute depression, low doses have been given for several months, followed by gradual tapering of the dose and drug discontinuation. However, recent studies indicate that full therapeutic doses (if clients can tolerate the adverse effects) for up to 5 years are effective in preventing recurrent episodes. The long-term effects of SSRIs and newer agents have not been studied. Monitoring and regular reassessment of the client's condition and response are often done in the home. Guidelines for strategies for ongoing evaluation and intervention are addressed in Home Care Considerations.

With lithium, long-term therapy is the usual practice because of a high recurrence rate if the drug is discontinued. When lithium is discontinued, most often because of adverse effects or the client's lack of adherence to the prescribed regimen, gradually tapering the dose over 2 to 4 weeks delays recurrence of symptoms.

## TYPES OF ANTIDEPRESSANTS AND INDIVIDUAL DRUGS

Additional characteristics of antidepressants and lithium are described in the following sections; names, indications for use, and dosage ranges of individual drugs are listed in Drugs at a Glance 10-1: Antidepressant Agents.

### Home Care Considerations: Use of Antidepressants

*ASSESS:* the client and family's knowledge of depression; the client for compliance with the prescribed regimen, for concurrent use of with MAOIs, thio-ridazine, or mesoridazine, for signs and symptoms of major depression or suicidal thoughts or plans, and quality of life; need for referral for treatment.

*MONITOR:* the therapeutic and adverse effects of the antidepressant, especially with changes in drugs or dosages; that client is keeping appointments for lab work, counseling (as indicated), and follow-up care.

*EDUCATE:* on safe use of the drugs (eg, that potentially hazardous activities should be avoided, and that it usually takes 2 to 4 weeks to feel better); on ways to minimize adverse effects. Reinforce additional teaching points (see Client Teaching Guidelines: Antidepressants and Lithium).

## Tricyclic Antidepressants

TCAs, of which **P** **amitriptyline** is the prototype, are similar drugs that produce a high incidence of adverse effects such as sedation, orthostatic hypotension, cardiac dysrhythmias, anticholinergic effects (eg, blurred vision, dry mouth, constipation, urinary retention), and weight gain (Prototype Profile 10-1). They are well absorbed after oral administration, but first-pass metabolism by the liver results in blood level variations of 10- to 30-fold among people given identical doses. Once absorbed, these drugs are widely distributed in body tissues and metabolized by the liver to active and inactive metabolites. Because of adverse effects on the heart, especially in overdose, baseline and follow-up ECGs are recommended for all clients. **Imipramine** (Tofranil) is a commonly used TCA.

Tricyclic antidepressants are also less readily metabolized with severe hepatic impairment (eg, severe cirrhosis). This increases the risk for adverse effects such as sedation and hypotension.

## Selective Serotonin Reuptake Inhibitors

SSRIs, of which **P** **fluoxetine** (Prozac, Sarafem) is the prototype, produce fewer serious adverse effects than the TCAs (Prototype Profile 10-2). They are well absorbed with oral administration, undergo extensive first-pass metabolism in the liver, are highly protein bound (95%), and have a half-life of 24 to 72 hours, which may lead to accumulation with chronic administration. Fluoxetine also forms an active metabolite with a half-life of 7 to 9 days. Thus, steady-state blood levels are achieved slowly, over several weeks, and drug effects decrease slowly (over 2 to 3 months) when fluoxetine is discontinued. Sertraline (Zoloft) and citalopram (Celexa) also have active metabolites, but fluoxetine and paroxetine (Paxil) are more likely to accumulate. Paroxetine, sertraline, and fluvoxamine (Luvox) reach steady-state concentrations in 1 to 2 weeks. SSRIs are usually given once daily.

Fluoxetine and sertraline are less readily metabolized to their active metabolites with hepatic impairment. In clients with cirrhosis, for example, the average half-life of fluoxetine may increase from 2 to 3 days to more than 7 days, and that of norfluoxetine, the active metabolite, from 7 to 9 days to 12 days. Clearance of sertraline is also decreased in clients with cirrhosis.

Because SSRIs are highly bound to plasma proteins, the drugs compete with endogenous compounds and other medications for binding sites. Because they are highly lipid soluble, they accumulate in the CNS and other adipose-rich tissue.

Adverse effects include a high incidence of gastrointestinal symptoms (eg, nausea, diarrhea, weight loss) and sexual dysfunction (eg, delayed ejaculation in men and impaired orgasmic ability in women). Most also cause

*(text continues on page 182)*

**DRUG TABLE 10-1**

*Drugs at a Glance*

## Antidepressant Agents

| Generic/Trade Name | Routes and Dosage Ranges | Comments |
|---|---|---|
| *Tricyclic Antidepressants* | | |
| **Amitriptyline** (Elavil) | See Prototype Profile 10-1: Amitriptyline | |
| **Clomipramine** (Anafranil) Pregnancy Category C | *Adults:* PO, 25 mg daily, increased to 100 mg daily by end of 2 weeks, in divided doses, with meals. Give maintenance dose in a single dose at bedtime. Maximum dose, 250 mg daily *Children and adolescents:* PO, 25 mg daily, increased to 3 mg/kg or 100 mg, whichever is smaller, over 2 weeks. Give maintenance dose in a single dose at bedtime. Maximum dose, 3 mg/kg or 200 mg, whichever is smaller | Indicated for obsessive-compulsive disorder (OCD) May cause seizures; risk increases with increasing doses; significant cardiotoxic and anticholinergic effects |
| **Desipramine** (Norpramin) Pregnancy Category C | *Adults:* PO, 100–200 mg daily in divided doses or as a single daily dose. Give maintenance dose once daily. Maximum dose, 300 mg/d *Adolescents and older adults:* PO, 25–100 mg daily in divided doses or as a single daily dose. Maximum dose, 150 mg/d | Use with caution in clients with cardiovascular disease or suicide risk |
| **Doxepin** (Sinequan, Prudoxin, Zonalon) Pregnancy Category C | *Adults:* PO, 75–150 mg daily, in divided doses or a single dose at bedtime. Maximum dose, 300 mg/d | Avoid unnecessary exposure to sunlight; may turn urine blue-green |
| **Imipramine** (Tofranil) Pregnancy Category D | *Adults:* PO, 75 mg daily in 3 divided doses gradually increased to 200 mg daily if necessary Maintenance dose, 75–150 mg daily *Adolescents and older adults:* PO, 30–40 mg daily in divided doses, increased to 100 mg daily if necessary *Children >6 y:* Enuresis, PO, 25 to 50 mg 1 h before bedtime | For depression and childhood enuresis |
| **Nortriptyline** (Aventyl, Pamelor) Pregnancy Category D | *Adults:* PO, 25 mg 3 or 4 times daily or in a single dose (75–100 mg) at bedtime. Maximum dose, 150 mg/d *Adolescents and older adults:* 30–50 mg/d, in divided doses or a single dose once daily | May increase appetite and craving for sweets |
| **Protriptyline** (Vivactil) Pregnancy Category C | *Adults:* PO, 15–40 mg daily in 3 or 4 divided doses. Maximum dose, 60 mg *Adolescents and older adults:* PO, 5 mg 3 times daily, increase gradually if necessary | May alter glucose metabolism; may be taken with food to decrease GI distress |
| **Trimipramine maleate** (Surmontil) Pregnancy Category C | *Adults:* PO, 75 mg daily, in divided doses or a single dose at bedtime, increased to 150 mg/d if necessary Maximum dose, 200 mg/d *Adolescents and older adults:* PO, 50 mg daily, increased to 100 mg/d if necessary | Significant sedative effect Valerian, St. John's wort, SAMe, and kava kava may increase the risk for excessive sedation and/or serotonin syndrome |

*(continued)*

**DRUG TABLE 10-1** *Drugs at a Glance*

## Antidepressant Agents (Continued)

| Generic/Trade Name | Routes and Dosage Ranges | Comments |
|---|---|---|
| **Selective Serotonin Reuptake Inhibitors (SSRIs)** | | |
| **Citalopram** (Celexa)<br>Pregnancy Category C | *Adults:* PO, 20 mg once daily, morning or evening, increased to 40 mg daily in 1 week, if necessary<br>*Elderly/hepatic impairment:* PO, 20 mg daily | Fatal reactions have occurred with concomitant use with monoamine oxidase inhibitors (MAOIs) |
| **Fluoxetine** (Prozac, Sarafem) | See Prototype Profile 10-2: Fluoxetine | |
| **Fluvoxamine** (Luvox)<br>Pregnancy Category C | *Adults:* PO, 50 mg once daily at bedtime, increased in 50-mg increments every 4–7 days if necessary. For daily amounts above 100 mg, give in 2 divided doses. Maximum dose, 300 mg/d<br>*Children 8–17 y:* PO, 25 mg once daily at bedtime, increased in 25-mg increments every 4–7 days if necessary. For daily amounts above 50 mg, give in 2 divided doses. Maximum dose 200 mg/d | Indicated for OCD<br>Use with MAOIs may potentate a serotonin syndrome |
| **Paroxetine** (Paxil, Paxil CR)<br>Pregnancy Category C | *Adults:* PO, 20 mg once daily in the morning, increased at 1 week or longer intervals, if necessary; usual range, 20–50 mg/d; maximum dose, 60 mg/d<br>Controlled-release tablets, PO, 25 mg once daily in the morning, increased up to 62.5 mg/d if necessary<br>*Elderly or debilitated adults:* PO, 10 mg once daily, increased if necessary. Maximum dose, 40 mg<br>*Severe renal or hepatic impairment:* Same as for older adults | Also indicated for generalized anxiety disorder; OCD; panic disorder; social anxiety disorder<br>Not recommended in children and adolescents due to associated increased risk for suicide ideation<br>Women may become anorgasmic while taking drug |
| **Sertraline** (Zoloft)<br>Pregnancy Category C | *Adults:* Depression, OCD: PO, 50 mg once daily morning or evening, increased at 1-week or longer intervals to a maximum daily dose of 200 mg<br>Panic, post-traumatic stress disorder (PTSD): PO, 25 mg once daily, increased after 1 week to 50 mg once daily<br>*Children, OCD: 6–12 y:* 25 mg once daily; *13–17 y:* 50 mg once daily | Also indicated for OCD; panic disorder; PTSD; premenstrual dysphoric disorder (PMDD) |
| **Monoamine Oxidase Inhibitors** | | |
| **Isocarboxazid** (Marplan)<br>Pregnancy Category C | *Adults:* PO, 10 mg twice daily, increased to 60 mg/d if necessary, in 2 to 4 divided doses | For depression refractory to the tricyclic antidepressants |
| **Phenelzine** (Nardil)<br>Pregnancy Category C | *Adults:* PO, 15 mg 3 times daily, increased to 90 mg/d if necessary | Observe for postural hypotension<br>Severe hypertension may occur if taken with tyramine, tryptophan, or dopamine-containing foods |

*(continued)*

*Drugs at a Glance*

**DRUG TABLE
10-1**

## Antidepressant Agents (Continued)

| Generic/Trade Name | Routes and Dosage Ranges | Comments |
|---|---|---|
| **Tranylcypromine** (Parnate) Pregnancy Category C | *Adults:* PO, 30 mg daily in divided doses, increased to 60 mg/d if necessary | Severe hypertension may occur if taken with tyramine, tryptophan, or dopamine-containing foods |
| *Miscellaneous Antidepressants* | | |
| **Amoxapine** (Asendin) Pregnancy Category C | *Adults:* PO, 50 mg 2 or 3 times daily, increased to 100 mg 2 or 3 times daily by end of 1 week. Give maintenance dose in a single dose at bedtime *Older adults:* PO, 25 mg 2 or 3 times daily, increased to 50 mg 2 or 3 times daily by end of 1 week. Give mainte- nance dose in a single dose at bedtime | A heterocyclic antidepressant; may cause extrapyramidal symptoms and orthostatic hypotension |
| **Bupropion** (Wellbutrin, Wellbutrin SR, Zyban) Pregnancy Category B | *Adults:* Immediate release tablets, PO, 100 mg twice daily, increased to 100 mg 3 times daily (at least 6 h apart) if necessary. Maximal single dose, 150 mg Sustained release tablets, PO, 150 mg once daily in the morning, increased to 150 twice daily (at least 8 hours apart). Maximum single dose, 150 mg | Zyban also indicated as adjunct in smoking cessation May cause seizures; risk increases with increasing doses |
| **Maprotiline** Pregnancy Category B | *Adults:* PO, 75 mg daily in single or divided doses, increased to a maxi- mum of 300 mg daily if necessary | Investigational use with the urinary symptoms associated with multiple sclerosis and with cocaine withdrawal |
| **Mirtazapine** (Remeron) Pregnancy Category C | *Adults:* PO, 15 mg/d, in a single dose, at bedtime. Increase by 15 mg/d (at least 1–2 weeks between incre- ments) up to 45 mg/d if necessary | The degree of sedation is moderate to high compared with other anti- depressants May increase appetite and cause weight gain |
| **Nefazodone** (Serzone) Pregnancy Category C | *Adults:* PO, 200 mg daily in 2 divided doses; increase at 1-week intervals in increments of 100–200 mg/d; usual range, 300–600 mg/d *Elderly or debilitated adults:* PO, initially 100 mg/d in 2 divided doses | Life-threatening liver failure has been reported with use |
| **Trazodone** (Desyrel) Pregnancy Category C | *Adults:* PO, 100–300 mg daily, increased to a maximum dose of 600 mg daily if necessary | May be taken at bedtime to decrease concern about sedative effects |
| **Venlafaxine** (Effexor, Effexor XR) Pregnancy Category C | *Adults:* Immediate release tablets, PO, initially 75 mg/d in 2 or 3 divided doses, with food. Increase by 75 mg/d (4 days or longer between incre- ments) up to 225 mg/d if necessary Extended release capsules, PO, initially 37.5 or 75 mg/d in a single dose morning or evening Increase by 75 mg/d (4 days or longer between increments) up to 225 mg/d if necessary *Hepatic or renal impairment:* reduce dose by 50% and increase very slowly | Extended release tablets also indicated for generalized anxiety disorder Does not cause sedation or cardiovas- cular concern |
| *Mood-stabilizing Agent* | | |
| **Lithium carbonate** (Eskalith, Lithobid) | See Prototype Profile 10-3: Lithium carbonate | |

## PROTOTYPE PROFILE 10-1

### *P* Amitriptyline (a mee TRIP ti leen)

### Drug Class
*Chemical:* Tricyclic antidepressant
*Functional:* Antidepressant

### Trade Name
Elavil

### Therapeutic Indications
Relief of symptoms of depression
Other uses/unlabeled: Migraine
prophylaxis, fibromyalgia, polyneuropathy, pain

### Pharmacokinetics
*Absorption*
Oral: Complete
Systemic availability is reduced by first-pass metabolism

*Distribution*
Crosses placenta, enters breast milk

*Metabolism*
Hepatic

*Excretion*
Urine (18% as unchanged drug)
Feces (small amounts)

### Pharmacodynamics
*Onset of Action*

*Depression*
4–6 wk

*Migraine Prophylaxis*
6 wk

*Duration*
*Half-life:* Adults 9–27 h (average, ~15 h)

### Contraindications/Precautions
*Contraindications*
Acute recovery period following myocardial infarction;
hypersensitivity to tricyclic antidepressants; use of
MAOIs within past 14 days

*Precautions*
History of seizures, urinary retention, cardiovascular
disorders, closed-angle glaucoma or intraocular pressure; hyperthyroidism; pregnancy; schizophrenic
patients; manic-depressive patients; potentially suicidal patients should not have access to large amounts;
concomitant electroshock therapy; impaired liver
function; start elderly on low doses

### Pregnancy Considerations
Category C
Crosses placenta, enters breast milk

### Dosage
*Depression*
Oral: 50–150 mg/d as a single dose at bedtime or in
2–3 divided doses, maximum of 300 mg/d
IM, 20–30 mg 4 times per day (switch to oral dosing
as soon as possible)

*Chronic Pain Management*
Oral: 10–25 mg at bedtime; may increase to maximum of 150–200 mg/d as tolerated

*Elderly*
Dosage adjustment necessary

### Adverse Effects
*Common*
Blurred vision, drowsiness, dizziness, weakness,
fatigue, headache, dry mouth, constipation, bloating,
weight gain

*Serious*
Arrhythmias, AV conduction changes, heart block
palpitations, orthostatic hypotension, syncope,
hypertension

*Serious but Rare*
Agranulocytosis, aplastic anemia, eosinophilia,
leukopenia, jaundice and hepatic dysfunction,
myocardial infarction, stroke, pancytopenia, purpura,
thrombocytopenia, seizures

### Drug Interactions
*Increased Effects*
Effect of warfarin, amphetamines, anticholinergics,
sedatives, alcohol, hypnotics, carbamazepine

*Decreased Effects*
Antidepressant effects with carbamazepine, phenobarbital, and rifampin
Antihypertensive response with clonidine, guanadrel,
guanethidine, guanabenz, or guanfacine
Cholestyramine and colestipol may bind TCAs and
reduce their absorption

### Herbal Supplements and Dietary Considerations
Avoid valerian, St John's wort (may decrease
amitriptyline levels), kava kava, gotu kola as they may
increase CNS depression
Avoid ethanol
Grapefruit juice may inhibit the metabolism of some
TCAs, and clinical toxicity may result

## PROTOTYPE PROFILE 10-2

### *P* Fluoxetine (floo OKS e teen)

**Drug Class**
*Chemical:* Selective serotonin reuptake inhibitor (SSRI)
*Functional:* Antidepressant agent

**Trade Names**
Prozac, Sarafem

**Therapeutic Indications**
Indicated for depression; obsessive-compulsive disorder (OCD), binge-eating in individuals with bulimia nervosa, panic disorder and premenstrual dysphoric disorder (Sarafem)

**Pharmacokinetics**
*Absorption*
Well absorbed; delayed 1 to 2 h with delayed-release capsules

*Distribution*
Plasma protein binding 95%; crosses the placenta

*Metabolism*
Hepatic to active metabolite

*Excretion*
Urine

**Pharmacodynamics**
*Onset of Action*
Peak antidepressant effect: 2–4 wk

*Duration*
2–3 months due to active metabolites

**Contraindications/Precautions**
Concurrent use (or within 14 days) with MAOIs, thioridazine, or mesoridazine

**Pregnancy Considerations**
Category C
Enters breast milk, not recommended

**Dosage**
*Adults:* PO, 20 mg once daily in the morning, increased after several weeks if necessary. Give doses larger than 20 mg once in the morning or in 2 divided doses, morning and noon; maximum daily dose 80 mg
Prozac weekly (delayed-release capsules), PO, 90 mg once each week, starting 7 days after the last 20 mg dose
*Children:* Depression:
*8–18 y:* 10 to 20 mg/d, increased as necessary to 20 mg/d after 1 week
OCD:
*7–18 y:* 10 to 20 mg/d; lower-weight children can be started at 10 mg/d; may be increased to 20 mg/d after 2 weeks; range 10–60 mg/d

**Adverse Effects**
Insomnia, restlessness, headache, dry mouth, GI distress, sexual dysfunction, seizures, ST-segment depression on ECG, pharyngitis, yawning

**Drug Interactions**
*Increased Effects*
CNS depression with alcohol
Effects of amphetamines, anticholinergics, other CNS depressants
Risk for neurotoxicity with lithium

*Decreased Effects*
Effects of SSRIs with cyproheptadine

**Herbal Supplements and Dietary Considerations**
Avoid valerian, kava kava, St. John's wort, gotu kola because they may increase CNS depression
May be taken with or without food

---

some degree of CNS stimulation (eg, anxiety, nervousness, insomnia), which is highest with fluoxetine.

Serious, sometimes fatal, reactions have occurred from combined therapy with an SSRI and an MAOI, and the drugs should not be given concurrently or within 2 weeks of each other. If a client on an SSRI is to be transferred to an MAOI, most SSRIs should be discontinued at least 14 days before starting the MAOI; fluoxetine should be discontinued at least 5 weeks before starting an MAOI.

## Monoamine Oxidase Inhibitors

MAOIs are infrequently used, mainly because they may interact with some foods and drugs to produce severe hypertension and possible heart attack or stroke. Foods that interact contain tyramine, a monoamine precursor of norepinephrine. Normally, tyramine is deactivated in the gastrointestinal tract and liver, so that large amounts do not reach the systemic circulation. However, when deactivation is blocked by MAOIs, tyramine is absorbed systemically and transported to adrenergic nerve terminals, where it causes a sudden release of large amounts of norepinephrine. Foods that should be avoided include aged cheeses and meats, concentrated yeast extracts, sauerkraut, and fava beans. Drugs that should be avoided include CNS stimulants (eg, amphetamines, cocaine), adrenergics (eg, pseudoephedrine), antidepressants (SSRIs, venlafaxine), buspirone, levodopa, and meperidine.

## Miscellaneous Antidepressants

**Bupropion** (Wellbutrin, Zyban) inhibits the reuptake of dopamine, norepinephrine, and serotonin. It was marketed with warnings related to seizure activity. Seizures are most likely to occur with doses above 450 mg/day and in clients known to have a seizure disorder.

After an oral dose, peak plasma levels are reached in about 2 hours. The average drug half-life is about 14 hours. The drug is metabolized in the liver and excreted primarily in the urine. Several metabolites are pharmacologically active. Dosage should be reduced with impaired hepatic or renal function. Acute episodes of depression usually require several months of drug therapy. Bupropion is also used as a smoking cessation aid.

Bupropion has few adverse effects on cardiac function and does not cause orthostatic hypotension or sexual dysfunction. In addition to seizures, however, the drug has CNS stimulant effects (agitation, anxiety, excitement, increased motor activity, insomnia, restlessness) that may require a sedative during the first few days of administration. These effects may increase the risk for abuse. Other common adverse effects include dry mouth, headache, nausea and vomiting, and constipation.

**Maprotiline** is similar to the TCAs in therapeutic and adverse effects.

**Mirtazapine** (Remeron) blocks presynaptic alpha$_2$-adrenergic receptors (which increases the release of norepinephrine), serotonin receptors, and histamine-$_1$ receptors. Consequently, the drug decreases anxiety, agitation, insomnia, and migraine headache as well as depression.

The drug is well absorbed after oral administration, and peak plasma levels occur within 2 hours after an oral dose. It is metabolized in the liver, mainly to inactive metabolites. Common adverse effects include drowsiness (with accompanying cognitive and motor impairment), increased appetite, weight gain, dizziness, dry mouth, and constipation. It does not cause sexual dysfunction.

Mirtazapine should not be taken concurrently with other CNS depressants (eg, alcohol or benzodiazepine antianxiety or hypnotic agents) because of additive sedation. In addition, it should not be taken concurrently with an MAOI or for 14 days after stopping an MAOI. An MAOI should not be started until at least 14 days after stopping mirtazapine.

**Nefazodone** (Serzone) inhibits the neuronal reuptake of serotonin and norepinephrine, thereby increasing the amount of these neurotransmitters in the brain. It is contraindicated in pregnancy and liver damage and should be used with caution in people with cardiovascular or cerebrovascular disorders, dehydration, hypovolemia, mania, hypomania, suicidal ideation, hepatic cirrhosis, electroconvulsive therapy, debilitation, and lactation. It has a long half-life (2 to 3 days) and crosses the placenta. It is metabolized in the liver and produces two active metabolites. It is excreted in breast milk, urine, and feces.

Adverse effects resemble those of SSRIs and TCAs, including agitation, confusion, dizziness, gastrointestinal (GI) symptoms (nausea, vomiting, diarrhea), headache,

insomnia, orthostatic hypotension, sedation, and skin rash. Because of its association with liver failure, serum levels of liver enzymes (eg, aspartate and alanine aminotransferases [AST and ALT]) should be measured before starting nefazodone therapy, periodically during therapy, and immediately when symptoms of liver dysfunction develop (eg, anorexia, nausea, vomiting, dark urine).

Nefazodone should not be taken with an MAOI because of the risk for severe toxic effects. If a client on nefazodone is to be transferred to an MAOI, the nefazodone should be discontinued at least 7 days before starting the MAOI; if a client on an MAOI is to be transferred to nefazodone, the MAOI should be discontinued at least 14 days before starting nefazodone. Other potentially serious drug interactions include increased CNS depression with general anesthetics and decreased metabolism of drugs metabolized by the cytochrome P450 3A4 enzymes, which are inhibited by nefazodone.

Nefazodone has been associated with a few cases of liver failure and should not be given to clients with severe liver impairment. In addition, blood levels of nefazodone are higher in clients with cirrhosis.

**Trazodone** (Desyrel) is used more often for sedation and sleep than for depression because high doses (>300 mg/day) are required for antidepressant effects, and these amounts cause excessive sedation for many clients. It is often given concurrently with a stimulating antidepressant, such as bupropion, fluoxetine, sertraline, or venlafaxine.

Trazodone is well absorbed with oral administration, and peak plasma concentrations are obtained within 30 minutes to 2 hours. It is metabolized by the liver and excreted primarily by the kidneys. Adverse effects include sedation, dizziness, edema, cardiac dysrhythmias, and priapism (prolonged and painful penile erection).

**Venlafaxine** (Effexor) inhibits the reuptake of norepinephrine, serotonin, and dopamine, thereby increasing the activity of these neurotransmitters in the brain. The drug crosses the placenta and may enter breast milk. It is metabolized in the liver and excreted in urine. It is contraindicated during pregnancy, and women should use effective birth control methods while taking this drug. Adverse effects include CNS (anxiety, dizziness, dreams, insomnia, nervousness, somnolence, tremors), GI (anorexia, nausea, vomiting, constipation, diarrhea), cardiovascular (hypertension, tachycardia, vasodilation), genitourinary (abnormal ejaculation, impotence, urinary frequency), and dermatologic (sweating, rash, pruritus) symptoms. Venlafaxine does not interact with drugs metabolized by the cytochrome P450 system, but it should not be taken concurrently with MAOIs because of increased serum levels and risks for toxicity. If a client on venlafaxine is to be transferred to an MAOI, the venlafaxine should be discontinued at least 7 days before starting the MAOI; if a client on an MAOI is to be transferred to venlafaxine, the MAOI should be discontinued at least 14 days before starting venlafaxine.

# MOOD-STABILIZING AGENTS

**Lithium carbonate** (Eskalith) is a naturally occurring metallic salt that is used in bipolar disorder, mainly to treat and prevent manic episodes. Prototype Profile 10-3 discusses lithium. It is well absorbed after oral administration, with peak serum levels in 1 to 3 hours after a dose and steady-state concentrations in 5 to 7 days. Serum lithium concentrations should be monitored frequently because they vary widely among clients taking similar doses and because of the narrow range between therapeutic and toxic levels.

Lithium is not metabolized by the body; it is entirely excreted by the kidneys and has a very narrow therapeutic range, so that adequate renal function is a prerequisite for lithium therapy. Approximately 80% of a lithium dose is reabsorbed in the proximal renal tubules. The amount of reabsorption depends on the concentration of sodium in the proximal renal tubules. A deficiency of sodium causes more lithium to be reabsorbed and increases the risk for lithium toxicity; excessive sodium intake causes more lithium to be excreted (ie, lithium diuresis) and may lower serum lithium levels to non-therapeutic ranges. If given to a client with renal impairment or unstable renal function, the dose must be markedly reduced, and plasma lithium levels must be closely monitored.

Before lithium therapy is begun, baseline studies of renal, cardiac, and thyroid status should be obtained because adverse drug effects involve these organ systems. Baseline electrolyte studies are also necessary.

**Anticonvulsants** (see Chap. 11) are also used as mood-stabilizing agents in bipolar disorder because they modify nerve cell function. Carbamazepine (Tegretol) and valproate (Depakene) are commonly used. Newer drugs (eg, gabapentin, lamotrigine, topiramate, oxcarbazepine)

---

## PROTOTYPE PROFILE 10-3
### *P* Lithium (LITH ee um)

**Drug Class**
*Chemical:* Metallic salt
*Functional:* Mood-stabilizing agent; antimanic agent

**Trade Names**
Eskalith, Lithobid

**Therapeutic Indications**
Indicated for bipolar disorder (mania)

**Pharmacokinetics**
*Absorption*
Oral: rapid and complete

*Distribution*
Not protein bound; complete distribution in 6 to 10 h

*Metabolism*
Not metabolized

*Excretion*
Urine (90%–98% as unchanged drug)

**Pharmacodynamics**
*Onset of Action*
5 to 7 d (antimanic effects)

*Duration*
Half-life: 21–30 h (>36 h in elderly or in renal impairment)

**Contraindications/Precautions**
Avoid in clients with severe cardiovascular or renal disease, those who are severely debilitated, dehydrated, or pregnant

**Pregnancy Considerations**
Category D
Enters breast milk, contraindicated

**Dosage**
*Adults:* PO, 600 mg 3 times daily or 900 mg twice daily (slow release forms)
Maintenance dose, PO, 300 mg 3 or 4 times daily to maintain a serum lithium level of 0.6–1.2 mEq/L
*Children <12 y:* safety not established

**Adverse Effects**
Dysrhythmias, dizziness, slurred speech, stupor, leuko-cytosis, blurred vision, urinary incontinence

**Drug Interactions**
*Increased Effect*
Risk for neurotoxicity with carbamazepine, SSRIs, TCAs, methyldopa, diltiazem, haloperidol, pheno-thiazines, phenytoin, and verapamil
Risk for lithium toxicity with nonsteroidal anti-inflammatory drugs (NSAIDs), angiotensin-converting enzyme (ACE) inhibitors, diuretics, angiotensin receptor antagonists, tetracycline, or cyclooxygenase II (COX-II) inhibitors
Risk for fatal malignant hyperpyrexia with MAOIs

*Decreased Effect*
Lower level of both drugs with concurrent use of chlorpromazine
Lower lithium levels with sodium bicarbonate, high sodium intake, or caffeine
Blunted pressor effects with sympathomimetics

**Herbal Supplements and Dietary Considerations**
Taking with food may increase serum concentration; limit caffeine intake
Have client drink 2–3 L of water daily

are being used and studied regarding their effects in bipolar disorder, but none is FDA-approved for this purpose. Thus far, most of the drugs seem to have some beneficial effects, but additional studies are needed.

## Herbal Supplement

**St. John's wort** (*Hypericum perforatum*) is an herb that is widely self-prescribed for depression. Several studies, most of which used about 900 mg daily of a standardized extract, indicate its usefulness in mild to moderate depression, with fewer adverse effects than antidepressant drugs. A 3-year, multicenter study by the National Institutes of Health concluded that the herb is not effective in major depression.

Antidepressant effects are attributed mainly to hypericin, although several other active components have also been identified. The mechanism of action is unknown, but the herb is thought to act similarly to antidepressant drugs by decreasing reuptake of the neurotransmitters serotonin and dopamine. Some herbalists refer to St. John's wort as "natural Prozac."

Adverse effects, which are usually infrequent and mild, include constipation, dizziness, dry mouth, fatigue, GI distress, nausea, photosensitivity, restlessness, skin rash, and sleep disturbances. Stopping the herb relieves these symptoms.

Drug interactions may be extensive. St. John's wort should not be combined with alcohol, antidepressant drugs (eg, MAOIs, SSRIs, TCAs), nasal decongestants or other over-the-counter cold and flu medications, bronchodilators, opioid analgesics, or amino acid supplements containing phenylalanine and tyrosine. All of these interactions may result in hypertension, possibly severe.

Most authorities agree that there is insufficient evidence to support the use of St. John's wort for mild to moderate depression and that more studies are needed to confirm the herb's safety and effectiveness. Most of the previous studies were considered flawed.

Overall, both consumers and health care professionals seem to underestimate the risks associated with taking this herbal supplement. For clients who report use of St. John's wort, teach them to purchase products from reputable sources because the amount and type of herbal content may vary among manufacturers; to avoid taking antidepressant drugs, alcohol, and cold and flu medications while taking St. John's wort; to avoid the herb during pregnancy because effects are unknown; and to use sunscreen lotions and clothing to protect themselves from sun exposure.

## ■ DRUG USE IN SPECIFIC SITUATIONS

### Concurrent Use of Antidepressants With Other Drugs

The SSRIs are strong inhibitors of the cytochrome P450 enzyme system that metabolizes many drugs, especially those metabolized by the 1A2, 2D6, and 3A4 groups of enzymes. Inhibiting the enzymes that normally metabolize or inactivate a drug produces the same effect as an excessive dose of the inhibited drug. As a result, serum drug levels and risks for adverse effects are greatly increased. Specific interactions include the following:

---

 **URSING PROCESS**

### Assessment

Assess the client's condition in relation to depressive disorders.

- Identify clients at risk for current or potential depression. Areas to assess include health status, family and social relationships, and work status. Severe or prolonged illness, impaired interpersonal relationships, inability to work, and job dissatisfaction may precipitate depression. Depression also occurs without an identifiable cause.
- Observe for signs and symptoms of depression. Clinical manifestations are nonspecific and vary in severity. For example, fatigue and insomnia may be caused by a variety of disorders and range from mild to severe. When symptoms are present, try to determine their frequency, duration, and severity.
- When a client appears depressed or has a history of depression, assess for suicidal thoughts and behaviors. Statements indicating a detailed plan, accompanied by the intent, ability, and method for carrying out the plan, place the client at high risk for suicide.

- Identify the client's usual coping mechanisms for stressful situations. Coping mechanisms vary widely, and behavior that may be helpful to one client may not be helpful to another. For example, one person may prefer being alone or having decreased contact with family and friends, whereas another may find increased contact desirable.

### Nursing Diagnoses

- Dysfunctional Grieving related to loss (of health, ability to perform usual tasks, job, significant other, and so forth)
- Self Care Deficit related to fatigue and self-esteem disturbance with depression or sedation with antidepressant drugs
- Sleep Pattern Disturbance related to mood disorder or drug therapy
- Risk for Injury related to adverse drug effects
- Risk for Violence: Self-Directed or Directed at Others
- Deficient Knowledge: Effects and appropriate use of antidepressant and mood stabilizing drugs

*(continued)*

**N**URSING PROCESS (Continued)

### Planning/Goals

*The client will:*

- Experience improvement of mood and depressive state
- Receive or self-administer the drugs correctly
- Remain safe while sedated during therapy with the TCAs and related drugs
- Not manifest suicidal tendencies. If present, caretakers will implement safety measures.
- Have needs met in areas of nutrition, hygiene, exercise, and social interactions even when unable to provide self-care
- Resume self-care and other usual activities
- Avoid preventable adverse drug effects

### Interventions

Use measures to prevent or decrease the severity of depression. General measures include supportive psychotherapy and reduction of environmental stress. Specific measures include the following:

- Support the client's usual mechanisms for handling stressful situations, when feasible. Helpful actions may involve relieving pain or insomnia, scheduling rest periods, and increasing or decreasing socialization.
- Call the client by name, encourage self-care activities, allow him or her to participate in setting goals and making decisions, and praise efforts to accomplish tasks. These actions promote a positive self-image.
- When signs and symptoms of depression are observed, initiate treatment before depression becomes severe. Institute suicide precautions for clients at risk. These usually involve close observation, often on a one-to-one basis, and removal of potential weapons from the environment. For clients hospitalized on medical-surgical units, transfer to a psychiatric unit may be needed.

### Evaluation

- Observe for behaviors indicating lessened depression.
- Interview regarding feelings and mood.
- Observe and interview regarding adverse drug effects.
- Observe and interview regarding suicidal thoughts and behaviors.

---

## CLIENT TEACHING GUIDELINES
## Antidepressants and Lithium

### General Considerations

✔ Take antidepressants as directed to maximize therapeutic benefits and minimize adverse effects. Do not alter doses when symptoms subside. Antidepressants are usually given for several months, perhaps years; lithium therapy may be lifelong.

✔ Therapeutic effects (relief of symptoms) may not occur for 2 to 4 weeks after drug therapy is started. As a result, it is very important not to think the drug is ineffective and stop taking it prematurely.

✔ Do not take other prescription or over-the-counter drugs without consulting a health care provider, including over-the-counter cold remedies. Potentially serious drug interactions may occur.

✔ Do not take the herbal supplement St. John's wort while taking a prescription antidepressant drug. Serious interactions may occur.

✔ Inform any physician, surgeon, dentist, or nurse practitioner about the antidepressant drugs being taken. Potentially serious adverse effects or drug interactions may occur if certain other drugs are prescribed.

✔ Avoid activities that require alertness and physical coordination (eg, driving a car, operating other machinery) until reasonably sure the medication does not make you drowsy or impair your ability to perform the activities safely.

✔ Avoid alcohol and other central nervous system depressants (eg, any drugs that cause drowsiness). Excessive drowsiness, dizziness, difficulty breathing, and low blood pressure may occur, with potentially serious consequences.

✔ Learn the name and type of a prescribed antidepressant drug to help avoid undesirable interactions with other drugs or a health care provider prescribing other drugs with similar effects. There are several different types of antidepressant drugs, with different characteristics and precautions for safe and effective usage.

✔ Bupropion is a unique drug prescribed for depression (brand name, Wellbutrin) and for smoking cessation (brand name, Zyban). It is extremely important not to increase the dose or take the two brand names at the same time (as might happen with different physicians or filling prescriptions at different pharmacies). Overdoses may cause seizures, as well as other adverse effects. When used for smoking cessation, Zyban is recommended for up to 12 weeks if progress is being made. If significant progress is not made by approximately 7 weeks, it is considered unlikely that longer drug use will be helpful.

✔ Do not stop taking any antidepressant drug without discussing it with a health care provider. If a problem occurs, the type of drug, the dose, or other aspects may be changed to solve the problem and allow continued use of the medication.

✔ Counseling, support groups, relaxation techniques, and other nonmedication treatments are recommended along with drug therapy.

*(continued)*

**CLIENT TEACHING GUIDELINES**
**Antidepressants and Lithium** (Continued)

**Self-administration**

✔ With a selective serotonin reuptake inhibitor (eg, Celexa, Paxil, Prozac, Zoloft), take in the morning because the drug may interfere with sleep if taken at bedtime. In addition, notify a health care provider if a skin rash or other allergic reaction occurs. Allergic reactions are uncommon but may require that the drug be discontinued.

✔ With a tricyclic antidepressant (eg, amitriptyline), take at bedtime to aid sleep and decrease side effects. Also, report urinary retention, fainting, irregular heartbeat, seizures, restlessness, and mental confusion. These are potentially serious adverse drug effects.

✔ With nefazodone (Serzone) and venlafaxine (Effexor), take as directed or ask for instructions. These drugs are often taken twice daily. Notify a health care provider if a skin rash or other allergic reaction occurs. An allergic reaction may require that the drug be discontinued.

✔ With bupropion, take two or three times daily, as prescribed.

✔ With lithium, several precautions are needed for safe use:
1. Take with food or milk or soon after a meal to decrease stomach upset.

2. Do not alter dietary salt intake. Decreased salt intake (eg, low-salt diet) increases risk of adverse effects from lithium. Increased intake may decrease therapeutic effects.
3. Drink 8 to 12 glasses of fluids daily; avoid excessive intake of caffeine-containing beverages. Caffeine has a diuretic effect and dehydration increases lithium toxicity.
4. Minimize activities that cause excessive perspiration. Loss of salt in sweat increases the risk of adverse effects from lithium.
5. Report for measurements of lithium blood levels as instructed, and do not take the morning dose of lithium until the blood sample has been obtained. Regular measurements of blood lithium levels are necessary for safe and effective lithium therapy. Accurate measurement of serum drug levels requires that blood be drawn approximately 12 hours after the previous dose of lithium.
6. If signs of overdose occur (eg, vomiting, diarrhea, unsteady walking, tremor, drowsiness, muscle weakness), stop taking lithium and contact the prescribing physician or other health care provider.

---

■ Fluvoxamine inhibits both 1A2 and 3A4 enzymes. Inhibition of 1A2 enzymes slows metabolism of acetaminophen, caffeine, clozapine, haloperidol, olanzapine, tacrine, theophylline, tricyclic antidepressants, and warfarin. Inhibition of 3A4 enzymes slows metabolism of benzodiazepines (alprazolam, midazolam, triazolam), calcium channel blockers (diltiazem, nifedipine, verapamil), cyclosporine, erythromycin, protease inhibitors (anti–acquired immunodeficiency syndrome [anti-AIDS] drugs, indinavir, ritonavir, saquinavir), steroids, tamoxifen, warfarin, and zolpidem.

■ Fluoxetine, paroxetine, and sertraline inhibit 2D6 enzymes and slow metabolism of bupropion, codeine, desipramine, dextromethorphan, flecainide, metoprolol, nortriptyline, phenothiazines, propranolol, risperidone, and timolol.

■ Nefazodone also inhibits 3A4 enzymes and slows the metabolism of many drugs (see fluvoxamine, above). If nefazodone is given with alprazolam or triazolam (benzodiazepines), dosage of the benzodiazepine should be reduced by 50% or more.

■ Mirtazapine and venlafaxine are not thought to have clinically significant effects on cytochrome P450 enzymes, but few studies have been done, and effects are unknown.

■ TCAs are metabolized by 2D6 enzymes and may inhibit the metabolism of other drugs metabolized by the 2D6 group (other antidepressants, phenothiazines, carbamazepine, flecainide, propafenone).

Lower-than-usual doses of both the TCA and the other drug may be needed.

## Toxicity of Antidepressants and Lithium: Recognition and Management

Some antidepressant drugs are highly toxic and potentially lethal when taken in large doses. Toxicity is most likely to occur in depressed clients who intentionally ingest large amounts of drug in suicide attempts and in young children who accidentally gain access to medication containers. Measures to prevent acute poisoning from drug overdose include dispensing only a few days' supply (ie, 5 to 7 days) to clients with suicidal tendencies and storing the drugs in places inaccessible to young children. General measures to treat acute poisoning include early detection of signs and symptoms, stopping the drug, and instituting treatment if indicated. Specific measures include the following:

**SSRI overdose:** Symptoms include nausea, vomiting, agitation, restlessness, hypomania, and other signs of CNS stimulation. Management includes symptomatic and supportive treatment, such as maintaining an adequate airway and ventilation and administering activated charcoal.

**TCA overdose:** Symptoms occur 1 to 4 hours after drug ingestion and consist primarily of CNS depression and cardiovascular effects (eg, nystagmus, tremor, restlessness, seizures, hypotension, dysrhythmias, myocardial depression). Death usually results from cardiac, respiratory, and circulatory failure. Management of TCA toxicity consists of performing gastric lavage and giving activated charcoal to reduce drug absorption, establishing and maintaining a patent airway, performing continuous ECG monitoring of comatose clients or those with respiratory insufficiency or wide QRS intervals, giving intravenous fluids and vasopressors for severe hypotension, and giving intravenous phenytoin (Dilantin) or fosphenytoin (Cerebyx), or a parenteral benzodiazepine (eg, lorazepam) if seizures occur.

**MAOI overdose:** Symptoms occur 12 hours or more after drug ingestion and consist primarily of adrenergic effects (eg, tachycardia, increased rate of respiration, agitation, tremors, convulsive seizures, sweating, heart block, hypotension, delirium, coma). Management consists of diuresis, acidification of urine, or hemodialysis to remove the drug from the body.

**Bupropion overdose:** Symptoms include agitation and other mental status changes, nausea and vomiting, and seizures. General treatment measures include hospitalization, decreasing absorption (eg, giving activated charcoal to conscious clients), and supporting vital functions. If seizures occur, an intravenous benzodiazepine (eg, lorazepam) is the drug of first choice.

**Nefazodone or venlafaxine overdose:** Symptoms include increased incidence or severity of adverse effects, with nausea, vomiting, and drowsiness most often reported. Hypotension and excessive sedation may occur with nefazodone; seizures and diastolic hypertension, with venlafaxine. There are no specific antidotes; treatment is symptomatic and supportive.

**Lithium overdose:** Toxic manifestations occur with serum lithium levels above 2.5 mEq/L and include nystagmus, tremors, oliguria, confusion, impaired consciousness, visual or tactile hallucinations, choreiform movements, convulsions, coma, and death. Treatment involves supportive care to maintain vital functions, including correction of fluid and electrolyte imbalances. With severe overdoses, hemodialysis is preferred because it removes lithium from the body.

## Prevention and Management of Withdrawal Symptoms

Withdrawal symptoms have been reported with sudden discontinuation of most antidepressant drugs. In general, symptoms occur more rapidly and may be more intense with drugs having a short half-life. As with other psychotropic drugs, these drugs should be tapered in dosage and discontinued gradually unless severe drug toxicity, anaphylactic reactions, or other life-threatening conditions are present. Most antidepressants may be tapered and discontinued over approximately 1 week

without serious withdrawal symptoms. For a client on maintenance drug therapy, the occurrence of withdrawal symptoms may indicate that the client has omitted doses or stopped taking the drug.

The most clearly defined withdrawal syndromes are associated with SSRIs and TCAs. With SSRIs, withdrawal symptoms include dizziness, nausea, and headache and last from several days to several weeks. More serious symptoms may include aggression, hypomania, mood disturbances, and suicidal tendencies. Fluoxetine has a long half-life and has not been associated with withdrawal symptoms. Other SSRIs have short half-lives and may cause withdrawal reactions if stopped abruptly. Paroxetine, which has a half-life of approximately 24 hours and does not produce active metabolites, may be associated with relatively severe withdrawal symptoms even when discontinued gradually, over 7 to 10 days. Symptoms may include a flulike syndrome with nausea, vomiting, fatigue, muscle aches, dizziness, headache, and insomnia. The short-acting SSRIs should be tapered in dosage and gradually discontinued to prevent or minimize withdrawal reactions.

With TCAs, the main concern is over those with strong anticholinergic effects. When stopped abruptly, especially with high doses, these drugs can cause symptoms of excessive cholinergic activity (ie, hypersalivation, diarrhea, urinary urgency, abdominal cramping, and sweating). A recommended rate for tapering TCAs is approximately 25 to 50 mg every 2 to 3 days.

## Genetic or Ethnic Considerations

Antidepressant drug therapy for nonwhite populations in the United States is based primarily on dosage recommendations, pharmacokinetic data, and adverse effects derived from white recipients. However, several studies document differences in drug effects in nonwhite populations. The differences are mainly attributed to genetic or ethnic variations in drug-metabolizing enzymes in the liver. Although all ethnic groups are genetically heterogeneous and individual members may respond differently, health care providers need to consider potential differences in responses to drug therapy.

1. *African Americans* tend to have higher plasma levels for a given dose, respond more rapidly, experience a higher incidence of adverse effects, and metabolize TCAs more slowly than whites. To decrease adverse effects, initial doses may need to be lower than those given to whites, and later doses should be titrated according to clinical response and serum drug levels. In addition, baseline and periodic ECGs are recommended to detect adverse drug effects on the heart. Studies have not been done with newer antidepressants. With lithium, African Americans report more adverse reactions than whites and may need smaller doses.

2. *Asians* tend to metabolize antidepressant drugs slowly and therefore have higher plasma drug levels for a given dose than whites. Most studies have been done with TCAs and a limited number of Asian subgroups. Thus, it cannot be assumed that all antidepressant drugs and all people of Asian heritage respond the same. To avoid drug toxicity, initial doses should be approximately half the usual doses given to whites, and later doses should be titrated according to clinical response and serum drug levels. This recommendation is supported by a survey from several Asian countries that reported the use of much smaller doses of TCAs than in the United States. In addition, in Asians as in African Americans, baseline and periodic ECGs are recommended to detect adverse drug effects on the heart. Studies have not been done with newer antidepressants. With lithium, there are no apparent differences between effects in Asians and whites.

3. *Hispanics'* responses to antidepressant drugs are largely unknown. Few studies have been done, with some reporting a need for lower doses of TCAs and greater susceptibility to anticholinergic effects, whereas others report no differences between Hispanics and whites.

## Use in Perioperative Periods

Antidepressants must be used very cautiously, if at all, perioperatively because of the risk for serious adverse effects and adverse interactions with anesthetics and

---

**? How Can You Avoid This Medication Error?**

Jane, a 17-year-old, was admitted to your psychiatric unit after a suicide attempt. When you approach her with her morning medications (including an antidepressant), she is lying on her bed in a fetal position. She opens her eyes when you call her name. She instructs you to just leave her medications on the table so she can take them later. You do so, leave the room, and chart the medications.

---

other commonly used drugs. MAOIs are contraindicated and should be discontinued at least 10 days before elective surgery. TCAs should be discontinued several days before elective surgery and resumed several days after surgery. SSRIs and miscellaneous antidepressants have not been studied in relation to perioperative use; however, it seems reasonable to discontinue the drugs when feasible because of potential adverse effects, especially on the cardiovascular system and CNS. It is usually recommended that antidepressants be tapered in dosage and gradually discontinued. Lithium should be stopped 1 to 2 days before surgery and resumed when full oral intake of food and fluids is allowed. Lithium may prolong the effects of anesthetics and neuromuscular-blocking drugs.

*(text continues on page 192)*

---

## *Nursing Actions*
## Antidepressants

| Nursing Actions | Rationale/Explanation |
|---|---|
| **1. Administer accurately.** | |
| a. Give most selective serotonin reuptake inhibitors (SSRIs) once daily in the morning; citalopram and sertraline may be given morning or evening. | To prevent insomnia |
| b. Mix sertraline oral concentrate (20 mg/mL) in 4 oz of water, ginger ale, lemon/lime soda, lemonade, or orange juice only; give immediately after mixing. | Manufacturer's recommendation |
| c. Give tricyclic antidepressants (TCAs) and mirtazapine at bedtime. | To aid sleep and decrease daytime sedation |
| d. Give venlafaxine and lithium with food. | To decrease gastrointestinal (GI) effects (eg, nausea and vomiting) |
| **2. Observe for therapeutic effects.** | Therapeutic effects occur 2 to 4 weeks after drug therapy is started. |
| a. With antidepressants for depression, observe for statements of feeling better or less depressed; increased appetite, physical activity, and interest in surroundings; improved sleep patterns; improved appearance; decreased anxiety; decreased somatic complaints. | |
| b. With antidepressants for anxiety disorders, observe for decreased symptoms of the disorders (see Chap. 8) | |

*(continued)*

## *Nursing Actions*
## Antidepressants (Continued)

| *Nursing Actions* | *Rationale/Explanation* |
|---|---|
| c. With lithium, observe for decreases in manic behavior and mood swings. | Therapeutic effects do not occur until approximately 7 to 10 days after therapeutic serum drug levels (1–1.5 mEq/L with acute mania; 0.6–1.2 mEq/L for maintenance therapy) are attained. In mania, a benzodiazepine or an antipsychotic drug is usually given to reduce agitation and control behavior until the lithium takes effect. |
| **3. Observe for adverse effects.** | |
| a. With SSRIs nefazodone and venlafaxine, observe for dizziness, headache, nervousness, insomnia, nausea, diarrhea, dizziness, dry mouth, sedation, skin rash, sexual dysfunction. | GI upset and diarrhea are common with SSRIs; GI upset, diarrhea, and orthostatic hypotension are common with nefazodone; GI upset, diarrhea, agitation, and insomnia are common with venlafaxine. Although numerous adverse effects may occur, they are usually less serious than those occurring with most other antidepressants. Compared with the TCAs, SSRIs and other newer drugs are less likely to cause significant sedation, hypotension, and cardiac arrhythmias but are more likely to cause nausea, nervousness, and insomnia. Most adverse effects result from anticholinergic or anti-adrenergic activity. Cardiovascular effects are most serious in overdose. |
| b. With TCAs, observe for: <br> (1) Central nervous system (CNS) effects—drowsiness, dizziness, confusion, poor memory <br> (2) Cardiovascular effects—cardiac arrhythmias, tachycardia, orthostatic hypotension <br> (3) GI effects—nausea, dry mouth, constipation <br> (4) Other effects—blurred vision, urinary retention, sexual dysfunction, weight gain | |
| c. With monoamine oxidase inhibitors (MAOIs), observe for blurred vision, constipation, dizziness, dry mouth, hypotension, urinary retention, hypoglycemia. | Anticholinergic effects are common. Hypoglycemia results from a drug-induced reduction in blood sugar. |
| d. With bupropion, observe for seizure activity, CNS stimulation (agitation, insomnia, hyperactivity, hallucinations, delusions), headache, nausea and vomiting, and weight loss. | Adverse effects are most likely to occur if recommended doses are exceeded. Note that bupropion has few, if any, effects on cardiac conduction and does not cause orthostatic hypotension. |
| e. With mirtazapine, observe for sedation, confusion, dry mouth, constipation, nausea and vomiting, hypotension, tachycardia, urinary retention, photosensitivity, skin rash, weight gain. | Common effects are drowsiness, dizziness, and weight gain. Has CNS depressant and anticholinergic effects. |
| f. With nefazodone, observe for: <br> (1) CNS effects—anxiety, drowsiness, dizziness, headache, insomnia <br> (2) GI effects—nausea, vomiting, diarrhea, dry mouth, anorexia, constipation <br> (3) Cardiovascular effect—orthostatic hypotension <br> (4) Hepatic effect—liver failure (anorexia, nausea, vomiting, abdominal pain, dark urine, jaundice) | |
| g. With lithium, observe for: <br> (1) Metallic taste, hand tremors, nausea, polyuria, polydipsia, diarrhea, muscular weakness, fatigue, edema, and weight gain <br> (2) More severe nausea and diarrhea, vomiting, ataxia, incoordination, dizziness, slurred speech, blurred vision, tinnitus, muscle twitching and tremors, increased muscle tone | Most clients who take lithium experience adverse effects. Symptoms listed in (1) are common, occur at therapeutic serum drug levels (0.8–1.2 mEq/L), and usually subside during the first few weeks of drug therapy. Symptoms listed in (2) occur at higher serum drug levels (1.5–2.5 mEq/L). Nausea may be decreased by giving lithium with meals. Propranolol (Inderal), 20–120 mg daily, may be given to control tremors. Severe adverse effects may be managed by decreasing lithium dosage, omitting a few doses, or discontinuing the drug temporarily. Toxic symptoms occur at serum drug levels above 2.5 mEq/L. |

*(continued)*

## Nursing Actions

### Antidepressants (Continued)

| Nursing Actions | Rationale/Explanation |
|---|---|
|     (3) Leukocytosis | Lithium mobilizes white blood cells (WBCs) from bone marrow to the bloodstream. Maximum increase in WBCs occurs in 7 to 10 days. |
| 4. Observe for drug interactions.<br>  a. Drugs that *increase* effects of SSRIs:<br>    (1) Cimetidine | Drug interactions with the SSRIs vary with individual drugs. May increase serum drug levels of SSRIs by slowing their metabolism |
|     (2) MAOIs | **SSRIs and MAOIs should not be given concurrently or close together because serious and fatal reactions have occurred.** The reaction, attributed to excess serotonin and called the *serotonin syndrome,* may cause hyperthermia, muscle spasm, agitation, delirium, and coma. To avoid this reaction, an SSRI should not be started for at least 2 weeks after an MAOI is discontinued, and an MAOI should not be started for at least 2 weeks after an SSRI has been discontinued (5 weeks with fluoxetine, because of its long half-life). |
|   b. Drugs that *decrease* effects of SSRIs:<br>    (1) Carbamazepine, phenytoin, rifampin | These drugs induce liver enzymes that accelerate the metabolism of the SSRIs. |
|     (2) Cyproheptadine | This is an antihistamine with antiserotonin effects. |
|   c. Drugs that *increase* the effects of mirtazapine, nefazodone, and venlafaxine:<br>    (1) MAOIs | See SSRIs, above. **These drugs and MAOIs should not be given concurrently or close together because serious and fatal reactions have occurred.** Mirtazapine should be stopped at least 14 days and nefazodone or venlafaxine at least 7 days before starting an MAOI, and an MAOI should be stopped at least 14 days before starting mirtazapine, nefazodone, or venlafaxine. |
|   d. Drugs that increase effects of TCAs:<br>    (1) Antiarrhythmics (eg, quinidine, disopyramide, procainamide) | Additive effects on cardiac conduction, increasing risk of heart block |
|     (2) Antihistamines, atropine, and other drugs with anticholinergic effects | Additive anticholinergic effects (eg, dry mouth, blurred vision, urinary retention, constipation) |
|     (3) Antihypertensives | Additive hypotension |
|     (4) Cimetidine | Increases risks of toxicity by decreasing hepatic metabolism and increasing blood levels of TCAs |
|     (5) CNS depressants (eg, alcohol, benzodiazepine antianxiety and hypnotic agents, opioid analgesics) | Additive sedation and CNS depression |
|     (6) MAOIs | **TCAs should not be given with MAOIs or within 2 weeks after an MAOI drug;** hyperpyrexia, convulsions, and death have occurred with concurrent use. |
|     (7) SSRIs | Inhibit metabolism of TCAs |
|   e. Drugs that *decrease* effects of TCAs:<br>    (1) Carbamazepine, phenytoin, rifampin, nicotine (cigarette smoking) | These drugs induce drug-metabolizing enzymes in the liver, which increases the rate of TCA metabolism and elimination from the body. |
|   f. Drugs that *increase* effects of MAOIs:<br>    (1) Anticholinergic drugs (eg, atropine, antipsychotic agents, TCAs) | Additive anticholinergic effects |
|     (2) Adrenergic agents (eg, epinephrine, phenylephrine), alcohol (some beers and wines), levodopa, meperidine | Hypertensive crisis and stroke may occur. |

*(continued)*

## Nursing Actions

### Antidepressants (Continued)

| Nursing Actions | Rationale/Explanation |
|---|---|
| g. Drugs that *increase* effects of lithium: | |
|   (1) Angiotensin-converting enzyme inhibitors (eg, captopril) | Decrease renal clearance of lithium and thus increase serum lithium levels and risks of toxicity. |
|   (2) Diuretics (eg, furosemide, hydrochlorothiazide) | Increase neurotoxicity and cardiotoxicity of lithium by increasing excretion of sodium and potassium and thereby decreasing excretion of lithium. |
|   (3) Nonsteroidal anti-inflammatory drugs | Decrease renal clearance of lithium and thus increase serum levels and risks of lithium toxicity. |
|   (4) Phenothiazines | Increased risk of hyperglycemia |
|   (5) TCAs | May increase effects of lithium and are sometimes combined with lithium for this purpose. These drugs also may precipitate a manic episode and increase risks of hypothyroidism. |
| h. Drugs that *decrease* effects of lithium: | |
|   (1) Acetazolamide, sodium chloride (in excessive amounts), drugs with a high sodium content (eg, ticarcillin), theophylline | Increase excretion of lithium |

### ? How Can You Avoid This Medication Error?

**Answer:** Do not leave medications at the bedside of a client. Often they can be forgotten or taken away with the food tray. Missing a dose of a medication can affect therapeutic blood levels. In this situation, special care should be taken to supervise all medications. Depressed clients could save up medication to commit suicide by overdosing. The risk for this increases as the antidepressant drugs start to work, giving the client more energy to carry out suicidal actions. Wake Jane up and firmly encourage her to take her medications as you watch.

## Critical Thinking Exercises

1. Hepatic impairment leads to reduced first-pass metabolism of most antidepressant drugs. This will result in:
   a. A need for higher doses
   b. Higher plasma levels of the drug
   c. Decreased plasma levels of the drug
   d. More rapid dose increases than usual

2. The classification of drugs that are considered first line for the treatment of depression is the:
   a. Tricyclic antidepressants
   b. Monoamine oxidase inhibitors
   c. Selective serotonin reuptake inhibitors
   d. Miscellaneous antidepressants

3. The drug of choice for clients with bipolar disorder is:
   a. Amoxapine
   b. Lithium
   c. Trazodone
   d. Bupropion

4. For most clients, the therapeutic range of serum lithium levels for maintenance therapy is:
   a. 0. to 0.8 mEq/L
   b. 0.6 to 1.2 mEq/L
   c. 1.0 to 1.8 mEq/L
   d. 1.5 to 2.0 mEq/L

5. A deficiency of sodium causes more lithium to be reabsorbed, which:
   a. May lower serum lithium levels to nontherapeutic ranges
   b. Leads to lithium diuresis
   c. Requires an increase in dosage
   d. Increases the risk for lithium toxicity

## SELECTED REFERENCES

American Psychiatric Association. (2000). *Diagnostic and statistical manual of mental disorders* (4th ed.). Text Revision (DSM-IV-TR). Washington, DC: Author.

Baldwin, D. S. (2000). Adverse drug reactions to newer antidepressants. *Adverse Drug Reaction Bulletin*, No. 200, ISSN 0044-6394, 763–766.

Barkin, R. L., & Barkin, D. (2001). Pharmacologic management of acute and chronic pain. *Southern Medical Journal*, 94(8), 756–812.

Beckman, S. E., Sommi, R. W., & Switzer, J. (2000). Consumer use of St. John's wort. *Pharmacotherapy, 20*(5), 568–574. [On-line.] Available: http://www.medscape.com/PP/Pharmacotherapy/2000/v20.n05/pharm2005.beck/pharm2005.08.beck-01.html. Accessed August 10, 2003.

Depression Guideline Panel. (1993). *Clinical practice guideline: Depression in primary care. 2. Treatment of major depression.* Rockville, MD: U.S. Department of Health and Human Services, Public Health Service, Agency for Health Care Policy and Research; AHCPR publication No. 93-0551.

DerMarderosian, A. (Ed.). (2001). *The review of natural products.* St. Louis: Facts and Comparisons.

*Drug facts and comparisons.* (Updated monthly). St. Louis: Facts and Comparisons.

Fetrow, C. W., & Avila, J. R. (1999). *Professional's handbook of complementary and alternative medicines.* Springhouse, PA: Springhouse Corporation.

Kim, R. B. (Ed.). (2001). *Handbook of adverse drug interactions.* New Rochelle, NY: The Medical Letter, Inc.

Lacy, C. F., Armstrong, L. L., Goldman, M. P., & Lance, L. L. (2003). *Lexi-Comp's drug information handbook* (11th ed.). Hudson, OH: American Pharmaceutical Association.

Sadek, N., & Nemeroff, C. B. (2000). Update on the neurobiology of depression. Medscape article. [On-line.] Available: http://www.medscape.com?Medscape/psychiatry/TreatmentUpdate/2000/tu03/public/toc-tu03.html. Accessed June 2003.

Stimmel, G. L. (2000). Mood disorders. In E. T. Herfindal & D. R. Gourley (Eds.), *Textbook of therapeutics: Drug and disease management* (7th ed., pp. 1203–1216). Philadelphia: Lippincott Williams & Wilkins.

Waddell, D. L., Hummel, M. E., & Sumners, A. D. (2001). Three herbs you should get to know: Kava, St. John's wort, ginkgo. *American Journal of Nursing, 101*(4), 48–54.

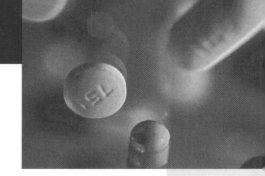

# 11

# Antiseizure Drugs

## OBJECTIVES

*After studying this chapter, the student will be able to:*

1 Identify types and potential causes of seizures.

2 Discuss major factors that influence choice of an antiseizure drug for a client with a seizure disorder.

3 Differentiate characteristics and effects of commonly used antiseizure drugs.

4 Explain differences between older and newer antiseizure drugs.

5 Compare advantages and disadvantages of monotherapy and combination drug therapy for seizure disorders.

6 Apply the nursing process with clients receiving antiepileptic drugs.

7 Describe strategies for prevention and treatment of status epilepticus.

## CRITICAL THINKING SCENARIO

*Y*ou are caring for 6-month-old Sean, who was just diagnosed with tonic-clonic seizures. He was started on valproic acid (Depakene), 30 mg PO four times daily, and has only had one seizure during his 4-day hospitalization. He will be discharged today to his single, teenaged mother, who will be the primary caregiver.

✔ How you would feel as a new parent if your infant were diagnosed with a seizure disorder. What would be your most significant fears?

✔ Given 15 minutes for discharge teaching, prioritize your teaching plan, considering the following: safe administration of an anticonvulsant medication to a 6-month-old; methods to avoid skipping doses, which could increase risk for seizures; and management of Sean during a seizure to ensure safety.

## PROTOTYPE PROFILE

phenytoin (Dilantin), p. 202

# SEIZURE DISORDERS

Antiseizure drugs are also called antiepileptic drugs (AEDs) or anticonvulsants. The terms *seizure* and *convulsion* are often used interchangeably, although they are not the same. A seizure involves a brief episode of abnormal electrical activity in nerve cells of the brain that may or may not be accompanied by visible changes in appearance or behavior. A convulsion is a tonic-clonic type of seizure characterized by spasmodic contractions of involuntary muscles.

Seizures may occur as single events in response to hypoglycemia, fever, electrolyte imbalances, overdoses of numerous drugs (eg, amphetamine, cocaine, isoniazid, lidocaine, lithium, methylphenidate, antipsychotics, theophylline), and withdrawal of alcohol or sedative-hypnotic drugs. In these instances, treatment of the underlying problem or temporary use of an AED may relieve the seizures.

## Epilepsy

When seizures occur in a chronic, recurrent pattern, the disorder is called *epilepsy*, and drug therapy is usually required. The etiology of epilepsy is outlined in At the Foundation: Epilepsy. It is diagnosed by clinical signs and symptoms of seizure activity and by the presence of abnormal brain wave patterns on the electroencephalogram. The cause is unknown in 60% to 80% of children and adolescents and 50% of older adults.

When epilepsy begins in infancy, causes include developmental defects, metabolic disease, or birth injury. Fever is a common cause during late infancy and early childhood, and inherited forms usually begin in childhood or adolescence.

When epilepsy begins in adulthood, it is often caused by an acquired neurologic disorder (eg, head injury, stroke, brain tumor) or alcohol and other drug effects. The incidence of epilepsy is higher in young children and older adults than in other age groups.

Epilepsy is broadly classified as partial and generalized seizures. *Partial seizures* begin in a specific area of the brain and often indicate a localized brain lesion such as birth injury, trauma, stroke, or tumor. They produce symptoms ranging from simple motor and sensory manifestations to more complex abnormal movements and bizarre behavior. Movements are usually automatic, repetitive, and inappropriate to the situation, such as chewing, swallowing, or aversive movements. Behavior is sometimes so bizarre that the person is diagnosed as psychotic or schizophrenic. In simple partial seizures, consciousness is not impaired; in complex partial seizures, the level of consciousness is decreased.

*Generalized seizures* are bilateral and symmetric and have no discernible point of origin in the brain. The most common type is the tonic-clonic or major motor seizure. The tonic phase involves sustained contraction of skeletal muscles; abnormal postures, such as opisthotonos; and absence of respiration, during which the person becomes cyanotic. The clonic phase is characterized by rapid rhythmic and symmetric jerking movements of the body. Tonic-clonic seizures are sometimes preceded by an aura, a brief warning, such as a flash of light or a specific sound. In children, febrile seizures (ie, tonic-clonic seizures that occur in the absence of other identifiable causes) are the most common form of epilepsy.

Another type of generalized seizure is the absence seizure, characterized by abrupt alterations in consciousness that last only a few seconds. The person may have a blank, staring expression with or without blinking of the eyelids, twitching of the head or arms, and other motor movements. Other types of generalized seizures include the myoclonic type (contraction of a muscle or group of muscles) and the akinetic type (absence of movement). Some people are subject to mixed seizures.

*Status epilepticus* is a life-threatening emergency characterized by generalized tonic-clonic convulsions lasting for several minutes or occurring at close intervals during which the client does not regain consciousness. Hypotension, hypoxia, and cardiac dysrhythmias may also occur. There

## AT THE FOUNDATION: *Epilepsy*

Epilepsy is characterized by abnormal and excessive electrical discharges in a group of nerve cells (epileptogenic focus), resulting in alterations in brain function. The neurons experience a paroxysmal shift in depolarization and abrupt changes in the typical membrane potential. The plasma membranes become more permeable and hypersensitive and thus are more easily stimulated by various clinical conditions (hypoxia, hyperthermia, hypoglycemia, hyponatremia, repetitive sensory stimulation, and certain phases of sleep).

The primary abnormality may result in (1) instability in the neuron's resting potential, (2) abnormalities in potassium conductance or calcium channels, (3) a defect in the GABA inhibitory system, or (4) irregularity in excitatory transmission enhancement.

The involved neurons fire with escalating frequency and amplitude, reach threshold, and spread to adjacent normal neurons through cortical stimulation. If uninhibited at this point, the excitation will spread to other parts of the nervous system. The seizure discharge produces changes typically resulting in altered level of arousal and motor, sensory, autonomic, or psychic clinical manifestations.

is a high risk for permanent brain damage and death unless prompt, appropriate treatment is instituted. In a person taking medications for a diagnosed seizure disorder, the most common cause of status epilepticus is abruptly stopping AEDs. In other clients, regardless of whether they have a diagnosed seizure disorder, causes of status epilepticus include brain trauma or tumors, systemic or central nervous system (CNS) infections, alcohol withdrawal, and overdoses of drugs (eg, cocaine, theophylline).

## ANTISEIZURE DRUGS

Antiseizure drugs can usually control seizure activity but do not cure the underlying disorder. Numerous difficulties, for both clinicians and clients, have been associated with antiepileptic drug therapy, including trials of different drugs, consideration of monotherapy versus two or more drugs, the need to titrate dosage over a period of time, lack of seizure control while drugs are being selected and dosages adjusted, a social stigma and adverse drug effects that often lead to poor client compliance, and undesirable drug interactions among AEDs and between AEDs and other drugs. Attempts to overcome these difficulties have led to the development of several new drugs in recent years.

Drug therapy of epilepsy is rapidly evolving as older, more toxic drugs are virtually eliminated from clinical use, and the roles of newer drugs are being defined. In this chapter, older drugs that are still commonly used (phenytoin, carbamazepine, ethosuximide, phenobarbital, valproate) and newer drugs (gabapentin, lamotrigine, levetiracetam, oxcarbazepine, tiagabine, topiramate, zonisamide) are discussed.

## Mechanisms of Action

Although the exact mechanism of action is unknown for most AEDs, the drugs are thought to suppress seizures by decreasing movement of ions into nerve cells, altering the activity of neurotransmitters (eg, gamma-aminobutyric acid [GABA], glutamate), or a combination of these mechanisms. Because movement of sodium and calcium ions is required for normal conduction of nerve impulses, blocking these ions decreases responsiveness to stimuli and results in stabilized, less excitable cell membranes. Increasing the activity of GABA, the major inhibitory neurotransmitter in the brain, and decreasing the activity of glutamate, the major excitatory neurotransmitter, also decrease nerve cell excitability. The actions of both sodium channel blockers (eg, phenytoin, oxcarbazepine) and GABA enhancers (eg, benzodiazepines and most of the newer AEDs) raise the amount of stimulation required to produce a seizure (called the *seizure threshold*). Overall, the drugs are thought to stabilize neuronal membranes and decrease neuronal firing in response to stimuli. Some seem able to suppress abnormal neuronal firing without suppressing normal neurotransmission.

## Indications for Use

The major clinical indication for AEDs is the prevention or treatment of seizures, especially the chronic recurring seizures of epilepsy. Indications for particular drugs depend on the types and severity of seizures involved. For example, most of the newer drugs are indicated for use with one or two other AEDs to treat more severe seizure disorders that do not respond to a single drug. However, oxcarbazepine is approved for monotherapy, and studies indicate that most of the other newer drugs may be effective as monotherapy in some types of seizures.

In addition to maintenance treatment of epilepsy, AEDs also are used to stop acute, tonic-clonic convulsions and status epilepticus. The drug of choice for this purpose is an intravenous (IV) benzodiazepine, usually lorazepam. Once acute seizure activity is controlled, a longer-acting drug, such as phenytoin or fosphenytoin, is given to prevent recurrence. AEDs also are used prophylactically in clients with brain trauma from injury or surgery.

In addition to treatment of seizure disorders, AEDs are used to treat bipolar disorder (eg, carbamazepine and valproate), although they are not approved by the U.S. Food and Drug Administration (FDA) for this purpose. They are also used in the management of chronic neuropathic pain, although few studies validate their effectiveness for this purpose. Carbamazepine is approved for treatment of the pain associated with trigeminal neuralgia. Gabapentin is also being used, but it is not approved for this indication and is not considered better than carbamazepine. Some of the newer AEDs are being tested for effectiveness in relation to bipolar, neuropathic pain, and other disorders. Because the drugs are being used for indications other than seizure disorders, some people suggest they be called neuromodulators or neurostabilizers rather than AEDs or anticonvulsants.

When an AED is started, a few weeks may be required to titrate the dosage and determine whether the chosen drug is effective in controlling seizures. Home care may be an essential component in the management of individuals taking AEDs. The nurse can play an important role by clinical assessment of the client, interviewing the family about the occurrence of seizures (a log of date, time, duration, and characteristics of seizures can be very helpful), and ensuring compliance with the prescribed regimen. Guidelines for ongoing evaluation and intervention are addressed in Home Care Considerations.

Seizure disorders are seen in children and commonly occur in older adults and require drug therapy. Age-specific considerations in the management of individuals taking AEDs are found in Age-related Considerations.

## Contraindications to Use

AEDs are contraindicated or must be used with caution in clients with CNS depression. Phenytoin, carbamazepine, gabapentin, lamotrigine, levetiracetam, oxcarbazepine, tiagabine, topiramate, and valproate are contraindicated

## Home Care Considerations: Use of Antiseizure Drugs

**ASSESS:** medication regime, serum drug levels, use of MedicAlert device, quality-of-life considerations.

**MONITOR:** client for compliance with the prescribed regimen, including driving restrictions as applicable; therapeutic and adverse drug effects, especially with changes in drugs or dosages; that client is keeping appointments for serum drug levels and follow-up care.

**EDUCATE:** how to use, store, and replace medications to ensure a constant supply. Discuss circumstances for which the client should seek emergency care. Stress the importance to women of consulting with health care provider if contemplating pregnancy (phenytoin and valproic acid have been associated with teratogenic effect). Reinforce additional teaching points (see Client Teaching Guidelines: Antiseizure Medications).

in clients who have experienced a hypersensitivity reaction to the particular drug (usually manifested by a skin rash, arthralgia, and other symptoms). Phenytoin, carbamazepine, ethosuximide, lamotrigine, topiramate, and zonisamide are contraindicated or must be used cautiously in clients with hepatic or renal impairment. Additional contraindications include phenytoin with sinus bradycardia or heart block; carbamazepine with bone marrow depression (eg, leukopenia, agranulocytosis); and tiagabine and valproic acid with liver disease. All of the drugs must be used cautiously during pregnancy because they are teratogenic in animals.

##  INDIVIDUAL ANTISEIZURE DRUGS

Most AEDs are well absorbed with oral administration and are usually given by this route. Most are metabolized in the liver; a few are eliminated mainly through the

## Age-related Considerations: Use of Antiseizure Drugs

### USE IN CHILDREN

Oral drugs are absorbed slowly and inefficiently in newborns. If an antiseizure drug is necessary during the first 7 to 10 days of life, IM phenobarbital is effective. Metabolism and excretion also are delayed during the first 2 weeks of life, but rates become more rapid than those of adults by 2 to 3 months of age. In infants and children, oral drugs are rapidly absorbed and have short half-lives. This produces therapeutic serum drug levels earlier in children than in adults. Rates of metabolism and excretion also are increased. Consequently, children require higher doses per kilogram of body weight than adults.

The rapid rate of drug elimination persists until approximately 6 years of age, then decreases until it stabilizes around the adult rate by age 10 to 14 years. Antiepileptic drugs (AEDs) must be used cautiously to avoid excessive sedation and interference with learning and social development.

There is little information about the effects of the newer AEDs in children. Most of the drugs (eg, gabapentin, lamotrigine, oxcarbazepine, tiagabine, and topiramate) are approved for use in children; levetiracetam and zonisamide are not approved for use in children. Oxcarbazepine is metabolized faster in children younger than 8 years of age; the rate of metabolism is similar to that in adults after 8 years. Several studies have indicated that oxcarbazepine is effective in monotherapy and combination therapy, with relatively few and mild adverse effects.

### USE IN OLDER ADULTS

Older adults often have multiple medical conditions, take multiple drugs, and have decreases in protein binding and liver and kidney function. As a result, older adults are at

high risk for adverse drug effects and adverse drug–drug interactions with AEDs. For example, reduced levels of serum albumin may increase the active portion of highly protein-bound AEDs (eg, phenytoin, valproic acid) and increase risk for adverse effects even when total serum drug concentrations are normal. Similarly, decreased elimination by the liver and kidneys may lead to drug accumulation, with subsequent risk for dizziness, impaired coordination, and injuries due to falls.

In addition to ataxia, confusion, dizziness, and drowsiness that may occur with most AEDs, older adults are more likely to develop some adverse effects associated with specific drugs. For example, with carbamazepine, they may develop hyponatremia, especially if they also take sodium-losing diuretics (eg, furosemide, hydrochlorothiazide) or cardiac dysrhythmias, especially if they have underlying heart disease. Older adults with preexisting heart disease should have a thorough cardiac evaluation before starting carbamazepine therapy. These effects may also occur with oxcarbazepine. With valproic acid, older adults may develop a tremor, which is difficult to diagnose because of its gradual onset and similarity to the tremor that occurs with Parkinson's disease. The tremor is often dose related and reverses when the drug is reduced in dosage or discontinued.

Most of these potential problems can be averted or minimized by using AEDs very cautiously in older adults. In general, small initial doses, slow titration to desired doses, and small maintenance doses are needed. Use of controlled-release formulations, when available, to minimize peak plasma concentrations may also be helpful. In addition, frequent assessment of clients for adverse effects and periodic monitoring of serum drug levels, liver function, and kidney function are indicated.

kidneys. Most produce ataxia (impaired muscular coordination, such as a staggering gait when trying to walk), confusion, dizziness, and drowsiness as common adverse effects; some may cause serious or life-threatening adverse effects such as cardiac dysrhythmias, bone marrow depression, or pancreatitis. Because the drugs are so diverse, they cannot be adequately discussed as groups. Consequently, the drugs are described individually; types of seizures for which the drugs are used and dosages are listed in Drugs at a Glance 11-1: Antiseizure Drugs.

*P* **Phenytoin** (Dilantin), the prototype, is one of the oldest and most widely used AEDs. It is often the initial drug of choice, especially in adults, and is highlighted in

*(text continues on page 201)*

**DRUG TABLE 11-1**

## *Drugs at a Glance*
## Antiseizure Drugs

| Generic/Trade Name | Types of Seizures Used to Treat | Routes and Dosage Ranges | Comments |
|---|---|---|---|
| **Carbamazepine** (Tegretol) Pregnancy Category D | Partial, generalized tonic-clonic, and mixed seizures | *Adults:* Epilepsy, PO, 200 mg twice daily, increased gradually to 600–1200 mg daily if needed, in 3 or 4 divided doses<br>Trigeminal neuralgia, PO, 200 mg daily, increased gradually to 1200 mg if necessary<br>*Children:* Epilepsy, >12 y: PO, 200 mg twice daily; may increase to 1000 mg daily for children 12–15 years and 1200 mg for children >15 y, if necessary<br>6–12 y: PO, 100 mg twice daily (tablet) or 50 mg 4 times daily (suspension), increase to 1000 mg daily if necessary, in 3 or 4 divided doses | Available in oral and chewable tablets, extended release tablets and capsules, and a suspension of 100 mg/5 mL<br>The suspension is absorbed more rapidly and produces higher peak drug levels than tablets<br>Therapeutic serum drug level is 4–12 mcg/mL (SI units, 17–51 μmol/L) |
| **Clonazepam** (Klonopin) Pregnancy Category D | Myoclonic or akinetic seizures, alone or with other AEDs; possibly effective in generalized tonic-clonic and psychomotor seizures | *Adults:* PO, 1.5 mg/d, increased by 0.5 mg/d every 3–7 days if necessary; maximum dose, 20 mg/d<br>*Children:* PO, 0.01–0.03 mg/kg/d, increased by 0.25–0.5 mg/d every 3–7 days if necessary; maximum dose, 0.2 mg/kg/d | Schedule IV drug |
| **Clorazepate** (Tranxene) Pregnancy Category D | Partial seizures, with other AEDs | *Adults:* PO, maximal initial dose 7.5 mg 3 times daily; increased by 7.5 mg every week, if necessary; maximum dose, 90 mg/d<br>*Children:* >12 y: PO, same as adults<br>9–12 y: PO, maximal initial dose 7.5 mg 2 times daily; increased by 7.5 mg every week, if necessary; maximum dose, 60 mg/d | Schedule IV drug |
| **Diazepam** (Valium) Pregnancy Category D | Acute convulsive seizures, status epilepticus | *Adults:* IV, 5–10 mg no faster than 2 mg/min; repeat every 5–10 min if needed; maximum dose, 30 mg<br>Repeat in 2–4 hours if necessary; maximum dose, 100 mg/24 h<br>*Children:* >30 d and <5 y: IV, 0.2–0.5 mg over 2–3 min, every 2–5 min up to a maximum of 5 mg<br>5 y and older: IV, 1 mg every 2–5 min up to a maximum of 10 mg. Repeat in 2–4 hours if necessary | Schedule IV drug<br>See Prototype Profile 8-1: Diazepam |

*(continued)*

**DRUG TABLE 11-1**

*Drugs at a Glance*

## Antiseizure Drugs (Continued)

| Generic/Trade Name | Types of Seizures Used to Treat | Routes and Dosage Ranges | Comments |
|---|---|---|---|
| **Ethosuximide** (Zarontin) Pregnancy Category C | Absence seizures; also may be effective in myoclonic and akinetic epilepsy | *Adults:* PO, initially 500 mg/d, increased by 250 mg weekly until seizures are controlled or toxicity occurs; maximum dose, 1500 mg/d<br>*Children:* PO, initially 250 mg/d, increased at weekly intervals until seizures are controlled or toxicity occurs; maximum dose, approximately 750–1000 mg/d | Available in oral capsules and syrup<br>Therapeutic serum drug level is 40–80 mcg/mL |
| **Fosphenytoin** (Cerebyx) Pregnancy Category D | Status epilepticus and short-term use in clients who cannot take oral phenytoin | *Adults:* Nonemergent seizures, IV, IM loading dose 10–20 mg PE/kg; maintenance dose 4–6 mg PE/kg/d; status epilepticus, IV, 15–20 mg PE/kg, at a rate of 100–150 mg PE/min<br>*Children:* Dosage not established | Much easier to give IV than phenytoin; can also be given IM |
| **Gabapentin** (Neurontin) Pregnancy Category C | Partial seizures, with other AEDs | *Adults:* PO, 900 mg daily, in 3 divided doses; increased up to 1800 mg/d if necessary. Intervals between doses should not exceed 12 h<br>Renal impairment: Crcl >60 mL/min, 400 mg 3 times daily (1200 mg/d); Crcl 30–60 mL/min, 300 mg 2 times daily (600 mg/d); Crcl 15–30 mL/min, 300 mg once daily; Crcl <15 mL/min, 300 mg every other day. For clients on hemodialysis, 200–300 mg after each 4 h of hemodialysis<br>*Children:* >12 y: PO, 900–1800 mg/d, in 3 divided doses (same as adults)<br>3–12 y: 10–15 mg/kg/d, in 3 divided doses, increased if necessary. Intervals between doses should not exceed 12 h | Does not cause significant drug–drug interactions |
| **Lamotrigine** (Lamictal) Pregnancy Category C | Partial seizures, with other AEDs<br>Lennox-Gastaut syndrome, with other AEDs | *Adults:* With AEDs other than valproic acid: PO, 50 mg once daily for 2 wk, then 50 mg twice daily (100 mg/d) for 2 wk, then increase by 100 mg/d at weekly intervals to a maintenance dose. Usual maintenance dose, 300–500 mg/d in 2 divided doses.<br>With AEDs including valproic acid: PO, 25 mg every other day for 2 wk, then 25 mg once daily for 2 wk, then increase by 25 to 50 mg/d every 1 to 2 wk to a maintenance dose. Usual maintenance dose, 100–150 mg/d in 2 divided doses<br>*Children:* 2–12 y: With enzyme-inducing AEDs, initially, PO, 0.15 mg/kg/d in 1 or 2 doses for 2 wk<br>If calculated dose is 2.5–5 mg, give 5 mg on alternate days for 2 wk, then 0.3 mg/kd/d in 1 or 2 doses, rounded to nearest 5 mg, for 2 wk<br>Maintenance dose, PO, 5–15 mg/kg/d in 2 divided doses | Valproic acid slows lamotrigine's metabolism by approximately 50%. If lamotrigine is combined with other AEDs plus valproic acid, dosage must be substantially reduced |

*(continued)*

**DRUG TABLE 11-1** *Drugs at a Glance*

## Antiseizure Drugs (Continued)

| Generic/Trade Name | Types of Seizures Used to Treat | Routes and Dosage Ranges | Comments |
|---|---|---|---|
| | | >12 y: With enzyme-inducing AEDs, initially, PO, 25 mg every other day for 2 wk, then 25 mg daily for 2 wk<br>Maintenance dose, PO, 100–400 mg daily in 1 or 2 divided doses<br>With valproic acid, PO, 50 mg daily for 2 wk, then 100 mg daily in 2 divided doses for 2 wk<br>Maintenance dose, PO, 300–500 mg daily in 1 or 2 doses | |
| **Levetiracetam** (Keppra)<br>Pregnancy Category C | Partial seizures, with other AEDs | *Adults:* PO, 500 mg twice daily initially, increased by 1000 mg/d every 2 wk, if necessary. Maximum dose, 3000 mg daily<br>Renal impairment: Crcl >80, 500–1500 mg; crcl 50–80, 500–1000 mg; crcl 30–50, 250–750 mg; crcl <30, 250–500 mg<br>End-stage renal disease, on hemodialysis, 500–1000 mg, with a supplemental dose of half the total daily dose (250–500 mg)<br>*Children:* Dosage not established | A newer drug that may have several advantages over older agents |
| **Lorazepam** (Ativan)<br>Pregnancy Category D | Acute convulsive seizures, status epilepticus | IV, 2–10 mg, diluted in an equal amount of sterile water for injection, 0.9% sodium chloride injection, or 5% dextrose in water, and injected over 2 min<br>*Children:* Dosage not established | Schedule IV Drug |
| **Oxcarbazepine** (Trileptal)<br>Pregnancy Category C | Partial seizures, as monotherapy or with other AEDs in adults, with other AEDs in children 4–16 years old | PO, 600 mg twice daily (1200 mg/d)<br>*Adults:* Severe renal impairment (Crcl <30 mL/min), PO, 300 mg twice daily (600 mg/d) and increased slowly until response achieved<br>*Children:* With other AEDs, PO, 8–10 mg/kg/d, not to exceed 600 mg twice daily. Titrate to reach target dose over 2 wk | A newer drug with possible advantages over older drugs<br>Available in 150-, 300-, and 600-mg scored tablets and a 60-mg/mL, fruit-flavored suspension |
| **Phenobarbital**<br>Pregnancy Category D | Generalized tonic-clonic and partial seizures | *Adults:* PO, 100–300 mg daily in 2 to 3 divided doses<br>*Children:* PO, 5 mg/kg daily in 2 to 3 divided doses | Serum drug levels of 10–25 mcg/mL are in the therapeutic range |
| **Phenytoin** (Dilantin) | See Prototype Profile 11-1: Phenytoin | | |
| **Tiagabine** (Gabitril)<br>Pregnancy Category C | Partial seizures, with other AEDs | *Adults:* PO, 4 mg daily for 1 wk, increased by 4–8 mg/wk until desired effect; maximum dose 56 mg/d in 2 to 4 divided doses<br>*Children:* 12–18 y: PO, 4 mg daily for 1 wk, increased to 8 mg/d in 2 divided doses for 1 wk; then increased by 4–8 mg/wk up to a maximum of 32 mg/d in 2 to 4 divided doses<br><12 y: not recommended | Most experience obtained in patients receiving at least one concomitant enzyme-inducing AED. Use in noninduced patients (eg, those receiving valproate monotherapy) may require lower doses or a slower dose titration |

*(continued)*

**DRUG TABLE 11-1**

## Drugs at a Glance

### Antiseizure Drugs (Continued)

| Generic/Trade Name | Types of Seizures Used to Treat | Routes and Dosage Ranges | Comments |
|---|---|---|---|
| **Topiramate** (Topamax) Pregnancy Category C | Partial seizures, with other AEDs | *Adults:* PO, 25–50 mg daily, increased by 25–50 mg per week until response. Usual dose, 400 mg daily in 2 divided doses<br>*Children:* 2–16 y: PO wk 1, 25 mg every PM, increase by 1–3 mg/kg/d at 1 or 2 wk intervals until response. Usual dose 5 to 9 mg/kg/d, in 2 divided doses | |
| **Valproic acid** (Depakene capsules); **sodium valproate** (Depakene syrup, Depacon injection); **divalproex sodium** (Depakote enteric-coated tablets) Pregnancy Category D | Absence, mixed, and complex partial seizures | *Adults:* PO, 10–15 mg/kg/d, increase weekly by 5–10 mg/kg/d, until seizures controlled, adverse effects occur, or the maximum dose (60 mg/kg/d) is reached. Give amounts >250 mg/d in divided doses. Usual daily dose, 1000–1600 mg, in divided doses<br>IV client's usual dose, diluted in 5% dextrose or 0.9% sodium chloride injection.<br>*Children:* PO, 15–30 mg/kg/d | Therapeutic serum levels are 50–100 mcg/mL (SI units, 350–700 μmol/L)<br>*Note:* Dosage ranges are the same for the different formulations; doses are in valproic acid equivalents.<br>Do not give IV >14 days; switch to oral product when possible. Several formulations of valproic acid are available in the United States. These products may contain valproic acid as the acid, as the sodium salt (sodium valproate), or a combination of the two (divalproex sodium) |
| **Zonisamide** (Zonegran) Pregnancy Category C | Partial seizures, with other AEDs | *Adults:* PO, 100–200 mg daily as a single dose or as 2–3 divided doses; increase by 100 mg/d every 1–2 wk if necessary; maximum dose, 600 mg daily<br>*Children:* <16 y: not recommended | |

AED, antiepileptic drug; IV, intravenous; PE, phenytoin equivalent; PO, oral; crcl, creatinine clearance.

Prototype Profile 11-1: Phenytoin. In addition to treatment of seizure disorders, it is sometimes used to treat cardiac dysrhythmias.

Phenytoin is available as a generic or trade-name capsule, a chewable tablet, an oral suspension, and an injectable solution. The injectable solution is highly irritating to tissues, and special techniques are required when the drug is given intravenously. *Clients should not switch between generic and trade-name formulations of phenytoin because of differences in absorption and bioavailability. If a client is stabilized on a generic formulation and switches to Dilantin, there is a risk for higher serum phenytoin levels and toxicity. If a client takes Dilantin and switches to a generic form, there is a risk for lower serum phenytoin levels, loss of therapeutic effectiveness, and seizures. There may also be differences in bioavailability among generic formulations manufactured by different companies.*

With renal impairment, protein binding is decreased, and the amount of free, active drug is higher than in clients with normal renal function.

**Fosphenytoin** (Cerebyx) is a prodrug formulation that is rapidly hydrolyzed to phenytoin after IV or IM injection. It is approved for treatment of status epilepticus and for short-term use in clients who cannot take oral phenytoin. In contrast to other preparations of injectable phenytoin, fosphenytoin causes minimal tissue irritation, can be diluted with 5% dextrose or 0.9% sodium chloride solution, and can be given intravenously more rapidly. The manufacturer recommends that all dosages be expressed in phenytoin equivalents (PE). Fosphenytoin is available in 2-mL and 10-mL vials with 50 mg PE/mL (fosphenytoin 50 mg PE = phenytoin 50 mg). For IV administration, fosphenytoin can be diluted to a concentration of 1.5 to 25 mg PE/mL and infused at a maximal rate of 150 mg PE/minute.

**Carbamazepine** (Tegretol) is used to treat, in addition to seizure disorders, trigeminal neuralgia and bipolar disorder. It is given orally, and peak blood levels are reached in about 1.5 hours with the liquid suspension, 4 to 5 hours with conventional tablets, and 3 to 12 hours

## PROTOTYPE PROFILE 11-1

### P Phenytoin (FEN i toyn)

### Drug Class
*Chemical:* Anticonvulsant, hydantoin, antiarrhythmic class Ib
*Functional:* Antiepileptic agent

### Trade Names
Dilantin, Phenytek

### Therapeutic Indications
Generalized tonic-clonic seizures (grand mal); complex partial seizures; prevention of seizures resulting from head trauma or neurosurgery

### Pharmacokinetics
*Absorption*
Oral: Slow

*Distribution*
Plasma protein binding: adults—90%–95%; neonates ≥80%; infants ≥85%
Decreased protein binding in disease states results in a decrease in albumin or decrease in affinity of phenytoin for serum albumin

*Metabolism*
Hepatic

*Excretion*
Urine (<5% unchanged)

### Pharmacodynamics
*Onset of Action*
IV: 0.5–1 h, immediate with loading dose
Time to peak: oral (extended release 4–12 h; immediate release 2–3 h)

*Duration*
Varies

### Contraindications/Precautions
*Contraindications*
Hypersensitivity to phenytoin/hydantoins; pregnancy

*Precautions*
IV: May cause hypotension; skin necrosis at site
Oral/IV: Impaired liver function; sinus bradycardia; SA block; AV block; caution in elderly and in patients with low serum albumin (increases pharmacologic response of phenytoin); porphyria
*Abrupt withdrawal may induce status epilepticus.*

### Pregnancy Considerations
Category D
Crosses placenta; cardiac defects and multiple malformations noted as "fetal hydantoin syndrome" have been reported
Consider benefit versus risk
Enters breast milk

### Dosage
Seizures: PO loading dose is 1000 mg divided into 3 doses given every 2 h (400 mg, 300 mg, 300 mg). Maintenance dose should begin 24 h after loading dose
Seizures (loading dose not necessary): 300–400 mg/d (initially in divided doses)
Antiarrhythmic: 50–100 mg IV every 10–15 minutes (maximum dose of 15 mg/kg with maximum rate of 50 mg/min)
Antineuralgic: 200–600 mg/day PO (divided doses)

### Adverse Effects
IV: Hypotension, bradycardia, cardiac arrhythmias, cardiovascular collapse, irritation/pain at site of infusion, thrombophlebitis

*Concentration-related effects (toxicity)*
Nystagmus, blurred vision, ataxia, slurred speech, dizziness, drowsiness, lethargy, nausea, vomiting, coma, rash, mood changes, folic acid depletion, hyperglycemia, gum tenderness, osteomalacia

*Adverse effects not related to concentration*
Gingival hyperplasia, carbohydrate intolerance, vitamin D deficiency, peripheral neuropathy, systemic lupus erythematosus, folic acid deficiency, osteomalacia

### Drug Interactions (consult pharmacist if of concern)
*Increased Effects*
Of phenytoin with isoniazid, cimetidine, chloramphenicol, valproic acid, nifedipine, omeprazole, ciprofloxacin, influenza vaccine and many others

*Decreased Effects*
Of oral contraceptives, antihistamines, anticoagulants, levodopa, furosemide, diazepam, theophylline, cyclosporine, dopamine, rifampin, quinidine, clozapine, methadone, and many others

### Herbal Supplements and Dietary Considerations
Evening primrose and borage decreases seizure threshold
Valerian, St. John's wort, kava kava, and gotu kula may increase central nervous system depression
Avoid or limit alcohol (inhibits phenytoin metabolism with acute use and stimulates metabolism with chronic use)
Tube feedings (decreased bioavailability)—hold 2 h before and 2 h after feeding; take on empty stomach with oral administration

with extended-release forms (tablets and capsules). It is metabolized in the liver to an active metabolite. Because it induces its own metabolism, its half-life shortens with chronic administration. Carbamazepine is contraindicated in clients with previous bone marrow depression or hypersensitivity to carbamazepine and in clients receiving monoamine oxidase inhibitors (MAOIs). MAOIs should be discontinued at least 14 days before carbamazepine is started.

**Clonazepam** (Klonopin), **clorazepate** (Tranxene), **diazepam** (Valium), and **lorazepam** (Ativan) are benzodiazepines (see Chap. 8) used in seizure disorders. Clonazepam and clorazepate are used in long-term treatment of seizure disorders, alone or with other AEDs. Tolerance to antiseizure effects develops with long-term use. Clonazepam has a long half-life and may require weeks of continued administration to achieve therapeutic serum levels. As with other benzodiazepines, clonazepam produces physical dependence and withdrawal symptoms. Because of clonazepam's long half-life, withdrawal symptoms may appear several days after administration is stopped. Abrupt withdrawal may precipitate seizure activity or status epilepticus.

Diazepam and lorazepam are used to terminate acute convulsive seizures, especially the life-threatening seizures of status epilepticus. Diazepam has a short duration of action and must be given in repeated doses. In status epilepticus, it is followed with a long-acting anticonvulsant, such as phenytoin. Lorazepam has become the drug of choice for status epilepticus because its effects last longer than those of diazepam.

**Ethosuximide** (Zarontin) is the AED of choice for absence seizures. It is well absorbed with oral administration and reaches peak serum levels in 3 to 7 hours; a steady-state serum concentration is reached in about 5 days. It is eliminated mainly by hepatic metabolism to inactive metabolites; about 20% is excreted unchanged through the kidneys. The elimination half-life is approximately 30 hours in children and 60 hours in adults. Ethosuximide may be used with other AEDs for treatment of mixed types of seizures.

**Gabapentin** (Neurontin) is used with other AEDs for treatment of partial seizures. It is 60% absorbed with usual doses, circulates largely in a free state because of minimal binding to plasma proteins, is not appreciably metabolized, and is eliminated by the kidneys as unchanged drug. The elimination half-life is 5 to 7 hours with normal renal function and up to 50 hours with impaired renal function, depending on creatinine clearance.

Adverse effects include dizziness, drowsiness, fatigue, loss of muscle coordination, tremor, nausea, vomiting, abnormal vision, gingivitis, and pruritus. Most adverse effects subside spontaneously or with dosage reduction. Gabapentin reportedly does not cause significant drug–drug interactions. Because the drug is eliminated only by the kidneys, dosage must be reduced in clients with renal impairment.

**Lamotrigine** (Lamictal) is used with other AEDs for treatment of partial seizures. It is thought to reduce the release of glutamate, an excitatory neurotransmitter, in the brain. It is well absorbed after oral administration, with peak plasma levels reached in 1.5 to 4.5 hours. Lamotrigine is about 55% bound to plasma proteins. It is metabolized in the liver to an inactive metabolite and eliminated mainly in the urine.

Adverse effects include dizziness, drowsiness, headache, ataxia, blurred or double vision, nausea and vomiting, and weakness. Because a serious skin rash may occur, especially in children, lamotrigine should not be given to children younger than 16 years of age and should be discontinued at the first sign of skin rash in an adult. Skin rash is more likely to occur with concomitant valproic acid therapy, high lamotrigine starting dose, and rapid titration rate. It may resolve if lamotrigine is discontinued, but it progresses in some clients to a more severe form, such as Stevens-Johnson syndrome.

Lamotrigine has little effect on the metabolism of other AEDs, but other AEDs affect lamotrigine's metabolism. Phenytoin, carbamazepine, and phenobarbital induce drug-metabolizing enzymes in the liver and accelerate lamotrigine's metabolism. Valproic acid inhibits those enzymes and thereby slows lamotrigine's metabolism by approximately 50%. If lamotrigine is combined with other AEDs plus valproic acid, the dosage must be substantially reduced. To discontinue, the dosage should be tapered over at least 2 weeks.

**Levetiracetam** (Keppra) is a newer drug approved for treatment of partial seizures, in combination with other AEDs. It is chemically unrelated to other AEDs, and its mechanism of action is unknown. It inhibits abnormal neuronal firing but does not affect normal neuronal excitability or function.

Levetiracetam is well and rapidly absorbed with oral administration; peak plasma levels occur in about 1 hour. Food reduces peak plasma levels by 20% and delays them to 1.5 hours, but does not affect the extent of drug absorption. The drug is minimally bound (10%) to plasma proteins and reaches steady-state plasma concentrations after 2 days of twice-daily administration. This rapid attainment of therapeutic effects is especially useful for clients with frequent or severe seizures.

Most of a dose (66%) is eliminated by the kidneys as unchanged drug. Dosage must be reduced with impaired renal function. The drug is not metabolized by the liver and does not affect the hepatic metabolism of other drugs. Thus, it has a low potential for drug interactions. It was well tolerated in clinical trials, and the incidence of adverse events was similar to that of placebo. Common adverse effects include drowsiness, dizziness, and fatigue; others include decreases in red and white blood cell counts, double vision, amnesia, anxiety, ataxia, emotional lability, hostility, nervousness, paresthesia, pharyngitis, and rhinitis.

Overall, levetiracetam has pharmacokinetic and other characteristics that may make it especially useful in clients who require combination antiepileptic drug therapy, who take drugs with increased potential for drug interactions, or who have impaired liver function.

**Oxcarbazepine** (Trileptal) is a newer drug that is structurally related to carbamazepine. It is approved for both monotherapy and adjunctive therapy (with other AEDs) in adults with partial seizures and for adjunctive therapy only in children. For clients receiving carbamazepine or oxcarbazepine, either drug may be substituted for the other without tapering the dose of one or gradually increasing the dose of the other. However, the equivalent dose of oxcarbazepine is 50% higher than the carbamazepine dosage. In older adults, the recommended equivalent oxcarbazepine dosage is 20% higher than the carbamazepine dosage.

The drug is well absorbed with oral administration, with peak plasma levels in about 5 hours. Most effects are attributed to an active metabolite produced during first-pass metabolism in the liver; the metabolite is 40% protein bound. The elimination half-life is 2 hours for oxcarbazepine and is 9 hours for the metabolite. The metabolite is conjugated with glucuronic acid in the liver and excreted in the urine, along with a small amount of unchanged drug. Dosage must be reduced in clients with severe renal impairment (ie, creatinine clearance less than 30 mL/min).

In clinical trials, adverse effects were similar in adult and pediatric clients and when oxcarbazepine was used alone or with other AEDs. They included cardiac dysrhythmias, drowsiness, dizziness, hypotension, nausea, vomiting, skin rash, and hyponatremia. Because of the risk for hyponatremia, oxcarbazepine should be used with caution in clients taking other drugs that decrease serum sodium levels, and serum sodium levels should be monitored periodically during maintenance therapy. Some studies indicate that skin reactions occur less often with oxcarbazepine than with carbamazepine.

Several drug–drug interactions may occur with oxcarbazepine. The drug inhibits cytochrome P450 2C19 enzymes and induces 3A4 enzymes to influence the metabolism of other drugs metabolized by these enzymes. For example, oxcarbazepine increases metabolism of estrogens and may decrease the effectiveness of oral contraceptives and postmenopausal estrogen replacement therapy. In addition, other drugs that induce cytochrome P450 enzymes, including phenytoin, may reduce plasma levels of the active metabolite by about one third; drugs that inhibit these enzymes (eg, cimetidine, erythromycin) do not significantly affect the elimination of oxcarbazepine or its metabolite.

**Phenobarbital** is a long-acting barbiturate that is used alone or with another AED (most often phenytoin). Its use has declined with the advent of other AEDs that cause less sedation and cognitive impairment. CNS depression and other adverse effects associated with barbiturates may occur, but drug dependence and barbiturate intoxication are unlikely with usual antiepileptic doses. Because phenobarbital has a long half-life (50 to 140 hours), it takes 2 to 3 weeks to reach therapeutic serum levels and 3 to

4 weeks to reach a steady-state concentration. It is metabolized in the liver; about 25% is eliminated unchanged in the urine. It induces drug-metabolizing enzymes in the liver and thereby accelerates the metabolism of most AEDs when given with them. Effects on other drugs begin 1 or 2 weeks after phenobarbital therapy is started.

**Tiagabine** (Gabitril), which may increase GABA levels in the brain, is used with other AEDs in clients with partial seizures. After oral administration, tiagabine is well absorbed; peak plasma levels occur in about 45 minutes if taken on an empty stomach and in 2.5 hours if taken with food. It is highly protein bound (96%) and is extensively metabolized in the liver, by the cytochrome P450 3A family of enzymes. Only 1% of the drug is excreted unchanged in the urine, and the metabolites are excreted in urine and feces. The elimination half-life is 4 to 7 hours in clients receiving enzyme-inducing AEDs (eg, phenytoin, carbamazepine). Clients with impaired liver function may need smaller doses because the drug is cleared more slowly. CNS effects (eg, confusion, drowsiness, impaired concentration or speech) are the most common adverse effects. GI upset and a serious skin rash may also occur.

**Topiramate** (Topamax), which has a broad spectrum of antiseizure activity, may act by increasing the effects of GABA and other mechanisms. It is rapidly absorbed and produces peak plasma levels in about 2 hours after oral administration. The average elimination half-life is about 21 hours, and steady-state concentrations are reached in about 4 days with normal renal function. It is 20% bound to plasma proteins. It is not extensively metabolized and is primarily eliminated unchanged through the kidneys. For clients with a creatinine clearance below 70 mL/minute, the dosage should be reduced by one half.

The most common adverse effects are ataxia, drowsiness, dizziness, and nausea. Renal stones may also occur. Interventions to help prevent renal stones include maintaining an adequate fluid intake, avoiding concurrent use of topiramate with other drugs associated with renal stone formation or increased urinary pH (eg, triamterene, zonisamide), and avoiding topiramate in people with conditions requiring fluid restriction (eg, heart failure) or a history of renal stones.

Additive CNS depression may occur with alcohol and other CNS depressant drugs.

**Valproic acid** preparations (Depakene, Depacon, Depakote) are chemically unrelated to other AEDs. They are thought to enhance the effects of GABA in the brain. They are also used to treat manic reactions in bipolar disorder and to prevent migraine headaches.

Valproic acid preparations are well absorbed after oral administration and produce peak plasma levels in 1 to 4 hours (15 minutes to 2 hours with the syrup). They are highly bound (90%) to plasma proteins. They are primarily metabolized in the liver, and metabolites are excreted through the kidneys.

These preparations produce less sedation and cognitive impairment than phenytoin and phenobarbital. Although they are uncommon, potentially serious adverse effects include hepatotoxicity and pancreatitis. The drugs are contraindicated in people who have had hypersensitivity reactions to any of the preparations and people with hepatic disease or impaired hepatic function.

Valproic acid (Depakene) is available in capsules; sodium valproate is a syrup formulation. Divalproex sodium (Depakote) contains equal parts of valproic acid and sodium valproate and is available as delayed-release tablets and sprinkle capsules. Depacon is an injectable formulation of valproate. Dosages of all formulations are expressed in valproic acid equivalents.

**Zonisamide** (Zonegran) is chemically a sulfonamide (and contraindicated for use in clients who are allergic to sulfonamides). It is approved for adjunctive treatment of partial seizures and may also be effective for monotherapy and generalized seizures. It is thought to act by inhibiting the entry of sodium and calcium ions into nerve cells.

Zonisamide is well absorbed with oral administration and produces peak plasma levels in 2 to 6 hours. It is 40% bound to plasma proteins and also binds extensively to red blood cells. Its elimination half-life is about 63 hours in plasma and more than 100 hours in red blood cells. It is metabolized by the cytochrome P450 3A enzymes and perhaps other pathways. It is excreted in the urine as unchanged drug (35%) and metabolites (65%). Clients with impaired renal function may require lower doses or a slower titration schedule.

Adverse effects include drowsiness, dizziness, ataxia, confusion, abnormal thinking, nervousness, and fatigue, which can be reduced by increasing the dosage gradually, over several weeks. There is also a risk for kidney stones, which is higher in clients with an inadequate fluid intake or who also take topiramate or triamterene. Skin rash, including the life-threatening Stevens-Johnson syndrome, has been observed.

Drugs that induce the cytochrome P450 enzymes (eg, carbamazepine, phenytoin) increase the metabolism of zonisamide and reduce its half-life. However, administration with cimetidine, which inhibits the cytochrome P450 enzymes, does not seem to inhibit zonisamide metabolism or increase its half-life. Zonisamide apparently does not induce or inhibit the cytochrome P450 enzymes and therefore has little effect on the metabolism of other drugs.

## ▓ MANAGEMENT CONSIDERATIONS

### Therapeutic Goal

Drug therapy is the main treatment of epilepsy for clients of all ages. The goal is to control seizure activity with minimal adverse drug effects. To meet this goal, therapy must be individualized. In most clients, treatment with a single AED is sufficient to meet this goal. In 20% to 30% of clients, however, two or more AEDs are required. In general, combination therapy is associated with more severe adverse effects, interactions between AEDs, poor compliance, and higher costs.

## Drug Selection

1. **Type of seizure** is a major factor. Therefore, an accurate diagnosis is essential before drug therapy is started. In general, AEDs with activity against both partial-onset and generalized seizures include lamotrigine, levetiracetam, topiramate, valproic acid, and zonisamide. Drugs considered most useful for partial seizures include carbamazepine, gabapentin, oxcarbazepine, phenobarbital, phenytoin, and tiagabine. For absence seizures, ethosuximide is the drug of choice; clonazepam and valproate are also effective. For mixed seizures, a combination of drugs is usually necessary.

   Guidelines for newer drugs are evolving as research studies are done and clinical experience with their use increases. Most of these agents are approved for combination therapy with other AEDs in clients whose seizures are not adequately controlled with a single drug. Oxcarbazepine is approved for monotherapy of partial seizures; some of the other drugs are also thought to be effective as monotherapy.

2. **Adverse drug effects** may be the deciding factor in choosing an AED because most types of seizures can be treated effectively by a variety of drugs. The use of carbamazepine and valproic acid increased largely because they cause less sedation and cognitive and psychomotor impairment than phenobarbital and phenytoin, although they may cause other potentially serious adverse effects. Most of the newer AEDs reportedly cause fewer adverse effects and are better tolerated than the older drugs, although they may also cause potentially serious adverse effects. Fewer and milder adverse effects can greatly increase a client's willingness to comply with the prescribed regimen and attain seizure control.

3. **Monotherapy versus combination therapy.** A single drug (monotherapy) is recommended when possible. If effective in controlling seizures, monotherapy has the advantages of fewer adverse drug effects, fewer drug–drug interactions, lower costs, and usually greater client compliance. If the first drug, in adequate dosage, fails to control seizures or causes unacceptable adverse effects, then another agent should be tried as monotherapy. Most practitioners recommend sequential trials of two to three agents as monotherapy before considering combination therapy.

   When substituting one AED for another, the second drug should be added and allowed to reach therapeutic blood levels before the first drug is gradually decreased in dosage and discontinued. This is not necessary when substituting oxcarbazepine for carbamazepine or vice versa because the drugs are similar.

   When monotherapy is ineffective, a second, and sometimes a third, drug may be added. If combination therapy is ineffective, the clinician may need to reassess the client for type of seizure, medical conditions or

*(text continues on page 208)*

# NURSING PROCESS

## Assessment

Assess client status in relation to seizure activity and other factors:

- If the client has a known seizure disorder and is taking antiseizure drugs, helpful assessment data can be obtained by interviewing the client. Some questions and guidelines include the following:
  - How long has the client had the seizure disorder?
  - How long has it been since seizure activity occurred, or what is the frequency of seizures?
  - Does any particular situation or activity precipitate a seizure?
  - How does the seizure affect the client? For example, what parts of the body are involved? Does he or she lose consciousness? Is he or she drowsy and tired afterward?
  - Which antiseizure drugs are taken? How do they affect the client? How long has the client taken the drugs? Is the currently ordered dosage the same as what the client has been taking? Does the client usually take the drugs as prescribed, or does he or she find it difficult to do so?
  - What other drugs are taken? This includes both prescription and nonprescription drugs, as well as those taken regularly or periodically. This information is necessary because many drugs interact with antiseizure drugs to decrease seizure control or increase drug toxicity.
  - What is the client's attitude toward the seizure disorder? Clues to attitude may include terminology, willingness or reluctance to discuss the seizure disorder, compliance or rejection of drug therapy, and others.
- Check reports of serum drug levels for abnormal values.
- Identify risk factors for seizure disorders. In people without previous seizure activity, seizure disorders may develop with brain surgery, head injury, hypoxia, hypoglycemia, drug overdosage (CNS stimulants, such as amphetamines or cocaine, or local anesthetics, such as lidocaine), and withdrawal from CNS depressants, such as alcohol and barbiturates.
- To observe and record seizure activity accurately, note the location (localized or generalized); specific characteristics of abnormal movements or behavior; duration; concomitant events, such as loss of consciousness and loss of bowel or bladder control; and postseizure behavior.
- Assess for risk of status epilepticus. Risk factors include recent changes in antiseizure drug therapy, chronic alcohol ingestion, use of drugs known to cause seizures, and infection.

## Nursing Diagnoses

- Ineffective Coping related to denial of the disease process and need for long-term drug therapy
- Deficient Knowledge: Disease process
- Deficient Knowledge: Drug effects
- Risk for Injury: Trauma related to ataxia, dizziness, confusion
- Risk for Injury: Seizure activity or drug toxicity
- Noncompliance: Underuse of medications

## Planning/Goals

*The client will:*

- Take medications as prescribed
- Experience control of seizures
- Avoid serious adverse drug effects
- Verbalize knowledge of the disease process and treatment regimen

- Avoid discontinuing antiseizure medications abruptly
- Keep follow-up appointments with health care providers

## Interventions

Use measures to minimize seizure activity. Guidelines include the following:

- Help the client identify conditions under which seizures are likely to occur. These precipitating factors, to be avoided or decreased when possible, may include ingestion of alcoholic beverages or stimulant drugs; fever; severe physical or emotional stress; and sensory stimuli, such as flashing lights and loud noises. Identification of precipitating factors is important because lifestyle changes (reducing stress, reducing alcohol and caffeine intake, increasing exercise, improving sleep and diet) and treatment of existing disorders can reduce the frequency of seizures.
- Assist the client in planning how to get enough rest and exercise and eat a balanced diet, if needed.
- Discuss the seizure disorder, the plan for treatment, and the importance of complying with prescribed drug therapy with the client and family members.
- Involve the client in decision making when possible.
- Inform the client and family that seizure control is not gained immediately when drug therapy is started. The goal is to avoid unrealistic expectations and excessive frustration while drugs and dosages are being changed in an effort to determine the best regimen for the client.
- Discuss social and economic factors that promote or prevent compliance.
- Protect a client experiencing a generalized tonic-clonic seizure by:
  - Placing a small pillow or piece of clothing under the head if injury could be sustained from the ground or floor.
  - Not restraining the client's movements; fractures may result.
  - Loosening tight clothing, especially around the neck and chest, to promote respiration.
  - Turning the client to one side so that accumulated secretions can drain from the mouth and throat when convulsive movements stop. The cyanosis, abnormal movements, and loss of consciousness that characterize a generalized tonic-clonic seizure can be quite alarming to witnesses. Most of these seizures, however, subside within 3 or 4 minutes, and the person starts responding and regaining normal skin color. If the person has one seizure after another (status epilepticus), has trouble breathing or continued cyanosis, or has sustained an injury, further care is needed, and a health care provider should be notified immediately.
- When risk factors for seizures, especially status epilepticus, are identified, try to prevent or minimize their occurrence.

## Evaluation

- Interview and observe for decrease in or absence of seizure activity.
- Interview and observe for avoidance of adverse drug effects, especially those that impair safety.
- When available, check laboratory reports of serum drug levels for therapeutic ranges or evidence of underdosing or overdosing.

## CLIENT TEACHING GUIDELINES
## Antiseizure Medications

### General Considerations

✔ Take the medications as prescribed. This is extremely important. These drugs must be taken regularly to maintain blood levels adequate to control seizure activity. At the same time, additional doses must not be taken because of increased risks of serious adverse reactions.

✔ Do not suddenly stop taking any antiseizure medication. Severe, even life-threatening, seizures may occur if the drugs are stopped abruptly.

✔ Discuss any problems (eg, seizure activity, excessive drowsiness, other adverse effects) associated with an antiseizure medication with the prescribing physician or other health care professional. Adjusting dosage or time of administration may relieve the problems.

✔ Do not drive a car, operate machinery, or perform other activities requiring physical and mental alertness when drowsy from antiseizure medications. Excessive drowsiness, decreased physical coordination, and decreased mental alertness increase the likelihood of injury.

✔ Do not take other drugs without the health care provider's knowledge and inform any other health care provider or dentist about taking antiseizure medications. There are many potential drug interactions in which the effects of the antiseizure drug or other drugs may be altered when drugs are given concomitantly.

✔ Do not take any other drugs that cause drowsiness, including over-the-counter antihistamines and sleep aids.

✔ Carry identification, such as a MedicAlert device, with the name and dose of the medication being taken. This is necessary for rapid and appropriate treatment in the event of a seizure, accidental injury, or other emergency situation.

✔ Notify your health care provider if you become pregnant or intend to become pregnant during therapy. Oxcarbazepine (Trileptal) decreases the effectiveness of oral contraceptive drugs.

✔ Notify your health care provider if you are breast-feeding or intend to breast-feed during therapy.

### Self-administration

✔ Take most antiseizure medications with food or a full glass of fluid. This will prevent or decrease nausea, vomiting, and gastric distress, which are adverse reactions to most of these drugs. Levetiracetam (Keppra), oxcarbazepine (Trileptal), topiramate (Topamax), and zonisamide (Zonegran) may be taken with or without food.

✔ When taking generic phenytoin or the Dilantin brand of phenytoin:

1. Do not switch from a generic to Dilantin, or vice versa, without discussing with the prescribing health care provider. There are differences in formulations that may upset seizure control and cause adverse effects.

2. Ask your health care provider if you should take (or give a child) supplements of folic acid, calcium, vitamin D, or vitamin K. These supplements may help to prevent some adverse effects of phenytoin.

3. Brush and floss your teeth and have regular dental care to prevent or delay a gum disorder called gingival hyperplasia.

4. If you have diabetes, you may need to check your blood sugar more often or take a higher dose of your antidiabetic medication. Phenytoin may inhibit the release of insulin and increase blood sugar.

5. Notify your health care provider or another health care professional if you develop a skin rash, severe nausea and vomiting, swollen glands, bleeding, swollen or tender gums, yellowish skin or eyes, joint pain, unexplained fever, sore throat, unusual bleeding or bruising, persistent headache, or any indication of infection or bleeding, and if you become pregnant.

6. If you are taking phenytoin liquid suspension or giving it to a child, mix it thoroughly immediately before use and measure it with a calibrated medicine cup or a measuring teaspoon. Do not use regular teaspoons because they hold varying amounts of medication.

✔ If you are taking oxcarbazepine liquid suspension or giving it to a child, mix it thoroughly immediately before use. Measure it with the syringe supplied by the manufacturer and squirt the medication directly into the mouth. Store the suspension at room temperature and use the bottle within 7 weeks or discard the amount remaining. It is helpful to write the date opened and the expiration date on the container.

✔ With valproic acid, the regular capsule should not be opened and the tablet should not be crushed for administration. The sprinkle capsule may be opened and the contents sprinkled on soft food for administration. The syrup formulation may be diluted in water or milk but should not be mixed in carbonated beverages.

✔ Swallow tablets or capsules of valproic acid (Depakene or Depakote) whole; chewing or crushing may cause irritation of the mouth and throat.

✔ Taking valproic acid at bedtime may reduce dizziness and drowsiness.

✔ Lamotrigine may cause photosensitivity. When outdoors, wear protective clothing and sunscreen.

✔ If taking lamotrigine, notify the health care provider immediately if a skin rash or decreased seizure control develops.

drug–drug interactions that aggravate the seizure disorder or decrease the effectiveness of AEDs, and compliance with the prescribed drug therapy regimen.

4. **Dosage forms** may increase seizure control, client convenience, and compliance. For example, extended-release or long-acting dosage forms can maintain more consistent serum drug levels and decrease frequency of administration. Most of the AEDs are available in oral tablets or capsules; a few are available as oral liquids or injectable solutions.

5. **Cost** should be considered because this may be a major factor in client compliance. Although the newer drugs are generally effective and better tolerated than older agents, they are also quite expensive. Costs, which depend on manufacturers' wholesale prices and pharmacies' markups, as well as prescribed dose amounts and other factors, may vary among pharmacies and change over time. However, the following lists of costs per month allow comparisons among AEDs and may be useful in clinical practice. Costs of older drugs are as follows: carbamazepine, $54 to $81; ethosuximide, $105 to $158; phenobarbital, $2 to $5; phenytoin, $26 to $35; and valproate, $80 to $280. Costs of newer drugs are as follows: gabapentin, $139 to $354; lamotrigine, $196 to $289; levetiracetam, $105 to $315; oxcarbazepine, $97 to $358; tiagabine, $99 to $190; topiramate, $88 to $354; and zonisamide, $100 to $201. When possible, prescribers can encourage compliance by choosing drugs that are covered by clients' insurance plans or, for uninsured clients, choosing less expensive drug therapy regimens.

6. **Pregnancy risk.** Sexually active adolescent girls and women of child-bearing potential who require an AED must be evaluated and monitored very closely because all of the drugs are considered teratogenic. In general, infants exposed to one AED have a significantly higher risk for birth defects than those not exposed, and infants exposed to two or more AEDs have a significantly higher risk than those exposed to one AED.

## Drug Dosage

The dosage of most drugs is determined empirically by observation of seizure control and adverse effects.

1. Usually, larger doses are needed for a single drug than for multiple drugs; for people with a large body mass (assuming normal liver and kidney function); and in cases involving trauma, surgery, and emotional stress.

2. Smaller doses are usually required when liver disease is present and when multiple drugs are being given. Smaller doses of gabapentin, levetiracetam, and topiramate must be given in the presence of renal impairment, and smaller doses of lamotrigine must be given when combined with valproic acid and another AED.

3. For most drugs, initial doses are relatively low; doses are gradually increased until seizures are controlled or adverse effects occur. Then, doses may be lowered to the minimum effective level, to decrease adverse effects. Adverse effects are more likely to occur during initiation of treatment, and if treatment is started too aggressively, clients may be unwilling to continue a particular medication even if doses are reduced in amount or frequency of administration.

   When one AED is being substituted for another, dosage of the one being added is gradually increased while the one being discontinued is gradually decreased. The first drug is usually stopped when therapeutic effects or therapeutic serum drug levels of the second drug are attained.

   When an AED is being discontinued, its dosage should always be tapered gradually, usually over 1 to 3 months. Abruptly stopping an AED may exacerbate seizures or cause status epilepticus.

4. When fosphenytoin is substituted for oral phenytoin, the same total daily dosage (in PE) may be given intravenously or intramuscularly.

5. For clients receiving carbamazepine or oxcarbazepine therapy, either agent may be substituted for the other without gradual reduction or titration of the dose. For most clients, the equivalent oxcarbazepine dosage is 50% higher than the carbamazepine dosage. When switching between agents in older adults, the recommended equivalent oxcarbazepine dosage is 20% higher than the carbamazepine dosage.

6. Dosages of most AEDs must be reduced with renal impairment. With phenytoin, for example, protein binding is decreased, and the amount of free, active drug is higher than in clients with normal renal function. The use of phenobarbital in clients with severe renal impairment requires markedly reduced dosage, close monitoring of plasma drug levels, and frequent observation for toxic effects. Smaller doses of gabapentin, levetiracetam, oxcarbazepine, topiramate, and zonisamide must be given because these drugs are eliminated primarily through the kidneys. Dosage of oxcarbazepine should be decreased by 50% in clients with creatinine clearance of less than 30 mL/minute. Zonisamide should not be given to clients with renal failure and should be discontinued in clients who develop acute renal failure or increased serum creatinine and blood urea nitrogen during therapy. Elimination of tiagabine is not significantly affected by renal

insufficiency, renal failure, or hemodialysis, and dose adjustment for renal dysfunction is not necessary. Renal stones have been reported with topiramate and zonisamide.

7. Tiagabine is cleared more slowly in clients with liver impairment. Increased plasma levels of unbound tiagabine, increased elimination half-life, and increased frequency of neurologic adverse effects (eg, ataxia, dizziness, drowsiness, tremor) have been observed in clients with mild and moderate hepatic insufficiency. Doses may need to be reduced or given at less frequent intervals. Topiramate may also be cleared more slowly, even though it is eliminated mainly through the kidneys and does not undergo significant hepatic metabolism. It should be used with caution in the presence of hepatic impairment. Valproic acid is a hepatotoxic drug and contraindicated for use in hepatic impairment. No dosage adjustment is indicated with levetiracetam, oxcarbazepine, or zonisamide.

## Monitoring Antiepileptic Drug Therapy

1. The effectiveness of drug therapy is evaluated primarily by client response in terms of therapeutic or adverse effects.

2. Periodic measurements of serum drug levels are recommended, especially when multiple AEDs are being given. This helps to document blood levels associated with particular drug dosages, seizure control, or adverse drug effects; to assess and document therapeutic failures; to assess for drug malabsorption or client noncompliance; to guide dosage adjustments; and to evaluate possible drug-related adverse effects.

   To be useful, serum drug levels must be interpreted in relation to clinical responses because there are wide variations among clients receiving similar doses, probably owing to differences in hepatic metabolism. In other words, doses should not be increased or decreased solely to maintain a certain serum drug level. In addition, the timing of blood samples in relation to drug administration is important. For routine monitoring, blood samples should generally be obtained in the morning, before the first daily dose of an AED.

3. Several antiseizure drugs have the potential for causing blood, liver, or kidney disorders. For this reason, it is usually recommended that baseline blood studies (complete blood count, platelet count) and liver function tests (eg, bilirubin, serum protein, aspartate aminotransferase) be performed before drug therapy starts and periodically thereafter.

4. When drug therapy fails to control seizures, there are several possible causes. A common one is the client's failure to take the antiseizure drug as prescribed. Other causes include incorrect diagnosis of the type of seizure, use of the wrong drug for the type of seizure, inadequate drug dosage, and too-

frequent changes or premature withdrawal of drugs. Additional causes may include drug overdoses (eg, theophylline) and severe electrolyte imbalances (eg, hyponatremia) or use of alcohol or recreational drugs.

## Duration and Discontinuation of Therapy

Antiseizure drug therapy may be discontinued for some clients, usually after a seizure-free period of at least 2 years. Although opinions differ about whether, when, and how the drugs should be discontinued, studies indicate that medications can be stopped in approximately two thirds of clients whose epilepsy is completely controlled with drug therapy. Advantages of discontinuation include avoiding adverse drug effects and decreasing costs; disadvantages include recurrence of seizures, with possible status epilepticus. Even if drugs cannot be stopped completely, periodic attempts to decrease the number or dosage of drugs are probably desirable to minimize adverse reactions. Discontinuing drugs, changing drugs, or changing dosage must be done gradually over 2 to 3 months for each drug and with close medical supervision because sudden withdrawal or dosage decreases may cause status epilepticus. Only one drug should be reduced in dosage or gradually discontinued at a time.

## ■ DRUG USE IN SPECIFIC SITUATIONS

### Drug Therapy for Status Epilepticus

An IV benzodiazepine (eg, lorazepam 0.1 mg/kg at 2 mg/minute) is the drug of choice for rapid control of tonic-clonic seizures. However, seizures often recur unless the benzodiazepine is repeated or another, longer-acting drug is given, such as IV phenytoin (20 mg/kg at 50 mg/minute) or fosphenytoin (20 mg/kg phenytoin equivalents at 150 mg/minute). Further treatments are based on the client's response to these medications. Because there is a risk for significant respiratory depression with IV benzodiazepines, personnel and supplies for emergency resuscitation must be readily available.

### Toxicity of Antiseizure Drugs: Recognition and Management

Signs and symptoms of overdose and toxicity are usually extensions of known adverse effects. Severe overdoses disturb vital functions (eg, CNS depression with confusion, impaired consciousness and possible coma, respiratory depression; cardiovascular problems such as dysrhythmias and hypotension) and are life threatening. Fatalities have been reported with most antiseizure drugs. If toxicity is suspected, a serum drug level is indicated for those drugs with established therapeutic ranges. There are no specific antidotes, and treatment is symptomatic and supportive (ie, gastric lavage and activated charcoal, if indicated, to prevent absorption of additional drug). An endotracheal tube should be inserted before lavage, to prevent aspiration. Activated charcoal is not effective in adsorbing topiramate and is not recommended for topiramate overdose. Hemodialysis is effective in removing drugs that are poorly bound to plasma proteins and that are excreted mainly or partly by the kidneys (eg, gabapentin, levetiracetam, topiramate, valproate). Vital signs, electrocardiogram, level of consciousness, pupillary reflexes, and urine output should be monitored.

## Effects of Antiepileptic Drugs on Non–antiepileptic Drugs

Antiepileptic drugs may have clinically significant interactions with many non-AEDs. Because the drugs depress the CNS and cause drowsiness, their combination with any other CNS depressant drugs may cause excessive sedation and other adverse CNS effects. They may also decrease the effects of numerous other drugs, mainly by inducing drug-metabolizing enzymes in the liver. Enzyme induction means the affected drugs are metabolized and eliminated more quickly. In some cases, larger doses of the affected drugs are needed to achieve therapeutic effects.

*Phenytoin* reduces the effects of cardiovascular drugs (eg, amiodarone, digoxin, disopyramide, dopamine, mexiletine, quinidine), female sex hormones (estrogens, oral contraceptives, levonorgestrel), adrenal corticosteroids, antipsychotic drugs (eg, phenothiazines, haloperidol), oral antidiabetic agents (eg, sulfonylureas), doxycycline, furosemide, levodopa, methadone, and theophylline. With acetaminophen, phenytoin decreases therapeutic effects but may increase the risk for hepatotoxicity by accelerating production of the metabolite that damages the liver. The consequence of increasing metabolism of oral contraceptives may be unintended pregnancy; the consequence of decreasing the effects of sulfonylureas may be greater difficulty in controlling blood sugar levels in diabetic clients who require both drugs.

*Carbamazepine* reduces the effects of tricyclic antidepressants, oral anticoagulants, oral contraceptives, bupropion, cyclosporine, doxycycline, felodipine, and haloperidol. The effects on acetaminophen are the same as those of phenytoin (see above).

*Topiramate* decreases effects of digoxin and oral contraceptives.

Few interactions have been reported with the newer drugs. *Levetiracetam* does not induce or inhibit hepatic metabolism of drugs, and risk for interactions are minimal. *Oxcarbazepine* decreases effectiveness of felodipine and oral contraceptives (a barrier type of contraception is recommended during oxcarbazepine therapy). *Zonisamide* interacts with other AEDs, but no interactions have been reported with non-AEDs. More interactions with these drugs may be observed with longer clinical use.

*(text continues on page 214)*

## Nursing Actions
### Antiseizure Drugs

| Nursing Actions | Rationale/Explanation |
| --- | --- |
| 1. Administer accurately. | |
| a. Give on a regular schedule about the same time each day. | To maintain therapeutic blood levels of drugs |
| b. Give most oral antiseizure drugs after meals or with a full glass of water or other fluid; levetiracetam, oxcarbazepine, topiramate, and zonisamide may be taken with or without food. | Most antiseizure drugs cause some gastric irritation, nausea, or vomiting. Taking the drugs with food or fluid helps decrease gastrointestinal side effects. |
| c. To give phenytoin: | |
| (1) Shake oral suspensions of the drug vigorously before pouring and always use the same measuring equipment. | In *suspensions*, particles of drug are suspended in water or other liquid. On standing, drug particles settle to the bottom of the container. Shaking the container is necessary to distribute drug particles in the liquid vehicle. If the contents are not mixed well every time a dose is given, the liquid vehicle will be given initially, and the concentrated drug will be given later. That is, underdosage will occur at first, and little if any therapeutic benefit will result. Overdosage will follow, and the risks of serious toxicity are greatly increased. Using the same measuring container ensures consistent dosage. Calibrated medication cups or measuring teaspoons or tablespoons are acceptable. Regular household teaspoons and tablespoons used for eating and serving are not acceptable because sizes vary widely. |

*(continued)*

## Nursing Actions
### Antiseizure Drugs (Continued)

| Nursing Actions | Rationale/Explanation |
|---|---|
| (2) Do not mix parenteral phenytoin in the same syringe with any other drug. | Phenytoin solution is highly alkaline (pH approximately 12) and physically incompatible with other drugs. A precipitate occurs if mixing is attempted. |
| (3) Give phenytoin as an undiluted (IV) bolus injection at a rate not exceeding 50 mg/min, then flush the IV line with normal saline or dilute in 50–100 mL of normal saline (0.9% NaCl) and administer over approximately 30–60 minutes. If "piggybacked" into a primary IV line, the primary IV solution must be normal saline or the line must be flushed with normal saline before and after administration of phenytoin. An in-line filter is recommended. | Phenytoin cannot be diluted or given in IV fluids other than normal saline because it precipitates within minutes. Slow administration and dilution decrease local venous irritation from the highly alkaline drug solution. Rapid administration must be avoided because it may produce myocardial depression, hypotension, cardiac arrhythmias, and even cardiac arrest. |
| d. To give IV fosphenytoin: | |
| (1) Check the prescriber's order and the drug concentration carefully. | The dose is expressed in phenytoin equivalents (PE; fosphenytoin 50 mg PE = phenytoin 50 mg). |
| (2) Dilute the dose in 5% dextrose or 0.9% sodium chloride solution to a concentration of 1.5 mg PE/mL to 25 mg PE/mL and infuse no faster than 150 mg PE/min. | The drug is preferably diluted in the pharmacy and labeled with the concentration and duration of the infusion. For a 100-mg PE dose, diluting with 4 mL yields the maximum concentration of 25 mg PE/mL; this amount could be infused in about 1 min at the maximal recommended rate. A 1-g loading dose could be added to 50 mL of 0.9% sodium chloride and infused in approximately 10 min at the maximal recommended rate. |
| (3) Consult a pharmacist or the manufacturer's literature if any aspect of the dose or instructions for administration are unclear. | To avoid error |
| e. To give carbamazepine and phenytoin suspensions by nasogastric (NG) feeding tube, dilute with an equal amount of water, and rinse the NG tube before and after administration. | Absorption is slow and decreased, possibly because of drug adherence to the NG tube. Dilution and tube irrigation decrease such adherence. |
| f. To give oxcarbazepine suspension, use the 10-mL oral dosing syringe provided by the manufacturer with each bottle. Also check expiration date. | For accurate measurement and a reminder that the suspension is given orally only. The suspension is stored at room temperature and must be used within 7 weeks after opening the bottle. |
| 2. Observe for therapeutic effects. | |
| a. When the drug is given on a long-term basis to prevent seizures, observe for a decrease in or absence of seizure activity. | Therapeutic effects begin later with antiseizure drugs than with most other drug groups because the antiseizure drugs have relatively long half-lives. Optimum therapeutic benefits of phenytoin occur approximately 7–10 days after drug therapy is started. |
| b. When the drug is given to stop an acute convulsive seizure, seizure activity usually slows or stops within a few minutes. | IV lorazepam is the drug of choice for controlling an acute convulsion. |
| 3. Observe for adverse effects. | |
| a. Central nervous system (CNS) effects—ataxia, dizziness, drowsiness, double vision | These effects are common, especially during the first week or two of drug therapy. |
| b. Gastrointestinal effects—anorexia, nausea, vomiting | These common effects of oral drugs can be reduced by taking the drugs with food or a full glass of water. |
| c. Hypersensitivity reactions—often manifested by skin disorders such as rash, urticaria, exfoliative dermatitis, Stevens-Johnson syndrome (a severe reaction accompanied by headache, arthralgia, and other symptoms in addition to skin lesions) | These may occur with almost all the antiseizure drugs. Some are mild; some are potentially serious but rare. These skin reactions are usually sufficient reason to discontinue the drug. About 25–30% of patients with allergic reactions to carbamazepine are likely to be allergic to oxcarbazepine. |

*(continued)*

## Nursing Actions

### Antiseizure Drugs (Continued)

| Nursing Actions | Rationale/Explanation |
|---|---|
| d. Blood dyscrasias—anemia, leukopenia, thrombocytopenia, agranulocytosis | Most antiseizure drugs decrease blood levels of folic acid, which may progress to megaloblastic anemia. The other disorders indicate bone marrow depression and are potentially life threatening. They do not usually occur with phenytoin, but may infrequently occur with most other antiseizure drugs. |
| e. Respiratory depression | This is not likely to be a significant adverse reaction except when a depressant drug, such as lorazepam, is given IV to control acute seizures, such as status epilepticus. Even then, respiratory depression can be minimized by avoiding overdosage and rapid administration. |
| f. Liver damage—hepatitis symptoms, jaundice, abnormal liver function test results | Hepatic damage may occur with phenytoin, and fatal hepatotoxicity has been reported with valproic acid. |
| g. Gingival hyperplasia | Occurs often with phenytoin, especially in children. It may be prevented or delayed by vigorous oral hygiene. |
| h. Hypocalcemia | May occur when antiseizure drugs are taken in high doses and over long periods |
| i. Hyponatremia | May occur with carbamazepine and oxcarbazepine, especially if taken concurrently with sodium-losing diuretics (eg, furosemide, hydrochlorothiazide). Usually transient and levels return to normal with fluid restriction or dose reduction. |
| j. Lymphadenopathy resembling malignant lymphoma | This reaction has occurred with several antiseizure drugs, most often with phenytoin. |
| k. Pancreatitis | Life-threatening pancreatitis has occurred after short- and long-term therapy with valproic acid. Patients should be monitored for the development of acute abdominal pain, nausea, and vomiting. |
| l. Kidney stones | May occur with topiramate and zonisamide. Inadequate fluid intake or concurrent administration of triamterene may increase risk. |
| **4. Observe for drug interactions.** | |
| a. Drugs that *increase* effects of antiseizure drugs: | |
| (1) CNS depressants—alcohol, sedating antihistamines, benzodiazepines, opioid analgesics, sedatives | Additive CNS depression |
| (2) Most other antiseizure drugs | Additive or synergistic effects. The drugs are often given in combination, to increase therapeutic effects. |
| b. Drugs that *decrease* effects of antiseizure drugs: | |
| (1) Tricyclic antidepressants, antipsychotic drugs | These drugs may lower the seizure threshold and precipitate seizures. Dosage of antiseizure drugs may need to be increased. |
| (2) Carbemazepine, phenytoin, and other enzyme inducers | These drugs inhibit themselves and other antiseizure drugs by activating liver enzymes and accelerating the rate of drug metabolism. |
| c. Additional drugs that alter effects of phenytoin and fosphenytoin: | |
| (1) Alcohol (acute ingestion), allopurinol, amiodarone, benzodiazepines, chlorpheniramine, cimetidine, fluconazole, fluoxetine, isoniazid, metronidazole, miconazole, omeprazole, paroxetine, sertraline, and trimethoprim increase effects. | These drugs *increase* phenytoin toxicity by inhibiting hepatic metabolism of phenytoin or by displacing it from plasma protein-binding sites. |
| (2) Alcohol (chronic ingestion), antacids, antineoplastics, folic acid, pyridoxine, rifampin, sucralfate, and theophylline decrease effects. | These drugs *decrease* effects of phenytoin by decreasing absorption, accelerating metabolism, or by unknown mechanisms. |

*(continued)*

## Nursing Actions

## Antiseizure Drugs (Continued)

| Nursing Actions | Rationale/Explanation |
|---|---|
| (3) Phenobarbital has variable interactions with phenytoin. | Phenytoin and phenobarbital have complex interactions with unpredictable effects. Although phenobarbital induces drug metabolism in the liver and may increase the rate of metabolism of other anticonvulsant drugs, its interaction with phenytoin differs. Phenobarbital apparently decreases serum levels of phenytoin and perhaps its half-life. Still, the anticonvulsant effects of the two drugs together are greater than those of either drug given alone. The interaction apparently varies with dosage, route, time of administration, the degree of liver enzyme induction already present, and other factors. Thus, whether a significant interaction will occur in a client is unpredictable. Probably the most important clinical implication is that close observation of the client is necessary when either drug is being added or withdrawn. |
| d. Additional drugs that alter effects of carbamazepine:<br>(1) Cimetidine, clarithromycin, diltiazem, erythromycin, isoniazid, valproic acid, and verapamil increase effects. | Most of these drugs inhibit the cytochrome P450 enzymes (1A2, 2C8, and/or 3A4 groups) that normally metabolize carbamazepine, thereby increasing blood levels of carbamazepine. Valproic acid inhibits an epoxide hydrolase enzyme and causes an active metabolite to accumulate. Toxicity may result even if carbamazepine blood levels are at therapeutic concentrations. |
| (2) Alcohol, phenytoin, and phenobarbital decrease effects. | These drugs increase activity of hepatic drug-metabolizing enzymes, thereby decreasing blood levels of carbamazepine. |
| e. Drugs that alter the effects of gabapentin:<br>(1) Antacids | Reduce absorption of gabapentin. Gabapentin should be given at least 2 hours after a dose of an antacid to decrease interference with absorption. |
| f. Drugs that alter effects of lamotrigine:<br>(1) Valproic acid increases effects. | Valproic acid inhibits the liver enzymes that metabolize lamotrigine, thereby increasing blood levels and slowing metabolism of lamotrigine. As a result, lamotrigine dosage must be substantially reduced when the drug is given in a multidrug regimen that includes valproic acid. |
| (2) Carbamazepine, phenytoin, and phenobarbital decrease effects. | These drugs induce drug-metabolizing enzymes in the liver and thereby increase the rate of metabolism of themselves and of lamotrigine. |
| g. Drugs that decrease effects of oxcarbazepine<br>(1) Phenobarbital, phenytoin, valproic acid, verapamil | These drugs induce drug-metabolizing enzymes in the liver and thereby increase the metabolism and hasten the elimination of oxcarbazepine. |
| h. Drug that increases the effects of phenobarbital:<br>(1) Valproic acid | May increase plasma levels of phenobarbital as much as 40%, probably by inhibiting liver metabolizing enzymes. |
| i. Additional drugs that increase effects of valproate:<br>(1) Cimetidine | Inhibits drug-metabolizing enzymes, thereby slowing elimination from the body and increasing blood levels of valproic acid |
| (2) Salicylates | Displace valproic acid from binding sites on plasma proteins, thereby increasing the serum level of unbound valproic acid |
| j. Drugs that decrease effects of zonisamide<br>(1) Carbamazepine, phenytoin, phenobarbital | These drugs induce drug-metabolizing enzymes in the liver and thereby increase the metabolism and hasten the elimination of zonisamide. |
| k. Interactions with clonazepam, lorazepam, and diazepam | These drugs are benzodiazepines, discussed in Chapter 8. |

## ? How Can You Avoid This Medication Error?

**Answer:** Blood levels need to remain within a therapeutic range to prevent seizures. Even missing two doses could affect this level. Frequently, surgery patients are permitted to take medications with a sip of water, even when they are NPO. Good judgment requires a nurse to check with the health care provider when significant medications are withheld.

## Critical Thinking Exercises

1. A health care provider prescribes carbamazepine (Tegretol) for tonic-clonic seizures. After 1 month, the client's serum level is 18 mcg/mL. The nurse interprets this level as:
   a. Subtherapeutic
   b. Within normal limits, but in the lower range
   c. Within normal limits, but in the upper range
   d. Toxic

2. A 50 kg client is brought to the emergency department by EMS with seizures. The health care provider orders lorazepam (Ativan), 5 mg IV initially. For which type of seizure is diazepam the drug of choice?
   a. Partial seizure
   b. Tonic-clonic seizure
   c. Absence seizure
   d. Status epilepticus

3. A child is started on phenytoin (Dilantin) after experiencing his first seizure. A teaching plan for the child and family should include strategies to reduce what common side effect?
   a. Hypoglycemia
   b. Photosensitivity
   c. Gingival hyperplasia
   d. Hyponatremia

4. The use of valproate sodium (Depakene) is limited because of which adverse reaction?
   a. Nausea
   b. Sedation
   c. Muscle tremors
   d. Hepatotoxicity

5. A client receiving phenytoin therapy develops nystagmus. The nurse recognizes that the development of this condition is likely:
   a. A sign of toxicity
   b. Unrelated to the phenytoin therapy
   c. An indication that serum levels are subtherapeutic
   d. A normal finding in clients receiving phenytoin

## SELECTED REFERENCES

Alldredge, B. K. (2000). Seizure disorders. In E. T. Herfindal & D. R. Gourley (Eds.), *Textbook of therapeutics: Drug and disease management* (7th ed., pp. 1107–1137). Philadelphia: Lippincott Williams & Wilkins.

Bourdet, S. V., Gidal, B. E., & Alldredge, B. K. (2001). Pharmacologic management of epilepsy in the elderly. *Journal of the American Pharmaceutical Association, 41*(3), 421–436.

Buck, M. L. (2001). Oxcarbazepine use in children and adolescents. *Pediatric Pharmacotherapy, 7*(11), 711–716. [On-line.] Available: http://pediatrics.medscape.com/UVA/PedPharm/2001/v07.n11/pp0711.01.buck/pp0711.01.buck-01.html. Accessed September 2003.

Delgado-Escueta, A. V. (2000). Approach to the patient with seizures. In H. D. Humes (Ed.), *Kelley's textbook of internal medicine* (4th ed., pp. 2865–2876). Philadelphia: Lippincott Williams & Wilkins.

*Drug facts and comparisons.* (Updated monthly). St. Louis: Facts and Comparisons.

Hovinga, C. A. (2001). Levetiracetam: A novel antiepileptic drug. *Pharmacotherapy, 21*(11), 1375–1388.

Kim, R. B. (Ed.) (2001). *Handbook of adverse drug interactions.* New Rochelle, New York: The Medical Letter, Inc.

Lacy, C. F., Armstrong, L. L., Goldman, M. P., & Lance, L. L. (2003). *Lexi-Comp's drug information handbook* (11th ed.). Hudson, OH: American Pharmaceutical Association.

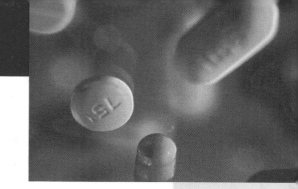

# 12

# Antiparkinson Drugs

## OBJECTIVES

*After studying this chapter, the student will be able to:*

1 Describe major characteristics of Parkinson's disease.

2 Differentiate between the types of commonly used antiparkinson drugs.

3 Identify therapeutic and adverse effects of dopaminergic and anticholinergic drugs.

4 Discuss the use of antiparkinson drugs in special populations.

5 Apply the nursing process with clients experiencing Parkinson's disease.

## CRITICAL THINKING SCENARIO

*R*ichard Rodgers was diagnosed with Parkinson's disease 1 week ago. His symptoms include slow, shuffling gait; stooped posture; fine tremor at rest; and masklike facial expression. His health care provider started him on levodopa, 500 mg PO three times daily, and benztropine (Cogentin), 1 mg at bedtime. You are a home health nurse visiting Mr. Rodgers.

✔ How can Parkinson's disease affect Mr. Rodgers' ability to function normally?

✔ How does each medication work to restore the balance of neurotransmitters?

✔ What assessment data will you collect to evaluate whether the antiparkinson medications are effective?

✔ What assessment data should be collected to detect adverse effects of antiparkinson drugs?

## PROTOTYPE PROFILE

**levodopa** (Larodopa, Dopar), p. 217

# PARKINSON'S DISEASE

Parkinson's disease (also called *parkinsonism*) is a chronic, progressive, degenerative disorder of the central nervous system (CNS) characterized by abnormalities in movement and posture (tremor, bradykinesia, joint and muscular rigidity). It occurs equally in men and women, usually between 50 and 80 years of age. Classic parkinsonism probably results from destruction or degenerative changes in dopamine-producing nerve cells. The cause of the nerve cell damage is unknown; age-related degeneration, genetics, and exposure to toxins (eg, carbon monoxide, organophosphate pesticides) are possible etiologic factors. Early-onset parkinsonism (before 45 years of age) is thought to have a genetic component. Signs and symptoms of the disease also may occur with other CNS diseases, brain tumors, and head injuries and with the use of typical or traditional antipsychotic drugs (eg, phenothiazines). Use of the newer "atypical" antipsychotic drugs may reduce the incidence of drug-induced parkinsonism. Discussion of the pathophysiology associated with this condition is described in At the Foundation: Parkinson's Disease.

# ANTIPARKINSON DRUGS

Drugs used in Parkinson's disease increase levels of dopamine (levodopa, dopamine agonists, monoamine oxidase [MAO] inhibitors, catechol-*O*-methyltransferase [COMT] inhibitors) or inhibit the actions of acetylcholine (anticholinergic agents) in the brain. Thus, the drugs help adjust the balance of neurotransmitters.

## Dopaminergic Drugs

Levodopa, carbidopa, amantadine, bromocriptine, pergolide, pramipexole, ropinirole, selegiline, entacapone, and tolcapone increase dopamine concentrations in the brain and exert dopaminergic activity, directly or indirectly. ⓟ **Levodopa** is the mainstay of drug therapy for idiopathic parkinsonism and serves as the prototype (see Prototype Profile 12-1: Levodopa). Carbidopa is used only in conjunction with levodopa. The other drugs are used as adjunctive agents, usually with levodopa.

## Anticholinergic Drugs

Anticholinergic drugs are discussed in Chapter 19 and are described here only in relation to their use in the treatment of Parkinson's disease. Only anticholinergic drugs that are centrally active (ie, those that penetrate the blood–brain barrier) are useful in treating parkinsonism. Atropine and scopolamine are centrally active but are not used because of a high incidence of adverse reactions. In addition to the primary anticholinergic drugs, an antihistamine (diphenhydramine) is used for parkinsonism because of its strong anticholinergic effects.

## Mechanisms of Action

Dopaminergic drugs increase the amount of dopamine in the brain by various mechanisms. Amantadine increases dopamine release and decreases dopamine reuptake by presynaptic nerve fibers. Bromocriptine, pergolide, pramipexole, and ropinirole are dopamine agonists that directly stimulate postsynaptic dopamine receptors. Levodopa is a precursor substance that is converted to dopamine. Selegiline blocks one of the enzymes (MAO-B) that normally inactivates dopamine. Entacapone and tolcapone block another enzyme (COMT) that normally inactivates dopamine and levodopa. Anticholinergic drugs decrease the effects of acetylcholine. This decreases the apparent excess of acetylcholine in relation to the amount of dopamine.

## Indications for Use

Entacapone, levodopa, pergolide, pramipexole, ropinirole, selegiline, and tolcapone are indicated for the treatment of idiopathic or acquired parkinsonism; carbidopa is used only to decrease peripheral breakdown of levodopa. Some of the other drugs have additional uses. For example, amantadine is also used to prevent and treat influenza A viral infections. Bromocriptine is also used in the treatment of amenorrhea and galactorrhea associated with hyperprolactinemia.

Anticholinergic drugs are used in idiopathic parkinsonism to decrease salivation, spasticity, and tremors. They are used primarily for people who have minimal symptoms or who cannot tolerate levodopa, or in combination with other antiparkinson drugs. Anticholinergic agents also are used to relieve symptoms of parkinsonism

**AT THE FOUNDATION:** *Neurotransmitter Imbalance*

The basal ganglia in the brain normally contain substantial amounts of the neurotransmitters dopamine and acetylcholine. The correct balance of dopamine and acetylcholine is important in regulating posture, muscle tone, and voluntary movement. Individuals with Parkinson's disease have an imbalance in these neurotransmitters, due to a lack of dopamine, resulting in a decrease in inhibitory brain dopamine and a relative increase in excitatory acetylcholine. Imbalances of other neurotransmitters (eg, gamma aminobutyric acid [GABA], glutamate, norepinephrine, and serotonin) also occur.

## PROTOTYPE PROFILE 12-1

### P Levodopa (lee voe DOE pa)

**Drug Class**
*Chemical:* Dopamine Agonist
*Functional:* Anti-Parkinson's Agent

**Trade Names**
Dopar; Larodopa

**Therapeutic Indications**
Treatment of Parkinson's disease

**Pharmacokinetics**
*Absorption*
Decreased absorption possible with a meal high in protein

*Distribution*
Total protein binding is minimal
Distributes to cerebrospinal fluid/brain in small amounts

*Metabolism*
Converted to dopamine by peripheral decarboxylation. Small amounts will reach the brain and be converted to active dopamine.

*Excretion*
Urine

**Pharmacodynamics**
*Onset of Action*
Time to peak (serum) 1–2 h; elimination half-life 1.3–2.3 h

*Duration*
Variable (typically, 6–12 hours)

**Contraindications/Precautions**
*Contraindications*
Hypersensitivity to levodopa; narrow-angle glaucoma; use of MAO inhibitors within previous 14 days (with selectivity for MAO type B). Levodopa may be administered concurrently with the manufacturer's recommended dosing); history of melanoma; undiagnosed skin lesions

*Precautions*
Cardiovascular disease; myocardial infarction, arrhythmias; pulmonary disease; psychosis; peptic ulcer disease; wide-angle glaucoma; renal, hepatic, endocrine disease. May cause or worsen dyskinesias

**Pregnancy Considerations**
Category C

**Dosage**
Oral: 500–1000 mg/d in divided doses (typically, every 6–12 hours). Maximum dose is 8000 mg/d. May increase by 100–750 mg/d every 3–7 days until a response is observed

**Adverse Effects**
Orthostatic hypotension, arrhythmias, hypertension, palpitations, dizziness, confusion, anxiety, nightmares, chest pain, hallucinations, decreased mental acuity, memory impairment, delusions, euphoria, somnolence, insomnia, gait abnormalities, nervousness, psychosis, anorexia, nausea, vomiting, constipation, GI bleed, diarrhea, urinary frequency, agranulocytosis, thrombocytopenia, discoloration of urine and sweat, hiccups

**Drug Interactions**
*Increased Effects*
MAO inhibitors (may result in hypertensive reactions)
*Decreased Effects*
Antipsychotics (may inhibit antiparkinsonian effects), benzodiazepines, phenytoin, pyridoxine, tacrine. Iron binds levodopa (separate doses)

**Herbal Supplements and Dietary Considerations**
Pyridoxine may decrease effectiveness; avoid ethanol; high protein foods may inhibit the effectiveness of levodopa

---

that can occur with the use of antipsychotic drugs. If used for this purpose, a course of therapy of approximately 3 months is recommended because symptoms usually subside by then even if the antipsychotic drug is continued.

## Contraindications to Use

Levodopa is contraindicated in clients with narrow-angle glaucoma, hemolytic anemia, severe angina pectoris, transient ischemic attacks, or a history of melanoma or undiagnosed skin disorders, and in clients taking MAO inhibitor drugs. In addition, levodopa must be used with caution in clients with severe cardiovascular, pulmonary, renal, hepatic, or endocrine disorders. Bromocriptine and pergolide are ergot derivatives and therefore are contraindicated in people hypersensitive to ergot alkaloids

and in those with uncontrolled hypertension. Selegiline, entacapone, and tolcapone are contraindicated in people with hypersensitivity reactions to the drugs. Tolcapone is contraindicated in people with impaired liver function.

Anticholinergic drugs are contraindicated in clients with glaucoma, gastrointestinal obstruction, prostatic hypertrophy, urinary bladder neck obstruction, and myasthenia gravis. The drugs must be used cautiously in clients with cardiovascular disorders (eg, tachycardia, dysrhythmias, hypertension) and liver or kidney disease.

## Management Considerations

### Goals of Treatment
The goals of antiparkinson drug therapy are to control symptoms, maintain functional ability in activities of

daily living, minimize adverse drug effects, and slow disease progression.

## Drug Selection

Choices of antiparkinson drugs depend largely on the type of parkinsonism (idiopathic or drug induced) and the severity of symptoms. In addition, because of difficulties with levodopa therapy (eg, adverse effects, loss of effectiveness in a few years, possible acceleration of the loss of dopaminergic neurons in the brain), several drug therapy strategies and combinations are used to delay the start of levodopa therapy and, once started, to reduce levodopa dosage.

1. For drug-induced parkinsonism or extrapyramidal symptoms, an anticholinergic agent is the drug of choice.

2. For early idiopathic parkinsonism, when symptoms and functional disability are relatively mild, several drugs may be used as monotherapy.
   - An anticholinergic agent may be the initial drug of choice in clients younger than 60 years of age, especially when tremor is the major symptom. An anticholinergic relieves tremor in approximately 50% of clients.
   - Amantadine may be useful in relieving bradykinesia or tremor.
   - A dopamine agonist may improve functional disability related to bradykinesia, rigidity, impaired physical dexterity, impaired speech, shuffling gait, and tremor.

3. For advanced idiopathic parkinsonism, a combination of medications is used. Two advantages of combination therapy are better control of symptoms and reduced dosage of individual drugs.
   - An anticholinergic agent may be given with levodopa alone or with a levodopa/carbidopa combination.
   - Amantadine may be given in combination with levodopa or other antiparkinson agents.
   - A dopamine agonist is usually given with levodopa/carbidopa. The combination provides more effective relief of symptoms and allows lower dosage of levodopa. Although all four of the available dopamine agonists are similarly effective, the newer agents (pramipexole and ropinirole) may cause fewer or less severe adverse effects than bromocriptine and pergolide.
   - The levodopa/carbidopa combination is probably the most effective drug when bradykinesia and rigidity become prominent. However, because levodopa becomes less effective after approximately 5 to 7 years, many clinicians use other drugs first and reserve levodopa for use when symptoms become more severe.
   - Selegiline may be given with levodopa/carbidopa. Although evidence is limited and opinions differ, selegiline may have a neuroprotective effect and slow the loss of dopaminergic neurons in the brain.
   - Entacapone is used only with levodopa/carbidopa. However, in contrast to amino acid decarboxylase (AADC) inhibitors, which increase the bioavailability of levodopa without increasing its plasma half-life, simultaneous administration of COMT and AADC inhibitors significantly increases the plasma half-life of levodopa. Tolcapone should be used only when other drugs are ineffective, because of its association with liver failure.
   - Selegiline and entacapone may both be used with levodopa/carbidopa because entacapone acts peripherally, and selegiline acts in the brain. Inhibition of levodopa-dopamine metabolism is a valuable addition to levodopa as an exogenous source of dopamine.

4. When changes are made in a drug therapy regimen, one change at a time is recommended so that effects of the change are clear.

## Drug Dosage

The dosage of antiparkinson drugs is highly individualized. The general rule is to start with a low initial dose and gradually increase the dosage until therapeutic effects, adverse effects, or maximum drug dosage is achieved. Age specific considerations are also important in the dosing and are highlighted in Age-related Considerations. Additional guidelines include the following:

1. The optimal dose is the lowest one that allows the client to function adequately. Optimal dosage may not be established for 6 to 8 weeks with levodopa.

2. Doses need to be adjusted as parkinsonism progresses.

3. Dosage must be individualized for levodopa and carbidopa. Only 5% to 10% of a dose of levodopa reaches the CNS, even with the addition of carbidopa. When carbidopa is given with levodopa, the dosage of levodopa must be reduced by approximately 75%. A daily dose of approximately 70 to 100 mg of carbidopa is required to saturate peripheral amino acid decarboxylase.

   A levodopa/carbidopa combination is available in three dosage formulations (10 mg carbidopa/100 mg levodopa, 25 mg carbidopa/100 mg levodopa, and 25 mg carbidopa/250 mg levodopa) of immediate-release tablets (Sinemet) and two dosage formulations (25 mg carbidopa/100 mg levodopa, 50 mg carbidopa/200 mg levodopa) of sustained-release tablets (Sinemet CR). Various preparations can be mixed to administer optimal amounts of each ingredient. Sinemet CR is not as well absorbed as the short-acting form, and a client being transferred to Sinemet CR needs a dosage increase of approximately one third.

4. With levodopa, dosage should be gradually increased to the desired therapeutic level. In addition, thera-

## Age-related Considerations: Use of Antiparkinson Drugs

### USE IN CHILDREN

Safety and effectiveness for use in children have not been established for most antiparkinson drugs, including the centrally acting anticholinergics (all ages), levodopa (<12 years), and bromocriptine (<15 years). However, anticholinergics are sometimes given to children who have drug-induced extrapyramidal reactions.

Because parkinsonism is a degenerative disorder of adults, antiparkinson drugs are most likely to be used for other purposes in children. Amantadine for influenza A prevention or treatment is not recommended for neonates or infants younger than 1 year of age but may be given to children 9 to 12 years of age.

### USE IN OLDER ADULTS

Dosage of amantadine may need to be reduced because the drug is excreted mainly through the kidneys, and renal function is usually decreased in older adults. Dosage of levodopa/carbidopa may need to be reduced because of an age-related decrease in peripheral AADC, the enzyme that carbidopa inhibits.

Anticholinergic drugs may cause blurred vision, dry mouth, tachycardia, and urinary retention. They also decrease sweating and may cause fever or heatstroke. Fever may occur in any age group, but heatstroke is more likely to occur in older adults, especially with cardiovascular disease, strenuous activity, and high environmental temperatures. When centrally active anticholinergics are given for Parkinson's disease, agitation, mental confusion, hallucinations, and psychosis may occur. In addition to the primary anticholinergics, many other drugs have significant anticholinergic activity. These include some antihistamines, including those in over-the-counter cold remedies and sleep aids; tricyclic antidepressants; and phenothiazine antipsychotic drugs. When an anticholinergic is needed by an older adult, dosage should be minimized, combinations of drugs with anticholinergic effects should be avoided, and clients should be closely monitored for adverse drug effects.

Older clients are at increased risk for hallucinations with dopamine agonist drugs. In addition, pramipexole dosage may need to be reduced in older adults with impaired renal function.

peutic effects may be increased and adverse effects decreased by frequent administration of small doses.

5. With pramipexole and ropinirole, dosage is started at low levels and gradually increased over several weeks. When the drugs are discontinued, they should be tapered in dosage over 1 week. With pramipexole, lower doses are indicated in older adults and those with renal impairment; with ropinirole, lower doses may be needed with hepatic impairment.

6. When combinations of drugs are used, dosage adjustments of individual components are often necessary. When levodopa is added to a regimen of anticholinergic drug therapy, for example, the anticholinergic drug need not be discontinued or reduced in dosage. However, when a dopaminergic drug is added to a regimen containing levodopa/carbidopa, dosage of levodopa/carbidopa must be reduced.

## ◼ INDIVIDUAL ANTIPARKINSON DRUGS

Dopaminergic antiparkinson drugs are described in this section; names, routes, and dosage ranges are listed in Drugs at a Glance 12-1: Antiparkinson Drugs.

**Levodopa** (Larodopa, Dopar) is the most effective drug available for the treatment of Parkinson's disease. It relieves all major symptoms, especially bradykinesia and rigidity. Although levodopa does not alter the underlying disease process, it may improve a client's quality of life.

Levodopa acts to replace dopamine in the basal ganglia of the brain. Dopamine cannot be used for replacement therapy because it does not penetrate the blood–brain barrier. Levodopa readily penetrates the CNS and is converted to dopamine by the enzyme AADC. The dopamine is stored in presynaptic dopaminergic neurons and functions like endogenous dopamine. In advanced stages of Parkinson's disease, there are fewer dopaminergic neurons and thus less storage capacity for dopamine derived from levodopa. As a result, levodopa has a shorter duration of action, and drug effects "wear off" between doses.

In peripheral tissues (eg, liver, kidney, gastrointestinal tract), levodopa is extensively metabolized by decarboxylase, whose concentration is greater in peripheral tissues than in the brain. It is metabolized to a lesser extent by the enzyme COMT. Consequently, most levodopa is metabolized in peripheral tissues, and large amounts are required to obtain therapeutic levels of dopamine in the brain. Peripheral metabolism of levodopa can be reduced (and the amounts reaching the brain can be increased) by giving the AADC inhibitor, carbidopa. The combination of levodopa and carbidopa greatly increases the amount of available levodopa, so that the levodopa dosage can be reduced by approximately 70%. The two drugs are usually given together in a fixed-dose formulation called Sinemet. When carbidopa inhibits the decarboxylase pathway of levodopa metabolism, the COMT pathway becomes more important (see entacapone and tolcapone, COMT inhibitors, below).

Levodopa is well absorbed from the small intestine after oral administration, but absorption is decreased by

**DRUG TABLE 12-1**

*Drugs at a Glance*

## Antiparkinson Drugs

| Generic/Trade Name | Routes and Dosage Ranges | Comments |
|---|---|---|
| *Dopaminergic Agents* | | |
| **Levodopa** (Larodopa) | See Prototype Profile: Levodopa | |
| **Carbidopa** (Lodosyn) Pregnancy Category C | PO, 70–100 mg/d, depending on dosage of levodopa; maximum dose, 200 mg/d | Has no effects without levodopa |
| **Levodopa/carbidopa** (Sinemet) Pregnancy Category C | *Clients not receiving levodopa:* PO 1 tab of 25 mg carbidopa/100 mg levodopa 3 times daily or 1 tab of 10 mg carbidopa/100 mg levodopa 3 or 4 times daily, increased by 1 tab every day or every other day until a dosage of 8 tablets daily is reached. Sinemet CR, PO, 1 tab twice daily at least 6 h apart initially, increased up to 8 tab daily and q4h intervals if necessary *Clients receiving levodopa:* Discontinue levodopa at least 8 h before starting Sinemet. PO, 1 tab of 25 mg carbidopa/250 mg levodopa 3 or 4 times daily for clients taking >1500 mg levodopa or 1 tab of 25 mg carbidopa/100 mg levodopa for clients taking <1500 mg levodopa | Sustained release products should not be crushed Should take on an empty stomach, if possible |
| **Amantadine** (Symmetrel) Pregnancy Category C | PO, 100 mg twice a day | If insomnia occurs, give 2nd dose several hours before bedtime |
| **Bromocriptine** (Parlodel) Pregnancy Category B | PO, 1.25 mg twice a day with meals, increased by 2.5 mg/d every 2–4 wk if necessary for therapeutic benefit | Reduce dose gradually if severe adverse effects occur |
| **Entacapone** (Comtan) Pregnancy Category C | PO, 200 mg with each dose of levodopa/carbidopa, up to 8 times (1600 mg) daily | Change in color of urine may occur (clinically irrelevant) |
| **Pergolide** (Permax) Pregnancy Category B | PO, 0.05–0.1 mg/d at bedtime, increased by 0.05–0.15 mg every 3 d to a maximum dose of 6 mg/d if necessary | Monitor closely for orthostasis (drop in blood pressure when assuming an upright position) and drowsiness |
| **Pramipexole** (Mirapex) Pregnancy Category C | PO wk 1, 0.125 mg 3 times daily; wk 2, 0.25 mg 3 times daily; wk 3, 0.5 mg 3 times daily; wk 4, 0.75 mg 3 times daily; wk 5, 1 mg 3 times daily; wk 6, 1.25 mg 3 times daily; wk 7, 1.5 mg 3 times daily Renal impairment: Creatinine clearance (Crcl) > 60 mL/min, 0.125 mg 3 times daily initially, up to a maximum of 1.5 mg 3 times daily; Crcl 35–59 mL/min, 0.125 mg 2 times daily initially, up to a maximum of 1.5 mg 2 times daily; Crcl 15–34 mL/min, 0.125 mg once daily, up to a maximum of 1.5 mg once daily | Can cause significant drowsiness; avoid alcohol |

*(continued)*

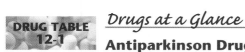

**DRUG TABLE 12-1**

*Drugs at a Glance*

## Antiparkinson Drugs (Continued)

| Generic/Trade Name | Routes and Dosage Ranges | Comments |
|---|---|---|
| **Ropinirole** (Requip) Pregnancy Category C | PO wk 1, 0.25 mg 3 times daily; wk 2, 0.5 mg 3 times daily; wk 3, 0.75 mg 3 times daily; wk 4, 1 mg 3 times daily | Hallucinations can occur, especially in elderly |
| **Selegiline** (Eldepryl) Pregnancy Category C | PO, 5 mg twice daily, morning and noon | Should not be a problem with tyramine-containing products within usual doses |
| **Tolcapone** (Tasmar) Pregnancy Category C | PO, 100–200 mg 3 times daily; maximum dose, 600 mg daily | Reports of fatal liver injury limit recommended usage for individuals who have not responded therapeutically to other treatments |
| *Anticholinergic Agents* | | |
| **Benztropine** (Cogentin) Pregnancy Category C | PO, 0.5–1 mg at bedtime initially, gradually increased to 4–6 mg daily if necessary | Use with caution in hot weather and with exercise Alcohol may increase CNS depression |
| **Biperiden** (Akineton) Pregnancy Category C | Parkinsonism, PO 2 mg 3–4 times daily Drug-induced extrapyramidal reactions, PO, 2 mg 1–3 times daily, IM 2 mg repeated q30min if necessary to a maximum of 8 mg in 24 h | |
| **Diphenhydramine** (Benadryl) Pregnancy Category B | PO, 25 mg 3 times daily, gradually increased to 50 mg 4 times daily if necessary *Adults:* Drug-induced extrapyramidal reactions, IM, IV 10–50 mg; maximal single dose, 100 mg; maximal daily dose, 400 mg *Children:* Drug-induced extrapyramidal reactions, IM 5 mg/kg per day; maximal daily dose, 300 mg | Observe for tolerance of anticholinergic effects |
| **Procyclidine** (Kemadrin) Pregnancy Category C | PO, 5 mg twice daily initially, gradually increased to 5 mg 3–4 times daily if necessary | Do not discontinue drug abruptly; avoid alcohol |
| **Trihexyphenidyl** (Trihexy) Pregnancy Category C | PO, 1–2 mg daily initially, gradually increased to 12–15 mg daily, until therapeutic or adverse effects occur *Adults:* Drug-induced extrapyramidal reactions, PO 1 mg initially, gradually increased to 5–15 mg daily if necessary | May tolerate best if given in 3 doses daily with food |

delayed gastric emptying, hyperacidity of gastric secretions, and competition with amino acids (from digestion of protein foods) for sites of absorption in the small intestine. Levodopa is metabolized to 30 or more metabolites, some of which are pharmacologically active and probably contribute to drug toxicity; the metabolites are excreted primarily in the urine, usually within 24 hours.

Because of side effects and recurrence of parkinsonian symptoms after a few years of levodopa therapy, levodopa is often reserved for clients with significant symptoms and functional disabilities. In addition to treating Parkinson's disease, levodopa also may be useful in other CNS disorders in which symptoms of parkinsonism occur (eg, juvenile Huntington's chorea, chronic manganese poisoning). Levodopa relieves only parkinsonian symptoms in these conditions.

**Carbidopa** (Lodosyn) inhibits the enzyme AADC. As a result, less levodopa is decarboxylated in peripheral tissues; more levodopa reaches the brain, where it is decarboxylated to dopamine; and much smaller doses of levodopa can be given. Carbidopa does not penetrate the blood–brain barrier. Although carbidopa is available alone, it is most often given in a levodopa/carbidopa fixed-dose combination product called Sinemet.

**Amantadine** (Symmetrel) is a synthetic antiviral agent initially used to prevent infection from influenza A virus. Amantadine increases the release and inhibits the reuptake of dopamine in the brain, thereby increasing dopamine levels. The drug relieves symptoms rapidly, within 1 to 5 days, but it loses efficacy with approximately 6 to 8 weeks of continuous administration. Consequently, it is usually given for 2- to 3-week periods during initiation of drug therapy with longer-acting agents (eg, levodopa), or when symptoms worsen. Amantadine is often given in conjunction with levodopa. Compared with other antiparkinson drugs, amantadine is considered less effective than levodopa but more effective than anticholinergic agents.

Amantadine is well absorbed from the gastrointestinal tract and has a relatively long duration of action. It is excreted unchanged in the urine. Dosage must be reduced with impaired renal function to avoid drug accumulation.

**Bromocriptine** (Parlodel) and **pergolide** (Permax) are ergot derivatives that directly stimulate dopamine receptors in the brain. They are used in the treatment of idiopathic Parkinson's disease, with levodopa/carbidopa, to prolong effectiveness and allow reduced dosage of levodopa. Pergolide has a longer duration of action than bromocriptine and may be effective in some clients unresponsive to bromocriptine. Adverse effects are similar for the two drugs.

**Entacapone** (Comtan) and **tolcapone** (Tasmar) are COMT inhibitors. COMT plays a role in brain metabolism of dopamine and metabolizes approximately 10% of peripheral levodopa. By inhibiting COMT, entacapone and tolcapone increase levels of dopamine in the brain and relieve symptoms more effectively and consistently. Although the main mechanism of action seems to be inhibiting the metabolism of levodopa in the bloodstream, the drugs may also inhibit COMT in the brain and prolong the activity of dopamine at the synapse. These drugs are used only in conjunction with levodopa/carbidopa, and dosage of levodopa must be reduced.

Entacapone is well absorbed with oral administration and reaches a peak plasma level in 1 hour. It is highly protein bound (98%), has a half-life of about 2.5 hours, and is metabolized in the liver to an inactive metabolite. Dosage must be reduced by 50% in the presence of impaired liver function. The parent drug and the metabolite are 90% excreted through the biliary tract and feces; 10% is excreted in the urine. Adverse effects include confusion, dizziness, drowsiness, hallucinations, nausea, and vomiting. These can be reduced by lowering the dose of either levodopa or entacapone. Although there were few instances of liver enzyme elevation or hemoglobin decreases during clinical trials, it is recommended that liver enzymes and red blood cell counts be done periodically.

Tolcapone is also well absorbed with oral administration. Its elimination half-life is 2 to 3 hours, and it is metabolized in the liver. Diarrhea was a common adverse effect during clinical trials. Because of several reports of liver damage and deaths from liver failure, tolcapone should be used only in clients who do not respond to other drugs. When used, liver aminotransferase enzymes (serum alanine aminotransferase [ALT] and aspartate aminotransferase [AST]) should be monitored every 2 weeks for 1 year, then every 4 weeks for 6 months, then every 2 months. Tolcapone should be discontinued if ALT and AST are elevated, if symptoms of liver failure occur (anorexia, abdominal tenderness, dark urine, jaundice, clay-colored stools), or if parkinsonian symptoms do not improve after 3 weeks of taking tolcapone.

**Pramipexole** (Mirapex) and **ropinirole** (Requip) are newer drugs that also stimulate dopamine receptors in the brain. They are approved for both beginning and advanced stages of Parkinson's disease. In early stages, one of the drugs can be used alone to improve motor performance, improve ability to participate in usual activities of daily living, and to delay levodopa therapy. In advanced stages, one of the drugs can be used with levodopa and perhaps other antiparkinson drugs to provide more consistent relief of symptoms between doses of levodopa and allow reduced dosage of levodopa. These drugs are not ergot derivatives and may not cause some adverse effects associated with bromocriptine and pergolide (eg, pulmonary and peritoneal fibrosis and constriction of coronary arteries).

Pramipexole is rapidly absorbed with oral administration. Peak serum levels are reached in 1 to 3 hours after a dose and steady-state concentrations in about 2 days. It is less than 20% bound to plasma proteins and has an elimination half-life of 8 to 12 hours. Most of the drug is excreted unchanged in the urine; only 10% of the drug is metabolized. As a result, renal failure may cause higher-than-usual plasma levels and possible toxicity, but hepatic disease is unlikely to alter drug effects.

Ropinirole is also well absorbed with oral administration. It reaches peak serum levels in 1 to 2 hours and steady-state concentrations within 2 days. It is 40% bound to plasma proteins and has an elimination half-life of 6 hours. It is metabolized by the cytochrome P450 enzymes in the liver to inactive metabolites, which are excreted through the kidneys. Less than 10% of ropinirole is excreted unchanged in the urine. Thus, liver failure may decrease metabolism, allow drug accumulation,

---

**?** **How Can You Avoid This Medication Error?**

Mr. Evans, a client with Parkinson's disease, has carbidopa/levodopa (Sinemet) 25/100 ordered tid. Your pharmacy supplies you with Sinemet 25/250. You administer 1 tablet to Mr. Evans for his morning dose.

and increase adverse effects. Renal failure does not appear to alter drug effects.

**Selegiline** (Eldepryl) increases dopamine in the brain by inhibiting its metabolism by MAO. MAO exists in two types, MAO-A and MAO-B, both of which are found in the CNS and peripheral tissues. They are differentiated by their relative specificities for individual catecholamines. MAO-A acts more specifically on tyramine, norepinephrine, epinephrine, and serotonin. It is the main subtype in gastrointestinal mucosa and the liver and is responsible for metabolizing dietary tyramine. If MAO-A is inhibited in the intestine, tyramine in various foods is absorbed systemically rather than deactivated. As a result, there is excessive stimulation of the sympathetic nervous system and severe hypertension and stroke can occur. This life-threatening reaction can also occur with medications that are normally metabolized by MAO.

MAO-B metabolizes dopamine; in the brain, most MAO activity is due to type B. At oral doses of 10 mg/day or less, selegiline inhibits MAO-B selectively and is unlikely to cause severe hypertension and stroke. At doses higher than 10 mg/day, however, selectivity is lost, and metabolism of both MAO-A and MAO-B is inhibited. Doses above 10 mg/day should be avoided in Parkinson's disease. Selegiline inhibition of MAO-B is irreversible, and drug effects persist until more MAO is synthesized in the brain, which may take several months.

In early Parkinson's disease, selegiline may be effective as monotherapy. In advanced disease, it is given to enhance the effects of levodopa. Its addition aids symptom control and allows the dosage of levodopa/carbidopa to be reduced.

*(text continues on page 227)*

---

### ? How Can You Avoid This Medication Error?

**Answer:** This medication error occurred because the wrong dose of levodopa was given to Mr. Evans. When administering a combination product, it is important that the dosage be correct for each medication. In this situation, the Sinemet provided contained 25 mg of carbidopa and 250 mg of levodopa. When administering Sinemet 25/250, you give the patient 250 mg of levodopa rather than the 100 mg that was ordered. Call the pharmacy and request that Sinemet 25/100 be provided.

---

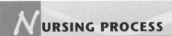

# NURSING PROCESS

## Assessment

Assess for signs and symptoms of Parkinson's disease and drug-induced extrapyramidal reactions. These may include the following, depending on the severity and stage of progression:

- Slow movements (bradykinesia) and difficulty in changing positions, assuming an upright position, eating, dressing, and other self-care activities
- Stooped posture
- Accelerating gait with short steps
- Tremor at rest (eg, "pill rolling" movements of fingers)
- Rigidity of arms, legs, and neck
- Mask-like, immobile facial expression
- Speech problems (eg, low volume, monotonous tone, rapid, difficult to understand)
- Excessive salivation and drooling
- Dysphagia
- Excessive sweating
- Constipation from decreased intestinal motility
- Mental depression from self-consciousness and embarrassment over physical appearance and activity limitations. The intellect is usually intact until the late stages of the disease process.

## Nursing Diagnoses

- Bathing/Grooming Self Care Deficit related to tremors and impaired motor function
- Impaired Physical Mobility related to alterations in balance and coordination
- Disturbed Body Image related to disease and disability
- Deficient Knowledge: Safe usage and effects of antiparkinson drugs
- Imbalanced Nutrition: Less Than Body Requirements related to difficulty in chewing and swallowing food
- Risk for Injury: Dizziness, hypotension related to adverse drug effects

## Planning/Goals

*The client will:*
- Experience relief of excessive salivation, muscle rigidity, spasticity, and tremors
- Experience improved motor function, mobility, and self-care abilities
- Experience improvement of self-concept and body image
- Increase knowledge of the disease process and drug therapy
- Take medications as instructed
- Avoid falls and other injuries from the disease process or drug therapy.

## Interventions

Use measures to assist the client and family in coping with symptoms and maintaining function. These include the following:

- Provide physical therapy for heel-to-toe gait training, widening stance to increase balance and base of support, other exercises.
- Encourage ambulation and frequent changes of position, assisted if necessary.

*(continued)*

## *N*URSING PROCESS (Continued)

- Help with active and passive range-of-motion exercises.
- Encourage self-care as much as possible. Cutting meat; opening cartons; giving frequent, small meals; and allowing privacy during mealtime may be helpful. If the client has difficulty chewing or swallowing, chopped or soft foods may be necessary. Velcro-type fasteners or zippers are easier to handle than buttons. Slip-on shoes are easier to manage than laced ones.
- Spend time with the client and encourage socialization with other people. Individuals with Parkinson's disease tend to become withdrawn, isolated, and depressed.

- Schedule rest periods. Tremor and rigidity are aggravated by fatigue and emotional stress.
- Provide facial tissues if drooling is a problem.

### Evaluation

- Interview and observe for relief of symptoms.
- Interview and observe for increased mobility and participation in activities of daily living.
- Interview and observe regarding correct usage of medications.

## Home Care Considerations: Use of Antiparkinson Drugs

**ASSESS:** for symptoms of dyskinesia and safety risks, serum drug levels and liver function tests, caregiver role strain, quality-of-life considerations.

**MONITOR:** vital signs and self-care abilities, compliance with the prescribed regimen; therapeutic and adverse drug effects, especially with changes in drugs or dosages; and that client is keeping appointments for lab work, physical therapy, and follow-up care.

**EDUCATE:** how to use, store, and replace medications to ensure a constant supply, discussing circumstances for which the client should seek emergency care; that urine as well as perspiration may be discolored, and although harmless, may stain clothes; that most activities (eg, eating, dressing) take longer and require considerable effort; not to stop taking medications abruptly because rebound parkinsonism may occur. Reinforce additional teaching points (see Client Teaching Guidelines: Antiparkinson Drugs).

## ✔ CLIENT TEACHING GUIDELINES
## Antiparkinson Drugs

### General Considerations

✔ Beneficial effects of antiparkinson drugs may not occur for a few weeks or months; do not stop taking them before they have had a chance to work.

✔ Do not take other drugs without the physician's knowledge and consent. This is necessary to avoid adverse drug interactions. Prescription and nonprescription drugs may interact with antiparkinson drugs to increase or decrease effects.

✔ Avoid driving an automobile or operating other potentially hazardous machinery if vision is blurred or drowsiness occurs with levodopa.

✔ Change positions slowly, especially when assuming an upright position, and wear elastic stockings, if needed, to prevent dizziness from a drop in blood pressure.

### Self-administration or Caregiver Administration

✔ Take antiparkinson drugs with or just after food intake to prevent or reduce anorexia, nausea, and vomiting.

✔ Do not crush or chew Sinemet CR. It is formulated to be released slowly; crushing or chewing destroys this feature.

✔ Take or give selegiline in the morning and at noon. This schedule decreases stimulating effects that may interfere with sleep if the drug is taken in the evening.

✔ Decrease excessive mouth dryness by maintaining an adequate fluid intake (2000–3000 mL daily if not contraindicated) and using sugarless chewing gum and hard candies. Both anticholinergics and levodopa may cause mouth dryness. This is usually a therapeutic effect in Parkinson's disease. However, excessive mouth dryness causes discomfort and dental caries.

✔ Report adverse effects. Adverse effects can often be reduced by changing drugs or dosages. However, some adverse effects usually must be tolerated for control of disease symptoms.

## Nursing Actions
## Antiparkinson Drugs

| Nursing Actions | Rationale/Explanation |
|---|---|
| **1. Administer accurately.** | |
| a. Give most antiparkinson drugs with or just after food; entacapone can be given without regard to meals. | To prevent or reduce nausea and vomiting |
| b. Do not crush Sinemet CR and instruct clients not to chew the tablet. | Crushing and chewing destroys the controlled-release feature of the formulation. |
| c. Do not give levodopa with iron preparations or multi-vitamin-mineral preparations containing iron. | Iron decreases absorption of levodopa. |
| d. Give selegiline in the morning and at noon. | To decrease central nervous system (CNS) stimulating effects that may interfere with sleep if the drug is taken in the evening |
| **2. Observe for therapeutic effects.** | |
| a. With anticholinergic agents, observe for decreased tremor, salivation, drooling, and sweating. | Decreased salivation and sweating are therapeutic effects when these drugs are used in Parkinson's disease, but they are adverse effects when the drugs are used in other disorders. |
| b. With levodopa and other dopaminergic agents, observe for improvement in mobility, balance, posture, gait, speech, handwriting, and self-care ability. Drooling and seborrhea may be abolished, and mood may be elevated. | Therapeutic effects are usually evident within 2–3 weeks, as levodopa dosage approaches 2–3 g/d, but may not reach optimum levels for 6 months. |
| **3. Observe for adverse effects.** | |
| a. With anticholinergic drugs, observe for atropine-like effects, such as: | |
| (1) Tachycardia and palpitations | These effects may occur with usual therapeutic doses but are not likely to be serious except in people with underlying heart disease. |
| (2) Excessive CNS stimulation (tremor, restlessness, confusion, hallucinations, delirium) | This effect is most likely to occur with large doses of tri-hexyphenidyl (Artane) or benztropine (Cogentin). It may occur with levodopa. |
| (3) Sedation and drowsiness | These are most likely to occur with benztropine. The drug has antihistaminic and anticholinergic properties, and sedation is attributed to the antihistamine effect. |
| (4) Constipation, impaction, paralytic ileus | These effects result from decreased gastrointestinal motility and muscle tone. They may be severe because decreased intestinal motility and constipation also are characteristics of Parkinson's disease; thus, additive effects may occur. |
| (5) Urinary retention | This reaction is caused by loss of muscle tone in the bladder and is most likely to occur in elderly men who have enlarged prostate glands. |
| (6) Dilated pupils (mydriasis), blurred vision, photophobia | Ocular effects are due to paralysis of accommodation and relaxation of the ciliary muscle and the sphincter muscle of the iris. |
| b. With levodopa, observe for: | |
| (1) Anorexia, nausea, and vomiting | These symptoms usually disappear after a few months of drug therapy. They may be minimized by giving levodopa with food, gradually increasing dosage, administering smaller doses more frequently, or adding carbidopa so that dosage of levodopa can be reduced. |
| (2) Orthostatic hypotension—check blood pressure in both sitting and standing positions q4h while the client is awake. | This effect is common during the first few weeks but usually subsides eventually. It can be minimized by arising slowly from supine or sitting positions and by wearing elastic stockings. |

*(continued)*

## *Nursing Actions*

## Antiparkinson Drugs (Continued)

| *Nursing Actions* | *Rationale/Explanation* |
|---|---|
| (3) Cardiac arrhythmias (tachycardia, premature ventricular contractions) and increased myocardial contractility | Levodopa and its metabolites stimulate beta-adrenergic receptors in the heart. People with pre-existing coronary artery disease may need a beta-adrenergic blocking agent (eg, propranolol) to counteract these effects. |
| (4) Dyskinesia—involuntary movements that may involve only the tongue, mouth, and face or the whole body | Dyskinesia eventually develops in most people who take levodopa. It is related to duration of levodopa therapy rather than dosage. Carbidopa may heighten this adverse effect, and there is no way to prevent it except by decreasing levodopa dosage. Many people prefer dyskinesia to lowering drug dosage and subsequent return of the parkinsonism symptoms. |
| (5) CNS stimulation—restlessness, agitation, confusion, delirium | This is more likely to occur with levodopa/carbidopa combination drug therapy. |
| (6) Abrupt swings in motor function (on–off phenomenon) | This fluctuation may indicate progression of the disease process. It often occurs after long-term levodopa use. |
| c. With amantadine, observe for: | |
| (1) CNS stimulation—insomnia, hyperexcitability, ataxia, dizziness, slurred speech, mental confusion, hallucinations | Compared with other antiparkinson drugs, amantadine produces few adverse effects. The ones that occur are mild, transient, and reversible. However, adverse effects increase if daily dosage exceeds 200 mg. |
| (2) Livedo reticularis—patchy, bluish discoloration of skin on the legs | This is a benign but cosmetically unappealing condition. It usually occurs with long-term use of amantadine and disappears when the drug is discontinued. |
| d. With bromocriptine and pergolide, observe for: | |
| (1) Nausea | These symptoms are usually mild and can be minimized by starting with low doses and increasing the dose gradually until the desired effect is achieved. If adverse effects do occur, they usually disappear with a decrease in dosage. These effects occurred more commonly than others during clinical trials. |
| (2) Confusion and hallucinations | |
| (3) Hypotension | |
| e. With pramipexole and ropinirole, observe for: | |
| (1) Nausea | |
| (2) Confusion, hallucinations | |
| (3) Dizziness, drowsiness | |
| (4) Dyskinesias | |
| (5) Orthostatic hypotension | |
| f. With selegiline, observe for: | |
| (1) CNS effects—agitation, ataxia, bradykinesia, confusion, dizziness, dyskinesias, hallucinations, insomnia | |
| (2) Nausea, abdominal pain | |
| g. With entocapone and tolcapone, observe for: | These effects occurred more commonly than others during clinical trials. |
| (1) Anorexia, nausea, vomiting, diarrhea, constipation | |
| (2) Dizziness, drowsiness | |
| (3) Dyskinesias and dystonias | |
| (4) Hallucinations | |
| (5) Orthostatic hypotension | |
| 4. Observe for drug interactions. | |
| a. Drugs that *increase* effects of anticholinergic drugs: | |
| (1) Antihistamines, disopyramide (Norpace), thiothixene (Navane), phenothiazines, and tricyclic antidepressants | These drugs have anticholinergic properties and produce additive anticholinergic effects. |
| b. Drugs that *decrease* effects of anticholinergic drugs: | |
| (1) Cholinergic agents | These drugs counteract the inhibition of gastrointestinal motility and tone, which is a side effect of anticholinergic drug therapy. |

*(continued)*

## Nursing Actions

### Antiparkinson Drugs (Continued)

| Nursing Actions | Rationale/Explanation |
|---|---|
| c. Drugs that *increase* effects of levodopa: | |
| (1) Amantadine, anticholinergic agents, bromocriptine, carbidopa, entacapone, pergolide, pramipexole, ropinirole, selegiline, tolcapone | These drugs are often used in combination for treatment of Parkinson's disease. |
| (2) Tricyclic antidepressants | These drugs potentiate levodopa effects and increase the risk of cardiac arrhythmias in people with heart disease. |
| (3) Monoamine oxidase type A (MAO-A) inhibitors, including isocarboxazid (Marplan), phenelzine (Nardil), and tranylcypromine (Parnate) | The combination of a catecholamine precursor (levodopa) and MAO-A inhibitors that decrease metabolism of catecholamines can result in excessive amounts of dopamine, epinephrine, and norepinephrine. Heart palpitations, headache, hypertensive crisis, and stroke may occur. Levodopa and MAO-A inhibitors should not be given concurrently. Also, levodopa should not be started within 3 weeks after an MAO-A inhibitor is discontinued. Effects of MAO-A inhibitors persist for 1–3 weeks after their discontinuation. These effects are unlikely to occur with selegiline, an MAO-B inhibitor, which more selectively inhibits the metabolism of dopamine. However, selectivity may be lost at doses higher than the recommended 10 mg/d. Selegiline is used with levodopa. |
| d. Drugs that *decrease* effects of levodopa: | |
| (1) Anticholinergics | Although anticholinergics are often given with levodopa for increased antiparkinson effects, they also may decrease effects of levodopa by delaying gastric emptying. This causes more levodopa to be metabolized in the stomach and decreases the amount available for absorption from the intestine. |
| (2) Alcohol, benzodiazepines (eg, diazepam [Valium]), antiemetics, antipsychotics such as phenothiazines, haloperidol (Haldol), and thiothixene (Navane) | The mechanisms by which most of these drugs decrease effects of levodopa are not clear. Phenothiazines block dopamine receptors in the basal ganglia. |
| (3) Oral iron preparations | Iron binds with levodopa and reduces levodopa absorption, possibly by as much as 50%. |
| (4) Pyridoxine (vitamin $B_6$) | Pyridoxine stimulates decarboxylase, the enzyme that converts levodopa to dopamine. As a result, more levodopa is metabolized in peripheral tissues, and less reaches the CNS, where antiparkinson effects occur. This interaction does not occur when carbidopa is given with levodopa. |
| e. Drugs that *decrease* effects of dopaminergic antiparkinson drugs: | |
| (1) Antipsychotic drugs | These drugs are dopamine antagonists and therefore inhibit the effects of dopamine agonists. |
| (2) Metoclopramide | |

## Critical Thinking Exercises

1. Which neurotransmitter is deficient and is primarily responsible for idiopathic and drug-induced parkinsonism?

   a. Tyramine
   b. Norepinephrine
   c. Serotonin
   d. Dopamine

2. A client with parkinsonism taking entacapone develops confusion, drowsiness, and hallucinations. These adverse effects are most likely observed if the client:

   a. Concomitantly takes levodopa
   b. Has a history of renal failure
   c. Stops the medication abruptly
   d. Has impaired liver function

**3.** When carbidopa is given with levodopa, the dosage of levodopa must be reduced by approximately:

a. 10%
b. 25%
c. 50%
d. 75%

**4.** At oral doses higher than 10 mg/day, selegiline (Eldepryl) metabolism of both MAO-A and MAO-B is inhibited. This could result in:

a. Little clinical significance
b. Life-threatening hypertension
c. Return of parkinsonian symptoms
d. Renal failure

**5.** The use of a combination of antiparkinson drugs over monotherapy with levodopa accomplishes all of the following except:

a. Reduction of adverse effects
b. Extension of the period of drug effectiveness
c. Delay in the possible acceleration of the loss of dopaminergic neurons in the brain
d. Reduction in the cost of drug therapy

## SELECTED REFERENCES

Chen, J. J., & Shimomura, S. K. (2000). Parkinsonism. In E. T. Herfindal & D. R. Gourley (Eds.), *Textbook of therapeutics: Drug and disease management* (7th ed., pp. 1139–1155). Philadelphia: Lippincott Williams & Wilkins.

*Drug facts and comparisons.* (Updated monthly). St. Louis: Facts and Comparisons.

Factor, S. A. (1999). Dopamine agonists. *Medical Clinics of North America, 83,* 415–443.

Hauser, R. A., & Zesiewicz, T. A. (1999). Management of early Parkinson's disease. *Medical Clinics of North America, 83,* 393–414.

Herndon, C. M., Young, K., Herndon, A. D., & Dole, E. J. (2000). Parkinson's disease revisited. *Journal of Neuroscience Nursing, 32*(4), 216–221.

Kuzel, M. D. (1999). Ropinirole: A dopamine agonist for the treatment of Parkinson's disease. *American Journal of Health-System Pharmacy, 56,* 217–224.

Lacy, C. F., Armstrong, L. L., Goldman, M. P., & Lance, L. L. (2003). *Lexi-Comp's drug information handbook* (11th ed.). Hudson, OH: American Pharmaceutical Association.

Porth, C. M., & Curtis, R. (2002). Alterations in motor function. In C. M. Porth (Ed.), *Pathophysiology: Concepts of altered health states* (6th ed., pp. 1123–1157). Philadelphia: Lippincott Williams & Wilkins.

Reich, S. G. (2000). Parkinson's disease and related disorders. In H. D. Humes (Ed.), *Kelley's textbook of internal medicine* (4th ed., pp. 2915–2918). Philadelphia: Lippincott Williams & Wilkins.

# 13

# Skeletal Muscle Relaxants

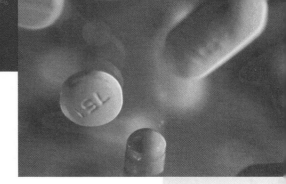

## OBJECTIVES

*After studying this chapter, the student will be able to:*

1 Discuss common symptoms and disorders for which skeletal muscle relaxants are used.

2 Differentiate uses and effects of selected skeletal muscle relaxants.

3 Describe nonpharmacologic interventions to relieve muscle spasm and spasticity.

4 Apply the nursing process with clients experiencing muscle spasm or spasticity.

## CRITICAL THINKING SCENARIO

*J*ohn Moore was in an automobile accident 5 days ago and sustained trauma to his back and left shoulder. Although no bones were broken, he continues to have pain and muscle spasms. His health care provider orders Tylox, as needed, for the pain and cyclobenzaprine (Flexeril) for muscle spasms.

✔ Why are two different medications ordered to manage John's discomfort?

✔ What nonpharmacologic treatments can be used to promote comfort?

✔ What teaching needs to be done before sending John home?

## SKELETAL MUSCLE RELAXANTS

Skeletal muscle relaxants are used to decrease muscle spasm or spasticity that occurs in certain neurologic and musculoskeletal disorders. (Neuromuscular blocking agents used as adjuncts to general anesthesia for surgery are discussed in Appendix D.) The conditions associated with the use of skeletal muscle relaxants, which serve as the focus of this chapter, are described in At the Foundation: Muscle Spasm and Spasticity.

Spasticity may be controlled with the use of baclofen, tizanidine, or dantrolene. In some cases, decreasing spasticity may not be desirable because clients with severe leg weakness may require some degree of spasticity to ambulate. In cases of severe spasticity, baclofen may be given intrathecally through an implanted subcutaneous pump.

## Mechanism of Action

All skeletal muscle relaxants except dantrolene are centrally active drugs. Pharmacologic action is usually attributed to general depression of the central nervous system (CNS) but may involve blockage of nerve impulses that cause increased muscle tone and contraction. It is unclear whether relief of pain results from sedative effects, muscular relaxation, or a placebo effect. In addition, although parenteral administration of some drugs (eg, diazepam, methocarbamol) relieves pain associated with acute musculoskeletal trauma or inflammation, it is uncertain whether oral administration of usual doses exerts a beneficial effect in acute or chronic disorders.

Baclofen and diazepam increase the effects of gamma-aminobutyric acid, an inhibitory neurotransmitter, and tizanidine inhibits motor neurons in the brain. Dantrolene is the only skeletal muscle relaxant that acts peripherally on the muscle itself. It inhibits the release of calcium in skeletal muscle cells and thereby decreases the strength of muscle contraction.

## Indications for Use

Skeletal muscle relaxants are used primarily as adjuncts to other treatment measures such as physical therapy. Occasionally, parenteral agents are given to facilitate orthopedic procedures and examinations. In spastic disorders, skeletal muscle relaxants are indicated when spasticity causes severe pain or inability to tolerate physical therapy, to sit in a wheelchair, or to participate in self-care activities of daily living (eg, eating, dressing). The drugs should not be given if they cause excessive muscle weakness and impair rather than facilitate mobility and function.

Dantrolene also is indicated for prevention and treatment of malignant hyperthermia, a rare but life-threatening complication of anesthesia characterized by hypercarbia, metabolic acidosis, skeletal muscle rigidity, fever, and cyanosis. For preoperative prophylaxis in people with previous episodes of malignant hyperthermia, the drug is given orally for 1 to 2 days before surgery. For intraoperative malignant hyperthermia, the drug is given intravenously. After an occurrence during surgery, the drug is given orally for 1 to 3 days to prevent recurrence of symptoms.

## Contraindications to Use

Most skeletal muscle relaxants cause CNS depression and have the same contraindications as other CNS depressants. They should be used cautiously in clients with impaired renal or hepatic function or respiratory depression and in clients who must be alert for activities of daily living (eg, driving a car, operating potentially hazardous machinery). Orphenadrine and cyclobenzaprine

---

### AT THE FOUNDATION: *Muscle Spasm and Spasticity*

**Muscle Spasm**
Muscle spasm or cramp is a sudden, involuntary, painful muscle contraction that occurs with trauma or an irritant. Spasms may involve alternating contraction and relaxation (clonic) or sustained contraction (tonic). Muscle spasm may occur with musculoskeletal trauma or inflammation (eg, sprains, strains, bursitis, arthritis). It is also encountered with acute or chronic low back pain, a common condition that is primarily a disorder of posture.

**Spasticity**
Spasticity involves increased muscle tone (hypertonia) or contraction with stiff, awkward movements. It is thought to result from increased excitability of the alpha motor neurons (stretch reflexes) in response to a stimulus without descending inhibition of the pyramidal systems. The exact mechanism is unclear. Increased deep tendon reflexes and clonus (increased spread of reflexes) typically accompany spasticity. It predominates in flexors of the upper extremities and extensors of the lower extremities and more frequently in pronators than supinators. Spasticity occurs with neurologic disorders such as spinal cord injury and multiple sclerosis.

have high levels of anticholinergic activity and therefore should be used cautiously with glaucoma, urinary retention, cardiac arrhythmias, or tachycardia.

## Management Considerations

### Goal of Treatment

The goal of treatment is to relieve pain, muscle spasm, and muscle spasticity without impairing the ability to perform self-care activities of daily living. Home care is an essential component in the management of individuals taking skeletal muscle relaxants for various health conditions because the symptoms are typically chronic in nature. Guidelines for ongoing evaluation and intervention are addressed in Home Care Considerations.

### Drug Selection

Choice of a skeletal muscle relaxant depends mainly on the disorder being treated:

1. For acute muscle spasm and pain, an oral or parenteral drug may be given. The drugs cause sedation and other adverse effects and are recommended for short-term use. Cyclobenzaprine should not be used longer than 3 weeks.
2. Parenteral agents are preferred for orthopedic procedures because they have greater sedative and pain-relieving effects.
3. Baclofen (Lioresal) is approved for treatment of spasticity in people with multiple sclerosis. It is variably effective, and its clinical usefulness may be limited by adverse reactions.
4. None of the skeletal muscle relaxants has been established as safe for use during pregnancy and lactation.
5. For children, the choice of drug should be limited to those with established pediatric dosages. Pediatric issues and pharmacologic management in the older adult are outlined in Age-related Considerations.

## Home Care Considerations: Use of Skeletal Muscle Relaxants

**ASSESS:** drug effects and the frequency and severity of spasticity and how successful it is managed, including nonpharmacologic alternatives to relieve discomfort.

**MONITOR:** the response to therapy, safe drug use, functional abilities, and quality of life.

**EDUCATE:** on safe use of drugs (eg, that the drugs decrease mental alertness, so potentially hazardous activities should be avoided), about nonpharmacologic methods of managing spasticity, and ways to prevent adverse effects of drugs. Reinforce additional teaching points (see Client Teaching Guidelines: Skeletal Muscle Relaxants).

## Drug Use in Specific Situations

### Spinal Cord Injury

In clients with spinal cord injury, spasticity requires treatment when it impairs safety, mobility, and the ability to perform activities of daily living (eg, self-care in hygiene, eating, dressing, and work or recreational activities). Stimuli that precipitate spasms vary from one individual to another and may include muscle stretching, bladder infections or stones, constipation and bowel distention, or infections. Each person needs to be assessed for personal precipitating factors, so that they can be avoided when possible. Treatment measures include passive range-of-motion and muscle-stretching exercises and antispasmodic medications (eg, baclofen, dantrolene).

### Multiple Sclerosis

Multiple sclerosis (MS) is a major cause of neurologic disability among young and middle-aged adults, occurs more often in women than in men, and has a pattern of exacerbations and remissions. It is considered an auto-immune disorder that occurs in genetically susceptible individuals, although its cause is unknown. It involves destruction of portions of the myelin sheath that covers nerves in the brain, spinal cord, and optic nerve. Myelin normally insulates the neuron from electrical activity and conducts electrical impulses rapidly along nerve fibers. When myelin is destroyed (a process called *demyelination*, which probably results from inflammation), fibrotic lesions are formed and nerve conduction is slowed or blocked around the lesions. Lesions in various states of development (eg, acute, subacute, and chronic) often occur at multiple sites in the CNS. Muscle weakness and other symptoms vary according to the location and duration of the myelin damage.

In recent years, researchers have discovered that nerve cells can be repaired (remyelinated) if the process that damaged the myelin is stopped before the oligodendrocytes (the cells that form myelin) are destroyed. Other researchers are trying to develop methods for enhancing nerve conduction velocity in demyelinated nerves. For example, exposure to cold by wearing a cooling vest or exercising in cool water temporarily increases the rate of nerve conduction and improves symptoms in some people. Avoiding environmental heat and conditions that cause fever may also help because an elevated body temperature slows nerve conduction and often aggravates MS symptoms.

The person with minimal symptoms does not require treatment but should be encouraged to maintain a healthy lifestyle. Those with more extensive symptoms should try to avoid emotional stress, environmental temperature extremes, infections, and excessive fatigue. Physical therapy may help maintain muscle tone, and occupational therapy may help maintain ability to perform activities of daily living.

## Age-related Considerations: Use of Skeletal Muscle Relaxants

### USE IN CHILDREN

For most of the drugs, safety and effectiveness for use in children 12 years of age and younger have not been established. The drugs should be used only when clearly indicated, for short periods, when close supervision is available for monitoring drug effects (especially sedation), and when mobility and alertness are not required.

### USE IN OLDER ADULTS

Any CNS depressant or sedating drugs should be used cautiously in older adults. Risks for falls, mental confusion, and other adverse effects are higher because of the potential for impaired drug metabolism and excretion.

Drug therapy for MS may also involve several types of medications for different types and stages of the disease. Acute exacerbations are treated with corticosteroids (see Chap. 35), interferon-beta (Avonex, Betaseron) or glatiramer (Copaxone) is given to prevent relapses, immunosuppressive drugs (eg, methotrexate) are used to treat progressive disease, and symptoms are treated with a variety of drugs, including antidepressants for depression and skeletal muscle relaxants for spasticity.

## ▨ INDIVIDUAL DRUGS

Individual skeletal muscle relaxants are described below; routes and dosage ranges are listed in Drugs at a Glance 13-1: Skeletal Muscle Relaxants. No prototype is identified within this group of drugs.

**Baclofen** (Lioresal) is used mainly to treat spasticity in multiple sclerosis and spinal cord injuries. It is contraindicated in people with hypersensitivity reactions to it and those with muscle spasm from rheumatic disorders. It can be given orally and intrathecally through an implanted, subcutaneous pump. Check the pump manufacturer's literature for information about pump implantation and drug infusion techniques.

The action of oral baclofen starts in 1 hour, peaks in 2 hours, and lasts 4 to 8 hours. It is metabolized in the liver and excreted in urine; its half-life is 3 to 4 hours. Dosage must be reduced in clients with impaired renal function. Common adverse effects include drowsiness, dizziness, confusion, constipation, fatigue, headache, hypotension, insomnia, nausea, and weakness. When discontinued, the dosage should be tapered and the drug withdrawn over 1 to 2 weeks.

**Carisoprodol** (Soma) is used to relieve discomfort from acute, painful, musculoskeletal disorders. It is not recommended for long-term use, and if used long-term or in high doses, it can cause physical dependence (ie, symptoms of withdrawal if stopped abruptly). The drug is contraindicated in clients with intermittent porphyria, a rare metabolic disorder characterized by acute abdominal pain and neurologic symptoms. Oral drug acts within 30 minutes, peaks in 1 to 2 hours, and lasts 4 to 6 hours.

It is metabolized in the liver and has a half-life of 8 hours. Common adverse effects include drowsiness, dizziness, and impaired motor coordination.

**Cyclobenzaprine** (Flexeril) has the same indication for use as carisoprodol and chlorphenesin, above. It is contraindicated in clients with cardiovascular disorders (eg, recent myocardial infarction, dysrhythmias, heart block) or hyperthyroidism. Oral drug acts in 1 hour, peaks in 4 to 6 hours, and lasts 12 to 24 hours; half-life is 1 to 3 days. Duration of use should not exceed 3 weeks. Common adverse effects are drowsiness, dizziness, and anticholinergic effects (eg, dry mouth, constipation, urinary retention, tachycardia).

**Dantrolene** (Dantrium) acts directly on skeletal muscle to inhibit muscle contraction. It is used to relieve spasticity in neurologic disorders (eg, multiple sclerosis, spinal cord injury) and to prevent or treat malignant hyperthermia, a rare but life-threatening complication of anesthesia characterized by hypercarbia, metabolic acidosis, skeletal muscle rigidity, fever, and cyanosis. For preoperative prophylaxis in people with previous episodes of malignant hyperthermia, the drug is given orally for 1 to 2 days before surgery. For intraoperative malignant hyperthermia, the drug is given intravenously. After an occurrence during surgery, the drug is given orally for 1 to 3 days to prevent recurrence of symptoms.

Oral drug acts slowly, peaks in 4 to 6 hours, and lasts 8 to 10 hours. Intravenous (IV) drug acts rapidly, peaks in about 5 hours, and lasts 6 to 8 hours. Common adverse effects include drowsiness, dizziness, diarrhea, and fatigue. The most serious adverse effect is potentially fatal hepatitis, with jaundice and other symptoms that usually occur within 1 month of starting drug therapy. Liver function tests should be monitored periodically in all clients receiving dantrolene. These adverse effects do not occur with short-term use of IV drug for malignant hyperthermia.

**Metaxalone** (Skelaxin) is used to relieve discomfort from acute, painful, musculoskeletal disorders. It is contraindicated in clients with anemia or severe renal or hepatic impairment. Oral drug acts within 60 minutes, peaks in 2 hours, and lasts 4 to 6 hours. It has a half-life of 2 to 3 hours, is metabolized in the liver, and is excreted in urine. Common adverse effects include drowsiness,

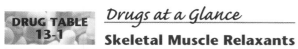

**DRUG TABLE
13-1**

*Drugs at a Glance*

## Skeletal Muscle Relaxants

| Generic/Trade Name | Routes and Dosage Ranges | Comments |
|---|---|---|
| **Baclofen** (Lioresal) Pregnancy Category C | *Adults:* PO, 5 mg 3 times daily for 3 days; 10 mg 3 times daily for 3 days; 15 mg 3 times daily for 3 days; then 20 mg 3 times daily, if necessary. Intrathecal via implanted pump: Dosage varies widely; see manufacturer's recommendations. *Children <12 years:* Safety not established | Avoid abrupt withdrawal |
| **Carisoprodol** (Soma) Pregnancy Category C | *Adults:* PO, 350 mg 3 or 4 times daily, with the last dose at bedtime *Children <12 years:* Not recommended | Can be compounded with aspirin and codeine |
| **Cyclobenzaprine** (Flexeril) Pregnancy Category B | *Adults:* PO, 10 mg 3 times daily. Maximal recommended duration, 3 weeks; maximal recommended dose, 60 mg daily *Children <15 years:* Safety and effectiveness have not been established. | Also used as supportive therapy in tetanus |
| **Dantrolene** (Dantrium) Pregnancy Category C | *Adults:* PO, 25 mg daily initially, gradually increased weekly (by increments of 50–100 mg/d) to a maximal dose of 400 mg daily in 4 divided doses *Children:* PO, 1 mg/kg per day initially, gradually increased to a maximal dose of 3 mg/kg 4 times daily, not to exceed 400 mg daily Preoperative prophylaxis of malignant hyperthermia: *Adults:* PO, 4–8 mg/kg per day in 3–4 divided doses for 1 or 2 days before surgery *Children:* Same as adults Intraoperative malignant hyperthermia: IV push 1 mg/kg initially, continued until symptoms are relieved or a maximum total dose of 10 mg/kg has been given Postcrisis follow-up treatment: PO, 4–8 mg/kg per day in 4 divided doses for 1–3 days | Used to manage spasticity associated with multiple sclerosis, spinal cord injury, stroke, cerebral palsy, and malignant hyperthermia |
| **Diazepam** (Valium) Pregnancy Category D | *Adults:* PO, 2–10 mg 3 or 4 times daily IM, IV 5–10 mg repeated in 3–4 hours if necessary *Children:* PO, 0.12–0.8 mg/kg per day in 3 or 4 divided doses IM, IV 0.04–0.2 mg/kg in a single dose, not to exceed 0.6 mg/kg within an 8-h period | See Prototype Profile 8-1: Diazepam |

*(continued)*

**DRUG TABLE 13-1**

*Drugs at a Glance*

## Skeletal Muscle Relaxants (Continued)

| Generic/Trade Name | Routes and Dosage Ranges | Comments |
|---|---|---|
| **Metaxalone** (Skelaxin)<br>Pregnancy Category C | *Adults:* PO 800 mg 3 or 4 times daily<br>*Children >12 years:* Same as adults<br>*Children <12 years:* Safety and effectiveness have not been established | Does not have direct skeletal muscle effects; beneficial effects result from actions on central nervous system |
| **Methocarbamol** (Robaxin)<br>Pregnancy Category C | *Adults:* PO, 1.5–2 g 4 times daily for 48–72 hours, reduced to 1.0 g 4 times daily for maintenance<br>IM, 500 mg q8h<br>IV, 1–3 g daily at a rate not to exceed 300 mg/min (3 mL of 10% injection). Do not give IV more than 3 days.<br>*Children:* Safety and effectiveness have not been established except for treatment of tetanus (IV 15 mg/kg every 6 hours as indicated) | May turn urine green, brown, or black; IV form may cause extravasation |
| **Orphenadrine citrate** (Norflex)<br>Pregnancy Category D | *Adults:* PO, 100 mg twice daily<br>IM, IV 60 mg twice daily<br>*Children:* Not recommended | Can be compounded with aspirin and caffeine |
| **Tizanidine** (Zanaflex)<br>Pregnancy Category C | *Adults:* PO, 4 mg q6–8h initially, increased gradually if needed. Maximum of 3 doses and 36 mg in 24 h<br>*Children:* Safety and effectiveness have not been established | Reduce dose in clients with renal or liver disease |

dizziness, and nausea; hepatotoxicity and hemolytic anemia may also occur. Liver function should be monitored during therapy.

**Methocarbamol** (Robaxin) is used to relieve discomfort from acute, painful, musculoskeletal disorders; it may also be used to treat tetanus. Parenteral drug is contraindicated in clients with renal impairment because the solution contains polyethylene glycol. Oral drug acts within 30 minutes and peaks in 2 hours; parenteral drug acts rapidly, but its peak and duration of action are unknown. The drug has a half-life of 1 to 2 hours, is metabolized in the liver, and is excreted in urine and feces. Common adverse effects with oral drug include drowsiness, dizziness, nausea, and urticaria; effects with injected drug also include fainting, incoordination, and hypotension. The drug may also discolor urine to a green, brown, or black. This is considered a harmless effect, but clients should be informed about it.

**Orphenadrine** (Norflex) is used to relieve discomfort from acute, painful, musculoskeletal disorders. Because of its strong anticholinergic effects, the drug is contraindicated in clients with glaucoma, duodenal obstruc-

tion, prostatic hypertrophy, bladder neck obstruction, and myasthenia gravis. It should be used cautiously in clients with cardiovascular disease (eg, heart failure, coronary insufficiency, dysrhythmias) and renal or hepatic impairment. The action of both oral and parenteral drug peaks in 2 hours and lasts 4 to 6 hours. The drug has a half-life of 14 hours, is metabolized in the liver, and is excreted in urine and feces. Common adverse effects include drowsiness, dizziness, constipation, dry mouth, nausea, tachycardia, and urinary retention.

**Tizanidine** (Zanaflex) is an alpha$_2$-adrenergic agonist, similar to clonidine, that is used to treat spasticity in clients with multiple sclerosis, spinal cord injury, or brain trauma. It should be used cautiously with renal or hepatic impairment and with hypotension. It is given orally, and its action starts within 30 to 60 minutes, peaks in 1 to 2 hours, and lasts 3 to 4 hours. Its half-life is 3 to 4 hours; it is metabolized in the liver and excreted in urine. Common adverse effects include drowsiness, dizziness, constipation, dry mouth, and hypotension. Hypotension may be significant and occur at usual doses. It may also cause psychotic symptoms, including hallucinations.

## NURSING PROCESS

### Assessment

Assess for muscle spasm and spasticity.

- With muscle spasm, assess for:
  - **Pain.** This is a prominent symptom of muscle spasm and is usually aggravated by movement. Try to determine the location as specifically as possible, as well as the intensity, duration, and precipitating factors (eg, traumatic injury, strenuous exercise).
  - **Accompanying signs and symptoms,** such as bruises (ecchymoses), edema, or signs of inflammation (redness, heat, edema, tenderness to touch)
- With spasticity, assess for pain and impaired functional ability in self-care (eg, eating, dressing). In addition, severe spasticity interferes with ambulation and other movement as well as exercises to maintain joint and muscle mobility.

### Nursing Diagnoses

- Pain related to muscle spasm
- Impaired Physical Mobility related to spasm and pain
- Bathing/Hygiene Self-Care Deficit related to spasm and pain
- Deficient Knowledge: Nondrug measures to relieve muscle spasm, pain, and spasticity and safe usage of skeletal muscle relaxants
- Risk for Injury: Dizziness, sedation related to CNS depression

### Planning/Goals

*The client will:*

- Experience relief of pain and spasm
- Experience improved motor function
- Increase self-care abilities in activities of daily living
- Take medications as instructed
- Use nondrug measures appropriately
- Be safeguarded when sedated from drug therapy

### Interventions

Use adjunctive measures for muscle spasm and spasticity:

- Physical therapy (massage, moist heat, exercises)
- Bed rest for acute muscle spasm
- Relaxation techniques
- Correct posture and lifting techniques (eg, stooping rather than bending to lift objects, holding heavy objects close to the body, *not* lifting excessive amounts of weight)
- Regular exercise and use of warm-up exercises. Strenuous exercise performed on an occasional basis (eg, weekly or monthly) is more likely to cause acute muscle spasm.

### Evaluation

- Interview and observe for relief of symptoms.
- Interview and observe regarding correct usage of medications and nondrug therapeutic measures.

## Nursing Actions

## Skeletal Muscle Relaxants

| Nursing Actions | Rationale/Explanation |
| --- | --- |
| 1. Administer accurately. | |
| a. Give baclofen, chlorphenesin, metaxalone with milk or food. | To decrease gastrointestinal distress |
| b. Do not mix parenteral diazepam in a syringe with any other drugs. | Diazepam is physically incompatible with other drugs. |
| c. Inject intravenous (IV) diazepam directly into a vein or the injection site nearest the vein (during continuous IV infusions) at a rate of approximately 2 mg/min. | Diazepam may cause a precipitate if diluted. Avoid contact with IV solutions as much as possible. A slow rate of injection minimizes the risks of respiratory depression and apnea. |
| d. Avoid extravasation with IV diazepam, and inject intramuscular (IM) diazepam deeply into a gluteal muscle. | To prevent or reduce tissue irritation |
| e. With IV methocarbamol, inject or infuse slowly. | Rapid administration may cause bradycardia, hypotension, and dizziness. |
| f. With IV methocarbamol, have the client lie down during and at least 15 minutes after administration. | To minimize orthostatic hypotension and other adverse drug effects |
| g. Avoid extravasation with IV methocarbamol, and give IM methocarbamol deeply into a gluteal muscle. (Dividing the dose and giving two injections is preferred.) | Parenteral methocarbamol is a hypertonic solution that is very irritating to tissues. Thrombophlebitis may occur at IV injection sites, and sloughing of tissue may occur at sites of extravasation or IM injections. |

*(continued)*

*Nursing Actions*

## Skeletal Muscle Relaxants (Continued)

| **Nursing Actions** | **Rationale/Explanation** |
|---|---|
| **2. Observe for therapeutic effects.**<br>a. When the drug is given for acute muscle spasm, observe for:<br>(1) Decreased pain and tenderness<br>(2) Increased mobility<br>(3) Increased ability to participate in activities of daily living<br>b. When the drug is given for spasticity in chronic neurologic disorders, observe for:<br>(1) Increased ability to maintain posture and balance<br>(2) Increased ability for self-care (eg, eating and dressing)<br>(3) Increased tolerance for physical therapy and exercises | Therapeutic effects usually occur within 30 minutes after IV injection of diazepam or methocarbamol. |
| **3. Observe for adverse effects.**<br>a. With centrally active agents, observe for:<br>(1) Drowsiness and dizziness<br>(2) Blurred vision, lethargy, flushing<br><br>(3) Nausea, vomiting, abdominal distress, constipation or diarrhea, ataxia, areflexia, flaccid paralysis, respiratory depression, tachycardia, hypotension<br>(4) Hypersensitivity—skin rash, pruritus<br><br><br>(5) Psychological or physical dependence with diazepam and other antianxiety agents<br>b. With a peripherally active agent (dantrolene), observe for:<br>(1) Drowsiness, fatigue, lethargy, weakness, nausea, vomiting<br>(2) Headache, anorexia, nervousness<br>(3) Hepatotoxicity | These are the most common adverse effects.<br>These effects occur more often with IV administration of drugs. They are usually transient.<br>These effects are most likely to occur with large oral doses.<br><br><br>The drug should be discontinued if hypersensitivity reactions occur. Serious allergic reactions (eg, anaphylaxis) are rare.<br>Most likely to occur with long-term use of large doses<br><br>Adverse effects are usually transient.<br><br>These effects are the most common.<br><br>Less common effects<br>This potentially serious adverse effect is most likely to occur in people older than 35 years of age who have taken the drug 60 days or longer. Women over age 35 years who take estrogens have the highest risk. Hepatotoxicity can be prevented or minimized by administering the lowest effective dose, monitoring liver enzymes (aspartate aminotransferase and alanine aminotransferase) during therapy, and discontinuing the drug if no beneficial effects occur within 45 days. |
| **4. Observe for drug interactions**<br>a. Drugs that *increase* effects of skeletal muscle relaxants:<br>(1) Central nervous system (CNS) depressants (alcohol, antianxiety agents, antidepressants, antihistamines, antipsychotic drugs, sedative-hypnotics)<br>(2) Monoamine oxidase inhibitors<br><br>(3) Antihypertensive agents | <br><br>Additive CNS depression with increased risks of excessive sedation and respiratory depression or apnea<br><br>May potentiate effects by inhibiting metabolism of muscle relaxants<br>Increased hypotension, especially with tizanidine |

## CLIENT TEACHING GUIDELINES
## Skeletal Muscle Relaxants

### General Considerations

✔ Use nondrug measures, such as exercises and applications of heat and cold, to decrease muscle spasm and spasticity.

✔ Avoid activities that require mental alertness or physical coordination (eg, driving an automobile, operating potentially dangerous machinery) if drowsy from medication.

✔ Do not take other drugs without the physician's knowledge, including nonprescription drugs. The major risk occurs with concurrent use of alcohol, antihistamines, sleeping aids, or other drugs that cause drowsiness.

✔ Avoid herbal preparations that cause drowsiness or sleep, including kava and valerian.

### Self-administration

✔ Take the drugs with milk or food, to avoid nausea and stomach irritation.

✔ Do not stop drugs abruptly. Dosage should be decreased gradually, especially with baclofen (Lioresal), carisoprodol (Soma), and cyclobenzaprine (Flexeril). Suddenly stopping baclofen may cause hallucinations; stopping the other drugs may cause fatigue, headache, and nausea.

## Critical Thinking Exercises

1. Which of the skeletal muscle relaxants is not a centrally active drug?
   a. Dantrolene (Dantrium)
   b. Carisoprodol (Soma)
   c. Cyclobenzaprine (Flexeril)
   d. Baclofen (Lioresal)

2. Tizanidine (Zanaflex) is an alpha₂-adrenergic agonist, similar to clonidine, that is used to treat spasticity. It should be used with caution in all of the following situations except:
   a. Renal impairment
   b. Hepatic impairment
   c. Hypotension
   d. Multiple sclerosis

3. Drug therapy for acute exacerbation of multiple sclerosis primarily includes the addition of:
   a. Interferon-beta (Avonex, Betaseron)
   b. Glatiramer (Copaxone)
   c. Corticosteroids
   d. Antidepressants

4. Adjunctive measures for muscle spasm and spasticity include all of the following except:
   a. Correct posture and lifting techniques
   b. Physical therapy (massage, moist heat, exercises)
   c. Moderate activity for acute muscle spasm
   d. Relaxation techniques

5. Which of the skeletal muscle relaxants is also used as supportive therapy in tetanus?
   a. Dantrolene (Dantrium)
   b. Carisoprodol (Soma)
   c. Baclofen (Lioresal)
   d. Cyclobenzaprine (Flexeril)

## SELECTED REFERENCES

*Drug facts and comparisons.* (Updated monthly). St. Louis: Facts and Comparisons.

Lacy, C. F., Armstrong, L. L., Goldman, M. P., & Lance, L. L. (2003). *Lexi-Comp's drug information handbook* (11th ed.). Hudson, OH: American Pharmaceutical Association.

Porth, C. M., & Curtis, R. L. (2002). Alterations in motor function. In C. M. Porth (Ed.), *Pathophysiology: Concepts of altered health states* (6th ed., pp. 1123–1157). Philadelphia: Lippincott Williams & Wilkins.

Richert, J. R. (2000). Demyelinating diseases. In H. D. Humes (Ed.), *Kelley's textbook of internal medicine* (4th ed., pp. 2912–2915). Philadelphia: Lippincott Williams & Wilkins.

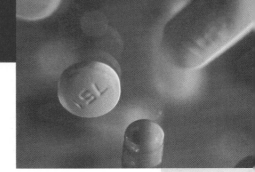

# 14

# Substance Abuse Disorders

## OBJECTIVES

*After studying this chapter, the student will be able to:*

1 Identify risk factors for development of drug dependence.

2 Describe the effects of alcohol, cocaine, marijuana, and nicotine on selected body organs.

3 Compare and contrast characteristics of dependence associated with alcohol, benzodiazepines, cocaine, and opiates.

4 Describe specific antidotes for overdoses of central nervous system (CNS) depressant drugs and the circumstances indicating their use.

5 Outline major elements of treatment for overdoses of commonly abused drugs that do not have antidotes.

6 Discuss interventions to prevent or manage withdrawal reactions associated with barbiturates, benzodiazepines, cocaine and other CNS stimulants, ethanol, and opiates.

## CRITICAL THINKING SCENARIO

*Y*ou are a school nurse working in a middle school. Just after lunch, an 8th grade student, Dan Powell, approaches you saying he is very worried about his friend. After lunch, on a dare, his friend drank more than half a bottle of vodka, and no one has been able to wake him up.

✔ Prioritize your assessment when you reach the intoxicated youth.

✔ List factors, especially during the adolescent period, that increase the likelihood a person will experiment with or abuse alcohol.

✔ Discuss important follow-up with this adolescent and his family after the incident.

# SUBSTANCE ABUSE

Abuse of alcohol and other drugs is a significant health, social, economic, and legal problem. Substance abuse is often associated with substantial damage to the abuser and society (eg, crime, child and spouse abuse, traumatic injury, death). As used in this chapter, the term *substance abuse* is defined as self-administration of a drug for prolonged periods or in excessive amounts to the point of producing physical or psychological dependence and reduced ability to function as a productive member of society.

Most drugs of abuse are those that affect the central nervous system (CNS) and alter the state of consciousness. These include prescription and nonprescription and legal and illegal drugs. Commonly abused drugs include CNS depressants (eg, alcohol, antianxiety/sedative-hypnotic agents, narcotic analgesics), CNS stimulants (eg, amphetamines, cocaine, nicotine), and other mind-altering drugs (eg, marijuana, "ecstasy"). Although these drugs produce different effects, they are associated with feelings of pleasure, positive reinforcement, and compulsive self-administration. Most are also associated with tolerance if used repeatedly. This means that the body adjusts to the drugs so that higher doses are needed to achieve feelings of pleasure or stave off withdrawal symptoms.

# DEPENDENCE

Characteristics of drug dependence include craving a drug, often with unsuccessful attempts to decrease its use; compulsive drug-seeking behavior; physical dependence (withdrawal symptoms if drug use is stopped); and continuing to take a drug despite adverse consequences (eg, drug-related illnesses, mental or legal problems, job loss or decreased ability to function in an occupation, impaired family relationships). A person may be dependent on more than one drug.

Many influencing factors are involved with drug dependence, including the specific drug and the amount, frequency, and route of administration. In addition to drug effects, other influencing factors include a person's psychological and physiologic characteristics and environmental or circumstantial characteristics. Characteristics of physical and psychological dependence are described in At the Foundation: Drug Dependence. Additional general characteristics of substance abuse and dependence include the following:

■ Substance abuse involves all socioeconomic levels and almost all age groups, from school-aged children to elderly adults. Patterns of abuse may vary among age groups. For example, adolescents and young adults may be more likely to use illicit drugs, and older adults are more likely to abuse alcohol and prescription drugs. Discussion of specific management considerations in children and older adults is found in Age-related Considerations. Health care professionals (eg, physicians, pharmacists, nurses) are also considered at high risk for development of substance abuse disorders, at least partly because of easy access.

■ A person who abuses one drug is likely to abuse others.

■ Multiple drugs are often abused concurrently. Alcohol, for example, is often used with other drugs of abuse, probably because it is legal and readily available. In addition, alcohol, marijuana, narcotics, and sedatives are often used to combat the anxiety and nervousness induced by cocaine and other CNS stimulants.

■ Drug effects vary according to the type of substance being abused, amount, route of administration, duration of use, and phase of substance abuse (eg, acute intoxication, withdrawal syndromes, organ damage, and medical illness). Thus, acute intoxication often produces profound behavioral changes, and chronic abuse often leads to serious organ damage and impaired ability to function in work, family, or social settings. Withdrawal symptoms are characteristic for particular types of drugs and are usually opposite the

---

**AT THE FOUNDATION:** *Drug Dependence*

Drug dependence is a complex phenomenon of unknown cause. One view is that drugs stimulate or inhibit neurotransmitters in the brain to produce pleasure and euphoria or to decrease unpleasant feelings such as anxiety.

*Psychological dependence* involves feelings of satisfaction and pleasure from taking the drug. These feelings, perceived as extremely desirable by the drug-dependent person, contribute to acute intoxication, development and maintenance of drug abuse patterns, and return to drug-taking behavior after periods of abstinence.

*Physical dependence* involves physiologic adaptation to chronic use of a drug so that unpleasant symptoms occur when the drug is stopped or its action is antagonized by another drug. The withdrawal or abstinence syndrome produces specific manifestations according to the type of drug and does not occur as long as adequate dosage is maintained. Attempts to avoid withdrawal symptoms reinforce psychological dependence and promote continuing drug use and relapses to drug-taking behavior. Tolerance is often an element of drug dependence, and increasing doses are therefore required to obtain psychological effects or avoid physical withdrawal symptoms.

## Age-related Considerations: Alcohol Abuse

### USE IN CHILDREN

Peer pressure is often an important factor in initial and continuing drug ingestion. A genetic factor seems evident in alcohol abuse: studies indicate that children of abusers are at risk for becoming abusers themselves, even if reared away from the abusing parent.

Parents can help prevent drug abuse in their children by positive role modeling. Children are more likely to use illegal drugs if their parents have a generally permissive attitude about drug taking, if either parent takes mind-altering drugs regularly, and if either parent is a heavy cigarette smoker.

### USE IN OLDER ADULTS

The abuse of substances in the older adult is not uncommon. In older adults, the pharmacokinetics of alcohol are essentially the same as for younger adults. However, equivalent amounts of alcohol produce higher blood levels in older adults because of changes in body composition (eg, a greater proportion of fatty tissue).

---

effects originally produced. For example, withdrawal symptoms of alcohol and sedative-type drugs are mainly agitation, nervousness, and hyperactivity.

- Alcohol and other drug abusers are not reliable sources of information about the types or amounts of drugs used. Most abusers understate the amount and frequency of substance use; heroin addicts may overstate the amount used in attempts to obtain higher doses of methadone. In addition, those who use illegal street drugs may not know what they have taken because of varying purity, potency, additives, names, and substitutions of one drug for another.

- Substance abusers rarely seek health care unless circumstances force the issue. Thus, most substance abuse comes to the attention of health care professionals when the abuser experiences a complication such as acute intoxication, withdrawal, or serious medical problems resulting from chronic drug overuse, misuse, or abuse.

- Smoking or inhaling drug vapors is a preferred route of administration for cocaine, marijuana, and nicotine because the drugs are rapidly absorbed from the large surface area of the lungs. Then, they rapidly circulate to the heart and brain without dilution by the systemic circulation or metabolism by enzymes. With crack cocaine, inhaling vapors from the heated drug produces blood levels comparable to those obtained with intravenous (IV) administration.

- Substance abusers who inject drugs intravenously are prey to serious problems because they use impure drugs of unknown potency, contaminated needles, poor hygiene, and other dangerous practices. Specific problems include overdoses, death, and numerous infections (eg, hepatitis, human immunodeficiency virus infection, endocarditis, phlebitis, and cellulitis at injection sites).

- Many drugs are abused for their mind-altering properties. Most of these have clinical usefulness and are discussed elsewhere (see Chap. 6, Narcotic Analgesics and Narcotic Antagonists; Chap. 8, Antianxiety and Sedative-Hypnotic Drugs; and Chap. 15, Central Nervous System Stimulants). This chapter describes commonly abused substances, characteristics and treatment of substance-related disorders, and drugs used to treat substance-related disorders (see Drugs at a Glance 14-1: Drugs Used to Treat Substance Abuse Disorders). No prototype is identified in this varied group.

## ■ CENTRAL NERVOUS SYSTEM DEPRESSANTS

CNS depressants are drugs that slow down or "depress" brain activity. They include alcohol, antianxiety and sedative-hypnotic agents, and opiates.

## Alcohol (Ethanol)

*Alcohol* is the most abused drug in the world. It is legal and readily available, and its use is accepted in most societies. There is no clear dividing line between use and abuse, but rather a continuum of progression over several years. Alcohol exerts profound metabolic and physiologic effects on all organ systems (Box 14-1). Some of these effects are evident with acute alcohol intake, whereas others become evident with chronic intake of substantial amounts. Alcohol is thought to exert its effects on the CNS by enhancing the activity of gamma-aminobutyric acid, an inhibitory neurotransmitter, or by inhibiting the activity of glutamate, an excitatory neurotransmitter.

When alcohol is ingested orally, a portion is inactivated in the stomach (by the enzyme alcohol dehydrogenase) and not absorbed systemically. Women have less enzyme activity than men and therefore absorb approximately 30% more alcohol than men when comparable amounts are ingested according to weight and size. As a result, women are especially vulnerable to adverse effects of alcohol, including more rapid intoxication from smaller amounts of alcohol and earlier development of hepatic cirrhosis and other complications of alcohol abuse.

## DRUG TABLE 14-1

*Drugs at a Glance*

## Drugs Used to Treat Substance Abuse Disorders

| Generic/ Trade Name | Indications for Use | Routes and Dosage Ranges: Adults | Comments |
|---|---|---|---|
| **Bupropion** (Zyban) Pregnancy Category B | Smoking cessation | PO, 150 mg once daily for 3 days, then increase to 150 mg twice daily, at least 8 hours apart. Maximum dose, 300 mg/d | May cause seizures |
| **Chlordiazepoxide** (Librium) Pregnancy Category D | Alcohol detoxification; benzo-diazepine withdrawal | PO, 50 mg q6–8h initially, then tapered over 1–2 wk | |
| **Clonidine** (Catapres) Pregnancy Category C | Alcohol withdrawal; opiate withdrawal | Alcohol withdrawal PO, 0.3–0.6 mg q6h Opiate withdrawal PO, 2 mcg/kg 3 times daily for 7–10 days | Unlabeled uses May cause hypotension |
| **Disulfiram** (Antabuse) Pregnancy Category C | Chronic alcohol abuse, to prevent continued alcohol ingestion | PO, 125–500 mg daily | Limited effectiveness because many alcoholics will not take the drug; should not be given until at least 12 h after alcohol ingestion |
| **Flumazenil** (Romazicon) Pregnancy Category C | Acute intoxication or overdose of benzodiazepine anti-anxiety or sedative-hypnotic drugs | IV, 0.1–0.2 mg/min up to 1 mg | May precipitate acute with-drawal symptoms |
| **Haloperidol** (Haldol) Pregnancy Category C | Psychotic symptoms associated with acute intoxication with cocaine and other central nervous system (CNS) stimulants | IM, 2–5 mg every 30 min to 6 h PRN for psychotic behavior | Other antipsychotic agents may also be used |
| **Levomethadyl** (LAAM) (ORLAAM) Pregnancy Category C | Maintenance therapy of heroin addiction | PO, 60–100 mg 3 times weekly | Reportedly as effective and well accepted by heroin addicts as methadone |
| **Lorazepam** (Ativan) Pregnancy Category D | Excessive CNS stimulation asso-ciated with acute intoxication with cocaine and other CNS stimulants, hallucinogens, marijuana, inhalants, and phencyclidine; alcohol withdrawal | *Agitation,* IM, q30 min–6 h PRN; *alcohol withdrawal hallucinations or seizures,* IM 2 mg, repeated if neces-sary; *benzodiazepine with-drawal,* PO 2 mg q6–8h initially, then tapered over 1–2 wk | 1 wk of tapering usually ade-quate for withdrawal from short-acting benzodiaze-pines; 2 wk needed for long-acting benzodiazepines |
| **Methadone** Pregnancy Category B; D prolonged use or high doses near term | Opiate withdrawal; mainte-nance therapy of heroin addiction | *Withdrawal,* PO, 20–80 mg daily initially, reduced by 5–10 mg daily over 7–10 days; *maintenance* PO 20–80 mg daily | Maintenance doses of 60–80 mg daily more effective than 20–30 mg daily in decreasing heroin use |
| **Naloxone** (Narcan) Pregnancy Category C | Acute intoxication or overdose of opiates (heroin, morphine, others) | IV, 0.4–2 mg q3min | May precipitate acute with-drawal symptoms |

*(continued)*

**DRUG TABLE 14-1**

*Drugs at a Glance*

## Drugs Used to Treat Substance Abuse Disorders (Continued)

| Generic/ Trade Name | Indications for Use | Routes and Dosage Ranges: Adults | Comments |
|---|---|---|---|
| **Naltrexone** (ReVia) Pregnancy Category C | Opiate dependence; alcohol dependence | PO, 50 mg daily | With opiate dependence, should not be started until patient is opioid-free for at least 7 d |
| **Nicotine** (Habitrol, Nicotrol, Nicoderm CQ, Nicorette, Nicotrol Inhaler, Nicotrol NS) Pregnancy Category D transdermal; X chewing gum | Aid smoking cessation by relieving nicotine withdrawal symptoms | *Transdermal patches, Habitrol, Nicoderm:* 21 mg/d for 6 wk; 14 mg/d for 2 wk; 7 mg/d for 2 wk *Nicotrol patch:* 15 mg/16 hours for 6 wk *Nicotrol chewing gum:* 1 piece every 1–2 h for wks 1–6; 1 piece every 2–4 h for wks 7–9; 1 piece every 4–8 h for wks 10–12 *Nicotrol inhaler,* 6–12 cartridges/d for 3 mo, then gradually taper dosage over 6–12 wk, then discontinue *Nicotrol nasal spray,* 1 spray to each nostril, every 1–2 h, to a maximum of 80 sprays (40 mg) per day for heavy smokers. Taper by using less often or spraying 1 nostril per dose. | Should not be used while continuing to smoke because of high risk of serious adverse effects Used patches contain enough nicotine to be toxic to children and pets; they should be discarded in a safe manner |

---

**BOX 14-1    Effects of Alcohol Abuse**

**Central and Peripheral Nervous System Effects**
Sedation ranging from drowsiness to coma; impaired memory, learning, and thinking processes; impaired motor coordination, with ataxia or staggering gait, altered speech patterns, poor task performance, and hypoactivity or hyperactivity; mental depression, anxiety, insomnia; impaired interpersonal relationships; brain damage, polyneuritis and Wernicke-Korsakoff syndrome.

**Hepatic Effects**
Induces drug-metabolizing enzymes that accelerate metabolism of alcohol and many other drugs and produces tolerance and cross-tolerance; eventually damages the liver enough to impair drug metabolism, leading to accumulation and toxic effects; decreases use and increases production of lactate, leading to lactic acidosis, decreased renal excretion of uric acid, and secondary hyperuricemia; decreases use and increases production of lipids, leading to hyperlipidemia and fatty liver. Fatty liver causes accumulation of fat and protein, leading to hepatomegaly; eventually produces severe liver

injury characterized by necrosis and inflammation (alcoholic hepatitis) or by fibrous bands of scar tissue that irreversibly alter structure and function (cirrhosis).

The incidence of liver disease correlates with the amount of alcohol consumed and the progression of liver damage is attributed directly to ethanol or indirectly to the metabolic changes produced by ethanol.

**Gastrointestinal Effects**
Slowed gastric emptying time; increased intestinal motility, which probably contributes to the diarrhea that often occurs with alcoholism; damage to the epithelial cells of the intestinal mucosa; multiple nutritional deficiencies, including protein and water-soluble vitamins, such as thiamine, folic acid, and vitamin $B_{12}$; pancreatic disease, which contributes to malabsorption of fat, nitrogen, and vitamin $B_{12}$.

**Cardiovascular Effects**
Damage to myocardial cells; cardiomyopathy manifested by cardiomegaly, edema, dyspnea, abnormal heart sounds, and

*(continued)*

BOX
14-1    **Effects of Alcohol Abuse** (Continued)

electrocardiographic changes indicating left ventricular hypertrophy, abnormal T waves, and conduction disturbances; possible impairment of coronary blood flow and myocardial contractility.

### Hematologic Effects

Bone marrow depression due to alcohol or associated conditions, such as malnutrition, infection, and liver disease; several types of anemia including *megaloblastic anemia* from folic acid deficiency, *sideroblastic anemia* (sideroblasts are precursors of red blood cells) probably from nutritional deficiency, *hemolytic anemia* from abnormalities in the structure of red blood cells, *iron deficiency anemia* usually from gastrointestinal bleeding, and anemias from hemodilution, chronic infection, and fatty liver and bone marrow failure associated with cirrhosis; thrombocytopenia and decreased platelet aggregation from folic acid deficiency, hypersplenism, and other factors; decreased numbers and impaired function of white blood cells, which lead to decreased resistance to infection.

### Endocrine Effects

Increased release of cortisol and catecholamines and decreased release of aldosterone from the adrenal glands; hypogonadism, gynecomastia, and feminization in men with cirrhosis due to decreased secretion of male sex hormones;

degenerative changes in the anterior pituitary gland; decreased secretion of antidiuretic hormone from the posterior pituitary; hypoglycemia due to impaired glucose synthesis or hyperglycemia due to glycogenolysis.

### Skeletal Effects

Impaired growth and development, which is most apparent in children born to alcoholic mothers. Fetal alcohol syndrome is characterized by low birth weight and length and by birth defects, such as cleft palate and cardiac septal defects. Impairment of growth and motor development persists in the postnatal period, and mental retardation becomes apparent. Other effects include decreased bone density, osteoporosis, and increased susceptibility to fractures; osteonecrosis due to obstructed blood supply; hypocalcemia, which leads to bone resorption and decreased skeletal mass; hypomagnesemia, which may further stimulate bone resorption; hypophosphatemia, probably from inadequate dietary intake of phosphorus.

### Muscular Effects

Acute myopathy, which may be manifested by acute pain, tenderness, edema, and hyperkalemia; chronic myopathy, which may involve muscle weakness, atrophy, episodes of acute myopathy associated with a drinking spree, and elevated creatine phosphokinase.

In men and women, alcohol is absorbed partly from the stomach but mostly from the upper small intestine. It is rapidly absorbed when the stomach and small intestine are empty. Food delays absorption by diluting the alcohol and delaying gastric emptying. Once absorbed, alcohol is quickly distributed to all body tissues, partly because it is lipid soluble and crosses cell membranes easily. The alcohol concentration in the brain rapidly approaches that in the blood, and CNS effects usually occur within a few minutes. These effects depend on the amount ingested, how rapidly it was ingested, whether the stomach was empty, and other factors. Effects with acute intoxication usually progress from a feeling of relaxation to impaired mental and motor functions to stupor and sleep. Excited behavior may occur because of depression of the cerebral cortex, which normally controls behavior. The person may seem more relaxed, talkative, and outgoing or more impulsive and aggressive because inhibitions have been lessened.

The rate of alcohol metabolism largely determines the duration of CNS effects. Most alcohol is oxidized in the liver to acetaldehyde, which can be used for energy or converted to fat and stored. When metabolized to acetaldehyde, alcohol no longer exerts depressant effects on the CNS. Although the rate of metabolism differs with acute ingestion or chronic intake and some other factors, it is approximately 120 mg/kg of body weight or 10 mL/hour. This is the amount of alcohol contained in approximately

2 to 3 oz of whiskey, 3 to 4 oz of wine, or 8 to 12 oz of beer. *Alcohol is metabolized at the same rate regardless of the amount present in body tissues.*

### Interactions With Other Drugs

Alcohol may cause several potentially significant interactions when used with other drugs. These interactions often differ between acute and chronic ingestion. *Acute ingestion* inhibits drug-metabolizing enzymes. This slows the metabolism of some drugs, thereby increasing their effects and the likelihood of toxicity. *Chronic ingestion* induces metabolizing enzymes. This increases the rate of metabolism and decreases drug effects. Long-term ingestion of large amounts of alcohol, however, causes liver damage and impaired ability to metabolize drugs.

Because so many variables influence alcohol's interactions with other drugs, it is difficult to predict effects of interactions in particular people. However, some important interactions include those with other CNS depressants, antihypertensive agents, antidiabetic agents, oral anticoagulants, and disulfiram. These are summarized as follows:

■ With other CNS depressants (eg, sedative-hypnotics, narcotic analgesics, antianxiety agents, antipsychotic agents, general anesthetics, and tricyclic antidepressants), alcohol potentiates CNS depression and increases risks for excessive sedation, respiratory depression, impaired mental and physical functioning, and other effects. Combining alcohol with these drugs may be lethal and should be avoided.

- With antihypertensive agents, alcohol potentiates vasodilation and hypotensive effects.
- With oral antidiabetic drugs, alcohol potentiates hypoglycemic effects.
- With oral anticoagulants (eg, warfarin), alcohol interactions vary. Acute ingestion increases anticoagulant effects and the risk for bleeding. Chronic ingestion decreases anticoagulant effects by inducing drug-metabolizing enzymes in the liver and increasing the rate of warfarin metabolism. However, if chronic ingestion has caused liver damage, metabolism of warfarin may be slowed. This increases the risk for excessive anticoagulant effect and bleeding.
- With disulfiram (Antabuse), alcohol produces significant distress (flushing, tachycardia, bronchospasm, sweating, nausea, and vomiting). This reaction may be used to treat alcohol dependence.
- A disulfiram-like reaction also may occur with other drugs, including several cephalosporin antibiotics (cefamandole, cefonicid, cefoperazone, ceforanide, cefotetan), chlorpropamide (Diabinese), tolbutamide (Orinase), and metronidazole (Flagyl).

## Alcohol Dependence

Alcohol dependence involves acute or chronic consumption of alcohol in excess of the limits accepted by the person's culture, at times considered inappropriate by that culture, and to the extent that physical health and social relationships are impaired. Psychological dependence, physical dependence, tolerance, and cross-tolerance (with other CNS depressants) are prominent characteristics.

Acute intoxication impairs thinking, judgment, and psychomotor coordination. These impairments lead to poor work performance, accidents, and disturbed relationships with other people. Conscious control of behavior is lost, and exhibitionism, aggressiveness, and assaultiveness often result. Chronic ingestion affects essentially all body systems and may cause severe organ damage and mental problems. Effects are summarized in Box 14-1.

Signs and symptoms of alcohol withdrawal include agitation, anxiety, tremors, sweating, nausea, tachycardia, fever, hyperreflexia, postural hypotension, and, if severe, convulsions and delirium. Confusion, disorientation, delusions, visual hallucinations, and other signs of acute psychosis characterize delirium tremens, the most serious form of alcohol withdrawal. The intensity of the alcohol withdrawal syndrome varies with the duration and amount of alcohol ingestion. Withdrawal symptoms start within a few hours after a person's last drink and last for several days.

## Treatment of Alcohol Dependence

Alcohol dependence is a progressive illness, and early recognition and treatment are desirable. The alcohol-dependent person is unlikely to seek treatment for alcohol abuse unless an acute situation forces the issue. He or she is likely, however, to seek treatment for other disorders, such as nervousness, anxiety, depression, insomnia, and gastroenteritis. Thus, health professionals may recognize alcohol abuse in its early stages if they are aware of indicative assessment data.

If the first step of treatment is recognition of alcohol abuse, the second step is probably confronting the client with evidence of alcohol abuse and trying to elicit cooperation. Unless the client admits that alcohol abuse is a problem and agrees to participate in a treatment program, success is unlikely. The client may fail to make return visits or may seek treatment elsewhere. If the client agrees to treatment, the three primary approaches are psychological counseling, referral to a self-help group such as Alcoholics Anonymous, and drug therapy.

Acute intoxication with alcohol does not usually require treatment. If the client is hyperactive and combative, a sedative-type drug may be given. The client must be closely observed because sedatives potentiate alcohol, and excessive CNS depression may occur. If the client is already sedated and stuporous, he or she can be allowed to sleep off the alcohol effects. If the client is comatose, supportive measures are indicated. For example, respiratory depression may require insertion of an artificial airway and mechanical ventilation.

Benzodiazepine antianxiety agents are the drugs of choice for treating alcohol withdrawal syndromes. They can help the client participate in rehabilitation programs and can be gradually reduced in dosage and discontinued. They provide adequate sedation and have a significant anticonvulsant effect. Some health care providers prefer a benzodiazepine with a long half-life (eg, diazepam or chlordiazepoxide), whereas others prefer one with a short half-life (eg, lorazepam or oxazepam). Lorazepam and oxazepam are less likely to accumulate and may be best for older adults or clients with hepatic disease. Alcoholic clients usually require high doses of benzodiazepines because of the drugs' cross-tolerance with alcohol.

Seizures require treatment if they are repeated or continuous. Antiseizure drugs need not be given for more than a few days unless the person has a preexisting seizure disorder. Clonidine may be given to reduce symptoms (eg, hyperactivity, tremors) associated with excessive stimulation of the sympathetic nervous system. Midazolam or propofol may be useful for treating delirium tremens because their doses can be easily titrated to manage the symptoms.

Drug therapy for maintenance of sobriety is limited, mainly because of poor compliance. The two drugs approved for this purpose are *disulfiram* (Antabuse) and *naltrexone* (ReVia). Disulfiram interferes with hepatic metabolism of alcohol and allows accumulation of acetaldehyde. If alcohol is ingested during disulfiram therapy, acetaldehyde causes nausea and vomiting, dyspnea, hypotension, tachycardia, syncope, blurred vision, headache, and confusion. Severe reactions include respiratory depression, cardiovascular collapse, cardiac arrhythmias, myocardial infarction, congestive heart failure, unconsciousness, convulsions, and death. The severity of reactions varies but is usually proportional to the amounts of alcohol and disulfiram taken. The duration of the reaction varies from a few minutes to several hours, as long as alcohol is present in the blood. Ingestion of prescription and over-the-counter medications that contain alcohol may cause a reaction in the disulfiram-treated alcoholic client. Disulfiram alone may produce adverse reactions of drowsiness, fatigue, impotence, headache, and dermatitis. These are more likely to occur during the first 2 weeks of treatment, after which they usually subside. Disulfiram also interferes with the metabolism of phenytoin and warfarin, which may increase blood levels of the drugs and increase their toxicity. Because of these reactions, disulfiram must be given only with the client's full consent, cooperation, and knowledge.

Naltrexone is an opiate antagonist that reduces craving for alcohol and increases abstinence rates when combined with psychosocial treatment. A possible mechanism is blockade of the endogenous opioid system, which is thought to reinforce alcohol craving and consumption. The most common adverse effect is nausea; others include anxiety, dizziness, drowsiness, headache, insomnia, nervousness, and vomiting. Naltrexone is hepatotoxic in high doses and contraindicated in clients with acute hepatitis or liver failure.

In addition to drug therapy to treat withdrawal and maintain sobriety, alcohol abusers often need treatment of coexisting psychiatric disorders, such as depression. Antidepressant drugs appear to decrease alcohol intake as well as relieve depression.

## Barbiturates and Benzodiazepines

Barbiturates are old drugs that are rarely used therapeutically but remain drugs of abuse. Overdoses may cause respiratory depression, coma, and death. Withdrawal is similar to alcohol withdrawal and may be more severe. Seizures and death can occur. With short-acting barbiturates such as pentobarbital (Nembutal) and secobarbital (Seconal), withdrawal symptoms begin 12 to 24 hours after the last dose and peak at 24 to 72 hours. With phenobarbital, symptoms begin 24 to 48 hours after the last dose and peak in 5 to 8 days.

Benzodiazepines are widely used for antianxiety and sedative-hypnotic effects (see Chap. 8) and are also widely abused, mainly by people who also abuse alcohol or other drugs. Benzodiazepines rarely cause respiratory depression or death, even in overdose, unless taken with alcohol or other drugs. They may, however, cause oversedation, memory impairment, poor motor coordination, and confusion. Withdrawal reactions can be extremely uncomfortable. Symptoms begin 12 to 24 hours after the last dose of a short-acting drug such as alprazolam

(Xanax) and peak at 24 to 72 hours. With long-acting drugs such as diazepam (Valium) and chlordiazepoxide (Librium), symptoms begin 24 to 48 hours after the last dose and peak within 5 to 8 days.

Combining any of these drugs with each other or with alcohol can cause serious depression of vital functions and death. Unfortunately, abusers often combine drugs in their quest for a greater "high" or to relieve the unpleasant effects of CNS stimulants and other street drugs.

### Barbiturate and Benzodiazepine Dependence
This type of dependence resembles alcohol dependence in symptoms of intoxication and withdrawal. Other characteristics include physical dependence, psychological dependence, tolerance, and cross-tolerance. Signs and symptoms of withdrawal include anxiety, tremors and muscle twitching, weakness, dizziness, distorted visual perceptions, nausea and vomiting, insomnia, nightmares, tachycardia, weight loss, postural hypotension, generalized tonic-clonic seizures, and delirium that resembles the delirium tremens of alcoholism or a major psychotic episode. Convulsions are more likely to occur during the first 48 hours of withdrawal and delirium after 48 to 72 hours. Signs and symptoms of withdrawal are less severe with the benzodiazepines than with the barbiturates.

### Treatment of Barbiturate or Benzodiazepine Abuse
Treatment may involve overdose and withdrawal syndromes. Overdose produces intoxication similar to that produced by alcohol. There may be a period of excitement and emotional lability followed by progressively increasing signs of CNS depression (eg, impaired mental function, muscular incoordination, and sedation). Treatment is unnecessary for mild overdose if vital functions are adequate. The client usually sleeps off the effects of the drug. The rate of recovery depends primarily on the amount of drug ingested and its rate of metabolism. More severe overdoses cause respiratory depression and coma.

There is no antidote for barbiturate overdose; treatment is symptomatic and supportive. The goals of treatment are to maintain vital functions until the drug is metabolized and eliminated from the body. Insertion of an artificial airway and mechanical ventilation often are necessary. Gastric lavage may help if started within approximately 3 hours of drug ingestion. If the person is comatose, a cuffed endotracheal tube should be inserted and the cuff inflated before lavage to prevent aspiration. Diuresis helps to eliminate the drugs and can be induced by IV fluids or diuretic drugs. Hemodialysis also removes most of these drugs and may be used with high serum drug levels or failure to respond to other treatment measures. Hypotension and shock are usually treated with IV fluids.

These treatments were formerly used for benzodiazepine overdoses and may still be needed in some cases (eg, overdoses involving multiple drugs). However, a specific antidote is now available to reverse sedation, coma, and respiratory depression. Flumazenil (Romazicon) competes with benzodiazepines for benzodiazepine receptors. The drug has a short duration of action, and repeated IV injections are usually needed. Recipients must be closely observed because symptoms of overdose may recur when the effects of a dose of flumazenil subside and because the drug may precipitate acute withdrawal symptoms (eg, agitation, confusion, seizures) in benzodiazepine abusers.

Treatment of withdrawal may involve administering a benzodiazepine or phenobarbital to relieve acute signs and symptoms, then tapering the dose until the drug can be discontinued. Barbiturate and benzodiazepine withdrawal syndromes can be life threatening. The person may experience cardiovascular collapse, generalized tonic-clonic seizures, and acute psychotic episodes. These can be prevented by gradually withdrawing the offending drug. If they do occur, each situation requires specific drug therapy and supportive measures. Withdrawal reactions should be supervised and managed by experienced people, such as health care professionals or staff at detoxification centers.

## Opiates

Opiates are potent analgesics and extensively used in pain management (see Chap. 6). They are also commonly abused. Because therapeutic opiates are discussed elsewhere, the focus here is heroin. Heroin, a semisynthetic derivative of morphine, is a common drug of abuse. It is a Schedule I drug in the United States and is not used therapeutically.

Heroin may be taken by IV injection, smoking, or nasal application (snorting). IV injection produces intense euphoria, which occurs within seconds, lasts a few minutes, and is followed by a period of sedation. Effects diminish over approximately 4 hours, depending on the dose. Addicts may inject several times daily, cycling between desired effects and symptoms of withdrawal. Tolerance to euphoric effects develops rapidly, leading to dosage escalation and continued use to avoid withdrawal. Like other opiates, heroin causes severe respiratory depression with overdose and produces a characteristic abstinence syndrome.

### Opiate Dependence

Opiates produce tolerance and high degrees of psychological and physical dependence. Most other drugs that produce dependence do so with prolonged use of large doses, but morphine-like drugs produce dependence with repeated administration of small doses. Medical use of these drugs produces physical dependence and tolerance but rarely leads to use or abuse for their mind-altering effects. Thus, "addiction" should not be an issue when the drugs are needed for pain management in clients with cancer or other severe illnesses.

Acute effects of opiate administration vary according to dosage, route of administration, and physical and mental characteristics of the user. They may produce euphoria, sedation, analgesia, respiratory depression, postural hypotension, vasodilation, pupil constriction, and constipation.

### Treatment of Opiate Dependence

Treatment may be needed for overdose or withdrawal syndromes. Overdose may produce severe respiratory depression and coma. Insertion of an endotracheal tube and mechanical ventilation may be required. Drug therapy consists of a narcotic antagonist to reverse narcotic effects. Giving a narcotic antagonist can precipitate withdrawal symptoms. If there is no response to the narcotic antagonist, the symptoms may be caused by depressant drugs other than opiates. In addition to profound respiratory depression, pulmonary edema, hypoglycemia, pneumonia, cellulitis, and other infections often accompany opiate overdose and require specific treatment measures.

Signs and symptoms of withdrawal can be reversed immediately by giving the drug producing the dependence. Therapeutic withdrawal, which is more comfortable and safer, can be managed by gradually reducing the dosage over several days. Clonidine, an antihypertensive drug, is sometimes used to relieve withdrawal symptoms associated with sympathetic nervous system overactivity.

Ideally, the goal of treatment for opiate abuse is abstinence from further opiate usage. Because this goal is rarely met, long-term drug therapy may be used to treat heroin dependence. One method uses narcotic substitutes to prevent withdrawal symptoms and improve a lifestyle that revolves around obtaining, using, and recovering from a drug. Methadone has long been used for this purpose, usually as a single, daily, oral dose given in a methadone clinic. Proponents say that methadone blocks euphoria produced by heroin, acts longer, and reduces preoccupation with drug use. This allows a more normal lifestyle for the client and reduces morbidity and mortality associated with the use of illegal and injected drugs. Also, because methadone is free, the heroin addict does not commit crimes to obtain drugs. Opponents say that methadone maintenance only substitutes one type of drug dependence for another. In addition, a substantial percentage of those receiving methadone maintenance therapy abuse other drugs, including cocaine.

Another drug approved for maintenance therapy is levomethadyl acetate hydrochloride, also called LAAM. LAAM (ORLAAM) is a synthetic, Schedule II narcotic indicated only for the treatment of opiate dependence. It is metabolized to long-acting, potent metabolites. After oral administration, effects occur within 90 minutes, peak in about 4 hours, and last about 72 hours. Its main advantage over methadone is that it can be given three times weekly rather than daily. However, if given on a Monday-Wednesday-Friday schedule, the Friday dose may need to be larger to prevent withdrawal symptoms until the Monday dose can be given. Also, initial dosage needs careful titration to prevent withdrawal symptoms but avoid overdosage when peak effects occur. Clients must be informed about the delayed effects of the drug and the risks for overdosage if they take other opiates. LAAM has prodysrhythmic effects, and an electrocardiogram should be done before starting the drug and periodically during therapy.

A third treatment option is naltrexone (ReVia), a narcotic antagonist that prevents opiates from occupying receptor sites and thereby prevents their physiologic effects. Used to maintain opiate-free states in the opiate addict, it is recommended for use in conjunction with psychological counseling to promote client motivation and compliance. If the client taking naltrexone has mild or moderate pain, non-narcotic analgesics (eg, acetaminophen or a nonsteroidal anti-inflammatory drug) should be given. If the client has severe pain and requires a narcotic, it should be given in a setting staffed and equipped for cardiopulmonary resuscitation because respiratory depression may be deeper and more prolonged than usual. In addition, clients needing elective surgery and narcotic analgesics should be instructed to stop taking naltrexone at least 72 hours before the scheduled procedure.

## CENTRAL NERVOUS SYSTEM STIMULANTS

### Amphetamines and Related Drugs

Amphetamines and related drugs (see Chap. 15) are used therapeutically for narcolepsy and attention deficit-hyperactivity disorder (ADHD). Except for the use of methylphenidate in treating ADHD, however, the drugs are more important as drugs of abuse than therapeutic agents.

#### Amphetamine Dependence

Amphetamines and related drugs (eg, methylphenidate) produce stimulation and euphoria, effects often sought by drug users. The user may increase the amount and frequency of administration to reach or continue the state of stimulation. One of the drugs, methamphetamine, may be chemically treated to produce potent crystals (called "ice"), which are then heated and the vapors smoked or inhaled. Psychological effects of amphetamines are similar to those produced by cocaine and are largely dose related. Small amounts produce mental alertness, wakefulness, and increased energy. Large amounts may cause psychosis (eg, hallucinations and paranoid delusions). Tolerance develops to amphetamines.

Acute ingestion of these drugs masks underlying fatigue or depression; withdrawal allows these conditions to emerge in an exaggerated form. The resulting exhaustion and depression reinforce the compulsion to continue using the drugs. Users may take them alone or to coun-

teract the effects of other drugs. In the latter case, these drugs may be part of a pattern of polydrug use in which CNS depressants, such as alcohol or sedative-type drugs ("downers"), are alternated with CNS stimulants, such as amphetamines ("uppers").

#### Treatment of Amphetamine Abuse

Treatment of amphetamine-type abuse is mainly concerned with overdosage because these drugs do not produce physical dependence and withdrawal as alcohol, opiates, and sedative-hypnotic drugs do. Because amphetamines delay gastric emptying, gastric lavage may be helpful even if several hours have passed since drug ingestion. The client is likely to be hyperactive, agitated, and hallucinating (toxic psychosis) and may have tachycardia, fever, and other symptoms. Symptomatic treatment includes sedation, lowering of body temperature, and administration of an antipsychotic drug. Sedative-type drugs must be used with great caution, however, because depression and sleep usually follow amphetamine use, and these aftereffects can be aggravated by sedative administration.

### Cocaine

Cocaine is a popular drug of abuse. It produces powerful CNS stimulation by preventing reuptake of neurotransmitters (eg, dopamine, norepinephrine, serotonin), which increases and prolongs neurotransmitter effects. Cocaine is commonly inhaled (snorted) through the nose; "crack" is heated and the vapors inhaled. Acute use of cocaine or crack produces intense euphoria, increased energy and alertness, sexual arousal, tachycardia, increased blood pressure, and restlessness followed by depression, fatigue, and drowsiness as drug effects wear off. Overdosage can cause cardiac dysrhythmias, convulsions, myocardial infarction, respiratory failure, stroke, and death, even in young, healthy adults and even with initial exposure. Both acute and chronic use produce numerous physiologic effects (Box 14-2).

#### Cocaine Abuse

Cocaine-induced euphoria is intense but brief and often leads to drug ingestion every few minutes as long as the drug is available. Cocaine is not thought to produce physical dependence, although fatigue, depression, drowsiness, dysphoria, and intense craving occur as drug effects dissipate. Crack is a strong, inexpensive, extremely addicting, and widely used form of cocaine. It is prepared by altering cocaine hydrochloride with chemicals and heat to form rocklike formations of cocaine base. The process removes impurities and results in a very potent drug. When the drug is heated and the vapors inhaled, crack acts within a few seconds. It reportedly can cause psychological dependence with one use.

#### Treatment of Cocaine Abuse

Drug therapy is largely symptomatic. Thus, agitation and hyperactivity may be treated with a benzodiazepine anti-

---

**BOX 14-2    Physiologic and Behavioral Effects of Cocaine Abuse**

**Central Nervous System Effects**

Cerebral infarct, subarachnoid and other hemorrhages; excessive central nervous system stimulation, manifested by anxiety, agitation, delirium, hyperactivity, irritability, insomnia, anorexia and weight loss; psychosis with paranoid delusions and hallucinations that may be indistinguishable from schizophrenia; seizures.

**Cardiovascular Effects**

Dysrhythmias, including tachycardia, premature ventricular contractions, ventricular tachycardia and fibrillation, and asystole; cardiopathy; myocardial ischemia and acute myocardial infarction; hypertension; stroke; rupture of the aorta; constriction of coronary and peripheral arteries.

**Respiratory Effects**

With snorting of cocaine, rhinitis, rhinorrhea, and damage (ulceration, perforation, necrosis) of the nasal septum from vasoconstriction and ischemia. With inhalation of crack cocaine vapors, respiratory symptoms occur in up to 25% of users and may include bronchitis, bronchospasm, cough, dyspnea, pneumonia, pulmonary edema, and fatal lung hemorrhage.

**Gastrointestinal Effects**

Nausea; weight loss; intestinal ischemia, possible necrosis.

**Genitourinary Effects**

Delayed orgasm for men and women; difficulty in maintaining erection.

**Effects of Intravenous Use**

Hepatitis; human immunodeficiency virus infection; endocarditis; cellulitis; abscesses.

---

anxiety agent; psychosis may be treated with haloperidol or other antipsychotic agent; cardiac dysrhythmias may be treated with usual antidysrhythmic drugs; myocardial infarction may be treated by standard methods; and so forth. Initial detoxification and long-term treatment are best accomplished in centers or units that specialize in substance abuse disorders.

Long-term treatment of cocaine abuse usually involves psychotherapy, behavioral therapy, and 12-step programs. In addition, many clients need treatment for coexisting psychiatric disorders.

## Nicotine

Nicotine, one of many active ingredients in tobacco products, is the ingredient that promotes compulsive use, abuse, and dependence. Inhaling smoke from a cigarette produces CNS stimulation in a few seconds. The average cigarette contains approximately 6 to 8 mg of nicotine and delivers approximately 1 mg of nicotine systemically to the smoker (most is burned or dissipated as "sidestream" smoke). Nicotine obtained from chewing tobacco produces longer-lasting effects because it is more slowly absorbed than inhaled nicotine. Nicotine produces its effects by increasing levels of dopamine and other substances in the brain.

Nicotine is readily absorbed through the lungs, skin, and mucous membranes. It is extensively metabolized, mainly in the liver, and its metabolites are eliminated by the kidneys. It is also excreted in breast milk of nursing mothers. Adverse effects include nausea in new smokers at low blood levels and in experienced smokers at blood levels higher than their accustomed levels. Nicotine poisoning can occur in infants and children from ingestion of tobacco products, skin contact with used nicotine trans-

dermal patches, or chewing nicotine gum. Poisoning may also occur with accidental ingestion of insecticide sprays containing nicotine. Oral ingestion usually causes vomiting, which limits the amount of nicotine absorbed. Toxic effects of a large dose may include hypertension, cardiac dysrhythmias, convulsions, coma, respiratory arrest, and paralysis of skeletal muscle. With chronic tobacco use, nicotine is implicated in the vascular disease and sudden cardiac death associated with smoking. However, the role of nicotine in the etiology of other disorders (eg, cancer and pulmonary disease) associated with chronic use of tobacco is unknown. Effects are summarized in Box 14-3.

### Nicotine Dependence

Like alcohol and opiate dependence, nicotine dependence is characterized by compulsive use and the development of tolerance and physical dependence. Mental depression is also associated with nicotine dependence. It is unknown whether depression leads to smoking or develops concomitantly with nicotine dependence. Cigarette smokers may smoke to obtain the perceived pleasure of nicotine's effects, avoid the discomfort of nicotine withdrawal, or both. Evidence indicates a compulsion to smoke when blood levels of nicotine become low. Abstinence from smoking leads to signs and symptoms of withdrawal (eg, anxiety, irritability, difficulty concentrating, restlessness, headache, increased appetite, weight gain, sleep disturbances), which usually begin within 24 hours of the last exposure to nicotine.

### Treatment of Nicotine Dependence

Most tobacco users who quit do so on their own. For those who are strongly dependent and unable or unwilling to quit on their own, there are two main methods of

> ## BOX 14-3    Effects of Nicotine
>
> **Central Nervous System Effects**
> Central nervous system stimulation with increased alertness, possibly feelings of enjoyment, decreased appetite, tremors, convulsions at high doses.
>
> **Cardiovascular Effects**
> Cardiac stimulation with tachycardia, vasoconstriction, increased blood pressure, increased force of myocardial contraction, and increased cardiac workload.
>
> **Gastrointestinal Effects**
> Increases secretion of gastric acid; increases muscle tone and motility; nausea and vomiting; aggravates gastroesophageal and peptic ulcer disease.

treatment. One method is the use of bupropion, an antidepressant (see Chap. 10). The antidepressant formulation is marketed as Wellbutrin; the smoking-cessation formulation is Zyban, a sustained-release tablet. The other method is nicotine replacement therapy with drug formulations of nicotine. These products prevent or reduce withdrawal symptoms, but they do not produce the subjective effects or peak blood levels seen with cigarettes.

Nicotine is available in transdermal patches, chewing gum, an oral inhaler, and a nasal spray. The gum, inhaler, and spray are used intermittently during the day; the transdermal patch is applied once daily. Transdermal patches produce a steady blood level of nicotine, and clients seem to use them more consistently than they use the other products. The patches and gum are available over the counter; the inhaler and nasal spray require a prescription. The products are contraindicated in people with significant cardiovascular disease (angina pectoris, dysrhythmias, or recent myocardial infarction). Adverse effects include soreness of mouth and throat (with gum), nausea, vomiting, dizziness, hypertension, dysrhythmias, confusion, and skin irritation at sites of transdermal patch application.

Nicotine products are intended to be used for limited periods of 3 to 6 months, with tapering of dosage and discontinuation. Although they are effective in helping smokers achieve abstinence, many resume smoking.

Overall, treatment regimens that combine counseling and behavioral therapy with drug therapy are more successful than those using drug therapy alone. In addition, a combination of Zyban and nicotine transdermal patches is sometimes used and may be more effective than either drug alone.

## Marijuana

Marijuana and other cannabis preparations are obtained from *Cannabis sativa*, the hemp plant, which grows in most parts of the world, including the entire United States. Marijuana and hashish are the two cannabis preparations used in the United States. Marijuana is obtained from leaves and stems; hashish, prepared from plant resin, is 5 to 10 times as potent as commonly available marijuana. These cannabis preparations contain several related compounds called *cannabinoids*. Delta-9-tetrahydrocannabinol (Δ-9-THC) is the main psychoactive ingredient, but metabolites and other constituents also may exert pharmacologic activity. The mechanism of action is unknown, although specific cannabinoid receptors have been identified in several regions of the brain. The endogenous substances that react with these receptors have not been determined.

Cannabis preparations are difficult to classify. Some people call them depressants; some call them stimulants; and others label them as mind-altering, hallucinogenic, psychotomimetic, or unique in terms of fitting into drug categories. It is also difficult to predict the effects of these drugs. Many factors apparently influence a person's response. One factor is the amount of active ingredients, which varies with the climate and soil where the plants are grown and with the method of preparation. Other factors include dose, route of administration, personality variables, and the environment in which the drug is taken.

Marijuana can be taken orally but is more often smoked and inhaled through the lungs. It is more potent and more rapid in its actions when inhaled. After smoking, subjective effects begin in minutes, peak in approximately 30 minutes, and last 2 to 3 hours. Low doses are mildly intoxicating and similar to small amounts of alcohol. Large doses can produce panic reactions and hallucinations similar to acute psychosis. Effects wear off as THC is metabolized to inactive products. Many physiologic effects (Box 14-4) and adverse reactions have been reported with marijuana use, including impaired ability to drive an automobile and perform other common tasks of everyday life.

Except for dronabinol (Marinol), marijuana and other cannabis preparations are illegal and not used therapeutically in the United States. Dronabinol, a formulation of Δ-9-THC, is used to treat nausea and vomiting associated with anticancer drugs and to stimulate appetite in clients with acquired immunodeficiency syndrome (AIDS). The risks for abuse are high, and the drug may cause physical and psychological dependence. It is a Schedule III controlled drug. Cannabinoids can also decrease intraocular pressure and may be useful in treating glaucoma. Some

---

**BOX 14-4    Effects of Marijuana**

**Central Nervous System Effects**
Impaired memory; perceptual and sensory distortions; disturbances in time perception; mood alteration; restlessness; depersonalization; panic reactions; paranoid ideation; impaired performance on cognitive, perceptual, and psychomotor tasks; drowsiness with high doses.

**Cardiovascular Effects**
Hypertension; bradycardia; peripheral vasoconstriction; orthostatic hypotension and tachycardia at high doses.

**Respiratory Effects**
Irritation and cellular changes in bronchial mucosa; bronchospasm; impaired gas exchange; aspergillosis in immuno-

compromised people; possibly increased risk of mouth, throat, and lung cancer (some known carcinogens are much higher in marijuana smoke than in tobacco smoke).

**Musculoskeletal Effects**
Ataxia; impaired coordination; increased reaction time.

**Miscellaneous Effects**
Constipation, decreased libido, thirst, decreased intraocular pressure.

---

people promote legalization of marijuana for medical uses. However, clinicians state that such use is no more effective than available legal treatments with less abuse potential.

## Marijuana Dependence

Tolerance and psychological dependence do not usually develop with occasional use but may occur with chronic use; physical dependence rarely occurs. There is no specific treatment other than abstinence.

## Hallucinogens

Hallucinogenic drugs include a variety of substances that cause mood changes, anxiety, distorted sensory perceptions, hallucinations, delusions, depersonalization, pupil dilation, elevated body temperature, and elevated blood pressure.

*LSD* is a synthetic derivative of lysergic acid, a compound in ergot and some varieties of morning glory seeds. It is very potent, and small doses can alter normal brain functioning. LSD is usually distributed as a soluble powder and ingested in capsule, tablet, or liquid form. The exact mechanism of action is unknown, and effects cannot be predicted accurately. LSD alters sensory perceptions and thought processes; impairs most intellectual functions, such as memory and problem-solving ability; distorts perception of time and space; and produces sympathomimetic reactions, including increased blood pressure, heart rate, body temperature, and pupil dilation. Adverse reactions include self-injury and possibly suicide, violent behavior, psychotic episodes, "flashbacks" (a phenomenon characterized by psychological effects and hallucinations that may recur days, weeks, or months after the drug is taken), and possible chromosomal damage resulting in birth defects.

*MDMA* (3,4 methylenedioxymethamphetamine), commonly called "ecstasy," is an illegal, Schedule I derivative of amphetamine that produces hallucinogenic and stim-

ulant effects when taken orally. It is usually taken by adolescents and young adults, often at dance parties called "raves," and its use is reportedly increasing. Users report increased energy and perception, euphoria, and feelings of closeness to others. These effects occur within an hour after oral ingestion and last 6 to 8 hours.

Although users apparently think this is a safe drug, evidence indicates it is extremely dangerous. Adverse effects include cardiac dysrhythmias, coma, dehydration, delirium, hypertension, hyperthermia, hyponatremia, rhabdomyolysis, seizures, tachycardia, and death. These effects have occurred with a single use. Even without these life-threatening adverse effects, drug use is usually followed by several days of depression, sadness, low energy, and a decreased ability to feel emotions or pleasure.

Another major concern is the drug's neurotoxicity. Early effects include spasmodic jerking, involuntary jaw clenching, and teeth grinding. Long-term or permanent changes may result from damage to the nerve cells in the brain that transmit serotonin. MDMA floods the brain with high amounts of serotonin, which is important in emotion, mood, and memory. As a result, repeated use of MDMA may lead to depression, insomnia, memory impairment, and low energy or passivity.

In addition to adverse effects of MDMA, users also need to be concerned about the actual product they are taking. There have been numerous reports of other drugs (eg, LSD, methamphetamine, ketamine, or phencyclidine [PCP]) being sold as ecstasy. All of these drugs may have serious adverse effects as well.

MDMA is not thought to cause dependence or withdrawal syndromes. Emergency treatment of MDMA abuse usually involves decreasing the high body temperature, replacing fluids and electrolytes, and monitoring for cardiovascular complications.

*Mescaline* is an alkaloid of the peyote cactus. It is the least active of the commonly used psychotomimetic agents but produces effects similar to those of LSD. It is usually ingested in the form of a soluble powder or capsule.

*Phencyclidine* (PCP) produces excitement, delirium, hallucinations, and other profound psychological and physiologic effects, including a state of intoxication similar to that produced by alcohol; altered sensory perceptions; impaired thought processes; impaired motor skills; psychotic reactions; sedation and analgesia; nystagmus and diplopia; and pressor effects that can cause hypertensive crisis, cerebral hemorrhage, convulsions, coma, and death. Death from overdose also has occurred as a result of respiratory depression. Bizarre murders, suicides, and self-mutilations have been attributed to the schizophrenic reaction induced by PCP, especially in high doses. The drug also produces flashbacks.

Phencyclidine is usually distributed in liquid or crystal form and can be ingested, inhaled, or injected. It is usually sprayed or sprinkled on marijuana or herbs and smoked. Probably because it is cheap, easily synthesized, and readily available, PCP is often sold as LSD, mescaline, cocaine, or THC (the active ingredient in marijuana). It is also added to low-potency marijuana without the user's knowledge. Consequently, the drug user may experience severe and unexpected reactions, including death.

### Hallucinogen Abuse

Tolerance develops, but there is no apparent physical dependence or abstinence syndrome. Psychological dependence probably occurs but is usually not intense. Users may prefer one of these drugs, but they apparently do without or substitute another drug if the one they favor is unavailable. A major danger with these drugs is their ability to impair judgment and insight, which can lead to panic reactions in which users may try to injure themselves (eg, by running into traffic).

### Treatment of Hallucinogen Abuse

There is no specific treatment for hallucinogen dependence. Those who experience severe panic reactions may be kept in a safe, supportive environment until drug effects wear off or may be given a sedative-type drug.

## Volatile Solvents (Inhalants)

Volatile solvents include acetone, toluene, and gasoline. These solvents may be constituents of some types of glue, plastic cements, aerosol sprays, and other products. Some general inhalation anesthetics, such as nitrous oxide, have also been abused to the point of dependence. Volatile solvents are most often abused by preadolescents and adolescents who squeeze glue into a plastic bag, for example, and sniff the fumes. Suffocation sometimes occurs when the sniffer loses consciousness while the bag covers the face.

These substances produce symptoms comparable with those of acute alcohol intoxication, including initial mild euphoria followed by ataxia, confusion, and disorientation. Some substances in gasoline and toluene also may produce symptoms similar to those produced by the

hallucinogens, including euphoria, hallucinations, recklessness, and loss of self-control. Large doses may cause convulsions, coma, and death. Substances containing gasoline, benzene, or carbon tetrachloride are especially likely to cause serious damage to the liver, kidneys, and bone marrow.

These substances produce psychological dependence, and some produce tolerance. There is some question about whether physical dependence occurs. If it does occur, it is considered less intense than the physical dependence associated with alcohol, barbiturates, and opiates.

## ■ MANAGEMENT CONSIDERATIONS

### Prevention of Alcohol and Other Drug Abuse

Use measures to prevent substance abuse. Although there are difficulties in trying to prevent conditions for which causes are not known, some of the following communitywide and individual measures may be helpful:

1. Decrease the supply or availability of commonly abused drugs. Most efforts at prevention have tried to reduce the supply of drugs. For example, laws designate certain drugs as illegal and provide penalties for possession or use of these drugs. Other laws regulate circumstances in which legal drugs, such as narcotic analgesics and barbiturates, may be used. Also, laws regulate the sale of alcoholic beverages.

2. Decrease the demand for drugs. Because this involves changing attitudes, it is very difficult but more effective in the long run. Many current attitudes seem to promote drug use, misuse, and abuse, including:
   a. The belief that a drug is available for every mental and physical discomfort and should be taken in preference to tolerating even minor discomfort. Consequently, society has a permissive attitude toward taking drugs, and health care providers who are quick to prescribe drugs and nurses who are quick to administer them probably perpetuate this attitude. Of course, there are many appropriate uses of drugs, and clients certainly should not be denied their benefits. The difficulties emerge when there is excessive reliance on drugs as chemical solutions to problems that are not amenable to chemical solutions.
   b. The widespread acceptance and use of alcohol. In some groups, alcoholic beverages of some kind accompany every social occasion.
   c. The apparently prevalent view that drug abuse refers only to the use of illegal drugs and that using alcohol or prescription drugs, however inappropriately, does not constitute drug abuse.
   d. The acceptance and use of illegal drugs in certain subgroups of the population. This is especially prevalent in high school and college students.

# Nursing Process

## Assessment

Assess clients for signs of alcohol and other drug abuse, including abuse of prescription drugs, such as antianxiety agents, opioids, and sedative-hypnotics. Some general screening-type questions are appropriate for any initial nursing assessment. The overall purpose of these questions is to determine whether a current or potential problem exists and whether additional information is needed. Some clients may refuse to answer or give answers that contradict other assessment data. Denial of excessive drinking and of problems resulting from alcohol use is a prominent characteristic of alcoholism; underreporting the extent of drug use is common in other types of drug abuse as well. Useful information includes each specific drug, the amount, the frequency of administration, and the duration of administration. If answers to general questions reveal problem areas, such as long-term use of alcohol or psychotropic drugs, more specific questions can be formulated to assess the scope and depth of the problem. It may be especially difficult to obtain needed information about illegal "street drugs," most of which have numerous, frequently changed names. For nurses who often encounter substance abusers, efforts to keep up with drug names and terminology may be helpful.

- Interview the client regarding alcohol and other drug use to help determine immediate and long-term nursing care needs. For example, information may be obtained that would indicate the likelihood of a withdrawal reaction, the risk of increased or decreased effects of a variety of drugs, and the client's susceptibility to drug abuse. People who abuse one drug are likely to abuse others, and abuse of multiple drugs is a more common pattern than abuse of a single drug. These and other factors aid effective planning of nursing care.
- Assess behavior that may indicate drug abuse, such as alcohol on the breath, altered speech patterns, staggering gait, hyperactivity or hypoactivity, and other signs of excessive central nervous system (CNS) depression or stimulation. Impairments in work performance and in interpersonal relationships also may be behavioral clues.
- Assess for disorders that may be caused by substance abuse. These disorders may include infections, liver disease, accidental injuries, and psychiatric problems of anxiety or depression. These disorders may be caused by other factors, of course, and are nonspecific.
- Check laboratory reports, when available, for abnormal liver function test results, indications of anemia, abnormal white blood cell counts, abnormal electrolytes (hypocalcemia, hypomagnesemia, and acidosis are common in alcoholics), and alcohol and drug levels in the blood.

## Nursing Diagnoses

- Ineffective Coping related to reliance on alcohol or other drugs
- Risk for Injury: Adverse effects of abused drug(s)
- Disturbed Thought Processes related to use of psychoactive drugs
- Risk for Other- or Self-Directed Violence related to disturbed thought processes, impaired judgment, and impulsive behavior
- Imbalanced Nutrition: Less Than Body Requirements related to drug effects and drug-seeking behavior
- Dysfunctional Family Processes: Alcoholism
- Risk for Injury: Infection, hepatitis, AIDS related to use of contaminated needles and syringes for IV drugs

## Planning/Goals

- Safety will be maintained for clients impaired by alcohol and drug abuse.
- Information will be provided regarding drug effects and treatment resources.
- The client's efforts toward stopping drug usage will be recognized and reinforced.

## Interventions

- Administer prescribed drugs correctly during acute intoxication or withdrawal.
- Decrease environmental stimuli for the person undergoing drug withdrawal.
- Record vital signs; cardiovascular, respiratory, and neurologic functions; mental status; and behavior at regular intervals.
- Support use of resources for stopping drug abuse (psychotherapy, treatment programs).
- Request patient referrals to psychiatric/mental health physicians, nurse clinical specialists, or self-help programs when indicated.
- Use therapeutic communication skills to discuss alcohol or other drug-related health problems, health-related benefits of stopping substance use or abuse, and available services or treatment options.
- Teach nondrug techniques for coping with stress and anxiety.
- Provide positive reinforcement for efforts toward quitting substance abuse.
- Inform smokers with young children in the home that cigarette smoke can precipitate or aggravate asthma and upper respiratory disorders in children.
- Inform smokers with nonsmoking spouses or other members of the household that "second-hand" smoke can increase the risks of cancer and lung disease in the nonsmokers as well as the smoker.
- For smokers who are concerned about weight gain if they quit smoking, emphasize that the health benefits of quitting far outweigh the disadvantages of gaining a few pounds, and discuss ways to control weight without smoking.

## Evaluation

- Observe for improved behavior (eg, less impulsiveness, improved judgment and thought processes, commits no injury to self or others).
- Observe for use or avoidance of nonprescribed drugs while hospitalized.
- Interview to determine the client's insight into personal problems stemming from drug abuse.
- Verify enrollment in a treatment program.
- Observe for appropriate use of drugs to decrease abuse of other drugs.

Efforts to change attitudes and decrease demand for drugs can be made through education and counseling about such topics as drug effects and non-drug ways to handle the stresses and problems of daily life.

3. Each person must take personal responsibility for drinking alcoholic beverages and taking mind-altering drugs. Initially, conscious, voluntary choices are made to drink or not to drink, to take a drug or not to take it. This period varies somewhat, but drug dependence develops in most instances only after prolonged use. When mind-altering drugs are prescribed for a legitimate reason, the client must use them in prescribed doses and preferably for a short time.

4. Health care providers can help prevent drug abuse by prescribing drugs appropriately, prescribing mind-altering drugs in limited amounts and for limited periods, using nondrug measures when they are likely to be effective, educating clients about the drugs prescribed for them, participating in drug education programs, and recognizing, as early as possible, clients who are abusing or are likely to abuse drugs.

5. Nurses can help prevent drug abuse by administering drugs appropriately, using nondrug measures when possible, teaching clients about drugs prescribed for them, and participating in drug education programs. Some resources for information and educational materials include the following:

National Institute on Drug Abuse
6001 Executive Blvd
Bethesda, MD 20892-9561
Phone: (301) 443-1124
www.nida.nih.gov
National Clearinghouse for Alcohol and Drug Abuse Information (NCADI)
Center for Substance Abuse Prevention
5600 Fishers Lane
Rockwall II
Rockville, MD 20857
Phone: (301) 443-0365
E-Mail: nnadal@samhsa.gov
www.health.org

6. Pregnant women should avoid alcohol, nicotine, and other drugs of abuse because of potentially harmful effects on the fetus.

## Treatment Measures for Substance Abuse

Treatment measures for alcohol and other drug abuse are not very successful. Even people who have been institutionalized and achieved a drug-free state for prolonged periods are apt to resume their drug-taking behavior when released from the institution. So far, voluntary, self-help groups, such as Alcoholics Anonymous and Narcotics Anonymous, have been more successful than health professionals in dealing with drug abuse. Health professionals are more likely to be involved in acute situations, such as intoxication or overdose, withdrawal syndromes, or various medical-surgical conditions. As a general rule, treatment depends on the type, extent, and duration of drug-taking behavior and the particular situation for which treatment is needed. Some general management principles include the following:

1. Psychological rehabilitation efforts should be part of any treatment program for a drug-dependent person. Several approaches may be useful, including psychotherapy, voluntary groups, and other types of emotional support and counseling.

2. Drug therapy is limited in treating drug dependence for several reasons. First, specific antidotes are available only for benzodiazepines (flumazenil) and narcotic narcotics (naloxone). Second, there is a high risk for substituting one abused drug for another. Third, there are significant drawbacks to giving CNS stimulants to reverse effects of CNS depressants, and vice versa. Fourth, there is often inadequate information about the types and amounts of drugs taken.

   Despite these drawbacks, however, there are some clinical indications for drug therapy, including treatment of overdose or withdrawal syndromes. Even when drug therapy is indicated, there are few guidelines for optimal use. Doses, for example, must often be estimated initially and then titrated according to response.

3. General care of clients with drug overdose is primarily symptomatic and supportive. The aim of treatment is usually to support vital functions, such as respiration and circulation, until the drug is metabolized and eliminated from the body. For example, respiratory depression from an overdose of a CNS depressant drug may be treated by inserting an artificial airway and mechanical ventilation. Removal of some drugs can be hastened by hemodialysis.

4. Treatment of substance abuse may be complicated by the presence of other disorders. For example, depression is common and may require antidepressant drug therapy.

## Critical Thinking Exercises

1. Chronic ingestion of alcohol induces metabolizing enzymes that increase the:
   a. Rate of metabolism
   b. Drug effects
   c. Likelihood of toxicity
   d. Anticonvulsant effect of alcohol

2. The drugs of choice for treating alcohol withdrawal syndromes are the:
   a. Benzodiazepines
   b. Opioids
   c. Antihistamines
   d. Catecholamines

3. Ingestion of alcohol while taking disulfiram (Antabuse) may result in:
   a. Bradycardia
   b. Bronchodilation
   c. Diaphoresis
   d. Headache

4. In individuals dependent on hallucinogenic drugs, such as LSD, there is a typical risk of:
   a. Tolerance
   b. Physical dependence
   c. Abstinence syndrome
   d. Intense psychological dependence

5. Naltrexone is an opiate antagonist that reduces craving for alcohol and increases abstinence rates when combined with psychosocial treatment. A possible mechanism is:
   a. Blockade of the endogenous opioid system
   b. Prevention of the reuptake of neurotransmitters
   c. Damage to the nerve cells in the brain that transmit serotonin
   d. Production of a sympathomimetic reaction

## SELECTED REFERENCES

Cooke, S. C., Lobo, B. L., & Eoff, J. C. III (2000). Substance abuse. In E. T. Herfindal & D. R. Gourley (Eds.), *Textbook of therapeutics: Drug and disease management* (7th ed., pp. 1313–1341). Philadelphia: Lippincott Williams & Wilkins.

DerMarderosian, A. (Ed.) (2001). Marijuana. In *The review of natural products* (pp. 391–393). St. Louis: Facts and Comparisons.

Enoch, M. A., & Goldman, D. (2002). Problem drinking and alcoholism: Diagnosis and treatment. *American Family Physician, 65*(3), 441–450.

Hashimoto, S. A., & Paty, D. W. (2000). The neurologic complications and consequences of ethanol use and abuse. In H. D. Humes (Ed.), *Kelley's textbook of internal medicine* (4th ed., pp. 2933–2936). Philadelphia: Lippincott Williams & Wilkins.

Henderson-Martin, B. (2000). No more surprises: Screening clients for alcohol abuse. *American Journal of Nursing, 100*(9), 26–32.

Lacy, C. F., Armstrong, L. L., Goldman, M. P., & Lance, L. L. (2003). *Lexi-Comp's drug information handbook* (11th ed.). Hudson, OH: American Pharmaceutical Association.

Lange, R. A. & Hillis, L. D. (2001). Cardiovascular complications of cocaine use. *New England Journal of Medicine, 345*(5), 351–358.

O'Brien, C. P. (2000). Approach to the problem of substance abuse. In H. D. Humes (Ed.), *Kelley's textbook of internal medicine* (4th ed., pp. 229–233). Philadelphia: Lippincott Williams & Wilkins.

Phipps, J. R. Jr., Baldwin, J. N., & Tong, T. G. (2000). Alcoholism. In E. T. Herfindal & D. R. Gourley (Eds.), *Textbook of therapeutics: Drug and disease management* (7th ed., pp. 1289–1312). Philadelphia: Lippincott Williams & Wilkins.

Sachse, D. S. (2000). Emergency: Delirium tremens. *American Journal of Nursing, 100*(5), 41–42.

Schwartz, R. H. (2002). Marijuana: A decade and a half later, still a crude drug with underappreciated toxicity. *Pediatrics, 109*(2), 284–289.

# 15

# Central Nervous System Stimulants

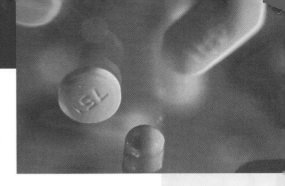

## OBJECTIVES

*After studying this chapter, the student will be able to:*

1 Describe general characteristics of central nervous system (CNS) stimulant drugs.

2 Discuss reasons for decreased use of amphetamines for therapeutic purposes.

3 Give the rationale for treating attention deficit-hyperactivity disorder with CNS stimulant drugs.

4 List effects and sources of caffeine.

5 Identify nursing interventions to prevent, recognize, and treat stimulant overdose.

## CRITICAL THINKING SCENARIO

*M*rs. Williams comes to your office with her 6-year-old son, Tom. She complains that he is a very active child who always seems to be getting into mischief. She likes a clean, orderly house, and he likes to make messes. He seems to be doing okay in school, although she would like to see his grades improve. She was talking to a neighbor, who encouraged her to talk with a health care provider about prescribing Ritalin, because her son may have attention deficit-hyperactivity disorder (ADHD).

✔ What advice would you have for Mrs. Williams?

✔ Identify possible therapeutic effects of prescribing Ritalin if the boy has ADHD.

✔ What are the possible negative effects of giving Tom Ritalin if he does not have ADHD?

# USES

Many drugs stimulate the central nervous system (CNS), but only a few are used therapeutically, and their indications for use are limited. Stimulant drugs are often misused and abused by people who want to combat fatigue and delay sleep, such as long-distance drivers, students, and athletes. Use of amphetamines or other stimulants for this purpose is not justified. These drugs are dangerous for drivers and those involved in similar activities, and they have no legitimate use in athletics. Two disorders treated with CNS stimulants are narcolepsy and attention deficit-hyperactivity disorder (ADHD); both disorders are described in At the Foundation: Narcolepsy and ADHD. Specific use in children and older adults is detailed in Age-related Considerations.

# TYPES OF STIMULANTS

Most CNS stimulants act by facilitating initiation and transmission of nerve impulses that excite other cells. The drugs are somewhat selective in their actions at lower doses but tend to involve the entire CNS at higher doses. The major groups are amphetamines and related drugs, analeptics, and xanthines.

*Amphetamines* increase the amounts of norepinephrine, dopamine, and possibly serotonin in the brain, thereby producing mood elevation or euphoria, increasing mental alertness and capacity for work, decreasing fatigue and drowsiness, and prolonging wakefulness. Larger doses, however, produce signs of excessive CNS stimulation, such as restlessness, hyperactivity, agitation, nervousness, difficulty concentrating on a task, and confusion. Overdoses can produce convulsions and psychotic behavior. Amphetamines also stimulate the sympathetic nervous system, resulting in increased heart rate and blood pressure, pupil dilation (mydriasis), slowed gastrointestinal motility, and other symptoms. In ADHD, the drugs reduce behavioral symptoms and may improve cognitive performance.

Amphetamines are Schedule II drugs under the Controlled Substances Act and have a high potential for drug abuse and dependence. Prescriptions for them are nonrefillable. These drugs are widely sold on the street and commonly abused (see Chap. 14).

*Amphetamine-related drugs* (methylphenidate and dexmethylphenidate) have essentially the same effects as the amphetamines and are also Schedule II drugs.

*Analeptics* are infrequently used (see doxapram and modafinil, below).

*Xanthines* stimulate the cerebral cortex, increasing mental alertness and decreasing drowsiness and fatigue. Other effects include myocardial stimulation with increased cardiac output and heart rate, diuresis, and increased secretion of pepsin and hydrochloric acid. Large doses can impair mental and physical functions by producing restlessness, nervousness, anxiety, agitation, insomnia, cardiac dysrhythmias, and gastritis.

---

## AT THE FOUNDATION: *Narcolepsy and ADHD*

### Narcolepsy
Narcolepsy is a sleep disorder characterized by daytime "sleep attacks" in which the victim goes to sleep at any place or any time. Signs and symptoms also include excessive daytime drowsiness, fatigue, muscle weakness and hallucinations at onset of sleep, and disturbances of nighttime sleep patterns. The hazards of drowsiness during normal waking hours and suddenly going to sleep in unsafe environments restrict activities of daily living.

Narcolepsy affects men and women equally and usually starts during teenage or young adult years. Its cause is unknown; sleep studies are required for an accurate diagnosis. In addition to drug therapy, prevention of sleep deprivation, regular sleeping and waking times, avoiding shift work, and short naps may be helpful in reducing daytime sleepiness.

### Attention Deficit-Hyperactivity Disorder (ADHD)
ADHD is reportedly the most common psychiatric or neurobehavioral disorder in children. It occurs before 7 years of age and is characterized by persistent hyperactivity, a short attention span, difficulty completing assigned tasks or schoolwork, restlessness, and impulsiveness. Such behaviors make it difficult for the child to get along with others (eg, family members, peer groups, teachers) and to function in situations requiring more controlled behavior (eg, classrooms).

Formerly thought to disappear with adolescence, ADHD is now thought to continue into adolescence and adulthood in up to two thirds of clients. In adolescents and adults, impulsiveness and inattention continue, but hyperactivity is not a prominent feature. A major criterion for diagnosing later ADHD is a previous diagnosis of childhood ADHD. Some studies indicate that children with ADHD are more likely to have learning disabilities, mood disorders, and substance abuse disorders as adolescents and adults as well as continuing difficulties in structured settings such as school or work.

## Age-related Considerations: Use of Central Nervous System Stimulants

### USE IN CHILDREN

Central nervous system stimulants are not recommended for ADHD in children younger than 6 years of age. When used, dosage should be carefully titrated and monitored to avoid excessive CNS stimulation, anorexia, and insomnia. Suppression of weight and height have been reported, and growth should be monitored at regular intervals during drug therapy. In children with psychosis or Tourette's syndrome, CNS stimulants may exacerbate symptoms.

In ADHD, careful documentation of baseline symptoms over approximately 1 month is necessary to establish the diagnosis and evaluate outcomes of treatment. This can be done by videotapes of behavior; observations and ratings by clinicians familiar with ADHD; and by interviewing the child, parents, or caretakers. Some authorities believe that this condition is overdiagnosed and that stimulant drugs are prescribed unnecessarily. Guidelines for treatment of ADHD include the following:

1. Counseling and psychotherapy (eg, parental counseling or family therapy) are recommended along with drug therapy for effective treatment and realistic expectations of outcomes.

2. Young children may not require treatment until starting school. Then, the goal of drug therapy is to control symptoms, facilitate learning, and promote social development.

3. Drug therapy is indicated when symptoms are moderate to severe; are present for several months; and interfere in social, academic, or behavioral functioning. When possible, drug therapy should be omitted or reduced in dosage when children are not in school.

4. Methylphenidate is the most commonly used drug. It is usually given daily, including weekends, for the first 3 to 4 weeks to allow caregivers to assess beneficial and adverse effects. Desirable effects may include improvement in behavior, attention span, and quality and quantity of schoolwork, and better relationships with other children and family members. Adverse effects include appetite suppression and weight loss, which may be worse during the first 6 months of therapy.

5. Drug holidays (stopping drug administration) are controversial. Some clinicians say they are indicated only if no significant problems occur during the drug-free period and are not recommended for most children. Other clinicians believe they are desirable when children are not in school (eg, summer) and necessary periodically to reevaluate the child's condition. Dosage adjustments are often needed at least annually as the child grows and hepatic metabolism slows. In addition, the drug-free periods decrease weight loss and growth suppression.

### USE IN OLDER ADULTS

CNS stimulants should be used cautiously in older adults. As with most other drugs, slowed metabolism and excretion increase the risks for accumulation and toxicity. Older adults are likely to experience anxiety, nervousness, insomnia, and mental confusion from excessive CNS stimulation. In addition, older adults often have cardiovascular disorders (eg, angina, dysrhythmias, hypertension) that may be aggravated by the cardiac-stimulating effects of the drugs, including dietary caffeine. In general, reduced doses are safer in older adults.

## Indications for Use

Amphetamines and methylphenidate are used in the treatment of narcolepsy and ADHD. Dexmethylphenidate is indicated only for ADHD. One analeptic is used occasionally to treat respiratory depression; the other one is approved only for treatment of narcolepsy. Caffeine (a xanthine) is an ingredient in nonprescription analgesics and stimulants that promote wakefulness (eg, NoDoz). A combination of caffeine and sodium benzoate is occasionally used as a respiratory stimulant in neonates.

## Contraindications to Use

CNS stimulants cause cardiac stimulation and thus are contraindicated in clients with cardiovascular disorders (eg, angina, dysrhythmias, hypertension) that are likely to be aggravated by the drugs. They also are contraindicated in clients with anxiety or agitation, glaucoma, or hyperthyroidism. They are usually contraindicated in clients with a history of drug abuse.

## ▨ INDIVIDUAL CENTRAL NERVOUS SYSTEM STIMULANTS

Individual drugs are described below; dosages are listed in Drugs at a Glance 15-1: Central Nervous System Stimulants. No prototype is identified in this group of drugs.

## Amphetamines and Related Drugs

**Amphetamine, dextroamphetamine** (Dexedrine), and **methamphetamine** (Desoxyn) are closely related drugs that share characteristics of the amphetamines as a group. They are more important as drugs of abuse than as therapeutic agents.

**Methylphenidate** (Ritalin) is chemically related to amphetamines and produces similar actions and adverse effects. It is well absorbed with oral administration. In children, peak plasma levels occur in about 2 hours with immediate-release tablets and about 5 hours with extended-release tablets. Half-life is 1 to 3 hours, but

**DRUG TABLE 15-1**

*Drugs at a Glance*

## Central Nervous System Stimulants

| Generic/Trade Name | Routes and Dosage Ranges | Comments |
|---|---|---|
| **Amphetamines** | | |
| **Amphetamine** Pregnancy Category C | *Adults:* Narcolepsy: PO, 5–60 mg/d in divided doses *Children:* Narcolepsy: >6 y: PO, 5 mg/d initially, increase by 5 mg/wk to effective dose ADHD: 3–5 y: PO, 2.5 mg/d initially, increase by 2.5 mg/d at weekly intervals until response; >6 y: PO, 5 mg once or twice daily initially, increase by 5 mg/d at weekly intervals until optimal response (usually no more than 40 mg/d) | As with all amphetamines, use lowest effective dose; administer first daily dose as soon as awake |
| **Dextroamphetamine** (Dexedrine) Pregnancy Category C | *Adults:* Narcolepsy: PO, 5–60 mg in divided doses *Children:* Narcolepsy: >6 y: PO, 5 mg/d initially, increase by 5 mg/wk to effective dose ADHD: 3–5 y: PO, 2.5 mg/d initially, increase by 2.5 mg/d at weekly intervals until optimal response; >6 y: PO, 5 mg once or twice daily initially, increase by 5 mg/d at weekly intervals until optimal response (usually no more than 40 mg/d) | |
| **Dextroamphetamine and amphetamine** (Adderall) Pregnancy Category C | *Adults:* Narcolepsy: PO, 10 mg daily initially, increase if necessary *Children:* ADHD: >6 y: PO, 5 mg 1–2 times daily, increased if necessary | |
| **Methamphetamine** (Desoxyn) Pregnancy Category C | *Children:* ADHD: PO, 5–10 mg daily initially. Usual dose, 15–25 mg daily, in 2 divided doses | Stimulant has been associated with growth suppression in children |
| **Amphetamine-related Drugs** | | |
| **Dexmethylphenidate** (Focalin) Pregnancy Category C | *Children:* ADHD: PO, 2.5–10 mg twice daily | Safety and effectiveness for long-term use has not been established |
| **Methylphenidate** (Ritalin, Ritalin SR, Concerta, Metadate) Pregnancy Category C | *Children:* Narcolepsy: PO, 10–60 mg/d in 2 or 3 divided doses 6 y and older: ADHD, PO, 5 mg twice a day initially, increase by 5–10 mg at weekly intervals to a maximum of 60 mg/d if necessary | Do not use in females of childbearing age unless benefits outweigh risks (teratogenic effects to fetus reported in animal studies) High potential for abuse |
| **Analeptics** | | |
| **Doxapram** (Dopram) Pregnancy Category B | *Adults:* IV, 0.5–1.5 mg/kg in single or divided doses; IV continuous infusion, 5 mg/min initially, decreased to 2.5 mg/min or more. Dose by infusion should not exceed 3 g | Also used for acute hypercapnia in clients with chronic lung disease |
| **Modafinil** (Provigil) Pregnancy Category C | *Adults:* Narcolepsy: PO, 200 mg once daily, in the morning. Dosage should be reduced by 50% with severe hepatic impairment. *Children:* Dosage not established for children <16 y | Avoid alcohol Immediately report suspected pregnancy to provider (no studies in humans evaluating teratogenic effects to fetus) A Schedule IV drug |

pharmacologic effects last 4 to 6 hours. Most of a dose is metabolized in the liver and excreted in urine.

**Dexmethylphenidate** (Focalin) is very similar to methylphenidate and the amphetamines. It is well absorbed with oral administration and reaches peak plasma levels in 1 to 1.5 hours. It is metabolized in the liver and excreted in urine.

## Analeptics

**Doxapram** (Dopram) is occasionally used by anesthesiologists and pulmonary specialists as a respiratory stimulant. Although it increases tidal volume and respiratory rate, it also increases oxygen consumption and carbon dioxide production. Limitations include a short duration of action (5 to 10 minutes after a single intravenous [IV] dose) and therapeutic dosages near or overlapping those that produce convulsions. Endotracheal intubation and mechanical ventilation are safer and more effective in relieving respiratory depression from depressant drugs or other causes.

**Modafinil** (Provigil) is a newer drug for treatment of narcolepsy. Its ability to promote wakefulness is similar to that of amphetamines and methylphenidate, but its mechanism of action is unknown. Like other CNS stimulants, it also has psychoactive and euphoric effects, which alter mood, perception, and thinking. It is rapidly absorbed (food may delay absorption), reaches peak plasma levels in 2 to 4 hours; is 60% bound to plasma proteins; and is 90% metabolized by the liver to metabolites, which are then excreted in urine. Steady-state concentrations are reached in 2 to 4 days, and half-life with chronic use is about 15 hours.

Modafinil is not recommended for clients with a history of left ventricular hypertrophy or ischemic changes on electrocardiograms. Adverse effects include anxiety, chest pain, dizziness, dyspnea, dysrhythmias, headache, nausea, nervousness, and palpitations. Interactions with other drugs include decreased effects of cyclosporine and oral contraceptives and increased effects of phenytoin, tricyclic antidepressants, and warfarin. Dosage should be reduced by 50% with severe hepatic impairment; effects of severe renal impairment are unknown.

## Xanthines

**Caffeine** has numerous pharmacologic actions, including CNS stimulation, diuresis, hyperglycemia, cardiac stimulation, coronary and peripheral vasodilation, cerebrovascular vasoconstriction, skeletal muscle stimulation, increased secretion of gastric acid and pepsin, and bronchodilation from relaxation of smooth muscle. In low to moderate amounts, caffeine increases alertness and capacity for work and decreases fatigue. Large amounts cause excessive CNS stimulation with anxiety, agitation, diarrhea, insomnia, irritability, nausea, nervousness, premature ventricular contractions, hyperactivity and restlessness, tachycardia, tremors, and vomiting. Toxic amounts may cause delirium and seizures. With large

amounts or chronic use, caffeine has been implicated as a causative or aggravating factor in cardiovascular disease (hypertension, dysrhythmias), gastrointestinal disorders (esophageal reflux, peptic ulcers), reproductive disorders, osteoporosis (may increase loss of calcium in urine), carcinogenicity, psychiatric disturbances, and drug abuse liability. Caffeine produces tolerance to its stimulating effects, and psychological dependence or habituation occurs.

Pharmaceutical preparations include an oral preparation and a solution for injection. Caffeine is usually prescribed as caffeine citrate for oral use and caffeine and sodium benzoate for parenteral use because these forms are more soluble than caffeine itself. It is an ingredient in some nonprescription analgesic preparations and may increase analgesia. It is combined with an ergot alkaloid to treat migraine headaches (eg, Cafergot) and is the active ingredient in nonprescription stimulant (anti-sleep) preparations. A combination of caffeine and sodium benzoate is used as a respiratory stimulant in neonatal apnea unresponsive to other therapies.

Caffeine is a frequently consumed CNS stimulant worldwide, and most is consumed from dietary sources (eg, coffee, tea, and cola drinks). The caffeine content of coffee and tea beverages is determined by the particular coffee bean or tea leaf and the method of preparation. Because of the widespread ingestion of caffeine-containing beverages and the wide availability of over-the-counter products that contain caffeine, toxicity may result from concomitant consumption of caffeine from several sources. Some authorities recommend that normal, healthy, nonpregnant adults consume no more than 250 mg of caffeine daily. Sources and amounts of caffeine are summarized in Table 15-1.

**Theophylline** preparations are xanthines used in the treatment of respiratory disorders, such as asthma and bronchitis. In these conditions, the desired effect is bronchodilation and improvement of breathing; CNS stimulation is then an adverse effect (see Chap. 36).

## Dietary and Herbal Supplement

**Guarana** is made from the seeds of a South American shrub. The main active ingredient is caffeine, which is present in greater amounts than in coffee beans or dried tea leaves. Guarana is widely used as a source of caffeine by soft drink manufacturers. It is also used as a flavoring agent and an ingredient in herbal stimulant and weight-loss products, usually in combination with ephedra (ma huang), energy drinks, vitamin supplements, candies, and chewing gums. The product, which may also contain theophylline and theobromine, is also available in teas, extracts, elixirs, capsules, and tablets of various strengths. In general, the caffeine content of a guarana product is unknown, and guarana may not be listed as an ingredient. As a result, consumers may not know how much caffeine they are ingesting in products containing guarana.

## TABLE 15-1    Sources of Caffeine

| Source | Amount (oz) | Caffeine (mg) | Remarks |
|---|---|---|---|
| *Coffee* | | | |
| Brewed, regular | 5–8 | 40–180 | Caffeine content varies with product |
| Instant | 5–8 | 30–120 | and preparation |
| Espresso | 2 | 120 | |
| *Tea* | | | |
| Brewed, leaf or bag | 8 | 80 | Caffeine content varies with product |
| Instant | 8 | 50 | and preparation |
| Iced | 12 | 70 | |
| *Soft Drinks* | | | |
| Coke, Diet Coke | 12 | 45 | Most other cola drinks contain |
| Pepsi, Diet Pepsi | 12 | 38 | 35–45 mg/12 oz |
| Mountain Dew | 12 | 54 | |
| Mr. Pibb, Diet | 12 | 57 | |
| *OTC Analgesics* | | | |
| Anacin, Vanquish | 1 tablet or caplet | 32–33 | |
| APAP-Plus, Excedrin, Midol | 1 tablet, caplet or geltab | 60–65 | |
| *OTC Antisleep Products* | | | |
| Caffedrine, NoDoz, Vivarin | 1 tablet or capsule | 200 | |
| *OTC Diuretic* | | | |
| Aqua-Ban | 1 tablet | 100 | Recommended dose 2 tablets 3 times daily (600 mg/d) |
| *Prescription Drugs* | | | |
| Cafergot | 1 tablet | 100 | Recommended dose 2 tabs at onset of migraine, then 1 tab every hour if needed, up to 6 tabs (600 mg/attack) |
| Fiorinal | 1 capsule | 40 | Recommended dose 1–2 cap every 4 hours, up to 6/d (240 mg/d) Also contains butalbital, a barbiturate, and is a Schedule III controlled drug |

As with caffeine from other sources, guarana may cause excessive nervousness and insomnia. It is contraindicated during pregnancy and lactation and should be used cautiously, if at all, in people who are sensitive to the effects of caffeine and in those with cardiovascular disease. Overall, the use of guarana as a CNS stimulant and weight-loss aid is not recommended and should be discouraged.

## ◼ DRUG USE IN SPECIFIC SITUATIONS

### Toxicity of Central Nervous System Stimulants: Recognition and Management

Overdoses may occur with acute or chronic ingestion of large amounts of a single stimulant, combinations of stimulants, or concurrent ingestion of a stimulant and another drug that slows the metabolism of the stimu-

lant. Signs of toxicity may include severe agitation, cardiac dysrhythmias, combativeness, confusion, delirium, hallucinations, high body temperature, hyperactivity, hypertension, insomnia, irritability, nervousness, panic states, restlessness, tremors, seizures, coma, circulatory collapse, and death.

Treatment is largely symptomatic and supportive. In general, place the client in a cool room, monitor cardiac function and temperature, and minimize external stimulation. Gastric lavage may be helpful if done within 4 hours of ingestion of the stimulant. After emptying the stomach, activated charcoal (1 g/kg) may be given. With amphetamines, urinary acidification, IV fluids, and IV diuretics (eg, furosemide or mannitol) hasten drug excretion. IV diazepam or lorazepam can be given to calm agitation, hyperactivity, or seizures; haloperidol may be given for symptoms of psychosis. If cardiovascular collapse occurs, fluid replacement and vasopressors may be used. If a long-acting form of the stimulant drug has

# NURSING PROCESS

## Assessment

- Assess use of stimulant and depressant drugs (prescribed, over-the-counter, or street drugs).
- Assess caffeine intake as a possible cause of nervousness, insomnia, or tachycardia, alone or in combination with other central nervous system (CNS) stimulants.
- Try to identify potentially significant sources of caffeine.
- Assess for conditions that are aggravated by CNS stimulants.
- For a child with possible attention deficit hyperactivity disorder (ADHD), assess behavior as specifically and thoroughly as possible.
- For any client receiving amphetamines or methylphenidate, assess behavior for signs of tolerance and abuse.

## Nursing Diagnoses

- Sleep Pattern Disturbance related to hyperactivity, nervousness, insomnia
- Risk for Injury: Adverse drug effects (excessive cardiac and CNS stimulation, drug dependence)
- Deficient Knowledge: Drug effects on children and adults
- Noncompliance: Overuse of drug

## Planning/Goals

*The client will:*
- Take drugs safely and accurately
- Improve attention span and task performance (children and adults with ADHD) and decrease hyperactivity (children with ADHD)
- Have fewer sleep episodes during normal waking hours (for clients with narcolepsy)

## Interventions

- For a child receiving CNS stimulants, assist parents in scheduling drug administration and drug holidays (eg, weekends, summers) to increase beneficial effects and help prevent drug dependence and stunted growth.
- Record weight at least weekly.
- Promote nutrition to avoid excessive weight loss.
- Provide information about the condition for which a stimulant drug is being given and the potential consequences of overusing the drug.

## Evaluation

- Reports of improved behavior and academic performance from parents and teachers of children with ADHD
- Self- or family reports of improved ability to function in work, school, or social environments for adolescents and adults with ADHD
- Reports of decreased inappropriate sleep episodes with narcolepsy

---

been ingested, saline cathartics may be useful to remove undissolved drug granules.

With caffeine, ingestion of 15 to 30 mg/kg (1 to 2 g for a person of 70 kg or 150 lb) may cause myocardial irritability, muscle tremors or spasms, and vomiting. Oral doses of 5 g or more may cause death. Signs of toxicity are correlated with serum levels of caffeine. Several cups of coffee may produce levels of 5 to 10 mcg/mL and symptoms of agitation and tremors. Cardiac dysrhythmias and seizures occur at higher levels. Additional

---

## CLIENT TEACHING GUIDELINES
## Methylphenidate and Dexmethylphenidate

### General Considerations

✔ These drugs may mask symptoms of fatigue, impair physical coordination, and cause dizziness or drowsiness. Use caution while driving or performing other tasks requiring alertness.

✔ Notify a health care provider of nervousness, insomnia, heart palpitations, vomiting, fever, or skin rash. These are adverse drug effects and dosage may need to be reduced.

✔ Avoid other central nervous system stimulants, including caffeine.

✔ Record weight at least weekly; report excessive losses.

✔ The drugs may cause weight loss; caloric intake (of nutritional foods) may need to be increased, especially in children.

✔ Take these drugs only as prescribed by a health care provider. These drugs have a high potential for abuse. The risks of drug dependence are lessened if they are taken correctly.

✔ Get adequate rest and sleep. Do not take stimulant drugs to delay fatigue and sleep; these are normal, necessary resting mechanisms for the body.

✔ Prevent nervousness, anxiety, tremors, and insomnia from excessive caffeine intake by decreasing consumption of coffee and other caffeine-containing beverages or by drinking decaffeinated coffee, tea, and cola. Sprite and 7-Up have no caffeine.

### Self-administration and Administration to Children

✔ Take regular tablets approximately 30 to 45 minutes before meals.

✔ Take the last dose of the day in the afternoon, before 6 PM, to avoid interference with sleep.

✔ Ritalin SR, Concerta, Metadate CD, and Metadate ER are long-acting forms of methylphenidate. They should be swallowed whole, without crushing or chewing.

✔ If excessive weight loss, nervousness, or insomnia develops, ask the prescribing physician if the dose can be reduced or taken on a different schedule to relieve these adverse effects.

manifestations of caffeine toxicity include opisthotonus, decerebrate posturing, muscle hypertonicity, rhabdomyolysis with subsequent renal failure, pulmonary edema, hyperglycemia, hypokalemia, leukocytosis, ketosis, and metabolic acidosis.

Treatment is symptomatic and supportive, with gastric lavage and activated charcoal if indicated. IV diazepam or lorazepam may be used to control seizures. Hemodialysis is indicated if the serum caffeine concentration is more than 100 mcg/mL or if life-threatening seizures or cardiac dysrhythmias occur.

Individuals are frequently followed up at home at discharge after toxicity of CNS stimulants. The Home Care Considerations display outlines assessment, monitoring, and education concerns with these clients.

## Effects of Central Nervous System Stimulants on Other Drugs

**Caffeine** may increase adverse effects of clozapine and theophylline by decreasing their metabolism and increasing their blood levels. It may increase effects of aspirin by increasing aspirin absorption. It may decrease effects of lithium by increasing lithium clearance. **Dexmethylphenidate** and **methylphenidate** may increase effects of phenytoin and antidepressants (selective serotonin reup-

take inhibitors and tricyclics). They may decrease effects of antihypertensive drugs. **Modafinil** may increase effects of clomipramine, phenytoin, tricyclic antidepressants, and warfarin. It may decrease effects of cyclosporine and oral contraceptives.

---

### Home Care Considerations: Use of Central Nervous System Stimulants

***ASSESS:*** for therapeutic effects of drugs (improved concentration and work product [ADHD], or improved wakefulness [narcolepsy]), adverse drug effects, overuse of the drugs, safety, and quality-of-life issues.

***MONITOR:*** the therapeutic and adverse effects of the drugs, correct dosing schedule, and client's need for additional information and provide that information.

***EDUCATE:*** regarding importance of reading and following instructions on labels of OTC stimulants, minimizing products containing caffeine, not exceeding recommended dosages without consulting a health care provider, and the use of drug holiday periods (ADHD). Reinforce additional teaching points (see Client Teaching Guidelines: Methylphenidate and Dexmethylphenidate).

---

## *Nursing Actions*
## Central Nervous System Stimulants

| ***Nursing Actions*** | ***Rationale/Explanation*** |
|---|---|
| 1. Administer accurately. | |
| a. Give amphetamines and methylphenidate early in the day, at least 6 hours before bedtime. | To avoid interference with sleep. If insomnia occurs, give the last dose of the day at an earlier time or decrease the dose. |
| b. For children with attention deficit-hyperactivity disorder (ADHD), give amphetamines and methylphenidate about 30 minutes before meals. | To minimize the drugs' appetite-suppressing effects and risks of interference with nutrition and growth. |
| c. Do not crush or open and instruct clients not to bite or chew long-acting forms of methylphenidate (Concerta, Metadate CD, Metadate ER, Ritalin SR). | Breaking the tablets or capsules destroys the extended-release feature and allows the drug to be absorbed faster. An overdose may result. |
| 2. Observe for therapeutic effects. | Therapeutic effects depend on the reason for use. |
| a. Fewer "sleep attacks" with narcolepsy | |
| b. Improved behavior and performance of cognitive and psychomotor tasks with ADHD | |
| c. Increased mental alertness and decreased fatigue | |
| 3. Observe for adverse effects. | Adverse effects may occur with acute or chronic ingestion of any CNS stimulant drugs. |
| a. Excessive central nervous system (CNS) stimulation—hyperactivity, nervousness, insomnia, anxiety, tremors, convulsions, psychotic behavior | These reactions are more likely to occur with large doses. |
| b. Cardiovascular effects—tachycardia, other dysrhythmias, hypertension | These reactions are caused by the sympathomimetic effects of the drugs. |
| c. Gastrointestinal effects—anorexia, gastritis, weight loss, nausea, diarrhea, constipation | |

*(continued)*

## Nursing Actions

### Central Nervous System Stimulants (Continued)

| Nursing Actions | Rationale/Explanation |
|---|---|
| 4. Observe for drug interactions. | |
| a. Drugs that *increase* the effects of CNS stimulants: | |
| (1) Other CNS stimulant drugs | Such combinations are potentially dangerous and should be avoided or minimized. |
| (2) Albuterol and related antiasthmatic drugs, pseudo-ephedrine | These drugs cause CNS and cardiac stimulating effects. |
| b. Drugs that *decrease* effects of CNS stimulants: | |
| (1) CNS depressants | IV diazepam or lorazepam may be used to decrease agitation, hyperactivity, and seizures occurring with stimulant overdose. |
| c. Drugs that *increase* effects of amphetamines: | |
| (1) Alkalinizing agents (eg, antacids) | Drugs that increase the alkalinity of the gastrointestinal tract increase intestinal absorption of amphetamines, and urinary alkalinizers decrease urinary excretion. Increased absorption and decreased excretion serve to potentiate drug effects. |
| (2) Monoamine oxidase (MAO) inhibitors | Potentiate amphetamines by slowing drug metabolism. These drugs thereby increase the risks of headache, subarachnoid hemorrhage, and other signs of a hypertensive crisis. The combination may cause death and should be avoided. |
| d. Drugs that *decrease* effects of amphetamines: | |
| (1) Acidifying agents | Urinary acidifying agents (eg, ammonium chloride) increase urinary excretion and lower blood levels of amphetamines. Decreased absorption and increased excretion serve to decrease drug effects. |
| (2) Antipsychotic agents | Decrease or antagonize the excessive CNS stimulation produced by amphetamines. Chlorpromazine (Thorazine) or haloperidol (Haldol) is sometimes used in treating amphetamine overdose. |
| e. Drugs that *increase* effects of modafinil: | |
| (1) Itraconazole, ketoconazole | These drugs inhibit cytochrome P450 3A4 enzymes that partly metabolize modafinil. |
| f. Drugs that *decrease* effects of modafinil: | |
| (1) Carbamazepine, phenytoin, rifampin | These drugs induce cytochrome P450 3A4 enzymes that partly metabolize modafinil. |
| g. Drugs that *increase* effects of caffeine: | |
| (1) Enoxacin, fluvoxamine, mexilitene, theophylline | These drugs inhibit the cytochrome P450 1A2 enzymes that participate in the metabolism of caffeine. Decreased metabolism may increase adverse effects. |
| (2) Cimetidine, oral contraceptives | May impair caffeine metabolism. |
| h. Drugs that *decrease* effects of caffeine: | |
| (1) Carbamazepine, phenytoin, rifampin | These drugs induce drug-metabolizing enzymes, thereby decreasing blood levels and increasing clearance of caffeine. |

## Critical Thinking Exercises

1. Amphetamines in large doses can create all of the following symptoms except:
   a. Restlessness
   b. Hyperactivity
   c. Confusion
   d. Increasing mental alertness and capacity for work

2. Doxapram (Dopram) is occasionally used by anesthesiologists as a respiratory stimulant. The drug has limited usefulness for this purpose because the drug:
   a. Decreases carbon dioxide production
   b. Has a long duration of action after a single intravenous dose
   c. Has therapeutic dosages near or overlapping those that produce convulsions
   d. Decreases oxygen consumption

3. Guarana is widely used as a flavoring agent and an ingredient in herbal stimulant and weight-loss products. Guarana may contain all of the following except:
   a. Amphetamines
   b. Caffeine
   c. Theophylline
   d. Theobromine

4. Which of the following substances contains the greatest amount of caffeine?
   a. Cola (12 ounces)
   b. Espresso coffee (2 ounces)
   c. Iced tea (12 ounces)
   d. Anacin (1 tablet)

5. For a child receiving CNS stimulants, parents should schedule drug holidays (eg, weekends, summers) to:
   a. Increase weight loss
   b. Foster drug dependence
   c. Eliminate the need for dosage adjustments during other times of the year
   d. Prevent stunted growth

## SELECTED REFERENCES

Carillo, J. A., & Benitez, J. (2000). Clinically significant pharmacokinetic interactions between dietary caffeine and medications. *Clinical Pharmacokinetics, 39*(2), 127–153.

*Drug facts and comparisons.* (Updated monthly). St. Louis: Facts and Comparisons.

Fetrow, C. W., & Avila, J. R. (1999). *Professional's handbook of complementary & alternative medicines.* Springhouse, PA: Springhouse Corporation.

Hovinga, C. A., & Phelps, S. J. (2000). Attention-deficit/hyperactivity disorder (ADHD). In E. T. Herfindal & D. R. Gourley (Eds.), *Textbook of therapeutics: Drug and disease management* (7th ed., pp. 1247–1270). Philadelphia: Lippincott Williams & Wilkins.

Kehoe, W. A. (2001). Treatment of attention deficit hyperactivity disorder in children. *Annals of pharmacotherapy, 35*(9), 1130–1134.

Kim, R. B. (Ed.). (2001). *The medical letter handbook of adverse drug interactions.* New Rochelle, NY: The Medical Letter, Inc.

Lacy, C. F., Armstrong, L. L., Goldman, M. P., & Lance, L. L. (2003). *Lexi-Comp's drug information handbook* (11th ed.). Hudson, OH: American Pharmaceutical Association.

Spencer, T., Biederman, J., Wilens, T., Faraone, S., Prince, J., Gerard, K., et al. (2001). Efficacy of a mixed amphetamine salts compound in adults with attention-deficit/hyperactivity disorder. *Archives of General Psychiatry, 58*(8), 775–782.

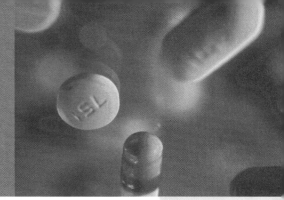

# Drugs Affecting the Autonomic Nervous System

## 16

# Adrenergic Drugs

## OBJECTIVES

*After studying this chapter, the student will be able to:*

1 Identify effects produced by stimulation of alpha- and beta-adrenergic receptors.

2 List characteristics of adrenergic drugs in terms of effects on body tissues, indications for use, adverse effects, nursing process implications, and observation of client responses.

3 Discuss use of epinephrine to treat anaphylactic shock, acute bronchospasm, and cardiac arrest.

4 Identify clients at risk for experiencing adverse effects with adrenergic drugs.

5 List commonly used over-the-counter (OTC) preparations and herbal preparations that contain adrenergic drugs.

6 Discuss nursing process for using adrenergic drugs in special populations.

7 Describe signs and symptoms of toxicity due to noncatecholamine adrenergic drugs.

8 Discuss treatment of overdose with noncatecholamine adrenergic drugs.

9 Teach the client about safe, effective use of adrenergic drugs.

## CRITICAL THINKING SCENARIO

Jennifer, 8 years old, is brought to the clinic for allergy desensitization. She is starting on a new concentration of allergy extract today. After her injection, as usual, you ask her to remain in the waiting room for 30 minutes. After 20 minutes, her mother comes to get you. Jennifer is restless, her voice is high-pitched, she feels odd, and her respiration rate has increased to 30 breaths per minute.

✔ What data would you collect next?

✔ How would you differentiate anaphylaxis from anxiety?

✔ If Jennifer were experiencing an anaphylactic reaction, what would be the treatment of choice?

## PROTOTYPE PROFILE

epinephrine (Adrenalin), p. 272

# DESCRIPTION

Adrenergic (sympathomimetic) drugs produce effects similar to those produced by stimulation of the sympathetic nervous system (SNS) and therefore have widespread effects on body tissues. Some of the drugs are exogenous formulations of naturally occurring neurotransmitters and hormones such as norepinephrine (Levophed), epinephrine (Adrenalin), and dopamine (Intropin). Other adrenergic medications such as phenylephrine (Neo-Synephrine), pseudoephedrine (Sudafed), and isoproterenol (Isuprel) are synthetic chemical relatives of naturally occurring neurotransmitters and hormones.

Specific effects of adrenergic medications depend mainly on the client's health status when a drug is given and the type of adrenergic receptor activated by the drug. Major therapeutic uses and adverse effects stem from drug effects on the heart, blood vessels, and lungs. An overview of the SNS is outlined in At the Foundation: Sympathetic Nervous System Effects found in Chapter 17. The drugs discussed in this chapter (epinephrine, ephedrine, pseudoephedrine, isoproterenol, and phenylephrine) are those with multiple effects and clinical uses (see Drugs at a Glance 16-1: Selected Adrenergic Drugs). Because epinephrine, ephedrine, and pseudoephedrine stimulate both alpha- and beta-adrenergic receptors, these drugs

**DRUG TABLE 16-1**

## Drugs at a Glance
### Selected Adrenergic Drugs

| Generic/Trade Name | Preparations, Routes, and Dosage Ranges | Comments/Clinical Use |
|---|---|---|
| **Epinephrine** (Adrenalin) Pregnancy Category C | See Prototype Profile 16-1: Epinephrine for further information | |
| | *Aqueous epinephrine* 1 mg/mL (1:1000): | Bronchodilator |
| | *Adults:* IM, Sub-Q, 0.1–0.5 mg q15min to q4h if needed | |
| | Do not exceed 1 mg in a single dose | |
| | IV injection (1:1000), dilute 1 mg with 10 mL NaCl injection for a final concentration of 1:10,000 or 0.1 mg/mL | |
| | Give 0.1–2.25 mg (1–2.5 mL) of this solution. Single dose maximum: 1 mg (10 mL) | |
| | *Children:* Sub-Q, 0.01 mg/kg q20min to q4h if needed. Do not exceed 0.5 mg in a single dose | |
| | *Sus-Phrine suspension* 5 mg/mL (1:200): | |
| | *Adults:* Sub-Q only: 0.1–0.3 mL or 0.5–1.5 mg | |
| | *Children:* Sub-Q only: 0.005 mL/kg | |
| | Maximum dose: 0.15 mL | |
| | *Epinephrine 1% aqueous solution* (1:100) for inhalation (nebulization): | |
| | *Adults:* Instill 8–15 drops into nebulizer reservoir. Administer 1–3 inhalations 4–6 times per day | |
| | *Epinephrine* by metered dose inhaler (MDI) (~200–275 mcg/puff): | |
| | *Adults:* 1 puff at onset of bronchospasm. Repeat if needed after 1–5 minutes. Dose is individualized to client's needs | |
| | *Aqueous epinephrine* 1 mg/mL (1:1000): | Cardiac arrest |
| | *Adults:* IV injection, 1 mg q3–5min. Higher doses (up to 0.2 mg/kg) may be used if 1-mg dose fails | |
| | *Continuous infusion:* Add 30 mg epinephrine to 250/mL NS or D5W, run at 100 mL/h and titrate to response | |
| | *Aqueous epinephrine* 0.1 mg/mL (1:10,000): | |
| | *Children:* Give 0.01 mg/kg (0.1 mL/kg) q3–5min | |
| | *Subsequent doses: Aqueous epinephrine* 1 mg/mL (1:1000): Give 0.1 mg/kg (0.1 mg/kg) up to 0.2 mg/kg (0.2 mL/kg) | |
| | *Adults:* Endotracheally, 2.0–2.5 mg of 1:1000 solution diluted in 10 mL NS | |
| | *Children:* Endotracheally, 0.1 mg/kg of 1:1000 solution q3–5min until IV access is established | |

*(continued)*

**DRUG TABLE 16-1**

*Drugs at a Glance*

## Selected Adrenergic Drugs (Continued)

| Generic/Trade Name | Preparations, Routes, and Dosage Ranges | Comments/Clinical Use |
|---|---|---|
| | *Aqueous epinephrine* 1 mg/mL (1:1000):<br>*Adults:* IM, Sub-Q, 0.1–0.5 mg q20min to q4h. Do not exceed 1 mg in a single dose<br>*Children:* IV, 0.01 mg q20min to q4h. Do not exceed 0.5 mg in a single dose | Allergic reaction, anaphylaxis |
| | *Adults:* Epinephrine HCl 0.1%, 0.5%, 1%, and 2%: 1–2 drops in eyes 1–2 times per day | Ophthalmic agent |
| | *Adults:* Epinephrine nasal solution 0.1% (1:1000): 1–2 drops per nostril q4–6h | Nasal agent for hemostasis |
| **Ephedrine**<br>Pregnancy Category C | *Adults:* PO, 25–50 mg q4h<br>*Children 6–12 y:* PO, 6.25–12.5 mg q4–6h. Children 2–6 y: PO, 0.3–0.5 mg/kg q4–6h | Asthma |
| | *Adults:* IM, Sub-Q, 25–50 mg. IV push: 5–25 mg/dose slowly, repeated q5–10min as needed, then q3–4h. Do not exceed 150 mg/24 h | Hypotension |
| | *Adults:* PO, 25–50 mg q4h<br>0.25% nasal spray or 1% nasal jelly | Nasal congestion |
| **Pseudoephedrine**<br> (Sudafed)<br>Pregnancy Category C | *Adults:* Give 30–60 mg PO q4–6h or 120 mg sustained release formula q12h. Do not exceed 240 mg/24 h<br>*Children:* 6–12 y: 30 mg PO q6h. Do not exceed 120 mg/24 h<br>2–5 y: 14 mg PO q6h. Do not exceed 60 mg/24 h | Nasal congestion |
| **Isoproterenol** (Isuprel)<br>Pregnancy Category C | *Adults:* Aerosol solutions: 0.2% (1:500), 0.25% (1:400): 1–2 metered doses 4–6 times/day. Second inhalation is given 2–5 minutes after the first<br>*Children:* Generally same as adult | Bronchodilator |
| | *Adults:* Nebulization solution: 0.031%, 0.062%, 0.25%, 0.5%, and 1%: 5–15 inhalations, repeated once in 10–30 min if needed. Treatments can be given up to 5 times/day<br>*Children:* Generally same as adult | |
| | *Adults:* Glossets: 10 and 15 mg; sublingually, 10–20 mg q3–4h not to exceed 60 mg/d<br>*Children:* Glossets: 10 mg; sublingually, 5–10 mg tid not to exceed 30 mg/d. Not a preferred route due to erratic absorption | |
| | *Adults:* IV, 20–60 mcg bolus initially, followed by IV infusion. Dilute 1 mg/250 mL D5W, NS, or LR, titrate to client response: 2–10 mcg/min | Cardiac dysrhythmias |
| | *Adults:* Dilute 1 mg/250 mL D5W, NS, or LR and infuse at 0.05–5 mcg/min. Titrate to client response | Shock |
| **Phenylephrine**<br> (Neo-Synephrine, others)<br>Pregnancy Category C | *Adults:* IM, Sub-Q, 2–5 mg q1–2h. Initial dose not to exceed 5 mg. IV bolus: 0.1–0.5 mg, diluted in NaCl injection, given slowly q10–15min as needed. Initial dose not to exceed 0.5 mg. IV infusion: 10 mg in 250 mL D5W or NS. Infuse at 100–180 mcg/min initially. When blood pressure is stable, reduce to maintenance rate of 40–60 mcg/min | Hypotension, shock |
| | *Adults:* Nasal decongestants: 0.25%, 0.5%, 1.0% solutions 1–2 drops or sprays q4h. Therapy should not exceed 5 days | Nasal congestion |
| | *Adults:* Ophthalmic preparations: 2.5% or 10% solutions Instill one drop. May be repeated in 10–60 min | Ophthalmic agent, mydriatic agent |

D5W, dextrose 5% in water; NS, 0.9% sodium chloride; LR, lactated Ringer's solution.

have widespread effects on body tissues and multiple clinical uses. Isoproterenol stimulates beta-adrenergic receptors (both $beta_1$ and $beta_2$) and may be used in the treatment of several clinical conditions. Phenylephrine stimulates alpha-adrenergic receptors and is used to induce vasoconstriction in several conditions.

Other adrenergic drugs are selective for specific adrenergic receptors or are given topically to produce more localized therapeutic effects and fewer systemic adverse effects. These drugs have relatively restricted clinical indications and are discussed more extensively elsewhere (see Chap. 37, Bronchodilating and Other Antiasthmatic Drugs; Chap. 42, Drugs Used in Hypotension and Shock; Appendix H, Nasal Decongestants, Antitussives, Mucolytics, and Cold Remedies; and Appendix G, Ophthalmics and Otics). Table 16-1 lists commonly used adrenergic drugs in relation to adrenergic receptor activity and their clinical use.

## Mechanisms of Action and Effects

Adrenergic (sympathomimetic) drugs have three mechanisms of action. For the most part, adrenergic drugs interact directly with *postsynaptic* alpha$_1$- or beta-adrenergic receptors on the surface membrane of body cells (Fig. 16-1). The drug–receptor complex then alters the cell membrane's permeability to ions or extracellular enzymes. The influx of these molecules stimulates intracellular metabolism and production of other enzymes, structural proteins, energy, and other products required for cell function and reproduction. Epinephrine, isoproterenol, norepinephrine, and phenylephrine are examples of direct-acting adrenergic drugs.

Some adrenergic drugs exert indirect effects on adrenergic receptors. Indirect adrenergic effects may be produced by drugs such as amphetamines that increase the amount of norepinephrine released into the synapse from storage sites in nerve endings (Fig. 16-2A). Norepinephrine then stimulates the alpha and beta receptors producing sympathetic effects in the body. Inhibition of norepinephrine reuptake from the synapse is another mechanism that will produce indirect adrenergic effects. Remember that norepinephrine reuptake is the major way that sympathetic nerve transmission is terminated. Drugs such as tricyclic antidepressants and cocaine block norepinephrine reuptake, resulting in stimulation of alpha- and beta-adrenergic receptors (see Fig. 16-2B). The third mechanism of adrenergic drug action is called *mixed acting* and is a combination of direct and indirect receptor stimulation. Ephedrine and pseudoephedrine are examples of mixed-acting adrenergic drugs. Drugs that activate alpha$_2$ receptors on *presynaptic* nerve fibers do not produce a sympathetic effect. These drugs inhibit the release of the neurotransmitter norepinephrine into synapses of the sympathetic nervous system and therefore exert a sympatholytic or antiadrenergic response in the body. Although activation of alpha$_2$

### TABLE 16-1 Commonly Used Adrenergic Drugs

| Generic/Trade Name | Major Clinical Uses |
|---|---|
| ***Alpha and Beta Activity*** | |
| **Dopamine** (Intropin) | Hypotension and shock |
| **Epinephrine** (Adrenalin) | Allergic reactions, cardiac arrest, hypotension and shock, local vasoconstriction, bronchodilation, cardiac stimulation, ophthalmic conditions |
| **Ephedrine** | Bronchodilation, cardiac stimulation, nasal decongestion |
| **Pseudoephedrine** (Sudafed) | Nasal decongestion |
| **Norepinephrine** (Levophed) | Hypotension and shock |
| ***Alpha Activity*** | |
| **Metaraminol** (Aramine) | Hypotension and shock |
| **Naphazoline hydrochloride** (Privine) | Nasal decongestion |
| **Oxymetazoline hydrochloride** (Afrin) | Nasal decongestion |
| **Phenylephrine** (Neo-Synephrine) | Hypotension and shock, nasal decongestion, ophthalmic conditions |
| **Propylhexedrine** (Benzedrex) | Nasal decongestion |
| **Tetrahydrozoline hydrochloride** (Tyzine, Visine) | Nasal decongestion, local vasoconstriction in the eye |
| **Tuaminoheptane** (Tuamine) | Nasal decongestion |
| **Xylometazoline hydrochloride** (Otrivin) | Nasal decongestion |
| ***Beta Activity*** | |
| **Albuterol** (Proventil) | Bronchodilation |
| **Bitolterol** (Tornalate) | Bronchodilation |
| **Dobutamine** (Dobutrex) | Cardiac stimulation |
| **Isoproterenol** (Isuprel) | Bronchodilation, cardiac stimulation |
| **Isoetharine** (Bronkosol) | Bronchodilation |
| **Metaproterenol** (Alupent) | Bronchodilation |
| **Pirbuterol** (Maxair) | Bronchodilation |
| **Salmeterol** (Serevent) | Bronchodilation |
| **Terbutaline** (Brethine) | Bronchodilation, preterm labor inhibition |

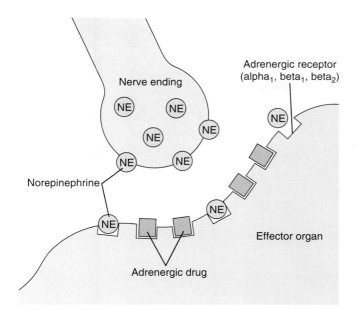

**FIGURE 16–1** Mechanism of direct adrenergic drug action. Adrenergic drugs interact directly with postsynaptic alpha$_1$ and beta receptors on target effector organs, activating the organ in a similar fashion as the neurotransmitter norepinephrine.

receptors in the periphery is not of clinical significance, activation of alpha$_2$ receptors in the central nervous system by medications is useful in treating hypertension (see Chap. 43).

Because most body tissues have both alpha and beta receptors, the effect produced by an adrenergic drug depends on the type of receptor activated and the number of affected receptors in a particular body tissue. Some drugs act on both types of receptors; some act more selec-

tively on certain subtypes of receptors. Activation of alpha$_1$ receptors in blood vessels results in vasoconstriction, which then raises blood pressure and decreases nasal congestion. Activation of beta$_1$ receptors in the heart results in cardiac stimulation (increased force of myocardial contraction and increased heart rate). Activation of beta$_2$ receptors in the lungs results in bronchodilation, and activation of beta$_2$ receptors in blood vessels results in vasodilation (increased blood flow to the heart, brain, and skeletal muscles, the tissues needed to aid the "fight-or-flight" response). Many newer adrenergic drugs (eg, beta$_2$ receptor agonists used as bronchodilators in asthma and other bronchoconstrictive disorders) were developed specifically to be more selective.

In addition to the cardiac, vascular, and pulmonary effects, other effects of adrenergic drugs include contraction of gastrointestinal (GI) and urinary sphincters, lipolysis, decreased GI tone, changes in renin secretion, uterine relaxation, hepatic glycogenolysis and gluconeogenesis, and decreased secretion of insulin.

## Indications for Use

Clinical indications for the use of adrenergic drugs stem mainly from their effects on the heart, blood vessels, and bronchi. They are often used as emergency drugs in the treatment of acute cardiovascular, respiratory, and allergic disorders. However, guidelines for safe and effective use of adrenergic drugs in children are not well established. Children and older adults are very sensitive to drug effects, including cardiac and central nervous system (CNS) stimulation, and recommended doses usually should not be exceeded. Specific use in children and older adults is detailed in Age-related Considerations. In cardiac arrest

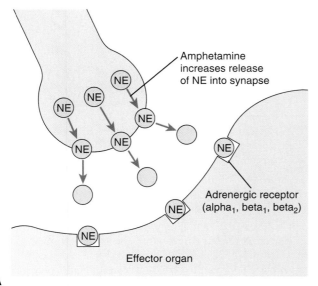

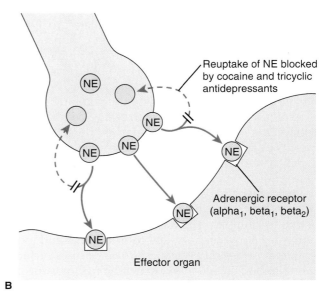

**A**               **B**

**FIGURE 16–2** Mechanisms of indirect adrenergic drug action. Stimulation of postsynaptic alpha$_1$, beta$_1$, and beta$_2$ receptors results from adrenergic medications that act indirectly, increasing the release of norepinephrine (NE) into the synapse (A) or inhibiting the reuptake of norepinephrine from the synapse (B).

## Age-related Considerations: Use of Adrenergic Drugs

### USE IN CHILDREN

The main use of epinephrine in children is for treatment of bronchospasm due to asthma or allergic reactions. Parenteral epinephrine may cause syncope when given to asthmatic children. Isoproterenol is rarely given parenterally, but if given, the first dose should be approximately half that of an adult's, and later doses should be based on the response to the first dose. There is little reason to use the inhalation route because in children, as in adults, selective beta$_2$ agonists such as albuterol are preferred for bronchodilation in asthma.

Phenylephrine is most often used to relieve congestion of the upper respiratory tract and may be given topically, as nose drops. Doses must be carefully measured. Rebound nasal congestion occurs with overuse.

### USE IN OLDER ADULTS

Adrenergic agents are used to treat asthma, hypotension, shock, cardiac arrest, and anaphylaxis in older adults. These drugs stimulate the heart to increase rate and force of contraction and blood pressure. Because older adults often have chronic cardiovascular conditions (eg, angina, dysrhythmias, congestive heart failure, coronary artery disease, hypertension, peripheral vascular disease) that are aggravated by adrenergic drugs, careful monitoring by the nurse is required.

Adrenergic drugs are often prescribed as bronchodilators and decongestants in older adults. Therapeutic doses increase the workload of the heart and may cause symptoms of impaired cardiovascular function; overdoses may cause severe cardiovascular dysfunction, including life-threatening dysrhythmias. The drugs also cause CNS stimulation. With therapeutic doses, anxiety, restlessness, nervousness, and insomnia often occur in older adults. Overdoses may cause hallucinations, convulsions, CNS depression, and death.

Adrenergics are ingredients in OTC asthma remedies, cold remedies, nasal decongestants, and appetite suppressants. Cautious use of these preparations is required for older adults. They should not be taken concurrently with prescription adrenergic drugs because of the high risk of overdose and toxicity.

Ophthalmic preparations of adrenergic drugs also should be used cautiously. For example, phenylephrine is used as a vasoconstrictor and mydriatic. Applying larger than recommended doses to the normal eye or usual doses to the traumatized, inflamed, or diseased eye may result in enough systemic absorption of the drug to cause increased blood pressure and other adverse effects.

---

and Stokes-Adams syndrome (heart block), they may be given as cardiac stimulants. In hypotension and shock, they may be given to increase blood pressure. In hemorrhagic or hypovolemic shock, the drugs are second-line agents that may be used if adequate fluid volume replacement does not restore sufficient blood pressure and circulation to maintain organ perfusion.

In bronchial asthma and other obstructive pulmonary diseases, the drugs are given as bronchodilators to relieve bronchoconstriction and bronchospasm. In upper respiratory infections, including the common cold and sinusitis, they may be given orally or applied topically to the nasal mucosa for decongestant effects.

In allergic disorders, the drugs are given for vasoconstricting or decongestant effects to relieve edema in the respiratory tract, skin, and other tissues. Thus, they may be used to treat allergic rhinitis, acute hypersensitivity (anaphylactoid reactions to drugs, animal serums, insect stings, and other allergens), serum sickness, urticaria, and angioneurotic edema.

Other clinical uses include relaxation of uterine musculature and inhibition of uterine contractions in preterm labor. They also may be added to intraspinal and local anesthetics to prolong anesthesia. Topical uses include application to skin and mucous membranes for vasoconstriction and hemostatic effects and to the eyes for vasoconstriction and mydriasis.

Adrenergic drugs are often used in the home setting. Frequently prescribed drugs include bronchodilators and nasal decongestants. OTC drugs with the same effects are also commonly used for asthma, allergic rhinitis, cold symptoms, and appetite suppression for weight control. Guidelines for strategies for ongoing evaluation and intervention are addressed in Home Care Considerations.

## Contraindications to Use

Contraindications to using adrenergic drugs include cardiac dysrhythmias, angina pectoris, hypertension,

## Home Care Considerations: Use of Adrenergic Drugs

**ASSESS:** the client for compliance with the prescribed regimen and for concurrent use with OTC drugs or herbal drugs containing similar ingredients.

**MONITOR:** for therapeutic and excessive adverse effects and client's need for additional information, and provide that information.

**EDUCATE:** on safe use of drugs (especially metered-dose inhalers), on ways to minimize adverse effects, to report excessive CNS or cardiac stimulation to a health care provider, and not to take OTC drugs or herbal preparations with the same or similar ingredients as prescription drugs. Reinforce additional teaching points (see Client Teaching Guidelines: Adrenergic Drugs).

hyperthyroidism, and cerebrovascular disease because stimulation of the SNS worsens these conditions. Adrenergic drugs are also contraindicated in persons with narrow-angle glaucoma because they result in mydriasis, closure of the filtration angle of the eye, and increased intraocular pressure. Hypersensitivity to an adrenergic drug or any component (some preparations contain sulfites, to which some people are allergic) is also a contraindication to their use. Adrenergic drugs are contraindicated with local anesthesia of distal areas with a single blood supply (e.g., fingers, toes, nose, ears) because of potential tissue damage and sloughing from vasoconstriction. They should not be given during the second stage of labor because they may delay progression. The drugs should be used with caution in clients with anxiety, insomnia, and psychiatric disorders because of their stimulant effects on the CNS and in older adults because of their cardiac- and CNS-stimulating effects. Adrenergic drugs exert effects on the renal system that may cause problems for clients with renal impairment. For example, adrenergic drugs with alpha$_1$ activity cause constriction of renal arteries, thereby diminishing renal blood flow and urine production. These drugs also constrict urinary sphincters, causing urinary retention and painful urination, especially in men with prostatic hyperplasia.

Many adrenergic drugs and their metabolites are eliminated by the renal system. In the presence of renal disease, these compounds may accumulate and cause increased adverse effects.

## ■ INDIVIDUAL ADRENERGIC DRUGS

P **Epinephrine** (Adrenalin) is the prototype of adrenergic drugs. When given systemically, the effects may be therapeutic or adverse, depending on the reason for use and route of administration. Specific effects include the following:

1. Increased systolic blood pressure, due primarily to increased force of myocardial contraction and vasoconstriction in skin, mucous membranes, and kidneys
2. Vasodilation and increased blood flow to skeletal muscles, heart, and brain
3. Vasoconstriction in peripheral blood vessels. This allows shunting of blood to the heart and brain, with increased perfusion pressure in the coronary and cerebral circulations. This action is thought to be the main beneficial effect in cardiac arrest and cardiopulmonary resuscitation (CPR).
4. Increased heart rate and possibly arrhythmias due to stimulation of conducting tissues in the heart. Reflex bradycardia may occur when blood pressure is raised.
5. Relaxation of GI smooth muscle
6. Relaxation or dilation of bronchial smooth muscle
7. Increased glucose, lactate, and fatty acids in the blood due to metabolic effects

8. Inhibition of insulin secretion
9. Miscellaneous effects, including increased total leukocyte count, increased rate of blood coagulation, and decreased intraocular pressure in wide-angle glaucoma. When given locally, the main effect is vasoconstriction.

Epinephrine stimulates both alpha and beta receptors. At usual doses, beta-adrenergic effects on the heart and vascular and other smooth muscles predominate. However, at high doses, alpha-adrenergic effects (eg, vasoconstriction) predominate. As the prototype of adrenergic drugs, effects and clinical indications for epinephrine are the same as for adrenergic drugs (see Prototype Profile 16-1: Epinephrine). In addition, epinephrine is the adrenergic drug of choice for relieving the acute bronchospasm and laryngeal edema of anaphylactic shock, the most serious allergic reaction. Epinephrine is used in cardiac arrest for its cardiac stimulant and peripheral vasoconstrictive effects. It also is added to local anesthetics for vasoconstrictive effects, which prolong the action of the local anesthetic drug, prevent systemic absorption, and minimize bleeding.

Epinephrine should be used with caution in infants and children; syncope has occurred with use in asthmatic children. Epinephrine is the active ingredient in OTC inhalation products for asthma (eg, AsthmaNefrin, Primatene Mist, Bronkaid Mist). People who have heart disease and elderly clients should not use these products on a regular basis. These preparations have a short duration of action, which promotes frequent and excessive use. Prolonged use may cause adverse effects and result in the development of tolerance to the therapeutic effects of the drug.

Epinephrine is not given orally because enzymes in the GI tract and liver destroy it. It may be given by inhalation, injection, or topical application. Numerous epinephrine solutions are available for various uses and routes of administration (Box 16-1). Solutions vary widely in the amount of drug they contain. They must be used correctly to avoid potentially serious hazards.

**Sus-Phrine** is an aqueous suspension of epinephrine that is given subcutaneously only. Some of the epinephrine is in solution and acts rapidly; some is suspended in crystalline form for slower absorption and relatively prolonged activity.

**Ephedrine** is a mixed-acting adrenergic drug that acts by stimulating alpha and beta receptors and causing release of norepinephrine. Its actions are less potent but longer lasting than those of epinephrine. Ephedrine produces more CNS stimulation than other adrenergic drugs. It may be used in the treatment of bronchial asthma to prevent bronchospasm, but it is less effective than epinephrine for acute bronchospasm and respiratory distress.

Ephedrine can be given orally or parenterally. When given orally, therapeutic effects occur within 1 hour and last 3 to 5 hours. When given subcutaneously, it acts in

## PROTOTYPE PROFILE 16-1

### P Epinephrine (ep I NEF rin)

**Drug Class**
*Chemical:* Alpha/beta agonist
*Functional:* Vasopressor, bronchodilator, antiasthmatic

**Trade Names**
Adrenalin, EpiPen

**Therapeutic Indications**
Treatment of bronchospasm, cardiac arrest, anaphylaxis
Management of open-angle glaucoma (additional uses outlined in Drug Table 16-1: Selected Adrenergic Drugs)

**Pharmacokinetics**
*Absorption*
Well absorbed

*Distribution*
Crosses placenta but not the blood–brain barrier

*Metabolism*
Hepatic

*Excretion*
Urine

**Pharmacodynamics**
*Onset of Action*
Inhalation, 3–5 min; IM, Sub-Q, 6–12 min; IV, rapid

*Duration*
Inhalation 1–3 h; IM, Sub-Q, 1–4 h; IV, 20–30 min

**Contraindications/Precautions**
Closed-angle glaucoma, cardiac dysrhythmias; with caution in the elderly, those with diabetes mellitus, cardiovascular or cerebrovascular disease, or thyroid disease

**Pregnancy Considerations**
Category C
Possible excretion in breast milk

**Dosage**
See Drugs at a Glance 16-1: Selected Adrenergic Drugs for dosage

**Adverse Effects**
Tachycardia, chest pain with increased myocardial oxygen consumption, nervousness, dizziness

**Drug Interactions**
*Increased Effects*
Cardiac irritability with beta-blocking or alpha-blocking agents, or halogenated inhalation anesthetics

*Decreased Effects*
Bronchodilation with beta blockers, reduced antihypertensive effect with concurrent use of guanethidine or methyldopa

**Herbal Supplements and Dietary Considerations**
Ephedra or ma huang contains derivatives of ephedrine; excessive central nervous system and cardiovascular stimulation may result with use

---

approximately 20 minutes, and effects last approximately 60 minutes; with intramuscular administration, it acts in approximately 10 to 20 minutes, and effects last less than 60 minutes. Ephedrine is excreted unchanged in the urine. Acidic urine increases the rate of drug elimination.

Ephedrine is a common ingredient in OTC antiasthma tablets (eg, Bronkaid, Primatene). The tablets contain 12.5 to 25 mg of ephedrine and 100 to 130 mg of theophylline, a xanthine bronchodilator. Other clinical uses include shock associated with spinal or epidural anesthesia, Stokes-Adams syndrome (sudden attacks of unconsciousness caused by heart block), allergic disorders, nasal congestion, and eye disorders.

**Pseudoephedrine** (Sudafed) is a related drug with similar actions. It is used for bronchodilating and nasal decongestant effects. Pseudoephedrine is given orally and is available OTC alone and as an ingredient in several multiple-ingredient sinus, allergy, and cold remedies. Pseudoephedrine is eliminated primarily in the urine. Its elimination may be slowed by alkaline urine, which promotes drug reabsorption in the renal tubules.

**Isoproterenol** (Isuprel) is a synthetic catecholamine that acts on beta$_1$- and beta$_2$-adrenergic receptors. Its main actions are to stimulate the heart, dilate blood vessels in skeletal muscle, and relax bronchial smooth muscle. Compared with epinephrine, its cardiac stimulant effects are similar, but it does not affect alpha receptors and therefore does not cause vasoconstriction. It is well absorbed when given by injection or as an aerosol. However, absorption is unreliable with sublingual and oral preparations; hence, their use is not recommended. It is metabolized more slowly than epinephrine by the enzyme catechol-*O*-methyltransferase (COMT). It is not

### BOX 16-1  Epinephrine Concentrations and Administration Routes

| Final Concentration | Route |
| --- | --- |
| 1% (1;100) | Inhalation |
| 0.5% (1;200) | Subcutaneous |
| 0.1% (1;1000) | Subcutaneous |
|  | Intramuscular |
| 0.01% (1;10,000) | Intravenous |
| 0.001% (1;100,000) | Intradermal (in combination with local anesthetics) |

well metabolized by monoamine oxidase (MAO), which may account for its slightly longer duration of action than epinephrine. Isoproterenol may be used as a cardiac stimulant in heart block and cardiogenic shock and as a bronchodilator in respiratory conditions characterized by bronchospasm. However, beta$_2$-selective agonists (eg, albuterol) are preferred for bronchodilating effects because they cause less cardiac stimulation. Too-frequent use of inhaled isoproterenol may lead to tolerance and decreased bronchodilating effects.

**Phenylephrine** (eg, Neo-Synephrine) is a synthetic drug that acts on alpha-adrenergic receptors to produce vasoconstriction. Vasoconstriction decreases cardiac output and renal perfusion and increases peripheral vascular resistance and blood pressure. There is little cardiac stimulation because phenylephrine does not activate beta$_1$ receptors in the heart or beta$_2$ receptors in blood vessels. Phenylephrine may be given to raise blood pressure in hypotension and shock. Compared with epinephrine, phenylephrine produces longer-lasting elevation of blood pressure (20 to 50 minutes with injection). When given systemically, phenylephrine produces a reflex bradycardia. This effect may be used therapeutically to relieve paroxysmal atrial tachycardia. However, other medications such as calcium channel blockers (see Chap. 41) are more likely to be used for this purpose. Other uses of phenylephrine include local application for nasal decongestant and mydriatic effects. Various preparations are available for different uses. Phenylephrine is often an ingredient in prescription and nonprescription cold and allergy remedies. It is excreted primarily in the urine.

**Phenylpropanolamine (PPA)** is an indirect-acting adrenergic drug that was a common ingredient in OTC cold and allergy remedies and appetite suppressants. The U.S. Food and Drug Administration (FDA) recently removed phenylpropanolamine from the market because of its association with severe hypertension and the occurrence of strokes. Nurses should instruct clients to check the labels on OTC medications and discard those containing PPA.

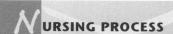

## NURSING PROCESS

### Assessment

Assess the client's status in relation to the following conditions:

- **Allergic disorders.** It is standard procedure to question a client about allergies on initial contact or admission to a health care agency. If the client reports a previous allergic reaction, try to determine what caused it and what specific symptoms occurred. It may be helpful to ask if swelling, breathing difficulty, or hives (urticaria) occurred. With anaphylactic reactions, severe respiratory distress (from bronchospasm and laryngeal edema) and profound hypotension (from vasodilation) may occur.

- **Asthma.** If the client is known to have asthma, assess the frequency of attacks, the specific signs and symptoms experienced, the precipitating factors, the actions taken to obtain relief, and the use of bronchodilators or other medications on a long-term basis. With acute bronchospasm, respiratory distress is clearly evidenced by loud, rapid, gasping, wheezing respirations. Acute asthma attacks may be precipitated by exposure to allergens or respiratory infections. When available, check arterial blood gas reports for the adequacy of oxygen–carbon dioxide gas exchange. Hypoxemia ($\downarrow$Po$_2$), hypercarbia ($\uparrow$Pco$_2$), and acidosis ($\downarrow$pH) may occur with acute bronchospasm.

- **Chronic obstructive pulmonary disorders.** Emphysema and chronic bronchitis are characterized by bronchoconstriction and dyspnea with exercise or at rest. Check arterial blood gas reports when available. Hypoxemia, hypercarbia, and acidosis are likely with chronic bronchoconstriction. Acute bronchospasm may be superimposed on the chronic bronchoconstrictive disorder, especially with a respiratory infection.

- **Cardiovascular status.** Assess for conditions that are caused or aggravated by adrenergic drugs (eg, angina, hypertension, tachyarrhythmias).

### Nursing Diagnoses

- Impaired Gas Exchange related to bronchoconstriction
- Ineffective Tissue Perfusion related to hypotension and shock or vasoconstriction with drug therapy
- Imbalanced Nutrition: Less than Body Requirements related to anorexia
- Disturbed Sleep Pattern: Insomnia, nervousness
- Noncompliance: Overuse
- Risk for Injury related to cardiac stimulation (arrhythmias, hypertension)
- Deficient Knowledge: Drug effects and safe usage

### Planning/Goals

*The client will:*
- Receive or self-administer drugs accurately
- Experience relief of symptoms for which adrenergic drugs are given
- Comply with instructions for safe drug use
- Demonstrate knowledge of adverse drug effects to be reported
- Avoid preventable adverse drug effects
- Avoid combinations of adrenergic drugs

### Interventions

Use measures to prevent or minimize conditions for which adrenergic drugs are required:

- Decrease exposure to allergens. Allergens include cigarette smoke, foods, drugs, air pollutants, plant pollens, insect

*(continued)*

## *N*URSING PROCESS (Continued)

venoms, and animal dander. Specific allergens must be determined for each person.

- For clients with chronic lung disease, use measures to prevent respiratory infections. These include interventions to aid removal of respiratory secretions, such as adequate hydration, ambulation, deep-breathing and coughing exercises, and chest physiotherapy. Immunizations with pneumococcal pneumonia vaccine (a single dose) and influenza vaccine (annually) are also strongly recommended.

- When administering substances known to produce hypersensitivity reactions (penicillin and other antibiotics, allergy extracts, vaccines, local anesthetics), observe the recipient carefully for at least 30 minutes after administration. Have adrenergic and other emergency drugs and equipment readily available in case a reaction occurs.

- Use noninvasive interventions in addition to adrenergic medications when treating shock and hypotension. These include applying external pressure over a bleeding site to control hemorrhage and placing the patient in modified Trendelenburg position (patient supine with legs markedly elevated and head and shoulders only slightly elevated) to improve venous return and blood pressure.

### Evaluation

- Observe for increased blood pressure and improved tissue perfusion when a drug is given for hypotension and shock or anaphylaxis.
- Interview and observe for improved breathing and arterial blood gas reports when a drug is given for bronchoconstriction or anaphylaxis.
- Interview and observe for decreased nasal congestion.

## CLIENT TEACHING GUIDELINES
## Adrenergic Drugs

### General Considerations

✔ Take no other medications without the physician's knowledge and approval. Many over-the-counter (OTC) cold remedies and appetite suppressants contain adrenergic drugs. Use of these along with prescribed adrenergic drugs can result in overdose and serious cardiovascular or central nervous system problems. In addition, adrenergic drugs interact with numerous other drugs to increase or decrease effects; some of these interactions may be life threatening.

✔ Herbal preparations of ephedra or ma huang contain derivatives of ephedrine and should not be taken with other adrenergic medications. Excessive central nervous system and cardiovascular stimulation may result.

✔ Tell your health care provider if you are pregnant, breastfeeding, taking any other prescription or OTC drugs, or if you are allergic to sulfite preservatives.

✔ Use these drugs only as directed. The potential for abuse is high, especially for the client with asthma or other chronic lung disease who is seeking relief from labored breathing. Some of these drugs are prescribed for long-term use, but excessive use does not increase therapeutic effects. Instead, it causes tolerance and decreased benefit from usual doses and increases the incidence and severity of adverse reactions.

✔ Frequent cardiac monitoring, checks of flow rate, blood pressure, and urine output are necessary if you are receiving intravenous adrenergic drugs to stimulate your heart or raise your blood pressure. These measures increase the safety and benefits of drug therapy rather than indicate the presence of a critical condition. Ask your nurse if you have concerns about your condition.

✔ You may feel anxious or tense; have difficulty sleeping; and experience palpitations, blurred vision,

headache, tremor, dizziness, and pallor. These are effects of the medication. Use of relaxation techniques to promote rest and decrease muscle tension may be helpful.

✔ Use caution when driving or performing activities requiring alertness, dexterity, and good vision.

✔ Report adverse reactions such as fast pulse, palpitations, and chest pain so that drug dosage can be reevaluated and therapy changed if needed.

### Self-administration

✔ Do not use topical decongestants longer than 3 to 5 days. Long-term use may be habit forming. Burning on use and rebound congestion after the dose wears off are common. Stop using the medication gradually.

✔ Stinging may occur when using ophthalmic preparations. Do not let the tip of the applicator touch your eye or anything else during administration of the medication, to avoid contamination. Do not wear soft contact lenses while using ophthalmic adrenergic drugs; discoloration of the lenses may occur. Report blurred vision, headache, palpitations, and muscle tremors to your health care provider.

✔ Follow guidelines for use of your inhaler. Do not increase the dosage or frequency; tolerance may occur. Report chest pain, dizziness, or failure to obtain relief of symptoms. Saliva and sputum may be discolored pink with isoproterenol.

✔ Learn to self-administer an injection of epinephrine if you have severe allergies. Always carry your injection kit with you. Seek immediate medical care after self-injection of epinephrine.

✔ If you are diabetic, monitor your glucose levels carefully because adrenergic medications may elevate them.

## ■ USE IN SPECIFIC SITUATIONS

Because adrenergic drugs are often used in crises, they must be readily available in all health care settings (eg, hospitals, long-term care facilities, health care providers' offices). All health care personnel should know where emergency drugs are stored.

### Anaphylaxis

Epinephrine is the drug of choice for the treatment of anaphylaxis. It relieves bronchospasm, laryngeal edema, and hypotension. In conjunction with its alpha (vasoconstriction) and beta (cardiac stimulation, bronchodilation) effects, epinephrine acts as a physiologic antagonist of histamine and other bronchoconstricting and vasodilating substances released during anaphylactic reactions. People susceptible to severe allergic responses should carry a syringe of epinephrine at all times. EpiPen and EpiPen Jr. are prefilled, autoinjection syringes for self-administration of epinephrine in an emergency situation.

Victims of anaphylaxis who have been taking beta-adrenergic blocking drugs (eg, propranolol [Inderal]) do not respond as readily to epinephrine as those not taking a beta blocker. Larger doses of epinephrine and large amounts of IV fluids may be required. Adjunct medications that may be useful in treating severe cases of anaphylaxis include corticosteroids, norepinephrine, and aminophylline. Antihistamines are not very useful because histamine plays a minor role in causing anaphylaxis, compared with leukotrienes and other inflammatory mediators.

### Cardiopulmonary Resuscitation

Epinephrine is often administered during CPR. Its most important action is constriction of peripheral blood vessels, which shunts blood to the central circulation and increases blood flow to the heart and brain. In the past, it was considered the drug of choice to treat cardiac arrest. Recent Advanced Cardiac Life Support (ACLS) guidelines for health professionals (2000) classify epinephrine as a class indeterminate for the treatment of defibrillation-resistant ventricular tachycardia and ventricular fibrillation during cardiac arrest. *Class indeterminate* means a treatment is promising but lacks research

evidence of benefit. Vasopressin is the alternative pressor to epinephrine that may be used in this situation. Vasopressin is listed as class IIb, which means the usefulness of the drug is supported by fair to good research. *Class IIb* drugs are considered optional or alternative interventions by most experts in treatment of cardiac arrest. When treating defibrillation-resistant ventricular tachycardia or ventricular fibrillation, vasopressin is given as a single dose of 40 units IV (see Chap. 40). Epinephrine is still considered the drug of choice to treat cardiac arrest in nonventricular tachycardia and fibrillation cases such as pulseless electrical activity (PEA) and asystole. Epinephrine is beneficial in these situations because it stimulates electrical and mechanical activity and produces myocardial contraction.

The specific effects of epinephrine depend largely on the dose and route of administration. The optimal dose in CPR has not been established. ACLS guidelines recommend epinephrine, 1 mg IV every 3 to 5 minutes. If this fails, higher doses of epinephrine (up to 0.2 mg/kg) are acceptable, but not recommended. In fact, there is growing evidence that higher doses of epinephrine may be harmful.

### Hypotension and Shock

In hypotension and shock, initial efforts involve identifying and treating the cause when possible. Such treatments include placing the client in the recumbent position, blood transfusions, fluid and electrolyte replacement, treatment of infection, and use of positive inotropic drugs to treat heart failure. If these measures are ineffective in raising the blood pressure enough to maintain perfusion to vital organs such as the brain, kidneys, and heart, vasopressor drugs may be used. The usual goal of vasopressor drug therapy is to maintain tissue perfusion and a mean arterial pressure of at least 80 to 100 mm Hg.

### Nasal Congestion

Adrenergic drugs are given topically and systemically to constrict blood vessels in nasal mucosa and decrease the nasal congestion associated with the common cold, allergic rhinitis, and sinusitis. Topical agents are effective, undergo little systemic absorption, are available OTC, and are widely used. However, overuse leads to decreased effectiveness (tolerance), irritation and ischemic changes in the nasal mucosa, and rebound congestion. These effects can be minimized by using small doses only when necessary and for no longer than 3 to 5 days.

Oral agents have a slower onset of action than topical ones but may last longer. They also may cause more adverse effects. Adverse effects may occur with usual therapeutic doses and are especially likely with high doses. The most problematic adverse effects are cardiac and CNS stimulation. Commonly used oral agents are pseudoephedrine and ephedrine. Pseudoephedrine seems to be the safest in relation to risks for hypertension and cerebral hemorrhage (stroke). Ephedrine may cause hypertension even in normotensive people, with higher risks in hypertensive people. Hypertensive clients should avoid these drugs if possible.

## Toxicity of Adrenergics: Recognition and Management

Unlike catecholamines, which are quickly cleared from the body, excessive use of noncatecholamine adrenergic drugs (phenylephrine, ephedrine, and pseudoephedrine) can lead to overdose and toxicity. These drugs are an ingredient in OTC products such as nasal decongestants, cold preparations, and appetite suppressants. Ephedrine and ephedra-containing herbal preparations (eg, ma huang and herbal ecstasy) are often abused as an alternative to amphetamines or to aid in rapid weight loss.

Phenylephrine and ephedrine have a narrow therapeutic index, with toxic doses only two to three times greater than the therapeutic dose. Pseudoephedrine toxicity occurs with doses four to five times greater than the normal therapeutic dose.

The primary clinical manifestation of noncatecholamine adrenergic drug toxicity is severe hypertension, which may lead to headache, confusion, seizures, and intracranial hemorrhage. Reflex bradycardia and atrioventricular block also have been associated with phenylephrine toxicity.

Treatment involves maintaining an airway and assisting with ventilation if needed. Activated charcoal may be administered early in treatment. Hypertension is aggressively treated with vasodilators such as phentolamine or nitroprusside. Beta blockers are not used alone to treat hypertension without first administering a vasodilator, to avoid a paradoxical increase in blood pressure.

Dialysis and hemoperfusion are not effective in clearing these drugs from the body. Urinary acidification may enhance elimination of ephedrine and pseudoephedrine; however, this technique is not routinely used because of the risk for renal damage from myoglobin deposition in the kidney.

Although adrenergic drugs may save the life of a client, they may result in a secondary health problem that requires monitoring and intervention. These include:

1. Potential for the vasopressor action of adrenergic drugs to result in diminished renal perfusion and decreased urine output
2. Potential for adrenergic drugs with beta$_1$ activity to induce irritable cardiac dysrhythmias
3. Potential for adrenergic drugs with beta$_1$ activity to increase myocardial oxygen requirement
4. Potential for adrenergic drugs with vasopressor action to decrease perfusion to the liver with subsequent liver damage
5. Hyperglycemia, hypokalemia, and hypophosphatemia due to beta$_1$-adrenergic effects
6. Severe hypertension and reflex bradycardia
7. Tissue necrosis after extravasation

Occurrence of any of these adverse effects may complicate the already complex care of the critically ill client. Careful assessment and prompt nursing intervention are essential in caring for the critically ill client experiencing these health problems.

## *Nursing Actions*
## Adrenergic Drugs

| Nursing Actions | Rationale/Explanation |
|---|---|
| 1. Administer accurately. | |
| a. Check package inserts or other references if not absolutely sure about the preparation, concentration, or method of administration for an adrenergic drug. | The many different preparations and concentrations available for various routes of administration increase the risk of medication error unless extreme caution is used. Preparations for intravenous, subcutaneous, inhalation, ophthalmic, or nasal routes must be used by the designated route only. |
| b. To give epinephrine subcutaneously, use a tuberculin syringe, aspirate, and massage the injection site. | The tuberculin syringe is necessary for accurate measurement of the small doses usually given (often less than 0.5 mL). Aspiration is necessary to avoid inadvertent IV administration of the larger, undiluted amount of drug intended for subcutaneous use. Massaging the injection site accelerates drug absorption and thus relief of symptoms. |
| c. Give Sus-Phrine subcutaneously only, and shake well before using (both vial and syringe). | Sus-Phrine is a suspension preparation of epinephrine, and suspensions must not be given IV. Rotating or shaking the container ensures that the medication is evenly distributed throughout the suspension. |
| d. For inhalation, be sure to use the correct drug concentration, and use the nebulizing device properly. | Inhalation medications are often administered by clients themselves or by respiratory therapists if intermittent positive-pressure breathing is used. The nurse may need to demonstrate and supervise self-administration initially. |

*(continued)*

## *Nursing Actions*

## Adrenergic Drugs (Continued)

| Nursing Actions | Rationale/Explanation |
|---|---|
| e. Do *not* give epinephrine and isoproterenol at the same time or within 4 hours of each other. | Both of these drugs are potent cardiac stimulants, and the combination could cause serious cardiac arrhythmias. However, they have synergistic bronchodilating effects, and doses can be alternated and given safely if the drugs are given no more closely together than 4 hours. |
| f. For IV injection of epinephrine, dilute 1 ml of 1;1000 solution with 10 mL of sodium chloride injection, or use a commercial preparation of 1;10,000 concentration. For IV infusion of epinephrine, dilute 1 mg in 250 mL D5W. Administer in intensive care, when possible, using an infusion pump and a central IV line. Use parenteral solutions of epinephrine only if clear. Epinephrine is unstable in alkaline solutions. | Dilution increases safety of administration. A solution that is brown or contains a precipitate should not be used. Discoloration indicates chemical deterioration of epinephrine. Do not administer at same time sodium bicarbonate is being administered. |
| g. For IV infusion of isoproterenol and phenylephrine:<br>(1) Administer in an intensive care unit when possible. | These drugs are given IV in emergencies, during which the client's condition must be carefully monitored. Frequent recording of blood pressure and pulse and continuous electrocardiographic monitoring are needed. |
| (2) Use only clear drug solutions. | A brownish color or precipitate indicates deterioration, and such solutions should not be used. |
| (3) Dilute isoproterenol in 500 mL of 5% dextrose injection. Phenylephrine can be diluted in 5% dextrose injection or 0.9% sodium chloride solution. Do not add the drug until ready to use. | Mixing solutions when ready for use helps to ensure drug stability. Note that drug concentration varies with the amount of drug and the amount of IV solution to which it is added. |
| (4) Use an infusion device to regulate flow rate accurately. | Flow rate usually requires frequent adjustment according to blood pressure measurements. An infusion device helps to regulate drug administration, so wide fluctuations in blood pressure are avoided. |
| (5) Use a "piggyback" IV apparatus. | Only one bottle contains an adrenergic drug, and it can be regulated or discontinued without disruption of the primary IV line. |
| (6) Start the adrenergic drug solution slowly and increase flow rate according to the client's response (eg, blood pressure, color, mental status). Slow or discontinue gradually as well. | To avoid abrupt changes in circulation and blood pressure |
| h. When giving adrenergic drugs as eye drops or nose drops, do not touch the dropper to the eye or nose. | Contaminated droppers can be a source of bacterial infection. |
| 2. **Observe for therapeutic effects.**<br>a. When the drug is used as a bronchodilator, observe for absence or reduction of wheezing, less labored breathing, and decreased rate of respirations. | These depend on the reason for use.<br>Indicates prevention or relief of bronchospasm. Acute bronchospasm is usually relieved within 5 minutes by injected or inhaled epinephrine or inhaled isoproterenol. |
| b. When epinephrine is given in anaphylactic shock, observe for decreased tissue edema and improved breathing and circulation. | Epinephrine injection usually relieves laryngeal edema and bronchospasm within 5 minutes and lasts for approximately 20 minutes. |
| c. When isoproterenol or phenylephrine is given in hypotension and shock, observe for increased blood pressure, stronger pulse, and improved urine output, level of consciousness, and color. | These are indicators of improved circulation. |
| d. When a drug is given nasally for decongestant effects, observe for decreased nasal congestion and ability to breathe through the nose. | The drugs act as vasoconstrictors to reduce engorgement of nasal mucosa. |
| e. When given as eye drops for vasoconstrictor effects, observe for decreased redness. When giving for mydriatic effects, observe for pupil dilation. | |

*(continued)*

## Nursing Actions

## Adrenergic Drugs (Continued)

| Nursing Actions | Rationale/Explanation |
|---|---|
| 3. Observe for adverse effects. | Adverse effects depend to some extent on the reason for use. For example, cardiovascular effects are considered adverse reactions when the drugs are given for bronchodilation. Adverse effects occur with usual therapeutic doses and are more likely to occur with higher doses. |
| a. Cardiovascular effects—cardiac dysrhythmias, hypertension | Tachycardia and hypertension are common; if severe or prolonged, myocardial ischemia or heart failure may occur. Premature ventricular contractions and other serious dysrhythmias may occur. Propranolol (Inderal) or another beta blocker may be given to decrease heart rate and hypertension resulting from overdosage of adrenergic drugs. Phentolamine (Regitine) may be used to decrease severe hypertension. |
| b. Excessive central nervous system (CNS) stimulation—nervousness, anxiety, tremor, insomnia | These effects are more likely to occur with ephedrine or high doses of other adrenergic drugs. Sometimes, a sedative-type drug is given concomitantly to offset these effects. |
| c. Rebound nasal congestion, rhinitis, possible ulceration of nasal mucosa | These effects occur with excessive use of nasal decongestant drugs. |
| 4. Observe for drug interactions. | |
| a. Drugs that *increase* effects of adrenergic drugs: | Most of these drugs increase incidence or severity of adverse reactions. |
| (1) Anesthetics, general (eg, halothane) | Increased risk of cardiac dysrhythmias. Potentially hazardous. |
| (2) Anticholinergics (eg, atropine) | Increased bronchial relaxation. Also increased mydriasis and therefore contraindicated with narrow-angle glaucoma. |
| (3) Antidepressants, tricyclic (eg, amitriptyline [Elavil]) | Increased pressor response with intravenous epinephrine |
| (4) Antihistamines | May increase pressor effects |
| (5) Cocaine | Increases pressor and mydriatic effects by inhibiting uptake of norepinephrine by nerve endings. Cardiac dysrhythmias, convulsions, and acute glaucoma may occur. |
| (6) Digoxin | Sympathomimetics, especially beta-adrenergics like epinephrine and isoproterenol, increase the likelihood of cardiac dysrhythmias due to ectopic pacemaker activity. |
| (7) Doxapram (Dopram) | Increased pressor effect |
| (8) Ergot alkaloids | Increased vasoconstriction. Extremely high blood pressure may occur. There also may be decreased perfusion of fingers and toes. |
| (9) Monoamine oxidase (MAO) inhibitors (eg, isocarboxazid [Marplan]) | Contraindicated. The combination may cause death. When these drugs are given concurrently with adrenergic drugs, there is danger of cardiac dysrhythmias, respiratory depression, and acute hypertensive crisis with possible intracranial hemorrhage, convulsions, coma, and death. Effects of MAO inhibitors may not occur for several weeks after treatment is started and may last up to 3 weeks after the drug is stopped. Every client taking MAO inhibitors should be warned against taking any other medication without the advice of a physician or pharmacist. |
| (10) Methylphenidate (Ritalin) | Increased pressor and mydriatic effects. The combination may be hazardous in glaucoma. |
| (11) Thyroid preparations (eg, Synthroid) | Increased adrenergic effects, resulting in increased likelihood of dysrhythmias |

*(continued)*

## Nursing Actions

### Adrenergic Drugs (Continued)

| Nursing Actions | Rationale/Explanation |
|---|---|
| (12) Xanthines (in caffeine-containing substances, such as coffee, tea, cola drinks; theophylline) | Synergistic bronchodilating effect. Sympathomimetics with CNS-stimulating properties (eg, ephedrine, isoproterenol) may produce excessive CNS stimulation with cardiac dysrhythmias, emotional disturbances, and insomnia. |
| (13) Beta-adrenergic blocking agents (eg, propranolol [Inderal])<br>b. Drugs that *decrease* effects of adrenergics: | May augment hypertensive response to epinephrine (see also b[4] below) |
| (1) Anticholinesterases (eg, neostigmine [Prostigmin], pyridostigmine [Mestinon]) and other cholinergic drugs | Decrease mydriatic effects of adrenergics; thus, the two groups should not be given concurrently in ophthalmic conditions. |
| (2) Antihypertensives (eg, methyldopa) | Generally antagonize pressor effects of adrenergics, which act to increase blood pressure while antihypertensives act to lower it. |
| (3) Antipsychotic drugs (eg, haloperidol [Haldol]) | Block the vasopressor action of epinephrine. Therefore, epinephrine should not be used to treat hypotension induced by these drugs. |
| (4) Beta-adrenergic blocking agents (eg, propranolol [Inderal]) | Decrease bronchodilating effects of adrenergics and may exacerbate asthma. Contraindicated with asthma. |
| (5) Phentolamine (Regitine) | Antagonizes vasopressor effects of adrenergics |

### ? How Can You Avoid This Medication Error?

**Answer:** In this situation, the wrong dose of epinephrine, which could be lethal, is being administered to the patient. IV epinephrine must be diluted to a concentration of 1;10,000 (0.1 mg/mL). In an emergency situation, it is easy to pick up the concentration of epinephrine that is intended for intramuscular or subcutaneous use. Labeling on these preparations should include "Not for IV Use" because there is not time to calculate dosage and dilute the solution in an emergency.

### Critical Thinking Exercises

1. Epinephrine stimulates both alpha and beta receptors. At high doses, what effects predominate?
   a. Alpha-adrenergic effects
   b. Vasodilatory effects
   c. Beta-adrenergic effects
   d. Cardiac effects

2. The adrenergic drug of choice to treat acute anaphylactic reactions is:
   a. Epinephrine (Adrenalin)
   b. Isoproterenol (Isuprel)
   c. Pseudoephedrine (Sudafed)
   d. Terbutaline (Brethine)

3. To administer epinephrine subcutaneously, all of the following considerations are necessary, except:
   a. Using a tuberculin syringe
   b. Aspirating before injection
   c. Massaging the injection site after administering
   d. Using the Z-track method for administration

4. The adrenergic drug of choice to treat nasal congestion is:
   a. Epinephrine (Adrenalin)
   b. Isoproterenol (Isuprel)
   c. Pseudoephedrine (Sudafed)
   d. Ephedrine

5. The adrenergic drug of choice to aid in preterm labor inhibition is:
   a. Isoproterenol (Isuprel)
   b. Pseudoephedrine (Sudafed)
   c. Terbutaline (Brethine)
   d. Epinephrine (Adrenalin)

## SELECTED REFERENCES

American Heart Association. (2000). *Handbook of emergency cardiovascular care for health care providers.* (M. F. Hazinski, R. O. Cummins, & J. M. Field, Eds.). Dallas, TX: Author.

DiPiro, J. T., Ownsby, D. R., & Schlesselman, L. S. (2002). Allergic and pseudoallergic drug reactions. In J. T. DiPiro, R. L. Talbert, G. C. Yee, G. R. Matzke, B. G. Wells, & L. M.

Posey (Eds.), *Pharmacotherapy: A pathophysiologic approach* (5th ed., pp. 1585–1597). New York: McGraw-Hill.

*Drug facts and comparisons.* (Updated monthly). St. Louis: Facts and Comparisons.

Fetrow, C. W., & Avila, J. R. (2001). *Complementary and alternative medicines* (2nd ed.). Springhouse, PA: Springhouse Corp.

Hoffman, B. B. (2001). Catecholamines, sympathomimetic drugs, and adrenergic receptor antagonists. In J. G. Hardman & L. E. Limbird (Eds.), *Goodman and Gilman's the pharmacological basis of therapeutics* (10th ed., pp. 215–268). New York: McGraw-Hill.

Hoffman, B. B. (2001). Adrenoreceptor-activating and other sympathomimetic drugs. In B. G. Katzung (Ed.), *Basic and clinical pharmacology* (8th ed., pp. 120–137). New York: McGraw-Hill.

Hoffman, B. B., & Taylor, P. (2001). Neurotransmission: The autonomic and somatic motor nervous systems. In J. G. Hardman & L. E. Limbird (Eds.), *Goodman and Gilman's the*

*pharmacological basis of therapeutics* (10th ed., pp. 115–153). New York: McGraw-Hill.

Kelly, H. W., & Sorkness, C. A. (2002). Asthma. In J. T. DiPiro, R. L. Talbert, G. C. Yee, G. R. Matzke, B. G. Wells, & L. M. Posey (Eds.), *Pharmacotherapy: A pathophysiologic approach* (5th ed., pp. 475–510). New York: McGraw-Hill.

Kuhn, M. A. (1999). *Complementary therapies for health care providers* (pp. 22–23). Philadelphia: Lippincott Williams & Wilkins.

Lacy, C. F., Armstrong, L. L., Goldman, M. P., & Lance, L. L. (2003). *Lexi-Comp's drug information handbook* (11th ed.). Hudson, OH: American Pharmaceutical Association.

Olson, K. R. (Ed.). (1999). *Poisoning and drug overdose* (3rd ed.). Stamford, CT: Appleton & Lange.

Piano, M. R., & Huether, S. E. (2002). Mechanisms of hormonal regulation. In K. L. McCance & S. E. Huether (Eds.), *Pathophysiology: The biologic basis for disease in adults and children* (4th ed., pp. 597–623). St. Louis: Mosby.

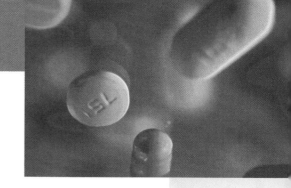

# 17

# Antiadrenergic Drugs

## OBJECTIVES

*After studying this chapter, the student will be able to:*

1 List characteristics of antiadrenergic drugs in terms of effects on body tissues, indications for use, nursing process implications, and observation of client response.

2 Discuss alpha$_1$-adrenergic blocking agents and alpha$_2$-adrenergic agonists in terms of indications for use, adverse effects, and selected other characteristics.

3 Compare and contrast beta-adrenergic blocking agents in terms of cardioselectivity, indications for use, adverse effects, and selected other characteristics.

4 Teach clients about safe, effective use of antiadrenergic drugs.

5 Discuss the nursing process for using antiadrenergic drugs in special populations.

## CRITICAL THINKING SCENARIO

Gary Griffith, 56 years of age, comes to the clinic complaining of chest pain with exertion. His vital signs are as follows: blood pressure, 194/88 mm Hg; pulse, 92 beats/minute; and respirations, 18 breaths/minute. His primary provider prescribes a selective beta-blocker, atenolol (Tenormin), and schedules a follow-up visit in 2 weeks.

✔ Why is a beta-blocker ordered for Mr. Griffith?

✔ What are the advantages of using a selective rather that a nonselective beta-blocker?

✔ What side effects are likely when a client is started on atenolol?

✔ Describe a teaching plan for Mr. Griffith.

## PROTOTYPE PROFILES

**prazosin** (Minipress), p. 290

**propranolol** (Inderal), Chap. 41, p. 759

## DESCRIPTION

Antiadrenergic or sympatholytic drugs decrease or block the effects of sympathetic nerve stimulation, endogenous catecholamines (eg, epinephrine), and adrenergic drugs. The drugs are chemically diverse and have a wide spectrum of pharmacologic activity, with specific effects depending mainly on the client's health status when a drug is given and the drug's binding with particular adrenergic receptors. Included here are clonidine and related centrally active antiadrenergic drugs, which are used primarily in the treatment of hypertension, and peripherally active agents (alpha- and beta-adrenergic blocking agents), which are used to treat various cardiovascular and other disorders. A few uncommonly used antiadrenergic drugs for hypertension are included in Chapter 43.

A basal level of sympathetic tone is necessary to maintain normal body functioning, including regulation of blood pressure, blood glucose, and stress response. Therefore, the goal of antiadrenergic drug therapy is to suppress pathologic stimulation, not the normal, physiologic response to activity, stress, and other stimuli. The consequences of sympathetic nervous system function on the body are outlined in At the Foundation: Sympathetic Nervous System Effects.

Antiadrenergic drugs are commonly used in the home setting, mainly to treat chronic disorders. Most clients probably take these medications for hypertension. However, some older men with benign prostatic hyperplasia (BPH) take one of these drugs to aid urinary elimination. Guidelines for strategies for ongoing evaluation and intervention in the home and with children and older adults are addressed in Home Care Considerations and Age-related Considerations, respectively.

## Mechanisms of Action and Effects

Antiadrenergic effects can occur either when alpha$_1$ receptors are blocked by adrenergic antagonists or when agonist drugs stimulate presynaptic alpha$_2$ receptors. Most antiadrenergic drugs have *antagonist* (blocking) *effects* in which they combine with alpha$_1$, beta$_1$, beta$_2$, or a combination of receptors in peripheral tissues and prevent adrenergic (sympathomimetic) effects. Clonidine and related drugs have *agonist effects* at presynaptic alpha$_2$ receptors in the brain. This means that some of the norepinephrine released by the presynaptic nerve cell into the synapse returns to the presynaptic site and activates alpha$_2$ receptors. This results in a negative feedback type of mechanism that decreases the release of additional norepinephrine. Thus, the overall effect is decreased sympathetic outflow from the brain and antiadrenergic effects on peripheral tissues (ie, decreased activation of alpha and beta receptors by norepinephrine throughout the body).

### Alpha–Adrenergic Agonists and Blocking Agents

*Alpha$_2$-adrenergic agonists* inhibit the release of norepinephrine in the brain, thereby decreasing the effects of sympathetic nervous system stimulation throughout the body. A major clinical effect is decreased blood pressure. Although clinical effects are attributed mainly to drug action at presynaptic alpha$_2$ receptors in the brain, post-

---

**AT THE FOUNDATION:** *Sympathetic Nervous System Effects*

The SNS is stimulated by physical or emotional stress, such as strenuous exercise or work, pain, hemorrhage, intense emotions, and temperature extremes. Increased capacity for vigorous muscle activity in response to a perceived threat, whether real or imaginary, is often called the *fight-or-flight* reaction. Specific body responses include the following:

• Increased arterial blood pressure and cardiac output
• Increased blood flow to the brain, heart, and skeletal muscles; decreased blood flow to viscera, skin, and other organs not needed for fight-or-flight response
• Increased rate of cellular metabolism—increased oxygen consumption and carbon dioxide production
• Increased breakdown of muscle glycogen for energy
• Increased blood sugar
• Increased mental activity and ability to think clearly
• Increased muscle strength
• Increased rate of blood coagulation
• Increased rate and depth of respiration
• Pupil dilation to aid vision

• Increased sweating. (Note that acetylcholine is the neurotransmitter for this sympathetic response. This is a deviation from the normal postganglionic neurotransmitter, which is norepinephrine.)

These responses are protective mechanisms designed to help the person cope with the stress or get away from it. The intensity and duration of responses depend on the amounts of norepinephrine and epinephrine secreted into the bloodstream by the adrenal medullae and transported to body tissues. Conversely, the amount of hormone present varies according to the degree of stress present and the ability of the adrenal medullae to respond to stimuli. The larger proportion of the circulating hormones (approximately 80%) is epinephrine. These catecholamines exert the same effects as those caused by direct stimulation of the SNS. However, the effects last longer because the hormones are removed from the blood more slowly. These hormones are metabolized mainly in the liver by the enzymes monoamine oxidase and catechol-*O*-methyltransferase.

## Home Care Considerations: Use of Antiadrenergic Drugs

**ASSESS:** for therapeutic and adverse drug effects, the reason for use, and client's ability to monitor for drug effects.

**MONITOR:** for alterations in blood sugar control, especially increased episodes of hypoglycemia if a client has diabetes mellitus; if wheezing respirations (indicating broncho-constriction) develop in a client taking a nonselective beta-blocker, consult the prescribing health care provider.

**EDUCATE:** client or other in the household to count and record the radial pulse daily, preferably about the same time interval before or after taking a beta-blocker; regarding ways to avoid orthostatic hypotension while talking alpha₁-adrenergic blocking agents. The home care nurse may need to teach the clients who have hypertension to avoid over-the-counter (OTC) asthma and cold remedies, decongestants, and appetite suppressants, and herbal preparations such as ma huang, black cohosh, and St. John's wort because these drugs act to increase blood pressure and may reduce the benefits of antiadrenergic medications. In addition, OTC analgesics such as ibuprofen, ketoprofen, and naproxen may raise blood pressure by causing retention of sodium and water.

synaptic alpha₂ receptors in the brain and peripheral tissues (eg, vascular smooth muscle) may also be involved. Activation of alpha₂ receptors in the pancreatic islets suppresses insulin secretion.

*Alpha₁-adrenergic blocking agents* occupy alpha₁-adrenergic receptor sites in smooth muscles and glands innervated by sympathetic nerve fibers. These drugs act primarily in the skin, mucosa, intestines, lungs, and kidneys to prevent alpha-mediated vasoconstriction. Specific effects include dilation of arterioles and veins, increased local blood flow, decreased blood pressure, constriction of pupils, and increased motility of the gastrointestinal tract. Alpha-adrenergic antagonists may activate reflexes that oppose the fall in blood pressure by increasing heart rate and cardiac output and causing fluid retention.

The drugs also can prevent alpha-mediated contraction of smooth muscle in nonvascular tissues. For example, BPH is characterized by obstructed urine flow because the enlarged prostate gland presses on the urethra. Alpha-blocking agents can decrease urinary retention and improve urine flow by inhibiting contraction of muscles in the prostate and urinary bladder.

*Nonselective alpha-adrenergic blocking agents* occupy peripheral alpha₁ receptors to cause vasodilation and

## Age-related Considerations: Use of Antiadrenergic Drugs

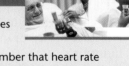

### USE IN CHILDREN

Most alpha-adrenergic agonists and blocking agents have not been established as safe and effective in children. Tolazoline (Priscoline), however, is an alpha-blocker that is useful in the treatment of persistent pulmonary hypertension of the newborn. The vasodilatory effects reduce pulmonary pressure and decrease the workload of the right ventricle. Vital signs should be carefully monitored because hypotension or hypertension, tachycardia, and dysrhythmias may occur. Ephedrine should be used in the treatment of hypotension, should it occur, rather than epinephrine or norepinephrine. The child should also be monitored for peptic ulcer formation. Prophylaxis against stress ulcers should be considered.

Beta-adrenergic blocking agents are used in children for disorders similar to those occurring in adults. However, safety and effectiveness have not been established, and manufacturers of most of the drugs do not recommend pediatric use or doses. The drugs are probably contraindicated in young children with resting heart rates below 60 beats/minute.

When a beta-blocker is given, general guidelines include the following:

1. Dosage should be adjusted for body weight.
2. Monitor responses closely. Children are more sensitive to adverse drug effects than adults.
3. If given to infants (up to 1 year of age) with immature liver function, blood levels may be higher, and accumu-

lation is more likely even when doses are based on weight.

4. When monitoring responses, remember that heart rate and blood pressure vary among children according to age and level of growth and development. They also differ from those of adults.
5. Children are more likely to have asthma than adults. Thus, they may be at greater risk for drug-induced bronchoconstriction.

Propranolol is probably the most frequently used beta-blocker in children. Intravenous administration is not recommended. The drug is given orally for hypertension, and dosage should be individualized. The usual dosage range is 2 to 4 mg/kg in two equal doses. Dosage calculated from body surface area is not recommended because of excessive blood levels of drug and greater risk of toxicity. As with adults, dosage should be tapered gradually over 1 to 3 weeks. The drug should not be stopped abruptly.

### USE IN OLDER ADULTS

Alpha₂-adrenergic agonists (clonidine and related drugs) may be used to treat hypertension in older adults; alpha₁-adrenergic antagonists (prazosin and related drugs) may be used to treat hypertension and benign prostatic hyperplasia. Dosage of these drugs should be reduced because older adults are more likely to experience adverse drug effects, especially with impaired renal or hepatic function.

*(continued)*

## Age-related Considerations: Use of Antiadrenergic Drugs (Continued)

As with other populations, these drugs should not be stopped suddenly. Instead, they should be tapered in dosage and discontinued gradually, over 1 to 2 weeks.

Beta-adrenergic blocking agents are commonly used in older adults for angina, dysrhythmias, hypertension, and glaucoma. With hypertension, beta-blockers are not recommended for monotherapy because older adults may be less responsive than younger adults. Thus, the drugs are probably most useful as second drugs (with diuretics) in clients who require multidrug therapy and in clients who also have angina pectoris or another disorder for which a beta-blocker is indicated.

Whatever the circumstances for using beta-blockers in older adults, use them cautiously and monitor responses closely. Older adults are likely to have disorders that place them at high risk for adverse drug effects, such as heart failure and other cardiovascular conditions, renal or hepatic impairment, and chronic pulmonary disease. Thus, they may experience bradycardia, bronchoconstriction, and hypotension to a greater degree than younger adults. Dosage usually should be reduced because of decreased hepatic blood flow and subsequent slowing of drug metabolism. As with administration in other populations, beta-blockers should be tapered in dosage and discontinued over 1 to 3 weeks to avoid myocardial ischemia and other potentially serious adverse cardiovascular effects.

---

alpha$_2$ receptors to cause cardiac stimulation. Consequently, decreased blood pressure is accompanied by tachycardia and perhaps other dysrhythmias.

### Beta-Adrenergic Blocking Drugs

*Beta-adrenergic blocking agents* occupy beta-adrenergic receptor sites and prevent the receptors from responding to sympathetic nerve impulses, circulating catecholamines, and beta-adrenergic drugs (see Figure 17-1). Specific effects include the following:

- Decreased heart rate (negative chronotropy)
- Decreased force of myocardial contraction (negative inotropy)
- Decreased cardiac output at rest and with exercise
- Slowed conduction through the atrioventricular (AV) node (negative dromotropy)
- Decreased automaticity of ectopic pacemakers
- Decreased renin secretion from the kidney
- Decreased blood pressure in supine and standing positions. This effect occurs primarily in people with hypertension.
- Bronchoconstriction from blockade of beta$_2$ receptors in bronchial smooth muscle. This effect occurs primarily in people with asthma or other chronic lung diseases.
- Less effective metabolism of glucose (decreased glycogenolysis) when needed by the body, especially in people taking beta-blocking agents along with antidiabetic drugs. These clients may experience more severe and prolonged hypoglycemia. In addition, early symptoms of hypoglycemia (eg, tachycardia) may be blocked, delaying recognition of the hypoglycemia.
- Decreased production of aqueous humor in the eye
- Chronic use of beta-blockers is associated with increased very–low-density lipoprotein (VLDL) and decreased high-density lipoprotein (HDL) cholesterol. These changes pose a potential risk for clients with cardiovascular disease.
- Diminished portal vein pressure in clients with cirrhosis

## Indications for Use

### Alpha–Adrenergic Agonists and Blocking Agents

Alpha$_2$ agonists are used in the treatment of hypertension. Clonidine, administered by the epidural route, is also approved for the relief of severe pain in cancer clients. Investigational uses of clonidine include treatment of alcohol withdrawal and opioid dependence, drug-induced akathisia, tic disorders, postmenopausal hot flashes, adjunct medication during anesthesia,

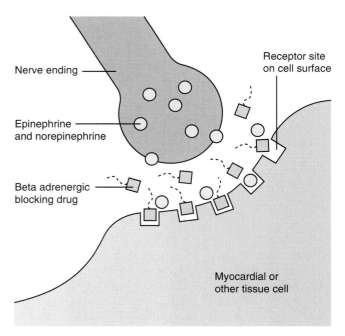

FIGURE 17–1 Beta-adrenergic blocking agents prevent epinephrine and norepinephrine from occupying receptor sites on cell membranes. This action alters cell functions normally stimulated by epinephrine and norepinephrine, according to the number of receptor sites occupied by the beta-blocking drugs. (Adapted by J. Harley from *Encyclopedia Britannica Medical and Health Annual.* [1983]. Chicago, Encyclopedia Britannica.)

migraines, and attention deficit-hyperactivity disorder. Clonidine has not received approval by the U.S. Food and Drug Administration (FDA) for these purposes.

Alpha$_1$-adrenergic blocking agents are used in the treatment of hypertension, BPH, vasospastic disorders, and persistent pulmonary hypertension in the newborn. Nonselective alpha-blocking agents are not used as antihypertensive drugs except in hypertension caused by excessive catecholamines. Excessive catecholamines may result from overdosage of adrenergic drugs or from pheochromocytoma, a rare tumor of the adrenal medulla that secretes epinephrine and norepinephrine and causes hypertension, tachycardia, and cardiac dysrhythmias. Although the treatment of choice for pheochromocytoma is surgical excision, alpha-adrenergic blocking drugs are useful adjuncts. They are given before and during surgery, usually in conjunction with beta-blockers. Nonselective alpha-blockers also are used in vascular diseases characterized by vasospasm, such as Raynaud's disease and frostbite, in which they improve blood flow. Phentolamine (Regitine) also can be used to prevent tissue necrosis from extravasation of potent vasoconstrictors (eg, norepinephrine, dopamine) into subcutaneous tissues.

### Beta–Adrenergic Blocking Drugs

Clinical indications for use of beta-blocking agents are mainly cardiovascular disorders (ie, angina pectoris, cardiac tachydysrhythmias, hypertension, myocardial infarction [MI], heart failure, and glaucoma).

In angina, beta-blockers decrease myocardial contractility, cardiac output, heart rate, and blood pressure. These effects decrease myocardial oxygen demand (cardiac workload), especially in response to activity, exercise, and stress. In dysrhythmias, drug effects depend on the sympathetic tone of the heart (ie, the degree of adrenergic stimulation of the heart that the drug must block or overcome). The drugs slow the sinus rate and prolong conduction through the AV node, thereby slowing the ventricular response rate to supraventricular tachydysrhythmias.

In hypertension, the actions by which the drugs lower blood pressure are unclear. Possible mechanisms include reduced cardiac output, inhibition of renin, and inhibition of sympathetic nervous system stimulation in the brain. However, the drugs effective in hypertension do not consistently demonstrate these effects—in other words, a drug may lower blood pressure without reducing cardiac output or inhibiting renin, for example. After MI, the drugs help protect the heart from reinfarction and decrease mortality rates over several years. A possible mechanism is preventing or decreasing the incidence of catecholamine-induced dysrhythmias. In heart failure (HF), beta-blockers have a limited role and require careful monitoring on the part of the prescriber and the nurse. Administration of beta-blockers may acutely worsen the condition of persons with HF by blocking the sympathetic stimulation that helps to maintain cardiac output. However, in selected clients who are able to tolerate the effects of beta-blockers, the drugs are beneficial. For these clients, beta-blockers decrease the risk for sudden cardiac death and may reduce ventricular

remodeling that accompanies HF and leads to further deterioration of cardiac function.

In glaucoma, the drugs reduce intraocular pressure by binding to beta-adrenergic receptors in the ciliary body of the eye and decreasing formation of aqueous humor.

**P Propranolol** (Inderal) is the prototype of beta-adrenergic blocking agents (see Prototype Profile 41-1: Propranolol, Chap. 41). It is also the oldest and most extensively studied beta-blocker. In addition to its use in the treatment of hypertension, dysrhythmias, angina pectoris, and MI, propranolol is used to treat a wide variety of other conditions. In hypertrophic obstructive cardiomyopathy, it is used to improve exercise tolerance by increasing stroke volume. In pheochromocytoma, it is used in conjunction with an alpha-blocking agent to counter the effect of excessive catecholamine secretion, preventing tachycardia and dysrhythmias. Propranolol is useful in treating dissecting aortic aneurysms by decreasing systolic blood pressure. Propranolol decreases heart rate, cardiac output, and tremor in clients with hyperthyroidism. It is also useful, by an unknown mechanism, for the prevention of migraine headaches. Propranolol is not helpful in acute attacks of migraine headaches. The drug also relieves palpitation and tremor associated with anxiety and stage fright, but it is not approved for clinical use as an antianxiety drug. Some clients experiencing alcohol withdrawal may also benefit from the administration of propranolol.

In cirrhosis of the liver, research indicates that propranolol may decrease the incidence of the initial episode of bleeding esophageal varices, prevent rebleeding episodes, and decrease the mortality rate due to hemorrhage.

## Contraindications to Use

Alpha$_2$ agonists are contraindicated in clients with hypersensitivity to the drugs, and methyldopa is also contraindicated in clients with active liver disease. Alpha-adrenergic blocking agents are contraindicated in angina pectoris, MI, and stroke. Beta-adrenergic blocking agents are contraindicated in bradycardia, heart block, and asthma and other allergic or pulmonary conditions characterized by bronchoconstriction. Although new research has shown that beta-blockers can be beneficial to selected clients with mild to moderate chronic heart failure, the drugs have not been proved safe for people older than 80 years of age or those with severe heart failure.

## ■ INDIVIDUAL ANTIADRENERGIC DRUGS

These drugs are described in the following sections. Trade names, clinical indications, and dosage ranges are listed in Drugs at a Glance 17-1: Antiadrenergics: Alpha-Adrenergic Agonists and Blocking Agents, and Drugs at a Glance 17-2: Antiadrenergics: Beta-Blocking Agents.

*(text continues on page 289)*

**DRUG TABLE 17-1**

*Drugs at a Glance*

## Antiadrenergics: Alpha-Adrenergic Agonists and Blocking Agents

| Generic/Trade Name | Routes and Dosage Ranges | Comments |
|---|---|---|
| **Alpha₂-Agonists** | | |
| **Clonidine** (Catapres)<br>Pregnancy Category C | *Adults:* PO, 0.1 mg 2 times daily initially, gradually increased if necessary. Average maintenance dose, 0.2–0.8 mg/d. Transdermal 0.1-mg patch every 7 d initially; increase every 7–14 d to 0.2 mg or 0.3 mg if necessary. Maximum dose, two 0.3-mg patches every 7 d | Treatment of hypertension |
| **Guanabenz** (Wytensin)<br>Pregnancy Category C | *Adults:* PO, 4 mg twice daily, increased by 4–8 mg/d every 1–2 wk if necessary to a maximal dose of 32 mg twice daily | Treatment of hypertension |
| **Guanfacine** (Tenex)<br>Pregnancy Category B | *Adults:* PO, 1 mg daily at bedtime, increased to 2 mg after 3–4 wk, then to 3 mg if necessary. | Treatment of hypertension |
| **Methyldopa** (Aldomet)<br>Pregnancy Category B | *Adults:* PO, 250 mg 2 or 3 times daily initially, increased gradually at intervals of not less than 2 d until blood pressure is controlled or a daily dose of 3 g is reached<br>*Children:* PO, 10 mg/kg/d in 2 to 4 divided doses initially, increased or decreased according to response. Maximal dose, 65 mg/kg/d or 3 g daily, whichever is less | Treatment of hypertension |
| **Alpha₁-Blocking Agents** | | |
| **Doxazosin** (Cardura)<br>Pregnancy Category C | *Adults:* PO, 1 mg once daily initially, increased to 2 mg, then to 4, 8, and 16 mg if necessary | Treatment of hypertension<br>Management of BPH |
| **Prazosin** (Minipress) | See Prototype Profile 17-1: Prazosin | |
| **Tamsulosin** (Flomax)<br>Pregnancy Category B | *Adults:* PO, 0.4 mg/d after same meal each day. Dose may be increased if needed after 2–4 wk trial period | Management of BPH |
| **Terazosin** (Hytrin)<br>Pregnancy Category C | *Adults:* PO, 1 mg at bedtime initially, increased gradually to maintenance dose, usually 1–5 mg once daily | Treatment of hypertension<br>Management of BPH |
| **Tolazoline HCl** (Priscoline)<br>Pregnancy Category C | *Adults:* (Sub-Q, IM, IV) 10–50 mg q 6 h | Treatment of vasospastic disorders |
| **Nonselective Alpha-Blocking Agents** | | |
| **Phenoxybenzamine** (Dibenzyline)<br>Pregnancy Category C | *Adults:* PO, 10 mg daily initially, gradually increased by 10 mg every 4 d until therapeutic effects are obtained or adverse effects become intolerable; optimum dosage level usually reached in 2 wk; usual maintenance dose 20–60 mg/d | Hypertension caused by pheochromocytoma<br>Raynaud's disorder<br>Frostbite |

*(continued)*

## *Drugs at a Glance*

**DRUG TABLE 17-1**

### Antiadrenergics: Alpha-Adrenergic Agonists and Blocking Agents (Continued)

| Generic/Trade Name | Routes and Dosage Ranges | Comments/Uses |
|---|---|---|
| **Phentolamine** (Regitine) <br> Pregnancy Category C | *Before and during surgery for pheochromocytoma:* IV, IM, 5–20 mg as needed to control blood pressure <br> *Prevention of tissue necrosis:* IV, 10 mg in each liter of IV solution containing a potent vasoconstrictor <br> *Treatment of extravasation:* Sub-Q 5–10 mg in 10 mL saline, infiltrated into the area within 12 h | Hypertension caused by pheochromocytoma <br><br> Prevention of tissue necrosis from extravasation of vasoconstrictive drugs |

BPH, benign prostatic hyperplasia.

## *Drugs at a Glance*

**DRUG TABLE 17-2**

### Antiadrenergics: Beta-Blocking Agents

| Generic/Trade Name | Routes and Dosage Ranges | Comments/Uses |
|---|---|---|
| *Nonselective Blocking Agents* | | |
| **Carteolol** (Cartrol, Ocupress) <br> Pregnancy Category C by manufacturer; D second and third trimesters by expert analysis | *Adults:* PO, Initially, 2.5 mg once daily, gradually increased to a maximum daily dose of 10 mg if necessary. Usual maintenance dose, 2.5–5 mg once daily <br> Extend dosage interval to 48 h for a creatinine clearance of 20–60 mL/min and to 72 h for a creatinine clearance below 20 mL/min | Treatment of hypertension |
| **Levobunolol** (Betagan) <br> Pregnancy Category C | Topically to affected eye, 1 drop twice daily | Management of glaucoma |
| **Metipranolol** (OptiPranolol) <br> Pregnancy Category C | Topically to each eye, 1 drop once or twice daily | Management of glaucoma |
| **Penbutolol** (Levatol) <br> Pregnancy Category C | *Adults:* PO, 20 mg once daily | Treatment of hypertension |
| **Propranolol** (Inderal) | See Prototype Profile 41-1: Propranolol | |
| **Nadolol** (Corgard) <br> Pregnancy Category C | *Adults:* PO, 40 mg once daily initially, gradually increased. Usual daily maintenance dose, 80–320 mg <br> PO, 40 mg once daily initially, increased by 40–80 mg at 3- to 7-d intervals. Usual daily maintenance dose, 80–240 mg | Treatment of hypertension <br><br> Management of angina pectoris |
| **Pindolol** (Visken) <br> Pregnancy Category B | *Adults:* PO, 5 mg twice daily initially, increased by 10 mg every 3–4 wk, to a maximal daily dose of 60 mg if necessary | Treatment of hypertension |

*(continued)*

**DRUG TABLE 17-2**

*Drugs at a Glance*

## Antiadrenergics: Beta-Blocking Agents (Continued)

| Generic/Trade Name | Routes and Dosage Ranges | Comments/Uses |
|---|---|---|
| **Sotalol** (Betapace) Pregnancy Category B | *Adults:* PO, 80–160 mg twice daily | Management of cardiac dysrhythmias |
| **Timolol** (Blocadren, Timoptic) Pregnancy Category C by manufacturer; D second and third trimesters by expert analysis | *Adults:* PO, 10 mg twice daily initially, increased at 7-d intervals to a maximum of 60 mg/d in 2 divided doses; usual maintenance dose, 20–40 mg daily | Treatment of hypertension |
| | PO, 10 mg twice daily | Myocardial infarction |
| | Topically to eye, 1 drop of 0.25% or 0.5% solution (Timoptic) in each eye twice daily | Management of glaucoma |
| ***Cardioselective Blocking Agents*** | | |
| **Acebutolol** (Sectral) Pregnancy Category B by manufacturer; D second and third trimesters by expert analysis | *Adults:* PO, 400 mg daily in 1 or 2 doses; usual maintenance dose, 400–800 mg daily | Management of hypertension |
| | PO, 400 mg daily in 2 divided doses; usual maintenance dose, 600–1200 mg daily | Treatment of ventricular dysrhythmias |
| **Atenolol** (Tenormin) Pregnancy Category D | *Adults:* PO, 50–100 mg daily | Management of hypertension |
| | PO, 50–100 mg daily, increased to 200 mg daily if necessary | Management of angina pectoris |
| | IV, 5 mg over 5 min, then 5 mg 10 min later, then 50 mg PO 10 min later, then 50 mg 12 h later. Thereafter, PO, 100 mg daily, in 1 or 2 doses, for 6–9 d or until discharge from hospital | Management of myocardial infarction |
| **Betaxolol** (Betoptic, Kerlone) Pregnancy Category C by manufacturer; D second and third trimesters by expert analysis | Topically to each eye, 1 drop twice daily | Treatment of glaucoma |
| | PO, 10–20 mg daily | Management of hypertension |
| **Bisoprolol** (Zebeta) Pregnancy Category C by manufacturer; D second and third trimesters by expert analysis | *Adults:* PO, 5–20 mg once daily | Management of hypertension |
| **Esmolol** (Brevibloc) Pregnancy Category C by manufacturer; D second and third trimesters by expert analysis | *Adults:* IV, 50–200 mcg/kg per minute; average dose, 100 mcg/kg per minute, titrated to effect with close monitoring of client's condition | Treatment of supraventricular tachydysrhythmias |
| **Metoprolol** (Lopressor) Pregnancy Category C by manufacturer; D second and third trimesters by expert analysis | *Adults:* PO, 100 mg daily in single or divided doses, increased at 7-d or longer intervals; usual maintenance dose, 100–450 mg/d | Management of hypertension |
| | *Early treatment of MI:* IV, 5 mg every 2 min for total of 3 doses (15 mg), then 50 mg PO q6h for 48 h, then 100 mg PO twice daily. | Used with myocardial infarction (MI) |
| | *Late treatment of MI:* PO, 100 mg twice daily, at least 3 months, up to 1–3 y | |

*(continued)*

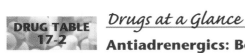

## Drugs at a Glance

**DRUG TABLE 17-2**

### Antiadrenergics: Beta-Blocking Agents (Continued)

| Generic/Trade Name | Routes and Dosage Ranges | Comments/Uses |
|---|---|---|
| *Alpha- and Beta-Blocking Agents* | | |
| **Carvedilol** (Coreg)<br>Pregnancy Category C by manufacturer; D second and third trimesters by expert analysis | *Adults:* PO, 6.25 mg twice daily for 7–14 d, then increase to 12.5 mg twice daily if necessary for 7–14 d, then increase to 25 mg twice daily if necessary (maximum dose) | Management of hypertension |
| **Labetalol** (Trandate, Normodyne)<br>Pregnancy Category C by manufacturer; D second and third trimesters by expert analysis | *Adults:* PO, 100 mg twice daily<br>IV, 20 mg over 2 min, then 40–80 mg every 10 min until desired blood pressure achieved or 300 mg given<br>IV infusion, 2 mg/min (eg, add 200 mg of drug to 250 mL 5% dextrose solution for a 2 mg/3 mL concentration) | Used for hypertension, including hypertensive emergencies |

## Alpha–Adrenergic Agonists and Blocking Agents

Alpha$_2$-adrenergic agonists include clonidine, guanabenz, guanfacine, and methyldopa. These drugs produce similar therapeutic and adverse effects but differ in their pharmacokinetics and frequency of administration. Oral **clonidine** reduces blood pressure within 1 hour, reaches peak plasma levels in 3 to 5 hours, and has a plasma half-life of approximately 12 to 16 hours (longer with renal impairment). Approximately half the oral dose is metabolized in the liver; the remainder is excreted unchanged in urine. With transdermal clonidine, therapeutic plasma levels are reached in 2 to 3 days and last 1 week. **Guanabenz** action occurs within 1 hour, peaks within 2 to 4 hours, and lasts 6 to 8 hours. It is metabolized extensively; very little unchanged drug is excreted in urine. **Guanfacine** is well absorbed and widely distributed, with approximately 70% bound to plasma proteins. Peak plasma levels occur in 1 to 4 hours, and the half-life is 10 to 30 hours. Approximately half is metabolized, and the metabolites and unchanged drug are excreted in urine. Because of its longer half-life, guanfacine can be given once daily. **Methyldopa** is an older drug with low to moderate absorption, peak plasma levels in 2 to 4 hours, and peak antihypertensive effects in approximately 2 days. When discontinued, blood pressure rises in approximately 2 days. Intravenous administration reduces blood pressure in 4 to 6 hours and lasts 10 to 16 hours. Methyldopa is metabolized to some extent in the liver but is largely excreted in urine. In clients with renal impairment, blood pressure–lowering effects may be pronounced and prolonged because of slower excretion. In addition to the adverse effects that occur with all these drugs, methyldopa also may cause hemolytic anemia and hepatotoxicity (eg, jaundice, hepatitis).

Alpha$_1$-adrenergic antagonists include doxazosin, prazosin, terazosin, tamsulosin, and tolazoline. **P** **Prazosin**, the prototype, is well absorbed after oral administration and reaches peak plasma concentrations in 1 to 3 hours; action lasts approximately 4 to 6 hours (see Prototype Profile 17-1). The drug is highly bound to plasma proteins, and the plasma half-life is approximately 2 to 3 hours. It is extensively metabolized in the liver, and its metabolites are excreted by the kidneys. **Doxazosin** and **terazosin** are similar to prazosin but have longer half-lives (doxazosin, 10 to 20 hours; terazosin, approximately 12 hours) and durations of action (doxazosin, up to 36 hours; terazosin, 18 hours or longer). Prazosin must be taken in multiple doses; doxazosin and terazosin may usually be taken once daily to control hypertension.

**Tamsulosin** is the first alpha$_1$ antagonist designed specifically to treat BPH. It blocks alpha$_1$ receptors in the male genitourinary system, producing smooth muscle relaxation in the prostate gland and bladder neck. Urinary flow rate is improved, and symptoms of BPH are reduced. Because of the specificity of tamsulosin for receptors in the genitourinary system, this drug causes less orthostatic hypotension than other alpha$_1$ antagonists. After oral administration, greater than 90% of tamsulosin is absorbed. Administration with food decreases bioavailability by 30%. Tamsulosin is highly protein bound and is metabolized by the liver; approximately 10% of the drug is excreted unchanged in the urine. An advantage of tamsulosin is the ability to start the drug at the recommended dosage. Most of the alpha$_1$ antagonists must be gradually increased to the recommended dosage. Common side effects include abnormal ejaculation and dizziness.

**Tolazoline** produces vasodilation in peripheral vessels as well as the pulmonary artery. It is used primarily to treat vasospastic disorders in adults and persistent pul-

**PROTOTYPE PROFILE 17-1**

**ⓟ Prazosin** (PRA zoe sin)

**Drug Class**
*Chemical:* Alpha-adrenergic blocking agent
*Functional:* Antihypertensive

**Trade Name**
Minipress

**Therapeutic Indications**
Treatment of hypertension (can benefit males with benign prostatic hypertrophy but not an FDA approved use)

**Pharmacokinetics**
*Absorption*
PO: 60%

*Distribution*
Widely distributed

*Metabolism*
Extensive hepatic

*Excretion*
Bile (90%), Renal (10%)

**Pharmacodynamics**
*Onset of Action*
2 h

*Duration*
10 h

**Contraindications/Precautions**
Hypersensitivity, with caution with angina pectoris, renal sufficiency, pregnancy, lactation, or in children

**Pregnancy Considerations**
Category C
Excretion in breast milk unknown; use with caution

**Dosage**
*Adults:* PO, 1 mg 2 to 3 times daily initially, increased if necessary to a total daily dose of 20 mg in divided doses
Average maintenance dose, 6–15 mg/d

**Adverse Effects**
Marked "first dose phenomenon" (orthostatic hypotension, syncope, loss of consciousness with first dose), dizziness, palpitations, headache, drowsiness, inhibition of ejaculation, nasal congestion, decreased energy, and dry mouth

**Drug Interactions**
*Increased Effects*
Enhanced hypotension with beta-blockers, angiotensin-converting enzyme inhibitors, calcium channel blockers, nitrates, diuretics, or other anti-hypertensive medications
Increased risk for orthostasis with tricyclic antidepressants, low potency antipsychotics, alcohol

*Decreased Effects*
Antihypertensive effect with nonsteroidal anti-inflammatory drugs

**Herbal Supplements and Dietary Considerations**
Ma huang, black cohosh, and St. John's wort increase blood pressure and may reduce the benefits of anti-adrenergic medications

---

monary hypertension in newborns. The vasodilation effect in the pulmonary artery may be pH dependent because it is decreased in the presence of acidosis. Tolazoline is excreted in the urine, and dosages should be modified in the presence of renal impairment. Tolazoline should not be used concurrently with ethanol because a disulfiram-like reaction may occur.

Nonselective alpha-adrenergic blocking agents include phenoxybenzamine and phentolamine. **Phenoxybenzamine** (Dibenzyline) is long acting; the effects of a single dose persist for 3 to 4 days. **Phentolamine** (Regitine) is similar to phenoxybenzamine but more useful clinically. Phentolamine is short acting; effects last only a few hours and can be reversed by an alpha-adrenergic stimulant drug, such as norepinephrine (Levophed).

## Beta–Adrenergic Blocking Drugs

Numerous beta-blocking agents are marketed in the United States. Although they produce similar effects,

they differ in several characteristics, including clinical indications for use, receptor selectivity, intrinsic sympathomimetic activity, membrane-stabilizing ability, lipid solubility, routes of excretion, routes of administration, and duration of action.

### Clinical Indications

Most beta-blockers are approved for the treatment of hypertension. A beta-blocker may be used alone or with another antihypertensive drug, such as a diuretic. Labetalol is also approved for treatment of hypertensive emergencies. Atenolol, metoprolol, nadolol, and propranolol are approved as antianginal agents; acebutolol, esmolol, propranolol, and sotalol are approved as antidysrhythmic agents. Atenolol, metoprolol, propranolol, and timolol are used to prevent MI or reinfarction. Betaxolol, carteolol, and timolol are used for hypertension and glaucoma; levobunolol and metipranolol are used only for glaucoma.

Beta-blockers have traditionally been considered contraindicated in clients with heart failure because of their ability to decrease cardiac function. A growing number of studies, however, are showing that beta-blockers are useful not only in the treatment of mild to moderate cases of chronic heart failure, but also in reducing the risk for sudden death in these clients. The only beta-blocker approved by the FDA to treat heart failure is carvedilol. Treatment should begin with a low dose of the beta-blocker, administered concurrently with an angiotensin-converting enzyme (ACE) inhibitor. The purpose of the ACE inhibitor is to counteract any initial worsening of the heart failure symptoms due to beta-blocker therapy. It is unclear exactly how beta-blockers benefit clients with heart failure. Possible mechanisms of action include blockade of the damaging effects of sympathetic stimulation on the heart, beta receptor up-regulation, decreased sympathetic stimulation due to decreased plasma norepinephrine and antiarrhythmic effects, and improved diastolic function by lengthening diastolic filling time. Research has shown that carvedilol demonstrates antioxidant activity. The clinical significance of this for clients with heart failure is not yet clear.

### Receptor Selectivity

Carteolol, levobunolol, metipranolol, penbutolol, nadolol, pindolol, propranolol, sotalol, and timolol are nonselective beta-blockers. The term *nonselective* indicates that the drugs block both beta$_1$ (cardiac) and beta$_2$ (mainly smooth muscle in the bronchi and blood vessels) receptors. Blockade of beta$_2$ receptors is associated with adverse effects such as bronchoconstriction, peripheral vasoconstriction, and interference with glycogenolysis.

Acebutolol, atenolol, betaxolol, bisoprolol, esmolol, and metoprolol are cardioselective agents, which means they have more effect on beta$_1$ receptors than on beta$_2$ receptors. As a result, they may cause less bronchospasm, less impairment of glucose metabolism, and less peripheral vascular insufficiency. These drugs are preferred when beta-blockers are needed by clients with asthma or other bronchospastic pulmonary disorders, diabetes mellitus, or peripheral vascular disorders. However, cardioselectivity is lost at higher doses because most organs have both beta$_1$ and beta$_2$ receptors rather than one or the other exclusively.

Labetalol and carvedilol block alpha$_1$ receptors to cause vasodilation and beta$_1$ and beta$_2$ receptors to cause all the effects of the nonselective agents. Both alpha- and beta-adrenergic blocking actions contribute to antihypertensive effects, but it is unclear whether these drugs have any definite advantage over other beta-blockers. They may cause less bradycardia but more postural hypotension than other beta-blocking agents, and they may cause less reflex tachycardia than other vasodilators.

### Intrinsic Sympathomimetic Activity

Drugs with this characteristic (ie, acebutolol, carteolol, penbutolol, and pindolol) have a chemical structure similar to that of catecholamines. As a result, they can block some beta receptors and stimulate others. Consequently, these drugs are less likely to cause bradycardia and may be useful for clients experiencing bradycardia with other beta-blockers.

### Membrane–Stabilizing Activity

Several beta-blockers have a membrane-stabilizing effect sometimes described as quinidine-like (ie, producing myocardial depression). Because the doses required to produce this effect are much higher than those used for therapeutic effects, this characteristic is considered clinically insignificant.

### Lipid Solubility

The more lipid-soluble beta-blockers were thought to penetrate the central nervous system (CNS) more extensively and cause adverse effects such as confusion, depression, hallucinations, and insomnia. Some clinicians state that this characteristic is important only in terms of drug use and excretion in certain disease states. Thus, a water-soluble, renally excreted beta-blocker may be preferred in clients with liver disease, and a lipid-soluble, hepatically metabolized drug may be preferred in clients with renal disease.

### Routes of Elimination

Most beta-blocking agents are metabolized in the liver. Atenolol, carteolol, nadolol, and an active metabolite of acebutolol are excreted by the kidneys; dosage must be reduced in the presence of renal failure.

### Routes of Administration

Most beta-blockers can be given orally. Atenolol, esmolol, labetalol, metoprolol, and propranolol also can be given intravenously, and ophthalmic solutions are applied topically to the eye. Betaxolol, carteolol, and timolol are available in oral and ophthalmic forms.

### Duration of Action

Acebutolol, atenolol, bisoprolol, carteolol, penbutolol, and nadolol have long serum half-lives and can usually be given once daily. Carvedilol, labetalol, metoprolol, pindolol, sotalol, and timolol are usually given twice daily. Propranolol required administration several times daily until development of a sustained-release capsule allowed once-daily dosing.

> **? How Can You Avoid This Medication Error?**
>
> Inderal, 40 mg PO bid, has been effectively controlling John Morgan's hypertension for 3 years. He is admitted to a medical unit for tests. In the morning he is NPO. The stock supply of intravenous (IV) Inderal provides 1 mg per 0.5 mL. You administer 20 cc of Inderal IV over 5 minutes for his morning dose.

# NURSING PROCESS

## Assessment

- Assess the client's condition in relation to disorders in which antiadrenergic drugs are used. Because most of the drugs are used to treat hypertension, assess blood pressure patterns over time, when possible, including antihypertensive drugs used and the response obtained. With other cardiovascular disorders, check blood pressure for elevation and pulse for tachycardia or arrhythmia, and determine the presence or absence of chest pain, migraine headache, or hyperthyroidism. If the client reports or medical records indicate one or more of these disorders, assess for specific signs and symptoms. With BPH, assess for signs and symptoms of urinary retention and difficulty voiding.
- Assess for conditions that contraindicate the use of antiadrenergic drugs.
- Assess vital signs to establish a baseline for later comparisons.
- Assess for use of prescription and nonprescription drugs that are likely to increase or decrease effects of antiadrenergic drugs.
- Assess for lifestyle habits that are likely to increase or decrease effects of antiadrenergic drugs (eg, ingestion of caffeine or nicotine).

## Nursing Diagnoses

- Decreased Cardiac Output related to drug-induced postural hypotension (alpha$_2$ agonists, alpha$_1$ and nonselective alpha-blocking agents, and beta blockers) and worsening heart failure (beta blockers)
- Impaired Gas Exchange related to drug-induced bronchoconstriction with beta blockers
- Sexual Dysfunction in men related to impotence and decreased libido
- Fatigue related to decreased cardiac output
- Noncompliance with drug therapy related to adverse drug effects or inadequate understanding of drug regimen
- Risk for Injury related to hypotension, dizziness, sedation
- Deficient Knowledge of drug effects and safe usage

## Planning/Goals

*The client will:*
- Receive or self-administer drugs accurately
- Experience relief of symptoms for which antiadrenergic drugs are given

- Comply with instructions for safe drug usage
- Avoid stopping antiadrenergic drugs abruptly
- Demonstrate knowledge of adverse drug effects to be reported
- Avoid preventable adverse drug effects
- Keep appointments for blood pressure monitoring and other follow-up activities

## Interventions

Use measures to prevent or decrease the need for antiadrenergic drugs. Because the sympathetic nervous system is stimulated by physical and emotional stress, efforts to decrease stress may indirectly decrease the need for drugs to antagonize sympathetic effects. Such efforts may include the following:

- Helping the client stop or decrease cigarette smoking. Nicotine stimulates the CNS and the sympathetic nervous system to cause tremors, tachycardia, and elevated blood pressure.
- Teaching measures to relieve pain, anxiety, and other stresses
- Counseling regarding relaxation techniques
- Helping the client avoid temperature extremes
- Helping the client avoid excessive caffeine in coffee or other beverages
- Helping the client develop a reasonable balance among rest, exercise, work, and recreation
- Recording vital signs at regular intervals in hospitalized clients to monitor for adverse effects
- Helping with activity or ambulation as needed to prevent injury from dizziness

## Evaluation

- Observe for decreased blood pressure when antiadrenergic drugs are given for hypertension.
- Interview regarding decreased chest pain when beta blockers are given for angina.
- Interview and observe for signs and symptoms of adverse drug effects (eg, edema, tachycardia with alpha agonists and blocking agents; bradycardia, congestive heart failure, bronchoconstriction with beta blockers).
- Interview regarding knowledge and use of drugs.

## ■ USE IN SPECIFIC CONDITIONS

## Alpha-Adrenergic Agonists and Blocking Agents

1. When an alpha$_1$-blocking agent (doxazosin, prazosin, or terazosin) is given for hypertension, "first-dose syncope" may occur from hypotension. This reaction can be prevented or minimized by starting with a low dose, increasing the dose gradually, and giving the first dose at bedtime. In addition, the decreased blood pressure stimulates reflex mechanisms to raise blood pressure (increase heart rate and cardiac output, fluid retention), so that a diuretic may be needed.

2. A client diagnosed with BPH should be evaluated for prostatic cancer before starting drug therapy because the signs and symptoms of the two conditions are similar. The two conditions may also coexist.

3. When an alpha$_2$ agonist is given for hypertension, it is very important not to stop the drug abruptly because of the risk for rebound hypertension. To discontinue

## CLIENT TEACHING GUIDELINES
### Alpha₂ Agonists and Alpha-Blocking Agents

**General Considerations**

✔ Have your blood pressure checked regularly. Report high or low values to your health care provider.

✔ The adverse reactions of palpitations, weakness, and dizziness usually disappear with continued use. However, they may recur with conditions promoting vasodilation (dosage increase, exercise, high environmental temperatures, ingesting alcohol or a large meal).

✔ To prevent falls and injuries, if the above reactions occur, sit down or lie down immediately and flex arms and legs. Change positions slowly, especially from supine to standing.

✔ Do not drive a car or operate machinery if drowsy or dizzy from medication.

✔ Do not stop the drugs abruptly. Hypertension, possibly severe, may develop.

✔ With methyldopa, report any signs of abdominal pain, nausea, vomiting, diarrhea, or jaundice to your health care provider. Regular blood tests are needed to make sure the medication is working as it should.

✔ Do not take over-the-counter or other medications without the physician's knowledge. Many drugs interact to increase or decrease the effects of antiadrenergic drugs.

**Self-administration**

✔ Sedation and first-dose syncope may be minimized by taking all or most of the prescribed dose at bedtime.

✔ When using the clonidine transdermal patch, select a hairless area on the upper arm or torso for the application. The patch is changed once a week.

✔ Avoid alcohol use with these medications because excessive drowsiness may occur.

---

clonidine, for example, the dose should be gradually reduced over 2 to 4 days.

4. When phenoxybenzamine is given on a long-term basis, dosage must be carefully individualized. Because the drug is long acting and accumulates in the body, dosage is small initially and gradually increased at intervals of approximately 4 days. Several weeks may be required for full therapeutic benefit, and drug effects persist for several days after the drug is discontinued. If circulatory shock develops from overdosage or hypersensitivity, norepinephrine (Levophed) can be given to overcome the blockade of alpha-adrenergic receptors in arterioles and to raise blood pressure. Epinephrine is contraindicated because it stimulates

both alpha- and beta-adrenergic receptors, resulting in increased vasodilation and hypotension.

## Beta–Adrenergic Blocking Drugs

1. For most people, a nonselective beta-blocker that can be taken once or twice daily is acceptable. For others, the choice of a beta-blocking agent depends largely on the client's condition and response to the drugs. For example, cardioselective drugs are preferred for clients with pulmonary disorders and diabetes mellitus; a drug with intrinsic sympathomimetic activity may be preferred for those who experience significant bradycardia with beta-blockers lacking this property.

## CLIENT TEACHING GUIDELINES
### Beta-Blocking Agents

**General Considerations**

✔ Count your pulse daily and report to a health care provider if under 50 for several days in succession. This information helps to determine if the drug therapy needs to be altered to avoid more serious adverse effects.

✔ Report weight gain (more than 2 pounds within a week), ankle edema, shortness of breath, or excessive fatigue. These are signs of heart failure. If they occur, the drug will be stopped.

✔ Report fainting spells, excessive weakness, or difficulty in breathing. Beta-blocking drugs decrease the usual adaptive responses to exercise or stress. Syncope may result from hypotension, bradycardia, or heart block; its occurrence probably indicates stopping or decreasing the dose of the drug.

✔ Do not stop taking the drugs abruptly. Stopping the drugs suddenly may cause or aggravate chest pain (angina).

✔ Do not take over-the-counter or other medications without the physician's knowledge. Many drugs interact to increase or decrease the effects of beta-blocking agents.

**Self-administration**

✔ Consistently take the drug at the same time each day with or without food. This maintains consistent therapeutic blood levels.

✔ Do not crush or chew long-acting forms of these medications.

2. Dosage of beta-blocking agents must be individualized because of wide variations in plasma levels from comparable doses. Variations are attributed to initial metabolism in the liver, the extent of binding to plasma proteins, and the degree of beta-adrenergic stimulation that the drugs must overcome. In general, low doses should be used initially and increased gradually until therapeutic or adverse effects occur. Adequacy of dosage or extent of beta blockade can be assessed by determining whether the heart rate increases in response to exercise.

3. When a beta-blocker is used to prevent MI, it should be started as soon as the client is hemodynamically stable after a definite or suspected acute MI. The drug should be continued for at least 2 years. Studies have shown that such use of a beta-blocker may reduce mortality by as much as 25%. However, many post-MI clients still do not receive a prescription for this medication.

4. Beta-blocking drugs should not be discontinued abruptly. Long-term blockade of beta-adrenergic receptors increases the receptors' sensitivity to epinephrine and norepinephrine when the drugs are discontinued. There is a risk for severe hypertension, angina, dysrhythmias, and MI from the increased or excessive sympathetic nervous system stimulation. Thus, dosage should be tapered and gradually discontinued to allow beta-adrenergic receptors to return to predrug density and sensitivity. An optimal tapering period has not been defined. Some authorities recommend 1 to 2 weeks; others recommend reducing dosage over approximately 10 days to 30 mg/day of propranolol (or an equivalent amount of other drugs) and continuing this amount at least 2 weeks before the drug is stopped completely.

5. Opinions differ regarding use of beta-blockers before anesthesia and major surgery. On the one hand, the drugs block arrhythmogenic properties of some general inhalation anesthetics; on the other hand, there is a risk for excessive myocardial depression. If feasible, the drug may be tapered gradually and discontinued (at least 48 hours) before surgery. If the drug is continued, the lowest effective dosage should be given. If emergency surgery is necessary, the effects of beta-blockers can be reversed by administration of beta-receptor stimulants, such as dobutamine or isoproterenol.

6. Various drugs may be used to treat adverse effects of beta-blockers. Atropine can be given for bradycardia, digoxin and diuretics for heart failure, vasopressors for hypotension, and bronchodilator drugs for bronchoconstriction.

## Genetic or Ethnic Considerations

Most studies involve adults with hypertension and compare drug therapy responses between African Americans and whites. Findings indicate that monotherapy with alpha$_1$-blockers and combination therapy with alpha- and beta-blockers is equally effective in the two groups. However, monotherapy with beta-blockers is less effective in African Americans than in whites. When beta-blockers are used in African Americans, they should usually be part of a multidrug treatment regimen, and higher doses may be required. In addition, labetalol, an alpha- and beta-blocker, has been shown to be more effective in the African-American population than propranolol, timolol, or metoprolol.

Several studies indicate that Asians achieve higher blood levels of beta-blockers with given doses and, in general, need much smaller doses than whites. This increased sensitivity to the drugs may result from slower metabolism and excretion.

> **?** **How Can You Avoid This Medication Error?**
>
> **Answer:** This would be a lethal mistake. Inderal is greatly affected by the first-pass effect, so the normal IV dose is significantly less than the normal oral dose. When a patient is NPO, an order must be obtained to change the route of administration. The nurse should question administering 20 cc of any medication IV push. Normal IV push doses are usually 1 to 2 cc.

## *Nursing Actions*
## Antiadrenergic Drugs

| *Nursing Actions* | *Rationale/Explanation* |
|---|---|
| 1. Administer accurately. | |
|   a. With alpha$_2$ agonists: | |
|     (1) Give all or most of a dose at bedtime, when possible. | To minimize daytime drowsiness and sedation |
|     (2) Apply the clonidine skin patch to a hairless, intact area on the upper arm or torso; then apply adhesive overlay securely. Do not cut or alter the patch. Remove a used patch and fold its adhesive edges together before discarding. Apply a new patch in a new site. | To promote effectiveness and safe usage |

*(continued)*

## Nursing Actions

### Antiadrenergic Drugs (Continued)

| Nursing Actions | Rationale/Explanation |
|---|---|
| **b.** With alpha₁-blocking agents: | |
| (1) Give the first dose of doxazosin, prazosin, or terazosin at bedtime. | To prevent fainting from severe orthostatic hypotension |
| **c.** With beta-adrenergic blocking agents: | |
| (1) Check blood pressure and pulse frequently, especially when dosage is being increased. | To monitor therapeutic effects and the occurrence of adverse reactions. Some clients with heart rates between 50 and 60 beats per minute may be continued on a beta blocker if hypotension or escape arrhythmias do not develop. Specific instructions vary with individual drugs. |
| (2) See Drugs at a Glance: Beta-Adrenergic Blocking Agents and manufacturers' literature regarding IV administration. | |
| **2. Observe for therapeutic effects.** | |
| **a.** With alpha₂ agonists and alpha-blocking agents: | |
| (1) With hypertension, observe for decreased blood pressure. | With most of the drugs, blood pressure decreases within a few hours. However, antihypertensive effects with clonidine skin patches occur 2–3 days after initial application (overlap with oral clonidine or other antihypertensive drugs may be needed) and persist 2–3 days when discontinued. |
| (2) With benign prostatic hyperplasia, observe for improved urination. | The client may report a larger stream, less nocturnal voiding, and more complete emptying of the bladder. |
| (3) In pheochromocytoma, observe for decreased pulse rate, blood pressure, sweating, palpitations, and blood sugar. | Because symptoms of pheochromocytoma are caused by excessive sympathetic nervous system stimulation, blocking stimulation with these drugs produces a decrease or absence of symptoms. |
| (4) In Raynaud's disease or frostbite, observe affected areas for improvement in skin color and temperature and in the quality of peripheral pulses. | These conditions are characterized by vasospasm, which diminishes blood flow to the affected part. The drugs improve blood flow by vasodilation. |
| **3. Observe for adverse effects.** | Adverse effects are usually extensions of therapeutic effects. |
| **a.** With alpha₂ agonists and alpha-blocking agents: | |
| (1) Hypotension | Hypotension may range from transient postural hypotension to a more severe hypotensive state resembling shock. "First-dose syncope" may occur with prazosin and related drugs. |
| (2) Sedation, drowsiness | Sedation can be minimized by increasing dosage slowly and giving all or most of the daily dose at bedtime. |
| (3) Tachycardia | Tachycardia occurs as a reflex mechanism to increase blood supply to body tissues in hypotensive states. |
| (4) Edema | These drugs promote retention of sodium and water. Concomitant diuretic therapy may be needed to maintain antihypertensive effects with long-term use. |
| **b.** With beta-blocking agents: | |
| (1) Bradycardia and heart block | These are extensions of the therapeutic effects, which slow conduction of electrical impulses through the atrioventricular node, particularly in clients with compromised cardiac function. |
| (2) Congestive heart failure—edema, dyspnea, fatigue | Caused by reduced force of myocardial contraction |
| (3) Bronchospasm—dyspnea, wheezing | Caused by drug-induced constriction of bronchi and bronchioles. It is more likely to occur in people with bronchial asthma or other obstructive lung disease. |
| (4) Fatigue and dizziness, especially with activity or exercise | These symptoms occur because the usual sympathetic nervous system stimulation in response to activity or stress is blocked by drug action. |
| (5) Central nervous system (CNS) effects—depression, insomnia, vivid dreams, and hallucinations | The mechanism by which these effects are produced is unknown. |

*(continued)*

## Nursing Actions

## Antiadrenergic Drugs (Continued)

| Nursing Actions | Rationale/Explanation |
|---|---|
| **4. Observe for drug interactions.** | |
| a. Drugs that *increase* effects of alpha-antiadrenergic agents: | |
| (1) Other antihypertensive drugs | Additive antihypertensive effects |
| (2) CNS depressants | Additive sedation and drowsiness |
| (3) Nonsteroidal anti-inflammatory drugs | Additive sodium and water retention, possible edema |
| (4) Epinephrine | Epinephrine increases the hypotensive effects of phenoxybenzamine and phentolamine and should not be given to treat shock caused by these drugs. Because epinephrine stimulates both alpha- and beta-adrenergic receptors, the net effect is vasodilation and a further drop in blood pressure. |
| b. Drugs that *decrease* effects of alpha-antiadrenergic agents: | |
| (1) Alpha adrenergics (eg, norepinephrine [Levophed]) | Norepinephrine is a strong vasoconstricting agent and is the drug of choice for treating shock caused by overdosage of, or hypersensitivity to, phenoxybenzamine or phentolamine. |
| (2) Estrogens, oral contraceptives, nonsteroidal anti-inflammatory drugs | These drugs may cause sodium and fluid retention and thereby decrease antihypertensive effects of alpha-antiadrenergic drugs. |
| c. Drugs that *increase* effects of beta-adrenergic blocking agents (eg, propranolol): | |
| (1) Other antihypertensives | Synergistic antihypertensive effects. Clients who do not respond to beta blockers or vasodilators alone may respond well to the combination. Also, beta blockers prevent reflex tachycardia, which usually occurs with vasodilator antihypertensive drugs. |
| (2) Phenoxybenzamine or phentolamine | Synergistic effects to prevent excessive hypertension before and during surgical excision of pheochromocytoma |
| (3) Cimetidine, furosemide | Increase plasma levels by slowing hepatic metabolism |
| (4) Digoxin | Additive bradycardia, heart block |
| (5) Phenytoin | Potentiates cardiac depressant effects of propranolol |
| (6) Quinidine | The combination may be synergistic in treating cardiac arrhythmias. However, additive cardiac depressant effects also may occur (bradycardia, decreased force of myocardial contraction [negative inotropy], decreased cardiac output). |
| (7) Verapamil, IV | IV verapamil and IV propranolol should never be used in combination because of additive bradycardia and hypotension. |
| d. Drugs that *decrease* effects of beta-adrenergic blocking agents: | |
| (1) Antacids | Decrease absorption of several oral beta blockers |
| (2) Atropine | Increases heart rate and may be used to counteract excessive bradycardia caused by beta blockers |
| (3) Isoproterenol | Stimulates beta-adrenergic receptors and therefore antagonizes effects of beta-blocking agents. Isoproterenol also can be used to counteract excessive bradycardia. |

## Critical Thinking Exercises

1. To minimize common side effects, alpha$_2$ agonists should have all or most of a dose administered:
   a. At bedtime
   b. With meals
   c. In the morning
   d. One hour before or 2 hours after meals

2. Adverse drug effects with beta-blockers include all of the following except:
   a. Bronchoconstriction
   b. Tachycardia
   c. Edema
   d. Heart failure

3. Chronic use of beta-blockers is associated with increased VLDL and decreased HDL cholesterol. These changes pose a potential risk for clients with:
   a. Glaucoma
   b. Hepatic encephalopathy
   c. Cardiovascular disease
   d. Renal disease

4. A client should be cautioned against abruptly stopping alpha$_2$ agonists and alpha$_1$-blocking agents because:
   a. Vasodilation of the arterioles may intensify
   b. Hypertension, possibly severe, may develop
   c. An increased heart rate and cardiac output may occur
   d. Cessation may cause hemolytic anemia

5. Which drug has been shown to be more effective when administering an alpha- and beta-blocker in the African-American population?
   a. Labetalol
   b. Propranolol
   c. Timolol
   d. Metoprolol

## SELECTED REFERENCES

*Drug facts and comparisons.* (Updated monthly). St. Louis: Facts and Comparisons.

Fetrow, C. W., & Avila, J. R. (2001). *Complementary and alternative medicines* (2nd ed.). Springhouse, PA: Springhouse.

Carter, B. L., & Saseen, J. L. (2002). Hypertension. In J. T. DiPiro, R. L. Talbert, G. C. Yee, G. R. Matzke, B. G. Wells, & L. M. Posey (Eds.), *Pharmacotherapy: A pathophysiologic approach* (5th ed., pp.157–183). New York: McGraw-Hill.

Hoffman, B. B. (2001a). Adrenoreceptor antagonist drugs. In B. G. Katzung (Ed.), *Basic and clinical pharmacology* (8th ed., pp. 138–154). New York: McGraw-Hill.

Hoffman, B. B. (2001b). Catecholamines, sympathomimetic drugs, and adrenergic receptor antagonists. In J. G. Hardman & L. E. Limbird (Eds.), *Goodman and Gilman's the pharmacological basis of therapeutics* (10th ed., pp. 215–268). New York: McGraw-Hill.

Johnson, J. A., Parker, R. B., & Patterson, J. H. (2002). Heart failure. In J. T. DiPiro, R. L. Talbert, G. C. Yee, G. R. Matzke, B. G. Wells, & L. M. Posey (Eds.), *Pharmacotherapy: A pathophysiologic approach* (4th ed., pp. 185–218). New York: McGraw-Hill.

Kudzma, E. C. (1999). Culturally competent drug administration. *American Journal of Nursing, 99*(8), 46–51.

Kuhn, M. A. (1999). *Complementary therapies for health care providers* (pp. 22–23). Philadelphia: Lippincott Williams & Wilkins.

Lacy, C. F., Armstrong, L. L., Goldman, M. P., & Lance, L. L. (2003). *Lexi-Comp's drug information handbook* (11th ed.). Hudson, OH: American Pharmaceutical Association.

Porth, C. M. (2002). *Pathophysiology: Concepts of altered health states* (6th ed., pp. 487–530). Philadelphia: Lippincott Williams & Wilkins.

Piano, M. R., & Huether, S. E. (2002). Mechanisms of hormonal regulation. In K. L. McCance & S. E. Huether (Eds.), *Pathophysiology: The biologic basis for disease in adults and children* (4th ed., pp. 597–623). St. Louis: Mosby.

Robinson, K. M., & McCance, K. L. (2002). Alterations of the reproductive system. In K. L. McCance & S. E. Huether (Eds.), *Pathophysiology: The biologic basis for disease in adults and children* (4th ed., pp. 597–623). St. Louis: Mosby.

Stringer, K. A., & Lopez, L. M. (2002). Acute myocardial infarction. In J. T. DiPiro, R. L. Talbert, G. C. Yee, G. R. Matzke, B. G. Wells, & L. M. Posey (Eds.), *Pharmacotherapy: A pathophysiologic approach* (5th ed., pp. 251–272). Stamford, CT: Appleton & Lange.

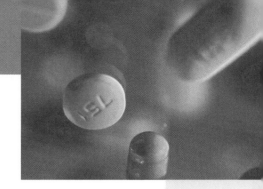

# 18

# Cholinergic Drugs

## OBJECTIVES

*After studying this chapter, the student will be able to:*

1 Identify effects and indications for use of selected cholinergic drugs.

2 Discuss drug therapy of myasthenia gravis.

3 Explain the use of cholinergic drug therapy for paralytic ileus and urinary retention.

4 Discuss drug therapy of Alzheimer's disease.

5 Describe major nursing care needs of clients receiving cholinergic drugs.

6 Explain signs, symptoms, and treatment of overdose with cholinergic drugs.

7 Discuss atropine and pralidoxime as antidotes for cholinergic drugs.

8 Discuss guidelines for using cholinergic drugs in special populations.

9 Teach clients about safe, effective use of cholinergic drugs.

## CRITICAL THINKING SCENARIO

Joe Mitchell, a 14-year-old, was diagnosed with myasthenia gravis 3 years ago and has been well managed on neostigmine (Prostigmin), an anticholinesterase agent. His mother calls the clinic and, clearly upset, reports the following symptoms that Joe is experiencing: severe headache, drooling, and one fainting episode. Joe states that he "just doesn't feel right."

✔ Review the underlying pathophysiology of myasthenia gravis. Explain how Prostigmin alters neurotransmitters to manage this condition. (Hint: think first how the parasympathetic nervous system is altered and how balance could be restored.)

✔ Contrast the symptoms of cholinergic crisis (too much Prostigmin) with myasthenic crisis (insufficient Prostigmin). Which seems to fit with Joe's symptoms?

✔ What additional data would you collect to help arrive at a diagnosis before treatment?

✔ Discuss appropriate medical and pharmacologic management of Joe.

## PROTOTYPE PROFILE

**neostigmine** (Prostigmin), p. 303

# CHOLINERGIC DRUGS

Cholinergic drugs, also called parasympathomimetics and cholinomimetics, stimulate the parasympathetic nervous system (PNS) in the same manner as acetylcholine (see At the Foundation: Acetylcholine). Additionally, the action of the PNS is further described in At the Foundation: Parasympathetic Nervous System in Chapter 19. Some drugs act directly to stimulate cholinergic receptors; others act indirectly by slowing acetylcholine metabolism (by the enzyme acetylcholinesterase) at autonomic nerve synapses and terminals. Selected drugs are discussed here in relation to their use in myasthenia gravis, Alzheimer's disease, and atony of the smooth muscle of the gastrointestinal (GI) and urinary systems, which results in paralytic ileus and urinary retention, respectively.

In normal neuromuscular function, acetylcholine is released from nerve endings and binds to nicotinic receptors on cell membranes of muscle cells to cause muscle contraction. Myasthenia gravis is an autoimmune disorder in which autoantibodies are thought to destroy nicotinic receptors for acetylcholine on skeletal muscle. As a result, acetylcholine is less able to stimulate muscle contraction, and muscle weakness occurs.

In normal brain function, acetylcholine is an essential neurotransmitter and plays an important role in cognitive functions, including memory storage and retrieval. Alzheimer's disease, the most common type of dementia in adults, is characterized by abnormalities in the cholinergic, serotonergic, noradrenergic, and glutamatergic neurotransmission systems. In the cholinergic system, there is a substantial loss of neurons that secrete acetylcholine in the brain and decreased activity of choline acetyltransferase, the enzyme required for synthesis of acetylcholine.

Acetylcholine stimulates cholinergic receptors in the gut to promote normal secretory and motor activity. Cholinergic stimulation results in increased peristalsis and relaxation of the smooth muscle in sphincters to facilitate movement of flatus and feces. The secretory functions of the salivary and gastric glands are also stimulated.

Acetylcholine stimulates cholinergic receptors in the urinary system to promote normal urination. Cholinergic stimulation results in contraction of the detrusor muscle and relaxation of the urinary sphincter to facilitate emptying the urinary bladder.

## Mechanisms of Action and Effects

*Direct-acting cholinergic drugs* are synthetic derivatives of choline. Most direct-acting cholinergic drugs are quaternary amines, carry a positive charge, and are lipid insoluble. They do not readily enter the central nervous system; thus, their effects occur primarily in the periphery. These drugs can exert their therapeutic effects because they are highly resistant to metabolism by acetylcholinesterase, the enzyme that normally metabolizes acetylcholine. Their action is longer than that of acetylcholine. They have widespread systemic effects when they combine with muscarinic receptors in cardiac muscle, smooth muscle, exocrine glands, and the eye (Fig. 18-1). Specific effects include the following:

1. Decreased heart rate, vasodilation, and unpredictable changes in blood pressure
2. Increased tone and contractility in GI smooth muscle, relaxation of sphincters, increased salivary gland and GI secretions
3. Increased tone and contractility of smooth muscle (detrusor) in the urinary bladder and relaxation of the sphincter

## AT THE FOUNDATION: *Acetylcholine*

One of the main neurotransmitters of the autonomic nervous system (ANS) is acetylcholine. Acetylcholine is synthesized from acetylcoenzyme A and choline and released at preganglionic fibers of both the sympathetic nervous system (SNS) and the parasympathetic nervous system (PNS) and at postganglionic fibers of the PNS. Acetylcholine is also released from postganglionic sympathetic neurons that innervate the sweat glands and from motor neurons of the somatic nervous system that innervate the skeletal muscles. The nerve fibers that secrete acetylcholine are called *cholinergic fibers*. The two divisions of the ANS are usually antagonistic in their actions on a particular organ. When the SNS excites a particular organ, the PNS often inhibits it. For example, sympathetic stimulation of the heart causes an increased rate and force of myocardial contraction; parasympathetic stimulation decreases rate and force of contraction, thereby resting the heart.

When acetylcholine acts on body cells that respond to parasympathetic nerve stimulation, it interacts with two types of cholinergic receptors: nicotinic and muscarinic. Nicotinic receptors are located in motor nerves and skeletal muscle. When they are activated by acetylcholine, the cell membrane depolarizes and produces muscle contraction. Muscarinic receptors are located in most internal organs, including the cardiovascular, respiratory, gastrointestinal, and genitourinary systems. When muscarinic receptors are activated by acetylcholine, the affected cells may be excited or inhibited in their functions.

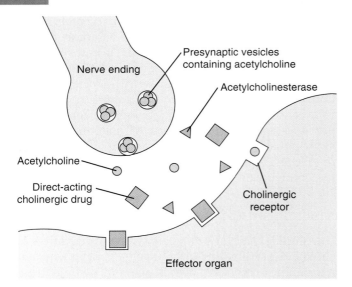

**FIGURE 18-1** Mechanism of direct cholinergic drug action. Direct-acting cholinergic drugs interact with postsynaptic cholinergic receptors on target effector organs, activating the organ in a similar fashion as the neurotransmitter acetylcholine.

4. Increased tone and contractility of bronchial smooth muscle
5. Increased respiratory secretions
6. Constriction of pupils (miosis) and contraction of ciliary muscle, resulting in accommodation for near vision

*Indirect-acting cholinergic* or *anticholinesterase drugs* decrease the inactivation of acetylcholine in the synapse by the enzyme acetylcholinesterase. Acetylcholine can then accumulate in the synapse and enhance the acti-

vation of postsynaptic muscarinic and nicotinic receptors (Fig. 18-2). This improves cholinergic neurotransmission in the brain and the force of muscle contraction in peripheral tissues.

Anticholinesterase drugs are classified as either reversible or irreversible inhibitors of acetylcholinesterase. The reversible inhibitors exhibit a moderate duration of action and have several therapeutic uses, as described later. The irreversible inhibitors produce prolonged effects and are highly toxic. These agents are used primarily as poisons (ie, insecticides and nerve gases). Their only therapeutic use is in the treatment of glaucoma (see Appendix G).

## Indications for Use

Cholinergic drugs have limited but varied uses. A direct-acting drug, bethanechol, is used to treat urinary retention due to urinary bladder atony and postoperative abdominal distention due to paralytic ileus. The anticholinesterase agents are used in the diagnosis and treatment of myasthenia gravis and to reverse the action of nondepolarizing neuromuscular blocking agents (eg, tubocurarine and related drugs) used in surgery (see Appendix D). The drugs do not reverse the neuromuscular blockade produced by depolarizing agents, such as succinylcholine. In addition, tacrine, donepezil, and rivastigmine are anticholinesterase agents approved for treatment of Alzheimer's disease. Cholinergic drugs may also be used to treat glaucoma (see Appendix G). Medications to treat long-term conditions such as myasthenia gravis or Alzheimer's disease are often administered in the home setting. The person using the drugs may have difficulty with self-administration; therefore, working with responsible family members in such cases ensures accurate drug administration. Addi-

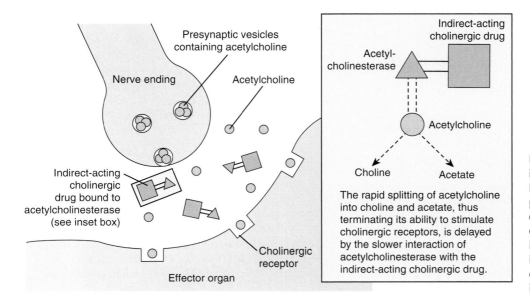

**FIGURE 18-2** Mechanism of indirect cholinergic drug action. Indirect-acting cholinergic drugs prevent the enzymatic breakdown of the neurotransmitter acetylcholine. The acetylcholine remains in the synapse and continues to interact with cholinergic receptors on target effector organs, producing a cholinergic response.

## Home Care Considerations: Use of Cholinergic Drugs

**ASSESS:** the client and family's knowledge of drug therapy and clinical condition; the client for compliance with the prescribed regimen, use of MedicAlert device, quality of life; and need for referral.

**MONITOR:** the therapeutic and adverse effects of the anti-cholinesterase drugs, especially with changes in drugs or dosages; that the client is keeping appointments for lab work and follow-up care.

**EDUCATE:** that a MedicAlert identification device should be worn if taking long-term cholinergic drug therapy for myasthenia gravis, hypotonic bladder, or Alzheimer's disease; that the drugs for myasthenia gravis should be administered on time as scheduled and that diplopia or diminished muscle strength may make it difficult to self-administer medications. The client with Alzheimer's disease may have problems with remembering to take medications and may easily underdose or overdose. The client with urinary retention should expect results from drug within 60 minutes, and bathroom facilities should be readily available. Reinforce additional teaching points (see Client Teaching Guidelines: Cholinergic Drugs).

tional interventions to promote safe and effective drug administration in the home are outlined in Home Care Considerations. In addition, most drugs in this class are most often administered to adults but Age-related Considerations address the use of these drugs in the child and older adult.

## Contraindications to Use

These drugs are contraindicated in urinary or GI tract obstruction, asthma, peptic ulcer disease, coronary artery disease, hyperthyroidism, pregnancy, and inflammatory abdominal conditions. Tacrine is also contraindicated in

previous users in whom jaundice or a serum bilirubin level above 3 mg/dL developed.

 ## INDIVIDUAL CHOLINERGIC DRUGS

See Drugs at a Glance 18-1: Selected Cholinergic Drugs.

### Direct–Acting Cholinergics

**Bethanechol** (Urecholine) is a synthetic derivative of choline. Because bethanechol and other cholinergic drugs increase pressure in the urinary tract by stimulating detrusor muscle contraction and relaxation of urinary sphincters, they are contraindicated for clients with urinary tract obstructions or weaknesses in the bladder wall. Administering a cholinergic drug to these people might result in rupture of the bladder.

Oral bethanechol is not well absorbed from the GI tract; therefore, oral doses are much larger than subcutaneous doses. Bethanechol is not given by the intramuscular (IM) or intravenous (IV) route because it results in severe adverse effects owing to excessive cholinergic stimulation.

### Reversible Indirect–Acting Cholinergics (Anticholinesterases)

**Neostigmine** (Prostigmin) is the prototype anti-cholinesterase agent (see Prototype Profile 18-1: Neostigmine). It is used for long-term treatment of myasthenia gravis and as an antidote for tubocurarine and other nondepolarizing skeletal muscle relaxants used in surgery. Neostigmine, like bethanecol, is a quaternary amine and carries a positive charge. This reduces its lipid solubility and results in poor absorption from the GI tract. Consequently, oral doses are much larger than parenteral doses. When it is used for long-term treatment of myasthenia gravis, resistance to its action may occur, and

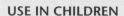 ## Age-related Considerations: Use of Cholinergic Drugs

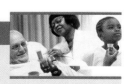

### USE IN CHILDREN

Bethanechol is occasionally used to treat urinary retention and paralytic ileus, but safety and effectiveness for children younger than 8 years of age have not been established. Neostigmine is used to treat myasthenia gravis and to reverse neuromuscular blockade after general anesthesia but is not recommended for urinary retention. Pyridostigmine may be used in the neonate of a mother with myasthenia gravis to treat difficulties with sucking, swallowing, and breathing. Other indirect-acting cholinergic drugs are used only in the treatment of myasthenia gravis. Pre-

cautions and adverse effects are the same for children as for adults.

### USE IN OLDER ADULTS

Indirect-acting cholinergic drugs may be used in myasthenia gravis, Alzheimer's disease, or overdoses of atropine and other centrally acting anticholinergic drugs (eg, those used for parkinsonism). Older adults are more likely to experience adverse drug effects because of age-related physiologic changes and superimposed pathologic conditions.

## Drugs at a Glance

## Selected Cholinergic Drugs

| Generic/Trade Name | Routes and Dosage Ranges | Comments |
|---|---|---|
| **Direct-Acting Cholinergics** | | |
| **Bethanechol** (Urecholine)<br>Pregnancy Category C | *Adults:* PO, 10–50 mg bid to qid, maximum single dose not to exceed 50 mg. Sub-Q, 2.5–5 mg tid or qid<br>*Children:* Safety and efficacy not established < 8 y. PO, 0.6 mg/kg tid to qid. Sub-Q, 0.2 mg/kg tid to qid | *Do not give IM or IV.*<br>Should be taken 1 h before or 2 h after meals to avoid nausea or vomiting |
| **Indirect-Acting Cholinergics (Anticholinesterase Drugs)** | | |
| **Ambenonium** (Mytelase)<br>Pregnancy Category C | *Adults:* PO, 5–25 mg tid to qid<br>*Children:* Safety and efficacy not established | |
| **Edrophonium** (Tensilon)<br>Pregnancy Category C | *For diagnosis of myasthenia gravis*<br>*Adults:* IV route preferred: 2 mg IV over 15–30 sec. 8 mg IV given 45 seconds later if no response.<br>Test dose may be repeated in 30 min.<br>IM route, 10 mg. May follow-up with an additional 2 mg 30 min later if no response<br>*Infants:* 0.5 mg IV<br><34 kg: 1 mg IV. May titrate up to 5 mg if no response<br>>34 kg: 2 mg IV. May titrate up to 10 mg if no response<br>IM, <34 kg: Give 2 mg<br>>34 kg: Give 5 mg<br>*Differentiation or myasthenic crisis from cholinergic crisis*<br>*Adults:* 1 mg IV, may repeat in 1 min. *Be prepared to intubate* | Used to diagnose myasthenia gravis, to differentiate myasthenic crisis from cholinergic crisis, and for reversal of non-depolarizing neuromuscular blockers |
| **Neostigmine** (Prostigmin) | See Prototype Profile 18-1: Neostigmine | |
| **Physostigmine** (Antilirium)<br>Pregnancy Category C | *Adults:* IM, IV, 0.5–2 mg | Give IV slowly, no faster than 1 mg/min to avoid adverse effects of bradycardia, hypersalivation, respiratory distress, and seizures |
| **Pyridostigmine** (Mestinon)<br>Pregnancy Category C | *Adults:* PO, 60 mg tid initially, individualize dose to control symptoms. Average dose in 24 h: 600 mg. Range in 24 h: 60–1500 mg. IM, IV slowly: 1/30 the oral dose<br>*Military:* PO, 30 mg several hours before soman exposure<br>*Children:* PO, 7 mg/kg/d divided into 5 or 6 doses<br>Neonates of mothers with myasthenia gravis who have difficulty with sucking, breathing, or swallowing: 0.05–0.15 mg/kg IM. Change to syrup as soon as possible | Do not crush sustained-release product<br><br>Has demonstrated increased survival after exposure to soman (nerve agent) |
| **Indirect-Acting Cholinergics for Alzheimer's Disease** | | |
| **Donepezil** (Aricept)<br>Pregnancy Category C | *Adults:* PO, 5 mg daily hs for 4–6 wk, then increase to 10 mg qd if needed | St. John's wort may decrease drug levels |
| **Galantamine** (Reminyl)<br>Pregnancy Category B | *Adults:* PO, 8 mg/d initially, increase to 8 mg/bid after 4 wk if needed. May continue to increase q4wk up to maximum dose 24 mg/d | Administer with breakfast and dinner |
| **Rivastigmine** (Exelon)<br>Pregnancy Category B | *Adults:* PO, 1.5 mg bid with food initially. May titrate to higher doses at 1.5 mg intervals q2wk to a maximum dose of 12 mg/d | Administer with breakfast and dinner; instruct client to swallow capsules whole |
| **Tacrine** (Cognex)<br>Pregnancy Category C | *Adults:* PO, 40 mg/d (10 mg qid) for 6 wk. If aminotransferase levels are satisfactory after weekly monitoring, may increase the dose to 80 mg/d (20 mg/qid)<br>If liver function remains normal, may increase daily dose by 10 mg q6wk to a total of 120–160 mg/d | Monitor liver function weekly for a minimum of 18 wk, then once every 3 months; administer with food only if client cannot tolerate gastrointestinal symptoms (will decrease absorption) |

## PROTOTYPE PROFILE 18-1

### P Neostigmine (nee o STIG meen)

**Drug Class**
*Chemical:* Acetylcholinesterase inhibitor
*Functional:* Diagnostic agent for myasthenia gravis; antidote for tubocurarine and other nondepolarizing skeletal muscle relaxants

**Trade Name**
Prostigmin

**Therapeutic Indications**
Diagnosis and treatment of myasthenia gravis; postoperative reversal of effects of nondepolarizing neuromuscular blocking agents; prevention and treatment of postoperative urinary retention and bladder distention

**Pharmacokinetics**
*Absorption*
PO, poor (so oral and parenteral doses are not interchangeable)

*Distribution*
Uncertain if crosses placenta or enters breast milk

*Metabolism*
By plasma cholinesterases and hepatic enzymes

*Excretion*
Urine

**Pharmacodynamics**
*Onset of Action*
PO, 45–75 min; IV, 1–20 min; IM, 20–30 min

*Duration*
PO, 2–4 h; IV, 1–2 h; IM, 2.5–4 h

**Contraindications/Precautions**
GI or GU obstruction; with caution in clients with bradycardia, dysrhythmias, epilepsy, asthma, hyperthyroidism, peptic ulcers

**Pregnancy Considerations**
Category C
Excretion in breast milk unknown; not recommended

**Dosage**
Treatment of myasthenia gravis:
*Adults:* Dosage individualized to client needs
PO, 15–375 mg/d in 3–4 divided doses. Sub-Q, IV, or IM, 0.5 mg initially. Individualize subsequent doses.
*Children:* PO, 0.3–0.6 mg/kg q3–4h Sub-Q, IV, IM, 0.01–0.04 mg/kg/dose q2–3h as needed
Diagnosis of myasthenia gravis:
*Adults:* 0.022 mg/kg IM
*Children:* 0.04 mg/kg IM
Antidote for nondepolarizing neuromuscular blockers:
*Adults:* Give atropine sulfate 0.6–1.2 mg IV several minutes before slow IV injection of neostigmine 0.5–2 mg. Repeat as needed, total dose not to exceed 5 mg
*Children:* Give 0.008–0.025 mg/kg atropine sulfate IV several minutes before slow IV injection of neostigmine, 0.07–0.08 mg/kg.
Prevention/treatment of postoperative distention and urinary retention:
*Adults:* 0.25–0.5 mg IM or Sub-Q q4–6h for 2–3 days
Prevention/treatment of postoperative retention:
*Children:* Safety and efficacy not established

**Adverse Effects**
Dysrhythmias (particularly bradycardia), seizures, bronchospasm, excessive salivation, abdominal cramps, diarrhea, sweating

**Drug Interactions**
*Increased Effects*
Neuromuscular blocking agents

*Decreased Effects*
Nondepolarizing muscle relaxants
Muscarinic effects of neostigmine with use of atropine

**Herbal Supplements and Dietary Considerations**
May be administered with food to minimize side effects; clients who have difficulty chewing should receive drug 30 min before meals

larger doses may be required. The hepatic metabolism of neostigmine may be impaired by liver disease, resulting in increased adverse effects.

**Edrophonium** (Tensilon) is a short-acting cholinergic drug used to diagnose myasthenia gravis, to differentiate between myasthenic crisis and cholinergic crisis, and to reverse the neuromuscular blockade produced by nondepolarizing skeletal muscle relaxants. It is given IM or IV by a health care provider who remains in attendance. Atropine, an antidote, and life support equipment, such as ventilators and endotracheal tubes, must be available when the drug is given.

**Ambenonium** (Mytelase) is a long-acting drug used for the treatment of myasthenia gravis. It is used less

often than neostigmine and pyridostigmine. It may be useful in clients who are allergic to bromides, however, because the other drugs are both bromide salts. Ambenonium may be useful for myasthenic clients on ventilators because it is less likely to increase respiratory secretions than other anticholinesterase drugs.

**Physostigmine salicylate** (Antilirium) is the only anticholinesterase capable of crossing the blood–brain barrier. Unlike other drugs in this group, physostigmine is not a quaternary amine, does not carry a positive charge, and therefore is more lipid soluble. It is sometimes used as an antidote for overdosage of anticholinergic drugs, including atropine, antihistamines, tricyclic antidepressants, and phenothiazine antipsychotics. However, its potential for causing serious adverse effects limits its usefulness. Some preparations of physostigmine are also used in the treatment of glaucoma (see Appendix G).

**Pyridostigmine** (Mestinon) is similar to neostigmine in actions, uses, and adverse effects. It may have a longer duration of action than neostigmine and is the maintenance drug of choice for clients with myasthenia gravis. An added advantage is the availability of a slow-release form, which is effective for 8 to 12 hours. When this form is taken at bedtime, the client does not have to take other medications during the night and does not awaken too weak to swallow. The hepatic metabolism of pyridostigmine may be impaired by liver disease, resulting in increased adverse effects.

**Donepezil** (Aricept) is used to treat mild to moderate Alzheimer's disease. In long-term studies, donepezil delayed the progression of the disease for up to 55 weeks. Donepezil increases acetylcholine in the brain by inhibiting its metabolism. The drug is well absorbed after oral administration, and absorption is unaffected by food. It is highly bound (96%) to plasma proteins. It is metabolized in the liver to several metabolites, some of which are pharmacologically active; metabolites and some unchanged drug are excreted mainly in urine. Adverse effects include nausea, vomiting, diarrhea, bradycardia, and possible aggravation of asthma, peptic ulcer disease, and chronic obstructive pulmonary disease. Unlike tacrine, donepezil does not cause liver toxicity.

**Galantamine (Reminyl)** is the newest long-acting anticholinesterase agent approved by the U.S. Food and Drug Administration (FDA) for the treatment of Alzheimer's disease. Its pharmacokinetics and side-effect profile are similar to those of donepezil and rivastigmine.

**Rivastigmine (Exelon)** is a long-acting central anticholinesterase agent approved for the treatment of Alzheimer's disease. It lasts 12 hours, making twice-a-day dosing possible. Like other drugs in this class, it is not a cure for Alzheimer's disease, but it does slow down progression of the symptoms. Rivastigmine is metabolized by the liver and excreted in the feces. It has a side-effect profile similar to that of donepezil.

**Tacrine** (Cognex) is a centrally acting anticholinesterase agent approved for treatment of clients with mild to moderate Alzheimer's disease. The drug does not cure the disease, but it may delay progression in some clients. Tacrine is well absorbed after oral administration and reaches peak plasma levels in 1 to 2 hours. It is approximately 50% protein bound, is extensively metabolized in the liver, is excreted in the urine, and has an elimination half-life of 2 to 4 hours. The initial enthusiasm for tacrine has declined because of inconsistent clinical trial results and the occurrence of hepatotoxicity. Approximately 30% of clients receiving low-dose tacrine therapy experience elevated alanine aminotransferase (ALT) values of three times normal. Most enzyme elevation occurs in the first 18 weeks of therapy and is more common in female clients. Immediate withdrawal of the medication usually restores liver enzymes to normal levels with no permanent liver injury. Tacrine is contraindicated in liver disease because of the occurrence of hepatotoxicity with use.

## ◼ USE IN SPECIFIC CONDITIONS

### Use in Myasthenia Gravis

Guidelines for the use of anticholinesterase drugs in myasthenia gravis include the following:

1. Drug dosage should be increased gradually until maximal benefit is obtained. Larger doses are often required with increased physical activity, emotional stress, and infections, and sometimes premenstrually.

2. Some clients with myasthenia gravis cannot tolerate optimal doses of anticholinesterase drugs unless atropine is given to decrease the severity of adverse reactions due to muscarinic activation. However, atropine should be given only if necessary because it may mask the sudden increase of side effects. This increase is the first sign of overdose.

3. Drug dosage in excess of the amount needed to maintain muscle strength and function can produce a cholinergic crisis. A cholinergic crisis is characterized by excessive stimulation of the PNS. If early symptoms are not treated, hypotension and respiratory failure may occur. At high doses, anticholinesterase drugs weaken rather than strengthen skeletal muscle contraction because excessive amounts of acetylcholine accumulate at motor end plates and reduce nerve impulse transmission to muscle tissue.

4. *Treatment for cholinergic crisis* includes withdrawal of anticholinesterase drugs, administration of atropine, and measures to maintain respiration. Endotracheal intubation and mechanical ventilation may be necessary because of profound skeletal muscle weakness (including muscles of respiration), which is not counteracted by atropine.

5. *Differentiating myasthenic crisis from cholinergic crisis* may be difficult because both are characterized by respiratory difficulty or failure. It is necessary to differentiate between them, however, because they require *opposite* treatment measures. Myasthenic crisis requires more anticholinesterase drug, whereas cholinergic crisis requires discontinuing any anticholinesterase drug the client has been receiving. The health care provider may be able to make an accurate diagnosis from signs and symptoms and their timing in relation to medication; that is, signs and symptoms having their onset within approximately 1 hour after a dose of anticholinesterase drug are more likely to be caused by cholinergic crisis (too much drug). Signs and symptoms beginning 3 hours or more after a drug dose are more likely to be caused by myasthenic crisis (too little drug).

# NURSING PROCESS

## Assessment

Assess the client's condition in relation to disorders for which cholinergic drugs are used:

- In clients known to have myasthenia gravis, assess for muscle weakness. This may be manifested by ptosis (drooping) of the upper eyelid and diplopia (double vision) caused by weakness of the eye muscles. More severe disease may be indicated by difficulty in chewing, swallowing, and speaking; accumulation of oral secretions, which the client may be unable to expectorate or swallow; decreased skeletal muscle activity, including impaired chest expansion; and eventual respiratory failure.
- In clients with possible urinary retention, assess for bladder distention, time and amount of previous urination, and fluid intake.
- In clients with possible paralytic ileus, assess for presence of bowel sounds, abdominal distention, and elimination pattern.
- In clients with Alzheimer's disease, assess for abilities and limitations in relation to memory, cognitive functioning, self-care activities, and preexisting conditions that may be aggravated by a cholinergic drug.

## Nursing Diagnoses

- Impaired gas exchange related to increased respiratory secretions, bronchospasm, and/or respiratory paralysis
- Ineffective Breathing Pattern related to bronchoconstriction
- Ineffective Airway Clearance related to increased respiratory secretions
- Self Care Deficit related to muscle weakness, cognitive impairment, or diplopia
- Deficient Knowledge: Drug administration and effects

## Planning/Goals

*The client will:*
- Verbalize or demonstrate correct drug administration
- Improve in self-care abilities
- Regain usual patterns of urinary and bowel elimination
- Maintain effective oxygenation of tissues
- Report adverse drug effects
- For clients with myasthenia gravis, at least one family member will verbalize or demonstrate correct drug administration, symptoms of too much or too little drug, and emergency care procedures.
- For clients with dementia, a caregiver will verbalize or demonstrate correct drug administration and knowledge of adverse effects to be reported to a health care provider.

## Interventions

- Use measures to prevent or decrease the need for cholinergic drugs. Ambulation, adequate fluid intake, and judicious use of opioid analgesics or other sedative-type drugs help prevent postoperative urinary retention. In myasthenia gravis, muscle weakness is aggravated by exercise and improved by rest. Therefore, scheduling activities to avoid excessive fatigue and to allow adequate rest periods may be beneficial.
- With drug therapy for Alzheimer's disease, assist and teach caregivers to:
  - Maintain a quiet, stable environment and daily routines to decrease confusion (eg, verbal or written reminders, simple directions, adequate lighting, calendars, and personal objects within view and reach).
  - Avoid altering dosage or stopping the drug without consulting the prescribing health care provider.
  - Be sure that clients keep appointments for supervision and blood tests.
  - Report signs and symptoms (ie, skin rash, jaundice, light-colored stools) that may indicate hepatotoxicity for clients taking tacrine.
  - Notify surgeons about tacrine therapy. Exaggerated muscle relaxation may occur if succinylcholine-type drugs are given.
- Do not give cholinergic drugs for bladder atony and urinary retention or paralytic ileus in the presence of an obstruction.
- For long-term use, assist clients and families to establish a schedule of drug administration that best meets the client's needs.
- With myasthenia gravis, recommend that one or more family members be trained in cardiopulmonary resuscitation.

## Evaluation

- Observe and interview about the adequacy of urinary elimination.
- Observe abilities and limitations in self-care.
- Question the client and at least one family member of clients with myasthenia gravis about correct drug usage, symptoms of underdosage and overdosage, and emergency care procedures.
- Question caregivers of clients with dementia about the client's level of functioning and response to medication.

---

6. If the differential diagnosis cannot be made on the basis of signs and symptoms, the client can be intubated, mechanically ventilated, and observed closely until a diagnosis is possible. Still another way to differentiate between the two conditions is for the health care provider to inject a small dose of IV edrophonium. If the edrophonium causes a dramatic improvement in breathing, the diagnosis is myasthenic crisis; if it makes the client even weaker, the diagnosis is cholinergic crisis. Note, however, that edrophonium or any other pharmacologic agent should be administered only after endotracheal intubation and controlled ventilation have been instituted.

7. Some people acquire partial or total resistance to anticholinesterase drugs after taking them for months or years. Therefore, do not assume that drug therapy

## CLIENT TEACHING GUIDELINES
## Cholinergic Drugs

### General Considerations

✔ Cholinergic drugs used for urinary retention usually act within 60 minutes after administration. Be sure bathroom facilities are available.

✔ Wear a medical alert identification device if taking long-term cholinergic drug therapy for myasthenia gravis, hypotonic bladder, or Alzheimer's disease.

✔ Atropine 0.6 mg IV may be administered for overdose of cholinergic drugs.

✔ Record symptoms of myasthenia gravis and effects of drug therapy, especially when drug therapy is initiated and medication doses are being titrated. The amount of medication required to control symptoms of myasthenia gravis varies greatly and the health care provider needs this information to adjust the dosage correctly.

✔ Do not overexert yourself if you have myasthenia gravis. Rest between activities. Although the dose of medication may be increased during periods of increased activity, it is desirable to space activities to obtain optimal benefit from the drug, at the lowest possible dose, with the fewest adverse effects.

✔ Report increased muscle weakness, difficulty breathing, or recurrence of myasthenic symptoms to the prescriber. These are signs of drug underdosage (myasthenic crisis) and indicate a need to increase or change drug therapy.

✔ Report adverse reactions, including abdominal cramps, diarrhea, excessive oral secretions, difficulty in breathing, and muscle weakness. These are signs of drug overdosage (cholinergic crisis) and require immediate discontinuation of drugs and treatment by the health

care provider. Respiratory failure can result if this condition is not recognized and treated properly.

✔ Clients taking tacrine need weekly monitoring of liver aminotransferase levels for 18 weeks when initiating therapy and weekly for 6 weeks after any increase in dose. Caregivers should report any signs or symptoms of adverse drug reactions such as nausea, vomiting, diarrhea, rash, jaundice, or change in the color of stools. The drug should not be suddenly discontinued.

✔ If dizziness or syncope occurs when taking tacrine, donepezil, or other anticholinesterase drugs, ambulation should be supervised to avoid injury.

✔ Caregivers should record observed effects of anticholinesterase medications given to treat Alzheimer's disease. These medications are often titrated upward to improve cognitive function and delay symptom progression, and this information will be helpful to the prescriber.

### Self- or Caregiver Administration

✔ Take drugs as directed on a regular schedule to maintain consistent blood levels and control of symptoms.

✔ Do not chew or crush sustained-release medications.

✔ Take oral cholinergics on an empty stomach to lessen nausea and vomiting. Also, food decreases absorption of tacrine by up to 40%.

✔ Ensure adequate fluid intake if vomiting or diarrhea occurs as a side effect of cholinergic medications.

✔ St. John's wort should be avoided because concurrent use may reduce blood levels of donepezil.

---

that is effective initially will continue to be effective over the long-term course of the disease.

## Toxicity of Cholinergic Drugs: Recognition and Management

Atropine, an anticholinergic (antimuscarinic) drug, is a specific antidote to cholinergic agents. The drug and equipment for injection should be readily available whenever cholinergic drugs are given. It is important to note that atropine reverses only the muscarinic effects of cholinergic drugs, primarily in the heart, smooth muscle, and glands. Atropine does not interact with nicotinic receptors and therefore cannot reverse the nicotinic effects of skeletal muscle weakness or paralysis due to overdose of the indirect cholinergic drugs.

## Management of Mushroom Poisoning

Muscarinic receptors in the parasympathetic nervous system were given their name because they can be stimulated

by muscarine, an alkaloid that is found in small quantities in the *amanita muscaria* mushroom. Some mushrooms found in North America, such as the *clitocybe* and *inocybe* mushrooms, however, contain much larger quantities of muscarine. Accidental or intentional ingestion of these mushrooms results in intense cholinergic stimulation (cholinergic crisis) and is potentially fatal. Atropine is the specific antidote for mushroom poisoning.

## Toxicity of Irreversible Anticholinesterase Agents: Recognition and Management

Most irreversible anticholinesterase agents are highly lipid soluble and can enter the body by a variety of routes, including the eye, skin, respiratory system, and GI tract. Because they readily cross the blood–brain barrier, their effects are seen peripherally as well as centrally.

Exposure to toxic doses of irreversible anticholinesterase agents, such as organophosphate insecticides (malathion, parathion) or nerve gases (sarin, tabun, soman), produces a cholinergic crisis characterized by excessive cholinergic (muscarinic) stimulation and neuromuscular blockade. This cholinergic crisis occurs because the irreversible anticholinesterase poison binds to the enzyme acetylcholinesterase and inactivates it. Consequently, acetylcholine remains in cholinergic synapses and causes excessive stimulation of muscarinic and nicotinic receptors.

Emergency treatment includes decontamination procedures such as removing contaminated clothing, flushing the poison from skin and eyes, and using activated charcoal and lavage to remove ingested poison from the GI tract. Pharmacologic treatment includes administering atropine to counteract the muscarinic effects of the poison (eg, salivation, urination, defecation, bronchial secretions, laryngospasm, bronchospasm).

To relieve the neuromuscular blockade produced by nicotinic effects of the poison, a second drug, pralidoxime,

is needed. Pralidoxime (Protopam), a cholinesterase reactivator, is a specific antidote for overdose with irreversible anticholinesterase agents. Pralidoxime treats toxicity by causing the anticholinesterase poison to release the enzyme acetylcholinesterase. The reactivated acetylcholinesterase can then degrade excess acetylcholine at the cholinergic synapses, including the neuromuscular junction. Pralidoxime cannot cross the blood–brain barrier and therefore is effective only in the peripheral areas of the body. Pralidoxime must be given as soon after the poisoning as possible. If too much time passes, the bond between the irreversible anticholinesterase agent and acetylcholinesterase becomes stronger, and pralidoxime is unable to release the enzyme from the poison. Treatment of anticholinesterase overdose may also require diazepam or lorazepam to control seizures. Mechanical ventilation may be necessary to treat respiratory paralysis.

## Nursing Actions
## Cholinergic Drugs

| Nursing Actions | Rationale/Explanation |
|---|---|
| 1. Administer accurately. | |
| a. Give oral bethanechol before meals. | If these drugs are given after meals, nausea and vomiting may occur because the drug stimulates contraction of muscles in the GI tract. |
| b. Give parenteral bethanechol by the subcutaneous route only. | IM and IV injections may cause acute, severe hypotension and circulatory failure. Cardiac arrest may occur. |
| c. With pyridostigmine and other drugs for myasthenia gravis, give at regularly scheduled intervals. | For consistent blood levels and control of symptoms |
| d. Give tacrine on an empty stomach, 1 hour before or 2 hours after a meal, if possible, at regular intervals around the clock (eg, q6h). Give with meals if GI upset occurs. | Food decreases absorption and decreases serum drug levels by 30% or more. Regular intervals increase therapeutic effects and decrease adverse effects. |
| 2. Observe for therapeutic effects. | |
| a. When the drug is given for postoperative hypoperistalsis, observe for bowel sounds, passage of flatus through the rectum, or a bowel movement. | These are indicators of increased GI muscle tone and motility. |
| b. When bethanechol or neostigmine is given for urinary retention, micturition usually occurs within approximately 60 minutes. If it does not, urinary catheterization may be necessary. | |
| c. When the drug is given in myasthenia gravis, observe for increased muscle strength as shown by: | |
| (1) Decreased or absent ptosis of eyelids | With neostigmine, onset of action is 2–4 hours after oral administration and 10–30 minutes after injection. Duration is approximately 3–4 hours. With pyridostigmine, onset of action is approximately 30–45 minutes after oral use, 15 minutes after IM injection, and 2–5 minutes after IV injection. Duration is approximately 4–6 hours. The long-acting form of pyridostigmine lasts 8–12 hours. |
| (2) Decreased difficulty with chewing, swallowing, and speech | |
| (3) Increased skeletal muscle strength, increased tolerance of activity, less fatigue | |
| d. With cholinergic drugs to treat Alzheimer's disease (tacrine, donepezil, galantamine, and rivastigmine) observe for improvement in memory and cognitive functioning in activities of daily living. | Improved functioning is most likely to occur in clients with mild to moderate dementia. |

(continued)

## Nursing Actions

### Cholinergic Drugs (Continued)

| Nursing Actions | Rationale/Explanation |
|---|---|
| 3. Observe for adverse effects. | Adverse effects occur with usual therapeutic doses but are more likely with large doses. They are caused by stimulation of the parasympathetic nervous system. |
| a. Central nervous system effects—convulsions, dizziness, drowsiness, headache, loss of consciousness | |
| b. Respiratory effects—increased secretions, broncho-spasm, laryngospasm, respiratory failure | |
| c. Cardiovascular effects—dysrhythmias (bradycardia, tachycardia, atrioventricular block), cardiac arrest, hypotension, syncope | These may be detected early by regular assessment of blood pressure and heart rate. Bradycardia is probably the most likely dysrhythmia to occur. GI effects commonly occur. |
| d. GI effects—nausea and vomiting, diarrhea, increased peristalsis, abdominal cramping, increased secretions (ie, saliva, gastric and intestinal secretions) | |
| e. Other effects—increased frequency and urgency of urination, increased sweating, miosis, skin rash | Skin rashes are most likely to occur from formulations of neostigmine or pyridostigmine that contain bromide. |
| 4. Observe for drug interactions. | |
| a. Drug that increases effects of tacrine: | |
| (1) Cimetidine | Slows metabolism of tacrine in the liver, thereby increasing risks of accumulation and adverse effects |
| b. Drugs that *decrease* effects of cholinergic agents: | |
| (1) Anticholinergic drugs (eg, atropine) | Antagonize effects of cholinergic drugs (miosis, increased tone and motility in smooth muscle of the GI tract, bronchi, and urinary bladder, bradycardia). Atropine is the specific antidote for overdosage with cholinergic drugs. |
| (2) Antihistamines | Most antihistamines have anticholinergic properties that antagonize effects of cholinergic drugs. |
| c. Drugs that *decrease* effects of anticholinesterase drugs | |
| (1) Corticosteroids | Steroids may antagonize anticholinesterase agents and increase muscle weakness in the patient with myasthenia gravis. |
| (2) Aminoglycoside antibiotics (eg, gentamicin) | Aminoglycoside antibiotics (eg, gentamicin) can produce a neuromuscular blockade that antagonizes the effects of anti-cholinesterase drugs and causes muscle weakness in patients with myasthenia gravis. |

## Critical Thinking Exercises

1. Accidental or intentional ingestion of *clitocybe* or *inocybe* mushrooms results in intense cholinergic stim-ulation and is potentially fatal. The specific antidote for mushroom poisoning is:
   a. Atropine
   b. Diazepam
   c. Pralidoxime
   d. Lorazepam

2. A client with myasthenia gravis is in cholinergic crisis. All of the following interventions are appropriate except:
   a. Administer additional anticholinesterase drug
   b. Provide ventilatory support
   c. Discontinue any anticholinesterase drug
   d. Administer atropine

3. Which neurotransmitter is involved in cholinergic (parasympathetic) stimulation?
   a. Norepinephrine
   b. Acetylcholine
   c. Dopamine
   d. Epinephrine

4. What is the desired effect when tacrine (Cognex) is given to treat Alzheimer's disease?
   a. Delay progression of the disease
   b. Cure the disease
   c. Prevent the side effects of anticholinesterase agents
   d. Decrease the exaggerated muscle relaxation that may occur

**5.** A client with myasthenia gravis is scheduled to receive a dose of medication at 9:00 AM. She misses that dose. The family should be instructed to:

a. Administer next dose at regularly scheduled time

b. Assess swallowing ability and adequacy of ventilation

c. Administer as soon as missed dose is recognized

d. Call the health care provider for directions on administration

## SELECTED REFERENCES

Brown, J. H., & Taylor, P. (2001). Muscarinic receptor agonists and antagonists. In J. G. Hardman & L. E. Limbird (Eds.), *Goodman and Gilman's the pharmacological basis of therapeutics* (10th ed., pp. 155–173). New York: McGraw-Hill.

Difilippi, J. L., Crismon, M. L., Clark, W. R. (2002). Alzheimer's disease. In J. T. DiPiro, R. L. Talbert, G. C. Yee, G. R. Matzke, B. G. Wells, & L. M. Posey (Eds.), *Pharmacotherapy: A pathophysiologic approach* (5th ed., pp. 1165–1182). New York: McGraw-Hill.

*Drug facts and comparisons.* (Updated monthly). St. Louis: Facts and Comparisons.

Girolami, U. D., Anthony, D. C., & Frosch, M. P. (1999). Peripheral nerve and skeletal muscle. In R. S. Cotran, V. Kumar, & T. Collins (Eds.), *Pathologic basis of disease* (6th ed., p. 1289). Philadelphia: W. B. Saunders.

Girolami, U. D., Anthony, D. C., & Frosch, M. P. (1999). The central nervous system. In R. S. Cotran, V. Kumar, & T. Collins (Eds.), *Pathologic basis of disease* (6th ed., pp. 1329–1333). Philadelphia: W. B. Saunders.

Karch, A. M. (2002). *Lippincott's nursing drug guide.* Philadelphia: Lippincott Williams and Wilkins.

Lacy, C. F., Armstrong, L. L., Goldman, M. P., & Lance, L. L. (2003). *Lexi-Comp's drug information handbook* (11th ed.). Hudson, OH: American Pharmaceutical Association.

Olson, K. R. (Ed.). (1999). *Poisoning and drug overdose* (3rd ed.). Stamford, CT: Appleton & Lange.

Pappano, A. J. (2001). Cholinoceptor-activating and cholinesterase-inhibiting drugs. In B. G. Katzung (Ed.), *Basic and clinical pharmacology* (8th ed., pp. 92–106). New York: McGraw-Hill.

Taylor, P. (2001). Anticholinesterase agents. In J. G. Hardman & L. E. Limbird (Eds.), *Goodman and Gilman's the pharmacological basis of therapeutics* (10th ed., pp. 175–191). New York: McGraw-Hill.

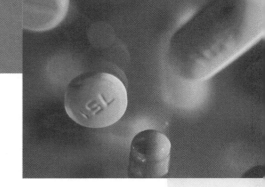

# 19

# Anticholinergic Drugs

## OBJECTIVES

*After studying this chapter, the student will be able to:*

1 List characteristics of anticholinergic drugs in terms of effects on body tissues, indications for use, nursing process implications, observation of client response, and teaching clients.

2 Discuss atropine as the prototype of anticholinergic drugs.

3 Identify clinical disorders and symptoms for which anticholinergic drugs are used.

4 Describe the mechanism by which atropine relieves bradycardia.

5 Review anticholinergic effects of antipsychotics, tricyclic antidepressants, and antihistamines.

6 Give principles of therapy and nursing process for using anticholinergic drugs in special populations.

7 Describe the signs and symptoms of atropine or anticholinergic drug overdose and its treatment.

8 Teach clients about the safe, effective use of anticholinergic drugs.

## CRITICAL THINKING SCENARIO

*G*eorge Wilson, 76 years of age, has been treated for depression with amitriptyline (Elavil) for 5 years. He is admitted to the hospital for elective surgery, after which he becomes acutely confused. The health care provider prescribes haloperidol (Haldol), as needed, to control severe agitation. You note in the drug reference text that both these medications have anticholinergic side effects.

✔ What important assessments are needed to detect anticholinergic effects?

✔ How are side effects of anticholinergic drugs especially significant for the elderly?

✔ How would you develop a plan to minimize or manage anticholinergic effects for this client?

## PROTOTYPE PROFILE

atropine, p. 312

# ANTICHOLINERGIC DRUGS

Anticholinergic drugs, also called cholinergic blocking and parasympatholytic agents, block the action of acetylcholine on the parasympathetic nervous system (PNS). The action of acetylcholine is detailed in the At the Foundation section of Chapter 18, and the PNS is further described here in At the Foundation: Parasympathetic Nervous System Effects. Most anticholinergic drugs interact with muscarinic cholinergic receptors in the brain, secretory glands, heart, and smooth muscle and are also called *antimuscarinic agents*. A few anticholinergic drugs, when given at high doses, are also able to block nicotinic receptors in autonomic ganglia and skeletal muscles. Glycopyrrolate (Robinul) is an example of such a medication. The prototype anticholinergic drug is ℗ atropine (see Prototype Profile 19-1: Atropine), and this drug class includes belladonna alkaloids, their derivatives, and many synthetic substitutes.

Most anticholinergic medications are either tertiary amines or quaternary amines in their chemical structure. Tertiary amines are uncharged lipid-soluble molecules. Atropine and scopolamine are tertiary amines and therefore are able to cross cell membranes readily. They are well absorbed from the gastrointestinal (GI) tract and conjunctiva, and they cross the blood–brain barrier. Tertiary amines are excreted in the urine. Some belladonna derivatives and synthetic anticholinergics are quaternary amines. These drugs carry a positive charge and are lipid insoluble. Consequently, they do not readily cross cell membranes. They are poorly absorbed from the GI tract and do not cross the blood–brain barrier. Quaternary amines are excreted largely in the feces and thus are better tolerated in clients with renal insufficiency. Table 19-1 lists common tertiary amine and quaternary amine anticholinergic drugs.

## Mechanism of Action and Effects

These drugs act by occupying receptor sites at parasympathetic nerve endings, thereby leaving fewer receptor sites free to respond to acetylcholine (Fig. 19-1). Parasympathetic response is absent or decreased, depending on the number of receptors blocked by anticholinergic drugs and the underlying degree of parasympathetic activity. Because cholinergic muscarinic receptors are widely distributed in the body, anticholinergic drugs produce effects in a variety of locations, including the central nervous system, heart, smooth muscle, glands, and eye.

Specific effects on body tissues and organs include the following:

1. **Central nervous system (CNS) stimulation followed by depression,** which may result in coma and death. This is most likely to occur with large doses of anticholinergic drugs that cross the blood–brain barrier (atropine, scopolamine, and antiparkinson agents).
2. **Decreased cardiovascular response to parasympathetic (vagal) stimulation that slows heart rate.** Atropine is the anticholinergic drug most often used for its cardiovascular effects. According to the advanced cardiac life support (ACLS) protocol (2000), atropine is the drug of choice to treat symptomatic sinus bradycardia. Low doses (<0.5 mg) may produce a slight and temporary decrease in heart rate; however,

---

**AT THE FOUNDATION:** *Parasympathetic Nervous System Effects*

Functions stimulated by the parasympathetic nervous system (PNS) are often described as resting, reparative, or vegetative functions. They include digestion, excretion, cardiac deceleration, anabolism, and near vision.

Approximately 75% of all parasympathetic nerve fibers are in the vagus nerves. These nerves supply the thoracic and abdominal organs; their branches go to the heart, lungs, esophagus, stomach, small intestine, proximal half of the colon, liver, gallbladder, pancreas, and upper portions of the ureters. Other parasympathetic fibers supply pupillary sphincters and circular muscles of the eye; lacrimal, nasal, submaxillary, and parotid glands; descending colon and rectum; lower portions of the ureters and bladder; and genitalia.

Specific body responses to parasympathetic stimulation include the following:

1. Dilation of blood vessels in the skin.
2. Release of nitrous oxide (NO) (previously called endothelium-derived relaxing factor [EDRF]) from the endothelium of blood vessels, resulting in decreased platelet aggregation, decreased inflammation, and relaxation of vascular endothelium and dilation of blood vessels.
3. Decreased heart rate, possibly bradycardia
4. Increased secretion of digestive enzymes and motility of the gastrointestinal tract
5. Constriction of smooth muscle of bronchi
6. Increased secretions from glands in the lungs, stomach, intestines, and skin (sweat glands)
7. Constricted pupils (from contraction of the circular muscle of the iris) and accommodation to near vision (from contraction of the ciliary muscle of the eye)
8. Contraction of smooth muscle in the urinary bladder
9. Contraction of skeletal muscle
10. No apparent effects on blood coagulation, blood sugar, mental activity, or muscle strength

These responses are regulated by acetylcholine, a neurotransmitter in the brain, autonomic nervous system, and neuromuscular junctions. Acetylcholine exerts excitatory effects at nerve synapses and nerve–muscle junctions and inhibitory effects at some peripheral sites, such as the heart.

## PROTOTYPE PROFILE 19-1

### P Atropine (AT ro peen)

**Drug Class**
*Chemical:* Anticholinergic (Antimuscarinic)
*Functional:* Antidysrhythmic

**Trade Name**
Atro-pen; as ophthalmic (Isopto-Atropine)

**Therapeutic Indications**
Treatment of bradycardia
Given to decrease oral and respiratory secretions; for reversal of muscarinic effects of anticholinesterase agents

**Pharmacokinetics**
*Absorption*
Well-absorbed

*Distribution*
Crosses placenta and enters breast milk; readily crosses blood–brain barrier

*Metabolism*
Primarily hepatic

*Excretion*
Urine

**Pharmacodynamics**
*Onset of Action*
PO, 30 min; IM, Sub-Q, rapid; IV, immediate

*Duration*
4–6 h

**Contraindications/Precautions**
Hypersensitivity, narrow-angle glaucoma, acute hemorrhage, tachycardia associated with thyrotoxicosis and cardiac insufficiency; with caution in chronic renal, cardiac, hepatic, and respiratory disease, pregnancy and lactation, prostatic hypertrophy

**Pregnancy Considerations**
Category C
Crosses placenta and enters breast milk

**Dosage**
Systemic use:
*Adults:* PO, IM, Sub-Q, IV, 0.4–0.6 mg.
*Children:* PO, IM, Sub-Q, IV:
7–16 lb: 0.1 mg

16–24 lb: 0.15 mg
24–40 lb: 0.2 mg
40–65 lb: 0.3 mg
65–90 lb: 0.4 mg
>90 lb: 0.4–0.6 mg
Surgery:
*Adults:* IM, Sub-Q, or IV, 0.4–0.6 mg before induction. Use 0.4 mg dose with cyclopropane anesthesia
*Children:* 0.1 mg (newborn) to 0.6 mg (12 y) given Sub-Q 30 min before surgery
Bradydysrhythmias:
*Adults:* IV, 0.4–1 mg (up to 2 mg) q1–2 h PRN
Antidote for cholinergic poisoning:
*Adults:* IV, titrate large doses of 2–3 mg as needed until signs of atropine toxicity appear and cholinergic crisis is controlled
Mydriatic/cycloplegia for refraction:
*Adults:* Instill 1–2 drops of 1% solution into eye 1 h before refraction
*Children:* Instill 1–2 drops of 0.5% solution bid for 1–3 days before procedure
For uveitis:
*Adults:* Instill 1–2 drops of 1% solution into eye qid

**Adverse Effects**
Tachycardia, palpitations, dry mouth (xerostomia), thickened respiratory secretions, constipation, blurred vision and photophobia, drowsiness, urinary hesitancy, and elevation in intraocular pressure (*physostigmine is the antidote*)

**Drug Interactions**
*Increased Effects*
Additive anticholinergic effects with antihistamines, tricyclic antidepressants, quinidine, phenothiazine antipsychotics, disopyramide, and other anticholinergic agents

*Decreased Effects*
Decreased motility and altered absorption of PO drugs
Decreased anticholinergic effects with antacids

**Herbal Supplements and Dietary Considerations**
Increased anticholinergic effects with scopolia, jimson weed, and angel's trumpet

moderate to large doses (0.5 to 1 mg) increase heart rate by blocking parasympathetic vagal stimulation. Although the increase in heart rate may be therapeutic in bradycardia, it can be an adverse effect in clients with other types of heart disease because atropine increases the myocardial oxygen demand. Atropine usually has little or no effect on blood pressure. Large doses cause facial flushing because of dilation of blood vessels in the neck.

3. **Bronchodilation and decreased respiratory tract secretions.** Bronchodilating effects result from blocking the bronchoconstrictive effects of acetylcholine. When anticholinergic drugs are given systemically, respiratory secretions decrease and may become viscous, resulting in mucus plugging of small respiratory passages. Administering the medications by inhalation decreases this effect while preserving the beneficial bronchodilation effect.

**TABLE 19-1 Common Tertiary Amine and Quaternary Amine Anticholinergic Drugs**

| Tertiary Amines | Quaternary Amines |
|---|---|
| Atropine | Glycopyrrolate (Robinul) |
| Benztropine (Cogentin) | Ipratropium (Atrovent) |
| Biperiden (Akineton) | Methscopolamine (Pamine) |
| Dicyclomine hydrochloride (Bentyl) | Propantheline bromide (Pro-Banthine) |
| Flavoxate (Urispas) | |
| *l*-Hyoscyamine (Anaspaz) | |
| Oxybutynin (Ditropan) | |
| Procyclidine (Kemadrin) | |
| Scopolamine | |
| Tolterodine (Detrol and Detrol LA) | |
| Trihexyphenidyl (Trihexy) | |

4. **Antispasmodic effects in the GI tract due to decreased muscle tone and motility.** The drugs have little inhibitory effect on gastric acid secretion with usual doses and insignificant effects on pancreatic and intestinal secretions.

5. **Mydriasis and cycloplegia in the eye.** Normally, anticholinergics do not change intraocular pressure, but with narrow-angle glaucoma, they may increase intraocular pressure and precipitate an episode of acute glaucoma. When the pupil is fully dilated, photophobia may be bothersome, and reflexes to light and accommodation may disappear.

6. **Miscellaneous effects** include decreased secretions from salivary and sweat glands; relaxation of ureters,

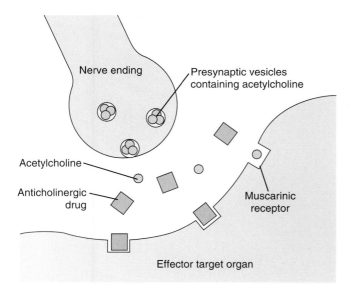

**FIGURE 19–1** Mechanism of action of anticholinergic drugs. Anticholinergic (antimuscarinic) blocking agents prevent acetylcholine from interacting with muscarinic receptors on target effector organs, thus blocking or decreasing a parasympathetic response in these organs.

urinary bladder, and the detrusor muscle; and relaxation of smooth muscle in the gallbladder and bile ducts.

The clinical usefulness of anticholinergic drugs is limited by their widespread effects. Consequently, several synthetic drugs have been developed in an effort to increase selectivity of action on particular body tissues, especially to retain the antispasmodic and antisecretory effects of atropine while eliminating its adverse effects. This effort has been less than successful—all the synthetic drugs produce atropine-like adverse effects when given in sufficient dosage.

One group of synthetic drugs is used for antispasmodic effects in GI disorders. Another group of synthetic drugs includes centrally active anticholinergics used in the treatment of Parkinson's disease (see Chap. 12). They balance the relative cholinergic dominance that causes the movement disorders associated with parkinsonism.

## Indications for Use

Anticholinergic drugs are used for disorders in many body systems. Clinical indications for use of anticholinergic drugs include GI, genitourinary, ophthalmic and respiratory disorders, bradycardia, and Parkinson's disease. They also are used before surgery and bronchoscopy. Drugs at a Glance: Selected Anticholinergic Drugs describes the therapeutic use, dosage, and route of administration of selected anticholinergic medications. Anticholinergic medications are commonly used in home care with children and adults (see Home Care Considerations). Children and older adults are probably most likely to experience adverse effects of these drugs and should be monitored carefully. Guidelines for ongoing evaluation and intervention are addressed in Age-related Considerations.

■ **GI disorders** in which anticholinergics have been used include peptic ulcer disease, gastritis, pylorospasm, diverticulitis, ileitis, and ulcerative colitis. These conditions are often characterized by excessive gastric acid and abdominal pain because of increased motility and spasm of GI smooth muscle. In peptic ulcer disease, more effective drugs have been developed, and anticholinergics are rarely used. The drugs are weak inhibitors of gastric acid secretion even in maximal doses (which usually produce intolerable adverse effects). Although they do not heal peptic ulcers, they may relieve abdominal pain by relaxing GI smooth muscle. Anticholinergics may be helpful in treating irritable colon or colitis, but they may be contraindicated in chronic inflammatory disorders (eg, diverticulitis, ulcerative colitis) or acute intestinal infections (eg, bacterial, viral, amebic). Other drugs are used to decrease diarrhea and intestinal motility in these conditions.

■ In **genitourinary disorders,** anticholinergic drugs may be given for their antispasmodic effects on smooth

**DRUG TABLE 19-1**

_Drugs at a Glance_

## Selected Anticholinergic Drugs

| Generic/Trade Name | Routes and Dosage Ranges | Comments |
|---|---|---|
| **Belladonna Alkaloids and Derivatives** | | |
| **Atropine** | See Prototype Profile 19-1: Atropine | |
| **Homatropine** (Homapin)<br>Pregnancy Category C | Mydriatic/cycloplegia for refraction:<br>_Adults:_ Instill 1–2 drops of 2% solution or 1 drop 5% solution into eye before procedure. May repeat at 5–10 min intervals as needed.<br>_Children:_ Instill 1 drop of 2% solution into eye before procedure. May repeat q10min as needed<br>For uveitis: _Adults:_ Instill 1–2 drops of 2% or 5% solution bid to tid or q3–4h as needed<br>_Children:_ Instill 1 drop of 2% solution bid to tid | Produces mydriasis and cycloplegia for refraction and for treatment of infections of the uveal tract; protect drug from light |
| **Hyoscyamine** (Anaspaz)<br>Pregnancy Category C | Antispasmodic antisecretory for GI and GU disorders: _Adults:_ PO, SL, 0.125–0.25 mg tid or qid, before meals and at bedtime; PO (timed release formula), 0.375–0.75 q12h.<br>IM, IV, Sub-Q, 0.25–0.5 mg q6h<br>_Children:_ 2–10 y: PO, 0.062–0.125 mg q6–8h. Children <2 y: Half the previous dose | Observe for tachycardia with administration; do not chew or crush extended release forms |
| **Ipratropium** (Atrovent)<br>Pregnancy Category B | Bronchodilation: _Adults:_ 2 puffs (36 mcg) of aerosol qid. Additional inhalations may be needed. Do not exceed 12 puffs/24 h. Solution for inhalation: 500 mcg, tid to qid.<br>Nasal spray for rhinorrhea:<br>_Adults:_ 2 sprays/nostril of 0.03% spray bid to tid.<br>2 sprays/nostril of 0.06% spray tid to qid<br>_Children:_ 2 sprays/nostril of 0.03% spray bid to tid. | Educate client on use of inhaler, particularly the importance of shaking inhaler before use |
| **Scopolamine**<br>Pregnancy Category C | Systemic use: _Adults:_ PO, 0.4–0.8 mg qd<br>Sub-Q, IM, 0.32–0.65 mg<br>IV, 0.32–0.65 mg diluted in sterile water for injection.<br>_Children:_ Not approved for PO use <6 y<br>Parenteral: 0.006mg/kg. Max dose: 0.3 mg<br>Antiemetic:<br>_Adults:_ Transdermal, Apply disc 4 h before antiemetic effect is needed. Replace q3d<br>Mydriatic/cycloplegia for refraction:<br>_Adults and children:_ Instill 1–2 drops into eye 1 h before refracting. For uveitis: Instill 1–2 drops into eye up to tid | Wash hands before or after administering; avoid contact of drug with eyes |

_(continued)_

**DRUG TABLE 19-1**

*Drugs at a Glance*

## Selected Anticholinergic Drugs (Continued)

| Generic/Trade Name | Routes and Dosage Ranges | Comments |
|---|---|---|
| **Antisecretory and Antispasmodic Anticholinergics for GI Disorders** | | |
| **Dicyclomine** (Bentyl) Pregnancy Category B | Antisecretory and antispasmodic: *Adults:* PO, 20–40 mg before meals and at bedtime IM, 20 mg before meals and at bedtime | Overdose may cause curare-like effects, such as respiratory paralysis |
| **Glycopyrrolate** (Robinul) Pregnancy Category B | Antisecretory and antispasmodic: *Adults:* PO, 1–2 mg bid to tid IM, IV, 0.1–0.2 mg *Children:* Not recommended <12 y Preanesthetic: *Adults:* IM, 0.004 mg/kg 30–60 min before anesthesia Children <2 y: 0.004 mg/lb IM, 30–60 min before anesthesia 2–12 y: 0.002–0.004 mg/lb IM 30–60 min before anesthesia | Monitor heart rate |
| **Propantheline bromide** (Pro-Banthine) Pregnancy Category C | PO, 7.5–15 mg 30 min before meals and at bedtime | Should increase fluid and fiber intake to minimize constipation as an adverse effect |
| **Anticholinergics Used in Parkinson's Disease** | | |
| **Benztropine** (Cogentin) Pregnancy Category C | Parkinsonism: *Adults:* PO, IM, IV, 0.5–1 mg at bedtime. May increase up to 6 mg given at bedtime or in 2–4 divided doses Drug-induced extrapyramidal symptoms: *Adults:* For acute dystonia: IM, IV, 1–2 mg. May repeat if needed. For prevention: PO, 1–2 mg | Administer after meals or with food if GI upset occurs; do not discontinue abruptly; may cause drowsiness; alcohol may increase CNS depression |
| **Biperiden** (Akineton) Pregnancy Category C | Parkinsonism: *Adults:* PO, 2 mg tid to qid. Drug-induced extrapyramidal symptoms *Adults:* Max dose 16 mg/d. PO, 2 mg tid to qid IM, IV, 2 mg. Repeat q12h until symptoms are resolved. Do not give more than 4 doses/24 h | May cause drowsiness; alcohol may increase CNS depression |
| **Procyclidine** (Kemadrin) Pregnancy Category C | Parkinsonism: *Adults:* PO, 2.5 mg tid after meals. May increase to 5 mg tid Drug-induced extrapyramidal symptoms: *Adults:* PO, 2.5 mg tid. Increase by 2.5 mg increments until symptoms are resolved. Usual maximum dose 10–20 mg/d | Do not discontinue drug abruptly; should be taken after meals to decrease GI upset |
| **Trihexyphenidyl** (Trihexy) Pregnancy Category C | *Adults:* PO, 1–2 mg. Increase by 2 mg increments at 3–5 d intervals until a total of 6–10 mg is given qd in divided doses 3–4 times daily at mealtimes and bedtime PO, 1 mg initially. Increase as needed to control symptoms | Alcohol may increase CNS depression |

*(continued)*

**DRUG TABLE 19-1**

*Drugs at a Glance*

**Selected Anticholinergic Drugs** (Continued)

| Generic/Trade Name | Routes and Dosage Ranges | Comments |
|---|---|---|
| **Urinary Antispasmodics** | | |
| **Flavoxate** (Urispas)<br>Pregnancy Category B | *Adults:* PO, 100–200 mg tid to qid. Reduce when symptoms improve<br>*Children:* <12 y: Safety and efficacy not established | Relief of dysuria, urgency, nocturia |
| **Oxybutynin** (Ditropan and Ditropan XL)<br>Pregnancy Category B | *Adults:* PO, 5 mg bid or tid. Maximum dose, 5 mg qid. Extended release: 5 mg PO qd up to 30 mg/d<br>*Children:* >5 y: 5 mg PO bid. Maximum dose 5 mg tid | Should be taken on an empty stomach with water; may cause drowsiness; do not crush or chew sustained-release forms |
| **Tolterodine** (Detrol and Detrol LA)<br>Pregnancy Category C | *Adults:* PO, 2 mg bid. May decrease to 1 mg when symptoms improve. Reduce doses to 1mg PO bid in presence of hepatic impairment<br>*Children:* Safety and efficacy not established | Treatment of overactive bladder; do not crush or chew sustained release forms |

muscle to relieve the symptoms of urinary incontinence and frequency that accompany an overactive bladder. In infections such as cystitis, urethritis, and prostatitis, the drugs decrease the frequency and pain of urination. The drugs are also given to increase bladder capacity in enuresis, paraplegia, or neurogenic bladder.

■ In **ophthalmology,** anticholinergic drugs are applied topically for mydriatic and cycloplegic effects to aid examination or surgery. They are also used to treat some inflammatory disorders. Anticholinergic prepa-rations used in ophthalmology are discussed further in Appendix G.

■ In **respiratory disorders** characterized by broncho-constriction (ie, asthma, chronic bronchitis), ipra-tropium (Atrovent) may be given by inhalation for bronchodilating effects (see Chap. 47).

■ In **cardiology,** atropine may be given to increase heart rate in bradycardia and heart block characterized by hypotension and shock.

■ In **Parkinson's disease,** anticholinergic drugs are given for their central effects in decreasing salivation, spas-ticity, and tremors. They are used mainly in clients who have minimal symptoms, who do not respond to levodopa, or who cannot tolerate levodopa because of adverse reactions or contraindications. An additional use of anticholinergic drugs is to relieve Parkinson's disease–like symptoms that occur with older anti-psychotic drugs.

■ **Before surgery,** anticholinergics are given to prevent vagal stimulation and potential bradycardia, hypoten-sion, and cardiac arrest. They are also given to reduce respiratory tract secretions, especially in head and neck surgery and bronchoscopy.

## Home Care Considerations: Use of Anticholinergic Drugs

**ASSESS:** the client and family's knowledge of drug therapy; the client for compliance with the prescribed regimen; for urinary hesitancy and retention (adverse effects of anti-cholinergics) in males with benign prostatic hypertrophy.

**MONITOR:** the therapeutic and adverse effects of the drugs and the client's need for additional information, and provide that information; that client is keeping appointments for follow-up care.

**EDUCATE:** regarding the importance of consulting the health care provider before taking OTC products, not to exceed recommended dosages and taking exactly as directed (do not take double doses); that sugarless gum or candy, oral rinses, and frequent oral hygiene may help relieve dry mouth; that changes in urinary stream should be reported to the health care provider. Reinforce addi-tional teaching points (see Client Teaching Guidelines: Anticholinergic Drugs).

## Contraindications to Use

Contraindications to the use of anticholinergic drugs include any condition characterized by symptoms that would be aggravated by the drugs. Some of these are prostatic hypertrophy, myasthenia gravis, hyperthy-roidism, glaucoma, tachydysrhythmias, myocardial infarc-tion, and heart failure unless bradycardia is present. They should not be given in hiatal hernia or other conditions

## Age-related Considerations: Use of Anticholinergic Drugs

### USE IN CHILDREN

Systemic anticholinergics, including atropine, glycopyrrolate (Robinul), and scopolamine, are given to children of all ages for essentially the same effects as for adults. Most of the antisecretory, antispasmodic agents for gastrointestinal disorders are not recommended for children. With the urinary antispasmodics, flavoxate is not recommended for children younger than 12 years, oxybutynin is not recommended for children younger than 5 years of age, and the safety and efficacy of tolterodine are not established in children.

The drugs cause the same adverse effects in children as in adults. However, they may be more severe because children are especially sensitive to the drugs. Facial flushing is common in children, and a skin rash may occur.

Ophthalmic anticholinergic drugs are used for cycloplegia and mydriasis before eye examinations and surgical procedures (see Appendix G). They should be used only with close medical supervision. Cyclopentolate (Cyclogyl) and tropicamide (Mydriacyl) have been associated with behavioral disturbances and psychotic reactions in children. Tropicamide has also been associated with cardiopulmonary collapse.

### USE IN OLDER ADULTS

Anticholinergic drugs are given for the same purposes as in younger adults. In addition to the primary anticholinergic drugs, many others that are commonly prescribed for older adults have high anticholinergic activity. These include many antihistamines (histamine-1 receptor antagonists), tricyclic antidepressants, and antipsychotic drugs.

Older adults are especially likely to have significant adverse reactions because of slowed drug metabolism and the frequent presence of several disease processes. Some common adverse effects and suggestions for reducing their impact are as follows:

- **Blurred vision.** The client may need help with ambulation, especially with stairs or other potentially hazardous environments. Remove obstacles and hazards when possible.

- **Confusion.** Provide whatever assistance is needed to prevent falls and other injuries.

- **Heat stroke.** Help to avoid precipitating factors, such as strenuous activity and high environmental temperatures.

- **Constipation.** Encourage or assist with an adequate intake of high-fiber foods and fluids and adequate exercise when feasible.

- **Urinary retention.** Encourage adequate fluid intake and avoid high doses of the drugs. Men should be examined for prostatic hypertrophy.

- **Hallucinations and other psychotic symptoms.** These are most likely to occur with the centrally active anticholinergics given for Parkinson's disease or drug-induced extrapyramidal effects, such as trihexyphenidyl or benztropine. Dosage of these drugs should be carefully regulated and supervised.

---

contributing to reflux esophagitis because the drugs delay gastric emptying, relax the cardioesophageal sphincter, and increase esophageal reflux.

## INDIVIDUAL ANTICHOLINERGIC DRUGS

### Belladonna Alkaloids and Derivatives

**Atropine,** the prototype of anticholinergic drugs, produces the same effects, has the same clinical indications for use, and has the same contraindications as those described earlier. In addition, it is used as an antidote for an overdose of cholinergic drugs and exposure to insecticides that have cholinergic effects.

Atropine is a naturally occurring belladonna alkaloid that can be extracted from the belladonna plant or prepared synthetically. It is usually prepared as atropine sulfate, a salt that is very soluble in water. It is well absorbed from the GI tract and distributed throughout the body. It crosses the blood–brain barrier to enter the CNS, where large doses produce stimulant effects and toxic doses produce depressant effects. Atropine is also absorbed systemically when applied locally to mucous membranes. The drug is rapidly excreted in the urine. Pharmacologic effects are of short duration, except for ocular effects, which may last for several days.

**Belladonna tincture** is a mixture of alkaloids in an aqueous-alcohol solution. It is most often used in GI disorders for antispasmodic effect. It is an ingredient in several drug mixtures.

**Homatropine hydrobromide** (Homapin) is a semisynthetic derivative of atropine used as eye drops to produce mydriasis and cycloplegia. Homatropine may be preferable to atropine because the ocular effects do not last as long.

**Hyoscyamine** (Anaspaz) is a belladonna alkaloid used in GI and genitourinary disorders characterized by spasm, increased secretion, and increased motility. It has the same effects as other atropine-like drugs.

**Ipratropium** (Atrovent) is an anticholinergic drug chemically related to atropine. When given as a nasal spray, it is useful in treating rhinorrhea due to allergy or the common cold. When given as an inhalation treatment or aerosol to clients with chronic obstructive pulmonary disease (COPD), it is beneficial as a bronchodilator. An advantage of administration of anticholinergic drugs by the respiratory route over systemic administration is less thickening of respiratory secretions and reduced incidence of mucus-plugged airways.

**Scopolamine** is similar to atropine in uses, adverse effects, and peripheral effects but different in central effects. When given parenterally, scopolamine depresses the CNS and causes amnesia, drowsiness, euphoria, relaxation, and sleep. Effects of scopolamine appear more quickly and disappear more readily than those of atropine. Scopolamine also is used in motion sickness. It is available as oral tablets and as a transdermal adhesive disc that is placed behind the ear. The disc (Transderm-V) protects against motion sickness for 72 hours.

## Centrally Acting Anticholinergics Used in Parkinson's Disease

Older anticholinergic drugs such as atropine are rarely used to treat Parkinson's disease because of their undesirable peripheral effects (eg, dry mouth, blurred vision, photophobia, constipation, urinary retention, and tachycardia). Newer, centrally acting synthetic anticholinergic drugs are more selective for muscarinic receptors in the CNS and are designed to produce fewer side effects.

**Trihexyphenidyl** (Trihexy) is used in the treatment of parkinsonism and extrapyramidal reactions caused by some antipsychotic drugs. Trihexyphenidyl relieves smooth muscle spasm by a direct action on the muscle and by inhibiting the PNS. The drug supposedly has fewer side effects than atropine, but approximately half the recipients report mouth dryness, blurring of vision, and other side effects common to anticholinergic drugs. Trihexyphenidyl requires the same precautions as other anticholinergic drugs and is contraindicated in glaucoma. **Biperiden** (Akineton) and **procyclidine** (Kemadrin) are chemical derivatives of trihexyphenidyl and have similar actions.

**Benztropine** (Cogentin) is a synthetic drug with both anticholinergic and antihistaminic effects. Its anticholinergic activity approximates that of atropine. A major clinical use is to treat acute dystonic reactions caused by antipsychotic drugs and to prevent their recurrence in clients receiving long-term antipsychotic drug therapy. It also may be given in small doses to supplement other antiparkinson drugs. In full dosage, adverse reactions are common.

## Urinary Antispasmodics

**Flavoxate** (Urispas) was developed specifically to counteract spasm in smooth muscle tissue of the urinary tract. It has anticholinergic, local anesthetic, and analgesic effects. Thus, the drug relieves dysuria, urgency, frequency, and pain with genitourinary infections, such as cystitis and prostatitis.

**Oxybutynin** (Ditropan and Ditropan XL) has direct antispasmodic effects on smooth muscle and anticholinergic effects. It increases bladder capacity and decreases frequency of voiding in clients with neurogenic bladder. Oxybutynin is now available in an extended release form for once-a-day dosing.

**Tolterodine** (Detrol and Detrol LA) is a competitive antimuscarinic, anticholinergic agent that inhibits bladder contraction, decreases detrusor muscle pressure, and delays the urge to void. It is used to treat urinary frequency, urgency, and urge incontinence. Tolterodine is more selective for muscarinic receptors in the urinary bladder than other areas of the body, such as the salivary glands, and therefore anticholinergic side effects are less marked. Reduced doses (of 1 mg) are recommended for those with hepatic dysfunction. Tolterodine is also available in an extended-release form.

## ■ USE IN SPECIFIC CONDITIONS

### Renal or Biliary Colic

Atropine is sometimes given with morphine or meperidine to relieve the severe pain of renal or biliary colic. It acts mainly to decrease the spasm-producing effects of the opioid analgesics. It has little antispasmodic effect on the involved muscles and is not used alone for this purpose.

### Preoperative Use in Clients With Glaucoma

Glaucoma is usually listed as a contraindication to anticholinergic drugs because the drugs impair outflow of aqueous humor and may cause an acute attack of glaucoma (increased intraocular pressure). However, anticholinergic drugs can be given safely before surgery to clients with open-angle glaucoma (80% of clients with primary glaucoma) if they are receiving miotic drugs, such as pilocarpine. If anticholinergic preoperative medication is needed in clients predisposed to angle closure, the hazard of causing acute glaucoma can be minimized by also giving pilocarpine eye drops and acetazolamide (Diamox).

### Gastrointestinal Disorders

When anticholinergic drugs are given for GI disorders, larger doses may be given at bedtime to prevent pain and awakening during sleep.

---

**?** **How Can You Avoid This Medication Error?**

Sam Miller is admitted for elective surgery. He has a history of heart disease, glaucoma, and benign prostatic hyperplasia (BPH). After surgery, a scopolamine patch is prescribed to control nausea. You administer the patch, as ordered, placing it on his chest in a nonhairy area.

## NURSING PROCESS

### Assessment

- Assess the client's condition in relation to disorders for which anticholinergic drugs are used (ie, check for bradycardia or heart block, diarrhea, dysuria, abdominal pain, and other disorders). If the client reports or medical records indicate a specific disorder, assess for signs and symptoms of that disorder (eg, Parkinson's disease).
- Assess for disorders in which anticholinergic drugs are contraindicated (eg, glaucoma, prostatic hypertrophy, reflux esophagitis, myasthenia gravis, hyperthyroidism).
- Assess use of other drugs with anticholinergic effects, such as antihistamines (histamine-1 receptor antagonists [see Chap. 48]), antipsychotic agents, and tricyclic antidepressants.

### Nursing Diagnoses

- Impaired Urinary Elimination: Decreased bladder tone and urine retention
- Constipation related to slowed GI function
- Disturbed Thought Processes: Confusion, disorientation, especially in older adults
- Deficient Knowledge: Drug effects and accurate usage
- Risk for Injury related to drug-induced blurred vision and photophobia
- Risk for Noncompliance related to adverse drug effects
- Risk for Altered Body Temperature: Hyperthermia

### Planning/Goals

*The client will:*
- Receive or self-administer the drugs correctly
- Experience relief of symptoms for which anticholinergic drugs are given
- Be assisted to avoid or cope with adverse drug effects on vision, thought processes, bowel and bladder elimination, and heat dissipation

### Interventions

Use measures to decrease the need for anticholinergic drugs. For example, with peptic ulcer disease, teach the client to avoid factors known to increase gastric secretion and GI motility (alcohol; cigarette smoking; caffeine-containing beverages, such as coffee, tea, and cola drinks; ulcerogenic drugs, such as aspirin). Late evening snacks also should be avoided because increased gastric acid secretion occurs approximately 90 minutes after eating and may cause pain and awakening from sleep. Although milk was once considered an "ulcer food," it contains protein and calcium, which promote acid secretion, and is a poor buffer of gastric acid. Thus, drinking large amounts of milk should be avoided.

### Evaluation

- Interview and observe in relation to safe, accurate drug administration.
- Interview and observe for relief of symptoms for which the drugs are given.
- Interview and observe for adverse drug effects.

## Parkinsonism

When these drugs are used in parkinsonism, small doses are given initially and gradually increased. This regimen decreases adverse reactions.

## Extrapyramidal Reactions

When used in drug-induced extrapyramidal reactions (parkinsonism-like symptoms), these drugs should be prescribed only if symptoms occur. They should not be used routinely to prevent extrapyramidal reactions because fewer than half the clients taking antipsychotic drugs experience such reactions. Most drug-induced reactions last approximately 3 months and do not recur if anticholinergic drugs are discontinued at that time. (An exception is tardive dyskinesia, which does not respond to anticholinergic drugs and may be aggravated by them.)

## Muscarinic Agonist Poisoning

Atropine is the antidote for poisoning by muscarinic agonists such as certain species of mushrooms, cholinergic agonist drugs, cholinesterase inhibitor drugs, and insecticides containing organophosphates. Symptoms of muscarinic poisoning include salivation, lacrimation, visual disturbances, bronchospasm, diarrhea, bradycardia, and hypotension. Atropine blocks the poison from interacting with the muscarinic receptor, thus reversing the toxic effects.

## Asthma

Oral anticholinergics are not used to treat asthma and other COPDs because of their tendency to thicken secretions and form mucus plugs in airways. Ipratropium (Atrovent) may be given by inhalation to produce bronchodilation without thickening of respiratory secretions.

## Toxicity of Anticholinergics: Recognition and Management

Overdosage of atropine or other anticholinergic drugs produces the usual pharmacologic effects in a severe and exaggerated form. The anticholinergic overdose syndrome is characterized by hyperthermia; hot, dry, flushed skin; dry mouth; mydriasis; delirium; tachycardia; ileus; and urinary retention. Myoclonic movements and choreoathetosis may be seen. Seizures, coma, and respiratory arrest may also occur. Treatment involves use of activated charcoal to absorb ingested poison. Hemodialysis, hemoper-

## CLIENT TEACHING GUIDELINES
### Anticholinergic Drugs

**General Considerations**

✔ Do not take other drugs without the health care provider's knowledge. In addition to some prescribed antiparkinson drugs, antidepressants, antihistamines, and antipsychotic drugs with anticholinergic properties, over-the-counter sleeping pills and antihistamines have anticholinergic effects. Taking any of these concurrently could cause overdosage or excessive anticholinergic effects.

✔ Use measures to minimize risks of heat exhaustion and heat stroke:

   ✔ Wear light, cool clothing in warm climates or environments.
   ✔ Maintain fluid and salt intake if not contraindicated.
   ✔ Limit exposure to direct sunlight.
   ✔ Limit physical activity.
   ✔ Take frequent cool baths.
   ✔ Ensure adequate ventilation, with fans or air conditioners if necessary.
   ✔ Avoid alcoholic beverages.

✔ Use sugarless chewing gum and hard candy, if not contraindicated, to relieve mouth dryness.

✔ Carry out good dental hygiene practices (eg, regular brushing of teeth) to prevent dental caries and loss of teeth that may result from drug-induced xerostomia (dry mouth from decreased saliva production). This is more likely to occur with long-term use of these drugs.

✔ To prevent injury due to blurring of vision or drowsiness, avoid potentially hazardous activities (eg, driving or operating machinery).

✔ To reduce sensitivity to light (photophobia), dark glasses can be worn outdoors in strong light.

✔ Contact lens wearers who experience dry eyes may need to use an ophthalmic lubricating solution.

✔ When using anticholinergic ophthalmic preparations, if eye pain occurs, stop using the medication and contact your physician or health care provider. This may be a warning sign of undiagnosed glaucoma.

✔ Notify your physician or health care provider if urinary retention or constipation occurs.

✔ Tell your physician or health care provider if you are pregnant or breast-feeding or allergic to sulfite preservatives or any other atropine compound.

**Self-administration**

✔ Take anticholinergic drugs for gastrointestinal disorders 30 minutes before meals and at bedtime.

✔ Safeguard anticholinergic medications from children because they are especially sensitive to atropine poisoning.

✔ To prevent constipation, use a diet high in fiber. Include whole grains, fruits, and vegetables in your daily menu. Also, drink 2 to 3 quarts of fluid a day and exercise regularly.

---

fusion, peritoneal dialysis, and repeated doses of charcoal are not effective in removing anticholinergic agents.

Physostigmine salicylate (Antilirium), an acetylcholinesterase inhibitor, is a specific antidote. It is usually given intravenously at a slow rate of injection. Adult dosage is 2 mg (no more than 1 mg/minute); child dosage is 0.5 to 1 mg (no more than 0.5 mg/minute). Rapid administration may cause bradycardia, hypersalivation (with subsequent respiratory distress), and seizures. Repeated doses may be given if life-threatening dysrhythmias, convulsions, or coma occur. Diazepam (Valium) or a similar drug may be given for excessive CNS stimulation (delirium, excitement). Ice bags, cooling blankets, and tepid sponge baths may help reduce fever. Artificial ventilation and cardiopulmonary resuscitative measures are used if excessive depression of the CNS causes coma and respiratory failure. Infants, children, and the elderly are especially susceptible to the toxic effects of anticholinergic agents.

## Abuse of Anticholinergic Agents

Anticholinergic drugs have potential intoxicating effects. Abuse of these drugs may produce euphoria, disorientation, hallucinations, and paranoia in addition to the classic anticholinergic adverse reactions.

---

## Nursing Actions
## Anticholinergic Drugs

| Nursing Actions | Rationale/Explanation |
|---|---|
| 1. Administer accurately. | |
| a. For gastrointestinal disorders, give most oral anticholinergic drugs approximately 30 min before meals and at bedtime. | To allow the drugs to reach peak antisecretory effects by the time ingested food is stimulating gastric acid secretion. Bedtime administration helps prevent awakening with abdominal pain. |

*(continued)*

## Nursing Actions

### Anticholinergic Drugs (Continued)

| Nursing Actions | Rationale/Explanation |
|---|---|
| b. When given before surgery, parenteral preparations of atropine can be mixed in the same syringe with several other common preoperative medications, such as meperidine (Demerol), morphine, oxymorphone (Numorphan), and promethazine (Phenergan). | The primary reason for mixing medications in the same syringe is to decrease the number of injections and thus decrease client discomfort. Note, however, that extra caution is required when mixing drugs to be sure that the dosage of each drug is accurate. Also, if any question exists regarding compatibility with another drug, it is safer not to mix the drugs, even if two or three injections are required. |
| c. When applying topical atropine solutions or ointment to the eye, be sure to use the correct concentration and blot any excess from the inner canthus. | Atropine ophthalmic preparations are available in several concentrations (usually 1%, 2%, and 3%). Excess medication should be removed so the drug will not enter the nasolacrimal (tear) ducts and be absorbed systemically through the mucous membrane of the nasopharynx or be carried to the throat and swallowed. |
| d. If propantheline is to be given intravenously, dissolve the 30-mg dose of powder in no less than 10 mL of sterile water for injection. | Parenteral administration is reserved for clients who cannot take the drug orally. |
| e. Instruct clients to swallow oral propantheline tablets, not to chew them. | The tablets have a hard sugar coating to mask the bitter taste of the drug. |
| f. Parenteral glycopyrrolate can be given through the tubing of a running intravenous infusion of physiologic saline or lactated Ringer's solution. | |
| g. Do not crush extended-release forms of anticholinergic drugs such as Detrol LA and Ditropan XL. | Crushing long-acting medications may result in high blood levels of the medication and increased adverse effects. |
| 2. Observe for therapeutic effects. | Therapeutic effects depend primarily on the reason for use. Thus, a therapeutic effect in one condition may be a side effect or an adverse reaction in another condition. |
| a. When a drug is given for *peptic ulcer disease* or other gastrointestinal disorders, observe for decreased abdominal pain. | Relief of abdominal pain is due to the smooth muscle relaxant or antispasmodic effect of the drug. |
| b. When the drug is given for *diagnosing or treating eye disorders,* observe for pupil dilation (mydriasis) and blurring of vision (cycloplegia). | Note that these ocular effects are side effects when the drugs are given for problems not related to the eyes. |
| c. When the drug is given for *symptomatic bradycardia,* observe for increased pulse rate. | These drugs increase heart rate by blocking action of the vagus nerve. |
| d. When the drug is given for *urinary tract disorders,* such as cystitis or enuresis, observe for decreased frequency of urination. When the drug is given for renal colic due to stones, observe for decreased pain. | Anticholinergic drugs decrease muscle tone and spasm in the smooth muscle of the ureters and urinary bladder. |
| e. When the centrally acting anticholinergics are given for *Parkinson's disease,* observe for decrease in tremor, salivation, and drooling. | Decreased salivation is a therapeutic effect with parkinsonism but an adverse reaction in most other conditions. |
| 3. Observe for adverse effects.<br>a. Tachycardia | These depend on reasons for use and are dose related. Tachycardia may occur with usual therapeutic doses because anticholinergic drugs block vagal action, which normally slows heart rate. Tachycardia is not likely to be serious except in clients with underlying heart disease. For example, in clients with angina pectoris, prolonged or severe tachycardia may increase myocardial ischemia to the point of causing an acute attack of angina (chest pain) or even myocardial infarction. In clients with congestive heart failure, severe or prolonged tachycardia can increase the workload of the heart to the point of causing acute heart failure or pulmonary edema. |

*(continued)*

## Nursing Actions

## Anticholinergic Drugs (Continued)

| Nursing Actions | Rationale/Explanation |
|---|---|
| b. Excessive central nervous system (CNS) stimulation (tremor, restlessness, confusion, hallucinations, delirium) followed by excessive CNS depression (coma, respiratory depression) | These effects are more likely to occur with large doses of atropine because atropine crosses the blood–brain barrier. Large doses of trihexyphenidyl (Trihexy) also may cause CNS stimulation. |
| c. Sedation and amnesia with scopolamine or benztropine (Cogentin) | This may be a therapeutic effect but becomes an adverse reaction if severe or if the drug is given for another purpose. Benztropine has anticholinergic and antihistaminic properties. Apparently, drowsiness and sedation are caused by the antihistaminic component. |
| d. Constipation or paralytic ileus | These effects are the result of decreased gastrointestinal motility and muscle tone. Constipation is more likely with large doses or parenteral administration. Paralytic ileus is not likely unless the drugs are given to clients who already have decreased gastrointestinal motility. |
| e. Decreased oral and respiratory tract secretions, which cause mouth dryness and thick respiratory secretions | Mouth dryness is more annoying than serious in most cases and is caused by decreased salivation. However, clients with chronic lung disease, who usually have excessive secretions, tend to retain them with the consequence of frequent respiratory tract infections. |
| f. Urinary retention | This reaction is caused by loss of bladder tone and is most likely to occur in elderly men with enlarged prostate glands. Thus, the drugs are usually contraindicated with prostatic hypertrophy. |
| g. Hot, dry skin; fever; heat stroke | These effects are due to decreased sweating and impairment of the normal heat loss mechanism. Fever may occur with any age group. Heat stroke is more likely to occur with cardiovascular disease, strenuous physical activity, and high environmental temperatures, especially in elderly people. |
| h. Ocular effects—mydriasis, blurred vision, photophobia | These are adverse effects when anticholinergic drugs are given for conditions not related to the eyes. |
| 4. Observe for drug interactions.<br>a. Drugs that *increase* effects of anticholinergic drugs: Antihistamines, disopyramide, phenothiazines, thioxanthene agents, tricyclic antidepressants and amantadine | These drugs have anticholinergic properties and produce additive anticholinergic effects. |
| b. Drugs that *decrease* effects of anticholinergic drugs: Cholinergic drugs | These drugs counteract the inhibition of gastrointestinal motility and tone induced by atropine. They are sometimes used in atropine overdose. |

## ? How Can You Avoid This Medication Error?

**Answer:** To prevent possible complications, more information must be obtained from Mr. Miller before the scopolamine patch can be safely administered. If Mr. Miller has closed-angle glaucoma, administering an anticholinergic agent could result in a significant rise in intraocular pressure and visual impairment. If it cannot be determined whether Mr. Miller has open-angle or closed-angle glaucoma, the drug should be held. Anticholinergic medications should be used cautiously with clients who have BPH because these drugs can cause urinary retention. Anticholinergic medications increase heart rate, which may not be advisable for many clients with heart disease.

## Critical Thinking Exercises

1. Ipratropium (Atrovent) is an anticholinergic drug useful in treating rhinorrhea due to allergy or the common cold when given as a nasal spray. An advantage of the administration of anticholinergic drugs by the respiratory route over systemic administration is:
   a. Increased thickening of respiratory secretions
   b. Reduced incidence of mucus-plugged airways
   c. Prevention of adverse effects
   d. Decreased risk for reflux esophagitis

**2.** An anticholinergic drug used to treat acute dystonic reactions caused by antipsychotic drugs and to prevent their recurrence in clients receiving long-term antipsychotic drug therapy is:

a. Biperiden (Akineton)
b. Procyclidine (Kemadrin)
c. Benztropine (Cogentin)
d. Flavoxate (Urispas)

**3.** A client receives atropine as a preanesthetic agent. What is the purpose of administering the drug to this client?

a. Reduce excessive gastric secretions and saliva
b. Decrease the risk for postoperative ileus
c. Reduce urinary retention postoperatively
d. Decrease the incidence of tachycardia on induction of anesthesia

**4.** A client complains of constipation during propantheline bromide (Pro-Banthine) therapy. The nurse should instruct the client to:

a. Increase milk intake
b. Avoid eating fresh fruits
c. Stop taking the drug and notify the health care provider
d. Increase fiber and fluid intake

**5.** A client manifests signs of anticholinergic overdose syndrome and is hyperthermic, delirious, and tachycardiac. The nurse should anticipate all of the following measures as treatment except:

a. Respiratory support
b. Administration of activated charcoal
c. Hemodialysis
d. Seizure precautions

## SELECTED REFERENCES

American Heart Association. (2000). *Handbook of emergency cardiovascular care for health care providers.* (M. F. Hazinski, R. O. Cummins, & J. M. Field, Eds.) Dallas, TX: Author.

Barletta, J. F. (2002). Pharmacotherapy of cardiopulmonary resuscitation. In J. T. Dipiro, R. L. Talbert, G. C. Yee, G. R. Matzke, B. G. Wells, & L. M. Posey (Eds.), *Pharmacotherapy: A pathophysiologic approach* (5th ed., pp. 145–156). New York: McGraw-Hill.

Brown, J. H., & Taylor, P. (2001). Muscarinic receptor agonists and antagonists. In J. G. Hardman & L. E. Limbird (Eds.), *Goodman & Gilman's the pharmacological basis of therapeutics* (10th ed., pp. 155–173). New York: McGraw-Hill.

*Drug facts and comparisons.* (Updated monthly). St. Louis: Facts and Comparisons.

Huether, S. E. (2004). Mechanisms of hormonal regulation. In S. E. Huether & K. L. McCance (Eds.), *Understanding pathophysiology* (3rd ed., pp. 449–472). St. Louis: Mosby.

Karch A. M. (2002). *Lippincott's nursing drug guide.* Philadelphia: Lippincott Williams and Wilkins.

Kelly, H. W., & Sorkness, C. A. (2002). Asthma. In J. T. Dipiro, R. L. Talbert, G. C. Yee, G. R. Matzke, B. G. Wells, and L. M. Posey (Eds.), *Pharmacotherapy: A pathophysiologic approach* (5th ed., pp. 475–510). New York: McGraw-Hill.

Lacy, C. F., Armstrong, L. L., Goldman, M. P., & Lance, L. L. (2003). *Lexi-Comp's drug information handbook* (11th ed.). Hudson, OH: American Pharmaceutical Association.

Olson, K. R. (Ed.). (1999). *Poisoning and drug overdose* (3rd ed.). Stamford, CT: Appleton & Lange.

Pappano, A. J., & Katzung, B. G. (2001). Cholinoceptor-blocking drugs. In B. G. Katzung (Ed.), *Basic and clinical pharmacology* (8th ed., pp. 107–119). New York: McGraw-Hill.

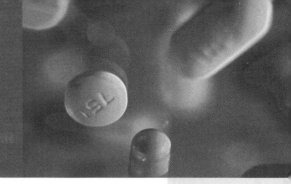

## 20

# Hypothalamic, Pituitary, Parathyroid, and Adrenal Hormones

## OBJECTIVES

*After studying this chapter, the student will be able to:*

1 Describe clinical uses of selected hormones.

2 Differentiate characteristics and functions of anterior and posterior pituitary hormones.

3 Discuss limitations of hypothalamic and pituitary hormones as therapeutic agents.

4 State the major nursing considerations in the care of clients receiving specific hypothalamic and pituitary hormones.

5 Describe the roles of parathyroid hormone, calcitonin, and vitamin D in regulating calcium metabolism.

6 Discuss recognition and management of hypercalcemia as a medical emergency.

7 Discuss the use of calcium and vitamin D supplements, calcitonin, and bisphosphonate drugs in the treatment of osteoporosis.

8 Describe the indications for use of mineralocorticoids.

## CRITICAL THINKING SCENARIO

*Y*ou are working at a community center, providing health promotion and disease prevention programs for older adults who live independently in the community. You are planning an osteoporosis prevention workshop.

✔ What are the risk factors for osteoporosis?

✔ Describe the nonpharmacologic management strategies to reduce osteoporosis risk.

✔ What methods are used to increase calcium intake through diet or medications?

✔ What are the benefits of estrogen replacement therapy for postmenopausal women?

✔ How do medication classes, such as bisphosphonates and selective estrogen receptor modulators, work to prevent osteoporosis in high-risk people?

## OVERVIEW

The endocrine system participates in the regulation of essentially all body activities, including metabolism of nutrients and water, reproduction, growth and development, and adaptation to changes in internal and external environments. The major organs of the endocrine system are the hypothalamus, pituitary, thyroid, parathyroids, pancreas, adrenals, ovaries, and testes. These tissues function through *hormones*, substances that are synthesized and secreted into body fluids by one group of cells and have physiologic effects on other body cells. Hormones act as chemical messengers to transmit information between body cells and organs. This chapter discusses drug therapy related to conditions affecting the hypothalamus, pituitary, parathyroids, and adrenals. Drug therapy related to the thyroid is discussed in Chapter 21 and therapy related to the pancreas in Chapter 22. The adrenal cortex produces about 30 steroid hormones, which are divided into glucocorticoids, mineralocorticoids, and adrenal sex hormones. Glucocorticoids are important in metabolic, inflammatory, and immune processes and, although produced by the adrenal cortex, are detailed in Chapter 36. Mineralocorticoids are important in maintaining

fluid and electrolyte balance and are discussed in this chapter. The adrenal sex hormones have little effect on normal body function and are briefly described in Chapter 36. Drug therapy associated with the ovaries and testes is discussed in Chapters 24 and 25, respectively.

The hypothalamus and pituitary gland (Fig. 20-1) interact to control most metabolic functions of the body and to maintain homeostasis. The hypothalamus controls secretions of the pituitary gland. The pituitary gland, in turn, regulates secretions or functions of other body tissues, called *target* tissues. The pituitary gland is actually two glands, each with different structures and functions. The anterior pituitary is composed of different types of glandular cells that synthesize and secrete different hormones. The posterior pituitary is anatomically an extension of the hypothalamus and is composed largely of nerve fibers. It does not manufacture any hormones itself but stores and releases the hormones oxytocin and antidiuretic hormone (ADH), which are synthesized in the hypothalamus.

Parathyroid hormone, also called parathormone or PTH, regulates calcium and phosphate metabolism. Along with calcitonin and vitamin D, PTH acts to maintain normal serum levels of calcium. When serum calcium levels

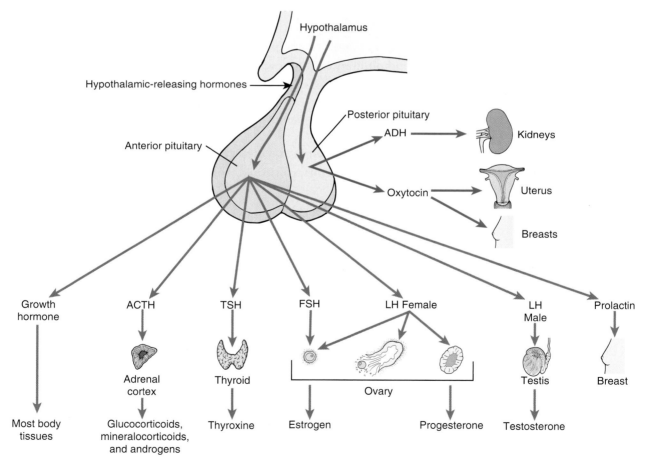

**FIGURE 20–1** Hypothalamic and pituitary hormones and their target organs. The hypothalamus produces hormones that act on the anterior pituitary or are stored in the posterior pituitary. The anterior pituitary produces hormones that act on various body tissues and stimulate production of other hormones.

are decreased, hormonal mechanisms are activated to raise them; when they are elevated, mechanisms act to lower them (Fig. 20-2). Overall, the hormones alter absorption of dietary calcium from the gastrointestinal tract, movement of calcium from bone to serum, and excretion of calcium through the kidneys. Calcium and phosphorus are discussed together because they are closely related physiologically. They are both required in cellular structure and function and, as calcium phosphate, in formation and maintenance of bones and teeth.

Drugs used to treat calcium and bone metabolism disorders are mainly those used to alter serum calcium levels or to strengthen bone. The role of bone in maintaining serum calcium levels takes precedence over its structural function (ie, bone may be weakened or destroyed as calcium leaves bone and enters serum). Hormonal deficiencies, some diseases, and some medications (eg, glucocorticoids) can contribute to loss of bone mass and osteoporosis. To aid understanding of these drugs, characteristics of the hormones, calcium, phosphorus, and bone metabolism are described in At the Foundation: Calcium and Phosphorus Regulation.

Mineralocorticoids play a vital role in maintaining fluid and electrolyte balance. *Aldosterone* is the main mineralo-corticoid and is responsible for approximately 90% of mineralocorticoid activity. Characteristics and physiologic effects of mineralocorticoids are summarized in Box 20-1.

## Hypothalamic Hormones

The hypothalamus produces a releasing hormone or an inhibiting hormone that corresponds to each of the major hormones of the anterior pituitary gland. These hormones include corticotropin-releasing hormone or factor (CRH or CRF), growth hormone–releasing hormone (GHRH), growth hormone release–inhibiting hormone (somatostatin), thyrotropin-releasing hormone (TRH), gonadotropin-releasing hormone (GnRH), follicle-stimulating hormone (FSH), luteinizing hormone (LH), prolactin-releasing factor (active during lactation after childbirth), and prolactin-inhibitory factor (PIF) (active at times other than during lactation).

## Anterior Pituitary Hormones

The anterior pituitary gland produces seven hormones. Two of these act directly on their target tissues, growth hormone, also called somatotropin, which stimulates

FIGURE 20-2 Hormonal regulation of serum calcium levels. When serum calcium levels are low (hypocalcemia), there is increased secretion of parathyroid hormone and increased activation of vitamin D. These mechanisms lead to decreased loss of calcium in the urine, increased absorption of calcium from the intestine, and increased resorption of calcium from bone. These mechanisms work together to raise serum calcium levels to normal.

When serum calcium levels are high (hypercalcemia), there is decreased secretion of parathyroid hormone and increased secretion of calcitonin. These mechanisms lead to increased loss of calcium in the urine, decreased absorption of calcium from the intestine, and decreased resorption of calcium from bone. These mechanisms lower serum calcium levels to normal.

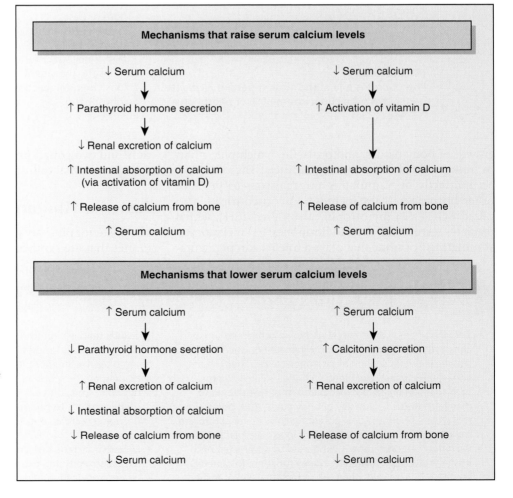

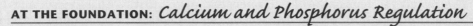

## AT THE FOUNDATION: *Calcium and Phosphorus Regulation*

### Calcium

Calcium is the most abundant cation in the body. Approximately 99% is located in the bones and teeth; the remaining portion is found in extracellular fluid and soft tissues. About half of serum calcium is bound, mostly to serum proteins, and is physiologically inactive. The other half is ionized and physiologically active. Ionized calcium can leave the vascular compartment and enter cells, where it participates in intracellular functions. An adequate amount of free (ionized) calcium is required for normal function of all body cells. Calcium is required for building and maintaining bones and teeth. Calcium is constantly shifting between bone and serum as bone is formed and broken down. When serum calcium levels become low, calcium moves into serum.

Calcium participates in many metabolic processes, including the regulation of:

- Cell membrane permeability and function
- Nerve cell excitability and transmission of impulses (eg, it is required for release of neurotransmitters at synapses)
- Contraction of cardiac, skeletal, and smooth muscle
- Conduction of electrical impulses in the heart
- Blood coagulation and platelet adhesion processes
- Hormone secretion
- Enzyme activity
- Catecholamine release from the adrenal medulla
- Release of chemical mediators (eg, histamine from mast cells)

### Phosphorus

Phosphorus is one of the most important elements in normal body function. About 80% of phosphorus is combined with calcium in bones and teeth as calcium phosphate. The remainder is distributed in every body cell and in extracellular fluid. It is combined with carbohydrates, lipids, proteins, and various other compounds.

Phosphorus is located within the cell as the phosphate ion, and performs many metabolic functions:

- It is an essential component of deoxyribonucleic acid, ribonucleic acid, and other nucleic acids in body cells. Thus, it is required for cell reproduction and body growth.
- It combines with fatty acids to form phospholipids, which are components of all cell membranes in the body. This reaction also prevents buildup of excessive amounts of free fatty acids.
- It forms a phosphate buffer system, which helps to maintain acid–base balance. When excess hydrogen ions are present in kidney tubules, phosphate combines with them and allows their excretion in urine. At the same time, bicarbonate is retained by the kidneys and contributes to alkalinity of body fluids. Although there are other buffering systems in the body, failure of the phosphate system leads to metabolic acidosis (retained hydrogen ions or acid and lost bicarbonate ions or base).
- It is necessary for cellular use of glucose and production of energy.
- It is necessary for proper function of several B vitamins (ie, the vitamins function as coenzymes in various chemical reactions only when combined with phosphate).

growth of body tissues, and prolactin, which play a part in milk production by nursing mothers. The other five act indirectly by stimulating target tissues to produce other hormones. They include (1) corticotropin, also called ACTH; (2) thyrotropin (also called TSH), which regulates secretion of thyroid hormones; (3) melanocyte-stimulating hormone that plays a role in skin pigmenta-tion; and two gonadotropins, (4) FSH, and (5) LH (also called interstitial cell–stimulating hormone).

## Posterior Pituitary Hormones

The posterior pituitary gland stores and releases two hormones that are synthesized by nerve cells in the hypo-

### BOX 20-1 Effects of Mineralocorticoids on Body Processes and Systems

- The overall physiologic effects of mineralocorticoids are to conserve sodium and water and eliminate potassium. Aldosterone increases sodium reabsorption from kidney tubules, and water is reabsorbed along with the sodium. When sodium is conserved, another cation must be excreted to maintain electrical neutrality of body fluids; thus, potassium is excreted. This is the only potent mechanism for controlling the concentration of potassium ions in extracellular fluids.
- Secretion of aldosterone is controlled by several factors, most of which are related to kidney function. In general, secretion is increased when the potassium level of extra-cellular fluid is high, the sodium level of extracellular fluid is low, the renin–angiotensin system of the kidneys is activated, or the anterior pituitary gland secretes corticotropin.
- Inadequate secretion of aldosterone causes hyperkalemia, hyponatremia, and extracellular fluid volume deficit (dehydration). Hypotension and shock may result from decreased cardiac output. Absence of mineralocorticoids causes death.
- Excessive secretion of aldosterone produces hypokalemia, hypernatremia, and extracellular fluid volume excess (water intoxication). Edema and hypertension may result.

thalamus. They include ADH, also called vasopressin, that functions to regulate water balance, and oxytocin, which functions in childbirth and lactation.

## Parathyroid Hormone

Parathyroid hormone secretion is stimulated by low serum calcium levels and inhibited by normal or high levels (a negative-feedback system). Because phosphate is closely related to calcium in body functions, PTH also regulates phosphate metabolism. In general, when serum calcium levels increase, serum phosphate levels decrease, and vice versa. Thus, an inverse relationship exists between calcium and phosphate.

## Calcitonin

Calcitonin is a hormone from the thyroid gland whose secretion is controlled by the concentration of ionized calcium in the blood flowing through the thyroid gland. When the serum level of ionized calcium is increased, secretion of calcitonin is increased. The function of calcitonin is to lower serum calcium in the presence of hypercalcemia, which it does by decreasing movement of calcium from bone to serum and increasing urinary excretion of calcium. The action of calcitonin is rapid but of short duration. Thus, it has little effect on long-term calcium metabolism.

## Vitamin D (Calciferol)

Vitamin D is a fat-soluble vitamin that functions as a hormone and plays an important role in calcium and bone metabolism. The main action of vitamin D is to raise serum calcium levels by increasing intestinal absorption of calcium and mobilizing calcium from bone. It also promotes bone formation by providing adequate serum concentrations of minerals. Vitamin D is not physiologically active in the body. It must be converted to an intermediate metabolite in the liver, then to an active metabolite (1,25-dihydroxyvitamin D or calcitriol) in the kidneys. PTH and adequate hepatic and renal function are required to produce the active metabolite.

## Adrenal Hormones

*Aldosterone* is the primary and most potent mineralocorticoid; it functions to conserve sodium through its action on the epithelial cells of the distal nephron. The secretion and synthesis of aldosterone is regulated by the renin-angiotensin-aldosterone system. Aldosterone is only 60% bound to plasma proteins. The large unbound portion of aldosterone contributes to its rapid turnover rate, short half-life of 20 minutes, and low plasma concentration. In general, protein binding functions as a storage area from which the hormone is released as needed. This promotes more consistent blood levels and more uniform distribution to the tissues. Additionally, an important variable in altered plasma concentration of aldosterone (and any active steroid) is the concentration of plasma proteins. Characteristics and physiologic effects of aldosterone are summarized in Box 20-1. Indication for use, route, and dosage range of drug affecting mineralocorticoid activity in the adrenals are listed later in Drug at a Glance 20-4: Mineralocorticoid Agent.

## INDIVIDUAL HORMONAL AGENTS

Selected drugs are described in the Drugs at a Glance tables. No prototype is identified within these groups owing to the wide range of actions and uses of the drugs. General considerations are described below.

Hypothalamic hormones are rarely used in most clinical practice settings and should be administered according to current manufacturers' literature.

Most drug therapy with pituitary hormones is given to replace or supplement naturally occurring hormones in situations involving inadequate function of the pituitary gland (hypopituitarism). Conditions resulting from excessive amounts of pituitary hormones (hyperpituitarism) are more often treated with surgery or irradiation. Because the hormones are proteins, they must be given by injection or nasal inhalation. If taken orally, proteolytic enzymes in the gastrointestinal (GI) tract would destroy them. Possible adverse effects, especially with high doses or chronic use, include acromegaly, diabetes, hypertension, and increased risk for serious cardiovascular disease (eg, heart failure). There is also concern about a possible link between growth hormone, which stimulates tumor growth, and cancer. Growth hormone stimulates the release of insulin-like growth factor-1 (IGF-1, also called somatomedin), a substance that circulates in the blood and stimulates cell division. Most tumor cells have receptors that recognize IGF-1, bind it, and allow it to enter the cell, where it could trigger uncontrolled cell division. This concern may be greater for middle-aged and older adults because malignancies are more common in these groups than in adolescents and young adults. Indications for use, routes, and dosage ranges of drugs affecting the hypothalamus and the anterior and posterior pituitary are listed later in Drugs at a Glance 20-1: Hypothalamic and Pituitary Agents.

Drugs from several groups are used to treat calcium and bone disorders. Calcium and vitamin D supplements are used to treat hypocalcemia and to prevent and treat osteoporosis. These agents are described in the following sections; names and dosages of individual drug preparations are listed later in Drugs at a Glance 20-3: Calcium and Vitamin D Preparations. Drugs used for hypercalcemia include bisphosphonates, calcitonin, corticosteroids, 0.9% sodium chloride intravenous (IV) infusion, and others. Those used for osteoporosis inhibit bone breakdown and demineralization and include bisphosphonates, calcitonin, estrogens, and antiestrogens. These drugs are described in the following sections.

Hypocalcemia is uncommon in any age group, and guidelines for treating hypercalcemia in children are essentially the same as those for adults, with drug dosages adjusted. Additional thoughts regarding this age group and older adults are found in Age-Related Considerations.

The home care nurse has an excellent opportunity to promote health and prevent illness related to calcium and bone disorders. All members of a household should be assessed in relation to calcium and vitamin D intake because an adequate amount of these nutrients is needed throughout life. Children, adolescent girls, and older women often have inadequate intakes, with risk for having or developing osteoporosis. Teaching may be needed about dietary and supplemental sources of these nutrients as well as the adverse effects of excessive amounts. Clients who are receiving medications to prevent or treat osteoporosis may also need teaching or other assistance. Guidelines for strategies for ongoing evaluation and intervention are addressed in Home Care Considerations.

## Hypothalamic Hormones

**Gonadorelin** (Factrel), **goserelin** (Zoladex), **histrelin** (Supprelin), **leuprolide** (Lupron), **nafarelin** (Synarel), and **triptorelin** (Trelstar) are equivalent to gonadotropin-releasing hormone. For information on hypothalamic and pituitary agents, see Drugs at a Glance 20-1: Hypothalamic and Pituitary Agents. After initial stimulation of LH and FSH secretion, chronic administration of therapeutic doses inhibits gonadotropin secretion. This action results in decreased production of testosterone and estrogen, which is reversible when drug administration is stopped. In males, testosterone is reduced to castration levels. In premenopausal females, estrogens are reduced to postmenopausal levels. These effects occur within 2 to 4 weeks after drug therapy is begun. In children with central precocious puberty (CPP), gonadotropins (testosterone in males, estrogen in females) are reduced to prepubertal levels.

## Age-related Considerations: Use of Drugs for Hypothalamus and Pituitary Disorders and Disorders of Calcium and Bone Metabolism

### USE IN CHILDREN

#### Drugs Associated With the Hypothalamus and Pituitary

An increasing concern in children and adolescents is the inappropriate use of growth hormone. Young athletes may use the drug for bodybuilding and to enhance athletic performance. If so, they are likely to use relatively high doses. In addition, the highest levels of physiologic hormone are secreted during adolescence. The combination of high pharmacologic and high physiologic amounts increases risks for health problems from excessive hormone. Also, there is little evidence that hormone use increases muscle mass or strength beyond that achieved with exercise alone.

#### Drugs Associated With Calcium and Bone Metabolism

Hypocalcemia is uncommon in children. However, inadequate calcium in the diet is thought to be common, especially in girls. Inadequate calcium and exercise in children are risk factors for eventual osteoporosis. If hypocalcemia or dietary calcium deficiency develops, principles of using calcium or vitamin D supplements are the same as those in adults. Children should be monitored closely for signs and symptoms of adverse effects, including hypercalcemia. Hypercalcemia is probably most likely to occur in children with a malignant tumor. Safety, effectiveness, and dosages of etidronate, pamidronate, and zoledronate have not been established.

### USE IN OLDER ADULTS

#### Drugs Associated With the Hypothalamus and Pituitary

Middle-aged and older adults may use growth hormone to combat the effects of aging, such as decreased energy, weaker muscles and joints, and wrinkled skin. One source

of the product is apparently "anti-aging" clinics. Although it is not illegal for health care providers to prescribe growth hormone for these populations, such use is unproved in safety and effectiveness. Endocrinologists emphasize that optimal adult levels of growth hormone are unknown and that using the drug to slow aging is unproved and potentially dangerous because the long-term effects are unknown.

#### Drugs Associated With Calcium and Bone Metabolism

Hypocalcemia is uncommon because calcium moves from bone to blood to maintain normal serum levels. However, calcium deficiency commonly occurs because of long-term dietary deficiencies of calcium and vitamin D, impaired absorption of calcium from the intestine, lack of exposure to sunlight, and impaired liver or kidney metabolism of vitamin D to its active form. These and other factors lead to demineralization and weakening of bone (osteoporosis) and an increased risk for fractures. Individuals who take corticosteroids are at risk for developing osteoporosis. The risk is higher with systemic corticosteroids but may also occur with oral or nasal inhalation, especially at higher doses. In general, all older adults need to continue their dietary intake of dairy products and other calcium-containing foods. Older adults with osteoporosis or risk factors for developing osteoporosis may need estrogen or testosterone replacement therapy, calcium supplements, and a bisphosphonate or calcitonin to prevent or treat the disorder.

With hypercalcemia, treatment usually requires large amounts of IV 0.9% sodium chloride (eg, 150 to 200 mL/hour). Older adults often have chronic cardiovascular disorders that may be aggravated by this treatment. They should be monitored closely for signs of fluid overload, congestive heart failure, pulmonary edema, and hypertension.

## Home Care Considerations: Use of Drugs for Hypothalamic, Pituitary, and Parathyroid Disorders and Osteoporosis

***ASSESS:*** adverse drug effects should be reviewed with clients, and clients should be assessed for characteristics (eg, older age group, renal impairment, overuse of the drugs) that increase the risks for adverse effects.

***MONITOR:*** the therapeutic and adverse effects of the drugs and client's need for additional information and provide that information.

***EDUCATE:*** regarding the importance of reading and following instructions, on ways to minimize adverse effects, and not exceeding recommended dosages without consulting a health care provider. Reinforce additional teaching points (see Client Teaching Guidelines: Drugs for Osteoporosis).

The drugs cannot be given orally because enzymes in the GI tract would destroy them. Most are given by injection and are available in depot preparations that can be given once monthly or less often. Adverse effects are basically those of testosterone or estrogen deficiency. When given for prostate cancer, the drugs may cause increased bone pain and increased difficulty in urinating during the first few weeks of treatment. The drugs may also cause or aggravate depression.

**Octreotide** (Sandostatin) has pharmacologic actions similar to those of somatostatin. Indications for use include acromegaly, in which it reduces blood levels of growth hormone and IGF-1; carcinoid tumors, in which it inhibits diarrhea and flushing; and vasoactive intestinal peptide tumors, in which it relieves diarrhea (by decreasing GI secretions and motility). It is also used to treat diarrhea in acquired immunodeficiency syndrome (AIDS) and other conditions. The drug is most often given subcutaneously and may be self-administered.

**DRUG TABLE 20-1**  *Drugs at a Glance*

## Hypothalamic and Pituitary Agents

| Generic/Trade Name | Routes and Dosage Ranges | Comments/Uses |
|---|---|---|
| ***Hypothalamic Hormones*** | | |
| **Gonadorelin** (Factrel) Pregnancy Category B | *Adults:* Sub-Q, IV, 100 mcg | As a diagnostic test of gonadotropic function of the anterior pituitary |
| **Goserelin** (Zoladex) Pregnancy Category X | *Adults:* Sub-Q implant into upper abdominal wall, 3.6 mg every 28 d or 10.8 mg every 3 mo | Used for endometriosis and metastatic breast and prostate cancer |
| **Leuprolide** (Lupron) Pregnancy Category X | *Adults:* Endometriosis, uterine fibroids: IM depot injection, 3.75 mg every mo or 11.25 every 3 mo for 6 mo<br>Prostate cancer: Sub-Q, 1 mg daily IM depot, 7.5 mg every mo, 22.5 mg every 3 mo, or 30 mg every 4 mo Implant (Viadur), one (72 mg) every 12 mo<br>*Children:* CPP Sub-Q, 50 mcg/kg/d IM Depot-Ped, weight ≤25 kg, 7.5 mg; >25 to 37.5 kg, 11.25 mg; >37.5 kg, 15 mg every month | Used in: Advanced prostatic cancer Central precocious puberty (CPP) in children Endometriosis Uterine fibroid tumors |
| **Nafarelin** (Synarel) Pregnancy Category X | *Adults:* Endometriosis: female, 1 spray (200 mcg) in 1 nostril each morning and 1 spray each evening in the other nostril starting on days 2 to 4 of the menstrual cycle for 6 months<br>*Children:* CPP: male and female, 2 sprays (400 mcg) into each nostril in the morning repeated into each nostril in the evening If inadequate suppression, the dose may increase to 3 sprays (600 mcg) into alternating nostrils 3 times/d | Endometriosis CPP in children |

*(continued)*

**DRUG TABLE
20-1**

*Drugs at a Glance*

## Hypothalamic and Pituitary Agents (Continued)

| Generic/Trade Name | Routes and Dosage Ranges | Comments/Uses |
|---|---|---|
| **Octreotide** (Sandostatin) Pregnancy Category B | *Adults:* Acromegaly, Sub-Q, 50–100 mcg three times daily<br>Carcinoid tumors: Sub-Q, 100–600 mcg daily (average 300 mcg) in 2 to 4 divided doses<br>Intestinal tumors: Sub-Q, 200–300 mcg daily in 2 to 4 divided doses<br>Diarrhea: IV, Sub-Q, 50 mcg 2 or 3 times daily initially, then adjusted according to response<br>*Children:* Dosage not established, but 1–10 mcg/kg reportedly well tolerated in young clients | Useful in the treatment of:<br>Acromegaly<br>Carcinoid tumors<br>Vasoactive intestinal peptide tumors<br>Diarrhea |
| ***Anterior Pituitary Hormones*** | | |
| **Corticotropin** (ACTH, Acthar Gel) Pregnancy Category C | *Adults:* Therapeutic use: IM, Sub-Q, 20 units four times daily<br>Diagnostic use: IV infusion, 10–25 units in 500 mL of 5% dextrose or 0.9% sodium chloride solution, over 8 hours<br>Acthar Gel, IM, 40–80 units q24–72h | Stimulate synthesis of hormones by the adrenal cortex<br>Diagnostic test of adrenal function |
| **Cosyntropin** (Cortrosyn) Pregnancy Category C | *Adults:* IM, IV, 0.25 mg (equivalent to 25 units ACTH) | Diagnostic test in suspected adrenal insufficiency |
| **Somatrem** (Protropin) Pregnancy Category C | *Children:* Somatrem IM, up to 0.1 mg/kg three times per week | Promote growth in children whose growth is impaired by a deficiency of endogenous growth hormone |
| **Somatropin** (Genotropin, Humatrope, Norditropin, Nutropin, Serostim) Pregnancy Category B/C depending on manufacturer | *Children:* Somatropin IM, up to 0.06 mg/kg three times per week | Promotes human growth |
| **Human chorionic gonadotropin** (Chorex, Choron, Pregnyl) Pregnancy Category C<br>**Choriogonadotropin alfa** (Ovidrel) Pregnancy Category X | *Adults:* Cryptorchidism and male hypogonadism, IM, 500–4000 units 2–3 times per week for several weeks<br>To induce ovulation, IM, 5000–10,000 units in one dose, 1 d after treatment with menotropins<br>*Children:* Preadolescent boys: Cryptorchidism and hypogonadism, IM, 500–4000 units 2–3 times per week for several weeks<br>To induce ovulation, IM, 5000–10,000 units in one dose, 1 d after treatment with menotropins | Cryptorchidism<br>Diagnostic test of testosterone production<br>Induce ovulation in the treatment of infertility |
| **Menotropins** (Pergonal) Pregnancy Category X | *Adults:* IM, 1 ampule (75 units FSH and 75 units LH) daily for 9–12 d, followed by HCG to induce ovulation | Combined with HCG to induce ovulation in treatment of infertility caused by lack of pituitary gonadotropins |
| **Thyrotropin alfa** (Thyrogen) Pregnancy Category C | *Adults:* IM, 0.9 mg every 24 h for 2 doses or every 72 h for 3 doses<br>*Children:* <16 y: Dosage not established | Diagnostic test of thyroid function |

*(continued)*

**DRUG TABLE 20-1**

## *Drugs at a Glance*

### Hypothalamic and Pituitary Agents (Continued)

| Generic/Trade Name | Routes and Dosage Ranges | Comments/Uses |
|---|---|---|
| ***Posterior Pituitary Hormones*** | | |
| **Desmopressin** (DDAVP, Stimate) Pregnancy Category B | *Adults:* Diabetes insipidus, intranasally, 0.1–0.4 mL/d, usually in two divided doses<br>Hemophilia A, von Willebrand's disease, IV, 0.3 mcg/kg in 50-mL sterile saline, infused over 15–30 min<br>*Children:* 3 mo–2 y: Diabetes insipidus, intranasally 0.05–0.3 mL/d in 1–2 doses<br>Weight >10 kg: Hemophilia A, von Willebrand's disease, same as adult dosage<br>Weight ≤10 kg: Hemophilia A, von Willebrand's disease, IV, 0.3 mcg/kg in 10 mL of sterile saline | Neurogenic diabetes insipidus<br>Hemostasis (parenteral only) in spontaneous, trauma-induced, and perioperative bleeding |
| **Lypressin** (Diapid) Pregnancy Category D | *Adults:* Intranasal spray, one or two sprays to one or both nostrils, 3–4 times per day | Diabetes insipidus |
| **Vasopressin** (Pitressin) Pregnancy Category C | *Adults:* IM, Sub-Q, intranasally on cotton pledgets, 0.25–0.5 mL (5–10 units) 2–3 times per day<br>*Children:* IM, Sub-Q, intranasally on cotton pledgets, 0.125–0.5 mL (2.5–10 units) 3–4 times per day | Diabetes insipidus |
| **Oxytocin** (Pitocin) Pregnancy Category C | *Adults:* Induction of labor, IV, 1-mL ampule (10 units) in 1000 mL of 5% dextrose injection (10 units/1000 mL = 10 milliunits/mL), infused at 0.2–2 milliunits/min initially, then regulated according to frequency and strength of uterine contractions<br>Prevention or treatment of postpartum bleeding, IV, 10–40 units in 1000 mL of 5% dextrose injection, infused at 125 mL/h (40 milliunits/min) or 0.6–1.8 units (0.06–0.18 mL) diluted in 3–5 mL sodium chloride injection and injected slowly; IM, 0.3–1 mL (3–10 units) | Induce labor<br>Control postpartum bleeding |

The long-acting formulation (Sandostatin LAR Depot) must be given intramuscularly in a gluteal muscle of the hip. Dosage should be reduced for older adults.

## Anterior Pituitary Hormones

**Corticotropin** (ACTH, Acthar), which is obtained from animal pituitary glands, is mainly of historical interest. For therapeutic purposes, it has been replaced by adrenal corticosteroids. It may be used occasionally as a diagnostic test to differentiate primary adrenal insufficiency (Addison's disease, which is associated with atrophy of the adrenal gland) from secondary adrenal insufficiency caused by inadequate pituitary secretion of corticotropin. However, **cosyntropin** (Cortrosyn), a synthetic formulation, is more commonly used to test for suspected adrenal insufficiency.

**Growth hormone** is synthesized from bacteria by recombinant DNA technology. Somatropin (Humatrope) and somatrem (Protropin) are therapeutically equivalent to endogenous growth hormone produced by the pituitary gland. The main clinical use of the drugs is for children whose growth is impaired by a deficiency of endogenous hormone. The drugs are ineffective when impaired growth results from other causes or after puberty, when epiphyses of the long bones have closed. They are also used to treat short stature in children that is associated with chronic renal failure or Turner's syndrome (a genetic disorder that occurs in girls). In adults, the drugs may be used to treat deficiency states (eg, those caused by disease, surgery, or radiation of the pituitary gland) or the tissue wasting associated with AIDS. In general, dosage should be individualized according to response. Excessive administration can cause excessive growth (gigantism).

**Human chorionic gonadotropin** (HCG; Chorex, others) produces physiologic effects similar to those of the naturally occurring LH. In males, it is used to evaluate the ability of Leydig's cells to produce testosterone, to treat hypogonadism due to pituitary deficiency, and to treat cryptorchidism (undescended testicle) in preadolescent boys. In women, HCG is used in combination with menotropins to induce ovulation in the treatment of infertility. Excessive doses or prolonged administration can lead to sexual precocity, edema, and breast enlargement caused by oversecretion of testosterone and estrogen.

**Menotropins** (Pergonal), a gonadotropin preparation obtained from the urine of postmenopausal women, contains both FSH and LH. It is usually combined with HCG to induce ovulation in the treatment of infertility caused by lack of pituitary gonadotropins.

**Thyrotropin** (Thytropar) is used as a diagnostic agent to distinguish between primary hypothyroidism (caused by a thyroid disorder) and secondary hypothyroidism (caused by pituitary malfunction). If thyroid hormones in serum are elevated after the administration of thyrotropin, then the hypothyroidism is secondary to inadequate pituitary function. Thyrotropin must be used cautiously in clients with coronary artery disease, congestive heart failure, or adrenocortical insufficiency. **Thyrotropin alfa** (Thyrogen) is a synthetic formulation of TSH used to treat thyroid cancer.

## Posterior Pituitary Hormones

**Desmopressin** (DDAVP, Stimate), lypressin, and vasopressin (Pitressin) are synthetic equivalents of ADH. A major clinical use is the treatment of neurogenic diabetes insipidus, a disorder characterized by a deficiency of ADH and the excretion of large amounts of dilute urine. Diabetes insipidus may be idiopathic, hereditary, or acquired as a result of trauma, surgery, tumor, infection, or other conditions that impair the function of the hypothalamus or posterior pituitary.

Lypressin is used only for controlling the excessive water loss of diabetes insipidus. Parenteral desmopressin is also used as a hemostatic agent in clients with hemo-

philia A or mild to moderate von Willebrand's disease (type 1). The drug is effective in controlling spontaneous or trauma-induced bleeding and intraoperative and postoperative bleeding when given 30 minutes before the procedure. Vasopressin is also used in the treatment of bleeding esophageal varices because of its vasoconstrictive effects. Desmopressin and lypressin may be inhaled intranasally; vasopressin must be injected.

**Oxytocin** (Pitocin) is a synthetic drug that exerts the same physiologic effects as the posterior pituitary hormone. Thus, it promotes uterine contractility and is used clinically to induce labor and in the postpartum period to control bleeding. Oxytocin must be used only when clearly indicated and when well-trained personnel, as in a hospital, can supervise the recipient.

## ◼ DRUGS USED FOR CALCIUM AND BONE DISORDERS

Indications for use and dosages are listed in Drugs at a Glance 20-2: Drugs Used in Hypercalcemia and Selected Bone Disorders.

### Bisphosphonates

**Alendronate** (Fosamax), **etidronate** (Didronel), **pamidronate** (Aredia), **risedronate** (Actonel), **tiludronate** (Skelid), and **zoledronate** (Zometa) are drugs that bind to bone and inhibit calcium resorption from bone. Although indications for use vary among the drugs, they are used mainly in the treatment of hypercalcemia and osteoporosis. Etidronate also inhibits bone mineralization and may cause osteomalacia. Newer bisphosphonates do not have this effect.

These drugs are poorly absorbed from the intestinal tract and must be taken on an empty stomach, with water, at least 30 minutes before any other fluid, food, or medication. The drugs are not metabolized. The drug bound to bone is slowly released into the bloodstream; most of the drug that is not bound to bone is excreted in the urine.

**Calcitonin-salmon** (Calcimar, Miacalcin) is used in the treatment of hypercalcemia, Paget's disease, and osteoporosis. In hypercalcemia, calcitonin lowers serum calcium levels by inhibiting bone resorption. It is most likely to be effective in hypercalcemia caused by hyperparathyroidism, prolonged immobilization, or certain malignant neoplasms. In acute hypercalcemia, calcitonin may be used along with other measures to lower serum calcium levels rapidly. A single injection of calcitonin decreases serum calcium levels in approximately 2 hours; effects last approximately 6 to 8 hours.

In Paget's disease, calcitonin slows the rate of bone turnover, improves bone lesions on radiologic examination, and relieves bone pain. In osteoporosis, calcitonin prevents further bone loss in the presence of adequate

## DRUG TABLE 20-2

*Drugs at a Glance*

### Drugs Used in Hypercalcemia and Selected Bone Disorders

| Generic/Trade Name | Routes and Dosage Ranges | Comments/Uses |
|---|---|---|
| *Bisphosphonates* | | |
| **Alendronate** (Fosamax) Pregnancy Category C | Osteoporosis: Postmenopausal women: Prevention, PO, 5 mg once daily or 35 mg once weekly; treatment, PO, 10 mg once daily or 70 mg once weekly Men: 10 mg once daily; glucocorticoid-induced, 5 mg once daily Paget's disease: PO, 40 mg daily for 6 mo; repeat if necessary | Osteoporosis: Prevention and treatment in post-menopausal women Treatment in men and men or women with glucocorticoid-induced osteo-porosis Paget's disease |
| **Etidronate** (Didronel) Pregnancy Category B (oral); C (parenteral) | Paget's disease, PO, 5–10 mg/kg/d up to 6 mo or 11–20 mg/kg/d up to 3 mo; may be repeated after 3 mo if symptoms recur Heterotopic ossification: with spinal cord injury, PO, 20 mg/kg/d for 2 wk, then 10 mg/kg/d for 10 wk; with total hip replacement, PO, 20 mg/kg/d for 1 mo before and 3 mo after surgery Hypercalcemia of malignancy: IV, 7.5 mg/kg/d, in at least 250 mL of 0.9% sodium chloride solution and infused over at least 2 h, daily for 3–7 d | Paget's disease Heterotopic ossification Hypercalcemia of malignancy |
| **Pamidronate** (Aredia) Pregnancy Category D | Hypercalcemia, IV, 60 mg over 4 h; 90 mg over 24 h Osteolytic bone lesions, breast cancer: IV, 90 mg over 2 h every 3–4 wk Multiple myeloma, IV, 90 mg over 4 h once monthly Paget's disease: IV, 30 mg over 4 h, daily for 3 doses | Hypercalcemia of malignancy Osteolytic lesions of breast cancer metastases or multiple myeloma Paget's disease |
| **Risedronate** (Actonel) Pregnancy Category C | Prevention and treatment of osteoporo-sis: PO, 5 mg once daily Paget's disease: PO, 30 mg once daily for 2 mo | Osteoporosis, postmenopausal and glucocorticoid-induced, prevention and treatment Paget's disease |
| **Tiludronate** (Skelid) Pregnancy Category C | PO, 400 mg once daily for 3 mo | Paget's disease |
| **Zoledronic acid** (Zometa) Pregnancy Category D | IV, 4 mg over 15 min or longer | Hypercalcemia of malignancy |

calcium and vitamin D. In addition, calcitonin helps to control pain in clients with osteoporosis or metastatic bone disease. Both subcutaneous injections and intranasal administration relieve pain within 1 to 12 weeks. The drug is given daily initially, then two to three times a week. The mechanism by which pain is reduced is unknown.

**Calcitonin-human** (Cibacalcin) is a synthetic prepa-ration used in Paget's disease. Compared with calcitonin-salmon, calcitonin-human is more likely to cause nausea and facial flushing and less likely to cause antibody for-mation and allergic reactions.

## Calcium Preparations

For acute, symptomatic hypocalcemia, a calcium salt (usually calcium gluconate) is given intravenously. For asymptomatic, less severe, or chronic hypocalcemia, an oral preparation (eg, calcium carbonate or citrate) is given.

These preparations differ mainly in the amounts of calcium they contain and the routes by which they may be given.

Even when serum calcium levels are normal, people who do not get enough calcium in their diets may need calcium supplements. Most diets are thought to be deficient in calcium for all age groups, but especially for young women and older adults. Calcium supplements are also used in the prevention and treatment of osteoporosis. Specific preparations and dosages are listed in Drugs at a Glance 20-3: Calcium and Vitamin D Preparations.

## Corticosteroids

Glucocorticoids (see Chap. 36) are used in the treatment of hypercalcemia due to malignancies or vitamin D intoxication. These drugs lower serum calcium by inhibiting cytokine release, by direct cytolytic effects on some tumor cells, by inhibiting calcium absorption from the intestine, and by increasing calcium excretion in the urine. Hydrocortisone or prednisone is often used; serum calcium levels decrease in approximately 5 to 10 days. After the serum calcium level stabilizes, dosage should be gradually reduced to the minimum needed to control symptoms of hypercalcemia. High dosage or prolonged administration leads to serious adverse effects.

## Estrogens and Antiestrogens

Estrogens are discussed here in relation to osteoporosis; see Chapter 24 for other uses and dosages. Estrogen replacement therapy (ERT) is a treatment for preventing postmenopausal osteoporosis. It is most beneficial immediately after menopause, when a period of accelerated bone loss occurs. Mechanisms by which ERT protects against bone loss and fractures are thought to include decreased bone breakdown, increased calcium absorption from the intestine, and increased calcitriol (the active form of vitamin D) concentration.

Progestins are used with estrogens in women with an intact uterus because of the increased risk for endometrial cancer with estrogen therapy alone. The combination is called hormone replacement therapy (HRT). Although progestins alone delay bone loss, HRT seems no more beneficial than estrogens alone. Raloxifene (Evista) and tamoxifen (Nolvadex) act like estrogen in some body tissues and prevent the action of estrogen in other body tissues. Raloxifene is classified as a selective estrogen receptor modulator and is approved for prevention of postmenopausal osteoporosis. It has estrogenic effects in bone tissue, thereby decreasing bone breakdown and increasing bone mass density. It has antiestrogen effects in uterine and breast tissue. Tamoxifen, which is classified as an antiestrogen, is used to prevent and treat breast cancer. It also has estrogenic effects and can be used to prevent osteoporosis and cardiovascular disease, although it is not approved for these uses. Tamoxifen may help prevent osteoporosis in clients with breast cancer. In postmenopausal osteoporosis, these drugs are recommended for those women who are unable or unwilling to take ERT or HRT.

## Parathyroid Hormone

Teriparatide (Forteo) is a recombinant DNA version of parathyroid hormone. It is approved for the treatment of osteoporosis in women. Other drugs for osteoporosis slow bone loss; teriparatide increases bone formation by increasing the number of bone-building cells (osteoblasts). It also increases serum levels of calcium and calcitriol (a metabolite of vitamin D that promotes absorption and use of calcium in bone building). In clinical trials, it increased vertebral bone mineral density and decreased vertebral fractures. It is recommended for use in clients with severe osteoporosis and those who have not responded adequately to other treatments, partly because osteosarcoma developed in some animals given high doses for long periods. None developed in humans during clinical trials, but the longest of these was 2 years.

Teriparatide is rapidly and well absorbed with subcutaneous injection. Bioavailability is 95%, and peak serum levels occur in 30 minutes. The drug is metabolized and excreted through the liver, kidneys, and bone. It is not expected to accumulate in bone or other tissues, to interact significantly with other drugs, or to require dosage adjustment with renal or hepatic impairment. Adverse effects include nausea, headache, back pain, dizziness, syncope, and leg cramps.

## Vitamin D Preparations

Vitamin D is used in chronic hypocalcemia if calcium supplements alone cannot maintain serum calcium levels within normal range. It is also used to prevent deficiency states and treat hypoparathyroidism and osteoporosis. Although authorities agree that dietary intake is better than supplements, some suggest a vitamin D supplement for people who ingest less than the recommended amount (400 IU daily for those aged 6 months to 24 years; 200 IU for those 25 years of age and older). In addition, the recommended amount for older adults may be too low, especially for those who receive little exposure to sunlight, and dosage needs for all age groups may be greater during winter, when there is less sunlight. If used, vitamin D supplements should be taken cautiously and not overused; excessive amounts can cause serious problems, including hypercalcemia. For information on specific preparations, see Drugs at a Glance 20-2: Drugs Used in Hypercalcemia and Selected Bone Disorders.

## Miscellaneous Drugs for Hypercalcemia

Furosemide (Lasix) is a loop diuretic (see Chap. 44) that increases calcium excretion in urine by preventing its reabsorption in renal tubules. Although it can be given

**DRUG TABLE 20-3**

*Drugs at a Glance*

## Calcium and Vitamin D Preparations

| Generic/Trade Name | Routes and Dosage Ranges | Comments/Uses |
|---|---|---|
| **Oral Calcium Products** | | |
| **Calcium acetate** (25% calcium) (PhosLo) Pregnancy Category C | *Adults:* PO, 2–4 tablets with each meal *Children:* Dosage not established | Compared with other calcium salts, calcium acetate binds to phosphorus better in the GI tract owing to its lower solubility |
| **Calcium carbonate, precipitated** (40% calcium) (Os-Cal, Tums) Pregnancy Category C | *Adults:* PO, 1–1.5 g three times daily with meals (maximal dose, 8 g daily) | As with all calcium products: Calcium products are not interchangeable |
| **Calcium citrate** (21% calcium) (Citracal) Pregnancy Category C | *Adults:* PO, 1–2 tablets (200 mg calcium per tablet) two to four times daily | Calcium may reduce iron absorption Foods containing phosphorus (milk and dairy products), oxalic acid (spinach, |
| **Calcium gluconate** (9% calcium) Pregnancy Category C | *Adults:* PO, 1–2 g three or four times daily *Children:* PO, 500 mg/kg/d in divided doses | rhubarb), or phytic acid (whole grain or bran) may interfere with calcium absorption |
| **Calcium lactate** (13% calcium) Pregnancy Category C | *Adults:* PO, 1 g three times daily with meals *Children:* PO, 500 mg/kg/d in divided doses | |
| **Tricalcium phosphate** (39% calcium) (Posture) Pregnancy Category C | *Adults:* PO, 1–2 tablets (600 mg calcium per tablet) two to four times daily | |
| **Parenteral Calcium Products** | | |
| **Calcium chloride** (10 mL of 10% solution contains 273 mg [13.6 mEq] of calcium) Pregnancy Category C | *Adults:* IV, 500 mg–1 g (5–10 mL of 10% solution) every 1–3 d, depending on clinical response or serum calcium measurements *Children:* IV, 0.2 mL/kg, up to 1–10 mL/d | Give only by IV route; more irritating to tissues than calcium gluconate; precipitation may occur with phosphorus or phosphate in parenteral fluids; use an in-line filter |
| **Calcium gluceptate** 1.1 g/5 mL (5 mL contains 90 mg [4.5 mEq] of calcium) Pregnancy Category C | *Adults:* IV, 5–20 mL (90–360 mg calcium); IM, 2–5 mL *Children:* IM, 2–5 mL (36–90 mg calcium) | Give IM injections in lateral thigh in infants and in gluteal region in adults; use IM route only in emergency as the calcium salts irritate tissue |
| **Calcium gluconate** (10 mL of 10% solution contains 93 mg [4.65 mEq] of calcium) Pregnancy Category C | *Adults:* IV, 5–20 mL of 10% solution *Children:* IV, 500 mg/kg/d in divided doses | Give only by IV route |
| **Vitamin D Preparations** | | |
| **Calcifediol** (Calderol) Pregnancy Category C | *Adults:* Dialysis clients, PO, 50–100 mcg daily | Colestipol and cholestyramine decrease absorption of vitamin D preparations; mineral oil interferes with absorption of fat-soluble vitamins |
| **Calcitriol (1,25-dihydroxycholecalciferol)** (Rocaltrol, Calcijex) Pregnancy Category C | *Adults:* Dialysis clients, hypoparathyroidism: PO, 0.25 mcg daily initially, then adjusted according to serum calcium levels (usual daily maintenance dose 0.5–1 mcg) *Children:* Hypoparathyroidism, ≥6 y: PO, 0.5–2 mcg daily *1–5 y:* PO, 0.25–0.75 mcg daily | Most potent form of vitamin D available |

*(continued)*

**DRUG TABLE 20-3**

*Drugs at a Glance*

## Calcium and Vitamin D Preparations (Continued)

| Generic/Trade Name | Routes and Dosage Ranges | Comments/Uses |
|---|---|---|
| **Cholecalciferol (vitamin D₃)** (Delta-D) Pregnancy Category A; C with dose exceeding RDA recommendations | *Adults:* PO, 400–1000 IU daily | |
| **Dihydrotachysterol** (Hytakerol) Pregnancy Category D | *Adults:* PO, 0.75–2.5 mg daily for several days, then decreased (average daily maintenance dose, 0.6 mg) | |
| **Doxercalciferol** (Hectorol) Pregnancy Category B | *Adults:* Dialysis clients, PO, 10 mcg three times weekly initially, increased if necessary. Maximum dose, 20 mcg three times weekly | |
| **Ergocalciferol (vitamin D₂)** (Calciferol, (Drisdol) Pregnancy Category A; C with dose exceeding RDA recommendations | *Adults:* Hypoparathyroidism, PO, 50,000–200,000 units daily initially (average daily maintenance dose, 25,000–100,000 units) | |
| **Paricalcitol** (Zemplar) Pregnancy Category C | *Adults:* Dialysis clients, 0.04–0.1 mcg/kg every other day initially; increased by 2–4 mcg at 2- to 4-week intervals, if necessary | Reduce dosage or stop therapy if hypercalcemia occurs |

intravenously for rapid effects in acute hypercalcemia, opinions seem divided regarding its use. Some recommend its use once extracellular fluid volume has been restored and saline diuresis occurs with IV infusion of several liters of 0.9% sodium chloride. Others recommend its use only if evidence of fluid overload or heart failure develops. Thiazide diuretics are contraindicated in clients with hypercalcemia because they *decrease* urinary excretion of calcium.

**Phosphate salts** (Neutra-Phos) inhibit intestinal absorption of calcium and increase deposition of calcium in bone. Oral salts are effective in the treatment of hypercalcemia of any etiology. A potential adverse effect of phosphates is calcification of soft tissues due to deposition of calcium phosphate. This can lead to severe impairment of function in the kidneys and other organs. Phosphates should be given only when hypercalcemia is accompanied by hypophosphatemia (serum phosphorus <3 mg/dL) and renal function is normal, to minimize the risk for soft tissue calcification. Serum calcium, phosphorus, and creatinine should be monitored frequently, and the dose should be reduced if serum phosphorus exceeds 4.5 mg/dL or the product of serum calcium and phosphorus (measured in milligrams per deciliter) exceeds 60. Neutra-Phos is an oral combination of sodium phosphate and potassium phosphate.

**Plicamycin** (Mithracin) lowers serum calcium levels by blocking calcium resorption from bone. It is used to treat malignancy-associated hypercalcemia that does not respond to hydration and diuretics. Calcium levels start to decline within 12 hours after a dose and reach their lowest levels in 2 to 4 days.

**Sodium chloride (0.9%) injection** (normal saline) is an IV solution containing water, sodium, and chloride. It is included here because it is the treatment of choice for hypercalcemia and is usually effective. The sodium contained in the solution inhibits the reabsorption of calcium in renal tubules and thereby increases urinary excretion of calcium. The solution also relieves the dehydration caused by vomiting and polyuria, and it dilutes the calcium concentration of serum and urine. Several liters are given daily. The client should be monitored closely for signs of fluid overload, and serum calcium, magnesium, and potassium levels should be measured every 6 to 12 hours. Large amounts of magnesium and potassium are lost in the urine, and adequate replacement is essential.

## Adrenal Agent

The adrenal cortex produces glucocorticoids, mineralocorticoids, and adrenal sex hormones. **Fludrocortisone** (Florinef, Apothecon) is the only mineralocorticoid agent described here. Indications for use, route, and dosage range of drug affecting mineralocorticoid activity in the adrenals are listed in Drug at a Glance 20-4: Mineralocorticoid Agent.

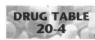

## DRUG TABLE 20-4

*Drug at a Glance*

## Mineralocorticoid Agent

| Generic/Trade Name | Route and Dosage Ranges | Comments/Uses |
|---|---|---|
| **Fludrocortisone** (Florinef, Apothecon)<br>Pregnancy Category C | *Adults:* Chronic adrenocortical insufficiency (Addison's disease): PO, 0.1 mg daily<br>Salt-losing adrenogenetal syndrome: PO, 0.1–0.2 mg daily<br>*Children:* PO, 0.05–0.1 mg daily | Used in conjunction with a glucocorticoid (prednisone, hydrocortisone, or cortisone); the addition of a mineralocorticoid reduces the risk for hyperkalemia |

 **URSING PROCESS**

## Assessment

Assess for disorders for which hypothalamic and pituitary hormones are given:

- For children with impaired growth, assess height and weight (actual and compared with growth charts) and diagnostic x-ray reports of bone age.
- For clients with diabetes insipidus, assess baseline blood pressure, weight, ratio of fluid intake to urine output, urine specific gravity, and laboratory reports of serum electrolytes.
- For clients with diarrhea, assess number and consistency of stools per day as well as hydration status.

Assess for disorders of calcium metabolism:

- Assess for risk factors and manifestations of hypocalcemia and calcium deficiency.
- Assess dietary intake of dairy products, other calcium-containing foods, and vitamin D.
- Check serum calcium reports for abnormal values. The normal total serum calcium level is approximately 8.5 to 10.5 mg/dL (SI units, 2.2 to 2.6 mmol/L). Approximately half of the total serum calcium (eg, 4 to 5 mg/dL) should be free ionized calcium, the physiologically active form. To interpret serum calcium levels accurately, serum albumin levels and acid–base status must be considered. Low serum albumin decreases the total serum level of calcium by decreasing the amount of calcium that is bound to protein. However, the ionized concentration is normal. Metabolic and respiratory alkalosis increase binding of calcium to serum proteins, thereby maintaining normal total serum calcium but decreasing the ionized values. Conversely, metabolic and respiratory acidosis decrease binding and therefore increase the concentration of ionized calcium.
- Check for *Chvostek's sign:* Tap the facial nerve just below the temple, in front of the ear. If facial muscles twitch, hyperirritability of the nerve and potential tetany are indicated.
- Check for *Trousseau's sign:* Constrict blood circulation in an arm (usually with a blood pressure cuff) for 3 to 5 minutes. This produces ischemia and increased irritability of peripheral nerves, which causes spasms of the lower arm and hand muscles (carpopedal spasm) if tetany is present.

- Assess for conditions in which hypercalcemia is likely to occur (eg, cancer, prolonged immobilization, vitamin D overdose).
- Observe for signs and symptoms of hypercalcemia in clients at risk. Electrocardiogram changes indicative of hypercalcemia include a shortened Q-T interval and an inverted T wave.
- Assess for risk factors and manifestations of osteoporosis, especially in postmenopausal women and men and women on chronic corticosteroid therapy.
- If risk factors are identified, determine whether preventive measures are being used (eg, increasing calcium intake, exercise, medications).
- If the client is known to have osteoporosis, ask about duration and severity of symptoms, age of onset, location, whether fractures have occurred, what treatments have been done, and response to treatments.
- If Paget's disease is suspected, assess for an elevated serum alkaline phosphatase level and abnormal bone scan reports.

## Nursing Diagnoses

For disorders for which hypothalamic and pituitary hormones are given:

- Deficient Knowledge: Drug administration and effects
- Anxiety related to multiple injections
- Risk for Injury: Adverse drug effects

For disorders of calcium metabolism:

- Deficient Knowledge: Recommended daily amounts and dietary sources of calcium and vitamin D
- Risk for Injury: Tetany, sedation, seizures from hypocalcemia
- Risk for Injury: Hypercalcemia related to overuse of supplements; hypocalcemia from aggressive treatment of hypercalcemia

## Planning/Goals

*The client will:*

For disorders for which hypothalamic and pituitary hormones are given:

- Experience relief of symptoms without serious adverse effects
- Take or receive the drug accurately
- Comply with procedures for monitoring and follow-up

*(continued)*

## NURSING PROCESS (Continued)

For disorders of calcium metabolism:

- Achieve and maintain normal serum levels of calcium
- Increase dietary intake of calcium-containing foods to prevent or treat osteoporosis
- Use calcium or vitamin D supplements in recommended amounts
- Comply with instructions for safe drug use
- Comply with procedures for follow-up treatment of hypocalcemia, hypercalcemia, or osteoporosis
- Avoid preventable adverse effects of treatment for acute hypocalcemia or hypercalcemia

### Interventions

For disorders for which hypothalamic and pituitary hormones are given:

- For children receiving growth hormone, assist the family to set reasonable goals for increased height and weight and to comply with accurate drug administration and follow-up procedures (periodic x-rays to determine bone growth and progress toward epiphyseal closure, recording height and weight at least weekly).
- For clients with diabetes insipidus, assist them to develop a daily routine to monitor their response to drug therapy (eg, weigh themselves, monitor fluid intake and urine output for approximately equal amounts, or check urine specific gravity [should be at least 1.015] and replace fluids accordingly).

For disorders of calcium metabolism:

- Assist all clients in meeting the recommended daily amounts of calcium and vitamin D. With an adequate protein and calcium intake, enough phosphorus also is obtained.
- Educate that the best dietary source is milk and other dairy products, including yogurt.
    1. Unless contraindicated by the client's condition, recommend that adults drink at least two 8-oz glasses of milk daily. This furnishes about half the daily calcium requirement; the remainder will probably be obtained from other foods.
    2. Children need about four glasses of milk or an equivalent amount of calcium in milk and other foods to support normal growth and development.

3. Pregnant and lactating women also need about four glasses of milk or their equivalents. Vitamin and mineral supplements are usually needed during these periods.
4. Postmenopausal women who take estrogens need 1000 mg daily; those who do not take estrogens need 1500 mg.
5. For clients who avoid or minimize their intake of dairy products because of the calories, identify low-calorie sources, such as skim milk and low-fat yogurt.
6. Milk that has been fortified with vitamin D is the best food source. Exposure of skin to sunlight is also needed to supply adequate amounts of vitamin D.
7. For people who are unable or unwilling to ingest sufficient calcium, a supplement may be needed to prevent osteoporosis.

- Assist clients with hypercalcemia to decrease formation of renal calculi by forcing fluids to approximately 3000 to 4000 mL/day and preventing urinary tract infections.

### Evaluation

For disorders for which hypothalamic and pituitary hormones are given:

- Interview and observe for compliance with instructions for taking the drugs.
- Observe for relief of symptoms for which pituitary hormones were prescribed.

For disorders of calcium metabolism:

- Check laboratory reports of serum calcium levels for normal values.
- Interview and observe for relief of symptoms of hypocalcemia, hypercalcemia, or osteoporosis.
- Interview and observe intake of calcium-containing foods.
- Question about normal calcium requirements and how to meet them.
- Interview and observe for accurate drug use and compliance with follow-up procedures.
- Interview and observe for therapeutic and adverse drug effects.

## ▢ USE IN SPECIFIC SITUATIONS

### Therapeutic Administration of Hypothalamic and Pituitary Hormones

There are few therapeutic uses for hypothalamic hormones and pituitary hormones. Most hypothalamic hormones are used to diagnose pituitary insufficiency. Pituitary hormones are not used extensively because most conditions in which they are indicated are uncommon; other effective agents are available for some uses; and deficiencies of target-gland hormones (eg, corticosteroids, thyroid hormones, male or female sex hormones) are usually more effectively treated with those hormones than with anterior pituitary hormones that stimulate their secretion. However, the hormones perform important functions when used in particular circumstances, and drug formulations of most hormones have been synthesized for these purposes.

### Management of Hypocalcemia

Treatment of hypocalcemia includes giving a calcium preparation and perhaps vitamin D.

## Nursing Actions

## Hypothalamic and Pituitary Hormones

| Nursing Actions | Rationale/Explanation |
|---|---|
| **1. Administer accurately.** | |
| a. Read the manufacturer's instructions and drug labels carefully before drug preparation and administration. | These hormone preparations are given infrequently and often require special techniques of administration. |
| **2. Observe for therapeutic effects.** | Therapeutic effects vary widely, depending on the particular pituitary hormone given and the reason for use. |
| a. With gonadorelin and related drugs, observe for ovulation or decreased symptoms of endometriosis and absence of menstruation. | Therapeutic effects depend on the reason for use. Note that different formulations are used to stimulate ovulation and treat endometriosis. |
| b. With corticotropin, therapeutic effects stem largely from increased secretion of adrenal cortex hormones, especially the glucocorticoids, and include anti-inflammatory effects (see Chap. 36). | Corticotropin is usually not recommended for the numerous nonendocrine inflammatory disorders that respond to glucocorticoids. Administration of glucocorticoids is more convenient and effective than administration of corticotropin. |
| c. With chorionic gonadotropin and menotropins given in cases of female infertility, ovulation and conception are therapeutic effects. | |
| d. With chorionic gonadotropin given in cryptorchidism, the therapeutic effect is descent of the testicles from the abdomen to the scrotum. | |
| e. With growth hormone, observe for increased skeletal growth and development. | Indicated by appropriate increases in height and weight. |
| f. With antidiuretics (desmopressin, lypressin, and vasopressin), observe for decreased urine output, increased urine specific gravity, decreased signs of dehydration, decreased thirst. | These effects indicate control of diabetes insipidus. |
| g. With oxytocin given to induce labor, observe for the beginning or the intensifying of uterine contractions. | |
| h. With oxytocin given to control postpartum bleeding, observe for a firm uterine fundus and decreased vaginal bleeding. | |
| i. With octreotide given for diarrhea, observe for decreased number and fluidity of stools. | Octreotide is often used to control diarrhea associated with a number of conditions. |
| **3. Observe for adverse effects.** | |
| a. With gonadorelin, observe for headache, nausea, lightheadedness, and local edema, pain, and pruritus after subcutaneous injections. | Systemic reactions occur infrequently. |
| b. With corticotropin, observe for sodium and fluid retention, edema, hypokalemia, hyperglycemia, osteoporosis, increased susceptibility to infection, myopathy, behavioral changes. | These adverse reactions are in general the same as those produced by adrenal cortex hormones. Severity of adverse reactions tends to increase with dosage and duration of corticotropin administration. |
| c. With human chorionic gonadotropin given to preadolescent boys, observe for sexual precocity, breast enlargement, and edema. | Sexual precocity results from stimulation of excessive testosterone secretion at an early age. |
| d. With growth hormone, observe for mild edema, headache, localized muscle pain, weakness, hyperglycemia. | Adverse effects are not common. Another adverse effect may be development of antibodies to the drug, but this does not prevent its growth-stimulating effects. |
| e. With menotropins, observe for symptoms of ovarian hyperstimulation, such as abdominal discomfort, weight gain, ascites, pleural effusion, oliguria, and hypotension. | Adverse effects can be minimized by frequent pelvic examinations to check for ovarian enlargement and by laboratory measurement of estrogen levels. Multiple gestation (mostly twins) is a possibility and is related to ovarian overstimulation. |

*(continued)*

## Nursing Actions
## Hypothalamic and Pituitary Hormones (Continued)

| Nursing Actions | Rationale/Explanation |
|---|---|
| f. With desmopressin, observe for headache, nasal congestion, nausea, and increased blood pressure. A more serious adverse reaction is water retention and hyponatremia. | Adverse reactions usually occur only with high dosages and tend to be relatively mild. Water intoxication (headache, nausea, vomiting, confusion, lethargy, coma, convulsions) may occur with any antidiuretic therapy if excessive fluids are ingested. |
| g. With lypressin, observe for headache and congestion of nasal passages, dyspnea and coughing (if the drug is inhaled), and water intoxication if excessive amounts of lypressin or fluid are taken. | Adverse effects are usually mild and occur infrequently with usual doses. |
| h. With vasopressin, observe for water intoxication; chest pain, myocardial infarction, increased blood pressure; abdominal cramps, nausea, and diarrhea. | With high doses, vasopressin constricts blood vessels, especially coronary arteries, and stimulates smooth muscle of the gastrointestinal tract. Special caution is necessary in clients with heart disease, asthma, or epilepsy. |
| i. With oxytocin, observe for excessive stimulation or contractility of the uterus, uterine rupture, and cervical and perineal lacerations. | Severe adverse reactions are most likely to occur when oxytocin is given to induce labor and delivery. |
| j. With octreotide, observe for arrhythmias, bradycardia, diarrhea, headache, hyperglycemia, injection site pain, and symptoms of gallstones. | These are more common effects, especially in those receiving octreotide for acromegaly. |
| **4. Observe for drug interactions.** | |
| a. Drugs that *increase* effects of vasopressin: General anesthetics, chlorpropamide (Diabinese) | Potentiate vasopressin |
| b. Drug that *decreases* effects of vasopressin: Lithium | Inhibits the renal tubular reabsorption of water normally stimulated by vasopressin |
| c. Drugs that *increase* effects of oxytocin: (1) Estrogens | With adequate estrogen levels, oxytocin increases uterine contractility. When estrogen levels are low, the effect of oxytocin is reduced. |
| (2) Vasoconstrictors or vasopressors (eg, ephedrine, epinephrine, norepinephrine) | Severe, persistent hypertension with rupture of cerebral blood vessels may occur because of additive vasoconstrictor effects. This is a potentially lethal interaction and should be avoided. |

1. Acute, severe hypocalcemia is a medical emergency and requires IV administration of calcium, usually 10 to 20 mL of 10% calcium gluconate (1 to 2 g of calcium). Doses may be repeated, a continuous infusion may be given, or oral supplements may be used to avoid symptoms of hypocalcemia and maintain normal serum calcium levels (as measured every 4 to 6 hours). Once stabilized, treatment is aimed toward the underlying cause or preventing recurrence. Serum magnesium levels should also be measured, and if hypomagnesemia is present, it must be treated before treatment of hypocalcemia can be effective.

2. For less acute situations or for long-term treatment of chronic hypocalcemia, oral calcium supplements are preferred. Vitamin D is also given if a calcium preparation alone cannot maintain serum calcium levels within a normal range.

3. Calcium deficits caused by inadequate dietary intake affect bone tissue rather than serum calcium levels. Calcium supplements can decrease bone loss and fractures, especially in women, including those who take replacement estrogens. Calcium carbonate contains the most elemental calcium by weight (40%) and is inexpensive. It is available in the nonprescription antacid called Tums. Calcium citrate is reportedly better absorbed than calcium carbonate.

4. If hypocalcemia is caused by diarrhea or malabsorption, treatment of the underlying condition decreases loss of calcium from the body and increases absorption.

5. When vitamin D is given to treat hypocalcemia, dosage is determined by frequent measurement of serum calcium levels. Usually, higher doses are given initially and lower doses for maintenance therapy.

6. Calcium salts and vitamin D are combined in many over-the-counter preparations promoted as dietary supplements (Table 20-1). These preparations contain variable amounts of calcium and vitamin D. Calcium, 600 mg, and vitamin D, 200 IU, once or twice daily are often recommended for postmenopausal women with osteoporosis. In general, intake of calcium should not exceed 2500 mg daily, from all sources, and intake of vitamin D should not exceed 400 IU daily. These mixtures are not indicated for maintenance therapy in chronic hypocalcemia.

7. Calcium preparations and digoxin have similar effects on the myocardium. Therefore, if calcium is given to a digitalized client, the risk for digitalis toxicity and cardiac dysrhythmia is increased. This combination must be used very cautiously.

8. Oral calcium preparations decrease effects of oral tetracycline drugs by combining with the antibiotic and preventing its absorption. They should not be given at the same time or within 2 to 3 hours of each other.

## Management of Hypercalcemia

Clients at risk for hypercalcemia should be monitored for early signs and symptoms so that treatment can be started before severe hypercalcemia develops. Treatment depends largely on the cause and severity.

1. When hypercalcemia is caused by a tumor of parathyroid tissue, the usual treatment is surgical excision. When it is caused by malignant tumor, treatment of the tumor with surgery, irradiation, or chemotherapy may reduce production of PTH. When it is caused by excessive intake of vitamin D, the vitamin D preparation should be stopped immediately.

2. Acute hypercalcemia is a medical emergency. It is treated with interventions that increase calcium excretion in the urine and decrease resorption of calcium from bone into the serum. For severe symptoms or a serum calcium level above 12 mg/dL, the priority is rehydration. This need can be met by IV saline infusion (0.9% or 0.45% NaCl), 4000 mL/day or more if kidney function is adequate. After rehydration, furosemide may be given intravenously to increase renal excretion of calcium and prevent fluid overload. Because sodium, potassium, and water are also lost in the urine, these must be replaced in the IV fluids.

With mild hypercalcemia, most clients respond to the aforementioned treatment, and further drug therapy is not needed. With moderate to severe hypercalcemia, pamidronate or zoledronate may be the drug of choice. When pamidronate is given in a single IV infusion containing 60 or 90 mg, serum calcium levels decrease within 2 days, reach their lowest levels in approximately 7 days, and remain lower for 2 weeks or longer. Treatment can be repeated if hypercalcemia recurs. Zoledronate can be given over 15 minutes, and its effects may last longer than those of pamidronate. Adverse effects of the two drugs are similar. Phosphates should not be used unless hypophosphatemia is present. They are also contraindicated in clients with persistent urinary tract infections and alkaline urine because calcium phosphate kidney stones are likely to form in such cases.

3. Chronic hypercalcemia requires treatment of the underlying disease process and measures to control serum calcium levels (eg, a high fluid intake and mobilization to help retain calcium in bone). Oral phosphate administration may help if other measures are ineffective.

4. Serum calcium levels should be measured periodically to monitor effects of therapy.

5. For clients with severely impaired renal function in whom hypercalcemia develops, hemodialysis or peritoneal dialysis with a calcium-free solution is effective and safe.

6. For clients receiving a calcium channel blocker (see Chap. 41), the drug may be less effective in the presence of hypercalcemia.

### TABLE 20-1 Selected Calcium/Vitamin D Combination Products

| Generic/ Trade Name | Calcium (mg)*/ Tablet or Capsule | Vitamin D (IU)*/ Tablet |
|---|---|---|
| Caltrate 600 + D and Caltrate Plus | 600 | 200 |
| Citracal caplets + D | 315 | 200 |
| Dical-D tablets | 117 | 133 |
| Dical-D Wafers | 233 | 200 |
| Os-Cal 250 + D | 250 | 125 |
| Os-Cal 500 + D | 500 | 125 |
| Posture-D | 600 | 125 |

*mg of elemental calcium; *IU, international units.

## Nursing Actions

## Drugs Used in Calcium and Bone Disorders

| Nursing Actions | Rationale/Explanation |
|---|---|
| 1. Administer accurately. | |
| a. With calcium preparations: | |
| (1) Give oral preparations with or after meals. | To increase absorption |
| (2) Give intravenous (IV) preparations slowly (0.5–2 mL/min), check pulse and blood pressure closely, and monitor the electrocardiogram (ECG) if possible. | These solutions may cause dysrhythmias and hypotension if injected rapidly. They are also irritating to tissues. |
| (3) Do not mix IV preparations with any other drug in the same syringe. | Calcium reacts with some other drugs and forms a precipitate. |
| b. With bisphosphonates: | |
| (1) Give alendronate and risedronate with 6–8 oz of plain water, at least 30 min before the first food, beverage, or medication of the day. | To promote absorption and decrease esophageal and gastric irritation |
| (2) Give oral etidronate on an empty stomach, as a single dose or in divided doses. Avoid giving within 2 h of ingesting dairy products, antacids, or vitamin or mineral preparations. | If gastrointestinal (GI) symptoms occur with the single dose, divided doses may relieve them. Substances containing calcium or other minerals decrease absorption of etidronate. |
| (3) Give IV etidronate, pamidronate, and zoledronate according to the manufacturers' instructions. | These drugs require reconstitution, diluting with IV fluids, and specific time intervals of administration. |
| c. Give calcitonin at bedtime. | To decrease nausea and discomfort from flushing |
| d. With phosphate salts, mix powder forms with water for oral administration. See package inserts for specific instructions. | |
| 2. Observe for therapeutic effects. | |
| a. With calcium preparations, observe for: | |
| (1) Relief of symptoms of neuromuscular irritability and tetany, such as decreased muscle spasms and decreased paresthesias | |
| (2) Serum calcium levels within the normal range (8.5–10.5 mg/dL) | |
| (3) Absence of Chvostek's and Trousseau's signs | |
| b. With alendronate or risedronate for osteoporosis, observe for improved bone mass density and absence of fractures. | Early osteopenia and osteoporosis are asymptomatic. Measurement of bone mass density is the only way to quantify bone loss. |
| c. With calcitonin, corticosteroids, pamidronate, or zoledronate for hypercalcemia, observe for: | |
| (1) Decreased serum calcium level | Calcitonin lowers serum calcium levels in about 2 h after injection and effects last 6–8 h. Corticosteroids require 10–14 days to lower serum calcium. Bisphosphonates lower serum calcium levels within 2 days, but may require a week or more to produce normal serum calcium levels. |
| (2) Decreased signs and symptoms of hypercalcemia | |
| 3. Observe for adverse effects. | |
| a. With calcium preparations, observe for hypercalcemia: | |
| (1) GI effects—anorexia, nausea, vomiting, abdominal pain, constipation | |
| (2) Central nervous system effects—apathy, poor memory, depression, drowsiness, disorientation | |
| (3) Other effects—weakness and decreased tone in skeletal and smooth muscles, dysphagia, polyuria, polydipsia, cardiac dysrhythmias | |
| (4) Serum calcium >10.5 mg/dL | |
| (5) ECG changes indicating hypercalcemia (a prolonged Q-T interval and an inverted T wave) | |

*(continued)*

*Nursing Actions*

## Drugs Used in Calcium and Bone Disorders (Continued)

| Nursing Actions | Rationale/Explanation |
|---|---|
| b. With vitamin D preparations, observe for hypervitaminosis D and hypercalcemia (see above). | This is most likely to occur with chronic ingestion of high doses daily. In children, accidental ingestion may lead to acute toxicity. |
| c. With alendronate and risedronate, observe for:<br>(1) GI effects—abdominal distention, acid regurgitation, dysphagia, esophagitis, flatulence<br>(2) Other effects—headache, musculoskeletal pain, decreased serum calcium and phosphate | Adverse effects are usually minor with the doses taken for prevention or treatment of osteoporosis, if the drugs are taken as directed. More severe effects may occur with the higher doses taken for Paget's disease. |
| d. With calcitonin, observe for nausea, vomiting, tissue irritation at administration sites, and allergic reactions. | Adverse effects are usually mild and transient. Nasal administration produces greater client compliance than injections, with few adverse effects. |
| e. With drug therapy of hypercalcemia, observe for hypocalcemia. | Hypocalcemia may occur with vigorous treatment of hypercalcemia. This can be minimized by monitoring serum calcium levels frequently and adjusting drug dosages and other treatments. |
| f. With pamidronate and zoledronate, observe for:<br>(1) GI effects—anorexia, nausea, vomiting, constipation<br>(2) Cardiovascular effects—fluid overload, hypertension<br>(3) Electrolyte imbalances—hypokalemia, hypomagnesemia, hypophosphatemia<br>(4) Musculoskeletal effects—muscle and joint pain<br>(5) Miscellaneous effects—fever, tissue irritation at IV insertion site, pain, anemia | |
| g. With etidronate, observe for anorexia, nausea, diarrhea, bone pain, fever, fluid overload, and increased serum creatinine. | Adverse effects are more frequent and more severe at higher doses. The drug is nephrotoxic and should not be used in clients with renal failure. |
| h. With phosphates, observe for nausea, vomiting, and diarrhea. | |
| **4. Observe for drug interactions.**<br>a. Drugs that *increase* effects of calcium:<br>(1) Vitamin D | Increases intestinal absorption of calcium from both dietary and supplemental drug sources |
| (2) Thiazide diuretics | Reduce calcium losses in urine |
| b. Drugs that *decrease* effects of calcium: Corticosteroids (prednisone, others), calcitonin, and phosphates | These drugs lower serum calcium levels by various mechanisms. They are used in the treatment of hypercalcemia. |
| c. Drugs that *increase* effects of vitamin D: Thiazide diuretics | Thiazide diuretics administered to hypoparathyroid clients may cause hypercalcemia (potentiate vitamin D effects) |
| d. Drugs that *decrease* effects of vitamin D:<br>(1) Phenytoin | Accelerates metabolism of vitamin D in the liver and may cause vitamin D deficiency, hypocalcemia, and rickets or osteomalacia. Increased intake of vitamin D may be needed. |
| (2) Cholestyramine resin (Questran)<br>(3) Mineral oil | May decrease intestinal absorption of vitamin D preparations<br>Mineral oil is a fat and therefore combines with fat-soluble vitamins, such as vitamin D, and prevents their absorption from the gastrointestinal tract. |
| e. Drugs that *decrease* effects of alendronate and other oral bisphosphonates: Antacids and calcium supplements | These drugs interfere with absorption of bisphosphonates and should be taken at least 2 h after a bisphosphonate. |
| f. Drugs that alter effects of calcitonin:<br>(1) Testosterone and other androgens *increase* effects. | Androgens and calcitonin have additive effects on calcium retention and inhibition of bone resorption (movement of calcium from bone to serum). |
| (2) Parathyroid hormone *decreases* effects. | Parathyroid hormone antagonizes or opposes calcitonin. |
| g. Drugs that *decrease* effects of phosphate salts: Antacids containing aluminum and magnesium | Aluminum and magnesium may combine with phosphate and thereby prevent its absorption and therapeutic effect. |

## Prevention of Osteoporosis

Preventive measures should be implemented for all age groups to avoid or slow bone loss.

1. In all age groups, preventive efforts include a consistently adequate dietary intake of calcium to promote normal bone development and maintenance. In children, adolescents, and young adults, an adequate calcium intake promotes bone growth and peak bone mass. A well-stocked "reservoir" means that, in later years when bone loss exceeds formation, more bone can be lost before osteoporosis develops. In postmenopausal women and men older than 40 years of age, an adequate calcium intake may slow the development of osteoporosis and fractures. Although dietary intake is much preferred, a supplement may be needed to ensure a daily intake of 1000 to 1500 mg, especially in adolescent girls, frail elderly clients, and those receiving corticosteroids.

2. Regular exercise is also important in all age groups. Vigorous, weight-bearing exercise helps to promote and maintain strong bone; inactivity promotes bone weakening and loss.

3. Women who smoke should be encouraged to stop. Smoking decreases the amount of active estrogen in the body and thus accelerates bone loss.

4. Estrogen replacement therapy (plus progesterone in those with an intact uterus) is being questioned as the best preventive measure for postmenopausal women. See Chapter 24 for further discussion. Conjugated estrogens (eg, Premarin) have been used in most studies; 0.625 mg daily is considered adequate for "bone protection." If ERT is stopped, the rate of bone loss accelerates. Thus, lifetime therapy may be needed. ERT is contraindicated in women with active estrogen-dependent cancers.

5. Alendronate (Fosamax) and risedronate (Actonel) are approved by the U.S. Food and Drug Administration (FDA) for prevention of osteoporosis. With alendronate, recommended dosage is smaller for prevention than for treatment.

6. Raloxifene (Evista) is approved for prevention of postmenopausal osteoporosis in women who are unable or unwilling to take ERT.

7. An adequate intake of vitamin D helps to prevent osteoporosis, but supplementation is probably not indicated unless a deficiency can be demonstrated. Serum calcitriol can be measured in clients at risk for vitamin D deficiency, including elderly adults and those on chronic corticosteroid therapy.

8. Preventive measures are needed for clients on chronic corticosteroid therapy (eg, prednisone, 7.5 mg daily, equivalent amounts of other systemic drugs, or high doses of inhaled drugs). For both men and women, most of the preceding guidelines apply (eg, calcium supplements, regular exercise, a bisphosphonate drug). In addition, low doses and nonsystemic routes help prevent osteoporosis and other adverse effects. For men, corticosteroids decrease testosterone levels by approximately one half, and replacement therapy may be needed.

## Management of Osteoporosis

Once bone loss is evident (from diagnostic tests of bone density or occurrence of fractures), several interventions may help slow further skeletal bone loss or prevent fractures. Most drugs used to treat osteoporosis decrease the rate of bone breakdown and thus slow the rate of bone loss; a newer drug, teriparatide (Forteo), actually increases bone formation.

1. As with prevention, those diagnosed with osteoporosis need adequate calcium and vitamin D (at least the recommended dietary allowance), whether obtained from the diet or from supplements. Pharmacologic doses of vitamin D are sometimes used to treat clients with serious osteoporosis. If such doses are used, caution should be exercised because excessive amounts of vitamin D can cause hypercalcemia and hypercalciuria.

2. Regular exercise is needed. Numerous studies indicate that regular physical activity helps to reduce bone loss and fractures.

3. Women who smoke should be encouraged to stop because smoking has effects similar to those of menopause (estrogen deficiency and accelerated bone loss).

4. In menopausal women, ERT is the most beneficial treatment and should usually be used along with any other measures (see Prevention of Osteoporosis, earlier). For women with an intact uterus, combined estrogen and progesterone therapy (HRT) is needed.

5. Alendronate (Fosamax), 10 mg daily or 70 mg weekly, and risedronate (Actonel), 5 mg daily, are FDA approved for treatment of osteoporosis in postmenopausal women. The drugs can increase bone mineral density, reduce the risk for vertebral fractures, and slow progression of vertebral deformities and loss of height. One of these drugs is often used in combination with estrogen and calcium and vitamin D supplements.

6. Treatment of men is similar to that of women except that testosterone replacement may be needed rather than estrogen.

7. With corticosteroid-induced osteoporosis, multiple treatment measures may be needed, including increased dietary and supplemental calcium and possibly vitamin D supplementation, hormone replacement, corticosteroid dosage reduction, exercise, and a bisphosphonate or calcitonin to slow skeletal bone loss.

## Disorders of the Adrenal Cortex

Disorders of the adrenal cortex involve increased or decreased production of corticosteroids (see Chap. 36) and aldosterone as the primary mineralocorticoid. Two

## CLIENT TEACHING GUIDELINES
### Drugs for Osteoporosis

**General Considerations**

✔ Osteoporosis involves weak bones that fracture easily and may cause pain and disability.

✔ Important factors in prevention and treatment include an adequate intake of calcium and vitamin D (from the diet, from supplements, or a combination of both sources), regular weight-bearing exercise, and drugs that can slow bone loss.

✔ It is better to obtain calcium and vitamin D from foods such as milk and other dairy products. Approximately 1000 to 1500 mg of calcium and 400 IU of vitamin D are recommended daily.

✔ If unable to get sufficient dietary calcium and vitamin D, consider supplements of these nutrients. Consult a health care provider about the types and amounts. For example, a daily multivitamin and mineral supplement may contain adequate amounts when added to dietary intake. If taking other supplements, avoid those containing bone meal because they may contain lead and other contaminants that are toxic to the human body. Do not take more than the recommended amounts of supplements; overuse can cause serious, life-threatening problems.

✔ The main drugs approved for prevention and treatment of osteoporosis are the bisphosphonates (eg, Fosamax, Actonel). These drugs help prevent the loss of calcium from bone, thereby strengthening bone and reducing the risks of fractures.

✔ For people at high risk for development of osteoporosis (eg, postmenopausal women, men and women who take an oral or inhaled corticosteroid such as prednisone or fluticasone [Flonase]), or those being treated for osteoporosis, a baseline measurement of bone mineral density and periodic follow-up measurements are needed. This is a noninvasive test that does not involve any injections or device insertions.

**Self-administration**

✔ If taking a calcium supplement, calcium carbonate 500 mg twice daily is often recommended. This can be obtained from an inexpensive over-the-counter antacid called Tums, which contains 200 mg of calcium per tablet.

✔ Do not take a calcium supplement with an iron preparation, tetracycline, ciprofloxacin, or phenytoin. Instead, take the drugs at least 2 hours apart to avoid calcium interference with absorption of the other drugs.

✔ If taking both a calcium supplement and a bisphosphonate, take the calcium at least 2 hours after the bisphosphonate. Calcium, antacids, and other drugs interfere with absorption of bisphosphonate.

✔ Take bisphosphonates with 6 to 8 oz of water at least 30 minutes before any food, other fluid, or other medication. Beverages other than water and foods decrease absorption and effectiveness.

✔ Take a bisphosphonate in an upright position and do not lie down for at least 30 minutes. This helps prevent esophageal irritation and stomach upset.

---

disorders in which mineralocorticoid secretion is significantly impaired are as follows:

- **Primary adrenocortical insufficiency (Addison's disease)** is associated with destruction of the adrenal cortex by disorders such as tuberculosis, cancer, or hemorrhage; with atrophy of the adrenal cortex caused by autoimmune disease or prolonged administration of exogenous corticosteroids; and with surgical excision of the adrenal glands. In this condition, there is inadequate production of both cortisol and aldosterone.
- **Hyperaldosteronism** is a rare disorder caused by adenoma or hyperplasia of the adrenal cortex cells that produce aldosterone. It is characterized by hypokalemia, hypernatremia, hypertension, thirst, and polyuria.

## Critical Thinking Exercises

1. A calcium preparation is started in a client currently taking digoxin. The nurse should be aware of the following potential effect on the myocardium:

   a. Congestive heart failure
   b. Dysrhythmias
   c. Decreased atrial natriuretic factor
   d. Increased hypercoagulability

2. A low serum albumin has what effect on the serum level of calcium?

   a. Increases the total serum level
   b. Decreases the ionized concentration
   c. Increases the ionized concentration
   d. Decreases the total serum level

3. The main drugs approved for prevention and treatment of osteoporosis include all of the following except:

   a. Estrogen replacement therapy
   b. Alendronate (Fosamax)
   c. Risedronate (Actonel)
   d. Tamoxifen (Nolvadex)

4. Drugs equivalent to gonadotropin-releasing hormone, such as leuprolide (Lupron), are given by intramuscular depot injections because the drugs cannot be given orally. This is because:

 a. Enzymes in the gastrointestinal tract would destroy them

 b. They undergo extensive first-pass metabolism by the liver

 c. They cause significant gastric ulcerations with oral administration

 d. They are unpalatable and are frequently refused by clients

5. Postmenopausal women who take estrogens have the following recommendation for calcium intake:

 a. Vitamin D, 200 IU, once or twice daily to supplement dietary calcium intake

 b. Calcium, 1000 mg daily

 c. Calcium, 1500 mg daily

 d. Calcium, 2500 mg daily, with vitamin D, 400 IU daily

## SELECTED REFERENCES

*Drug facts and comparisons.* (Updated monthly). St. Louis: Facts and Comparisons.

Guyton, A. C., & Hall, J. E. (2000). *Textbook of medical physiology* (10th ed.). Philadelphia: W. B. Saunders.

Lacy, C. F., Armstrong, L. L., Goldman, M. P., & Lance, L. L. (2003). *Lexi-Comp's drug information handbook* (11th ed.). Hudson, OH: American Pharmaceutical Association.

Lobaugh, B. L., & Drezner, M. K. (2000). Approach to hypercalcemia and hypocalcemia. In H. D. Humes (Ed.), *Kelley's textbook of internal medicine* (4th ed., pp. 2652–2662). Philadelphia: Lippincott Williams & Wilkins.

Marshall, J. C., & Barkan, A. L. (2000). Disorders of the hypothalamus and anterior pituitary. In H. D. Humes (Ed.), *Kelley's textbook of internal medicine* (4th ed., pp. 2663–2683). Philadelphia: Lippincott Williams & Wilkins.

Parent-Stevens, L. (2000) Osteoporosis and osteomalacia. In E. T. Herfindal & D. R. Gourley (Eds.), *Textbook of therapeutics: Drug and disease management* (7th ed., pp. 709–723). Philadelphia: Lippincott Williams & Wilkins.

Porth, C. M. (Ed.). (2002). *Pathophysiology: Concepts of altered health states* (6th ed.). Philadelphia: Lippincott Williams & Wilkins.

Prestwood, K. M. (2000). Diagnosis and management of osteoporosis in older adults. In H. D. Humes (Ed.), *Kelley's textbook of internal medicine* (4th ed., pp. 3074–3082). Philadelphia: Lippincott Williams & Wilkins.

Robinson, A. G. (2000). Disorders of posterior pituitary function. In H. D. Humes (Ed.), *Kelley's textbook of internal medicine* (4th ed., pp. 2684–2691). Philadelphia: Lippincott Williams & Wilkins.

Shoback, D., & Gross, C. (2000). Metabolic bone disease. In H. D. Humes (Ed.), *Kelley's textbook of internal medicine* (4th ed., pp. 2769–2784). Philadelphia: Lippincott Williams & Wilkins.

Singh, R. F., & Dong, B. J. (2000). Parathyroid disorders. In E. T. Herfindal & D. R. Gourley (Eds.), *Textbook of therapeutics: Drug and disease management* (7th ed., pp. 359–375). Philadelphia: Lippincott Williams & Wilkins.

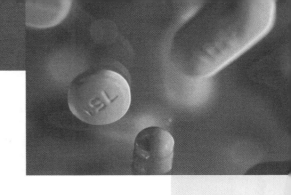

# 21

# Thyroid and Antithyroid Drugs

## OBJECTIVES

*After studying this chapter, the student will be able to:*

1 Describe physiologic effects of thyroid hormone.

2 Identify subclinical, symptomatic, and severe effects of inadequate or excessive thyroid hormone.

3 Give characteristics, uses, and effects of thyroid drugs.

4 Describe characteristics, uses, and effects of antithyroid drugs.

5 Discuss the influence of thyroid and antithyroid drugs on the metabolism of other drugs.

6 Teach clients self-care activities related to the use of thyroid and antithyroid drugs.

## CRITICAL THINKING SCENARIO

$\mathcal{M}$ary Sanchez, 55 years of age, is diagnosed with chronic (Hashimoto's) thyroiditis and is to begin treatment with levothyroxine (Synthroid), 0.1 mg daily. You are the nurse in the clinic and are responsible for teaching Ms. Sanchez about her hypothyroidism and thyroid replacement therapy.

✔ What are the signs and symptoms of hypothyroidism, and what is its impact on the client's functional abilities?

✔ What priority information should be given to Ms. Sanchez during the brief (10-minute) time allotted?

✔ How will you need to individualize teaching if Ms. Sanchez's ability to speak and read English is limited?

✔ Describe the necessary follow-up for Ms. Sanchez's hypothyroidism and drug management.

## PROTOTYPE PROFILES

**levothyroxine** (Synthroid, Levothroid), p. 356

**propylthiouracil** (PTU), p. 357

## OVERVIEW

The thyroid gland produces three hormones: thyroxine, triiodothyronine, and calcitonin. Thyroxine contains four atoms of iodine and is also called $T_4$. Triiodothyronine contains three atoms of iodine and is called $T_3$. Compared with thyroxine, triiodothyronine is more potent and has a more rapid onset but shorter duration of action. Despite these minor differences, the two hormones produce the same physiologic effects and have the same actions and uses; they are discussed in At the Foundation: Thyroid Hormone Production. Calcitonin functions in calcium metabolism and is discussed in Chapter 20.

Thyroid hormones control the rate of cellular metabolism and thereby influence the functioning of virtually every cell in the body. The heart, skeletal muscle, liver, and kidneys are especially responsive to the stimulating effects of thyroid hormones. The brain, spleen, and gonads are less responsive. Thyroid hormones are required for normal growth and development and are considered especially critical for brain and skeletal development and maturation. These hormones are thought to act mainly by controlling intracellular protein synthesis. Some specific physiologic effects include the following:

- Increased rate of cellular metabolism and oxygen consumption with a resultant increase in heat production
- Increased heart rate, force of contraction, and cardiac output (increased cardiac workload)
- Increased carbohydrate metabolism
- Increased fat metabolism, including increased lipolytic effects of other hormones and metabolism of cholesterol to bile acids
- Inhibition of pituitary secretion of thyroid-stimulating hormone (TSH)

## THYROID DISORDERS

Thyroid disorders requiring drug therapy are goiter, hypothyroidism, and hyperthyroidism. Hypothyroidism and hyperthyroidism produce opposing effects on body tissues, depending on the levels of circulating thyroid hormone. Signs and symptoms of thyroid disorders may mimic those of other disorders that often occur in older adults (eg, congestive heart failure). Therefore, a thorough physical examination and diagnostic tests of thyroid function are necessary before starting any type of treatment. Guidelines for strategies for ongoing evaluation and intervention in the home and with children and older adults are addressed in Home Care Considerations and Age-related Considerations, respectively. Specific effects and clinical manifestations are listed in Table 21-1.

### Simple Goiter

Simple goiter is an enlargement of the thyroid gland resulting from iodine deficiency. Inadequate iodine decreases thyroid hormone production. To compensate, the anterior pituitary gland secretes more TSH, which causes the thyroid to enlarge and produce more hormone. If the enlarged gland secretes enough hormone, thyroid function is normal, and the main consequences of the goiter are disfigurement, psychological distress, dyspnea, and dysphagia. If the gland cannot secrete enough hormone despite enlargement, hypothyroidism results. Simple or endemic goiter is a common condition in some geographic areas. It is uncommon in the United States, largely because of the widespread use of iodized table salt.

Treatment of simple goiter involves giving iodine preparations and thyroid hormones to prevent further enlargement and to promote regression in gland size. Large goiters may require surgical excision.

---

**AT THE FOUNDATION: *Thyroid Hormone Production***

Production of thyroxine and triiodothyronine depends on the presence of iodine and tyrosine in the thyroid gland. Plasma iodide is derived from dietary sources and from the metabolic breakdown of thyroid hormone, which allows some iodine to be reused. The thyroid gland extracts iodide from the circulating blood, concentrates it, and secretes enzymes that change the chemically inactive iodide to free iodine atoms. Tyrosine is an amino acid derived from dietary protein. It forms the basic structure of thyroglobulin. In a series of chemical reactions, iodine atoms become attached to tyrosine to form the thyroid hormones $T_3$ and $T_4$. Once formed, the hormones are stored within the chemically inactive thyroglobulin molecule.

Thyroid hormones are released into the circulation when the thyroid gland is stimulated by thyroid-stimulating hormone (thyrotropin or TSH) from the anterior pituitary gland. Because the thyroglobulin molecule is too large to cross cell membranes, proteolytic enzymes break down the molecule so that the active hormones can be released. After their release from thyroglobulin, the hormones become largely bound to plasma proteins. Only the small amounts left unbound are biologically active. The bound thyroid hormones are released to tissue cells very slowly. Once in the cells, the hormones combine with intracellular proteins so that they are again stored. They are released slowly within the cell and used over a period of days or weeks. Once used by the cells, the thyroid hormones release the iodine atoms. Most of the iodine is reabsorbed and used to produce new thyroid hormones; the remainder is excreted in the urine.

## Home Care Considerations: Use of Thyroid and Antithyroid Drugs

**ASSESS:** the client and family's knowledge of disease process; the client for compliance with the prescribed regimen, for quality of life; and need for referral for treatment.

**MONITOR:** the therapeutic and adverse effects of medications, especially with changes in drugs or dosages; that client is keeping appointments for lab work and follow-up care; the client's understanding of the importance of compliance and not stopping drugs inappropriately.

**EDUCATE:** on safe use of the drugs (eg, avoiding OTC medications without first consulting provider), on ways to minimize adverse effects, on not switching brands (liotrix), and to take medication at the same time each day (preferably in the morning) to maintain a constant serum level and avoid sleep disturbances. Reinforce additional teaching points (see Client Teaching Guidelines: Levothyroxine; Propylthiouracil or Methimazole).

## Hypothyroidism

Primary hypothyroidism occurs when disease or destruction of thyroid gland tissue causes inadequate production of thyroid hormones. Common causes of primary hypothyroidism include chronic (Hashimoto's) thyroiditis, an autoimmune disorder, and treatment of hyperthyroidism with antithyroid drugs, radiation therapy, or surgery. Other causes include previous radiation to the thyroid area of the neck and treatment with amiodarone, lithium, or iodine. Secondary hypothyroidism occurs when there is decreased TSH from the anterior pituitary gland.

Congenital hypothyroidism (cretinism) occurs when a child is born without a thyroid gland or with a poorly functioning gland. Cretinism is uncommon in the United States but may occur with a lack of iodine in the mother's diet. Symptoms are rarely present at birth, but develop gradually during infancy and early childhood and include poor growth and development, lethargy and inactivity, feeding problems, slow pulse, subnormal temperature, and constipation. If the disorder is untreated until the child is several months old, permanent mental retardation is likely to result.

Adult hypothyroidism (myxedema) may be subclinical or clinical and occurs much more often in women than in men. Subclinical hypothyroidism, which is the most common thyroid disorder, involves mildly elevated serum TSH and normal serum thyroxine levels. It is usually asymptomatic. Clinical hypothyroidism produces variable signs and symptoms, depending on the amount of

## Age-related Considerations: Use of Thyroid and Antithyroid Drugs

### USE IN CHILDREN

For *hypothyroidism* in children, replacement therapy is required because thyroid hormone is essential for normal growth and development. As in adults, levothyroxine is the drug of choice in children, and dosage needs may change with growth. Infants requiring thyroid hormone replacement need relatively large doses. After thyroid drugs are started, the maintenance dosage is determined by periodic radioimmunoassay of serum thyroxine levels and by periodic radiographs to follow bone development. For congenital hypothyroidism (cretinism), drug therapy should be started within 6 weeks of birth and continued for life. Initially, the recommended dose is 10 to 15 mcg/kg per day. Then, maintenance doses for long-term therapy vary with the child's age and weight, usually decreasing over time to a typical adult dose at 11 to 20 years of age. To monitor drug effects on growth, height and weight should be recorded and compared with growth charts at regular intervals. Adverse drug effects are similar to those seen in adults, and children should be monitored closely.

For *hyperthyroidism* in children, propylthiouracil or methimazole is used. Potential risks for adverse effects are similar to those in adults. Because radioactive iodine may cause cancer and chromosome damage in children, it should be used only for hyperthyroidism that cannot be controlled by other antithyroid drugs or surgery.

### USE IN OLDER ADULTS

For *hypothyroidism*, levothyroxine is given. Thyroid replacement hormone increases the workload of the heart and may cause serious adverse effects in older adults, especially those with cardiovascular disease. Cardiac effects also may be increased in clients receiving bronchodilators or other cardiac stimulants. To decrease adverse effects, the drugs should be given in small initial dosages (eg, 25 mcg/day) and increased by 25 mcg/day at monthly intervals until euthyroidism is attained and a maintenance dose established. Periodic measurements of serum TSH levels are indicated to monitor drug therapy, and doses can be adjusted when indicated.

Blood pressure and pulse should be monitored regularly. As a general rule, the drug should not be given if the resting heart rate is more than 100 beats/minute.

For *hyperthyroidism*, propylthiouracil or methimazole may be used, but radioactive iodine is often preferred because it is associated with fewer adverse effects than other antithyroid drugs or surgery. Clients should be monitored closely for hypothyroidism, which usually develops within a year after receiving treatment for hyperthyroidism.

Clients who are elderly or have cardiovascular disease require cautious treatment because of a high risk for adverse effects on the cardiovascular system. Thus, they are given smaller initial doses and smaller increments at longer intervals than younger adults.

## TABLE 21-1    Thyroid Disorders and Their Effects on Body Systems

| Hypothyroidism | Hyperthyroidism |
| --- | --- |
| **Cardiovascular Effects** | |
| Increased capillary fragility | Tachycardia |
| Decreased cardiac output | Increased cardiac output |
| Decreased blood pressure | Increased blood volume |
| Decreased heart rate | Increased systolic blood pressure |
| Cardiac enlargement | Cardiac dysrhythmias |
| Congestive heart failure | Congestive heart failure |
| Anemia | |
| More rapid development of atherosclerosis and its complications (eg, coronary artery and peripheral vascular disease) | |
| **Central Nervous System Effects** | |
| Apathy and lethargy | Nervousness |
| Emotional dullness | Emotional instability |
| Slow speech, perhaps slurring and hoarseness as well | Restlessness |
| Hypoactive reflexes | Anxiety |
| Forgetfulness and mental sluggishness | Insomnia |
| Excessive drowsiness and sleeping | Hyperactive reflexes |
| **Metabolic Effects** | |
| Intolerance of cold | Intolerance of heat |
| Subnormal temperature | Low-grade fever |
| Increased serum cholesterol | Weight loss despite increased appetite |
| Weight gain | |
| **Gastrointestinal Effects** | |
| Decreased appetite | Increased appetite |
| Constipation | Abdominal cramps |
| | Diarrhea |
| | Nausea and vomiting |
| **Muscular Effects** | |
| Weakness | Weakness |
| Fatigue | Fatigue |
| Vague aches and pains | Muscle atrophy |
| | Tremors |
| **Integumentary Effects** | |
| Dry, coarse, and thickened skin | Moist, warm, flushed skin due to vasodilation and increased sweating |
| Puffy appearance of face and eyelids | |
| Dry and thinned hair | Hair and nails soft |
| Thick and hard nails | |
| **Reproductive Effects** | |
| Prolonged menstrual periods | Amenorrhea or oligomenorrhea |
| Infertility or sterility | |
| Decreased libido | |
| **Miscellaneous Effects** | |
| Increased susceptibility to infection | Dyspnea |
| Increased sensitivity to narcotics, barbiturates, and anesthetics owing to slowed metabolism of these drugs | Polyuria |
| | Hoarse, rapid speech |
| | Increased susceptibility to infection |
| | Excessive perspiration |
| | Localized edema around the eyeballs, which produces characteristic eye changes, including exophthalmos |

circulating thyroid hormone. Initially, manifestations are mild and vague. They usually increase in incidence and severity over time as the thyroid gland gradually atrophies and functioning glandular tissue is replaced by nonfunctioning fibrous connective tissue (see Table 21-1).

Myxedema coma is severe, life-threatening hypothyroidism characterized by coma, hypothermia, cardiovascular collapse, hypoventilation, and severe metabolic disorders such as hyponatremia, hypoglycemia, and lactic acidosis. Predisposing factors include exposure to cold, infection, trauma, respiratory disease, and administration of central nervous system (CNS) depressant drugs (eg, anesthetics, analgesics, sedatives). A person with severe hypothyroidism cannot metabolize and excrete the drugs.

### Treatment

Regardless of the cause of hypothyroidism and the age at which it occurs, the specific treatment is replacement of thyroid hormone from an exogenous source. Synthetic levothyroxine is the drug of choice. In clients with subclinical hypothyroidism, levothyroxine should be given if the serum TSH level is higher than 10 microunits/L. There is some difference of opinion about treatment for TSH values between 5 and 10 microunits/L. Two arguments for treatment of subclinical hypothyroidism are the high rate of progression to symptomatic hypothyroidism and improvement of cholesterol metabolism (eg, low-density lipoprotein [LDL] or "bad" cholesterol is reduced).

In clients with symptomatic hypothyroidism, levothyroxine therapy is definitely indicated. In addition to improvement of metabolism, treatment may also improve cardiac function, energy level, mood, muscle function, and fertility. In myxedema coma, levothyroxine or liothyronine is given intravenously, along with interventions to relieve precipitating factors and to support vital functions until the thyroid hormone becomes effective, often within 24 hours.

## Hyperthyroidism

Hyperthyroidism is characterized by excessive secretion of thyroid hormone. It may be associated with Graves' disease, nodular goiter, thyroiditis, overtreatment with thyroid drugs, functioning thyroid carcinoma, and pituitary adenoma that secretes excessive TSH. Hyperthyroidism usually involves an enlarged thyroid gland that has an increased number of cells and an increased rate of secretion. The hyperplastic thyroid gland may secrete 5 to 15 times the normal amount of thyroid hormone. As a result, body metabolism is greatly increased. Specific physiologic effects and clinical manifestations of hyperthyroidism are listed in Table 21-1. These effects vary, depending on the amount of circulating thyroid hormone, and they usually increase in incidence and severity with time if hyperthyroidism is not treated.

Subclinical hyperthyroidism is defined as a reduced TSH (below 0.1 microunit/L) and normal thyroxine and triiodothyronine levels. The most common cause is excess thyroid hormone therapy. Subclinical hyperthyroidism is a risk factor for osteoporosis in postmenopausal women who do not take estrogen replacement therapy because it leads to reduced bone mineral density. It also greatly increases the risk for atrial fibrillation in clients older than 60 years of age.

Thyroid storm or thyrotoxic crisis is a rare but severe complication characterized by extreme symptoms of hyperthyroidism, such as severe tachycardia, fever, dehydration, heart failure, and coma. It is most likely to occur in clients with hyperthyroidism that has been inadequately treated, especially when stressful situations occur (eg, trauma, infection, surgery, emotional upsets).

### Treatment

Treatment of hyperthyroidism depends on the cause. If the cause is an adenoma or multinodular goiter, surgery or radioactive iodine therapy is recommended, especially in older clients. If the cause is excessive levothyroxine dosage for hypothyroidism, the dose should be reduced. If the cause is Graves' disease, treatment may involve antithyroid drugs, radioactive iodine, surgery, or a combination of these methods. The drugs act by decreasing production or release of thyroid hormones. Radioactive iodine emits rays that destroy thyroid gland tissue. Subtotal thyroidectomy involves surgical excision of thyroid tissue. All these methods reduce the amount of thyroid hormones circulating in the bloodstream.

The antithyroid drugs include the thioamide derivatives (propylthiouracil and methimazole) and iodine preparations. The thioamide drugs inhibit synthesis of thyroid hormone, are inexpensive and relatively safe, and do not damage the thyroid gland. These drugs may be used as the primary treatment (for which they may be given 6 months to 2 years) or to decrease blood levels of thyroid hormone before radioactive iodine therapy or surgery.

Radioactive iodine is a frequently used treatment. It is safe, effective, inexpensive, and convenient. One disadvantage is hypothyroidism, which usually develops within a few months and requires lifelong thyroid hormone replacement therapy. Another disadvantage is the delay in therapeutic benefits. Results may not be apparent for 3 months or longer, during which time severe hyperthyroidism must be brought under control with one of the thioamide antithyroid drugs. Other iodine preparations are not used in long-term treatment of hyperthyroidism. They are indicated when a rapid clinical response is needed, as in thyroid storm and acute hyperthyroidism, or to prepare a hyperthyroid person for thyroidectomy. A thioamide drug is given to produce a euthyroid state, and an iodine preparation is given to reduce the size and vascularity of the thyroid gland to reduce the risk for excessive bleeding, often called involution of the thyroid.

Iodine preparations inhibit the release of thyroid hormones and cause them to be stored within the gland. They reduce blood levels of thyroid hormones more quickly than thioamide drugs or radioactive iodine. Maximal effects are reached in approximately 10 to 15 days of continuous therapy, and this is probably the primary advantage. Disadvantages, however, include the following:

- Iodine preparations may produce goiter, hyperthyroidism, or both.
- Iodine preparations cannot be used alone. Therapeutic benefits are temporary, and symptoms of hyperthyroidism may reappear and even be intensified if other treatment methods are not also used.
- Radioactive iodine cannot be used effectively for a prolonged period in a client who has received iodine preparations. Even if the iodine preparation is discontinued, the thyroid gland is saturated with iodine and does not attract enough radioactive iodine for treatment to be effective. Also, if radioactive iodine is given later, acute hyperthyroidism is likely to result because the radioactive iodine causes the stored hormones to be released into the circulation.
- Although giving a thioamide drug followed by an iodine preparation is standard preparation for thyroidectomy, the opposite sequence of administration is unsafe. If the iodine preparation is given first and followed by propylthiouracil or methimazole, the client is likely to experience acute hyperthyroidism because the thioamide causes release of the stored thyroid hormones.

Subtotal thyroidectomy is effective in relieving hyperthyroidism but also has several disadvantages. First, preparation for surgery requires several weeks of drug therapy. Second, there are risks involved in anesthesia and surgery and potential postoperative complications. Third, there is a high risk for eventual hypothyroidism. For these reasons, surgery is usually used for clients with large goiters or contraindications to other treatments.

Propranolol is used as an adjunctive drug in the treatment of hyperthyroidism. It relieves tachycardia, cardiac palpitations, excessive sweating, and other symptoms. Propranolol is especially helpful during the several weeks required for therapeutic results from antithyroid drugs or from radioactive iodine administration.

## ▓ INDIVIDUAL DRUGS

The drugs are described below; dosages are listed in Drugs at a Glance 21-1: Drugs for Hypothyroidism and Hyperthyroidism.

## Thyroid Agents (Drugs Used in Hypothyroidism)

**℗ Levothyroxine** (Synthroid, Levothroid), a synthetic preparation of thyroxine ($T_4$), is the drug of choice for long-term treatment of hypothyroidism because of uni-

form potency, once-daily dosing, and low cost and serves as the prototype of the group (see Prototype Profile 21-1: Levothyroxine). It is a potent form that contains a uniform amount of hormone and can be given parenterally. Compared with liothyronine, levothyroxine has a slower onset and longer duration of action.

Most (99%) of the circulating levothyroxine is bound to serum proteins, including thyroid-binding globulin, thyroid-binding prealbumin, and albumin. Levothyroxine has a long half-life of about 6 to 7 days in euthyroidism, but it is prolonged to 9 to 10 days in hypothyroidism and shortened to 3 to 4 days in hyperthyroidism.

Much of the levothyroxine is converted to liothyronine ($T_3$) in peripheral tissues. This conversion (ie, removal of an iodine atom, called deiodination) occurs at several locations, including the liver, kidneys, and other tissues. Some of the hormone is conjugated with glucuronide or sulfate and excreted in the bile and intestine.

**Liothyronine** (Cytomel, Triostat) is a synthetic preparation of $T_3$. Compared with levothyroxine, liothyronine has a more rapid onset and a shorter duration of action. Consequently, it may be more likely to produce high concentrations in blood and tissues and cause adverse reactions. Also, it requires more frequent administration if used for long-term treatment of hypothyroidism. Only the IV formulation (Triostat) is used in treating myxedema coma.

**Liotrix** (Euthroid, Thyrolar) contains levothyroxine and liothyronine in a 4:1 ratio, resembling the composition of natural thyroid hormone. Euthroid and Thyrolar are available in strengths ranging from 15 to 180 mg in thyroid equivalency.

## Antithyroid Agents (Drugs Used in Hyperthyroidism)

**℗ Propylthiouracil** (PTU) is the prototype of the thioamide antithyroid drugs and is described in Prototype Profile 21-2: Propylthiouracil. It can be used alone to treat hyperthyroidism, as part of the preoperative preparation for thyroidectomy, before or after radioactive iodine therapy, and in the treatment of thyroid storm or thyrotoxic crisis. Propylthiouracil acts by inhibiting production of thyroid hormones and peripheral conversion of $T_4$ to the more active $T_3$. It does not interfere with release of thyroid hormones previously produced and stored. Thus, therapeutic effects do not occur for several days or weeks until the stored hormones have been used.

PTU is well absorbed with oral administration, and peak plasma levels occur within 30 minutes. Plasma half-life is 1 to 2 hours. However, duration of action depends on the half-life within the thyroid gland rather than plasma half-life. Because this time is relatively short also, the drug must be given every 8 hours. PTU is metabolized in the liver and excreted in urine.

**Methimazole** (Tapazole) is similar to propylthiouracil in actions, uses, and adverse reactions. It is also well

**DRUG TABLE 21-1**

*Drugs at a Glance*

## Drugs for Hypothyroidism and Hyperthyroidism

| Generic/Trade Name | Routes and Dosage Ranges | Comments |
|---|---|---|
| **Drugs for Hypothyroidism** | | |
| **Levothyroxine** (Synthroid, Levothroid) Pregnancy Category A | See Prototype Profile 21-1: Levothyroxine | |
| **Liothyronine** (Cytomel, Triostat) Pregnancy Category A | *Adults:* PO, 25 mcg/d initially, increased by 12.5–25 mcg every 1–2 wk until desired response. Myxedema coma: IV, 25–50 mcg initially, then adjust dosage according to clinical response. Usual dosage, 65–100 mcg/d, with doses at least 4 h apart and no more than 12 h apart. *Older adults:* PO, 2.5–5 mcg/d for 3–6 wk, then doubled every 6 wk until desired response. Myxedema coma: IV, 10–20 mcg initially, then adjusted according to clinical response. *Children:* PO, 5 mcg/d initially, increased by 5 mcg/d every 3–4 d until desired response. Doses as high as 20–80 mcg/d may be required in congenital hypothyroidism | Dosage should be adjusted on the basis of clinical response and laboratory parameters |
| **Liotrix** (Euthroid, Thyrolar) Pregnancy Category A | *Adults:* PO, 15–30 mg/d initially, increased gradually every 2–3 wk until response is obtained. Usual maintenance dose, 60–120 mg/d. *Older adults, clients with cardiac disorders, and clients with hypothyroidism of long duration:* PO, one fourth to one half the usual adult dose initially, doubled every 8 wk if necessary | Combination product; instruct clients that the two brands of liotrix contain different amounts of levothyroxine and liothyronine |
| **Drugs for Hyperthyroidism** | | |
| **Potassium iodine** (Lugol's solution; SSKI) Pregnancy Category D | *Adults and children:* PO, 1–5 drops of SSKI or 2–6 drops of Lugol's solution three times per day for 10 d before thyroidectomy | Iodine crosses the placenta and may cause hypothyroidism and goiter in newborn |
| **Propylthiouracil** (PTU) | See Prototype Profile 21-2: Propylthiouracil | |
| **Methimazole** (Tapazole) Pregnancy Category D | *Adults:* PO, 15–60 mg/d initially, in divided doses q8h until the client is euthyroid; maintenance, 5–15 mg/d in two or three doses. *Children:* PO, 0.4 mg/kg/d initially, in divided doses q8h; maintenance dose, one half initial dose | Take with meals around-the-clock |
| **Sodium iodide** $^{131}$I (Iodotope) Pregnancy Category X | *Adults and children:* PO, IV, dosage as calculated by a radiologist trained in nuclear medicine | Institute full radiation precautions |
| **Propranolol** (Inderal) Pregnancy Category C by manufacturer; D second and third trimester by expert analysis | PO, 40–160 mg/d in divided doses | Nonselective beta-blocker; See Prototype Profile 41-1: Propranolol |

## PROTOTYPE PROFILE 21-1

### P Levothyroxine (lee voe thye ROKS een)

**Drug Class**

*Chemical:* Thyroid hormone replacement product
*Functional:* Thyroid product

**Trade Names**

Synthroid, Levothroid

**Therapeutic Indications**

Replacement of thyroid hormone in hypothyroidism; suppression of TSH from pituitary; treatment of myxedema coma

**Pharmacokinetics**

*Absorption*
PO: erratic (40%–80%); decreases with increasing age

*Distribution*
Plasma protein binding: 99%

*Metabolism*
Hepatic to triiodothyronine ($T_3$)

*Excretion*
Urine and feces; decreases with increasing age

**Pharmacodynamics**

*Onset of Action*
Therapeutic: PO, 3–5 d; IV, 6–8 h (peak effect IV, about 24 h)

*Duration*
PO, IV, unknown

**Contraindications/Precautions**

Hypersensitivity to drug, recent MI, thyrotoxicosis, untreated adrenal insufficiency; with caution in elderly clients or for weight reduction

**Pregnancy Considerations**

Category A
Enters breast milk; compatible

**Dosage**

*Adults:* PO, 0.05 mg/d initially, increased by 0.025 mg every 2–3 wk until desired response obtained; usual maintenance dose, 0.1–0.2 mg/d (100–200 mcg/d)
Myxedema coma: IV, 0.4 mg in a single dose; then 0.1–0.2 mg daily
TSH suppression in thyroid cancer, nodules, and euthyroid goiters: PO, 2.6 mcg/kg/d for 7–10 days
*Older adults, clients with cardiac disorders, and clients with hypothyroidism of long duration:* PO,

0.0125–0.025 mg/d for 6 wk, then dose is doubled every 6–8 wk until the desired response is obtained
Myxedema coma: same as adult dosage
*Children:* Congenital hypothyroidism, PO, as follows:
*Birth–6 mo:* 25–50 mcg/d (or 8–10 mcg/kg/d)
*6–12 mo:* 50–75 mcg/d (or 6–8 mcg/kg/d)
*1–5 y:* 75–100 mcg/d (or 5–6 mcg/kg/d)
*6–12 y:* 100–150 mcg/d (or 4–5 mcg/kg/d)
*>12 y:* >150 mcg/d (or 2–3 mcg/kg/d)

**Adverse Effects**

Arrhythmias, nervousness, insomnia, tremor, angina pectoris, heat intolerance, menstrual irregularities, diarrhea, vomiting, weight loss

**Drug Interactions**

*Increased Effects*
Hypoprothrombinemic effects with warfarin and other anticoagulants
Risk for toxicity of both drugs when used concomitantly with tricyclic antidepressants
Hypertension and tachycardia with concomitant administration with ketamine

*Decreased Effects*
Absorption of levothyroxine with cholestyramine, colestipol, antacids, phenytoin, carbamazepine, phenobarbital, rifampin
Serum levels of theophylline and digoxin may be altered with thyroid function
Decreased free thyroxine concentrations with concomitant use of estrogens
Decreased effects of oral sulfonylureas with concomitant use

**Herbal Supplements and Dietary Considerations**

Lemon balm has antithyroid effects
Should take on an empty stomach at least 30 min before food
Limit intake of goitrogenic foods: cabbage, peas, broccoli, asparagus, turnip greens, spinach, lettuce, soy beans, Brussels sprouts
Walnuts and dietary fiber may decrease absorption of levothyroxine as will soybean flour in infant formula
Taking with enteral nutrition may decrease absorption of levothyroxine

---

absorbed with oral administration and rapidly reaches peak plasma levels.

**Strong iodine solution** (Lugol's solution) and **saturated solution of potassium iodide** (SSKI) are iodine preparations sometimes used in short-term treatment of hyperthyroidism. The drugs inhibit release of thyroid hormones, causing them to accumulate in the thyroid

gland. Lugol's solution is usually used to treat thyrotoxic crisis and to decrease the size and vascularity of the thyroid gland before thyroidectomy. SSKI is more often used as an expectorant but may be given as preparation for thyroidectomy. Iodine preparations should not be followed by propylthiouracil, methimazole, or radioactive iodine because the latter drugs cause release

## PROTOTYPE PROFILE 21-2

### Ⓟ Propylthiouracil (proe pil thye oh YOOR a sil)

**Drug Class**
*Chemical:* Antithyroid agent
*Functional:* Antithyroid agent

**Trade Name**
PTU

**Therapeutic Indications**
Treatment of hyperthyroidism; management of thyrotoxicosis

**Pharmacokinetics**
*Absorption*
Well-absorbed (bioavailability 80%–95%)

*Distribution*
Concentrated in the thyroid gland

*Metabolism*
Hepatic

*Excretion*
Urine (35%)

**Pharmacodynamics**
*Onset of Action*
Therapeutic: 24–36 h

*Duration*
2–3 h

**Contraindications/Precautions**
Hypersensitivity, pregnancy, with caution in clients with agranulocytosis, hepatitis

**Pregnancy Considerations**
Category D
Enters breast milk; use with caution
May cross placenta and induce cretinism (hypothyroidism) in fetus

**Dosage**
*Adults:* PO, 300–400 mg/d in divided doses q8h, until the client is euthyroid; then 100–150 mg/d in three divided doses, for maintenance
*Children:* >10 y: PO, 150–300 mg/d in divided doses q8h; usual maintenance dose, 100–300 mg/d in two divided doses, q12h
*6–10 y:* 50–150 mg/d in divided doses q8h
*<6 y:* safety and efficacy not established

**Adverse Effects**
Nausea, vomiting, agranulocytosis, rash, urticaria, fever, headache, loss of taste

**Drug Interactions**
*Increased Effects*
Anticoagulant effect with warfarin

*Decreased Effects*
With correction of hyperthyroidism, drug dosages of other drugs, such as digoxin, theophylline, and beta-blockers, may need to be reduced

**Herbal Supplements and Dietary Considerations**
Lemon balm has antithyroid effects
Levels may be altered if taken with food; take consistently with or between meals

---

of stored thyroid hormone and may precipitate acute hyperthyroidism.

**Sodium iodide** [131]I (Iodotope) is a radioactive isotope of iodine. The thyroid gland cannot differentiate between regular iodide and radioactive iodide; thus, it picks up the radioactive iodide from the circulating blood. As a result, small amounts of radioactive iodide can be used as a diagnostic test of thyroid function, and larger doses are used therapeutically to treat hyperthyroidism. Therapeutic doses act by emitting beta and gamma rays, which destroy thyroid tissue and thereby decrease production of thyroid hormones. It is also used to treat thyroid cancer.

Radioactive iodide is usually given in a single dose on an outpatient basis. For most clients, no special radiation precautions are necessary. If a very large dose is given, the client may be isolated for 8 days, which is the half-life of radioactive iodide. Therapeutic effects are delayed for several weeks or up to 6 months. During this time, symptoms may be controlled with thioamide drugs or propranolol. Radioactive iodide is usually given to middle-aged and elderly people; it is contraindicated during pregnancy and lactation.

**Propranolol** (Inderal) is an antiadrenergic, not an antithyroid, drug. It does not affect thyroid function, hormone secretion, or hormone metabolism. It is most often used to treat cardiovascular conditions, such as arrhythmias, angina pectoris, and hypertension. When given to clients with hyperthyroidism, propranolol blocks beta-adrenergic receptors in various organs and thereby controls symptoms of hyperthyroidism resulting from excessive stimulation of the sympathetic nervous system. These symptoms include tachycardia, palpitations, excessive sweating, tremors, and nervousness. Propranolol is useful for controlling symptoms during the delayed response to thioamide drugs and radioactive iodine, before thyroidectomy, and in treating thyrotoxic crisis.

**?** **How Can You Avoid**
**This Medication Error?**

Jennifer Binggeli takes Synthroid, 0.1 mg once daily. The drug label lists Synthroid 100 mcg per tablet. To administer the morning dose, the nurse gives Ms. Binggeli 10 tablets.

When the client becomes euthyroid and hyperthyroid symptoms are controlled by definitive treatment measures, propranolol should be discontinued.

## ▓ USE IN SPECIAL CONDITIONS

### Thyroid Drugs

#### Hypothyroidism and the Metabolism of Other Drugs

Changes in the rate of body metabolism affect the metabolism of many drugs. Most drugs given to a client with hypothyroidism have a prolonged effect because drug metabolism in the liver is delayed and the glomerular filtration rate of the kidneys is decreased. Also, drug absorption from the intestine or a parenteral injection site may be slowed. As a result, dosage of many other drugs should be reduced, including digoxin and insulin. In addition, people with hypothyroidism are especially likely to experience respiratory depression and myxedema coma with opioid analgesics and other sedating drugs. These drugs should be avoided when possible. However, when necessary, they are given very cautiously and in dosages of approximately one third to one half the usual dose. Even then, clients must be observed very closely for respiratory depression.

Once thyroid replacement therapy is started and stabilized, the client becomes euthyroid, has a normal rate of metabolism, and can tolerate usual doses of most drugs if other influencing factors are not present. On the other hand, excessive doses of thyroid drugs may produce hyperthyroidism and a greatly increased rate of metabolism. In this instance, larger doses of most other drugs are necessary to produce the same effects. Rather than increasing dosage of other drugs, however, dosage

## ᴎURSING PROCESS

### Assessment

- Assess for signs and symptoms of thyroid disorders (see Table 25-1). During the course of treatment with thyroid or antithyroid drugs, the client's blood level of thyroid hormone may range from low to normal to high. At either end of the continuum, signs and symptoms may be dramatic and obvious. As blood levels change toward normal as a result of treatment, signs and symptoms become less obvious. If presenting signs and symptoms are treated too aggressively, they may change toward the opposite end of the continuum and indicate adverse drug effects. Thus, *each client receiving a drug that alters thyroid function must be assessed for indicators of hypothyroidism, euthyroidism, and hyperthyroidism.*
- Check laboratory reports for serum TSH (normal = 0.5 to 4.1 μU/mL) when available. An elevated serum TSH is the first indication of primary hypothyroidism and commonly occurs in middle-aged women, even in the absence of other signs and symptoms. Serum TSH is used to monitor response to drugs that alter thyroid function.

### Nursing Diagnoses

- Decreased Cardiac Output related to disease- or drug-induced thyroid disorders
- Imbalanced Nutrition: Less Than Body Requirements with hyperthyroidism
- Imbalanced Nutrition: More Than Body Requirements with hypothyroidism
- Ineffective Thermoregulation related to changes in metabolism rate and body heat production
- Deficient Knowledge: Disease process and drug therapy

### Planning/Goals

*The client will:*
- Achieve normal blood levels of thyroid hormone
- Receive or take drugs accurately
- Experience relief of symptoms of hypothyroidism or hyperthyroidism
- Be assisted to cope with symptoms until therapy becomes effective
- Avoid preventable adverse drug effects
- Be monitored regularly for therapeutic and adverse effects of drug therapy

### Interventions

Use nondrug measures to control symptoms, increase effectiveness of drug therapy, and decrease adverse reactions. Some areas for intervention include the following:

- **Environmental temperature.** Regulate for the client's comfort, when possible. Clients with *hypothyroidism* are very intolerant of cold owing to their slow metabolism rate. Chilling and shivering should be prevented because of added strain on the heart. Provide blankets and warm clothing as needed. Clients with *hyperthyroidism* are very intolerant of heat and perspire excessively owing to their rapid metabolism rate. Provide cooling baths and lightweight clothing as needed.
- **Diet.** Despite a poor appetite, *hypothyroid* clients are often overweight because of slow metabolism rates. Thus, a low-calorie, weight-reduction diet may be indicated. In addition, an increased intake of high-fiber foods is usually needed to prevent constipation as a result of decreased gastrointestinal secretion and motility. Despite a good appetite, *hyperthyroid*

*(continued)*

## NURSING PROCESS (Continued)

clients are often underweight because of rapid metabolism rates. They often need extra calories and nutrients to prevent tissue breakdown. These can be provided by extra meals and snacks. The client may wish to avoid highly seasoned and high-fiber foods because they may increase diarrhea.

- **Fluids.** With *hypothyroidism*, clients need an adequate intake of low-calorie fluids to prevent constipation. With *hyperthyroidism*, clients need large amounts of fluids (3000–4000 mL/day) unless contraindicated by cardiac or renal disease. The fluids are needed to eliminate heat and waste products produced by the hypermetabolic state. Much of the client's fluid loss is visible as excessive perspiration and urine output.
- **Activity.** With *hypothyroidism*, encourage activity to maintain cardiovascular, respiratory, gastrointestinal, and musculoskeletal function. With *hyperthyroidism*, encourage rest and quiet, nonstrenuous activity. Because clients differ in what they find restful, this must be determined with each one. A quiet room, reading, and soft music may be helpful. Mild sedatives are often given. The client is caught in the dilemma of needing rest because of the high metabolic rate but being unable to rest because of nervousness and excitement.
- **Skin care.** *Hypothyroid* clients are likely to have edema and dry skin. When edema is present, inspect pressure points, turn often, and avoid trauma when possible. Edema increases risks of skin breakdown and decubitus ulcer formation. Also, increased capillary fragility increases the likelihood of bruising from seemingly minor trauma. When skin is dry, use soap sparingly and lotions and other lubricants freely.
- **Eye care.** *Hyperthyroid* clients may have exophthalmos. In mild cases, use measures to protect the eye. For example, dark glasses, local lubricants, and patching of the eyes at night may be needed. Diuretic drugs and elevating the head of the bed may help reduce periorbital edema and eyeball protrusion. If the eyelids cannot close, they are sometimes taped shut to avoid corneal abrasion. In severe exophthalmos, the preceding measures are taken and large doses of corticosteroids are usually given.

### Evaluation

- Interview and observe for compliance with instructions for taking medications.
- Observe for relief of symptoms.
- Check laboratory reports for normal blood levels of TSH or thyroid hormones.
- Interview and observe for adverse drug effects.
- Check appointment records for compliance with follow-up procedures.

---

of thyroid drugs should be reduced so that the client is euthyroid again.

### Adrenal Insufficiency

When hypothyroidism and adrenal insufficiency coexist, the adrenal insufficiency should be treated with a corticosteroid drug before starting thyroid replacement. Thyroid hormones increase tissue metabolism and tissue demands for adrenocortical hormones. If adrenal insufficiency is not treated first, administration of thyroid hormone may cause acute adrenocortical insufficiency, a life-threatening condition.

---

## CLIENT TEACHING GUIDELINES
## Levothyroxine

### General Considerations

✔ Thyroid hormone is required for normal body functioning and for life. When a person's thyroid gland is unable to produce enough thyroid hormone, levothyroxine is used as a synthetic substitute. Thus, levothyroxine therapy for hypothyroidism is lifelong; stopping it may lead to life-threatening illness.

✔ Periodic tests of thyroid function are needed.

✔ Dosage adjustments are made according to clinical response and results of thyroid function tests.

✔ Do not switch from one brand name to another; effects may be different.

✔ Levothyroxine stimulates the central nervous system and the heart; excessive stimulation may occur if it is taken with other stimulating drugs. Thus, you should consult a health care provider before taking over-the-counter drugs that stimulate the heart or cause nervousness (eg, asthma remedies, cold remedies, decongestants). In addition, you should avoid the herb ephedra (also called ma huang and not recommended for anyone to take; it may increase blood pressure and cause heart attack or stroke) and probably limit your intake of caffeine-containing beverages to 2 to 3 servings daily.

### Self-administration

✔ Take every morning, on an empty stomach, for best absorption. Also, do not take the drug with an antacid (eg, Tums, Maalox), an iron preparation, or sucralfate (Carafate). These drugs decrease absorption of levothyroxine. If necessary to take one of these drugs, take levothyroxine 2 hours before or 4 to 6 hours after the other drug.

✔ Take about the same time each day for more consistent blood levels and more normal body metabolism.

✔ Report chest pain, heart palpitations, nervousness, or insomnia. These adverse effects result from excessive stimulation and may indicate that drug dosage or intake of other stimulants needs to be reduced.

## CLIENT TEACHING GUIDELINES
### Propylthiouracil or Methimazole

#### General Considerations

✔ These drugs are sometimes called antithyroid drugs because they are given to decrease the production of thyroid hormone by an overactive thyroid gland.

✔ These drugs must be taken for 1 year or longer to decrease thyroid hormone levels to normal.

✔ Periodic tests of thyroid function and drug dosage adjustments are needed.

✔ Ask the prescribing physician if it is necessary to avoid or restrict amounts of seafood or iodized salt. These sources of iodide may need to be reduced or omitted during antithyroid drug therapy.

#### Self-administration

✔ Take at regular intervals around the clock, usually every 8 hours.

✔ Report fever, sore throat, unusual bleeding or bruising, headache, skin rash, yellowing of the skin, or vomiting. If these adverse effects occur, drug dosage may need to be reduced or the drug may need to be discontinued.

✔ Consult a health care provider before taking over-the-counter drugs. Some drugs contain iodide, which can increase the likelihood of goiter and the risk of adverse effects from excessive doses of iodide (eg, some cough syrups, asthma medications, and multivitamins may contain iodide).

## Antithyroid Drugs

### Use in Pregnancy

Iodine preparations and thioamide antithyroid drugs are contraindicated during pregnancy because they can lead to goiter and hypothyroidism in the fetus or newborn.

### Hyperthyroidism and the Metabolism of Other Drugs

Treatment of hyperthyroidism changes the rate of body metabolism, including the rate of metabolism of many drugs. During the hyperthyroid state, drug metabolism may be very rapid, and higher doses of most drugs may be necessary to achieve therapeutic results. When the client becomes euthyroid, the rate of drug metabolism is decreased. Consequently, doses of all medications should be evaluated and probably reduced to avoid severe adverse effects.

### Iodine Ingestion and Hyperthyroidism

Iodine is present in foods (especially seafood) and in contrast dyes used for gallbladder and other radiologic procedures. Ingestion of large amounts of iodine from these sources may result in goiter and hyperthyroidism.

## Nursing Actions
### Thyroid and Antithyroid Drugs

| Nursing Actions | Rationale/Explanation |
|---|---|
| 1. Administer accurately. | |
| a. With thyroid drugs: | |
| (1) Administer in a single daily dose, on an empty stomach (eg, before breakfast). | Fasting increases drug absorption; early administration allows peak activity during daytime hours and is less likely to interfere with sleep. |
| (2) Check the pulse rate before giving the drug. If the rate is over 100 per minute or if any changes in cardiac rhythm are noted, consult the physician before giving the dose. | Tachycardia or other cardiac dysrhythmias may indicate adverse cardiac effects. Dosage may need to be reduced or the drug stopped temporarily. |
| (3) To give levothyroxine to an infant or young child, the tablet may be crushed and a small amount of formula or water added. Once mixed, administer soon, by spoon or dropper. Do *not* store the liquid very long. The crushed tablet may also be sprinkled on a small amount of food (eg, cereal or applesauce). | Accurate and consistent administration is vital to promoting normal growth and development. |
| (4) Do not switch among various brands or generic forms of the drug. | Differences in bioavailability have been identified among products. Changes in preparations may alter dosage and therefore symptom control. |

*(continued)*

## *Nursing Actions*

### Thyroid and Antithyroid Drugs (Continued)

| *Nursing Actions* | *Rationale/Explanation* |
|---|---|
| b. With antithyroid and iodine drugs:<br>(1) Administer q8h. | All these drugs have rather short half-lives and must be given frequently and regularly to maintain therapeutic blood levels. In addition, if iodine preparations are not given every 8 h, symptoms of hyperthyroidism may recur. |
| (2) Dilute iodine solutions in a full glass of fruit juice or milk, if possible, and have the client drink the medication through a straw. | Dilution of the drug reduces gastric irritation and masks the unpleasant taste. Using a straw prevents staining the teeth. |
| 2. **Observe for therapeutic effects.**<br>a. With thyroid drugs, observe for:<br>(1) Increased energy and activity level, less lethargy and fatigue<br>(2) Increased alertness and interest in surroundings<br>(3) Increased appetite<br>(4) Increased pulse rate and temperature<br>(5) Decreased constipation<br>(6) Reversal of coarseness and other changes in skin and hair<br>(7) With cretinism, increased growth rate (record height periodically)<br>(8) With myxedema, diuresis, weight loss, and decreased edema | Therapeutic effects result from a return to normal metabolic activities and relief of the symptoms of hypothyroidism. Therapeutic effects may be evident as early as 2 or 3 d after drug therapy is started or delayed up to approximately 2 wk. All signs and symptoms of myxedema should disappear in approximately 3 to 12 wk. |
| (9) Decreased serum cholesterol and possibly decreased creatine phosphokinase, lactate dehydrogenase, and aspartate aminotransferase | These tests are often elevated with myxedema and may return to normal when thyroid replacement therapy is begun. |
| b. With antithyroid and iodine drugs, observe for:<br>(1) Slower pulse rate<br>(2) Slower speech | With propylthiouracil and methimazole, some therapeutic effects are apparent in 1 or 2 wk, but euthyroidism may not occur for 6 or 8 wk. |
| (3) More normal activity level (slowing of hyperactivity)<br>(4) Decreased nervousness<br>(5) Decreased tremors<br>(6) Improved ability to sleep and rest<br>(7) Weight gain | With iodine solutions, therapeutic effects may be apparent within 24 h. Maximal effects occur in approximately 10 to 15 d. However, therapeutic effects may not be sustained. Symptoms may reappear if the drug is given longer than a few weeks, and they may be more severe than initially. |
| 3. **Observe for adverse effects.**<br>a. With thyroid drugs, observe for tachycardia and other cardiac dysrhythmias, angina pectoris, myocardial infarction, congestive heart failure, nervousness, hyperactivity, insomnia, diarrhea, abdominal cramps, nausea and vomiting, weight loss, fever, intolerance to heat. | Most adverse reactions stem from excessive doses, and signs and symptoms produced are the same as those occurring with hyperthyroidism. Excessive thyroid hormones make the heart work very hard and fast in attempting to meet tissue demands for oxygenated blood and nutrients. Symptoms of myocardial ischemia occur when the myocardium does not get an adequate supply of oxygenated blood. Symptoms of congestive heart failure occur when the increased cardiac workload is prolonged. Cardiovascular problems are more likely to occur in clients who are elderly or who already have heart disease. |
| b. With propylthiouracil and methimazole, observe for:<br>(1) Hypothyroidism—bradycardia, congestive heart failure, anemia, coronary artery and peripheral vascular disease, slow speech and movements, emotional and mental dullness, excessive sleeping, weight gain, constipation, skin changes, and others | |

*(continued)*

*Nursing Actions*

## Thyroid and Antithyroid Drugs (Continued)

| Nursing Actions | Rationale/Explanation |
|---|---|
| (2) Blood disorders—leukopenia, agranulocytosis, hypoprothrombinemia | Leukopenia may be difficult to evaluate because it may occur with hyperthyroidism and with antithyroid drugs. Agranulocytosis occurs rarely but is the most severe adverse reaction; the earliest symptoms are likely to be sore throat and fever. If these occur, report them to the physician immediately. |
| (3) Integumentary system—skin rash, pruritus, alopecia | |
| (4) Central nervous system (CNS)—headache, dizziness, loss of sense of taste, drowsiness, paresthesias | |
| (5) Gastrointestinal system—nausea, vomiting, abdominal discomfort, gastric irritation, cholestatic hepatitis | |
| (6) Other—lymphadenopathy, edema, joint pain, drug fever | |
| c. With iodine preparations, observe for: | Adverse effects are uncommon with short-term use. |
| (1) Iodism—metallic taste, burning in mouth, soreness of gums, excessive salivation, gastric or respiratory irritation, rhinitis, headache, redness of conjunctiva, edema of eyelids | |
| (2) Hypersensitivity—acneiform skin rash, pruritus, fever, jaundice, angioedema, serum sickness | Allergic reactions rarely occur. |
| (3) Goiter with hypothyroidism | Uncommon but may occur in adults and newborns whose mothers have taken iodides for long periods |
| **4. Observe for drug interactions.** | |
| a. Drugs that *increase* effects of thyroid hormones: | |
| (1) Activating antidepressants (eg, bupropion, venlafaxine), adrenergic antiasthmatic drugs (eg, albuterol, epinephrine), nasal decongestants | These drugs may cause CNS and cardiovascular stimulation when taken alone. When combined with thyroid hormones, excessive cardiovascular stimulation may occur and cause myocardial ischemia, cardiac dysrhythmias, hypertension, and other adverse cardiovascular effects. Excessive CNS stimulation may produce anxiety, nervousness, hyperactivity, and insomnia. |
| b. Drugs that *decrease* effects of thyroid hormones: | |
| (1) Antacids, cholestyramine, iron, sucralfate | Decrease absorption of levothyroxine; give levothyroxine 2 hours before or 4 to 6 hours after one of these drugs |
| (2) Antihypertensives | Decrease cardiac stimulating effects |
| (3) Estrogens, including oral contraceptives containing estrogens | Estrogens increase thyroxine-binding globulin, thereby increasing the amount of bound, inactive levothyroxine in clients with hypothyroidism. This decreased effect does not occur in clients with adequate thyroid hormone secretion because the increased binding is offset by increased T4 production. Women taking oral contraceptives may need larger doses of thyroid hormone replacement than would otherwise be needed. |
| (4) Propranolol (Inderal) | This drug decreases cardiac effects of thyroid hormones. It is used in hyperthyroidism to reduce tachycardia and other symptoms of excessive cardiovascular stimulation. |
| (5) Phenytoin, rifampin | Induce enzymes that metabolize (inactivate) levothyroxine more rapidly |
| c. Drug that *increases* effects of antithyroid drugs: | |
| (1) Lithium | Acts synergistically to produce hypothyroidism |

## ? How Can You Avoid This Medication Error?

**Answer:** To convert from milligrams to micrograms, use the conversion factor of 1 mg = 1000 mcg. When doing the computation, 0.1 mg converts to 100 mcg, and thus 1 tablet should have been administered. Always question the dosage when more than 2 tablets are given.

## Critical Thinking Exercises

1. An iodine preparation is given before a thyroidectomy to accomplish all of the following except:
   a. Reduce the size of the thyroid gland
   b. Decrease the vascularity of the thyroid gland
   c. Reduce the risk for excessive bleeding
   d. Inhibit production of thyroid hormones

2. Which of the following clients with Graves' disease would be an appropriate candidate for sodium iodide $^{131}$I (Iodotope) therapy?
   a. An 8-year-old boy
   b. A 28-year-old breast-feeding mother
   c. A 35-year-old pregnant female
   d. A 40-year-old man

3. When propranolol (Inderal) is used in the treatment of hyperthyroidism, which of the following symptoms can be relieved?
   a. Heat intolerance
   b. Exophthalmos
   c. Dry skin
   d. Tachycardia

4. A newborn is recently diagnosed with congenital hypothyroidism and is started on levothyroxine (Synthroid). The mother asks how long the child will need to take this medication. The most accurate response by the nurse is:
   a. "Your child will need to take the medication for life."
   b. "Your health care provider will be best able to give you that information."
   c. "Your son will need to take the medication until he can have a stable intake of iron in his formula."
   d. "Let's start with this medication and see how your child responds to it."

5. Which of the following orders should a nurse question in a client with hypothyroidism?
   a. Psyllium (Metamucil)
   b. Levothyroxine (Synthroid)
   c. Morphine sulfate
   d. Liothyronine (Cytomel)

## SELECTED REFERENCES

Dong, B. J. (2000). Thyroid disorders. In E. T. Herfindal & D. R. Gourley (Eds.), *Textbook of therapeutics: Drug and disease management* (7th ed., pp. 325–358). Philadelphia: Lippincott Williams & Wilkins.

*Drug facts and comparisons.* (Updated monthly). St. Louis: Facts and Comparisons.

Fatourechi, V. (2001). Subclinical thyroid disease. *Mayo Clinic Proceedings, 76*(4), 413–417.

Guyton, A. C., & Hall, J. E. (2000). *Textbook of medical physiology* (10th ed.). Philadelphia: W. B. Saunders.

Lacy, C. F., Armstrong, L. L., Goldman, M. P., & Lance, L. L. (2003). *Lexi-Comp's drug information handbook* (11th ed.). Hudson, OH: American Pharmaceutical Association.

Matfin, G., Guven, S., & Kuenzi, J. A. (2002). Alterations in endocrine control of growth and metabolism. In C. M. Porth (Ed.), *Pathophysiology: Concepts of altered health states* (6th ed., pp. 903–923). Philadelphia: Lippincott Williams & Wilkins.

Wartofsky, L. (2000). Disorders of the thyroid gland. In H. D. Humes (Ed.), *Kelley's textbook of internal medicine* (4th ed., pp. 2693–2719). Philadelphia: Lippincott Williams & Wilkins.

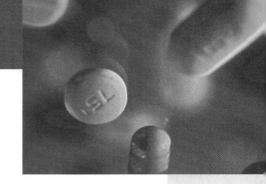

# 22

# Antidiabetic Drugs

## OBJECTIVES

*After studying this chapter, the student will be able to:*

1 Describe major effects of endogenous insulin on body tissues.

2 Discuss the characteristics and uses of the insulins and insulin analogs.

3 Discuss the relationships among diet, exercise, and drug therapy in controlling diabetes.

4 Differentiate types of oral antidiabetic agents in terms of mechanisms of action, indications for use, adverse effects, and nursing process implications.

5 Explain the benefits of maintaining glycemic control in preventing complications of diabetes.

6 State reasons for combinations of insulin and oral agents or different types of oral agents.

7 Assist clients or caregivers in learning how to manage diabetes care, including administration of antidiabetic medications.

8 Collaborate with nurse diabetes educators, dietitians, and others in teaching self-care activities to clients with diabetes.

9 Assess and monitor clients' conditions in relation to diabetes and their compliance with prescribed management strategies.

10 Discuss dietary and herbal supplements that affect blood sugar and diabetes control.

## CRITICAL THINKING SCENARIO

*Y*ou are assigned to care for Ellen Rodriguez, a 13-year-old client, who was admitted to the intensive care unit 12 hours ago in acute ketoacidosis. Her blood glucose level has stabilized after emergency treatment. She lives with her mother (a single parent) and five younger siblings in public housing within the Latino community. The diagnosis of diabetes mellitus is completely unexpected. Her mother asks why Ellen has to take shots because her aunt did just fine on pills.

Ellen will be discharged in 2 to 3 days on insulin, glucose monitoring before meals and at bedtime, and a diabetic diet. Use the following questions to think about and plan Ellen's care.

✔ Visualize yourself as Ellen and try to verbalize how you might feel. Now visualize yourself as Ellen's mother and again try to explain how you are feeling. Compare and contrast these two pictures.

✔ Reflect on developmental and socioeconomic factors that need to be considered when planning Ellen's care.

✔ Role-play how you might answer Ellen's mother's question concerning why her daughter needs to inject insulin rather than take pills to manage her diabetes.

✔ Before discharge, you have three teaching sessions of approximately 30 minutes each. Prioritize essential teaching and describe your teaching plan for Ellen.

✔ Discuss appropriate postdischarge follow-up to continue diabetic teaching and monitor compliance with prescribed management strategies.

# OVERVIEW

Insulin and oral agents are the two types of drugs used to lower blood glucose in diabetes mellitus. To assist readers in understanding the clinical use of these drugs, characteristics of endogenous insulin, diabetes mellitus, and the individual drugs are described in this chapter.

# ENDOGENOUS INSULIN

Insulin, the only hormone that decreases blood sugar, regulates the amount of glucose available for cellular metabolism and energy needs, during both fasting and feeding. Insulin secretion involves coordination of various nutrients, hormones, the autonomic nervous system, and other factors. The effects of insulin on carbohydrate, protein, and fat metabolism are described in At the Foundation: Effects of Insulin on Metabolism.

Glucose is the major stimulus of insulin secretion; others include amino acids, fatty acids, ketone bodies, and stimulation of beta$_2$-adrenergic receptors or vagal nerves. Oral glucose is more effective than intravenous glucose because glucose or food in the digestive tract induces the release of gastrointestinal (GI) hormones (eg, gastrin, secretin, cholecystokinin, gastric inhibitory peptide) and stimulates vagal activity. Other hormones that raise blood glucose levels and stimulate insulin secretion include cortisol, glucagon, growth hormone, epinephrine, estrogen, and progesterone. Excessive, prolonged endogenous secretion or administration of pharmacologic preparations of these hormones can exhaust the ability of pancreatic beta cells to produce insulin and thereby cause or aggravate diabetes mellitus.

## AT THE FOUNDATION: *Effects of Insulin on Metabolism*

Insulin is a protein hormone secreted by beta cells in the pancreas. At the cellular level, insulin binds with and activates receptors on the cell membranes of about 80% of body cells (Fig 22-1). Liver, muscle, and fat cells have many insulin receptors and are primary tissues for insulin action. After insulin receptor binding occurs, cell membranes become highly permeable to glucose and allow rapid entry of glucose into the cells. The cell membranes also become more permeable to amino acids, fatty acids, and electrolytes such as potassium, magnesium, and phosphate ions. Cellular metabolism is altered by the movement of these substances into the cells, activation of some enzymes and inactivation of others, movement of proteins between intracellular compartments, changes in the amounts of proteins produced, and perhaps other mechanisms. Overall, the changes in cellular metabolism stimulate anabolic effects (eg, use and storage of glucose, amino acids, and fatty acids) and inhibit catabolic processes (eg, breakdown of glycogen, fat, and protein). After binding to insulin and entering the cell, receptors may be degraded or recycled back to the cell surface.

Insulin plays a major role in metabolism of carbohydrate, fat, and protein. These foodstuffs are broken down into molecules of glucose, lipids, and amino acids, respectively.

### Carbohydrate Metabolism
• Insulin increases glucose transport into the liver, skeletal muscle, adipose tissue, the heart, and some smooth muscle organs, such as the uterus; it must be present for muscle and fat tissues to use glucose for energy.
• Insulin regulates glucose metabolism to produce energy for cellular functions. If excess glucose is present after this need is met, it is converted to glycogen and stored for future energy needs or converted to fat and stored. The excess glucose transported to liver cells is converted to fat only after glycogen stores are saturated. When insulin is absent or blood glucose levels are low, these stored forms of glucose can be reconverted. The liver is especially important in restoring blood sugar levels by breaking down glycogen or by forming new glucose.

### Fat Metabolism
• Insulin promotes transport of glucose into fat cells, where it is broken down. One of the breakdown products is alpha-glycerophosphate, which combines with fatty acids to form triglycerides. This is the mechanism by which insulin promotes fat storage.
• When insulin is lacking, fat is released into the bloodstream as free fatty acids. Blood concentrations of triglycerides, cholesterol, and phospholipids are also increased. The high blood lipid concentration probably accounts for the atherosclerosis that tends to develop early and progress more rapidly in people with diabetes mellitus. Also, when more fatty acids are released than the body can use as fuel, some fatty acids are converted into ketones. Excessive amounts of ketones produce acidosis and coma.

### Protein Metabolism
• Insulin increases the total amount of body protein by increasing transport of amino acids into cells and synthesis of protein within the cells. The basic mechanism of these effects is unknown.
• Insulin potentiates the effects of growth hormone.
• Lack of insulin causes protein breakdown into amino acids, which are released into the bloodstream and transported to the liver for energy or gluconeogenesis. The lost proteins are not replaced by synthesis of new proteins and protein wasting causes abnormal functioning of many body organs, severe weakness, and weight loss.

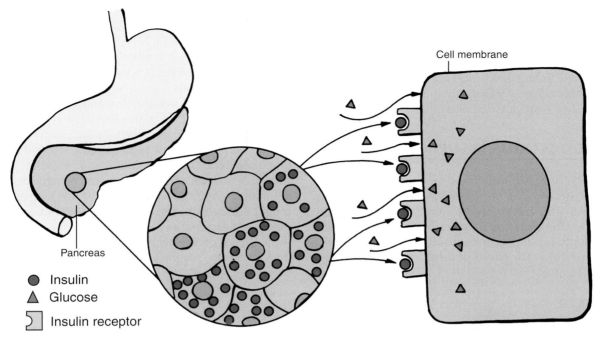

**FIGURE 22-1** Normal glucose metabolism. Once insulin binds with receptors on the cell membrane, glucose can move into the cell, promoting cellular metabolism and energy production.

Factors that inhibit insulin secretion include stimulation of pancreatic $alpha_2$-adrenergic receptors and stress conditions such as hypoxia, hypothermia, surgery, or severe burns.

## DIABETES MELLITUS

Diabetes mellitus is a chronic systemic disease characterized by metabolic and vascular abnormalities. Metabolic problems occur early in the disease process, are common and potentially disabling, and are related to changes in the metabolism of carbohydrate, fat, and protein. These result from hyperglycemia and other metabolic abnormalities that accompany a lack of effective insulin. The metabolic abnormalities associated with hyperglycemia can cause early, acute complications, such as diabetic ketoacidosis (DKA) or hyperosmolar hyperglycemic nonketotic coma (HHNC; Box 22-1). Eventually, metabolic abnormalities lead to damage to blood vessels and other body tissues. Microvascular changes result in nephropathy, retinopathy, and peripheral neuropathy. Other complications include musculoskeletal disorders, increased numbers and severity of infections, and complications of pregnancy. There is strong evidence that strict control of blood sugar delays the onset and slows progression of complications of diabetes. For most clients, the goals of treatment are to maintain blood glucose at normal or near-normal levels; promote normal metabolism of carbohydrate, fat, and protein; prevent acute and long-term complications; and prevent hypoglycemic episodes.

Diabetes is one of the most common chronic disorders of childhood and older adults, often requiring drug therapy. Age-specific considerations in the management of diabetes are found in Age-related Considerations. Most diabetes care is delivered in ambulatory care settings or in the home, and any client with diabetes may need home care. Hospitalization usually occurs only for complications, and clients are quickly discharged if possible. Guidelines for ongoing evaluation and intervention are addressed in Home Care Considerations.

## Classification

The two major classes are type 1 and type 2. Although both are characterized by hyperglycemia, they differ in onset, course, pathology, and treatment. Disease processes, certain drugs, and pregnancy may induce other types of diabetes. Gestational (pregnancy-induced) diabetes is described in Chapter 23.

### Type 1

Type 1 diabetes, a common chronic disorder of childhood, results from an autoimmune disorder that destroys pancreatic beta cells. Symptoms usually develop when 10% to 20% of functioning beta cells remain, but they may occur at any time if acute illness or stress increases the body's demand for insulin beyond the capacity of the remaining beta cells to secrete insulin. Eventually, all the beta cells are destroyed, and no insulin is produced.

Type 1 may occur at any age but usually begins between 4 and 20 years of age. The peak incidence for girls is 10 to 12 years, for boys, 12 to 14 years. Type 1 usually

# BOX 22-1 Acute Complications of Diabetes Mellitus

## Diabetic Ketoacidosis (DKA)

This life-threatening complication occurs with severe insulin deficiency. In the absence of insulin, glucose cannot be used by body cells for energy and fat is mobilized from adipose tissue to furnish a fuel source. The mobilized fat circulates in the bloodstream, from which it is extracted by the liver and broken down into glycerol and fatty acids. The fatty acids are further changed in the liver to ketones (eg, acetoacetic acid, acetone), which then enter the bloodstream and are circulated to body cells for metabolic conversion to energy, carbon dioxide, and water.

The ketones are produced more rapidly than body cells can use them and their accumulation produces acidemia (a drop in blood pH and an increase in blood hydrogen ions). The body attempts to buffer the acidic hydrogen ions by exchanging them for intracellular potassium ions. Hydrogen ions enter body cells, and potassium ions leave the cells to be excreted in the urine. Another attempt to remove excess acid involves the lungs. Deep, labored respirations, called Kussmaul respirations, eliminate more carbon dioxide and prevent formation of carbonic acid. A third attempt to regain homeostasis involves the kidneys, which excrete some of the ketones, thereby producing acetone in the urine.

DKA worsens as the compensatory mechanisms fail. Clinical signs and symptoms become progressively more severe. Early ones include blurred vision, anorexia, nausea and vomiting, thirst, and polyuria. Later ones include drowsiness, which progresses to stupor and coma, Kussmaul breathing, dehydration and other signs of fluid and electrolyte imbalances, and decreased blood pressure, increased pulse, and other signs of shock.

Two major causes of DKA are omission of insulin and illnesses such as infection, trauma, myocardial infarction, or stroke.

## Hyperosmolar Hyperglycemic Nonketotic Coma (HHNC)

HHNC is another type of diabetic coma that is potentially life threatening. It is relatively rare and carries a high mortality rate. The term *hyperosmolar* refers to an excessive amount of glucose, electrolytes, and other solutes in the blood in relation to the amount of water.

Like DKA, HHNC is characterized by hyperglycemia, which leads to osmotic diuresis and resultant thirst, polyuria, dehydration, and electrolyte losses, as well as neurologic signs ranging from drowsiness to stupor to coma. Additional clinical problems may include hypovolemic shock, thrombosis, renal problems, or stroke. In contrast to DKA, hyperosmolar coma occurs in people with previously unknown or mild diabetes, usually after an illness; occurs in hyperglycemic conditions other than diabetes (eg, severe burns, corticosteroid drug therapy); and does not cause ketosis.

# Age-related Considerations: Use of Antidiabetic Drugs

## USE IN CHILDREN

### Type 1 Diabetes

Insulin is the only drug indicated for use and is required as replacement therapy because affected children cannot produce insulin. Factors that influence management and insulin therapy include the following:

• Effective management requires a consistent schedule of meals, snacks, blood glucose monitoring, insulin injections and dose adjustments, and exercise. Insulin injections must be given three or four times per day. A healthful, varied diet, rich in whole grains, fruits, and vegetables and limited in simple sugars, is recommended. In addition, food intake must be synchronized with insulin injections and usually involves three meals and three snacks, all at regularly scheduled times.

Such a schedule is difficult to maintain in children, but extremely important in promoting normal growth and development. A major factor in optimal treatment is a supportive family in which at least one member is thoroughly educated about the disease and its management. Less-than-optimal treatment can lead to stunted growth; delayed puberty; and early development of complications such as retinopathy, nephropathy, or neuropathy.

• Infections and other illnesses may cause wide fluctuations in blood glucose levels and interfere with metabolic control. For example, some infections cause hypoglycemia; others, especially chronic infections, may cause hyperglycemia and insulin resistance and may precipitate ketoacidosis. As a result, insulin requirements may vary widely during illness episodes and should be based on blood glucose and urine ketone levels. Hypoglycemia often develops in young children, partly because of anorexia and smaller glycogen reserves.

• During illness, children are highly susceptible to dehydration, and an adequate fluid intake is very important. Many clinicians recommend sugar-containing liquids (eg, regular sodas, clear juices, regular gelatin desserts) if blood glucose values are lower than 250 mg/dL. When blood glucose values are above 250 mg/dL, diet soda, unsweetened tea, and other fluids without sugar should be given.

• For infants and toddlers who weigh less than 10 kg or require less than 5 units of insulin per day, a diluted insulin can be used because such small doses are hard to measure in a U-100 syringe. The most common dilution is U-10, and a diluent is available from insulin manufacturers. Vials

*(continued)*

## Age-related Considerations: Use of Antidiabetic Drugs (Continued)

of diluted insulin should be clearly labeled and discarded after 1 month.
- Rotation of injection sites is important in infants and young children because of the relatively small areas for injection at each anatomic site and to prevent lipodystrophy.
- Young children usually adjust to injections and blood glucose monitoring better when the parents express less anxiety about these vital procedures.
- Avoiding hypoglycemia is a major goal in infants and young children because of potentially damaging effects on growth and development. For example, the brain and spinal cord do not develop normally without an adequate supply of glucose. Animal studies indicate that prolonged hypoglycemia results in decreased brain weight, numbers of neurons, and protein content. Myelinization of nerve cells is also decreased. Because complex motor and intellectual functions require an intact central nervous system, frequent, severe, or prolonged hypoglycemia can be a serious problem in infants, toddlers, and preschoolers. In addition, recognition of hypoglycemia may be delayed because signs and symptoms are vague and the children may be unable to communicate them to parents or caregivers. Because of these difficulties, most pediatric diabetologists recommend maintaining blood glucose levels between 100 and 200 mg/dL to prevent hypoglycemia. In addition, *the bedtime snack and blood glucose measurement should never be skipped.*
- Signs and symptoms of hypoglycemia in older children are similar to those in adults (eg, hunger, sweating, tachycardia). In young children, hypoglycemia may be manifested by changes in behavior, including severe hunger, irritability, and lethargy. In addition, mental functioning may be impaired in all age groups, even with mild hypoglycemia. Whenever hypoglycemia is suspected, blood glucose should be tested.
- Adolescents may resist adhering to their prescribed treatment regimens, and effective management may be especially difficult during this developmental period. Adolescents and young adults may delay, omit, or decrease dosage of insulin to fit in socially (eg, by eating more, sleeping in, or drinking alcohol) or to control their weight. Omitting or decreasing insulin dosage may lead to repeated episodes of ketoacidosis. Also, adolescent females may develop eating disorders.
- A good resource is the Juvenile Diabetes Foundation (1-800-JDF-CURE), a not-for-profit health agency with support groups and other activities for families affected by diabetes.

### TYPE 2 DIABETES

Type 2 diabetes is being increasingly identified in children. This trend is attributed mainly to obesity and inadequate exercise because most children with type 2 are seriously overweight and have poor eating habits. In addition, most are members of high-risk ethnic groups (eg, African American, Native American, or Hispanic) and have relatives with diabetes. These children are at high risk for development of serious complications during early adulthood, such as myocardial infarction during their fourth decade. Management involves exercise, weight loss, and a more healthful diet.

### USE IN OLDER ADULTS

General precautions for safe and effective use of antidiabetic drugs apply to older adults, including close monitoring of blood glucose levels. In addition, older adults may have impaired vision or other problems that decrease their ability to perform needed tasks (eg, self-administration of insulin, monitoring blood glucose levels, managing diet and exercise). They also may have other disorders and may take other drugs that complicate management of diabetes. For example, renal insufficiency may increase risks for adverse effects with antidiabetic drugs and treatment with thiazide diuretics, corticosteroids, estrogens, and other drugs may cause hyperglycemia, thereby increasing dosage requirements for antidiabetic drugs.

With oral sulfonylureas, drugs with a short duration of action and inactive metabolites are considered safer, especially with impaired liver or kidney function. Therapy usually should start with a low dose, which is then increased or decreased according to blood glucose levels and clinical response.

Few guidelines have been developed for the use of newer antidiabetic drugs in older adults. Insulin analogs appear to have some advantages over conventional insulin. Acarbose, miglitol, and metformin may not be as useful in older adults as in younger ones because of the high prevalence of impaired renal function. These drugs are relatively contraindicated in clients with renal insufficiency because they have a longer half-life and may accumulate. With metformin, dosage should be based on periodic tests of renal function, and the drug should be stopped if renal impairment occurs or if serum lactate increases. In addition, dosage should not be titrated to the maximum amount recommended for younger adults. With the glitazones, older adults are more likely to have cardiovascular disorders that increase risks for fluid retention and congestive heart failure. With meglitinides, effects were similar in younger and older adults during clinical trials.

---

has a sudden onset; produces severe symptoms; is difficult to control; produces a high incidence of complications, such as DKA and renal failure; and requires administration of exogenous insulin. About 10% of people with diabetes have type 1.

**Type 2**

Type 2 is characterized by hyperglycemia and insulin resistance. The hyperglycemia results from increased production of glucose by the liver and decreased uptake of glucose in liver, muscle, and fat cells. Insulin resistance

## Home Care Considerations: Use of Antidiabetic Drugs

**ASSESS:** client's ability to prevent or solve problems and learn self-care and caregivers' ability to support clients' efforts to participate actively in diabetes management; caregiver role strain, and quality-of-life considerations with living with this disease on a day-to-day basis

**MONITOR:** client's health status; progress in disease management; self-care abilities in terms of diet, exercise, medication administration, blood glucose monitoring, and prevention, recognition, and treatment of complications; compliance with the prescribed regimen; therapeutic and adverse drug effects, especially with changes in drugs or dosages; that client is keeping appointments for lab work and follow-up care; need, and mobilize and coordinate health care providers and community resources

**EDUCATE:** with initial teaching or reinforcement and follow-up of teaching done by others regarding how to use, store, and replace medications to ensure a constant supply; circumstances for which the client should seek emergency care; interventions for "sick days"; and signs and symptoms of hyper and hypoglycemia. Reinforce additional teaching points (see Client Teaching Guidelines: Antidiabetic Drugs).

means that higher-than-usual concentrations of insulin are required. Thus, insulin is present but unable to work effectively (ie, inhibit hepatic production of glucose and cause glucose to move from the bloodstream into liver, muscle, and fat cells). Most insulin resistance is attributed to impaired insulin action at the cellular level, possibly related to postreceptor, intracellular mechanisms.

Type 2 may occur at any age but usually starts after 40 years. Compared with type 1, it usually has a gradual onset; produces less severe symptoms initially; is easier to control; causes less DKA and renal failure but more myocardial infarctions and strokes; and does not necessarily require exogenous insulin because endogenous insulin is still produced. About 90% of people with diabetes have type 2; 20% to 30% of them require exogenous insulin.

Type 2 is a heterogenous disease, and etiology probably involves multiple factors such as a genetic predisposition and environmental factors. Obesity is a major cause. With obesity and chronic ingestion of excess calories, along with a sedentary lifestyle, more insulin is required. The increased need leads to prolonged stimulation and eventual "fatigue" of pancreatic beta cells. As a result, the cells become less responsive to elevated blood glucose levels and less able to produce enough insulin to meet metabolic needs. Thus, insulin is secreted but is inadequate or ineffective, especially when insulin demand is increased by obesity, pregnancy, aging, or other factors.

## HYPOGLYCEMIC DRUGS

### Insulin

Insulin is described in this section, and individual insulins are listed in Drugs at a Glance 22-1: Insulins. Regular insulin is the prototype (see Prototype Profile 22-1).

- Exogenous insulin used to replace endogenous insulin has the same effects as the pancreatic hormone.
- Insulin and its analogs (structurally similar chemicals) lower blood glucose levels by increasing glucose uptake by body cells, especially skeletal muscle and fat cells, and by decreasing glucose production in the liver.
- The main clinical indication for insulin is treatment of diabetes mellitus. Insulin is the only effective treatment for type 1 because pancreatic beta cells are unable to secrete endogenous insulin and metabolism is severely impaired. Insulin is required for clients with type 2 who cannot control their disease with diet, weight control, and oral agents. It may be needed by anyone with diabetes during times of stress, such as illness, infection, or surgery. Insulin also is used to control diabetes induced by chronic pancreatitis, surgical excision of pancreatic tissue, hormones and other drugs, and pregnancy (gestational diabetes). In nondiabetic clients, insulin is used to prevent or treat hyperglycemia induced by total parenteral nutrition (TPN) solutions and to treat hyperkalemia. In hyperkalemia, an intravenous (IV) infusion of insulin and dextrose solution causes potassium to move from the blood into the cells; it does not alter total body potassium because it does not eliminate the electrolyte from the body.
- The only clearcut contraindication to the use of insulin is hypoglycemia, because of the risk for brain damage (Box 22-2). Pork insulin is contraindicated in clients allergic to the animal protein.
- Available insulins are pork insulin and human insulin. Pork insulin differs from human insulin by one amino acid. Human insulin is synthesized in the laboratory with recombinant DNA techniques using strains of *Escherichia coli* or by modifying pork insulin to replace the single different amino acid. The name *human insulin* means that the synthetic product is identical to endogenous insulin (ie, has the same number and sequence of amino acids). It is not derived from the human pancreas.

Insulin analogs are synthesized in the laboratory by altering the type or sequence of amino acids in insulin molecules. *Insulin lispro* (Humalog) and *insulin aspart* (NovoLog) are short-acting products. Lispro, the first analog to be marketed, is identical to human insulin except for the reversal of two amino acids (lysine and proline). It is similar to physiologic insulin secretion after a meal, more effective at decreasing postprandial hyperglycemia, and less likely to cause

*(text continues on page 373)*

**DRUG TABLE 22-1**

*Drugs at a Glance*

**Insulins**

| Generic/ Trade Name | Routes and Dosage Ranges | Comments/ Characteristics | Action (h) | | |
|---|---|---|---|---|---|
| | | | Onset | Peak | Duration |
| *Short-acting Insulin* | | | | | |
| **Insulin injection** (Regular Iletin II, Humulin R, Novolin R) Pregnancy Category B | Sub-Q, dosage individualized according to blood glucose levels. For sliding scale, 5–20 units before meals and bedtime, depending on blood glucose levels<br>IV, dosage individualized. For ketoacidosis, regular insulin may be given by direct injection, intermittent infusion, or continuous infusion. One regimen involves an initial bolus injection of 10–20 units followed by a continuous low-dose infusion of 2–10 units/h, based on hourly blood and urine glucose levels | 1. A clear liquid solution with the appearance of water<br>2. The hypoglycemic drug of choice for diabetics experiencing acute or emergency situations, diabetic ketoacidosis, hyperosmolar nonketotic coma, severe infections or other illnesses, major surgery, and pregnancy<br>3. The only insulin preparation that can be given IV<br>4. See Prototype Profile 22-1 | ½–1 | 2–3 | 5–7 |
| *Intermediate-acting Insulins* | | | | | |
| **Isophane insulin suspension** (NPH, NPH Iletin II, Humulin N, Novolin N) Pregnancy Category B | Sub-Q, dosage individualized. Initially, 7–26 units may be given once or twice daily. | 1. Commonly used for long-term administration<br>2. Modified by addition of protamine (a protein) and zinc<br>3. A suspension with a cloudy appearance when correctly mixed in the drug vial<br>4. Given *only* Sub-Q<br>5. Not recommended for use in acute situations<br>6. Hypoglycemic reactions are more likely to occur during mid-to-late afternoon | 1–1½ | 8–12 | 18–24 |
| **Insulin zinc suspension** (Lente Iletin II, Lente L, Humulin L, Novolin L) Pregnancy Category B | Sub-Q, dosage individualized. Initially, 7–26 units may be given once or twice daily. | 1. Modified by addition of zinc<br>2. May be used interchangeably with NPH insulin<br>3. A suspension with a cloudy appearance when correctly mixed in the drug vial<br>4. Given only Sub-Q | 1–2 | 8–12 | 18–24 |
| *Long-acting Insulin* | | | | | |
| **Extended insulin zinc suspension** (Humulin U, Ultralente) Pregnancy Category B | Sub-Q, dosage individualized. Initially, 7–26 units may be given once daily | 1. Modified by addition of zinc and formation of large crystals, which are slowly absorbed<br>2. Hypoglycemic reactions are frequent and likely to occur during sleep. | 4–8 | 10–30 | 36 plus |

*(continued)*

**DRUG TABLE 22-1**

## Drugs at a Glance

### Insulins (Continued)

| Generic/ Trade Name | Routes and Dosage Ranges | Comments/ Characteristics | Action (h) | | |
|---|---|---|---|---|---|
| | | | Onset | Peak | Duration |
| *Insulin Mixtures* | | | | | |
| **NPH 70%** **Regular 30%** (Humulin 70/30, Novolin 70/30) | Sub-Q, dosage individualized | 1. Stable mixture 2. Onset, peak, and duration of action same as individual components | | | |
| **NPH 50%** **Regular 50%** (Humulin 50/50) Pregnancy Category B | Sub-Q, dosage individualized | See Humulin 70/30, above | | | |
| *Insulin Analogs* | | | | | |
| **Insulin lispro** (Humalog) Pregnancy Category B | Sub-Q, dosage individualized, 15 min before meals | 1. A synthetic insulin of recombinant DNA origin, created by reversing two amino acids 2. Has a faster onset and a shorter duration of action than human regular insulin 3. Intended for use with a longer-acting insulin | 1/4 | 1/2–1 1/2 | 6–8 |
| **Insulin aspart** (NovoLog) | Sub-Q, dosage individualized | Similar to lispro | 1/4 | 1–3 | 3–5 |
| **Insulin glargine** (Lantus) Pregnancy Category C | Sub-Q, dosage individualized, once daily at bedtime | 1. Long-acting 2. Provides basal amount of insulin 3. Must not be diluted or mixed with any other insulin or solutions | 1.1 | None | 24 |

**BOX 22-2**

## Hypoglycemia: Characteristics and Management

Hypoglycemia may occur with insulin or oral sulfonylureas. When hypoglycemia is suspected, the blood glucose level should be measured if possible, although signs and symptoms and the plasma glucose level at which they occur vary from person to person. Hypoglycemia is a blood glucose below 60 to 70 mg/dL and is especially dangerous at approximately 40 mg/dL or below. Central nervous system effects may lead to accidental injury or permanent brain damage; cardiovascular effects may lead to cardiac dysrhythmias or myocardial infarction. Causes of hypoglycemia include:

- Intensive insulin therapy (ie, continuous subcutaneous [SC] infusion or three or more injections daily).
- Omitting or delaying meals
- An excessive or incorrect dose of insulin or an oral agent that causes hypoglycemia
- Altered sensitivity to insulin
- Decreased clearance of insulin or an oral agent (eg, with renal insufficiency)
- Decreased glucose intake
- Decreased production of glucose in the liver

- Giving an insulin injection intramuscularly (IM) rather than Sub-Q
- Drug interactions that decrease blood glucose levels
- Increased physical exertion
- Ethanol ingestion

### Hormones That Raise Blood Sugar

Normally, when hypoglycemia occurs, several hormones (glucagon, epinephrine, growth hormone, and cortisol) work to restore and maintain blood glucose levels. Glucagon and epinephrine, the dominant counter-regulatory hormones, act rapidly because they are activated as soon as blood glucose levels start declining. Growth hormone and cortisol act more slowly, about 2 hours after hypoglycemia occurs.

People with diabetes who develop hypoglycemia may have impaired secretion of these hormones, especially those with type 1 diabetes. Decreased secretion of glucagon is often evident in clients who have had diabetes for 5 years or longer. Decreased secretion of epinephrine also occurs in people who have been treated with insulin for several years. Decreased

*(continued)*

## BOX 22-2  Hypoglycemia: Characteristics and Management (Continued)

epinephrine decreases tachycardia, a common sign of hypo-glycemia, and may delay recognition and treatment.

### The Conscious Client

Treatment of hypoglycemic reactions consists of immediate administration of a rapidly absorbed carbohydrate. For the conscious client who is able to swallow, the carbohydrate is given orally. Foods and fluids that provide approximately 15 g of carbohydrate include:

- Two sugar cubes or 1 to 2 teaspoons of sugar, syrup, honey, or jelly
- Two or three small pieces of candy or eight Lifesaver candies
- 4 oz of fruit juice, such as orange, apple, or grape
- 4 oz of ginger ale
- Coffee or tea with 2 teaspoons of sugar added
- Commercial glucose products (eg, Glutose, B-D Glucose). These products must be swallowed to be effective.

Symptoms usually subside within 15 to 20 minutes. If they do not subside, the client should take another 10 to 15 g of oral carbohydrate. *If acarbose or miglitol has been taken with insulin or a sulfonylurea and a hypoglycemic reaction occurs, glucose (oral or intravenous [IV]) or glucagon must be given for treatment.* Sucrose (table sugar) and other oral carbohydrates do not relieve hypoglycemia because the presence of acarbose or miglitol prevents their digestion and absorption from the gastrointestinal tract.

### The Unconscious Client

For the unconscious client, carbohydrate cannot be given orally because of the risks of aspiration. Therefore, the treatment choices are parenteral glucose or glucagon.

If the client is in a health care facility where medical help is readily available, IV glucose in a 25% or 50% solution is the treatment of choice. It acts rapidly to raise blood glucose levels and arouse the client. If the client is at home or elsewhere, glucagon may be given if available and there is someone to inject it. A family member or roommate may be taught to give glucagon Sub-Q or IM. It can also be given IV. The usual adult dose is 0.5 to 1 mg. Glucagon is a pancreatic hormone that increases blood sugar by converting liver glycogen to glucose. It is effective only when liver glycogen is present. Some clients cannot respond to glucagon because glycogen stores are depleted by such conditions as starvation, adrenal insufficiency, or chronic hypoglycemia. The hyperglycemic effect of glucagon occurs more slowly than that of IV glucose and is of relatively brief duration. If the client does not respond to one or two doses of glucagon within 20 minutes, IV glucose is indicated.

Caution is needed in the treatment of hypoglycemia. Although the main goal of treatment is to relieve hypoglycemia and restore the brain's supply of glucose, a secondary goal is to avoid overtreatment and excessive hyperglycemia. The client having a hypoglycemic reaction should not use it as an excuse to eat high-caloric foods or large amounts of food. Health care personnel caring for the client should avoid giving excessive amounts of glucose.

### Posthypoglycemia Care

Once hypoglycemia is relieved, the person should have a snack or a meal. Slowly absorbed carbohydrate and protein foods, such as milk, cheese, and bread, are needed to replace glycogen stores in the liver and to prevent secondary hypoglycemia from rapid use of the carbohydrates given earlier. In addition, the episode needs to be evaluated for precipitating factors so that these can be minimized to prevent future episodes. Repeated episodes mean that the therapeutic regimen and client compliance must be re-evaluated and adjusted if indicated.

## PROTOTYPE PROFILE 22-1

### ℗ Insulin Regular (IN su lin)

**Drug Class**
**Chemical:** Insulins
**Functional:** Antidiabetic agent; hypoglycemic agent

**Trade Name**
Humulin R, and others

**Therapeutic Indications**
To lower blood glucose; management of diabetes mellitus

**Pharmacokinetics**
*Absorption*
Sub-Q, IV rapid
*Distribution*
Based on the adequacy of blood circulation; does not cross placenta

**Metabolism**
Half-life, 5–9 minutes

**Excretion**
Urine

**Pharmacodynamics**
*Onset of Action*
Sub-Q, ⅓–1h (peak 2–3 h); IV, 10–15 min (peak 15–30 min)
*Duration*
Sub-Q, 5-7 h; IV, 1–2 h

**Contraindications/Precautions**
Hypoglycemia; with caution with renal and hepatic impairment

*(continued)*

## PROTOTYPE PROFILE 22-1
### P Insulin Regular (Continued)

**Pregnancy Considerations**
Category B
Does not cross placenta or enter breast milk

**Dosage**
Varies with serum glucose level

**Adverse Effects**
Hypoglycemia, shock, Somogyi effect, tachycardia, hunger, headache

**Drug Interactions**
*Increased Effects*
Increased hypoglycemic effect with alcohol, oral hypoglycemics, anabolic steroids, beta blockers, tricyclic antidepressants, monoamine oxidase inhibitors, tetracycline, aspirin, oral anticoagulants

*Decreased Effects*
Decreased hypoglycemic effect with smoking, thyroid hormone, corticosteroids, epinephrine, diltiazem, oral contraceptives, thiazide diuretics, niacin

**Herbal Supplements and Dietary Considerations**
Alcohol, garlic, chromium, and gymnema may increase hypoglycemia, Dietary considerations based on American Diabetic Association recommendations Evaluate serum potassium levels

---

hypoglycemia before the next meal. Injection just before a meal produces hypoglycemic effects similar to those of an injection of conventional regular insulin given 30 minutes before a meal. Aspart has an even more rapid onset and shorter duration of action. In contrast, *insulin glargine* is a long-acting preparation used to provide a basal amount of insulin through 24 hours, similar to normal, endogenous insulin secretion.

■ Insulin cannot be given orally because it is a protein that is destroyed by proteolytic enzymes in the GI tract. It is given only parenterally, most often subcutaneously. However, a nasal spray formulation is being developed.

■ Insulins differ in onset and duration of action. They are usually categorized as short, intermediate, or long acting. Short-acting insulins have a rapid onset and a short duration of action. Intermediate- and long-acting insulins (except for insulin glargine) are modified by adding protamine (a large, insoluble protein), zinc, or both to slow absorption and prolong drug action. Several mixtures of an intermediate- and a short-acting insulin are available and commonly used.

■ U-100, the main insulin concentration in the United States, contains 100 units of insulin per milliliter of solution. *It can be accurately measured only in a syringe designed for use with U-100 insulin.*

■ Subcutaneous insulin is absorbed most rapidly when injected into the abdomen, followed by the upper arm, thigh, and buttocks. Absorption is delayed or decreased by injection into subcutaneous tissue with lipodystrophy or other lesions, by circulatory problems such as edema or hypotension, by insulin-binding antibodies (which develop after 2 or 3 months of insulin administration), and by injecting cold (ie, refrigerated) insulin.

■ Temperature extremes can cause loss of potency. Insulin retains potency up to 36 months under refrigeration and for 18 to 24 months at room temperature. At high temperatures (eg, 100°F, or 37.7°C), insulin loses potency in about 2 months. If frozen, insulin clumps or precipitates, cannot be measured accurately, and should be discarded.

■ Factors that increase insulin requirements include weight gain; increased caloric intake; pregnancy; decreased activity; acute infections; hyperadrenocorticism (Cushing's disease); primary hyperparathyroidism; acromegaly; hypokalemia; and drugs such as corticosteroids, epinephrine, levothyroxine, and thiazide diuretics. Clients who are obese may require 2 units/kg per day because of resistance to insulin in peripheral tissues.

■ Factors that decrease insulin requirements include weight reduction; decreased caloric intake; increased physical activity; development of renal insufficiency; stopping administration of corticosteroids, epinephrine, levothyroxine, and diuretics; hypothyroidism; hypopituitarism; recovery from hyperthyroidism; recovery from acute infections; and the "honeymoon period," which may occur with type 1 diabetes.

## Oral Hypoglycemic Drugs

There are five types of oral antidiabetic agents, all of which may be used to treat type 2 diabetes that is uncontrolled by diet and exercise. The drugs lower blood sugar by different mechanisms (Fig. 22-2) and may be used in various combinations for additive effects. Some are also combined with insulin. These drugs are further described below and in Drugs at a Glance 22-2: Oral Drugs for Diabetes Mellitus.

### Sulfonylureas

■ The sulfonylureas are the oldest and largest group of oral agents. They lower blood glucose mainly by increasing secretion of insulin. They may also increase peripheral

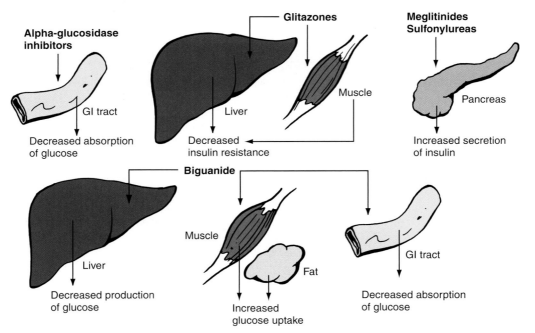

**FIGURE 22-2** Actions of oral antidiabetic drugs. The drugs lower blood sugar by decreasing absorption or production of glucose, by increasing secretion of insulin, or by increasing the effectiveness of available insulin (decreasing insulin resistance).

**DRUG TABLE 22-2**    *Drugs at a Glance*

## Oral Drugs For Diabetes Mellitus

| Generic/Trade Name | Routes and Dosage Ranges | Comments/Characteristics |
|---|---|---|
| *Sulfonylureas, Second Generation* | | |
| **Glimepiride** (Amaryl) Pregnancy Category C | PO, initially 1–2 mg once daily, with breakfast or first main meal. Maximum starting dose 2 mg or less. Maintenance dose 1–4 mg once daily. After a dose of 2 mg is reached, increase dose in increments of 2 mg or less at 1- to 2-week intervals, based on blood glucose levels. Maximum recommended dose, 8 mg once daily. In combination with insulin, PO 8 mg once daily with the first main meal. | Onset of action about 1 h; peak, 2–3 h |
| **Glipizide** (Glucotrol) Pregnancy Category C | PO, initially 5 mg daily in a single dose, 30 min before breakfast. Maximum dose, 40 mg daily. In elderly, may start with 2.5 mg daily | Onset of action, approximately 1–1.5 h; duration 10–16 h |
| **Glyburide** (DiaBeta, Micronase, Glynase Pres Tab) Pregnancy Category C | PO, initially 2.5–5 mg daily in a single dose, with breakfast. Maximum dose, 20 mg daily. Glynase PO initially 1.5–3 mg daily with breakfast. Maximum dose, 12 mg daily. | Onset of action approximately 2–4 h; duration 24 h. Glynase is better absorbed, acts faster (onset about 1 h; duration 24 h), and is given in smaller doses than other forms of glyburide. |

*(continued)*

**DRUG TABLE 22-2**

*Drugs at a Glance*

## Oral Drugs For Diabetes Mellitus (Continued)

| Generic/Trade Name | Routes and Dosage Ranges | Comments/Characteristics |
|---|---|---|
| **Alpha-Glucosidase Inhibitors** | | |
| **Acarbose** (Precose)<br>Pregnancy Category B | PO, initially 25 mg, three times daily with first bite of main meals; increase at 4- to 8-week intervals to a maximum dose of 50 mg three times daily (for patients weighing under 60 kg) if necessary, depending on 1-h postprandial blood glucose levels and tolerance. Clients weighing more than 60 kg may need doses up to 100 mg three times daily (the maximum dose). | Delays digestion of carbohydrate foods when acarbose and food are present in gastrointestinal (GI) tract at the same time |
| **Miglitol** (Glyset)<br>Pregnancy Category B | PO, initially 25 mg three times daily with the first bite of each main meal, gradually increased if necessary. Maximum dose, 100 mg three times daily | Delays digestion of carbohydrates in the GI tract |
| **Biguanide** | | |
| **Metformin** (Glucophage)<br>Pregnancy Category B | PO, initially 500 mg twice daily, with morning and evening meals; increase dose in increments of 500 mg/d every 2–3 weeks if necessary, up to a maximum of 3000 mg daily, based on patient tolerance and blood glucose levels. In elderly patients, do not increase to maximum dose. | Older adults are at higher risk for development of lactic acidosis, a rare but potentially fatal reaction. Thus, smaller doses and monitoring of renal function are recommended. |
| **Glitazones** | | |
| **Pioglitazone** (Actos)<br>Pregnancy Category C | PO, 15–30 mg once daily | Increases effects of insulin; may be used alone or with insulin, metformin, or a sulfonylurea |
| **Rosiglitazone** (Avandia)<br>Pregnancy Category C | PO, 4–8 mg once daily, in one dose or two divided doses | Increases effects of insulin; may be used alone or with metformin |
| **Meglitinides** | | |
| **Nateglinide** (Starlix)<br>Pregnancy Category C | PO, 120 mg three times daily, 1–30 min before meals. Omit dose if skip a meal. | Onset of action, within 20 min; peak, 1 h; duration, 3–4h |
| **Repaglinide** (Prandin)<br>Pregnancy Category C | PO, 1–2 mg 15–30 min before each meal; increased to 4 mg before meals if necessary. Maximum dose, 16 mg daily. Omit a dose if skip a meal; add a dose if add a meal. | Onset of action, within 30 min; peak, 1 h; duration approximately 3–4 h |
| **Combination Drug\*** | | |
| **Glyburide/metformin**<br>(Glucovance)<br>Pregnancy Category B (manufacturer); C (expert analysis) | Initially, PO, 1.25 mg/250 mg once or twice daily with meals. Patients previously treated with glyburide or other sulfonylurea plus metformin: Initially, PO 2.5 or 5 mg/500 mg twice daily with meals, not to exceed previous doses of separate drugs. | Available in preparations with 1.25 mg glyburide and 250 mg metformin; 2.5 mg glyburide and 500 mg metformin; or 5 mg glyburide and 500 mg metformin |

\*See Appendix A for additional combination drugs.

use of glucose, decrease production of glucose in the liver, increase the number of insulin receptors, or alter postreceptor actions to increase tissue responsiveness to insulin. Because the drugs stimulate pancreatic beta cells to produce more insulin, they are effective only when functioning pancreatic beta cells are present.

■ First-generation drugs (eg, acetohexamide, chlorpropamide, tolazamide, and tolbutamide) have largely been replaced by the second-generation agents and are not discussed further. The second-generation drugs—glipizide, glyburide, and glimepiride—are similar in therapeutic and adverse effects; none serves as the prototype. The main adverse effect is hypoglycemia (see Box 22-1).

■ The sulfonylureas are chemically related to sulfonamide antibacterial drugs; well absorbed with oral administration; more than 90% bound to plasma proteins; and metabolized in the liver to inactive metabolites, which are excreted mainly by the kidneys (except for glyburide, which is excreted about equally in urine and bile).

■ A sulfonylurea may be given alone or with most other antidiabetic drugs in the treatment of type 2 diabetes, including insulin, acarbose, miglitol, metformin, pioglitazone, or rosiglitazone.

■ Sulfonylureas are contraindicated in clients with hypersensitivity to them, with severe renal or hepatic impairment, and during pregnancy. They are unlikely to be effective during periods of stress, such as major surgery, severe illness, or infection. Insulin is usually required in these circumstances.

### Guidelines for Using Sulfonylureas

■ Sulfonylureas are not effective in all clients with type 2 diabetes, and many clients experience primary or secondary treatment failure. Primary failure involves a lack of initial response to the drugs. Secondary failure means that a therapeutic response occurs when the drugs are first given, but the drugs eventually become ineffective. Reasons for secondary failure may include decreased compliance with diet and exercise instructions, failure to take the drugs as prescribed, or decreased ability of the pancreatic beta cells to produce more insulin in response to the drugs.

■ These drugs must be used cautiously in clients with impaired renal or hepatic function.

■ Dosage of sulfonylureas is usually started low and increased gradually until the fasting blood glucose is 110 mg/dL or less. The lowest dose that achieves normal fasting and postprandial blood sugar levels is recommended.

■ Sulfonylureas are not recommended for use during pregnancy because of risks for fetal hypoglycemia and death, congenital anomalies, and overt diabetes in women with gestational diabetes (because the drugs stimulate an already overstimulated pancreas).

## Alpha–Glucosidase Inhibitors

■ Acarbose and miglitol inhibit alpha-glucosidase enzymes (eg, sucrase, maltase, amylase) in the GI tract and thereby delay digestion of complex carbohydrates into glucose and other simple sugars. As a result, glucose absorption is delayed, and there is a smaller increase in blood glucose levels after a meal.

■ The drugs are metabolized in the GI tract by digestive enzymes and intestinal bacteria. Some of the metabolites are absorbed systemically and excreted in urine; plasma concentrations are increased in the presence of renal impairment.

■ One of the drugs may be combined with insulin or an oral agent, usually a sulfonylurea.

■ These drugs are contraindicated in clients with hypersensitivity, DKA, hepatic cirrhosis, inflammatory or malabsorptive intestinal disorders, and severe renal impairment.

### Guidelines for Using Alpha-Glucosidase Inhibitors

■ These drugs do not alter insulin secretion or cause hypoglycemia.

■ Acarbose and miglitol should be taken at the beginning of a meal so that they will be present in the GI tract with food and able to delay digestion of carbohydrates.

■ Low initial doses and gradual increases decrease GI upset (eg, bloating, diarrhea) and promote client compliance.

■ Clients taking acarbose or miglitol should continue their diet, exercise, and blood glucose testing routines.

## Biguanide

■ Metformin increases the use of glucose by muscle and fat cells, decreases hepatic glucose production, and decreases intestinal absorption of glucose. It is preferably called an antihyperglycemic rather than a hypoglycemic agent because it does not cause hypoglycemia, even in large doses, when used alone.

■ It is absorbed from the small intestine, circulates without binding to plasma proteins, and has a serum half-life of 1.3 to 4.5 hours. It is not metabolized in the liver and is excreted unchanged in the urine.

■ Metformin may be used alone or in combination with insulin or other oral agents. It is widely prescribed as the initial drug in obese clients with newly diagnosed type 2 diabetes, largely because it does not cause weight gain as most other oral agents do.

■ It is contraindicated in clients with diabetes complicated by fever, severe infections, severe trauma, major surgery, acidosis, or pregnancy (insulin is indicated in these conditions). It is also contraindicated in clients with serious hepatic or renal impairment, cardiac or respiratory insufficiency, hypoxia, or a history of lactic acidosis because these conditions may increase production of lactate and the risk for potentially fatal lactic acidosis.

## Guidelines for Using Biguanide

- Renal function should be assessed before starting metformin and at least annually during long-term therapy. The drug should not be given initially if renal impairment is present; it should be stopped if renal impairment occurs during treatment.
- As with other antidiabetic drugs, clients taking metformin should continue their diet, exercise, and blood glucose testing regimens.
- Parenteral radiographic contrast media containing iodine (eg, Cholografin, Hypaque) may cause renal failure, and they have been associated with lactic acidosis in clients receiving metformin. Metformin should be discontinued at least 48 hours before diagnostic tests are performed with these materials and should not be resumed for at least 48 hours after the tests are done and tests indicate that renal function is normal.

## Glitazones

- These drugs, pioglitazone and rosiglitazone, are also called thiazolidinediones or TZDs and insulin sensitizers.
- They decrease insulin resistance, a major factor in the pathophysiology of type 2 diabetes. The drugs stimulate receptors on muscle, fat, and liver cells. This stimulation increases or restores the effectiveness of circulating insulin and results in increased uptake of glucose by peripheral tissues and decreased production of glucose by the liver.
- The drugs may be used as monotherapy with diet and exercise or in combination with insulin, metformin, or a sulfonylurea.
- The drugs are contraindicated in clients with active liver disease or a serum alanine aminotransferase (ALT) level more than 2.5 times the upper limit of normal. They are also contraindicated in clients who are hypersensitive to them.
- The drugs should be used very cautiously, if at all, in clients at risk for congestive heart failure. Glitazones increase plasma volume and may cause fluid retention and heart failure. In one study, heart failure developed in 4.5% of glitazone users within 10 months and in 12.4% within 36 months. In people who did not take a glitazone, 2.6% developed heart failure within 10 months and 8.4% within 36 months.

## Guidelines for Using Glitazones

Liver function tests (eg, serum aminotransferase enzymes) should be checked before starting therapy and periodically thereafter. In addition, clients should be monitored closely for edema and other signs of congestive heart failure.

## Meglitinides

- Nateglinide and repaglinide are nonsulfonylureas that lower blood sugar by stimulating pancreatic secretion of insulin.
- They can be used as monotherapy with diet and exercise or in combination with metformin.
- The drugs are well absorbed from the GI tract; peak plasma level occurs within 1 hour. They have a plasma half-life of 1 to 1.5 hours and are highly bound (>98%) to plasma proteins. They are metabolized in the liver; metabolites are excreted in urine and feces.
- Repaglinide is metabolized and removed from the bloodstream within 3 to 4 hours after a dose, nateglinide within about 6 hours. This decreases the workload of pancreatic beta cells (ie, decreases duration of beta-cell stimulation), allows serum insulin levels to return to normal before the next meal, and decreases risks for hypoglycemic episodes.
- These drugs should be taken just before or up to 30 minutes before a meal. If a meal is skipped, the drug dose should be skipped; if a meal is added, a drug dose should be added.

## Guidelines for Using Meglitinides

- As with other antidiabetic drugs, clients taking one of these drugs should continue their diet, exercise, and blood glucose testing regimens.
- Dosage is flexible, depending on food intake, but clients should eat within a few minutes after taking a dose, to avoid hypoglycemia.

## HERBAL AND DIETARY SUPPLEMENTS THAT AFFECT BLOOD GLUCOSE LEVELS

With most herbs and dietary supplements, even the commonly used ones (eg, echinacea, St. John's wort), the effects on blood glucose levels are unknown; well-controlled, long-term studies of effects have not been done; and interactions with antidiabetic drugs are unknown. Thus, anyone with diabetes who wishes to take an herbal or dietary supplement should consult a health care provider, read product labels carefully, seek the most authoritative information available, and monitor blood glucose closely when starting the supplement. Described below are some prod-

---

**? How Can You Avoid This Medication Error?**

Jean Watson, a 52-year-old type 2 diabetic, has been managed for the last 3 years on 500 mg of metformin (Glucophage) bid. Her blood glucose usually is under 200 mg/dL. Mrs. Watson is scheduled for an intravenous pyelogram (IVP) to evaluate a series of recent urinary tract infections. When Mrs. Watson comes in for her test, she mentions that her blood glucose was elevated that morning, so she took her metformin as usual with a sip of water but did not eat breakfast as instructed. You note this in the chart and proceed to prepare her for the IVP.

ucts that reportedly affect blood sugar and should be used cautiously, if at all, by clients with diabetes.

## Supplements That May Increase Blood Glucose Levels

**Bee pollen** may cause hyperglycemia and decrease the effects of antidiabetic medications. It should *not* be used by people with diabetes.

**Ginkgo biloba** extract is thought to increase blood sugar in clients with diabetes by increasing hepatic metabolism of insulin and oral hypoglycemic drugs, thereby making the drugs less effective. It is not recommended for use.

**Glucosamine** in animal studies has demonstrated impaired beta-cell function and insulin secretion similar to that observed in humans with type 2 diabetes. Long-term effects in humans are unknown, but the product is considered potentially harmful to people with diabetes or impaired glucose tolerance (prediabetes). Adverse effects on blood sugar and drug interactions with antidiabetic medications have not been reported. However, blood sugar should be monitored carefully. With chondroitin, which is often taken with glucosamine for osteoarthritis, there is no information about effects on blood sugar, use by diabetic clients, or interactions with antidiabetic drugs.

## Supplements That May Decrease Blood Glucose Levels

**Basil,** commonly used in cooking, is also available as an herbal supplement. The amounts used in cooking are unlikely to affect blood sugar, but larger amounts may cause hypoglycemia or increase the hypoglycemic effects of insulin and oral antidiabetic drugs. The use of supplemental amounts should probably be avoided by people with diabetes. If used, blood glucose levels should be closely monitored.

**Bay leaf** is commonly used in cooking (it should be removed from the food before eating) and is also available as an extract made with ground leaves. It increases the effects of insulin and is sometimes recommended by nutritionists for diabetic diets. If used, blood glucose levels should be monitored closely.

**Chromium** is a trace mineral required for normal glucose metabolism. It may increase production of insulin receptors and insulin binding to the receptors, thereby increasing insulin effectiveness, lowering blood glucose levels, and decreasing insulin requirements in people with diabetes. It also may have beneficial effects on serum cholesterol levels. However, evidence for these effects is inconsistent, with some supporting and some negating the use of chromium supplements.

Chromium deficiency, considered rare in the United States, may play a role in the development of diabetes and atherosclerosis. If so, beneficial effects of a supplement may be more evident in a deficiency state. In one study of pregnant women and older adults with marginal levels of chromium, administration of a supplement improved glucose tolerance. At present, there is insufficient evidence to recommend routine chromium supplementation in diabetic clients. In nondiabetic clients, chromium supplements do not have hypoglycemic effects.

**Echinacea.** Some clinical trials have been done, but people with diabetes were excluded. A conclusion was that diabetic clients should not take the drug.

**Garlic.** Some sources report no known effects on blood glucose; others report a decrease in animals and humans. Some researchers also reported increased serum insulin and improvement in liver glycogen storage after garlic administration. There is a potential for additive hypoglycemic effects with antidiabetic drugs, although no apparent interactions have been reported.

**Ginseng.** Several studies (generally small and not well designed) indicate that ginseng lowers blood glucose levels in both diabetic and nondiabetic subjects. It may be useful in preventing diabetes or complications of diabetes. However, larger and longer studies are needed before general use can be recommended for diabetic or nondiabetic clients. For nondiabetic clients who use ginseng, the herb may need to be taken with a meal to prevent unintentional hypoglycemia. For diabetic clients, use of ginseng should be very cautious (if at all), with frequent monitoring of blood glucose and signs of hypoglycemia, because of possible additive effects with antidiabetic medications. Its use should also be accompanied by proper diet, physical activity, and antidiabetic medication.

**Glucomannan,** which is promoted as a diet aid and laxative, has hypoglycemic effects and should be avoided or used very cautiously by people with diabetes. If used, blood sugar should be monitored closely, and lower doses of antidiabetic drugs may be needed.

**Guar gum** is a type of fiber that becomes gel-like upon contact with liquids (eg, like Metamucil). It is used as a thickening agent in foods and drugs and is an ingredient in some over-the-counter weight-loss products. It should be used cautiously, if at all, by people with diabetes because it has hypoglycemic effects and slows GI motility. Several cases of esophageal and intestinal obstruction have been reported with weight-loss products.

## ■ DRUG USE IN SPECIFIC SITUATIONS

## Management of Diabetic Ketoacidosis

Insulin therapy is a major component of any treatment for DKA. Clients with DKA have a deficiency in the total amount of insulin in the body and a resistance to the action of the insulin that is available, probably owing to acidosis, hyperosmolality, infection, and other factors. To be effective, insulin therapy must be individualized according to frequent measurements of blood glucose.

# NURSING PROCESS

## Assessment

Assess the client's knowledge, attitude, and condition in relation to diabetes, the prescribed treatment plan, and complications. Assessment data should include past manifestations of the disease process and the client's response to them, present status, and potential problem areas.

- *Historic data* include age at onset of diabetes, prescribed control measures and their effectiveness, the ease or difficulty of complying with the prescribed treatment, occurrence of complications such as ketoacidosis, and whether other disease processes have interfered with diabetes control.
- *Assess the client's current status*, in relation to the following areas:
  - **Diet.** Ask about the prescribed nutritional plan, who prepares the food, what factors help in following the diet, what factors interfere with following the diet, the current weight, and whether there has been a recent weight change. Also ask if herbal or other dietary supplements are used. If so, list each one by name and frequency of use. If a nutritionist is available, ask one to assess the client's dietary practice and needs.
  - **Activity.** Ask the client to describe usual activities of daily living, including those related to work, home, and recreation and whether he or she participates in a regular exercise program. If so, ask for more information about what, how often, how long, and so forth. If not, teaching is needed because exercise is extremely important in diabetes management.
  - **Medication.** If the client takes insulin, ask what kind, how much, who administers it, usual time of administration, sites used for injections, if a hypoglycemic reaction to insulin has ever been experienced, and if so, how it was handled. This information helps to assess knowledge, usual practices, and teaching needs. If the client takes an oral antidiabetic drug, ask the name, dosage, and time taken.
  - **Monitoring methods.** Testing the blood for glucose and the urine for ketones (eg, when blood sugar is elevated or when ill and unable to eat) are the two main methods of self-monitoring glycemic control. Ask about the method used, the frequency of testing, and the pattern of results. If possible, observe the client performing and interpreting an actual test to assess accuracy.
  - **Skin and mucous membranes.** Inspect for signs of infection and other lesions. Infections often occur in the axillary and groin areas because these areas have large numbers of microorganisms. Periodontal disease (pyorrhea) may be manifested by inflammation and bleeding of the gums. Women with diabetes are susceptible to monilial vaginitis and infections under the breasts. Check the sites of insulin injection for atrophy (dimpling or indentation), hypertrophy (nodules or lumps), and fibrosis (hardened areas). Check the lower leg for brown spots; these are caused by small hemorrhages into the skin and may indicate widespread changes in the blood vessels.

Problems are especially likely to develop in the feet from infection, trauma, pressure, vascular insufficiency, and neuropathy. Therefore, inspect the feet for calluses, ulcers, and signs of infection. When such problems develop, sensory impairment from neuropathy may delay detection and impaired circulation may delay healing. Check pedal pulses, color, and temperature in both feet to evaluate arterial blood flow. Ankle edema may indicate venous insufficiency or impaired cardiac function.

- **Eyes.** Ask about difficulties with vision and if eyes are examined regularly. Diabetic clients are prone to development of retinopathy, cataracts, and possibly glaucoma.
- **Cardiovascular system.** Clients with diabetes have a high incidence of atherosclerosis, which makes them susceptible to hypertension, angina pectoris, myocardial infarction, peripheral vascular disease, and stroke. Therefore, check blood pressure and ask about chest pain and pain in the legs with exercise (intermittent claudication).
- **Genitourinary system.** People with diabetes often have kidney and bladder problems. Assess for signs of urinary tract infection; albumin, white blood cells, or blood in urine; edema; increased urination at night; difficulty voiding; generalized itching; fatigue; and muscular weakness. Impotence may develop in men and is attributed to neuropathy.
- Assess blood sugar reports for abnormal levels. Two or more fasting blood glucose levels greater than 126 mg/dL or two random levels greater than 200 mg/dL are diagnostic of diabetes. Decreased blood sugar levels are especially dangerous at 40 mg/dL or below.
- Assess the glycosylated hemoglobin (also called glycated hemoglobin and $HbA_{1c}$) level when available. This test indicates glucose bound to hemoglobin in red blood cells (RBCs) when RBCs are exposed to hyperglycemia. The binding is irreversible and lasts for the lifespan of RBCs (approximately 120 days). The test reflects the average blood sugar during the previous 2 to 3 months. The goal is usually less than 7% (the range for people without diabetes is approximately 4% to 6%). The test should be done every 3 to 6 months.

Test results are not affected by several factors that alter blood sugar levels, such as time of day, food intake, exercise, recently administered antidiabetic drugs, emotional stress, or client cooperation. The test is especially useful with children, those whose diabetes is poorly controlled, those who do not test blood glucose regularly, and those who change their usual habits before a scheduled appointment with a health care provider so that their blood sugar control appears better than it actually is.

## Nursing Diagnoses

- Ineffective Tissue Perfusion, peripheral, related to atherosclerosis and vascular impairment
- Disturbed Sensory Perception, visual and tactile, related to impaired vision or neuropathy
- Ineffective Coping related to chronic illness and required treatment

*(continued)*

## *N*URSING PROCESS (Continued)

- Anxiety: Managing a chronic illness, finger sticks, insulin injections
- Risk for Injury: Trauma, infection, hypoglycemia, hyperglycemia
- Noncompliance related to inability or unwillingness to manage the disease process and required treatment
- Deficient Knowledge: Disease process and management; administration and effects of antidiabetic drugs; interrelationships among diet, exercise, and antidiabetic drugs; and management of hypoglycemia, "sick days," and other complications

### Planning/Goals

*The client will:*

- Learn self-care activities
- Manage drug therapy to prevent or minimize hypoglycemia and other adverse effects
- Develop a consistent pattern of diet and exercise
- Use available resources to learn about the disease process and how to manage it
- Take antidiabetic drugs accurately
- Self-monitor blood glucose and urine ketones appropriately
- Keep appointments for follow-up and monitoring procedures by a health care provider

### Interventions

Use nondrug measures to improve control of diabetes and to help prevent complications.

- Assist the client in maintaining the prescribed diet. Specific measures vary but may include teaching the client and family about the importance of diet, referring the client to a dietitian, and helping the client identify and modify factors that decrease compliance with the diet. If the client is obese, assist in developing a program to lose weight and then maintain weight at a more nearly normal level.
- Assist the client to develop and maintain a regular exercise program.
- Perform and interpret blood tests for glucose accurately, and assist clients and family members to do so. Self-monitoring of blood glucose levels allows the client to see the effects of diet, exercise, and hypoglycemic medications on blood glucose levels and may promote compliance.

    Several products are available for home glucose monitoring. All involve obtaining a drop of capillary blood from a finger with a sterile lancet. The blood is placed on a

semipermeable membrane that contains a reagent. The amount of blood glucose can be read with various machines (eg, glucometers).

- Test urine for ketones when the client is sick, when blood glucose levels are above 200 mg/dL, and when episodes of nocturnal hypoglycemia are suspected. Also teach clients and family members to test urine when indicated.
- Promote early recognition and treatment of problems by observing for signs and symptoms of urinary tract infection, peripheral vascular disease, vision changes, ketoacidosis, hypoglycemia, and others. Teach clients and families to observe for these conditions and report their occurrence.
- Discuss the importance of regular visits to health care facilities for blood sugar measurements, weights, blood pressure measurements, and eye examinations.
- Perform and teach correct foot care. Have the client observe the following safeguards: avoid going barefoot, to prevent trauma to the feet; wear correctly fitted shoes; wash the feet daily with warm water, dry well, inspect for any lesions or pressure areas, and apply lanolin if the skin is dry; wear cotton or wool socks because they are more absorbent than synthetic materials; cut toenails straight across and only after the feet have been soaked in warm water and washed thoroughly. Teach the client to avoid use of hot water bottles or electric heating pads, cutting toenails if vision is impaired, use of strong antiseptics on the feet, and cutting corns or calluses. Also teach the client to report any lesions on the feet to the physician.
- Help clients keep up with newer developments in diabetes care by providing information, sources of information, consultations with specialists, and other resources. However, do not overwhelm a newly diagnosed diabetic client with excessive information or assume that a long-term diabetic client does not need information.

### Evaluation

- Check blood sugar reports regularly for normal or abnormal values.
- Check glycosylated hemoglobin reports when available.
- Interview and observe for therapeutic and adverse responses to antidiabetic drugs.
- Interview and observe for compliance with prescribed treatment.
- Interview clients and family members about the frequency and length of hospitalizations for diabetes mellitus.

---

Low doses, given by continuous IV infusion, are preferred in most circumstances.

Additional measures include identification and treatment of conditions that precipitate DKA, administration of IV fluids to correct hyperosmolality and dehydration, administration of potassium supplements to restore and maintain normal serum potassium levels, and administration of sodium bicarbonate to correct metabolic acidosis. Infection is one of the most common causes of DKA. If no obvious source of infection is identified, cul-

tures of blood, urine, and throat swabs are recommended. When infection is identified, antibacterial drug therapy may be indicated.

IV fluids, the first step in treating DKA, usually consist of 0.9% sodium chloride, an isotonic solution. Hypotonic solutions are usually avoided because they allow intracellular fluid shifts and may cause cerebral, pulmonary, and peripheral edema.

Although serum potassium levels may be normal at first, they fall rapidly after insulin and IV fluid therapy

## CLIENT TEACHING GUIDELINES
## Antidiabetic Drugs

### General Considerations

✔ Wear or carry diabetic identification (eg, a Medic-Alert necklace or bracelet) at all times, to aid treatment if needed.

✔ Learn as much as you can about diabetes and its management. Few other diseases require as much adaptation in activities of daily living, and you must be well informed to control the disease, minimize complications, and achieve an optimal quality of life. Although much information is available from health care providers (physicians, nurses, nurse diabetes educators, nutritionists), an additional major resource is the

American Diabetes Association
1660 Duke St.
Alexandria, VA 22314
1-800-ADA-DISC
*http://www.diabetes.org*

✔ In general, a consistent schedule of diet, exercise, and medication produces the best control of blood sugar levels and the least risk of complications.

✔ Diet, weight control, and exercise are extremely important in managing diabetes. Maintaining normal weight and avoiding excessive caloric intake decrease the need for medication and decrease the workload of the pancreas. Exercise helps body tissues use insulin better, which means that glucose moves out of the bloodstream and into muscles and other body tissues. This promotes more normal blood glucose levels and decreases long-term complications of diabetes.

✔ Take any antidiabetic medication as prescribed. If unable to take a medication, notify a health care provider. To control blood sugar most effectively, medications are balanced with diet and exercise. If you take insulin, you need to know what type(s) you are taking, how to obtain more, and how to store it. Regular and NPH insulins and mixtures (eg, Humulin) are available over-the-counter; Humalog, NovoLog, and Lantus require a prescription. Keep several days' supply of insulin and syringes on hand to allow for weather or other conditions that might prevent replacement of insulin or other supplies when needed.

✔ You need to know the signs and symptoms of high blood sugar (hyperglycemia): increased blood glucose and excessive thirst, hunger, and urine output. Persistent hyperglycemia may indicate a need to change some aspect of the treatment program, such as diet or medication.

✔ You need to know the symptoms of low blood sugar (hypoglycemia): sweating, nervousness, hunger, weakness, tremors, and mental confusion. Hypoglycemia may indicate too much medication or exercise or too little food. Treatment is a rapidly absorbed source of sugar, which usually reverses symptoms within 10 to 20 minutes. If you are alert and able to swallow, take 4 oz of fruit juice, 4 to 6 oz of a sugar-containing soft drink, a

piece of fruit or ⅓ cup of raisins, two to three glucose tablets (5 grams each), a tube of glucose gel, 1 cup of skim milk, tea or coffee with 2 teaspoons of sugar, or eight Lifesaver candies. Avoid taking so much sugar that hyperglycemia occurs.

*If you take acarbose (Precose) or miglitol (Glyset) along with insulin, glimepiride (Amaryl), glipizide (Glucotrol), or glyburide (DiaBeta, Glynase, Micronase) and a hypoglycemic reaction occurs, you must take some form of glucose (or glucagon) for treatment.* Sucrose (table sugar) and other oral carbohydrates do not relieve hypoglycemia because the presence of acarbose or miglitol prevents their digestion and absorption from the gastrointestinal (GI) tract.

✔ You need to have a family member or another person able to recognize and manage hypoglycemia in case you are unable to obtain or swallow a source of glucose. If you take insulin, glucagon should be available in the home and a caregiver should know how to give it.

✔ The best way to prevent, delay, or decrease the severity of diabetes complications is to maintain blood sugar at a normal or near-normal level. Other measures include regular visits to health care providers, preferably a team of specialists in diabetes care; regular vision and glaucoma testing; and special foot care. In addition, if you have hypertension, treatment can help prevent heart attacks and strokes.

✔ Take only drugs prescribed by a physician who knows you have diabetes. Avoid other prescriptions and over-the-counter drugs unless these are discussed with the physician treating the diabetes because adverse reactions and interactions may occur. For example, nasal decongestants (alone or in cold remedies) and asthma medications may cause tachycardia and nervousness, which may be interpreted as hypoglycemia. In addition, liquid cold remedies and cough syrups may contain sugar and raise blood glucose levels.

✔ If you wish to take any kind of herbal or dietary supplement, you should discuss this with the health care provider who is managing your diabetes. There has been little study of these preparations in relation to diabetes; many can increase or decrease blood sugar and alter diabetes control. If you start a supplement, you need to check your blood sugar frequently to see how it affects your blood glucose level.

✔ Test blood regularly for glucose. A schedule individualized to your needs is best. Testing should be done more often when medication dosages are changed or when you are ill.

✔ Reduce insulin dosage or eat extra food if you expect to exercise more than usual. Specific recommendations should be individualized and worked out with health care providers in relation to the type of exercise.

✔ Ask for written instructions about managing "sick days" and call your physician if unsure about what you

*(continued)*

need to do. Although each person needs individualized instructions, some general guidelines include the following:

✔ Continue your antidiabetic medications unless instructed otherwise. Additional insulin also may be needed, especially if ketosis develops. Ketones (acetone) in the urine indicate insulin deficiency or insulin resistance.

✔ Check blood glucose levels at least four times daily; test urine for ketones when the blood glucose level exceeds 250 mg/dL or with each urination. If unable to test urine, have someone else do it.

✔ Rest, keep warm, do not exercise, and keep someone with you if possible.

✔ If unable to eat solid food, take easily digested liquids or semiliquid foods. About 15 g of carbohydrate every 1 to 2 hours is usually enough and can be provided by ¹/₂ cup of apple juice, applesauce, cola, cranberry juice, eggnog, Cream of Wheat cereal, custard, vanilla ice cream, regular gelatin, or frozen yogurt.

✔ Drink 2 to 3 quarts of fluids daily, especially if you have a fever. Water, tea, broths, clear soups, diet soda, or carbohydrate-containing fluids are acceptable.

✔ Record the amount of fluid intake as well as the number of times you urinate, vomit, or have loose stools.

✔ Seek medical attention if a premeal blood glucose level is more than 250 mg/dL, if urine acetone is present, if you have fever above 100°F, if you have several episodes of vomiting or diarrhea, or if you have difficulty in breathing, chest pain, severe abdominal pain, or severe dehydration.

**Self-administration**

✔ Use correct techniques for injecting insulin:

✔ Follow instructions for times of administration as nearly as possible. Different types of insulin have different onsets, peaks, and durations of action. Accurate timing (eg, in relation to meals), can increase beneficial effects and decrease risks of hypoglycemic reactions.

✔ Wash hands; wash injection site, if needed.

✔ Draw up insulin in a good light, being very careful to draw up the correct dose. If you have trouble seeing the syringe markers, get a magnifier or ask someone else to draw up the insulin. Prefilled syringes or cartridges for pen devices are also available.

✔ Instructions may vary about cleaning the top of the insulin vial and the injection site with an alcohol swab and about pulling back on the plunger after injection to see if any blood enters the syringe. These techniques have been commonly used, but many diabetes experts do not believe they are necessary.

✔ Inject straight into the fat layer under the skin, at a 90-degree angle. If very thin, pinch up a skin-fold and inject at a 45-degree angle.

✔ Rotate injection sites. Your health care provider may suggest a rotation plan. Many people rotate between the abdomen and the thighs. Insulin is absorbed fastest from the abdomen. Do not inject insulin within 2 inches of the "belly button" or into any skin lesions.

✔ If it is necessary to mix two insulin preparations, ask for specific instructions about the technique and then follow it consistently. There is a risk of inaccurate dosage of both insulins unless measured very carefully. Commercial mixtures are also available for some combinations.

✔ Change insulin dosage only if instructed to do so and the circumstances are specified.

✔ Carry sugar, candy, or a commercial glucose preparation for immediate use if a hypoglycemic reaction occurs.

✔ Take oral drugs as directed. Recommendations usually include the following:

✔ Take glipizide or glyburide approximately 30 minutes before meals; take glimepiride with breakfast or the first main meal.

✔ Take acarbose or miglitol with the first bite of each main meal. The drugs need to be in the GI tract with food because they act by decreasing absorption of sugar in the food. Starting with a small dose and increasing it gradually helps to prevent bloating, "gas pains," and diarrhea.

✔ Take metformin (Glucophage) with meals to decrease stomach upset.

✔ Take repaglinide (Prandin) or nateglinide (Starlix) about 15 to 30 minutes before meals (2, 3, or 4 times daily). Doses may vary from 0.5 to 4.0 mg, depending on fasting blood glucose levels. Dosage changes should be at least 1 week apart. If you skip a meal, you should skip that dose of repaglinide or nateglinide; if you eat an extra meal, you should take an extra dose.

✔ Take pioglitazone (Actos) and rosiglitazone (Avandia) without regard to meals.

✔ If you take glimepiride, glipizide, glyburide, or repaglinide, alone or in combination with other antidiabetic drugs, be prepared to handle hypoglycemic reactions (as with insulin, above). Acarbose, miglitol, metformin, pioglitazone, and rosiglitazone do not cause hypoglycemia when taken alone. Do not skip meals and snacks. This increases the risk of hypoglycemic reactions.

✔ If you exercise vigorously, you may need to decrease your dose of antidiabetic drug or eat more. Ask for specific instructions related to the type and frequency of the exercise.

are begun. Decreased serum potassium levels are caused by expansion of extracellular fluid volume, movement of potassium into cells in the presence of insulin, and continued loss of potassium in the urine as long as hyperglycemia persists. For these reasons, potassium supplements are usually added to IV fluids. Because both hypokalemia and hyperkalemia can cause serious cardiovascular disturbances, dosage of potassium supplements must be based on frequent measurements of serum potassium levels. Also, continuous or frequent electrocardiogram monitoring is recommended.

Severe acidosis can cause serious cardiovascular disturbances, which usually stem from peripheral vasodilation and decreased cardiac output with hypotension and shock. Acidosis usually can be corrected by giving fluids and insulin; sodium bicarbonate may be given if the pH is less than 7.2. If used, sodium bicarbonate should be given slowly and cautiously. Rapid alkalinization can cause potassium to move into body cells faster than it can be replaced intravenously. The result may be severe hypokalemia and cardiac dysrhythmias. Also, giving excessive amounts of sodium bicarbonate can produce alkalosis.

## Treatment of the Unconscious Client

When a person with diabetes becomes unconscious and it is unknown whether the unconsciousness is caused by DKA or by hypoglycemia, the client should be treated for hypoglycemia. If hypoglycemia is the cause, giving glucose may avert brain damage. If DKA is the cause, giving glucose does not harm the client. Sudden unconsciousness in a client who takes insulin is most likely to result from an insulin reaction; DKA usually develops gradually over several days or weeks.

## Hyperosmolar Hyperglycemic Nonketotic Coma

Treatment of HHNC is similar to that of DKA in that insulin, IV fluids, and potassium supplements are major components. Regular insulin is given by continuous IV infusion, and dosage is individualized according to frequent measurements of blood glucose levels. IV fluids are given to correct the profound dehydration and hyperosmolality, and potassium is given IV to replace the large amounts lost in urine during a hyperglycemic state.

## Perioperative Insulin Therapy

Clients with diabetes who undergo major surgery have increased risks for both surgical and diabetic complications. The risks associated with surgery and anesthesia are greater if diabetes is not well controlled and complications of diabetes (eg, hypertension, nephropathy, vascular damage) are already evident. Hyperglycemia and poor metabolic control are associated with increased susceptibility to infection, poor wound healing, and fluid and electrolyte imbalances. Risks for diabetic complications are increased because the stress of surgery increases insulin requirements and may precipitate DKA. Metabolic responses to stress include increased secretion of catecholamines, cortisol, glucagon, and growth hormone, all of which increase blood glucose levels. In addition to hyperglycemia, protein breakdown, lipolysis, ketogenesis, and insulin resistance occur. The risk for hypoglycemia is also increased.

The goals of treatment are to avoid hypoglycemia, severe hyperglycemia, ketoacidosis, and fluid and electrolyte imbalances. In general, mild hyperglycemia (eg, blood glucose levels between 150 and 250 mg/dL) is considered safer for the client than hypoglycemia, which may go unrecognized during anesthesia and surgery. Because surgery is a stressful event that increases blood glucose levels and the body's need for insulin, insulin therapy is usually required.

The goal of insulin therapy is to avoid ketosis from inadequate insulin and hypoglycemia from excessive insulin. Specific actions depend largely on the severity of diabetes and the type of surgical procedure. Diabetes should be well controlled before any type of surgery. Minor procedures usually require little change in the usual treatment program; major operations usually require a different medication regimen.

In general, regular, short-acting insulin is used with major surgery or surgery requiring general anesthesia. For clients who use an intermediate-acting insulin, a different regimen using regular insulin in doses approximating the usual daily requirement is needed. For clients who usually manage their diabetes with diet alone or with diet and oral medications, insulin therapy may be started. Human insulin is preferred for temporary use to minimize formation of insulin antibodies. Small doses are usually required.

For elective major surgery, clients should be scheduled early in the day to avoid prolonged fasting. In addition, most authorities recommend omitting usual doses of insulin on the day of surgery and oral antidiabetic medications for 1 or 2 days before surgery. While the client is receiving nothing by mouth, before and during surgery, IV insulin is usually given. One important consideration with IV insulin therapy is that 30% or more of a dose may adsorb into containers of IV fluid or infusion sets. Along with the insulin, clients need adequate sources of carbohydrate. This is usually supplied by IV solutions of 5% or 10% dextrose.

After surgery, IV insulin and dextrose may be continued until the client is able to eat and drink. Regular insulin also can be given subcutaneously every 4 to 6 hours, with frequent blood glucose measurements. Oral fluids and foods that contain carbohydrate should be resumed as soon as possible. When meals are fully tolerated, the preoperative insulin or oral medication regimen can be resumed. Additional regular insulin can be given for elevated blood glucose and ketones, if indicated.

## Use of Insulin with Oral Antidiabetic Drugs

Insulin has been used successfully with all currently available types of oral agents (alpha-glucosidase inhibitors, biguanide, glitazones, meglitinides, and sulfonylureas).

## Combination Drug Therapy for Type 2 Diabetes

Combination drug therapy is an increasing trend in type 2 diabetes uncontrolled by diet, exercise, and single-drug therapy. Useful combinations include drugs with different mechanisms of action, and several rational combinations are currently available. Most studies have involved combinations of two drugs; some three-drug combinations are also being used. All combination therapy should be monitored with periodic measurements of fasting plasma glucose and glycosylated (HbA$_{1c}$) hemoglobin levels. If adequate glycemic control is not achieved, oral drugs may need to be discontinued and insulin therapy started. Two-drug combinations include the following:

- **Insulin plus a sulfonylurea.** Advantages include lower fasting blood glucose levels, decreased glycosylated hemoglobin levels, increased secretion of endogenous insulin, smaller daily doses of insulin, and no significant change in body weight. The role of insulin analogs in combination therapy is not clear. One regimen, called BIDS, uses bedtime insulin, usually NPH, with a daytime sulfonylurea, usually glyburide.
- **Insulin plus a glitazone.** Glitazones increase the effectiveness of insulin, whether endogenous or exogenous.
- **Sulfonylurea plus acarbose or miglitol.** This combination is approved by the U.S. Food and Drug Administration (FDA) for clients who do not achieve adequate glycemic control with one of the drugs alone.
- **Sulfonylurea plus metformin.** Glimepiride is FDA approved for this combination.
- **Sulfonylurea plus a glitazone.** The sulfonylurea increases insulin, and the glitazone increases insulin effectiveness.
- **Metformin plus a meglitinide.** If one of the drugs alone does not produce adequate glycemic control, the other one may be added. Dosage of each drug should be titrated to the minimal dose required to achieve the desired effects.

## Effects of Illness on Diabetes Care

Illness may affect diabetes control in several ways. First, it causes a stress response. Part of the stress response is increased secretion of glucagon, epinephrine, growth hormone, and cortisol, hormones that raise blood glucose levels (by stimulating gluconeogenesis and inhibiting insulin action) and cause ketosis (by stimulating lipolysis and ketogenesis). Second, if the illness makes a person unable or unwilling to eat, hypoglycemia can occur. Third, if the illness affects GI function (eg, causes vomiting or diarrhea), the person may be unable to drink enough fluids to prevent dehydration and electrolyte imbalance. In addition, hyperglycemia induces an osmotic diuresis that increases dehydration and electrolyte imbalances.

As a result of these potentially serious effects, an illness that would be minor in people without diabetes may become a major illness or medical emergency in people with diabetes. Everyone involved should be vigilant about recognizing and seeking prompt treatment for any illness. In addition, clients with diabetes (or their caregivers) should be taught how to adjust their usual regimens to maintain metabolic balance and prevent severe complications. The main goal during illness is to prevent complications such as severe hyperglycemia, dehydration, and DKA.

## Use of Insulin Pumps

Insulin pumps are being increasingly used, especially by adolescents and young adults who want flexibility in diet and exercise. These devices allow continuous subcutaneous administration of regular insulin or insulin aspart. A basal amount of insulin is injected (eg, 1 unit/hour or a calculated fraction of the dose used previously) continuously, with bolus injections before meals. This method of insulin administration maintains more normal blood glucose levels and avoids wide fluctuations. Candidates for insulin pumps include clients with diabetes that is poorly controlled with other methods and those who are able and willing to care for the devices properly.

## Prevention of End–Stage Renal Disease in Diabetic Clients

In addition to glycemic control, other measures can be used to help prevent end-stage renal disease. Administration of angiotensin-converting enzyme (ACE) inhibitors (eg, captopril) has protective effects on the kidneys in both type 1 and type 2 diabetes and in both normotensive and hypertensive people. Although ACE inhibitors are also used in the treatment of hypertension, their ability to delay nephropathy seems to be independent of antihypertensive effects. Additional measures to preserve renal function include effective treatment of hypertension, limited intake of dietary protein, prompt treatment of urinary tract infections, and avoidance of nephrotoxic drugs when possible.

## Use of Insulin or Oral Hypoglycemic Agents in Renal Impairment

**Insulin.** Frequent monitoring of blood glucose levels and dosage adjustments may be needed. It is difficult to predict dosage needs because, on the one hand, less insulin is degraded by the kidneys (normally about 25%), and this may lead to higher blood levels of insulin if dosage is not reduced. On the other hand, muscles and possibly other tissues are less sensitive to insulin, and this insulin resistance may result in an increased blood glucose level if dosage is not increased. Overall, vigilance is required to prevent dangerous hypoglycemia, especially in clients whose renal function is unstable or worsening.

**Oral drugs. Sulfonylureas** and their metabolites are excreted mainly by the kidneys; renal impairment may lead to accumulation and hypoglycemia. They should be used cautiously, with close monitoring of renal function, in clients with mild to moderate renal impairment, and are contraindicated in severe renal impairment. **Alpha-glucosidase inhibitors** are excreted by the kidneys and accumulate in clients with renal impairment. However, dosage reduction is not helpful because the drugs act locally, within the GI tract. **Metformin** requires assessment of renal function before starting and at least annually during long-term therapy. It should not be given initially if renal impairment is present; it should be stopped if renal impairment occurs during treatment. **Meglitinides** do not require initial dosage adjustments, but increments should be made cautiously in clients with renal impairment or renal failure requiring hemodialysis.

## Use of Insulin or Oral Hypoglycemic Agents in Hepatic Impairment

**Insulin.** There may be higher blood levels of insulin in clients with hepatic impairment because less insulin may be degraded. Careful monitoring of blood glucose levels and insulin dosage reductions may be needed to prevent hypoglycemia.

**Oral drugs. Sulfonylureas** should be used cautiously, and liver function should be monitored. They are metabolized in the liver, and hepatic impairment may result in higher serum drug levels and inadequate release of hepatic glucose in response to hypoglycemia. With glipizide, initial dosage should be reduced in clients with liver failure. Glyburide may cause hypoglycemia in clients with liver disease. **Alpha-glucosidase inhibitors** require no precautions with hepatic impairment because acarbose is metabolized in the GI tract and miglitol is not metabolized. **Metformin** is not recommended for use in clients with clinical or laboratory evidence of hepatic impairment because risks for lactic acidosis may be increased. **Meglitinides** should be used cautiously and dosage increments made very slowly because serum drug levels are higher, for a longer period of time, in clients with moderate to severe hepatic impairment. **Glitazones** have been associated with hepatotoxicity and require monitoring of liver enzymes. The drugs should not be given to clients with active liver disease or an ALT level more than 2.5 times the upper limit of normal. Once glitazone therapy is initiated, liver enzymes should be measured every 2 months for 1 year, then periodically.

*(text continues on page 390)*

## Nursing Actions
### Antidiabetic Drugs

| Nursing Actions | Rationale/Explanation |
|---|---|
| 1. Administer accurately.<br> a. With insulin:<br> (1) Store the insulin vial in current use and administer insulin at room temperature. Refrigerate extra vials. | Cold insulin is more likely to cause lipodystrophy, local sensitivity reactions, discomfort, and delayed absorption. Insulin preparations are stable for months at room temperature if temperature extremes are avoided. |
| (2) Avoid freezing temperatures (32°F) or high temperatures (95°F or above). | Extremes of temperature decrease insulin potency and cause clumping of the suspended particles of modified insulins. This clumping phenomenon causes inaccurate dosage even if the volume is accurately measured. |
| (3) Use only an insulin syringe calibrated to measure U-100 insulin. | For accurate measurement of the prescribed dose. |
| (4) With NPH and Lente insulins, be sure they are mixed to a uniform cloudy appearance before drawing up a dose. | These insulin preparations are suspensions, and the components separate on standing. Unless the particles are resuspended in the solution and distributed evenly, dosage will be inaccurate. |

*(continued)*

## *Nursing Actions*
## Antidiabetic Drugs (Continued)

| Nursing Actions | Rationale/Explanation |
|---|---|
| (5) When regular and NPH insulins must be mixed, prepare as follows:<br>  (a) Draw into the insulin syringe the amount of air equal to the total amount of both insulins.<br>  (b) Draw up the regular insulin first. Inject the equivalent portion of air, and aspirate the ordered dose.<br>  (c) With the NPH vial, insert the remaining air (avoid injecting regular insulin into the NPH vial), and aspirate the ordered dose.<br>  (d) Expel air bubbles, if present, and verify that the correct dosage is in the syringe. | The insulins must be drawn up in the same sequence every time. Regular insulin should *always* be drawn up first, to avoid contamination of the regular insulin with the NPH. Because regular insulin combines with excess protamine in NPH, the concentration of regular insulin is changed when they are mixed. Following the same sequence also leaves the same type of insulin in the needle and syringe (dead space) every time. Although dead space is not usually a significant factor with available insulin syringes, it may be with small doses. |
| (e) Administer combined insulins *consistently* within 15 min of mixing or after a longer period; that is, do not give one dose within 15 min of mixing and another 2 h or days after mixing. | Regular insulin combines with excess protamine when mixed with NPH insulin. This reaction occurs within 15 min of mixing and alters the amount of regular insulin present. After 15 min, the mixture is stable for approximately 1 month at room temperature and 3 months when refrigerated. Thus, to administer the same dose consistently, the mixture must be given at approximately the same time interval after mixing. |
| (6) Rotate injection sites systematically, within the same anatomic area (eg, abdomen) until all sites are used. Avoid random rotation between the abdomen and thigh or arm, for example. | Frequent injection in the same site can cause tissue fibrosis, erratic absorption, and deposits of unabsorbed insulin. Also, if insulin is usually injected into fibrotic tissue where absorption is slow, injection into healthy tissue may result in hypoglycemia because of more rapid absorption. Further, deposits of unabsorbed insulin may initially lead to hyperglycemia. If dosage is increased to control the apparent hyperglycemia, hypoglycemia may occur. Rates of absorption differ among anatomic sites, and random rotation increases risks of hypoglycemic reactions. |
| (7) Inject insulin at a 90-degree angle into a subcutaneous pocket created by raising subcutaneous tissue away from muscle tissue. Avoid intramuscular injection. | Injection into a subcutaneous pocket is thought to produce less tissue irritation and better absorption than injection into subcutaneous tissue. Intramuscular injection should not be used because of rapid absorption. |
| (8) With insulin analogs, give aspart within 5 to 10 minutes of starting a meal; give lispro within 15 minutes before or immediately after a meal; give glargine once daily at bedtime. | Manufacturers' recommendations. Aspart and lispro act rapidly; glargine is long-acting. |
| b. With oral sulfonylureas: Give glipizide or glyburide 30 minutes before breakfast and the evening meal. Give glimepiride with breakfast. | To promote absorption and effective plasma levels. Most of these drugs are given once or twice daily. |
| c. With acarbose and miglitol: Give at the beginning of each main meal, three times daily. | These drugs must be in the gastrointestinal (GI) tract when carbohydrate foods are ingested because they act by decreasing absorption of sugar in the foods. |
| d. With metformin: Give with meals. | To decrease GI upset |
| e. With pioglitazone and rosiglitazone: Give once daily, without regard to meals. | Manufacturers' recommendations |
| f. With repaglinide and nateglinide: Give 15 to 30 min before meals (2, 3, or 4 times daily). If the client does not eat a meal, omit that dose; if the client eats an extra meal, give an extra dose. | Dosage is individualized according to the levels of fasting blood glucose and glycosylated hemoglobin. |

*(continued)*

## Nursing Actions

## Antidiabetic Drugs (Continued)

| Nursing Actions | Rationale/Explanation |
|---|---|
| **2. Observe for therapeutic effects.**<br>a. Improved blood glucose levels (fasting, preprandial, and postprandial) and glycosylated hemoglobin levels | The general goal is normal or near-normal blood glucose levels. However, specific targeted levels for individuals vary depending on intensity of treatment, risks of hypoglycemia, and other factors. Improved metabolic control can prevent or delay complications. |
| b. Absent or decreased ketones in urine (N = none) | In diabetes, ketonuria indicates insulin deficiency and impending diabetic ketoacidosis if preventive measures are not taken. Thus, always report the presence of ketones. In addition, when adequate insulin is given, ketonuria decreases. Ketonuria does not often occur with type 2 diabetes. |
| c. Absent or decreased pruritus, polyuria, polydipsia, polyphagia, and fatigue<br>d. Decreased complications of diabetes | These signs and symptoms occur in the presence of hyperglycemia. When blood sugar levels are lowered with antidiabetic drugs, they tend to subside. |
| **3. Observe for adverse effects.**<br>a. With insulin, sulfonylureas, and meglitinides:<br>(1) Hypoglycemia | Hypoglycemia is more likely to occur with insulin than with oral agents and at peak action times of the insulin being used (eg, 2 to 3 h after injection of regular insulin; 8 to 12 h after injection of NPH or Lente insulin). |
| (a) Sympathetic nervous system (SNS) activation—tachycardia, palpitations, nervousness, weakness, hunger, perspiration | The SNS is activated as part of the stress response to low blood glucose levels. Epinephrine and other hormones act to raise blood glucose levels. |
| (b) Central nervous system impairment—mental confusion, incoherent speech, blurred or double vision, headache, convulsions, coma | There is an inadequate supply of glucose for normal brain function. |
| (2) Weight gain | This effect may decrease compliance with drug therapy, especially in adolescent and young adult females. |
| b. With insulin:<br>(1) Local insulin allergy—erythema, induration, itching at injection sites | Uncommon with human insulin |
| (2) Systemic allergic reactions—skin rash, dyspnea, tachycardia, hypotension, angioedema, anaphylaxis | Uncommon; if a severe systemic reaction occurs, skin testing and desensitization are usually required. |
| (3) Lipodystrophy—atrophy and "dimpling" at injection site; hypertrophy at injection site | These changes in subcutaneous fat occur from too-frequent injections into the same site. They are uncommon with human insulin. |
| c. With sulfonylureas:<br>(1) Hypoglycemia and weight gain—see above | Hypoglycemia occurs less often with oral agents than with insulin. It is more likely to occur in patients who are elderly, debilitated, or who have impaired renal and hepatic function. |
| (2) Allergic skin reactions—skin rash, urticaria, erythema, pruritus | These reactions may subside with continued use of the drug. If they do not subside, the drug should be discontinued. |
| (3) GI upset—nausea, heartburn | These are the most commonly reported adverse effects. If severe, reducing drug dosage usually relieves them. |
| (4) Miscellaneous—fluid retention and hyponatremia; facial flushing if alcohol is ingested; hematologic disorders (hemolytic or aplastic anemia, leukopenia, thrombocytopenia, others) | These are less common adverse effects. |
| d. With acarbose and miglitol: GI symptoms—bloating, flatulence, diarrhea, abdominal pain | These are commonly reported. They are caused by the presence of undigested carbohydrate in the lower GI tract. They can be decreased by low doses initially and gradual increases. |

*(continued)*

## Nursing Actions
## Antidiabetic Drugs (Continued)

| Nursing Actions | Rationale/Explanation |
|---|---|
| e. With metformin: | |
| (1) GI effects—anorexia, nausea, vomiting, diarrhea, abdominal discomfort, decreased intestinal absorption of folate and vitamin B$_{12}$ | GI symptoms are common adverse effects. They may be minimized by taking the drug with meals and increasing dosage slowly. |
| (2) Allergic skin reactions—eczema, pruritus, erythema, urticaria | |
| (3) Lactic acidosis—drowsiness, malaise, respiratory distress, bradycardia and hypotension (if severe), blood lactate levels above 5 mmol/L, blood pH below 7.35 | A rare but serious adverse effect (approximately 50% fatal). Most likely with renal or hepatic impairment, advanced age, or hypoxia. This is a medical emergency that requires hospitalization for treatment. Hemodialysis is effective in correcting acidosis and removing metformin. Lactic acidosis may be prevented by monitoring plasma lactate levels and stopping the drug if they exceed 3 mmol/L. Other reasons to stop the drug include decreased renal or hepatic function, a prolonged fast, or a very low calorie diet. The drug should be stopped immediately if a patient has a myocardial infarction or septicemia. |
| f. With pioglitazone and rosiglitazone: | |
| (1) Upper respiratory infections—pharyngitis, sinusitis | |
| (2) Liver damage or failure | Few cases of liver failure have been reported, but the drugs are related to troglitazone (Rezulin), a drug that was taken off the market because of hepatotoxicity. Monitoring of liver enzymes is recommended during therapy. |
| (3) Fluid retention, edema, and congestive heart failure | Several reports indicate increased risks of developing or worsening heart failure. |
| (4) Weight gain | |
| (5) Headache | |
| (6) Anemia | |
| g. With nateglinide and repaglinide: | |
| (1) Hypoglycemia | If occurs, usually of mild to moderate intensity |
| (2) Rhinitis, respiratory infection, influenza symptoms | These were the most commonly reported during clinical drug trials. |
| **4. Observe for drug interactions.** | |
| a. Drugs that *increase* effects of insulin: | |
| (1) ACE inhibitors (eg, captopril) | |
| (2) Alcohol | Increased hypoglycemia. Ethanol inhibits gluconeogenesis (in people with or without diabetes). |
| (3) Anabolic steroids | |
| (4) Antidiabetic drugs, oral | Oral agents are increasingly being used with insulin in the treatment of type 2 diabetes. The risks of hypoglycemia are greater with the combination but depend on the dosage of each drug and other factors that affect blood glucose levels. |
| (5) Antimicrobials (sulfonamides, tetracyclines) | |
| (6) Beta-adrenergic blocking agents (eg, propranolol) | Increase hypoglycemia by inhibiting the effects of catecholamines on gluconeogenesis and glycogenolysis (effects that normally raise blood glucose levels in response to hypoglycemia). They also may mask signs and symptoms of hypoglycemia (eg, tachycardia, tremors) that normally occur with a hypoglycemia-induced activation of the SNS. |

*(continued)*

## Nursing Actions
### Antidiabetic Drugs (Continued)

| Nursing Actions | Rationale/Explanation |
|---|---|
| b. Drugs that *decrease* effects of insulin:<br>(1) Adrenergics (eg, albuterol, epinephrine, others)<br>(2) Corticosteroids (eg, prednisone)<br>(3) Estrogens and oral contraceptives<br>(4) Glucagon<br>(5) Levothyroxine (Synthroid)<br>(6) Phenytoin (Dilantin)<br>(7) Propranolol (Inderal)<br>(8) Thiazide diuretics (eg, hydrochlorothiazide) | These *diabetogenic* drugs may cause or aggravate diabetes because they raise blood sugar levels. Insulin dosage may need to be increased. Except with glucagon, hyperglycemia is an adverse effect of the drugs. Phenytoin and propranolol raise blood sugar by inhibiting insulin secretion; glucagon, a treatment for hypoglycemia, raises blood glucose by converting liver glycogen to glucose. |
| c. Drugs that *increase* effects of sulfonylureas:<br>(1) Acarbose, miglitol, metformin, pioglitazone, rosiglitazone | One of these drugs may be used concomitantly with a sulfonylurea to improve glycemic control in patients with type 2 diabetes. There is an increased risk of hypoglycemia with the combinations. |
| (2) Alcohol (acute ingestion) | Additive hypoglycemia |
| (3) Cimetidine (Tagamet) | May inhibit metabolism of sulfonylureas, thereby increasing and prolonging hypoglycemic effects |
| (4) Insulin | Additive hypoglycemia |
| d. Drugs that *decrease* effects of sulfonylureas:<br>(1) Alcohol | Heavy, chronic intake of alcohol induces metabolizing enzymes in the liver. This accelerates metabolism of sulfonylureas, shortens their half-lives, and may produce hyperglycemia. |
| (2) Beta-blocking agents | Decrease hypoglycemic effects, possibly by decreasing release of insulin in the pancreas |
| (3) Corticosteroids, diuretics, epinephrine, estrogens, and oral contraceptives | These drugs have hyperglycemic effects. |
| (4) Glucagon | Raises blood glucose levels. It is used to treat severe hypoglycemia induced by insulin or oral antidiabetic agents. |
| (5) Nicotinic acid | Large doses have a hyperglycemic effect. |
| (6) Phenytoin (Dilantin) | Inhibits insulin secretion and has hyperglycemic effects |
| (7) Rifampin | Increases the rate of metabolism of sulfonylureas by inducing liver metabolizing enzymes |
| (8) Thyroid preparations | Antagonize the hypoglycemic effects of oral antidiabetic drugs |
| e. Drugs that *decrease* effects of acarbose and miglitol:<br>(1) Digestive enzymes | Decrease effects and should not be used concomitantly |
| (2) Intestinal adsorbents (eg, charcoal) | Decrease effects and should not be used concomitantly |
| f. Drugs that *increase* effects of metformin:<br>(1) Alcohol | Increases risk of hypoglycemia and lactic acidosis. Patients should avoid acute and chronic ingestion of excessive alcohol. |
| (2) Cimetidine | Increases risk of hypoglycemia. Cimetidine interferes with metabolism and increases blood levels of metformin. |
| (3) Furosemide | Increases blood levels of metformin |
| (4) Sulfonylurea hypoglycemic agents | The combination of these drugs is used to improve control of hyperglycemia in type 2 diabetes but it also increases risk of hypoglycemia. |
| g. Drugs that *increase* effects of pioglitazone:<br>(1) Erythromycin, ketoconazole, and related drugs | Inhibit cytochrome P450 3A4 enzymes that partially metabolize pioglitazone and may increase adverse effects. This interaction not reported with rosiglitazone, which is metabolized mainly by 2C8 and 2C9 enzymes. |

*(continued)*

## Nursing Actions
### Antidiabetic Drugs (Continued)

| Nursing Actions | Rationale/Explanation |
|---|---|
| h. Drugs that *increase* effects of nateglinide and repaglinide: | |
| (1) Nonsteroidal anti-inflammatory drugs and other agents that are highly bound to plasma proteins | May displace drugs from binding sites, therefore increasing their blood levels |
| (2) Beta blockers | |
| (3) Cimetidine, erythromycin, ketoconazole, miconazole | May inhibit hepatic metabolism of repaglinide and nateglinide and increase their blood levels |
| (4) Sulfonamides | |
| i. Drugs that *decrease* effects of nateglinide and repaglinide: | |
| (1) Adrenergics, corticosteroids, estrogens, niacin, oral contraceptives, thiazide diuretics | May cause hyperglycemia |
| (2) Carbamazepine, rifampin | Induce drug-metabolizing enzymes in the liver, which leads to faster inactivation |

### ? How Can You Avoid This Medication Error?

**Answer:** Metformin (Glucophage) should be discontinued a few days before any diagnostic procedure involving a contrast medium to decrease the chance of lactic acidosis, a potentially lethal side effect. The incidence of lactic acidosis increases when renal insufficiency is present. Urinary tract infections can contribute to renal damage. Documenting in Mrs. Watson's chart that she has taken her metformin is good but this is not enough because the physician may overlook reading it in the chart. The physician should be notified because it would be prudent to reschedule Mrs. Watson's IVP.

## Critical Thinking Exercises

1. Individuals with type 2 diabetes during periods of stress, such as major surgery, severe illness, or infection, usually require what hypoglycemic agent for effective control?
   a. Sulfonylurea
   b. Insulin
   c. Glitazone
   d. Alpha-glucosidase inhibitor

2. A client is receiving NPH insulin at 7:00 AM. The nurse would need to instruct the client to watch for signs of a hypoglycemic reaction:
   a. Midafternoon
   b. Before breakfast
   c. Before lunch
   d. At bedtime

3. A client receives sliding scale regular insulin before her breakfast at 7:00 AM. The nurse can anticipate that the client would be at the greatest risk for developing hypoglycemia from this dose at:
   a. 10:00 AM
   b. 12:00 noon
   c. 5:00 PM
   d. 9:00 PM

4. Which of the following types of oral hypoglycemic agent act to inhibit carbohydrate digestion, thereby delaying glucose absorption?
   a. Sulfonylureas
   b. Biguanides
   c. Meglitinides
   d. Alpha-glucosidase inhibitors

5. The absorption of insulin is delayed or decreased by injection into subcutaneous tissue in all of the following situations, except:
   a. With lipodystrophy
   b. With hypotension
   c. By insulin-binding antibodies
   d. By injecting room-temperature insulin

## SELECTED REFERENCES

American Diabetes Association. (2002). Insulin administration. *Diabetes Care, 25* (Suppl. 1, Clinical Practice Recommendations 2002, January), S112–S115.

DerMarderosian, A. (Ed.) (2001). *The review of natural products.* St. Louis: Facts and Comparisons.

*Drug facts and comparisons.* (Updated monthly). St. Louis: Facts and Comparisons.

Fetrow, C. W., & Avila, J. R. (1999). *Professional's handbook of complementary and alternative medicines.* Springhouse, PA: Springhouse Corporation.

Guven, S., Kuenzi, J. A., & Matfin, G. (2002). Diabetes mellitus. In C. M. Porth (Ed.), *Pathophysiology: Concepts of altered health states* (6th ed., pp. 930–952). Philadelphia: Lippincott Williams & Wilkins.

Guyton, A. C. & Hall, J. E. (2000). *Textbook of medical physiology* (10th ed.). Philadelphia: W. B. Saunders.

Halter, J. B. (2000). Approach to the elderly patient with diabetes. In H. D. Humes (Ed.), *Kelley's textbook of internal medicine* (4th ed., pp. 3032–3037). Philadelphia: Lippincott Williams & Wilkins.

Hoffman, R. P. (2001). Eating disorders in adolescents with type 1 diabetes. *Postgraduate Medicine, 109*(4), 67–69, 73–74.

Hu, F. B., Manson, J. E., Stampfer, M. J., Colditz, G., Liu, S., Solomon, C. G., et al. (2001). Diet, lifestyle, and the risk of type 2 diabetes mellitus in women. *New England Journal of Medicine, 345*(11), 790–797.

Inzucchi, S. E. (2002). Oral antihyperglycemic therapy for type 2 diabetes. *Journal of the American Medical Association, 287*(3), 360–372.

Kudolo, G. B. (2001). The effect of 3-month ingestion of ginkgo biloba extract (EGb761) on pancreatic beta-cell function in response to glucose loading in individuals with non-insulin-dependent diabetes mellitus. *Journal of Clinical Pharmacology, 411*(6), 600–611.

Lacy, C. F., Armstrong, L. L., Goldman, M. P., & Lance, L. L. (2003). *Lexi-Comp's drug information handbook* (11th ed.). Hudson, OH: American Pharmaceutical Association.

Ludwig, D. S., & Ebbeling, C. B. (2001). Type 2 diabetes mellitus in children. *Journal of the American Medical Association, 286*(12), 1427–1430.

Massey, P. B. (2002). Dietary supplements. *Medical Clinics of North America, 86*(1), 127–147.

Mautz, H. (2001). Undiagnosed diabetes common among Mexican-Americans. *Diabetes Care, 24*(7), 1204–1209.

Rocchini, A. P. (2002). Childhood obesity and a diabetes epidemic (Editorial). *New England Journal of Medicine, 346*(11), 854–855.

Setter, S. M., White, J. R., Jr., & Campbell, R. K. (2000). Diabetes. In E. T. Herfindal & D. R. Gourley (Eds.), *Textbook of therapeutics: Drug and disease management* (7th ed., pp. 377–406).

Silverstein, J. H., & Rosenbloom, A. L. (2000). New developments in type 1 (insulin-dependent) diabetes. *Clinical Pediatrics 39*, 257–266.

Sinha, R., Fisch, G., Teague, B., Tamborlane, W. V., Banyas, B., Allen, K., et al. (2002). Prevalence of impaired glucose tolerance among children and adolescents with marked obesity. *New England Journal of Medicine 346*(11), 802–810.

Skyler, J. S. (2000). Approach to hyperglycemia in the client with diabetes mellitus. In H. D. Humes (Ed.), *Kelley's textbook of internal medicine* (4th ed., pp. 2635–2648). Philadelphia: Lippincott Williams & Wilkins.

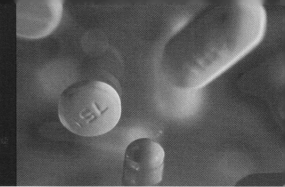

# Drugs Affecting Reproductive Health

# 23

# Drug Use During Pregnancy and Lactation

## OBJECTIVES

*After studying this chapter, the student will be able to:*

1 Provide reasons for avoiding or minimizing drug therapy during pregnancy and lactation.

2 Describe selected teratogenic drugs.

3 Give guidelines for drug therapy of pregnancy-associated signs and symptoms.

4 Discuss guidelines for drug therapy of selected chronic disorders during pregnancy and lactation.

5 Discuss the safety of immunizations given during pregnancy.

6 Teach adolescent and young adult women to avoid prescribed and over-the-counter drugs when possible and to inform physicians and dentists if there is a possibility of pregnancy.

7 Discuss the role of the home care nurse working with the pregnant mother.

8 Discuss drugs used during labor and delivery in terms of their effects on the mother and newborn infant.

9 Describe abortifacients in terms of characteristics and nursing process implications.

## CRITICAL THINKING SCENARIO

*T*hirty-eight-year-old Susan Williams comes in for her first prenatal visit. Mrs. Williams works as a corporate lawyer and is married to a university professor. Mrs. Williams is very excited about this planned pregnancy but also seems somewhat anxious because she asks lots of questions.

✔ What are the effects of drug use by the mother on the fetus during pregnancy?

✔ Do you make any assumptions about Mrs. Williams's knowledge level based on her profession and social class?

✔ How might such judgments assist you to individualize teaching? How might such judgments impair the teaching process?

✔ What essential information do you need to provide to Mrs. Williams regarding the use of any prescription, nonprescription, or herbal drugs during pregnancy?

## PROTOTYPE PROFILE

oxytocin (Pitocin), p. 405

## ▣ INTRODUCTION

Drug use during pregnancy and lactation requires special consideration because both the mother and the fetus, or nursing infant, are affected. Few drugs are considered safe, and drug use is generally contraindicated. However, many pregnant or lactating women take drugs for various reasons, including acute disorders that may or may not be associated with pregnancy, chronic disorders that require continued treatment during pregnancy or lactation, and habitual use of nontherapeutic drugs (eg, alcohol, tobacco, others). The main purpose of this chapter is to describe potential drug effects on the fetus and maternal drug therapy to protect the fetus while providing therapeutic effects to the pregnant woman.

## Pregnancy and Lactation

Pregnancy is a dynamic state: mother and fetus undergo physiologic changes that influence drug effects. In the pregnant woman, physiologic changes alter drug pharmacokinetics (Table 23-1), and drug effects are less predictable than in the nonpregnant state. Most of the drugs in this chapter are described elsewhere; they are discussed here in relation to pregnancy and lactation. Other drugs included in this chapter are used mainly to influence some aspect of pregnancy. These drugs are discussed in greater detail and include drugs used to induce abortion (abortifacients), drugs used to stop preterm labor (tocolytics), and drugs used during labor and delivery.

## Maternal–Placental–Fetal Circulation

Drugs ingested by the pregnant woman reach the fetus through the maternal–placental–fetal circulation, which is completed about the third week after conception. On the maternal side, arterial blood pressure carries blood and drugs to the placenta. In the placenta, a few thin layers of tissue over a large surface area separate maternal and fetal blood. Drugs readily cross the placenta, mainly by passive diffusion. Placental transfer begins approximately the fifth week after conception. When drugs are given on a regular schedule, serum levels reach equilibrium, with fetal blood usually containing 50% to 100% of the amount in maternal blood. Drug metabolism and distribution in the fetus are described in At the Foundation: Fetal Drug Metabolism.

| TABLE 23-1   Pregnancy: Physiologic and Pharmacokinetic Changes | |
|---|---|
| **Physiologic Change** | **Pharmacokinetic Change** |
| Increased plasma volume and body water, approximately 50% in a normal pregnancy | Once absorbed into the bloodstream, a drug (especially if water soluble) is distributed and "diluted" more than in the nonpregnant state. Drug dosage requirements may increase. However, this effect may be offset by other pharmacokinetic changes of pregnancy. |
| Increased weight (average 25 lb) and body fat | Drugs (especially fat-soluble ones) are distributed more widely. Drugs that are distributed to fatty tissues tend to linger in the body because they are slowly released from storage sites into the bloodstream. |
| Decreased serum albumin. The rate of albumin production is increased. However, serum levels fall because of plasma volume expansion. Also, many plasma protein-binding sites are occupied by hormones and other endogenous substances that increase during pregnancy. | The decreased capacity for drug binding leaves more free or unbound drug available for therapeutic or adverse effects on the mother and for placental transfer to the fetus. Thus, a given dose of a drug is likely to produce greater effects than it would in the nonpregnant state. Some commonly used drugs with higher unbound amounts during pregnancy include dexamethasone (Decadron), diazepam (Valium), lidocaine (Xylocaine), meperidine (Demerol), phenobarbital, phenytoin (Dilantin), propranolol (Inderal), and sulfisoxazole (Gantrisin). |
| Increased renal blood flow and glomerular filtration rate secondary to increased cardiac output | Increased excretion of drugs by the kidneys, especially those excreted primarily unchanged in the urine. These include penicillins, digoxin (Lanoxin), and lithium. |
| | In late pregnancy, the increased size and weight of the uterus may decrease renal blood flow when the woman assumes a supine position. This may result in decreased excretion and prolonged effects of renally excreted drugs. |

# Drug Effects on the Fetus

The fetus, which is exposed to any drugs circulating in maternal blood, is very sensitive to drug effects because it is small, has few plasma proteins that can bind drug molecules, and has a weak capacity for metabolizing and excreting drugs. Once drug molecules reach the fetus, they may cause teratogenicity (anatomic malformations) or other adverse effects. The teratogenicity of many drugs is unknown. However, since 1984, the U.S. Food and Drug Administration (FDA) has required that new drugs be assigned a risk category (see Chapter 2, Box 2-1). In review, these Pregnancy Categories include the following:

**A.** Adequate studies in pregnant women demonstrate no risk to the fetus.
**B.** Animal studies indicate no risk to the fetus, but there are no adequate studies in pregnant women; or animal studies show adverse effects, but adequate studies in pregnant women have not demonstrated a risk.
**C.** A potential risk, usually because animal studies have either not been performed or indicated adverse effects, and there are no data from human studies. These drugs may be used when potential benefits outweigh the potential risks.
**D.** There is evidence of human fetal risk, but the potential benefits to the mother may be acceptable despite the potential risk.
**X.** Studies in animals or humans, adverse reaction reports, or both have demonstrated fetal abnormalities; the risk of use in a pregnant woman clearly outweighs any possible benefit.

Drug teratogenicity is most likely to occur when drugs are taken during the first trimester of pregnancy, when fetal organs are formed (Fig. 23-1). For drugs taken during the second and third trimesters, adverse effects are usually manifested in the neonate (birth to 1 month) or infant (1 month to 1 year) as growth retardation, respiratory problems, infection, or bleeding. Overall, effects are determined mainly by the type and amount of drugs, the duration of exposure, and the level of fetal growth and development when exposed to the drugs. Both therapeutic and nontherapeutic drugs may affect the fetus.

Fetal effects of commonly used *therapeutic* drugs are listed in Box 23-1. Effects of *nontherapeutic* drugs are described in the following paragraphs.

**Alcohol** is contraindicated during pregnancy; no amount is considered safe. Heavy intake may cause fetal alcohol syndrome, a condition characterized by multiple congenital defects and mental retardation.

**Caffeine** is the most commonly ingested nontherapeutic drug during pregnancy. It is present in coffee, tea, cola drinks, over-the-counter analgesics, antisleep preparations, and chocolate. Although ingestion of moderate amounts has not been associated with birth defects, spontaneous abortions, preterm births, and low birth weights have occurred. In addition, high doses may cause cardiac dysrhythmias in the fetus.

**Cigarette smoking** (nicotine and carbon monoxide ingestion) is one of the few preventable causes of perinatal morbidity and mortality and is contraindicated. Effects include increased fetal, neonatal, and infant mortality; decreased birth weight and length; shortened gestation; and increased complications of pregnancy (eg, placental abruption, spontaneous abortion; preterm delivery). These effects are attributed to decreased flow of blood and oxygen to the placenta and uterus. Nicotine causes vasoconstriction and decreases blood flow to the fetus; carbon monoxide decreases the oxygen available to the fetus. Chronic fetal hypoxia from heavy smoking has been associated with mental retardation and other long-term effects on physical and intellectual development. Overall, effects of smoking are dose related, with light smoking (<1 pack/day) estimated to increase fetal deaths by 20% and heavy smoking (1 or more packs/day) increasing deaths by 35%.

**Cocaine, marijuana,** and **heroin** are illegal drugs of abuse, and their use during pregnancy is particularly

## AT THE FOUNDATION: *Fetal Drug Metabolism*

After drugs enter the fetal circulation, relatively large amounts are pharmacologically active because the fetus has low levels of serum albumin and thus low levels of drug binding. Drug molecules are distributed in two ways. Most are transported to the liver, where they are metabolized. Metabolism occurs slowly because the fetal liver is immature in quantity and quality of drug-metabolizing enzymes. Drugs metabolized by the fetal liver are excreted by the fetal kidneys into amniotic fluid. Excretion also is slow and inefficient owing to immature development of fetal kidneys. In addition,

the fetus swallows some amniotic fluid, and some drug molecules are recirculated.

Other drug molecules are transported directly to the heart, which then distributes them to the brain and coronary arteries. Drugs enter the brain easily because the blood–brain barrier is poorly developed in the fetus. Approximately half of the drug-containing blood is then transported through the umbilical arteries to the placenta, where it reenters the maternal circulation. Thus, the mother can metabolize and excrete some drug molecules for the fetus.

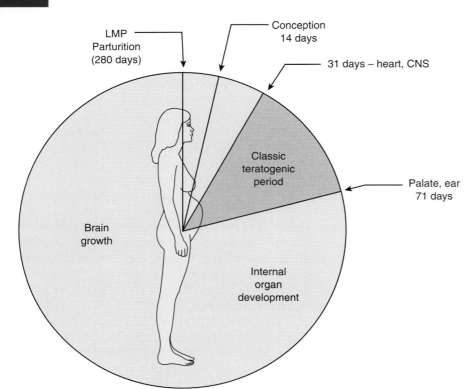

**FIGURE 23-1** The gestational clock showing the classic teratogenic risk assessment. (Adapted from Niebyl, J. [1999]. Drugs and related areas in pregnancy. In J. Sciarra [Ed.], *Obstetrics and gynecology*. Philadelphia: Lippincott Williams & Wilkins.)

serious. **Cocaine** may cause maternal vasoconstriction, tachycardia, hypertension, cardiac dysrhythmias, and seizures. These effects may impair fetal growth, impair neurologic development, and increase the risk for spontaneous abortion during the first and second trimesters. During the third trimester, cocaine causes increased uterine contractility, vasoconstriction, and decreased blood flow in the placenta, fetal tachycardia, and increased risk for fetal distress and abruptio placentae. These life-threatening effects on mother and fetus are even more likely to occur with "crack" cocaine, a highly purified and potent form.

**Marijuana** impairs formation of DNA and RNA, the basic genetic material of body cells. It also may decrease the oxygen supply of mother and fetus. **Heroin** ingestion increases the risks for pregnancy-induced hypertension, third-trimester bleeding, complications of labor and delivery, and postpartum morbidity.

## ■ FETAL THERAPEUTICS

Although the major concern about drugs ingested during pregnancy is adverse effects on the fetus, a few drugs are given to the mother for their therapeutic effects on the fetus. These include digoxin for fetal tachycardia or heart failure, levothyroxine for hypothyroidism, penicillin for exposure to maternal syphilis, and prenatal corticosteroids to promote surfactant production to improve lung function and decrease respiratory distress syndrome in preterm infants.

## ■ MATERNAL THERAPEUTICS

Thus far, the main emphasis on drug use during pregnancy has related to actual or potential adverse effects on the fetus. Despite the general principle that drug use should be avoided when possible, pregnant women may require drug therapy for various illnesses, increased nutritional needs, pregnancy-associated problems, chronic disease processes, treatment of preterm labor, induction of labor, and pain management during labor. The age of the mother during the pregnancy plays a role in the use of maternal therapeutics and is discussed in Age-related Considerations.

### General Guidelines: Pregnancy

1. Give medications only when clearly indicated, weighing anticipated benefits to the mother against the risk for harm to the fetus.
2. When drug therapy is required, the choice of drug should be based on the stage of pregnancy and available drug information (see Box 23-1). During the first trimester, for example, an older drug that has not been associated with teratogenic effects is usually preferred over a newer drug of unknown teratogenicity.
3. Any drugs used during pregnancy should be given in the lowest effective doses and for the shortest effective time.
4. Counsel pregnant women about the use of immunizations during pregnancy. Live virus vaccines

## BOX 23-1  Drug Effects in Pregnancy

All drugs are relatively contraindicated and should be used only if necessary. For most drugs, adequate studies have not been done in pregnant women and effects on the fetus are unknown. They should be used only if potential benefit to the mother justifies potential harm to the fetus.

### Adrenergics
Adrenergics are cardiac stimulants that increase rate and force of contractions and may increase blood pressure. Several were teratogenic and embryocidal in animal studies. These drugs are common ingredients in over-the-counter decongestants, cold remedies, and appetite suppressants.

Oral and parenteral adrenergics may inhibit uterine contractions during labor; cause hypokalemia, hypoglycemia, and pulmonary edema in the mother; and cause hypoglycemia in the neonate. These effects are unlikely with inhaled adrenergics (eg, albuterol). Oral *albuterol* and oral or intravenous *terbutaline* relax uterine muscles and inhibit preterm labor.

### Analgesics, Opioid
Opioids rapidly cross the placenta and reach the fetus. Maternal addiction and neonatal withdrawal symptoms result from regular use. Use of codeine during the first trimester has been associated with congenital defects.

When given to women in labor, opioids may decrease uterine contractility and slow progress toward delivery. They may also cause respiratory depression in the neonate. *Meperidine* reportedly causes less neonatal respiratory depression than other opioids. *Butorphanol* is also used. If respiratory depression occurs, it can be reversed by administration of *naloxone,* an opioid antagonist.

### Angiotensin-Converting Enzyme (ACE) Inhibitors
These drugs can cause fetal and neonatal morbidity and death; several dozen cases have been reported worldwide. Adverse fetal effects apparently do not occur during first trimester exposure. With exposure during the second and third trimesters, however, effects may include fetal and neonatal injury such as hypotension, neonatal skull hypoplasia, anuria, renal failure, and death. As a result, the drugs should be discontinued as soon as pregnancy is detected. Infants exposed to the drugs in utero should be closely observed for hypotension, oliguria, and hyperkalemia.

### Angiotensin II Receptor Blockers (ARBs)
See ACE inhibitors, above. These drugs should be discontinued when pregnancy is detected.

### Antianginal Agents (Nitrates)
The drugs lower blood pressure and may decrease blood supply to the fetus. Thus, they should be used only if necessary.

### Antianxiety and Sedative-Hypnotic Agents (Benzodiazepines)
These drugs should generally be avoided. They and their metabolites cross the placenta freely and accumulate in fetal blood. If taken during the first trimester, they may cause physical malformations. If taken during labor, they may cause sedation, respiratory depression, hypotonia, lethargy, tremors, irritability, and sucking difficulties in the neonate.

### Antibacterials
*Beta lactams. Penicillins* cross the placenta but apparently produce no adverse effects on the fetus. They are considered safer than other antibiotics. *Cephalosporins* cross the placenta and seem to be safe, although they have not been studied extensively in pregnancy. They have shorter half-lives, lower serum concentrations, and a faster rate of elimination in pregnancy. *Carbapenems* and *aztreonam* have not been studied and fetal effects are unknown.

*Aminoglycosides* (FDA category D) cross the placenta and fetal serum levels may reach 15% to 50% of maternal levels. Ototoxicity may occur with gentamicin. Serious adverse effects on the fetus or neonate have not been reported with other aminoglycosides, but there is potential harm because the drugs are nephrotoxic and ototoxic.

*Clindamycin* (Cleocin) should be used only when infection with *Bacteroides fragilis* is suspected.

*Fluoroquinolones* are contraindicated in pregnancy.

*Macrolides.* Erythromycin crosses the placenta to reach fetal serum levels up to 20% of maternal levels, but no fetal abnormalities have been reported. In animal studies, adverse fetal effects were reported with clarithromycin and dirithromycin but not with azithromycin. Clarithromycin is contraindicated if a safer alternative is available.

*Nitrofurantoin* should not be used during late pregnancy because of possible hemolytic anemia in the neonate.

*Sulfonamides* should not be used during the last trimester because they may cause kernicterus in the neonate.

*Tetracyclines* are contraindicated. They cross the placenta and interfere with development of teeth and bone in the fetus. Animal studies indicate embryotoxicity.

*Trimethoprim,* often given in combination with sulfamethoxazole (Bactrim), is contraindicated during the first trimester. It crosses the placenta to reach levels in fetal serum that are similar to those in maternal serum. It is a folate antagonist and may interfere with folic acid metabolism in the fetus. It was teratogenic in animals, but a few studies in pregnant women have not indicated teratogenic effects.

*Vancomycin* is not recommended because fetal effects are unknown.

### Antifungals
Systemic antifungals are generally contraindicated.

### Anticholinergics
*Atropine* crosses the placenta rapidly with IV injection; effects on the fetus depend on the maturity of its parasympathetic nervous system. *Scopolamine* may cause respiratory depression in the neonate and may contribute to neonatal hemorrhage by reducing vitamin K–dependent clotting factors in the neonate.

### Anticoagulants
*Heparin* does not cross the placenta and has not been associated with congenital defects. It is the anticoagulant of choice during pregnancy. However, its use has been associated with 13% to 22% unfavorable outcomes, including stillbirths and

*(continued)*

BOX
23-1   **Drug Effects in Pregnancy** (Continued)

prematurity. *Warfarin* crosses the placenta and fetal hemorrhage, spontaneous abortion, prematurity, stillbirth, and congenital anomalies may occur. Approximately 31% of fetuses exposed to warfarin may experience a problem related to the anticoagulant. If a woman becomes pregnant during warfarin therapy, inform her of the potential risks to the fetus, and discuss the possibility of terminating the pregnancy.

## Anticonvulsants

Although more than 90% of women receiving antiseizure drugs deliver normal infants, the drugs (eg, carbamazepine, phenytoin, valproate) are known teratogens. After years of questioning whether teratogenesis resulted from epilepsy or antiepileptic drugs, a recent study confirms that anticonvulsant drug therapy in pregnant women causes physical abnormalities in their offspring. Moreover, infants exposed to one drug had a much higher rate of abnormalities than infants not exposed (20.6% vs. 8.5%) and infants exposed to two or more drugs had a still higher rate (28%). Infants whose nonepileptic mothers took the drugs for bipolar disorder also had higher rates of birth defects. In general, the fetal effects of newer drugs (eg, *gabapentin, lamotrigine, oxcarbazepine, tiagabine,* and *topiramate*) (Topamax) are unknown. They are FDA category C.

## Antidepressants

Tricyclic antidepressants (eg, *amitriptyline*) have been associated with teratogenicity and embryotoxicity when given in large doses, and there have been reports of congenital malformations and neonatal withdrawal syndrome. Monoamine oxidase inhibitors (eg, *phenelzine*), were associated with fewer viable offspring and growth retardation in animal studies with large doses. The selective serotonin reuptake inhibitors were teratogenic in animals and, in one study of 228 women who took *fluoxetine* during the first trimester, 5.5% of the infants had major birth defects. In addition, late exposure to fluoxetine resulted in more preterm births than early exposure (14.3% vs. 4.1%).

## Antidiabetic Drugs

Insulin is the only antidiabetic drug recommended for use during pregnancy. Sulfonylureas except glyburide are teratogenic in animals; fetal effects of other oral agents are largely unknown. Acarbose, metformin, and miglitol are FDA category B; nateglinide, pioglitazone, repaglinide, and rosiglitazone are category C.

## Antiemetics

None of the available antiemetic drugs has been proven safe for use and nondrug measures are preferred for controlling nausea and vomiting when possible. If drug therapy is necessary, some antihistamines (eg, *cyclizine, dimenhydrinate*) are considered safer for the fetus than other drugs.

## Antihistamines

Histamine-1 receptor blocking agents (eg, *diphenhydramine*), have been associated with teratogenic effects, but the extent is unknown. The drugs should generally not be used during

the third trimester because of possible adverse effects in the neonate. With histamine-2 receptor blocking agents, *cimetidine* and *ranitidine* are considered acceptable for treatment of gastroesophageal reflux disease that does not respond to dietary and other lifestyle changes.

## Antihypertensives

*Methyldopa* crosses the placenta and reaches fetal concentrations similar to those of maternal serum. However, no teratogenic effects have been reported despite widespread use during pregnancy. Neonates of mothers receiving methyldopa may have decreased blood pressure for about 48 h. *Hydralazine* is considered safe. *Clonidine, guanabenz,* and *guanfacine* are not recommended because effects in pregnant women are unknown.

## Antimanic Agent

*Lithium* crosses the placenta and fetal concentrations are similar to those of the mother. Cardiac and other birth defects may occur. In the neonate, lithium is eliminated slowly and may cause bradycardia, cyanosis, diabetes insipidus, hypotonia, hypothyroidism, and electrocardiogram (ECG) abnormalities. Most of these effects resolve within 1 to 2 wk.

## Antipsychotics

Phenothiazines (eg, *chlorpromazine*) readily cross the placenta. Studies indicate that the drugs are not teratogenic, but animal studies indicate potential embryotoxicity, increased neonatal mortality, and decreased performance. The possibility of permanent neurologic damage cannot be excluded. Use near term may cause abnormal movements, abnormal reflexes, and jaundice in the neonate and hypotension in the mother. Fetal effects of newer drugs are unknown.

## Antitubercular Drugs

These drugs are recommended for treatment of active tuberculosis; use for prophylaxis can usually be delayed until after delivery. Isoniazid, ethambutol, and rifampin were embryocidal or teratogenic in animal studies. The effects of drug combinations on the fetus are unknown.

## Antivirals

Most systemic antivirals were teratogenic in animal studies. No well-controlled studies support their use in pregnancy, except for *zidovudine* and other anti–human immunodeficiency virus (HIV) drugs to prevent transmission of HIV infection to the fetus.

## Aspirin

*Aspirin* is contraindicated because of potential adverse effects on the mother and fetus. Maternal effects include prolonged gestation, prolonged labor, and antepartum and postpartum hemorrhage. Fetal effects include constriction of the ductus arteriosus, low birth weight, and increased incidence of stillbirth and neonatal death. The drug is FDA category D.

## Beta-Adrenergic Blocking Agents

Safety for use of these drugs (eg, *propranolol*) has not been established. Teratogenicity has not been reported in humans,

*(continued)*

**BOX 23-1    Drug Effects in Pregnancy (Continued)**

but problems may occur during delivery. These include maternal bradycardia and neonatal bradycardia, hypoglycemia, apnea, low Apgar scores, and low birth weight. Neonatal effects may last up to 72 h.

### Calcium Channel Blocking Agents

Teratogenic and embryotoxic effects occurred in small animals given large doses. *Diltiazem* caused fetal death, skeletal abnormalities, and increased incidence of stillbirths. *Nifedipine* caused developmental toxicity in animals. Fetal effects of most of the drugs are unknown. Because the drugs decrease maternal blood pressure, there is a potential risk of inadequate blood flow to the placenta and the fetus.

### Corticosteroids

Systemic corticosteroids cross the placenta. Animal studies indicate that large doses of cortisol early in pregnancy may produce cleft palate, stillbirths, and decreased fetal size. Chronic maternal ingestion during the first trimester has shown a 1% incidence of cleft palate in humans. Infants of mothers who received substantial amounts of corticosteroids during pregnancy should be closely observed for signs of adrenal insufficiency. Betamethasone is used to promote fetal production of surfactant to increase lung maturity in the preterm infant. Inhaled corticosteroids (eg, those used to treat allergic rhinitis or asthma) are less likely to cause adverse effects in the fetus because of less systemic absorption.

### Digoxin

*Digoxin* is apparently safe for use during pregnancy. It crosses the placenta to reach fetal serum levels that are 50% to 80% those of maternal serum. Fetal toxicity and neonatal death have occurred with maternal overdose. Dosage requirements may be less predictable during pregnancy, and serum drug levels and other assessment parameters must be closely monitored. Digoxin also has been administered to the mother for treatment of fetal tachycardia and heart failure.

### Diuretics

Thiazides (eg, *hydrochlorothiazide*) cross the placenta. They are not associated with teratogenesis, but they may cause other adverse effects. Because the drugs decrease plasma volume, decreased blood flow to the uterus and placenta may occur with resultant impairment of fetal nutrition and growth. Other adverse effects may include fetal or neonatal jaundice, thrombocytopenia, hyperbilirubinemia, hemolytic jaundice, fluid and electrolyte imbalances, and impaired carbohydrate metabolism. These drugs are not indicated for treatment of dependent edema caused by uterine enlargement and restriction of venous blood flow. They also are not effective in prevention or treatment of pregnancy-induced hypertension (preeclampsia). They may be used for treatment of pathologic edema.

Loop diuretics (eg, *furosemide*) are not considered teratogenic, but animal studies indicated fetal toxicity and death. Like the thiazides, loop diuretics may decrease plasma volume and blood flow to the placenta and fetus.

Potassium-conserving diuretics (eg, *triamterene,* an ingredient in Dyazide and Maxide) cross the placenta in animal studies, but effects on the human fetus are unknown.

### Dyslipidemics

*Cholestyramine* and *colestipol* are considered safe because they are not absorbed systemically. HMG-CoA reductase inhibitors or "statins" (eg, *lovastatin*) are FDA category X and contraindicated during pregnancy. They should be given to women of childbearing age only if they are highly unlikely to become pregnant and are informed of potential hazards. If a woman becomes pregnant while taking one of these drugs, the drug should be stopped and the patient informed of possible adverse drug effects on the fetus.

### Nonsteroidal Anti-Inflammatory Drugs (NSAIDs)

Use of NSAIDs (eg, *ibuprofen*) should generally be avoided, especially during the third trimester. All of the drugs are FDA category D in the third trimester or near delivery. If these drugs are taken in the third trimester, effects on human fetuses include constriction of the ductus arteriosus prenatally, nonclosure of the ductus arteriosus postnatally, impaired function of the tricuspid valve in the heart, pulmonary hypertension, degenerative changes in the myocardium, impaired platelet function with resultant bleeding, intracranial bleeding, renal impairment or failure, oligohydramnios, gastrointestinal (GI) bleeding or perforation, and increased risk of necrotizing enterocolitis, a life-threatening disorder. If taken near delivery, maternal effects include delayed onset of labor and delivery and increased risk of excessive bleeding. The newer COX-2 inhibitors (eg, *celecoxib*) have not been studied in pregnant women; *diclofenac* is contraindicated in pregnant women.

### Thyroid Hormone

Levothyroxine does not readily cross the placenta and it seems safe in appropriate dosages. However, it may cause tachycardia in the fetus. When given as replacement therapy in hypothyroid women, the drug should be continued through pregnancy.

---

(eg, measles, mumps, polio, rubella, yellow fever) should be avoided because of possible harmful effects to the fetus. Inactive virus vaccines, such as influenza, rabies, and hepatitis B (if the mother is high risk and negative for hepatitis B antigen) and toxoids (eg, diphtheria, tetanus) are considered safe for use. In addition, hyperimmune globulins can be given to pregnant women who are exposed to hepatitis B, rabies, tetanus, or varicella.

## Herbal and Dietary Supplements

Pregnancy increases nutritional needs, and vitamin and mineral supplements are commonly used. **Folic acid** supplementation is especially important to prevent neural tube birth defects (eg, spina bifida). Such defects occur early in pregnancy, often before the woman realizes she is pregnant. For this reason, it is recommended that all women of childbearing potential ingest at least 400 mcg

## Age-related Considerations: Drug Use During Pregnancy and Lactation

### USE IN CHILDREN

The effects of drugs on the fetus and nursing infant are well described in the chapter. Adolescent pregnancy poses additional risks to mother and baby. The complications of adolescent pregnancy include greater incidence of pregnancy-induced hypertension, preterm labor, iron-deficiency anemia, cephalopelvic disproportion, and conflicting developmental crises. Many of these concerns may require drug therapy.

### USE IN OLDER WOMEN (>35 YEARS OF AGE)

With the exception of greater incidence of chromosomal abnormality in women older than 35 years of age, little evidence supports increasing complications of pregnancy for the fetus in this age group provided that prenatal care was started early in the pregnancy. Women older than 35 years of age had no increased risk for preterm delivery or for delivering an infant who was small for gestational age, had a low Apgar at birth, or died during the perinatal period.

Women older than 40 years of age may have greater circulatory disturbances; varicose veins are more common. The incidence of pregnancy-induced hypertension is higher than in younger women, possibly related to inelasticity of blood vessels or because this age group may have an already elevated blood pressure. Complications related to labor, birth, and the postpartum period might also result from inelasticity of the blood vessels and include failure to progress in labor and postpartum hemorrhage. Additionally, the older mother may have difficulty accepting the reality of a new baby. These issues may require drug therapy.

---

daily from food, a supplement, or both. In addition, pregnancy increases folic acid requirements 5- to 10-fold, and deficiencies are common. A supplement is usually needed to supply adequate amounts. For deficiency states, 1 mg or more daily may be needed.

**Herbal** supplements are not recommended during pregnancy. **Ginger** has been used to relieve nausea and vomiting during pregnancy, with a few studies supporting its use. Overall, it has not been proved effective, although it is probably safe for use.

## Pregnancy-associated Symptoms and Their Management

Many obstetric clients with pregnancy-associated and chronic health conditions are now being managed in the home. The home care nurse who assists in managing these clients should be an obstetric specialist who is knowledgeable about normal pregnancy and potential complications. The overall goal of home care is to maintain the pregnancy to the most advanced gestational age possible. Guidelines for ongoing evaluation and intervention are addressed in Home Care Considerations. Home care follow-up by a nurse has been demonstrated to affect the outcome of a high-risk pregnancy positively.

### Anemias

Three types of anemia are common during pregnancy. One is physiologic anemia, which results from expanded blood volume. A second is iron-deficiency anemia, which is often related to long-term nutritional deficiencies. Iron supplements are usually given for prophylaxis (eg, ferrous sulfate, 300 mg, or ferrous gluconate, 600 mg, three times daily). Iron preparations should be given with food to decrease gastric irritation. Citrus juices enhance absorp-

tion. A third type is megaloblastic anemia, caused by folic acid deficiency. A folic acid supplement is often prescribed for prophylaxis.

### Constipation

Constipation often occurs during pregnancy, probably from decreased peristalsis. Preferred treatment, if effective, is to increase exercise and intake of fluids and high-fiber foods. If a laxative is required, a bulk-producing agent (eg, Metamucil) is the most physiologic for the mother and safest for the fetus because it is not absorbed systemically. A stool softener (eg, docusate) or an occasional saline laxative (eg, milk of magnesia) may also be

## Home Care Considerations: Drug Use During Pregnancy and Lactation

***ASSESS:*** maternal and fetal responses and compliance with the proposed management plan.

***MONITOR:*** drugs being used to treat the complicated obstetric client as well as maternal use of any non-prescription and nontherapeutic drugs, the therapeutic and adverse effects of the drugs and client's need for additional information, and provide that information.

***EDUCATE:*** regarding importance of reading and following instructions and restrictions on labels of OTC medications, not exceeding recommended dosages without consulting a health care provider, keeping appointments for lab work and follow-up care, and the importance of recognizing the danger signs and symptoms that may necessitate seeking professional help. Reinforce additional teaching points (see Client Teaching Guidelines: Drug Use During Pregnancy and Lactation).

used. Mineral oil should be avoided because it interferes with absorption of fat-soluble vitamins. Reduced absorption of vitamin K can lead to bleeding in newborns. Castor oil should be avoided because it can cause uterine contractions. Strong laxatives or any laxative used in excess may initiate uterine contractions and labor.

## Gastroesophageal Reflux Disease

Gastroesophageal reflux disease (GERD), of which heartburn (pyrosis) is the main symptom, often occurs in the later months of pregnancy. It develops when increased abdominal pressure and a relaxed esophageal sphincter allow gastric acid to splash into the esophagus and cause irritation, discomfort, and esophagitis.

Nonpharmacologic interventions include eating small meals; not eating for 2 to 3 hours before bedtime; avoiding caffeine, gas-producing foods, and constipation; and sitting in an upright position. For clients who do not obtain adequate relief with these measures, drug therapy may be needed. Antacids may be used if necessary. Because little systemic absorption occurs, the drugs are unlikely to harm the fetus if used in recommended doses. Cimetidine, ranitidine, or sucralfate may also be used.

## Gestational Diabetes

Some women first show signs of diabetes during pregnancy. This is called *gestational diabetes*. Women with risk factors (eg, obesity, family history of diabetes, being Hispanic, Native American, Asian, or African American) should be screened at the first prenatal visit. Most women without risk factors, or whose initial test was normal, should be tested between 24 and 28 weeks of gestation.

For women with gestational diabetes, initial management includes nutrition and exercise interventions, calorie restriction for obese women, and daily self-monitoring of blood glucose levels. If these interventions are ineffective, recombinant human insulin is needed to keep blood sugar levels as nearly normal as possible. Oral antidiabetic drugs are generally contraindicated, although acarbose, metformin, and miglitol appear to cause minimal fetal risk.

These women may revert to a nondiabetic state when pregnancy ends, but they are at increased risk for development of overt diabetes within 5 to 10 years. Gestational diabetes usually subsides within 6 weeks after delivery.

## Nausea and Vomiting

Nausea and vomiting often occur, especially during early pregnancy. Dietary management (eg, eating a few crackers when awakening and waiting a few minutes before arising) and maintaining fluid and electrolyte balance are recommended. Antiemetic drugs should be given only if nausea and vomiting are severe enough to threaten the mother's nutritional or metabolic status. Meclizine, 25 to 50 mg daily, and dimenhydrate, 50 mg every 3 to 4 hours, are thought to have low teratogenic risks. Pyridoxine (vitamin $B_6$) also may be helpful. If used, recommended dosage is 10 to 25 mg daily.

## Pregnancy-induced Hypertension

Pregnancy-induced hypertension includes preeclampsia and eclampsia, conditions that endanger the lives of mother and fetus. Preeclampsia is most likely to occur during the last 10 weeks of pregnancy, during labor, or within the first 48 hours after delivery. It is manifested by edema, hypertension, and proteinuria. Drug therapy includes intravenous hydralazine or labetalol for blood pressure control and magnesium sulfate for prevention or treatment of seizures. Eclampsia, characterized by severe symptoms and convulsions, occurs if preeclampsia is not treated effectively. Delivery of the fetus is the only known cure for preeclampsia or eclampsia. For women at risk for developing preeclampsia, aspirin, 60 mg daily, from 24 to 28 weeks of gestation until onset of labor, may be used for prophylaxis.

## Selected Infections

**Group B streptococcal infections** may affect the pregnant woman and the neonate. During late pregnancy, urinary tract infections (UTIs) or amnionitis may occur. After cesarean delivery, endometritis, bacteremia, or wound infection may occur. In the infant, sepsis, meningitis, or pneumonia may occur.

Because of the potentially serious consequences of infection with group B streptococci, pregnant women should have a vaginal culture at 35 to 37 weeks of gestation. A positive culture indicates infection that should be treated. However, antibiotics given at this time may not provide coverage during labor and delivery. Treatment should be initiated during labor, often with ampicillin, 2 g IV as a loading dose, then 1 g IV every 4 hours until delivery.

**Human immunodeficiency virus (HIV) infection** and **acquired immunodeficiency syndrome (AIDS)** can be transmitted to the fetus and neonate, and treatment is needed to reduce transmission. Oral zidovudine (AZT) monotherapy has been used for several years, after 14 weeks of gestation. During labor, IV AZT is given until delivery. After delivery, the infant should be given AZT for 6 weeks, with or without other anti-AIDS drugs. Increasingly, highly active antiretroviral therapy (HAART) is being used for pregnant women. HAART is a combination of drugs that may include a nucleoside reverse transcriptase inhibitor (eg, zidovudine, lamivudine, or didanosine), a non-nucleoside reverse transcriptase inhibitor (eg, nevirapine), and a protease inhibitor (eg, ritonavir, saquinavir, nelfinavir).

Women with HIV infection or AIDS should be encouraged to avoid pregnancy.

**Urinary tract infections** commonly occur during pregnancy and may include asymptomatic bacteriuria, cystitis, and pyelonephritis. Although treatment of asymptomatic bacteriuria is controversial in some populations, the condition should be treated in pregnant women because of its association with cystitis and pyelonephritis. Asymptomatic bacteriuria and UTIs are also associated with increased preterm deliveries and low birth weights. Amoxicillin, cephalexin, and nitrofurantoin are commonly used drugs. Hospitalization and an intravenous cephalosporin may be needed for management of pyelonephritis.

## Management of Chronic Diseases During Pregnancy

### Asthma

Asthma is associated with a variety of complications in pregnancy, including preeclampsia, perinatal death, low birth weights, and congenital malformations. Poor asthma control during pregnancy is considered more detrimental to a fetus than treatment with available drugs. Thus, good control is essential. Commonly used drugs include orally inhaled beta$_2$ agonists (eg, albuterol or metaproterenol) and anti-inflammatory agents (eg, cromolyn or beclomethasone).

### Diabetes Mellitus

Diabetes increases the risks of pregnancy for both mother and fetus, and the hormonal changes of pregnancy have diabetogenic effects that may cause or aggravate diabetes. Some women first show signs of diabetes during pregnancy (gestational diabetes). Others, who were previously able to control diabetes with diet alone, may become insulin dependent during pregnancy. Still others, already insulin dependent, are likely to need larger doses as pregnancy advances. Overall, pregnancy makes diabetes more difficult to control. In addition, insulin requirements fluctuate during pregnancy. For diabetic women who become pregnant, maintaining normal or near-normal blood sugar levels is required for successful outcomes because poor glycemic control increases the risks for birth defects. Recommendations for management include the following:

■ If oral antidiabetic drugs are taken by a woman of childbearing potential, they should be discontinued before conception, if possible (eg, for a planned pregnancy attempt), or as soon as pregnancy is suspected. Oral antidiabetic drugs are contraindicated in pregnancy, mainly because of fetal hypoglycemia. This recommendation may change in the future because acarbose, miglitol, and metformin are thought to carry little risk to the fetus. Glyburide has been used in some women after 11 weeks of gestation. However, its use is not recommended during the last few weeks of pregnancy. Most oral agents have not been studied in pregnant women.

■ Insulin is the antidiabetic drug of choice during pregnancy. Human insulin should be used because it is least likely to cause an allergic response. Because insulin requirements vary according to the stage of pregnancy, the diabetic client's blood glucose levels must be monitored closely and insulin therapy individualized. It is

especially important that sufficient insulin is given to prevent maternal acidosis. Uncontrolled acidosis is likely to interfere with neurologic development of the fetus. At the same time, careful dietary control and other treatment measures are necessary.

■ Insulin requirements usually decrease during the first trimester and increase during the second and third trimesters.

■ During labor and delivery, short-acting insulin and frequent blood glucose tests are used to control diabetes, as during other acute situations.

■ During the postpartum period, insulin requirements fluctuate because stress, trauma, infection, surgery, or other factors associated with delivery tend to increase blood glucose levels and insulin requirements. At the same time, termination of the pregnancy reverses the diabetogenic hormonal changes and decreases insulin requirements. Short-acting insulin is given, and dosage is based on frequent measurements of blood glucose. Once the insulin requirement is stabilized, the client may be able to return to the prepregnancy treatment program.

### Hypertension

Chronic hypertension (hypertension beginning before conception or up to 20 weeks of pregnancy) is associated with increased maternal and fetal risks. Thus, appropriate management is mandatory. Nonpharmacologic interventions (eg, avoiding excessive weight gain, sodium restriction, increased rest) should be emphasized. If drug therapy is required, methyldopa is the drug of first choice because it has not been associated with adverse effects on the fetus or neonate. Alternatives include labetalol and other beta blockers, clonidine, hydralazine, isradipine, nifedipine, and prazosin. With beta blockers, fetal and neonatal bradycardia, hypotension, hypoglycemia, and respiratory depression have been reported. As a result, some authorities recommend avoiding the drugs during the first trimester and stopping them 2 to 3 days before delivery.

Opinions seem divided on the use of angiotensin-converting enzyme (ACE) inhibitors. Some sources say the drugs are contraindicated during pregnancy; others say they can be used during the first trimester but should then be discontinued because of potential renal damage in the fetus. The same effects would probably occur with angiotensin II receptor blockers (ARBs) because they also act on the renin-angiotensin system.

Although diuretics are commonly used in the treatment of hypertension, they should not be given during pregnancy. They decrease blood volume, cardiac output, and blood pressure and may cause fluid and electrolyte imbalances, all of which may have adverse effects on the fetus.

### Seizure Disorders

Although antiepileptic drugs (AEDs) are known teratogens, they must often be taken during pregnancy because seizures may also be harmful to mother and fetus. Fortunately, most pregnancies (90% to 95%) result in normal infants. Despite the usually good outcomes, the incidence of birth defects is 2 to 3 times higher in fetuses exposed to AEDs than in those not exposed. If an AED is required, monotherapy with the lowest dose that stops seizures should be used, and plasma drug levels should be checked monthly. Women with epilepsy should take a folic acid supplement (at least 400 mcg daily) all the time and 800 mcg or more during pregnancy. Supplemental vitamin K is usually needed during the last month of pregnancy to prevent bleeding in neonates. An injection of vitamin K is also given to the infant immediately after birth.

There has been controversy regarding whether teratogenic effects stemmed from epilepsy or AEDs. A newer study indicates that the drugs are responsible. Moreover, the rate of birth defects in infants exposed to one AED was significantly higher than those not exposed (20.6% versus 8.5%) and was 28% in infants exposed to two or more AEDs. Infants whose mothers took AEDs for bipolar disorder rather than epilepsy also had higher rates of birth defects.

## ABORTIFACIENTS

Abortion is the termination of pregnancy before 20 weeks of gestation. It may occur spontaneously or be intentionally induced. Medical abortion may be induced by prostaglandins and an antiprogestin (see Drugs at a Glance 23-1: Abortifacients, Tocolytics, and Oxytocics). Prostaglandins may be used to terminate pregnancy during the second trimester. In the female reproductive system, prostaglandins E and F are found in the ovaries, myometrium, and menstrual fluid. They stimulate uterine contraction and are probably important in initiating and maintaining the normal birth process. Drug preparations of prostaglandins are capable of inducing labor at any time during pregnancy. Misoprostol, a prostaglandin developed to prevent nonsteroidal anti-inflammatory drug–induced gastric ulcers (see Chap. 46), is being given orally or intravaginally for first or second trimester termination. However, it is not FDA approved for this use.

Mifepristone is a progesterone antagonist used to terminate pregnancy during the first trimester. A prostaglandin is given approximately 48 hours after the mifepristone to augment uterine contractions and ensure expulsion of the conceptus.

## TOCOLYTICS

Drugs given to inhibit labor and maintain the pregnancy are called *tocolytics*. Uterine contractions with cervical changes between 20 and 37 weeks of gestation are con-

sidered premature labor. Nonpharmacologic treatment includes bed rest, hydration, and sedation. Drug therapy is most effective when the cervix is dilated less than 4 cm and membranes are intact.

Ritodrine, terbutaline, magnesium sulfate, and nifedipine) are used as tocolytics (see Drugs at a Glance 23-1). Ritodrine and terbutaline are beta-adrenergic agents that relax uterine smooth muscle and thereby slow or stop uterine contractions. Terbutaline is not FDA approved for use in premature labor but is used widely for that purpose. Magnesium sulfate is most often used as an anticonvulsant in the treatment of preeclampsia, but it also inhibits preterm labor. Hypermagnesemia may occur because tocolytic serum levels (4 to 7 mEq/L) are higher than normal levels (1.5 to 2.5 mEq/L). Close monitoring of serum levels and signs of hypermagnesemia (eg, decreased respiratory rate and loss of deep tendon reflexes) is required.

## DRUGS USED DURING LABOR AND DELIVERY AT TERM

At the end of gestation, labor usually begins spontaneously and proceeds through delivery of the neonate. In some instances, prostaglandin preparations (eg, Prepidil or Cervidil formulations of dinoprostone) are administered intravaginally to promote cervical ripening and induce labor. Drugs often used during labor, delivery, and the immediate postpartum period include oxytocics, analgesics, and anesthetics.

### Oxytocics

Oxytocic drugs include oxytocin (Pitocin) and methylergonovine (see Table 23-1). **P Oxytocin** is a hormone produced in the hypothalamus and released by the posterior pituitary gland (see Chap. 20). Oxytocin stimulates uterine contractions to initiate labor and promotes letdown of breast milk to the nipples in lactation. Pitocin is a synthetic form used to induce labor at or near full-term gestation and to augment labor when uterine contractions are weak and ineffective. It also can be used to prevent or control uterine bleeding after delivery or to complete an incomplete abortion. It is contraindicated for antepartum use in the presence of fetal distress, cephalopelvic disproportion, preterm labor, placenta previa, previous uterine surgery, and severe preeclampsia. Methergine is used for management of postpartum hemorrhage related to uterine atony.

Oxytocin is usually the drug of choice for induction or augmentation of labor because physiologic doses produce a rhythmic uterine contraction–relaxation pattern that approximates the normal labor process. It is also the drug of choice for prevention or control of postpartum uterine bleeding because it is less likely to cause hypertension than the ergot alkaloids. It is therefore

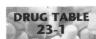
## Drugs at a Glance
## Abortifacients, Tocolytics, and Oxytocics

| Generic/Trade Name | Routes and Dosage Ranges (Adults) | Comments |
| --- | --- | --- |
| **Abortifacients** | | |
| *Progesterone Antagonist* | | |
| **Mifepristone** (Mifeprex) Pregnancy Category X | PO, 600 mg as a single dose or smaller amounts for 4–7 d | To terminate pregnancy <49 d |
| *Prostaglandins* | | |
| **Carboprost** (tromethamine, Hemabate) Pregnancy Category X | IM, 250 mcg q1.5–3.5h, depending on uterine response, increased to 500 mcg per dose if uterine contractility is inadequate after several 250-mcg doses | |
| **Dinoprostone** (Prostin E$_2$; Cervidil, Prepidil) Pregnancy Category C | Intravaginally 20 mg, repeated q3–5h until abortion occurs | Gel promotes cervical ripening Suppositories used to terminate pregnancy from 12 through 28 weeks of gestation Vaginal suppository also used for initiation and ripening of cervix at term or near term |
| **Misoprostol** (Cytotec) Pregnancy Category X | PO or intravaginally 200–400 mcg q12h for second trimester termination. Termination usually complete within 48 h | Administering the PO form with food may decrease the incidence of diarrhea |
| **Tocolytics** | | |
| **Ritodrine** (Yutopar) Pregnancy Category B | IV infusion, 0.1 mg/min initially, increased by 50 mcg/min every 10 min to a maximum dose of 350 mcg/min if necessary to stop labor. The infusion should be continued for 12 h after uterine contractions cease. PO, 10 mg 30 min before discontinuing the IV infusion, then 10 mg q2h for 24 h, then 10–20 mg q4–6h as long as necessary to maintain the pregnancy. Maximum oral dose, 120 mg daily | Maternal pulmonary edema has been noted with administration |
| **Terbutaline** (Brethine) Pregnancy Category B | IV infusion, 10 mcg/min, titrated up to a maximum dose of 80 mcg/min until contractions cease PO, 2.5 mg q4–6h as maintenance therapy until term | Terbutaline is not FDA approved for use in premature labor, but is used widely for that purpose |
| **Magnesium sulfate** Pregnancy Category B | IV infusion, loading dose 3–4 g mixed in 5% dextrose injection and administered over 15–20 min. Maintenance dose, 1–2 g/h, according to serum magnesium levels and deep tendon reflexes PO, 250–450 mg q3h, to maintain a serum level of 2.0–2.5 mEq/L | Hypotension or asystole may result from rapid administration; administer with an IV infusion pump Assess for respiratory depression and loss of deep tendon reflexes |
| **Nifedipine** (Procardia) Pregnancy Category C | PO, 10 mg every 20 min for two to three doses; maximum dose, 40 mg in 1 h | No information is available about whether drug crosses the placenta |
| **Oxytocics** | | |
| **Oxytocin** (Pitocin) | See Prototype Profile 23-1: Oxytocin | |
| **Methylergonovine maleate** (Methergine) Pregnancy Category C | After delivery of the placenta, IM, IV, 0.2 mg; repeat in 2–4 h if bleeding is severe To prevent excessive postpartum bleeding, PO, 0.2 mg 2–4 times daily for 2–7 d, if necessary | May cause increased blood pressure, headache, GI symptoms Routine IV administration should be avoided because risk for sudden hypertension and cerebrovascular accident (CVA) is increased with this route |

considered the prototype of the oxytocics (see Prototype Profile 23-1: Oxytocin).

## Analgesics

Parenteral opioid analgesics are used to control discomfort and pain during labor and delivery. They may prolong labor and cause sedation and respiratory depression in the mother and neonate. Meperidine may cause less neonatal depression than other opioid analgesics. Butorphanol is widely used. If neonatal respiratory depression occurs, it can be reversed by naloxone (Narcan).

Duramorph is a long-acting form of morphine that provides analgesia up to 24 hours after injection into the epidural catheter at the completion of a cesarean section.

Regional analgesia is achieved by the epidural injection of opioids (eg, fentanyl) or preservative-free morphine. Possible side effects include maternal urinary retention, but no significant effects on the fetus.

## Anesthetics

Local anesthetics also are used to control discomfort and pain. They are injected by physicians for regional anesthesia in the pelvic area. Epidural blocks involve injection into the epidural space of the spinal cord. Bupivacaine is commonly used. With regional anesthesia, the mother is usually conscious and comfortable, and the neonate is rarely depressed. Fentanyl may be combined with a small amount of an anesthetic drug for both analgesia and anesthesia. No significant effects on the fetus occurred in clinical studies.

## ■ NEONATAL THERAPEUTICS

In the neonate, any drug must be used cautiously. Drugs are usually given less often because they are metabolized and excreted slowly. Immature liver and kidney function prolongs drug action and increases risk for toxicity. Also,

---

### PROTOTYPE PROFILE 23-1
### *P* Oxytocin (oxs i TOE sin)

**Drug Class**
*Chemical:* Oxytocic drug
*Functional:* Labor-inducing agent

**Trade Names**
Pitocin, Syntocinon

**Therapeutic Indications**
To induce or augment labor contractions, to prevent or control postpartum hemorrhage, and to promote milk ejection

**Pharmacokinetics**
*Absorption*
PO, poorly absorbed

*Distribution*
Distributed widely into extracellular fluid; small amounts reach fetal circulation

*Metabolism*
Rapidly by liver

*Excretion*
Urine

**Pharmacodynamics**
*Onset of Action*
IV, Uterine contractions within 1 minute

*Duration*
Less than 30 min

**Contraindications/Precautions**
Significant cephalopelvic disproportion, fetal distress, undesirable fetal positioning that is undeliverable without conversion before delivery, hypertonic uterus, prolapse, total placenta previa

**Pregnancy Considerations**
Category X

**Dosage**
During labor and delivery, IV with infusion device; 2 milliunits/min, gradually increased to 20 milliunits/min, if necessary, to produce three or four contractions within 10-min periods. Prepare solution by adding 10 units (1 mL) of oxytocin to 1000 mL of 0.9% sodium chloride or 5% dextrose in 0.45% sodium chloride
To control postpartum hemorrhage: IV with infusion device; 10–40 units added to 1000 mL of 0.9% sodium chloride, infused at a rate to control bleeding
To prevent postpartum bleeding: IM, 3–10 units (0.3–1 mL) as a single dose
To promote milk ejection: topically: 1 spray of nasal solution to one or both nostrils 2–3 min before nursing

**Adverse Effects**
*Maternal*
Tetanic uterine contractions, fatal afibrinogenemia, uterine rupture, dysrhythmias, hypotension, anaphylaxis, antidiuretic effect, coma, death
*Fetal*
Dysrhythmias, neonatal jaundice, intracranial hemorrhage, hypoxia, brain damage, death

**Drug Interactions**
Incompatible with norepinephrine and prochlorperazine

**Herbal Supplements and Dietary Considerations**
None noted

drug therapy should be initiated with low doses, especially with drugs that are highly bound to plasma proteins. Neonates have few binding proteins, which leads to increased amounts of free, active drug and increased risk for toxicity. When assessing the neonate, drugs received by the mother during pregnancy, labor and delivery, and lactation must be considered.

At birth, some drugs are routinely administered to prevent hemorrhagic disease of the newborn and ophthalmia neonatorum. Hemorrhagic disease of the newborn occurs because the intestinal tract lacks the bacteria that normally synthesize vitamin K. Vitamin K is required for liver production of several clotting factors, including prothrombin. Thus, the neonate is at increased risk for bleeding during the first week of life. One dose of phytonadione, 0.5 to 1 mg, is injected at delivery or on admission to the nursery.

Ophthalmia neonatorum is a form of bacterial conjunctivitis that may cause ulceration and blindness. It may be caused by several bacteria, most commonly *Chlamydia trachomatis*, a sexually transmitted organism. Erythromycin ointment 0.5% is applied to each eye at delivery. It is effective against both chlamydial and gonococcal infections.

## GENERAL GUIDELINES: LACTATION

1. Most systemic drugs taken by the mother reach the infant in breast milk. For some, the amount of drug is too small to cause significant effects; for others, effects on the nursing infant are unknown or potentially adverse. Drugs that are considered safe, those to be used with caution, and those that are contraindicated are listed in Box 23-2.
2. Give medications only when clearly indicated, weighing potential benefit to the mother against possible harm to the nursing infant. For contraindicated drugs, it is usually recommended that the mother stop the drug or stop breast-feeding.
3. Any drugs used during lactation should be given in the lowest effective dose for the shortest effective time.
4. The American Academy of Pediatrics (AAP) supports breast-feeding as optimal nutrition for in-

---

### BOX 23-2 Drug Effects in Lactation

**Overview**

The American Academy of Pediatrics (AAP) recommends breast-feeding for optimal nutrition during the first year of life and is considered the most authoritative source of information about drug effects in lactation. Most drugs have not been tested in nursing women and no one knows exactly how a given drug will affect a nursing infant. Even the clinical practice guidelines from the AAP emphasize that the reported effects of drug safety or nonsafety are often anecdotal and based on observations in a single infant or a few infants rather than well-designed studies.

In general, maternal drug use during lactation should be cautious and based on the following assumptions:

1. There is some degree of risk with any systemic medication ingested by the mother. Some of the drug reaches the nursing infant, with the amount usually proportional to the amount in the mother's bloodstream. However, in many instances, the infant may not receive sufficient drug to produce adverse effects.
2. The lowest dose and the shortest effective duration are recommended.
3. Potential drug effects on nursing infants should be considered and the infants' health care providers should be consulted when indicated.
4. Most over-the-counter and prescription drugs, taken in moderation and only when needed, are thought to be safe.

**Drugs Generally Considered Safe During Lactation**

Acetaminophen, antibacterials (penicillins and cephalosporins), anticoagulants (heparin or warfarin), antiepilepsy medications, antihistamines, antihypertensives (angiotensin-converting enzyme [ACE] inhibitors, calcium channel blockers), butorphanol, caffeine (in moderate amounts), corticosteroids (prednisolone or inhaled products), cromolyn, decongestants (oxymetolazine nose drops or spray), digoxin, famotidine, ibuprofen, insulin, levothyroxine, progestin-only birth control pills (the "mini-pill"), sucralfate

**Drugs To Be Used With Caution During Lactation**

Alcohol (within 2 hours of breast-feeding), aluminum-containing antacids, amantadine, antianxiety agents (benzodiazepines), antibacterials (chloramphenicol, metronidazole, nitrofurantoin, sulfonamides), antidepressants (bupropion, tricyclics, and selective serotonin receptor inhibitors), antihistamine (clemastine), antipsychotics (older or typical agents), aspirin, beta blockers (acebutolol, atenolol), corticosteroids (systemic drugs may suppress growth, interfere with endogenous corticosteroid production, or cause other adverse effects in nursing infants), diuretics, dyslipidemics (cholestyramine [may cause severe constipation in the infant], statins), methadone, metoclopramide, theophylline

**Drugs That Are Contraindicated During Lactation**

If these drugs are required, breast-feeding should usually be stopped: Amiodarone, antibacterials (fluoroquinolones, tetracyclines, trimethoprim [may interfere with folic acid metabolism in the infant]), antineoplastics (cyclophosphamide, doxorubicin, methotrexate, most others), bromocriptine (decreases milk production), caffeine (large amounts), cyclosporine, drugs of abuse (amphetamines, cocaine, heroin, marijuana, phencyclidine, nicotine), ergotamine, isotretinoin, lithium, phenytoin

fants and does not recommend stopping during maternal drug therapy unless necessary. In some instances, mothers may pump and discard breast milk while receiving therapeutic drugs, to maintain lactation.

5. Women with human immunodeficiency virus (HIV) infection should not breast-feed. The virus can be transmitted to the nursing infant.

## NURSING PROCESS

### Assessment

Assess each female client of reproductive age for possible pregnancy. If the client is known to be pregnant, assess status in relation to pregnancy, as follows:

- Length of gestation
- Use of prescription, over-the-counter, herbal, non-therapeutic, and illegal drugs
- Acute and chronic health problems that may influence the pregnancy or require drug therapy
- With premature labor, assess length of gestation, the frequency and quality of uterine contractions, the amount of vaginal bleeding or discharge, and the length of labor. Also determine whether any tissue has been expelled from the vagina. When abortion is inevitable, oxytocics may be given. When stopping labor is possible or desired, a tocolytic may be given.
- When spontaneous labor occurs in normal, full-term pregnancy, assess frequency and quality of uterine contractions, amount of cervical dilatation, fetal heart rate and quality, and maternal blood pressure.
- Assess antepartum women for intention to breastfeed.

### Nursing Diagnoses

- Risk for Injury: Damage to fetus or neonate from maternal ingestion of drugs
- Noncompliance related to ingestion of nonessential drugs during pregnancy
- Risk for Injury related to possible damage to mother or infant during the birth process
- Deficient Knowledge: Drug effects during pregnancy and lactation

### Planning/Goals

*The client will:*

- Avoid unnecessary drug ingestion when pregnant or likely to become pregnant

- Use nonpharmacologic measures to relieve symptoms associated with pregnancy or other health problems when possible
- Obtain optimal care during pregnancy, labor and delivery, and the postpartum period
- Avoid behaviors that may lead to complications of pregnancy and labor and delivery
- Breast-feed safely and successfully if desired

### Interventions

- Use nondrug measures to prevent the need for drug therapy during pregnancy.
- Provide optimal prenatal care and counseling to promote a healthy pregnancy (eg, regular monitoring of blood pressure, weight, blood sugar, urine protein, and counseling about nutrition and other health-promoting activities).
- Help clients and families cope with complications of pregnancy, including therapeutic abortion.
- Counsel candidates for therapeutic abortion about methods and expected outcomes; counsel abortion clients about contraceptive techniques.

### Evaluation

- Observe and interview regarding actions taken to promote reproductive and general health.
- Observe and interview regarding compliance with instructions for promoting and maintaining a healthy pregnancy.
- Interview regarding ingestion of therapeutic and non-therapeutic drugs during prepregnant, pregnant, and lactating states.
- Observe and interview regarding the health status of the mother and neonate.

## Nursing Actions
## Abortifacients, Tocolytics, and Oxytocics

| Nursing Actions | Rationale/Explanation |
|---|---|
| 1. Administer accurately. | |
| a. Give abortifacients orally (PO), intramuscularly (IM), or intravaginally. | |
| b. Give tocolytics intravenously (IV) initially, via an infusion pump, then PO. With IV ritodrine, have the client lie in the left lateral position. | The side-lying position decreases risks of hypotension. |

*(continued)*

## *Nursing Actions*
## Abortifacients, Tocolytics, and Oxytocics (Continued)

| *Nursing Actions* | *Rationale/Explanation* |
|---|---|
| c. For IV oxytocin, dilute the drug in an IV sodium chloride solution, and piggyback the solution into a primary IV line. Use an infusion pump to administer. | Oxytocin may cause water intoxication, which is less likely to occur if the drug is given in a saline solution. Piggybacking allows regulation of the oxytocin drip without interrupting the main IV line. Infusion pumps deliver more accurate doses and minimize the risk of overdosage. |
| d. Give IM oxytocin immediately after delivery of the placenta. | To prevent excessive postpartum bleeding |
| **2. Observe for therapeutic effects.** | |
| a. When an abortifacient is given, observe for the onset of uterine bleeding and the expulsion of the fetus and placenta. | Abortion usually occurs within 24 h after a prostaglandin is given and approximately 5 d after mifepristone administration. |
| b. When a tocolytic drug is given in threatened abortion or premature labor, observe for absent or decreased uterine contractions. | The goal of drug therapy is to stop the labor process. |
| c. When oxytocin is given to induce or augment labor, observe for firm uterine contractions at a rate of three to four per 10 min. Each contraction should be followed by a palpable relaxation period. Examine periodically for cervical dilatation and effacement. | Oxytocin is given to stimulate the normal labor process. Contractions should become regular and increase in duration and intensity. |
| d. When oxytocin or an ergot alkaloid is given to prevent or control postpartum bleeding, observe for a small, firm uterus and minimal vaginal bleeding. | These agents control bleeding by causing strong uterine contractions. The uterus can be palpated in the lower abdomen. |
| **3. Observe for adverse effects.** | |
| a. With mifepristone, observe for excessive uterine bleeding and abdominal pain | These effects are uncommon but may occur. |
| b. With prostaglandins, observe for: | |
| (1) Nausea, vomiting, diarrhea | These are the most common adverse effects. They result from drug-induced stimulation of gastrointestinal smooth muscle. |
| (2) Fever, cardiac dysrhythmias, bronchospasm, convulsions, chest pain, muscle aches | These effects occur less often. Bronchospasm is more likely to occur in clients with asthma; seizures are more likely in clients with known epilepsy. |
| c. With ritodrine, observe for: | |
| (1) Change in fetal heart rate | This is a common adverse effect and may be significant if changes are extreme or prolonged. |
| (2) Maternal effects (eg, palpitations, dysrhythmias, changes in blood pressure, nausea and vomiting, hyperglycemia, dyspnea, chest pain, anaphylactic shock). | |
| d. With oxytocin, observe for: | |
| (1) Excessive stimulation of uterine contractility (hypertonicity, tetany, rupture, cervical and perineal lacerations, fetal hypoxia, dysrhythmias, death or damage from rapid, forceful propulsion through the birth canal) | Most likely to occur when excessive doses are given to initiate or augment labor |
| (2) Hypotension or hypertension | Usual obstetric doses do not cause significant change in blood pressure. Large doses may cause an initial drop in blood pressure, followed by a sustained elevation. |
| (3) Water intoxication (convulsions, coma) | |
| e. With ergot preparations, observe for: | |
| (1) Nausea, vomiting, diarrhea | These drugs stimulate the vomiting center of the brain and stimulate contraction of gastrointestinal smooth muscle. |
| (2) Symptoms of ergot poisoning—coolness, numbness and tingling of extremities, headache, vomiting, dizziness, thirst, convulsions, weak pulse, confusion, chest pain, and muscle weakness and pain | The ergot alkaloids are highly toxic. Circulatory impairments may result from vasoconstriction and vascular insufficiency. Large doses also damage capillary endothelium and may cause thrombosis and occlusion. |
| (3) Hypertension | Hypertension may result from generalized vasoconstriction. |

*(continued)*

## *Nursing Actions*

### Abortifacients, Tocolytics, and Oxytocics (Continued)

| Nursing Actions | Rationale/Explanation |
|---|---|
| 4. **Observe for drug interactions.** | |
| a. Drugs that alter effects of prostaglandins: | |
| (1) Aspirin and other nonsteroidal anti-inflammatory agents, such as ibuprofen | These drugs inhibit effects of prostaglandins. When given concurrently with abortifacient prostaglandins, the abortive process is prolonged. |
| b. Drugs that alter effects of ritodrine: | |
| (1) Beta-adrenergic blocking agents (eg, propranolol) | Decreased effectiveness of ritodrine, which is a beta-adrenergic stimulating (agonist) agent |
| (2) Corticosteroids | Increased risk of pulmonary edema |
| c. Drugs that alter effects of oxytocin: | |
| (1) Vasoconstrictors, such as epinephrine and other adrenergic drugs | Additive vasoconstriction with risks of severe, persistent hypertension and intracranial hemorrhage |
| d. Drugs that alter effects of ergot alkaloids: | |
| (1) Propranolol (Inderal) | Additive vasoconstriction |
| (2) Vasoconstrictors | See oxytocin, above. |

## CLIENT TEACHING GUIDELINES
### Drug Use During Pregnancy and Lactation

✔ Any systemic drug ingested by a pregnant woman reaches the fetus and may interfere with fetal growth and development. For most drugs, safety during pregnancy has not been established, and all drugs are relatively contraindicated. Therefore, any drug use must be cautious and minimal to avoid potential damage to the fetus.

✔ Avoid drugs when possible and use them very cautiously when necessary. If women who are sexually active and not using contraception take any drugs, there is a high risk that potentially harmful agents may be ingested before pregnancy is suspected or confirmed.

✔ Lifestyle or nontherapeutic drugs associated with problems during pregnancy include alcohol, caffeine, and cigarette smoking. Women should completely avoid alcohol when trying to conceive and throughout pregnancy; no amount is considered safe. Caffeine intake should be limited to about three caffeinated beverages per day; excessive intake should be avoided. Women who smoke should quit if possible during pregnancy, to avoid the effects of nicotine, carbon monoxide, and other chemicals on the fetus.

✔ Herbal supplements are not recommended; their effects during pregnancy are largely unknown.

✔ Measures to prevent the need for drug therapy include a healthful lifestyle (adequate nutrition, exercise, rest and sleep; avoiding alcohol and cigarette smoking) and avoiding infection (personal hygiene, avoiding contact with people known to have infections, maintaining indicated immunizations).

✔ Nondrug measures to relieve common health problems include positioning, adequate food and fluid intake, and deep breathing.

✔ See a health care provider as soon as pregnancy is suspected.

✔ Inform any health care provider from whom treatment is sought if there is a possibility of pregnancy.

✔ Many drugs are excreted in breast milk to some extent and reach the nursing infant. The infant's health care provider should be informed about medications taken by the nursing mother and consulted about potential drug effects on the infant. Before taking over-the-counter medications, consult a health care provider. In regard to nontherapeutic drugs, recommendations include the following:

1. Alcohol should be used in moderation and nursing should be withheld temporarily after alcohol consumption (1–2 hours per drink). Alcohol reaches the baby through breast milk, with the highest concentration about 30 to 60 minutes after drinking (60–90 minutes if taken with food). The effects of alcohol on the baby are directly related to the amount of alcohol the mother consumes. Moderate to heavy drinking (2 or more drinks per day) can interfere with the ability to breast-feed, harm the baby's motor development, and slow the baby's weight gain. If you plan to drink (eg, wine with dinner), you can avoid breast-feeding for a few hours (until the alcohol has time to leave your system) or you can pump your milk before drinking and give it to the baby after you have had the alcohol. You can also pump and discard the milk that is most affected by the ingested alcohol.

2. Caffeine is considered compatible with breast-feeding. However, large amounts should be avoided because infants may be jittery and have difficulty sleeping.

*(continued)*

CLIENT TEACHING GUIDELINES
## Drug Use During Pregnancy and Lactation (Continued)

3. Cigarette smoking is contraindicated. Nicotine and an active metabolite are concentrated in milk and the amounts reaching the infant are proportional to the number of cigarettes smoked by the mother. Ideally, the mother who smokes would stop. If unable or unwilling to stop, she should decrease the number of cigarettes as much as possible, avoid smoking before nursing, and avoid smoking (or allowing other people to smoke) in the same room with the infant. The risk for sudden infant death syndrome (SIDS) is greater when a mother smokes or when the baby is around secondhand (or passive) smoke. Maternal smoking and passive smoke may also increase respiratory and ear infections in infants.

## Critical Thinking Exercises

1. An antibacterial agent that crosses the placenta but apparently produces no adverse effects on the fetus is:
   a. Ciprofloxacin
   b. Penicillin
   c. Tetracycline
   d. Vancomycin

2. Counseling about the use of immunizations during pregnancy is an important nursing consideration. A pregnant women should be instructed to avoid receiving:
   a. Measles vaccines
   b. Tetanus toxoid
   c. Hyperimmune globulins
   d. Influenza vaccine

3. Drugs given to inhibit labor and maintain the pregnancy are called:
   a. Abortifacients
   b. Prostaglandins
   c. Tocolytics
   d. Oxytocics

4. The anticoagulant of choice during pregnancy is:
   a. Heparin
   b. Warfarin
   c. Vitamin K
   d. Protamine sulfate

5. Nontherapeutic drugs may negatively affect the fetus. Cigarette smoking is contraindicated during pregnancy because it produces which of the following fetal effects?
   a. Increased risk for cardiac dysrhythmias
   b. Decreased flow of blood and oxygen to the placenta and uterus
   c. Increased risk for intracranial bleeding
   d. Increased uterine contractility

## SELECTED REFERENCES

Briggs, G., Freeman, R., & Yaffee, S. (1998). *Drugs in pregnancy and lactation* (5th ed.). Baltimore: Williams & Wilkins.

Creinin, M. (1999). Medical termination of pregnancy. In J. Sciarra (Ed.), *Obstetrics and gynecology*. Philadelphia: Lippincott Williams & Wilkins.

*Drug facts and comparisons.* (Updated monthly). St. Louis: Facts and Comparisons.

Harding, J. (1999). The use of psychotropic medications during pregnancy and lactation. In J. Sciarra (Ed.), *Obstetrics and gynecology.* Philadelphia: Lippincott Williams & Wilkins.

Jain, J. K., Kuo, J., & Mishell, D. R. (1999). A comparison of two dosing regimens of intravaginal misoprostol for second trimester pregnancy termination. *Obstetrics and Gynecology, 93*, 571–575.

Lacy, C. F., Armstrong, L. L., Goldman, M. P., & Lance, L. L. (2003). *Lexi-Comp's drug information handbook* (11th ed.). Hudson, OH: American Pharmaceutical Association.

Niebyl, J. (1999). Drugs and related areas in pregnancy. In J. Sciarra (Ed.), *Obstetrics and gynecology*. Philadelphia: Lippincott Williams & Wilkins.

Olds, S., London, M., & Ladewig, P. (2000). *Maternal-newborn nursing* (6th ed.). Upper Saddle River, NJ: Prentice Hall.

Pangle, B. L. (2000). Drugs in pregnancy and lactation. In E. T. Herfindal & D. R. Gourley (Eds.), *Textbook of therapeutics: Drug and disease management* (7th ed., pp. 2037–2050). Philadelphia: Lippincott Williams & Wilkins.

Pigarelli, D. L., & Kraus, C. K. (2002). Pregnancy and lactation: Therapeutic considerations. In J. T. DiPiro, R. L. Talbert, G. C. Yee, G. R. Matzke, B. G. Wells, & L. M. Posey (Eds.), *Pharmacotherapy: A pathophysiologic approach* (5th ed., pp. 1413–1429). New York: McGraw-Hill.

Porth, C. M. (2002). *Pathophysiology: Concepts of altered health states* (6th ed.). Philadelphia: Lippincott Williams & Wilkins.

Reisner, L. A. (2000). Pain management. In E. T. Herfindal & D. R. Gourley (Eds.), *Textbook of therapeutics: Drug and disease management* (7th. ed., pp. 1157–1183). Philadelphia: Lippincott Williams & Wilkins.

Ressel, G. (2002). Practice guidelines: AAP updates statement for transfer of drugs and other chemicals into breast milk. *American Family Physician, 65*(5), 979–980.

Schroeder, B. M. (2002). Practice guidelines: ACOG practice bulletin on diagnosing and managing preeclampsia and eclampsia. *American Family Physician, 66*(2), 330–331.

Watts, D. H. (2002). Management of human immunodeficiency virus infection in pregnancy. *New England Journal of Medicine, 346*(24), 1879–1891.

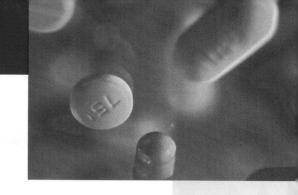

# 24

# Drugs Affecting Female Reproductive Health

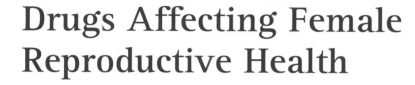

## OBJECTIVES

*After studying this chapter, the student will be able to:*

1 Discuss effects of endogenous estrogens and progestins.

2 Describe benefits and risks of postmenopausal hormone replacement therapy.

3 Identify adverse effects associated with estrogens, progestins, and hormonal contraceptives.

4 Apply nursing process with clients taking estrogens, progestins, and hormonal contraceptives.

5 Apply nursing process with clients dealing with infertility.

6 Outline recommended drug regimens for common sexually transmitted diseases.

## CRITICAL THINKING SCENARIO

*S*ally Chow, a perimenopausal woman, has concerns about hormone replacement therapy (HRT). She seeks information from you to help her make an informed choice about whether to use HRT.

✔ What are the benefits of HRT for the postmenopausal woman?

✔ What are the possible adverse effects of HRT for the postmenopausal woman?

✔ Devise teaching strategies helpful in teaching Ms. Chow about HRT.

✔ Define your role as a nurse in assisting Ms. Chow in her decision-making process.

## PROTOTYPE PROFILE

**clomiphene** (Clomid, Serophene), p. 427

# OVERVIEW

This chapter brings together drug regimens for several broad areas of female reproductive health: (1) estrogens, progestins, and hormonal contraceptives; (2) infertility; and (3) sexuality transmitted diseases. The major focus of this chapter is on estrogens, progestins, and hormonal contraceptives.

Although infertility is a condition that affects both a male and female as a couple, it is addressed in the section on female reproductive disorders. Although a brief discussion of infertility in males is outlined, fertility-promoting drugs in women are the emphasis.

The prevalence of sexually transmitted diseases (STDs) is a major health concern worldwide. The list of STDs continues to expand as an increasing number of organisms are identified through improved diagnostic techniques. Changing sexual attitudes and practices have played a key role in the risk for acquiring an STD. The drugs used to treat some of the more common STDs are described in Section 7, Drugs Used to Treat Infections; they are outlined here in table format in relation to specific STDs and their recommended drug therapy.

# ENDOGENOUS ESTROGENS AND PROGESTINS

Estrogens and progestins are female sex hormones produced primarily by the ovaries and secondarily by the adrenal cortices in nonpregnant women. Small amounts of estrogens are also synthesized in the liver, kidney, brain, skeletal muscle, testes, and adipose tissue. In normal premenopausal women, estrogen synthesis in adipose tissue may be a significant source of the hormone. Some evidence indicates that a minimum body weight (about 105 lb) and fat content (16% to 24%) are required for initiation and maintenance of the menstrual cycle. This view is supported by the observation that women with anorexia nervosa, chronic disease, or malnutrition and those who are long-distance runners usually have amenorrhea. With anorexia nervosa, regaining weight and body mass usually reestablishes normal menstrual patterns. Estrogen and progestin production is described in At the Foundation: Estrogens and Progestins.

## Estrogens

Three ovarian estrogens (estradiol, estrone, and estriol) are secreted in significant amounts. Estradiol is the major estrogen because it exerts more estrogenic activity than the other two combined. The main function of the estrogens is to promote growth in tissues related to reproduction and sexual characteristics in women. More specific effects of estrogens on body tissues are described in Box 24-1.

In nonpregnant women, between puberty and menopause, estrogens are secreted in a monthly cycle called the *menstrual cycle*. During the first half of the cycle, before ovulation, estrogens are secreted in progressively larger amounts. During the second half of the cycle, estrogens and progesterone are secreted in increasing amounts until 2 to 3 days before the onset of menstruation. At that time, secretion of both hormones decreases abruptly. When the endometrial lining of the uterus loses its hormonal stimulation, it is discharged vaginally as menstrual flow.

During pregnancy, the placenta produces large amounts of estrogen, mainly estriol. The increased estrogen causes enlargement of the uterus and breasts, growth of glandular tissue in the breasts, and relaxation of ligaments and joints in the pelvis. All these changes are necessary for growth and birth of the fetus.

Finally, estrogens are inactivated in the liver, partly or mainly by cytochrome P450 3A4 enzymes. Then, they are conjugated with glucuronic acid or sulfuric acid, which makes them water soluble and readily excreted through the kidneys. Metabolites are also formed in the gastrointestinal tract, brain, skin, and other steroid target tissues. Most of the conjugates are excreted in urine; some

## AT THE FOUNDATION: *Estrogens and Progestins*

The testes and adrenal glands secrete small amounts of progesterone. In men and postmenopausal women, the peripheral sites produce all endogenous estrogen. Almost no progesterone is synthesized in postmenopausal women.

Like other steroid hormones, estrogens and progestins are synthesized from cholesterol. The ovaries and adrenal glands can manufacture cholesterol or extract it from the blood. Through a series of chemical reactions, cholesterol is converted to progesterone, then to the androgens, testosterone and androstenedione. These male sex hormones are used by the ovaries to produce estrogens. After formation, the hormones are secreted into the bloodstream in response to stimulation by the anterior pituitary gonadotropic hormones, follicle-stimulating hormone (FSH), and luteinizing hormone (LH). In the bloodstream, the hormones combine with serum proteins and are transported to target tissues, where they enter body cells. They cross cell membranes easily because of their steroid structure and lipid solubility. Once inside the cells, they bind to estrogen or progestin receptors and regulate intracellular protein synthesis. Estrogen can enhance target tissue responses to progesterone by increasing progesterone receptors. Progesterone seems to inhibit tissue responses to estrogen by decreasing estrogen receptors.

## Effects of Endogenous Estrogens

### Breasts
- Stimulate growth at puberty by causing deposition of fat, formation of connective tissue, and construction of ducts. These ducts become part of the milk-producing apparatus after additional stimulation by progesterone.

### Sexual Organs
- Enlarge the fallopian tubes, uterus, vagina, and external genitalia at puberty, when estrogen secretion increases greatly.
- Cause the endometrial lining of the uterus to proliferate and develop glands that later nourish the implanted ovum when pregnancy occurs.
- Increase resistance of the epithelial lining of the vagina to trauma and infection.

### Skeleton
- Stimulate skeletal growth so that, beginning at puberty, height increases rapidly for several years. Estrogen then causes the epiphyses to unite with the shafts of the long bones, and linear growth is halted. This effect of estrogen is stronger than the similar effect of testosterone in the male. Consequently, women stop growing in height several years earlier than men and on the average are shorter than men.
- Conserve calcium and phosphorus for healthy bones and teeth. This action promotes bone formation and decreases bone loss.
- Broaden the pelvis in preparation for childbirth.

### Skin and Subcutaneous Tissue
- Increase vascularity in the skin. This leads to greater skin warmth and likelihood of bleeding in women.

- Cause deposition of fat in subcutaneous tissue, especially in the breasts, thighs, and buttocks, which produces the characteristic female figure.

### Anterior Pituitary Gland
- Decrease pituitary secretion of follicle-stimulating hormone and increase secretion of luteinizing hormone when blood levels are sufficiently high (negative feedback mechanism).

### Metabolism
- Affect metabolism of both reproductive and nonreproductive tissues. Estrogen receptors are found in female reproductive organs, breast tissue, bone, the brain, liver, heart, and blood vessels. They are also found in various tissues in men.
- Increase protein anabolism, bone growth, and epiphyseal closure in young girls.
- Decrease bone resorption.
- Increase sodium and water retention, serum triglycerides, and high-density lipoproteins (HDL or "good" cholesterol).
- Decrease low-density lipoproteins (LDL or "bad" cholesterol).
- Increase the amount of cholesterol in bile and thereby increase gallstone formation.

### Blood Coagulation
- Enhance coagulation by increasing blood levels of several clotting factors, including prothrombin and factors VII, IX, and X, and probably increase platelet aggregation.

are excreted in bile and recirculated to the liver or excreted in feces.

## Progesterone

Progesterone is a progestin concerned almost entirely with reproduction. In the nonpregnant woman, progesterone is secreted by the corpus luteum during the last half of the menstrual cycle, after ovulation. This hormone continues the changes in the endometrial lining of the uterus begun by estrogens during the first half of the menstrual cycle. These changes provide for implantation and nourishment of a fertilized ovum. When fertilization does not take place, the levels of estrogen and progesterone decrease, and menstruation occurs.

If the ovum is fertilized, progesterone acts to maintain the pregnancy. The corpus luteum produces progesterone during the first few weeks of gestation. Then, the placenta produces the progesterone needed to maintain the endometrial lining of the uterus. In addition to its effects on the uterus, progesterone prepares the breasts for lactation by promoting development of milk-producing cells. Milk is not secreted, however, until the cells are further stim-

ulated by prolactin from the anterior pituitary gland. Progesterone also may help maintain pregnancy by decreasing uterine contractility. This, in turn, decreases the risk for spontaneous abortion.

Progesterone, in general, has opposite effects on lipid metabolism compared with estrogen. That is, progestins decrease high-density lipoprotein (HDL) cholesterol and increase low-density lipoprotein (LDL) cholesterol, both of which increase risks for cardiovascular disease. Physiologic progesterone increases insulin levels but does not usually impair glucose tolerance. However, long-term administration of potent synthetic progestins such as norgestrel may decrease glucose tolerance and make diabetes mellitus more difficult to control. Like estrogen, progesterone is metabolized in the liver.

## ESTROGENS AND PROGESTINS USED AS DRUGS

- When exogenous estrogens and progestins are given for therapeutic purposes, they produce the same effects as endogenous (naturally occurring) hormones.

■ Several preparations of estrogens and progestins are available for various purposes and routes of administration:

■ *Naturally occurring, nonconjugated estrogens* (estradiol, estrone) *and natural progesterone* are given intramuscularly because they are rapidly metabolized if given orally. Some crystalline suspensions of estrogens and oil solutions of both estrogens and progesterone prolong drug action by slowing absorption.

■ *Conjugated estrogens* (eg, Premarin) and some synthetic derivatives of natural estrogens (eg, ethinyl estradiol) and natural progesterone (eg, norethindrone) are chemically modified to be effective with oral administration. The most widely used synthetic steroidal estrogen is ethinyl estradiol, which is used in hormonal contraceptives. Ethinyl estradiol is well absorbed with oral administration and reaches peak plasma levels within 2 hours. It is 98% bound to plasma proteins, and its half-life varies from 6 to 20 hours. It undergoes extensive first-pass hepatic metabolism and is further metabolized and conjugated in the liver, and the conjugates are excreted in bile and urine.

■ *Nonsteroidal, synthetic preparations* are usually given orally or topically. They are chemically altered to slow their metabolism in the liver. They are also less bound to serum proteins than the naturally occurring hormones.

■ Most hormonal contraceptives consist of a synthetic estrogen (eg, ethinyl estradiol) and a synthetic progestin (eg, norethindrone). Norethindrone undergoes first-pass metabolism so that it is only 65% bioavailable. It reaches peak plasma levels in 0.5 to 4 hours and has a half-life of 5 to 14 hours. It is metabolized in the liver and excreted in urine and feces.

■ Monophasic contraceptives contain fixed amounts of both estrogen and progestin components. Biphasics and triphasics contain either fixed amounts of estrogen and varied amounts of progestin or varied amounts of both estrogen and progestin. Biphasic and triphasic preparations mimic normal variations of hormone secretion, decrease the total dosage of hormones, and may decrease adverse effects.

These contraceptives are dispensed in containers with color-coded tablets that must be taken in the correct sequence. Dispensers with 28 tablets contain seven inactive or placebo tablets of a third color. A few contraceptive products contain a progestin only. These are not widely used because they are less effective in preventing pregnancy and are more likely to cause vaginal bleeding, which makes them less acceptable to many women.

■ Several combination products and alternative dosage forms are available to help individualize treatment and promote compliance. For example, several noncontraceptive combination oral tablets are available for treatment of menopausal symptoms and osteoporosis. Two combination products (Combi-Patch and Ortho Evra) are available in transdermal patches for topical application to skin. Also, along with several cream formulations, a vaginal tablet (Vagifem) and a vaginal ring (Estring) of estrogen are available for topical application in treating atrophic vaginitis. Estrogens, progestins, and hormonal contraceptives are usually self-administered at home. The home care nurse may encounter clients or family members taking one of the drugs when visiting the home for another purpose. Guidelines for strategies for ongoing evaluation and intervention are addressed in Home Care Considerations.

## Mechanisms of Action

The precise mechanisms by which estrogens and progestins produce their effects are unknown. Estrogens circulate in the bloodstream to target cells, where they enter the cells and combine with receptor proteins in cell cytoplasm. The estrogen–receptor complex is then transported to the cell nucleus where it interacts with deoxyribonucleic acid (DNA) to produce ribonucleic acid (RNA) and new DNA. These substances stimulate cell reproduction and production of various proteins. Progestins also diffuse freely into cells, where they bind to progesterone receptors.

Hormonal contraceptives act by several mechanisms. First, they inhibit hypothalamic secretion of gonadotropin-releasing hormone, which inhibits pituitary secretion of follicle-stimulating hormone (FSH) and luteinizing hormone (LH). When these gonadotropic hormones are absent, ovulation and therefore conception cannot occur. Second, the drugs produce cervical

## Home Care Considerations: Use of Estrogens and Progestin Drugs

*ASSESS:* medication regimen; assess for characteristics (eg, older age group, family history, thromboembolic disorders, known or suspected cancers of breast) that increase the risks for adverse effects.

*MONITOR:* the therapeutic and adverse effects of the drugs and the client's need for additional information and provide that information.

*EDUCATE:* to take the drugs as prescribed. In addition, clients may need encouragement to keep appointments for follow-up supervision and monitoring of blood pressure. When visiting families that include adolescent girls or young women, the nurse may need to teach about birth control or preventing osteoporosis by improving diet and exercise patterns. With families that include postmenopausal women, the nurse may need to teach about nonhormonal strategies for preventing or treating osteoporosis and cardiovascular disease. Reinforce additional teaching points (see Client Teaching Guidelines: Oral Contraceptives; Hormone Replacement Therapy; Infertility Agents).

mucus that resists penetration of spermatozoa into the upper reproductive tract. Third, the drugs interfere with endometrial maturation and reception of ova that are released and fertilized. These overlapping mechanisms make the drugs highly effective in preventing pregnancy.

## Indications for Use

### Estrogens

- **As replacement therapy in deficiency states.** Deficiency states usually result from hypofunction of the pituitary gland or the ovaries and may occur anytime during the life cycle. For example, in the adolescent girl with delayed sexual development, estrogen can be given to produce the changes that normally occur at puberty. In the woman of reproductive age (approximately 12 to 45 years of age), estrogens are sometimes used in menstrual disorders, including amenorrhea and abnormal uterine bleeding due to estrogen deficiency.
- **As a component in birth control pills and other contraceptive preparations.** An estrogen, combined with a progestin, is used widely in the 12- to 45-year-old group to control fertility. If pregnancy does occur, estrogens are contraindicated because their use during pregnancy has been associated with the occurrence of vaginal cancer in female offspring and possible harmful effects on male offspring.
- **Menopause.** Estrogens are given to relieve symptoms of estrogen deficiency (eg, atrophic vaginitis and vasomotor instability, which produces "hot flashes") and to prevent or treat osteoporosis. When estrogen is given to women with a uterus, a progestin is also given to prevent endometrial cancer. Such use is usually called ERT (estrogen replacement therapy) or HRT (hormone replacement therapy).

In addition, ERT and HRT have been used long-term for cardioprotective effects because it was thought that the drugs decreased myocardial infarctions and death from cardiovascular disease. This view was based largely on observational studies that indicated that postmenopausal women had a much higher risk for heart disease than premenopausal women. The difference was attributed to decreased hormone production at menopause. Now, the drugs are recommended for short-term use (eg, 2 years) to relieve menopausal symptoms, but not for long-term use for cardioprotective effects. A recent, well-done study indicated that risks are greater than benefits for combined estrogen-progestin therapy (Box 24-2). The part of the study concerned with estrogen replacement solely was stopped in February 2004 due to a slight stroke risk with estrogen replacement after hysterectomy.

Estrogens are contraindicated in impaired liver function, liver disease, or liver cancer. Impaired liver function may lead to impaired estrogen metabolism with resultant accumulation and adverse effects. In addition, women who have had jaundice during pregnancy have

an increased risk for recurrence if they take an estrogen-containing contraceptive. Any client in whom jaundice develops while taking estrogen should stop the drug. Because jaundice may indicate liver damage, the cause should be investigated.

### Progestins

Progestins are most often used in combination with an estrogen, in contraceptive products. They also are used to suppress ovarian function in dysmenorrhea, endometriosis, and uterine bleeding. These uses of progestins are extensions of the physiologic actions of progesterone on the neuroendocrine control of ovarian function and on the endometrium. For 20 to 25 years, approximately, they were used in combination with estrogen for long-term HRT in postmenopausal women with intact uteri. With HRT, the purpose of a progestin is to prevent endometrial cancer, which can occur with unopposed estrogenic stimulation. Currently, however, the combination is not recommended for long-term use because a research study indicated that the adverse effects outweigh the beneficial effects (see Box 24-2). Progestins are contraindicated in clients with impaired liver function or liver disease.

### Hormonal Contraceptives

The primary clinical indication for the use of hormonal contraceptives is to control fertility and prevent pregnancy. Some products are used for contraception after unprotected sexual intercourse. These preparations also are used to treat menstrual disorders (eg, amenorrhea, dysmenorrhea).

## Contraindications to Use

Because of their widespread effects on body tissues and reported adverse reactions, estrogens, progestins, and hormonal contraceptives are contraindicated in:

- Known or suspected pregnancy, because damage to the fetus may result
- Thromboembolic disorders, such as thrombophlebitis, deep vein thrombosis, or pulmonary embolism
- Known or suspected cancers of breast or genital tissues, because the drugs may stimulate tumor growth. An exception is the use of estrogens for treatment of metastatic breast cancer in women at least 5 years postmenopause.
- Undiagnosed vaginal or uterine bleeding
- Fibroid tumors of the uterus
- Active liver disease or impaired liver function
- History of cerebrovascular disease, coronary artery disease, thrombophlebitis, hypertension, or conditions predisposing to these disease processes
- Women older than 35 years of age who smoke cigarettes. These women have a greater risk for thromboembolic disorders if they take hormonal contraceptives, possibly because of increased platelet aggregation with

## BOX 24-2  Hormone Replacement Therapy in Postmenopausal Women

### Background

For many years, postmenopausal women have been treated with estrogen replacement therapy (ERT) to manage symptoms of menopause. In addition, estrogen was thought to have cardioprotective effects, partly because the incidence of heart attacks in women increased substantially after menopause and became similar to the incidence in men. Several studies also indicated beneficial effects in preventing osteoporosis, a common disorder in postmenopausal women. As a result of these observations, the use of ERT evolved from management of menopausal symptoms to prevention of cardiovascular disease and osteoporosis. Other benefits were also attributed to ERT. Because estrogen alone increases risks of endometrial cancer in women with an intact uterus, a progestin was added.

### Estrogen-Progestin Combinations

Combined estrogen/progestin hormone replacement therapy became the standard of care for women with an intact uterus and was widely prescribed for its perceived benefits in maintaining women's health. In 2002, the prevailing opinion changed dramatically to indicate that combined estrogen/progestin therapy should not be used to prevent cardiovascular disease in healthy postmenopausal women, because risks were greater than benefits.

This opinion resulted largely from the Women's Health Initiative (WHI), a randomized, controlled study involving >16,000 women with an intact uterus. The published report of the Writing Group for the Women's Health Initiative Investigators revealed that risks from long-term use of an estrogen-progestin combination (Prempro) outweighed its benefits. This part of the study was stopped after an average follow-up period of 5 years (8 years planned), because of a higher incidence of invasive breast cancer. Results also indicated increased risks of heart attacks, strokes, and blood clotting disorders and decreased risks of osteoporotic fractures and colon cancers.

Data analysis indicated that in 10,000 women taking the drug combination, there would be seven more coronary heart disease events, eight more strokes, eight more pulmonary emboli, eight more invasive breast cancers, six fewer colorectal cancers, and five fewer hip fractures. Although these numbers are not large and the risk is relatively small,

the investigators concluded that the drug combination produced more harm than benefit and should not be started or continued to prevent coronary heart disease (CHD) in healthy women.

The WHI study was done with healthy women, to see if the drugs would prevent CHD from developing. The Heart and Estrogen/Progestin Replacement Studies, HERS and HERS II, involved postmenopausal women with intact uteri who already had CHD. Results indicated that the drug combination (estrogen 0.625 mg and medroxyprogesterone 2.5 mg) conferred no benefit in relation to preventing serious cardiovascular events and actually increased risks during the first year of therapy. As with healthy women, the conclusion was that the hormones should not be started or continued in women with CHD for preventive purposes.

For individual women, the benefits in reducing symptoms of menopause, fractures from osteoporosis, and colon cancer must be weighed against the increased risks of CHD, thromboembolic stroke, venous thromboembolism, breast cancer, and cholecystitis. Thromboembolic disorders are most likely to occur during the first year of use; risks of developing breast cancer and gallbladder disease increase with the duration of drug use. If the combined drugs are prescribed to relieve menopausal symptoms in women who have not had a hysterectomy, they should probably be used for 1 to 2 years, then discontinued.

### Estrogen Alone

The part of the WHI study that explored the use of estrogen-alone therapy in post-hysterectomy women was stopped a year early because the hormone increased the risk of stroke and offered no protection against heart disease. The increased risk was small, estimated at about eight extra strokes per year for every 10,000 women taking estrogen. The study also found that estrogen-alone therapy significantly increased the hazard of deep vein thrombosis, but had no significant effect on the risk of colorectal or breast cancer. A reduced risk of hip and other fractures was reported. A related study also found that the hormone might also increase the risk of dementia and mild cognitive impairment in older women. As recommended for the other group, individual women and their health care providers must weigh risks versus benefits.

---

estrogen ingestion and cigarette smoking. In addition, estrogen increases hepatic production of blood clotting factors.

■ Family history of breast or reproductive system cancer

## INDIVIDUAL ESTROGENS, PROGESTINS, AND COMBINATION PRODUCTS

Clinical indications, routes of administration, and dosages are discussed in Drugs at a Glance 24-1: Estrogens, and

Drugs at a Glance 24-2: Progestins. Common noncontraceptive products are listed in Drugs at a Glance 24-3: Noncontraceptive Estrogen-Progestin Combinations, and hormonal contraceptive agents are listed in Table 24-1. Given the wide range of estrogen and combination products, there is no prototype identified.

## Herbal and Dietary Supplement

**Black cohosh** is an herb used to self-treat symptoms of menopause. It is reportedly effective in relieving vaso-

*(text continues on page 421)*

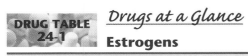

**DRUG TABLE 24-1**

*Drugs at a Glance*

**Estrogens**

| | Routes and Dosage Ranges for Various Indications | | | |
|---|---|---|---|---|
| Generic/ Trade Name | Menopausal Symptoms | Female Hypogonadism | Prevention of Osteoporosis | Other |
| **Conjugated estrogens** (synthetic) (Cenestin) | PO 0.625–1.25 mg daily | | | |
| **Conjugated estrogens** (Premarin) Pregnancy Category X | PO 0.3–1.25 mg daily for 21 d followed by 7 d without the drug | PO 2.5–7.5 mg daily in divided doses, cyclically, 20 d on, 10 d off the drug | PO 0.625 mg daily for 21 d, then 7 d without the drug | Dysfunctional uterine bleeding: IM or intravenous for emergency use, 25 mg, repeated in 6–12 h if necessary Atrophic vaginitis: topically, 2.4 g of vaginal cream inserted daily |
| **Dienestrol** (DV) | | | | Atrophic or senile vaginitis: topically, vaginal cream applied two or three times daily for approximately 2 wk, then reduced to 3 times weekly |
| **Esterified estrogens** (Estratab) Pregnancy Category X | PO 0.3–1.25 mg daily for 21 d, then 7 d without the drug | PO 2.5–7.5 mg daily in divided doses, for 21 d, then 7 d without the drug | | |
| **Estradiol** (Estrace) Pregnancy Category X | PO 1–2 mg daily for 3 wk, then 1 wk off or daily Monday through Friday, none on Saturday or Sunday | | PO 0.5 mg daily for 23 d and no drug for 5 d each month | Atrophic vaginitis, cream, 2–4 g daily for 2 wk, then 1–2 g daily for 2 wk, then 1 g 1–3 times weekly; vaginal ring (Estring), 1 every 3 mo |
| **Estradiol cypionate** (Depo-Estradiol) Pregnancy Category X | IM 1–5 mg every 3–4 wk | IM 1.5–2 mg at monthly intervals | | |
| **Estradiol hemihydrate** (Vagifem) Pregnancy Category X | | | | Atrophic vaginitis, 1 tablet, inserted into vagina, daily for 2 wk, then twice weekly |
| **Estradiol transdermal system** (Estraderm) Pregnancy Category X | Topically to skin, 1 patch one or two times weekly for 3 wk followed by 1 wk off (cyclically) | Same as for menopause | 0.05 mg daily | |
| **Estradiol valerate** (Delestrogen) Pregnancy Category X | IM 10–20 mg every 4 wk | IM 10–20 mg every 4 wk | | |
| **Estrone** Pregnancy Category X | IM 0.1–0.5 mg weekly in single or divided doses | IM 0.1–2 mg weekly | | Dysfunctional uterine bleeding: IM 2–4 mg daily for several days until bleeding is controlled, followed by progestin for 1 wk |

*(continued)*

**DRUG TABLE 24-1**

## Drugs at a Glance
### Estrogens (Continued)

| Generic/ Trade Name | Routes and Dosage Ranges for Various Indications | | | |
| | Menopausal Symptoms | Female Hypogonadism | Prevention of Osteoporosis | Other |
| --- | --- | --- | --- | --- |
| **Estropipate** (Ogen) Pregnancy Category X | PO 0.625–5 mg daily, cyclically | PO 1.25–7.5 mg daily for 3 wk, followed by an 8- to 10-d rest period. Repeat as needed. | PO 0.625 mg daily 25 d, no drug 6 d each month | Ovarian failure: same dosage as for female hypogonadism |
| **Ethinyl estradiol** (Estinyl) Pregnancy Category X | PO 0.02–0.05 mg daily, cyclically | PO 0.05 mg one to three times daily for 2 wk with addition of progestin for last 2 wk of month | | Atrophic vaginitis: topically, 1–2 g vaginal cream daily |

**DRUG TABLE 24-2**

## Drugs at a Glance
### Progestins

| Generic/ Trade Name | Routes and Dosage Ranges for Various Indications | | | |
| | Menopausal Disorders | Endometriosis | Endometrial Cancer | Other |
| --- | --- | --- | --- | --- |
| **Hydroxyprogesterone caproate** (Hylutin) Pregnancy Category X | Amenorrhea, dysfunctional uterine bleeding: IM 375 mg. If no bleeding after 21 d, begin cyclic therapy with estradiol and repeat every 4 wk for 4 cycles | | | Uterine adenocarcinoma: IM 1 g or more initially; repeat one or more times each week (maximum, 7 g/wk). Stop when relapse occurs or after 12 wk with no response. Test for endogenous estrogen production: IM 250 mg, repeated in 4 wk. Bleeding 7–14 d after injection indicates endogenous estrogen. |
| **Medroxyprogesterone acetate** (Depo-Provera, Provera) Pregnancy Category X | Dysfunctional uterine bleeding: PO 5–10 mg daily for 5–10 d beginning on 16th or 21st d of cycle | | IM 400–1000 mg weekly until improvement, then 400 mg monthly | |
| **Megestrol acetate** (Megace) Pregnancy Category X | Amenorrhea: PO 5–10 mg daily for 5–10 d | | PO 40–320 mg daily in 4 divided doses for at least 2 mo | Breast cancer:  PO 160 mg daily in 4 divided doses for at least 2 mo |
| **Norethindrone acetate** (Aygestin) Pregnancy Category X | Amenorrhea, dysfunctional uterine bleeding: PO 2.5–10 mg daily, starting on 5th d of menstrual cycle and ending on 25th d | PO 5 mg daily for 2 wk, increased by 2.5 mg daily every 2 wk to dose of 15 mg. Then give 10–15 mg daily for maintenance. | | Contraception:  See Table 24–3 |

*(continued)*

### DRUG TABLE 24-2

*Drugs at a Glance*

## Progestins (Continued)

| | Routes and Dosage Ranges for Various Indications | | | |
|---|---|---|---|---|
| Generic/ Trade Name | Menopausal Disorders | Endometriosis | Endometrial Cancer | Other |
| **Progesterone** Pregnancy Category X (injection) | Amenorrhea, dysfunctional uterine bleeding: IM 5–10 mg for 6–8 consecutive d | | | |

### DRUG TABLE 24-3

*Drugs at a Glance*

## Noncontraceptive Estrogen-Progestin Combinations

| Trade Name | Estrogen | Progestin | Indications for Use | Routes and Dosage Ranges |
|---|---|---|---|---|
| *Pregnancy Category X for all estrogens* | | | | |
| Activelle | Estradiol, 1 mg | Norethindrone, 0.5 mg | Menopausal symptoms Prevention of osteoporosis | PO, 1 tablet daily |
| Combi-Patch | Estradiol, 0.05 mg | Norethindrone, 0.14 mg or 0.25 mg | Estrogen deficiency states due to menopause, hypogonadism, castration, or primary ovarian failure | 1 transdermal patch twice weekly |
| Femhrt | Ethinyl estradiol, 5 mcg | Norethindrone, 1 mg | Menopausal symptoms Prevention of osteoporosis | PO, 1 tablet daily |
| Ortho-Prefest | Estradiol, 1 mg* | Norgestimate, 0.09 mg | Menopausal symptoms Prevention of osteoporosis | PO, 1 tablet estrogen-only (pink) daily for 3 days, then 1 combination tablet (white) daily for 3 days. Repeat this 6-d regimen continuously, without interruption |
| Premphase | Conjugated estrogens, 0.625 mg* | Medroxyprogesterone, 5 mg | Menopausal symptoms Prevention of osteoporosis | PO, 1 tablet of estrogen-only once daily on days 1–14, then 1 combination tablet once daily on days 15–28 |
| Prempro | Conjugated estrogens, 0.625 mg | Medroxyprogesterone, 2.5 or 5 mg | Menopausal symptoms Prevention of osteoporosis | PO, 1 tablet once daily |

*Also available with estrogen only.

## TABLE 24-1    Oral and Other Contraceptives

| Trade Name | Phase | Estrogen (mcg) | Progestin (mg) |
|---|---|---|---|
| *Monophasics* | | | |
| Alesse | | Ethinyl estradiol 20 | Levonorgestrel 0.1 |
| Apri | | Ethinyl estradiol 30 | Desogestrel 0.15 |
| Aviane | | Ethinyl estradiol 20 | Levonorgestrel 0.1 |
| Brevicon | | Ethinyl estradiol 35 | Norethindrone 0.5 |
| Demulen 1/35 | | Ethinyl estradiol 35 | Ethynodiol 1 |
| Demulen 1/50 | | Ethinyl estradiol 50 | Ethynodiol 1 |
| Desogen | | Ethinyl estradiol 30 | Desogestrel 0.15 |
| Levlen | | Ethinyl estradiol 30 | Levonorgestrel 0.15 |
| Levlite | | Ethinyl estradiol 20 | Levonorgestrel 0.1 |
| Levora | | Ethinyl estradiol 30 | Levonorgestrel 0.15 |
| Loestrin 21 1.5/30 | | Ethinyl estradiol 30 | Norethindrone 1.5 |
| Loestrin Fe 1/20 | | Ethinyl estradiol 20 | Norethindrone 1 |
| Loestrin Fe 1.5/30 | | Ethinyl estradiol 30 | Norethindrone 1.5 |
| Lo/Ovral | | Ethinyl estradiol 30 | Norgestrel 0.3 |
| Low-Orgestrel | | Ethinyl estradiol 30 | Norgestrel 0.3 |
| Microgestin Fe 1/20 | | Ethinyl estradiol 20 | Norethindrone 1 |
| Microgestin Fe 1.5/30 | | Ethinyl estradiol 30 | Norethindrone 1.5 |
| Modicon | | Ethinyl estradiol 35 | Norethindrone 0.5 |
| Necon 0.5/35 | | Ethinyl estradiol 35 | Norethindrone 0.5 |
| Necon 1/35 | | Ethinyl estradiol 35 | Norethindrone 1 |
| Necon 1/50 | | Mestranol 50 | Norethindrone 1 |
| Nordette | | Ethinyl estradiol 30 | Levonorgestrel 0.15 |
| Norinyl 1 + 35 | | Ethinyl estradiol 35 | Norethindrone 1 |
| Norinyl 1 + 50 | | Mestranol 50 | Norethindrone 1 |
| Nortrel 0.5/35 | | Ethinyl estradiol 35 | Norethindrone 0.5 |
| Nortrel 1/35 | | Ethinyl estradiol 35 | Norethindrone 1 |
| Ogestrel | | Ethinyl estradiol 50 | Norgestrel 0.5 |
| Ortho-Cept | | Ethinyl estradiol 30 | Desogestrel 0.15 |
| Ortho-Cyclen | | Ethinyl estradiol 35 | Norgestimate 0.25 |
| Ortho-Novum 1/35 | | Ethinyl estradiol 35 | Norethindrone 1 |
| Ortho-Novum 1/50 | | Mestranol 50 | Norethindrone 1 |
| Ovcon-35 | | Ethinyl estradiol 35 | Norethindrone 0.4 |
| Ovcon-50 | | Ethinyl estradiol 50 | Norethindrone 1 |
| Ovral-28 | | Ethinyl estradiol 50 | Norgestrel 0.5 |
| Yasmin | | Ethinyl estradiol 30 | Drospirenone 3 |
| Zovia 1/35E | | Ethinyl estradiol 35 | Ethynodiol 1 |
| Zovia 1/50E | | Ethinyl estradiol 50 | Ethynodiol 1 |
| *Biphasics* | | | |
| Jenest-28 | I: 10 d | Ethinyl estradiol 35 | Norethindrone 0.5 |
| | II: 11 d | Ethinyl estradiol 35 | Norethindrone 1 |
| Mircette | I: 21 d | Ethinyl estradiol 20 | Desogestrel 0.15 |
| | II: 5 d | Ethinyl estradiol 10 | |
| Necon 10/11 | I: 10 d | Ethinyl estradiol 35 | Norethindrone 0.5 |
| | II: 11 d | Ethinyl estradiol 35 | Norethindrone 1 |
| Ortho-Novum 10/11 | I: 10 d | Ethinyl estradiol 35 | Norethindrone 0.5 |
| | II: 11 d | Ethinyl estradiol 35 | Norethindrone 1 |
| *Triphasics* | | | |
| Estrostep 21 | I: 5 d | Ethinyl estradiol 20 | Norethindrone 1 |
| | II: 7 d | Ethinyl estradiol 30 | Norethindrone 1 |
| | III: 9 d | Ethinyl estradiol 35 | Norethindrone 1 |
| Estrostep Fe | I: 5 d | Ethinyl estradiol 20 | Norethindrone 1 |
| | II: 7 d | Ethinyl estradiol 30 | Norethindrone 1 |
| | III: 9 d | Ethinyl estradiol 35 | Norethindrone 1 |

*(continued)*

## TABLE 24-1  Oral and Other Contraceptives (Continued)

| Trade Name | Phase | Estrogen (mcg) | Progestin (mg) |
|---|---|---|---|
| Ortho-Novum 7/7/7 | I: 7 d | Ethinyl estradiol 35 | Norethindrone 0.5 |
| | II: 7 d | Ethinyl estradiol 35 | Norethindrone 0.75 |
| | III: 7 d | Ethinyl estradiol 35 | Norethindrone 1 |
| Ortho Tri-Cyclen | I: 7 d | Ethinyl estradiol 35 | Norgestimate 0.18 |
| | II: 9 d | Ethinyl estradiol 35 | Norgestimate 0.215 |
| | III: 5 d | Ethinyl estradiol 35 | Norgestimate 0.25 |
| Tri-Levlen | I: 6 d | Ethinyl estradiol 30 | Levonorgestrel 0.05 |
| | II: 5 d | Ethinyl estradiol 40 | Levonorgestrel 0.075 |
| | III: 10 d | Ethinyl estradiol 30 | Levonorgestrel 0.125 |
| Tri-Norinyl | I: 7 d | Ethinyl estradiol 35 | Norethindrone 0.5 |
| | II: 9 d | Ethinyl estradiol 35 | Norethindrone 1 |
| | III: 5 d | Ethinyl estradiol 35 | Norethindrone 0.5 |
| Triphasil | I: 6 d | Ethinyl estradiol 30 | Levonorgestrel 0.05 |
| | II: 5 d | Ethinyl estradiol 40 | Levonorgestrel 0.075 |
| | III: 10 d | Ethinyl estradiol 30 | Levonorgestrel 0.125 |
| Trivora-28 | I: 6 d | Ethinyl estradiol 30 | Levonorgestrel 0.05 |
| | II: 5 d | Ethinyl estradiol 40 | Levonorgestrel 0.075 |
| | III: 10 d | Ethinyl estradiol 30 | Levonorgestrel 0.125 |
| *Progestin-Only Products* | | | |
| Depo-Provera | | | Medroxyprogesterone 1.5 |
| Micronor | | | Norethindrone 0.35 |
| Norplant Subdermal System | | | Levonorgestrel 216 |
| Nor-QD | | | Norethindrone 0.35 |
| Ovrette | | | Norgestrel 0.075 |
| Progestasert intrauterine | | | Progesterone 38 |
| *Transdermal Preparation* | | | |
| Ortho Evra | | Ethinyl estradiol 0.02 mg/ 24 h (0.75 mg/wk) | Norelgestromin 0.15 mg/ 24 h (6 mg/wk) |
| *Emergency Contraceptive* | | | |
| Preven | | Ethinyl estradiol 0.05 mg/ tablet | Levonorgestrel 0.25 mg/ tablet |

motor instability. Most information is derived from small German studies using Remifemin, the brand name of a standardized extract that is marketed as an alternative to estrogen therapy for menopausal symptoms. The product apparently does not affect the endometrium or estrogen-dependent cancers; its effects on bone and osteoporosis are unknown. Animal studies indicate binding to estrogen receptors and suppression of LH. A study of post-hysterectomy clients indicated no advantage of the herb over conventional estrogen replacement therapy. Other trade names include Estroven, Femtrol, and GNC Menopause Formula.

Adverse effects may include nausea, vomiting, dizziness, hypotension, and visual disturbances. Blood pressure should be monitored closely in hypertensive clients because the herb may increase the hypotensive effects of antihypertensive drugs. Black cohosh is contraindicated in pregnancy and not recommended for use longer than 6 months for menopausal symptoms.

Overall, this herb may be useful in clients who refuse estrogen or have conditions in which estrogen is contraindicated. If Remifemin is taken, the recommended dose is 1 tablet (standardized to contain 20 mg of herbal drug) twice daily. Other dosage forms are available, and dosage depends on the method of preparation.

## ■ MANAGEMENT CONSIDERATIONS

### Need for Continuous Supervision

Because estrogens, progestins, and contraceptives are often taken for years and may cause adverse reactions, clients taking these drugs need continued supervision by a health care provider. Before the drugs are given, a complete medical history; a physical examination, including breast and pelvic examinations and a Pap smear; urinalysis; and weight and blood pressure measurements are recommended. These examinations should be repeated at least annually as long as the client is taking the drugs. See Age-related Considerations.

## NURSING PROCESS

### Assessment

Before drug therapy is started, clients need a thorough history and physical examination, including measurements of blood pressure, serum cholesterol, and triglycerides. These parameters must be monitored periodically as long as the drugs are taken.

- Assess for conditions in which estrogens and progestins are used.
- Assess for conditions that increase risks of adverse effects or are contraindications for hormonal therapy (eg, thromboembolic disorders, pregnancy).
- Record blood pressure with each outpatient contact or regularly with hospitalized clients.
- Check laboratory reports of cholesterol and triglyceride levels when available.
- Assess diet and presence of cigarette smoking. A high-fat diet increases the risks of gallbladder disease and perhaps other problems; cigarette smoking increases risks of thromboembolic disorders in women older than 35 years of age who take oral contraceptives.
- Assess the client's willingness to comply with instructions about drug therapy and follow-up procedures.
- Assess for signs and symptoms of thromboembolic disorders regularly. These are most likely to occur in women older than 35 years of age who take oral contraceptives, women who are postmenopausal who take hormone replacement therapy, and women or men who take large doses for cancer.
- Assess the infertile couple's reproductive and sexual history and their perception of their infertility, its cause, and its impact on their lives.

### Nursing Diagnoses

- Disturbed Body Image in women, related to effects of hormone deficiency states
- Disturbed Body Image in men, related to feminizing effects and impotence from female hormones

- Excess Fluid Volume related to sodium and water retention
- Deficient Knowledge: Effects of hormonal therapy
- Risk for Injury related to increased risks of hypertension and gallbladder disease
- Ineffective sexuality patterns related to inability to conceive and deliver a viable birth

### Planning/Goals

**The client will:**

- Be assisted to cope with self-concept and body image changes
- Take the drugs accurately, for the length of time prescribed
- Experience relief of symptoms for which the drugs are given
- Avoid preventable adverse drug effects
- Keep appointments for monitoring of drug effects
- Adhere to the medical regimen and achieve pregnancy with minimal adverse effects for the infertile couple

### Interventions

- Assist clients of childbearing age to choose an appropriate contraceptive method. If the choice is an estrogen–progestin combination, help the client take it accurately.
- Help postmenopausal women plan for adequate calcium and vitamin D in the diet and adequate weight-bearing exercise to maintain bone strength and prevent osteoporosis.
- Assist clients in obtaining follow-up health care when indicated.
- Assist the infertile couple to support the relationship, maintain self-esteem, and understand the treatment plan.

### Evaluation

- Interview and observe for compliance with instructions for taking the drugs.
- Interview and observe for therapeutic and adverse drug effects.

## Drug Selection Factors

Choice of preparation depends on the reason for use, desired route of administration, and duration of action. Conjugated estrogen (eg, Premarin) is a commonly used oral estrogen, and medroxyprogesterone (eg, Provera) is a commonly used oral progestin.

The choice of combination contraceptive product may be determined by the progestin component. Some progestins are more likely to cause weight gain, acne, and changes in blood lipids that increase risks for myocardial infarction or stroke. These adverse effects are attributed mainly to the androgenic activity of the progestin, and some progestins have more androgenic effects than others. Progestins with minimal androgenic activity are desogestrel and norgestimate; those with intermediate activity include norethindrone and ethynodiol; and norgestrel has high androgenic effects. In addition, there are long-

acting progestin contraceptive preparations such as intramuscular depot medroxyprogesterone (Depo-Provera) that lasts 3 months per injection, intrauterine progesterone that lasts 1 year, and levonorgestrel subcutaneous implants (Norplant) that last 5 years.

## Dosage Factors

Although dosage needs vary with clients and the conditions for which the drugs are prescribed, a general rule is to use the smallest effective dose for the shortest effective time. Estrogens are often given cyclically. In one regimen, the drug is taken for 3 weeks, and then omitted for 1 week; in another, it is omitted the first 5 days of each month. These regimens more closely resemble normal secretion of estrogen and avoid prolonged stimulation of body tissues. A progestin may be added for 10 days each month.

## Age-related Considerations: Use of Estrogen Preparations

### USE IN CHILDREN

There is little information about effects of estrogens in children, and the drugs are not indicated for use. Because the drugs cause epiphyseal closure, they should be used with caution before completion of bone growth and attainment of adult height. When hormonal contraceptives are given to adolescent girls, the smallest effective doses should be used, as in other populations.

### USE IN OLDER ADULTS

The short-term use (1–2 years) of estrogens or estrogens and progestins in postmenopausal women may be indicated for management of menopausal symptoms. Long-term use of an estrogen-alone or estrogen-progestin combination is no longer recommended for most women, because of potentially serious adverse effects.

## Effects of Estrogens and Oral Contraceptives on Other Drugs

These drugs may interact with several drugs or drug groups to increase or decrease their effects. Most interactions have been reported with oral contraceptives.

**Estrogens** may *decrease* the effectiveness of sulfonylurea antidiabetic drugs (probably by increasing their metabolism); warfarin, an oral anticoagulant (by increasing hepatic production of several clotting factors); and phenytoin, an anticonvulsant (possibly by increasing fluid retention). Estrogens may *increase* the adverse effects and risks for toxicity with corticosteroids, ropinirole, and tacrine by inhibiting their metabolism. Ropinirole and tacrine should not be used concurrently with an estrogen.

**Oral contraceptives** *decrease* effects of some benzodiazepines (eg, lorazepam, oxazepam, temazepam), insulin, sulfonylurea antidiabetic drugs, and warfarin. If one of these drugs is taken concurrently with an oral contraceptive, increased dosage may be needed for therapeutic effects. Contraceptives *increase* effects of several drugs by inhibiting their metabolism. These include alcohol, some benzodiazepines (eg, alprazolam, triazolam), tricyclic antidepressants, beta-blockers (eg, metoprolol), caffeine, corticosteroids, and theophylline (a xanthine bronchodilator). If one of these drugs is taken concurrently with an oral contraceptive, the drug may accumulate to toxic levels. Dosage may need to be reduced.

### ? How Can You Avoid This Medication Error?

Tami Smithford, a 19-year-old college student, comes into the college health clinic to renew her prescription for oral contraceptives. When she is there, she complains of a sore throat and having a fever for the last 2 days. A culture for streptococcus is performed, she is placed on ampicillin, and her oral contraceptives are renewed. The nurse provides the following patient teaching: "Take ampicillin 500 mg (1 capsule) 4 times a day for 10 days. Call the office in 2 days to see whether the results of your culture are positive. Drink lots of fluids and get plenty of rest."

## Use in Specific Situations

### Contraception

Estrogen and progestin contraceptive preparations are nearly 100% effective in preventing pregnancy. Some guidelines for their use include the following:

■ Numerous preparations are available, with different components and different doses of components, so that a preparation can be chosen to meet individual needs. Most oral contraceptives contain an estrogen and a progestin. The estrogen dose is usually 30 to 35 mcg. Smaller amounts (eg, 20 mcg) may be adequate for small or underweight women; larger amounts (eg, 50 mcg) may be needed for large or overweight women. When estrogen is contraindicated, a progestin-only contraceptive may be used.

■ Current products contain small amounts of estrogen and cause fewer adverse effects than earlier products. Despite the decreased estrogen dosage, oral contraceptives may still be safest when given to nonsmoking women younger than 35 years of age who do not have a history of thromboembolic problems, diabetes mellitus, hypertension, or migraine.

■ Assess each client's need and desire for contraception as well as her willingness to comply with the prescribed regimen. Assessment information includes the client's knowledge about pharmacologic and other methods of birth control. Compliance involves the willingness to take the drugs as prescribed and to have examinations of breasts and pelvis and blood pressure measurements every 6 to 12 months. Assessment also includes identifying clients in whom hormonal contraceptives are contraindicated or who are at increased risk for adverse drug effects.

■ The most effective and widely used contraceptives are estrogen-progestin combinations (see Drugs at a Glance 24-1). Effects of estrogen components are similar when prescribed in equipotent doses, but progestins differ in progestogenic, estrogenic, antiestrogenic, and androgenic activity. Consequently, adverse effects may differ to some extent, and a client may be able to tolerate one contraceptive better than another.

## CLIENT TEACHING GUIDELINES
### Oral Contraceptives

**General Considerations**

✔ Seek information about the use of oral contraceptives.

✔ Oral contraceptives are very effective at preventing pregnancy, but they do not prevent transmission of sexually transmitted diseases (eg, acquired immunodeficiency syndrome, chlamydia, gonorrhea).

✔ See a health care provider every 6 to 12 months for blood pressure measurement, breast and pelvic examinations, and other care as indicated. This is very important to monitor for adverse drug effects such as high blood pressure, gallbladder disease, and blood clotting disorders.

✔ Do not smoke cigarettes. Cigarette smoking increases risks of blood clots in the legs, lungs, heart, or brain. The blood clots may cause heart attack, stroke, or other serious diseases.

✔ Several medications may reduce the effectiveness of oral contraceptives (ie, increase the likelihood of pregnancy). These include several antibiotics (eg, ampicillin, clarithromycin and similar drugs, rifampin, penicillin V, sulfonamides [eg, Bactrim], tetracyclines), and antiseizure medications (eg, carbamazepine, oxcarbazepine, phenytoin, topiramate). Inform all health care providers who prescribe medications for you that you are taking a birth control pill.

✔ Be prepared to use an additional or alternative method of birth control if a dose is missed, if you are unable to take the oral contraceptive because of illness, or if you have an infection for which an antibiotic is prescribed. For example, use a different method of birth control while taking an antibiotic and for the remainder of that cycle.

✔ Avoid pregnancy for approximately 3 to 6 months after the drugs are stopped.

**Self-administration**

✔ Read, keep, and follow instructions in the package inserts that are dispensed with the drugs. These inserts provide information about safe and effective use of the drugs.

✔ Take oral contraceptives with meals or food or at bedtime to decrease nausea. (If using Ortho Evra, a contraceptive skin patch that lasts a week, follow package instructions for correct application.)

✔ Take about the same time every day to maintain effective blood levels and establish a routine so that missed doses are less likely. Missing one dose may allow pregnancy to occur. If you forget to take one pill, take it as soon as you remember. If you do not remember until the next scheduled pill, you can take two pills at once. If you miss two pills in a row, you may take two pills for the next 2 days. If you miss more than two pills, notify your health care provider.

✔ Use sunscreen and protective clothing when outdoors. The drugs may cause photosensitivity, with increased likelihood of sunburn after short periods of exposure.

✔ Weigh weekly and report sudden weight gain. The drugs may cause fluid retention; decreasing salt intake may be helpful.

✔ Report any unusual vaginal bleeding; calf tenderness, redness, or swelling; chest pain; weakness or numbness in an arm or leg; or sudden difficulty with seeing or talking.

## Emergency (Postcoital) Contraception

Emergency contraception (ie, high doses of estrogen and progestin) may be used to avoid pregnancy after unprotected sexual intercourse, especially for victims of rape or incest or women whose physical or mental health is threatened by pregnancy. It is very effective if started within 24 hours and no later than 72 hours after exposure. The drugs are thought to act mainly by inhibiting ovulation.

Although Preven (levonorgestrel 0.25 mg, and ethinyl estradiol 0.05 mg) is the only drug approved by the U.S. Food and Drug Administration (FDA) for postcoital contraception, multiple tablets of several birth control pills are also effective. The drugs are given in two doses, 12 hours apart. Amounts include 4 tablets of Levlen, Lo-Ovral, Nordette, Triphasil, or Tri-Levlen; 2 tablets of Ovral; and 5 tablets of Alesse. These are high doses, and common adverse effects are nausea and vomiting. Antiemetic medication or repeating vomited doses may be needed. Women who take a hormonal contraceptive should probably ask the prescriber about possible postcoital use.

## Menopause

Menopause usually occurs when women are 48 to 55 years of age. A women who has not menstruated for a full year is considered menopausal, although symptoms of estrogen deficiency and irregular periods start approximately 4 years before final cessation. Physiologic menopause results from the gradual cessation of ovarian function and the resultant decrease in estrogen levels. Surgical menopause results from excision of both ovaries and the sudden loss of ovarian estrogen. Although estrogens from the adrenal cortex and other sites are still produced, the amount is insufficient to prevent estrogen deficiency.

Estrogen replacement therapy prevents vasomotor instability (hot flashes/flushes) and other menopausal symptoms. A commonly prescribed regimen is a conjugated estrogen (eg, Premarin), 0.625 mg to 1.25 mg daily for 25 days of each month, with a progestin, such as Provera, 10 mg daily for 10 days of each month, on days 15 to 25 of the cycle. The main function of the progestin is to decrease the risk for endometrial cancer; thus, it is not needed by women who have had a hysterectomy. Another regimen uses estradiol as a transdermal patch (Estraderm), which releases the drug slowly, provides more consistent blood levels than oral formulations, and is applied weekly. A newer synthetic conjugated estrogen (Cenestin) is also approved for short-term treatment of hot flashes and sweating; it is not approved for long-term use in preventing osteoporosis in postmenopausal women.

### Prevention and Treatment of Osteoporosis

Estrogen or estrogen-progestin therapy is effective and has been widely used to prevent or treat osteoporosis and prevent fractures in postmenopausal women (see Chap. 20). Estrogenic effects in preventing bone loss include decreased bone resorption (breakdown), increased intestinal absorption of calcium, and increased calcitriol concentration. Calcitriol is the active form of vitamin D, which is required for absorption of calcium.

These hormones may be used less often for osteoporosis in the future, for two main reasons. First, recent evidence (see Box 24-2) indicates that the risks of estrogen-progestin hormonal therapy outweigh the benefits. The effects of estrogen alone are not yet known. Second, there are other effective measures for prevention and treatment of osteoporosis, including calcium and vitamin D supplements, bisphosphonate drugs (eg, alendronate and risedronate), and weight-bearing exercise.

## ◼ INFERTILITY

Infertility is the inability to conceive after 12 months of contraceptive-free sexual intercourse. Failure to conceive may be the result of reproductive dysfunction in either the male or female partner, or both. Approximately 1 in 10 couples desiring children experience some degree of infertility.

Multiple causes of infertility exist in the female and can be the result of dysfunction during any phase of the reproductive cycle. Causes of infertility are numerous, but most problems can be identified as problems with follicular maturation, ovulation, ovum transport through the fallopian tubes, ovum fertilization, implantation, and maturity of the developing fetus. Factors that contribute to these causes include an increased incidence of pelvic inflammatory disease and the delay of childbearing for many women until after the age of 35 years.

Male reproductive dysfunction may contribute to infertility in approximately 30% of couples. The primary causes of male infertility are related to decreased sperm motility or inadequate sperm count or to semen that is of abnormal quality or volume. Males may also have erectile dysfunction that creates a problem with ejaculation; the condition is described in Chapter 25.

A thorough history from both partners and various diagnostic procedures, including semen analysis, basal body temperature patterns, serum hormone levels, endometrial biopsy, and evaluation of fallopian tubes patency, can significantly enhance the likelihood of successful management. Management of infertility focuses on correcting the underlying problem, such as chronic illness, infection, insufficient hormone production, endometriosis, or inadequate sperm count or motility. Treatment includes surgery and assisted reproductive techniques, such as artificial insemination, in vitro fertilization, and embryo transfer. The goal of treatment of infertility is to produce a pregnancy that results in a healthy infant. The focus of this chapter is management through hormone therapy.

---

### CLIENT TEACHING GUIDELINES
### Hormone Replacement Therapy

#### General Considerations

✔ Estrogen replacement therapy relieves symptoms of menopause and helps to prevent or treat osteoporosis.

✔ Maintain medical supervision at least annually to check blood pressure, breasts, pelvis, and other areas for possible adverse reactions when these drugs are taken for long periods.

✔ Women who have not had a hysterectomy should take both estrogen and progestin; the progestin component (eg, Provera) prevents endometrial cancer, an adverse effect of estrogen-only therapy in this group. However, a well-done study concluded that risks of adverse effects with estrogen-only therapy and estrogen-progestin combinations are greater than previously believed. Women who are considering hormone replacement therapy (eg, for severe symptoms of menopause) should discuss their individual risks and potential benefits with their health care providers.

✔ Combined estrogen-progestin therapy may increase blood sugar levels in women with diabetes. This effect is attributed to progestin and is unlikely to occur with estrogen only therapy.

✔ Women with diabetes should report increased blood glucose levels.

#### Self-administration

✔ Take estrogens and progestins with food or at bedtime to decrease nausea, a common adverse reaction.

✔ Apply skin patch estrogen (eg, Estraderm) to clean, dry skin, preferably the abdomen. Press the patch tightly for 10 seconds to get a good seal and rotate sites so that at least a week passes between applications to a site.

✔ Weigh weekly and report sudden weight gain. Fluid retention and edema may occur and produce weight gain.

✔ Report any unusual vaginal bleeding.

Ovulation induction can be used as a pharmacologic means to produce ovulation for natural or artificial conception. Fertility-promoting drugs used for infertility include clomiphene, menotropins, human chorionic gonadotropin (hCG), bromocriptine, gonadotropin-releasing hormone (GnRH), and gonadorelin. They are discussed in Drugs at a Glance 24-4: Drugs used for Infertility.

## FERTILITY-PROMOTING DRUGS

**Clomiphene (Clomid, Serophene)** is a nonsteroidal estrogen receptor modulator that inhibits the negative feedback mechanism in the hypothalamus by bonding to estrogen receptors. By decreasing the number of available receptors, the drug makes it seem that estrogen levels are low and falsely signals the hypothalamus to increase the release of GnRH, with subsequent increases in FSH and LH. This promotes follicular maturation and ovulation if the pituitary is capable of producing FSH and LH and the ovaries are capable of responding to these hormones. Clomiphene is the most frequently used drug in this category and serves as the prototype (see Prototype Profile 24-1: Clomiphene). Common adverse effects include hot flashes/flushes, abdominal discomfort, bloating, and breast engorgement. These symptoms typically resolve on cessation of clomiphene therapy.

**Menotropins (Pergonal, Humegon)** are a purified preparation of the human gonadotropins FSH and LH that produce ovarian follicular maturation. Once the follicles have ripened, hCG is administered to induce ovulation. This drug is administered when gonadotropin secretion is insufficient by the anterior pituitary to produce ovarian stimulation. For ovulation to result after menotropins therapy, the ovaries must be able to respond to FSH and LH; no response is elicited in women with primary ovarian failure.

The most common adverse events are ovarian enlargement, hyperstimulation syndrome, multiple births, spontaneous abortion, and febrile reactions.

**Human chorionic gonadotropin (hCG)** is a hormone produced by the placenta that is alike in structure and identical in action to LH. Exogenous use of hCG induces ovulation in women who are infertile because of ovulatory failure. As stated previously, hCG promotes ovulation after follicular maturation is induced with drugs such as menotropins.

Adverse effects include hyperstimulation syndrome, pain at the injection site, headache, irritability, and restlessness.

**Gonadorelin (Lutrepulse, Factrel)** is a synthetic peptide identical to human GnRH. The drug is used to treat infertility resulting from failure of the hypothalamus to secrete GnRH. For the drug to be effective, it must be administered in a pulsatile pattern that follows the normal patterns of normal pulsatile GnRH secretion.

Adverse effects may be associated with the route of administration, including the risk for phlebitis and hematoma formation at the intravenous insertion site. Multiple births may occur. Hyperstimulation syndrome with the drug has been reported, although the incidence is less than with menotropins and hCG.

**Bromocriptine (Parlodel)** is used in individuals with excessive prolactin levels to correct amenorrhea and infertility. If a pituitary tumor is triggering the prolactin secretion, the drug can produce regression of the adenoma and produce prolactin levels. Reduced prolactin level may result in return of a normal menstrual cycle and fertility.

Adverse effects include nausea, dizziness, headache, and abdominal cramps. Taking the medication with food may minimize some of the gastrointestinal adverse effects.

---

## CLIENT TEACHING GUIDELINES
### Infertility Agents

#### General Considerations

✔ Ensure that client understands how the drug is administered; with use of infusion devices, client should understand how to administer and monitor.

✔ Reinforce teaching about potential risks and benefits of drug therapy.

✔ Continue medical supervision as long as the drugs are being taken.

✔ Alert couple to risk for multiple births.

✔ Educate on evaluating basal body temperature patterns.

✔ Refer to local support groups; acknowledge feelings of grief, disappointment, and failure.

#### Self-administration

✔ Take the drugs only if prescribed and as prescribed.

✔ Monitor ovulation and discontinue drug, as instructed, when ovulation is suspected.

✔ Recognize the importance of discontinuing drug when pregnancy is suspected.

✔ Monitor blood pressure for the first few days of therapy (bromocriptine).

✔ Take drug with food and exactly as prescribed.

✔ Observe for drug-specific adverse effects (dizziness, nausea, headache and abdominal cramps, hot flashes/flushes, blurring of vision and other visual symptoms).

✔ Pattern sexual intercourse as directed (ie, with menotropins, intercourse should occur daily beginning the day before hCG therapy to maximize desired response).

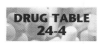

**DRUG TABLE 24-4**

*Drugs at a Glance*

## Drugs Used for Infertility

| Generic/Trade Name | Routes and Dosage Ranges | Comments |
|---|---|---|
| **Bromocriptine** (Parlodel)<br>Pregnancy Category B | Hyperprolactinemia: PO, 2.5 mg 2 to 3 times daily<br>Prolactin-secreting adenomas: PO, 1.25–2.5 mg/day; daily range 2.5–10 mg | May cause postural hypotension and dizziness |
| **Clomiphene** (Clomid, Serophene) | See Prototype Profile 24-1: Clomiphene | |
| **Gonadorelin** (Lutrepulse, Factrel)<br>**Gonadotropin-releasing hormone**<br>Pregnancy Category B | Primary hypothalamic amenorrhea: IV, 5 mcg every 90 min via Lutrepulse pump kit at intervals of 21 d | Pump will pulsate every 90 min for 7 d<br>Antipsychotic agents may decrease the effects of gonadorelin |
| **Human chorionic gonadotropin** (Novarel, Pregnyl, Profasi)<br>Pregnancy Category C | IM, 5000–10,000 units 1 day following last dose of menotropins | Use with menotropins; can only be administered by IM injection |
| **Menotropins** (Pergonal, Repronex)<br>Pregnancy Category X | IM, Sub-Q, Initial: 150 IU daily for first 5 days; adjustments should not exceed 75–150 IU per adjustment<br>Maximum daily dose should not exceed 450 IU; dosing beyond 12 days is not recommended | Instruct on appropriate method of measuring basal body temperature to indicate ovulation; instruct on appropriate injection technique and needle/vial/syringe disposal |

IU, International Units

---

## PROTOTYPE PROFILE 24-1

### ℗ Clomiphene (KLOE mi feen)

**Drug Class**

*Chemical:* Ovulation stimulator
*Functional:* Ovulation stimulator

**Trade Names**

Clomid, Serophene

**Therapeutic Indications**

Induction of ovulation in individuals desiring pregnancy

**Pharmacokinetics**

*Absorption*
Readily absorbed

*Distribution*
Unknown

*Metabolism*
Undergoes enterohepatic recirculation

*Excretion*
Primarily feces; small amount in urine

**Pharmacodynamics**

*Onset of Action*
LH and FSH levels peak 5 to 9 days after completing of course

*Duration*
Unknown

**Contraindications/Precautions**

Undiagnosed vaginal bleeding, pregnancy, uncontrolled adrenal or thyroid dysfunction, or ovarian cysts; if pregnancy is suspected, drug should be discontinued and health care provider notified

**Pregnancy Considerations**

Category X
Excretion in breast milk unknown; contraindicated

**Dosage**

PO, 50 mg/d for days 5 to 9 of cycle; if ovulation does not occur, the dose is increased to 100 mg/d in the next course; long-term therapy is not recommended beyond a total of 6 cycles

**Adverse Effects**

Hot flashes/flushes, ovarian enlargement, blurring of vision and other visual symptoms, abdominal pain, thromboembolism

**Drug Interactions**

*Increased Effects*
None reported

*Decreased Effects*
Estradiol response with clomiphene
Clomiphene response with danazol

**Herbal Supplements and Dietary Considerations**

None noted

**TABLE 24-2   Common Sexually Transmitted Diseases and Drug Therapy**

| Causative Agent | Drug Therapy |
|---|---|
| *Candida* species | Nystatin or miconazole (Monistat) suppositories or fluconazole (Diflucan) |
| *Chlamydia trachomatis* | Tetracycline or macrolides; ofloxacin, erythromycin during pregnancy |
| Herpes virus type II | Acyclovir (Zovirax), famciclovir, valacyclovir |
| Human immunodeficiency virus (HIV) infection and acquired immunodeficiency syndrome (AIDS) | See Drugs at a Glance 33-1: Drugs for Human Immunodeficiency Virus Infection and Acquired Immunodeficiency Syndrome |
| *Neisseria gonorrhoeae* | Cephalosporins, fluoroquinolones, azithromycin, doxycycline |
| *Treponema pallidum* (syphilis) | Parenteral penicillin G |
| *Trichomonas* species | Metronidazole (Flagyl) |

## SEXUALLY TRANSMITTED DISEASES

STDs are those diseases spread through sexual contact. STDs constitute a major health problem in the United States. Despite a higher reported incidence of STDs in males, the complications are overall more frequent and severe in females. Significant concerns with maternal and fetal health during pregnancy are well known. STDs are increasingly more difficult to treat because these organisms are becoming more resistant with changing drug susceptibility patterns to antibiotics.

Pathogens contributing to the development of STDs are highlighted in Table 24-2. An expanded discussion of the corresponding drug therapy is found in Section 7, Drugs Used to Treat Infections. Additional information on recommended treatment guidelines is available on line from the Centers for Disease Control and Prevention (CDC) at www.cdc.gov/std/treatment/1-2002TG.htm. The 2002 recommendations from the CDC for the treatment of STDs include updated guidelines with new alternative regimens, information regarding the emergence of drug-resistant pathogens, and inclusion of hepatitis C as a sexually transmitted infection.

## Nursing Actions
## Estrogens, Progestins, and Hormonal Contraceptives

| Nursing Actions | Rationale/Explanation |
|---|---|
| **1. Administer accurately.** | |
| a. Give oral estrogens, progestins, and contraceptive preparations after meals or at bedtime. | To decrease nausea, a common adverse reaction |
| b. With aqueous suspensions to be given intramuscularly, roll the vial between the hands several times. | To be sure that drug particles are evenly distributed through the liquid vehicle |
| c. Give oil preparations deeply into a large muscle mass, preferably gluteal muscles. | |
| d. With estradiol skin patches, apply to clean dry skin of the abdomen, buttocks, upper inner thigh, or upper arm. Avoid breasts, waistline areas, and areas exposed to sunlight. Press with palm of hand for about 10 seconds. Rotate sites. | To facilitate effective absorption and adherence to the skin and avoid skin irritation |
| e. With Combi-Patch, apply to clean dry skin of the lower abdomen; rotate sites. | Manufacturer's recommendation. Rotating sites decreases skin irritation. |
| f. With Ortho Evra patch, apply to abdomen, buttocks, upper torso (except breasts), or upper outer arm. | Manufacturer's recommendation |
| **2. Observe for therapeutic effects.** | Therapeutic effects vary, depending on the reason for use. |
| a. With estrogens: | |
| (1) When given for menopausal symptoms, observe for decrease in hot flashes and vaginal problems. | |

*(continued)*

## Nursing Actions

### Estrogens, Progestins, and Hormonal Contraceptives (Continued)

| Nursing Actions | Rationale/Explanation |
|---|---|
| (2) When given for amenorrhea, observe for menstruation. | |
| (3) When given for female hypogonadism, observe for menstruation, breast enlargement, axillary and pubic hair, and other secondary sexual characteristics. | |
| (4) When given to prevent or treat osteoporosis, observe for improved bone density tests and absence of fractures. | |
| b. With progestins: | |
| (1) When given for menstrual disorders, such as abnormal uterine bleeding, amenorrhea, dysmenorrhea, premenstrual discomfort, and endometriosis, observe for relief of symptoms. | |
| **3. Observe for adverse effects.** | |
| a. With estrogens: | |
| (1) Menstrual disorders—breakthrough bleeding, dysmenorrhea, amenorrhea | Estrogen drugs may alter hormonal balance. |
| (2) Gastrointestinal system—nausea, vomiting, abdominal cramps, bloating | Nausea commonly occurs but usually subsides within 1 to 2 wk of continued therapy. When high doses of estrogens are used as postcoital contraceptives, nausea and vomiting may be severe enough to require administration of antiemetic drugs. |
| (3) Gallbladder disease | Postmenopausal women taking an estrogen are 2 to 4 times more likely than nonusers to require surgery for gallbladder disease. |
| (4) Cardiovascular system—thromboembolic conditions such as thrombophlebitis, pulmonary embolism, cerebral thrombosis, and coronary thrombosis; edema and weight gain | Estrogens promote blood clotting by stimulating hepatic production of four clotting factors (II, VII, IX, X). Thromboembolic disorders are most likely to occur in women older than 35 y who take oral contraceptives and smoke cigarettes, postmenopausal women taking long-term estrogen and progestin therapy, and men or women who receive large doses of estrogens for cancer treatment. Edema and weight gain are caused by fluid retention. |
| (5) Central nervous system—headache, migraine, dizziness, mental depression | Estrogens may cause or aggravate migraine in some women; the mechanism is unknown. |
| (6) Cancer—endometrial and possibly breast cancer | When estrogens are used alone in postmenopausal women, they cause endometrial hyperplasia and may cause endometrial cancer. Women with an intact uterus should also be given a progestin, which opposes the effects of estrogen on the endometrium. |
| | Opinions differ regarding estrogens as a cause of breast cancer. Most studies indicate little risk; a few indicate some risk, especially with high doses for prolonged periods (ie, 10 y or longer). However, estrogens do stimulate growth in breast cancers that have estrogen receptors. |
| b. With progestins: | |
| (1) Menstrual disorders—breakthrough bleeding | Irregular vaginal bleeding is a common adverse effect that decreases during the first year of use. This is a major reason that some women do not want to take progestin-only contraceptives. |
| (2) Cardiovascular system—decreased high-density lipoprotein and increased low-density lipoprotein cholesterol | These adverse effects on plasma lipids potentially increase the risks of cardiovascular disease. |

*(continued)*

## Nursing Actions

### Estrogens, Progestins, and Hormonal Contraceptives (Continued)

| Nursing Actions | Rationale/Explanation |
|---|---|
| (3) Gastrointestinal system—nausea, increased or decreased weight | Nausea may be decreased by taking with food. |
| (4) Central nervous system—drowsiness, insomnia, mental depression | |
| (5) Miscellaneous effects—edema, weight gain | |
| c. Combined estrogen and progestin oral contraceptives: | |
| (1) Gastrointestinal effects—nausea, others | Nausea can be minimized by taking the drugs with food or at bedtime. |
| (2) Cardiovascular effects—thromboembolism, myocardial infarction, stroke, hypertension | These effects occurred with earlier oral contraceptives, which contained larger amounts of estrogen than those currently used, and are much less common in most people who take low-dose preparations. However, for women older than 35 y who smoke, there is an increased risk of myocardial infarction and other cardiovascular disorders even with low-dose pills. |
| (3) Gallbladder disease—cholelithiasis and cholecystitis | Women who use oral contraceptives or estrogen–progestin hormone replacement therapy are several times more likely to develop gallbladder disease than nonusers. This is attributed to increased concentration of cholesterol in bile acids, which leads to decreased solubility and increased precipitation of stones. |
| (4) Miscellaneous—edema, weight gain, headache | |
| 4. **Observe for drug interactions.** | |
| a. Drugs that *decrease* effects of estrogens, progestins, and oral contraceptives: | |
| (1) Anticonvulsants—carbamazepine, oxcarbazepine, phenytoin, topiramate | Decrease effects by inducing enzymes that accelerate metabolism of estrogens and progestins. |
| (2) Antimicrobials | Most interactions with antimicrobials have been reported with oral contraceptives. Rifampin induces drug-metabolizing enzymes that accelerate drug inactivation. Other antimicrobials act mainly by disrupting the normal bacterial flora of the gastrointestinal tract and decreasing enterohepatic recirculation of estrogens. This action may decrease effectiveness of contraceptives or cause breakthrough bleeding. To prevent pregnancy from occurring during antimicrobial therapy, a larger dose of oral contraceptive or an additional or alternative form of birth control is probably advisable. |
| (a) Antibacterials—ampicillin, macrolides (erythromycin, clarithromycin, dirithromycin), metronidazole, penicillin V, rifampin, sulfonamides, tetracyclines, trimethoprim | |
| (b) Antifungals—fluconazole, itraconazole, ketoconazole | |
| (c) Antivirals—efavirenz, ritonavir, lopinavir/ ritonavir combination | |

### ? How Can You Avoid This Medication Error?

**Answer:** The nurse has provided adequate patient teaching concerning Tami's antibiotic, but the nurse has not advised her regarding the drug–drug interaction between ampicillin and oral contraceptives. Taking both of these drugs together will decrease the effectiveness of the oral contraceptives and could result in an unplanned pregnancy. Tami needs to use additional contraceptive protection during the month she is taking the antibiotic. She also needs to know that birth control pills will not protect against sexually transmitted disease.

## Critical Thinking Exercises

1. Estrogen replacement therapy prevents menopausal symptoms. Hot flashes/flushes are the result of:

   a. Insufficient gonadotropin secretion
   b. Vasomotor instability
   c. High levels of estrogen
   d. Decreased progesterone

**2.** Progesterone is a progestin concerned almost entirely with reproduction. In the nonpregnant woman, progesterone is secreted by the:

  a. Corpus luteum
  b. Hypothalamus
  c. Anterior pituitary
  d. Adrenal cortex

**3.** Gonadorelin (Lutrepulse, Factrel) is useful in the treatment of infertility resulting from what mechanism?

  a. Failure of the hypothalamus to secrete GnRH
  b. Inhibited negative feedback mechanism on the pituitary
  c. Reduced sperm motility
  d. Inadequate sperm count

**4.** Black cohosh has been used to self-treat symptoms of menopause. Because of the risk for adverse effects, the client should be monitored closely for:

  a. Dysrhythmias
  b. Hypertension
  c. Hypotension
  d. Bradycardia

**5.** Emergency contraception may be used to avoid pregnancy after unprotected sexual intercourse, especially for victims of rape or incest and for women whose physical or mental health is threatened by pregnancy. Although multiple tablets of several birth control pills are effective, the only drug approved by the FDA for postcoital contraception is:

  a. Preven
  b. Nortrel
  c. Norinyl
  d. Triphasil

## SELECTED REFERENCES

Anonymous. (2002). Ortho-Evra—A contraceptive patch. *The Medical Letter, 44*(1122), 8.

Barbieri, R. L. (2000). Disorders of the reproductive cycle in women. In H. D. Humes (Ed.), *Kelley's textbook of internal medicine* (4th ed., pp. 2740–2743). Philadelphia: Lippincott Williams & Wilkins.

Brinton, L.A., Lamb, E. J., Moghissi, K. S., Scoccia, B., Althuis, M.D., Mabie, J. E., et al. (2004) Ovarian cancer risk after the use of ovulation-stimulating drugs. *Obstetrics & Gynecology, 200*(103), 1194–1203.

DerMarderosian, A. (Ed.) (2001). *The review of natural products.* St Louis: Facts and Comparisons.

*Drug facts and comparisons.* (Updated monthly). St. Louis: Facts and Comparisons.

Fetrow, C. W., & Avila, J. R. (1999). *Professional's handbook of complementary and alternative medicines.* Springhouse, PA: Springhouse Corporation.

Fletcher, S. W., & Colditz, G. A. (2002). Failure of estrogen plus progestin therapy for prevention (Editorial). *Journal of the American Medical Association, 288*(3), 366–367.

Gruber, C. J., Tschugguel, W., Schneeberger, C., & Huber, J. C. (2002). Production and actions of estrogens. *New England Journal of Medicine, 346*(5), 340–351.

Guyton, A. C., & Hall, J. E. (2000). *Textbook of medical physiology* (10th ed.). Philadelphia: W. B. Saunders.

Kim, R. B. (2001). *Handbook of adverse drug interactions.* New Rochelle, NY: The Medical Letter, Inc.

Lacy, C. F., Armstrong, L. L., Goldman, M. P., & Lance, L. L. (2003). *Lexi-Comp's drug information handbook* (11th ed.). Hudson, OH: American Pharmaceutical Association.

Lieu, C. L., & Yoshida, T. (2002). Infertility. In J. T. DiPiro, R. L. Talbert, G. C. Yee, G. R. Matzke, B. G. Wells, & L. M. Posey (Eds.), *Pharmacotherapy: A pathophysiologic approach* (5th ed., pp. 273–304). New York: McGraw-Hill.

Lynch, A., McDuffie, R. Murphy, J., Faber, K., Leff, M., & Orleans, M. (2001). Assisted reproductive interventions and multiple birth. *Obstetrics & Gynecology, 97,* 195–200.

Marcus, E. N. (2000). Principles of women's medicine. In H. D. Humes (Ed.), *Kelley's textbook of internal medicine* (4th ed., pp. 299–303). Philadelphia: Lippincott Williams & Wilkins.

Mehring, P. M. (2002). Structure and function of the female reproductive system. In C. M. Porth (Ed.), *Pathophysiology: Concepts of altered health states* (6th ed., pp. 983–995). Philadelphia: Lippincott Williams & Wilkins.

Morelli, V., & Naquin, C. (2002). Alternative therapies for traditional disease states: Menopause. *American Family Physician, 66*(1), 129–134.

Morris, B. J., & Young, C. (2000). Emergency contraception. *American Journal of Nursing, 100*(9), 46–48.

Nelson, H. D., Humphrey, L. L., Nygren, P., Teutsch, S.U., allan, J. D. (2002). Postmenopausal hormone replacement therapy. *Journal of the American Medical Association, 288*(7), 872–881.

Petitti, D. B. (2002). Hormone replacement therapy for prevention: More evidence, more pessimism (Editorial). *Journal of the American Medical Association, 288*(1), 99–101.

Scholtz, D., & Carmichael, J. M. (2000). Contraception. In E. T. Herfindal & D. R. Gourley (Eds.), *Textbook of therapeutics: Drug and disease management* (7th ed., pp. 2019–2036).

Smith, S., Pfeifer, S. M., & Collins, J. A. (2003). Diagnosis and management of female infertility. *JAMA, 290,* 1767–1770.

Writing Group for the Women's Health Initiative Investigators. (2002). Risks and benefits of estrogen plus progestin in healthy postmenopausal women; Principal results from the Women's Health Initiative Randomized Controlled Trial. *Journal of the American Medical Association, 288*(3), 321–333.

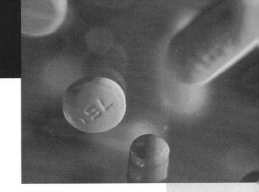

# 25

# Drugs Affecting Male Reproductive Health

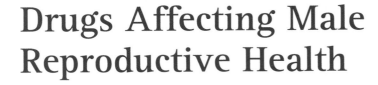

## OBJECTIVES

*After studying this chapter, the student will be able to:*

1 Discuss effects of endogenous androgens.

2 Give uses and effects of exogenous androgens and anabolic steroids.

3 Describe potential consequences of abusing androgens and anabolic steroids.

4 Counsel clients about the physiologic effects of the dietary supplements androstenedione, dehydroepiandrosterone (DHEA), and yohimbine.

5 Apply nursing process with clients using androgens.

6 Outline client teaching guidelines for clients with erectile dysfunction.

## CRITICAL THINKING SCENARIO

*Y*ou are a nurse working in a rural high school. The wrestling coach asks you to speak with his wrestling team about anabolic steroids.

✔ Why might adolescents want to use anabolic steroids?

✔ What are the potential dangers of anabolic steroid use?

✔ What is the basis for confusion regarding the difference between anabolic steroids and corticosteroids?

✔ Describe strategies that might be effective in limiting the use of anabolic steroids among young athletes.

## PROTOTYPE PROFILE

sildenafil (Viagra), p. 441

# OVERVIEW

Androgens are male sex hormones secreted by the testes in men, the ovaries in women, and the adrenal cortices of both sexes. Like the female sex hormones, the naturally occurring male sex hormones are steroids synthesized from cholesterol. The sex organs and adrenal glands can produce cholesterol or remove it from the blood. Cholesterol then undergoes a series of conversions to progesterone, androgenic prehormones, and testosterone. The androgens produced by the ovaries have little androgenic activity and are used mainly as precursor substances for the production of naturally occurring estrogens. The adrenal glands produce several androgens, including androstenedione and dehydroepiandrosterone (DHEA). Androstenedione and DHEA are weak androgens with little masculinizing effect that are mainly converted to estrogens. This chapter highlights the effects of endogenous testosterone and exogenous replacement of testosterone and the use of androgens and anabolic steroids as drugs. Additionally, the pharmacologic management of erectile dysfunction is addressed.

# TESTOSTERONE

**Testosterone** is normally the only important male sex hormone. It is secreted by Leydig's cells in the testes in response to stimulation by luteinizing hormone (LH) from the anterior pituitary gland. The main functions of testosterone are related to the development of male sexual characteristics, reproduction, and metabolism and are described in At the Foundation: Testosterone.

About 97% of the testosterone secreted by the testes binds to plasma albumin or to sex hormone–binding globulin and circulates in the blood for 30 minutes to several hours. The bound testosterone is either transferred to the tissues or broken down into inactive products that are excreted. Much of the testosterone that transfers to tissues undergoes intracellular conversion to dihydrotestosterone, especially in the external genitalia of the male fetus and the prostate gland in the adult male. The dihydrotestosterone combines with receptor proteins in the cytosol; the steroid–receptor combination then migrates to the cell nucleus, where it induces transcription of DNA and RNA and stimulates production of proteins. Almost all testosterone effects result from the increased formation of proteins throughout the body, especially in the cells of target organs and tissues responsible for development of male sexual characteristics.

The portion of testosterone that does not become attached to tissues is converted into androsterone and DHEA by the liver. These are conjugated with glucuronic or sulfuric acid and excreted in the bile or urine.

The association of testosterone with erectile dysfunction is a complex one. Testosterone stimulates libido in males. With a decreased libido, or sexual drive, a male may not develop an erection. Individuals with erectile dysfunction may have normal testosterone levels; conversely, individuals with normal sexual function may have decreased testosterone levels.

# ANABOLIC STEROIDS

Anabolic steroids are synthetic drugs with increased anabolic activity and decreased androgenic activity compared with testosterone. They were developed during attempts to modify testosterone so that its tissue-building and growth-stimulating effects could be retained while its masculinizing effects could be eliminated or reduced.

# ABUSE OF ANDROGENIC AND ANABOLIC STEROID DRUGS

Androgens and anabolic steroids are widely abused in attempts to enhance muscle development, muscle strength, and athletic performance. Because of their abuse potential, the drugs are Schedule III controlled substances. Although nonprescription sales of the drugs are illegal, they are apparently easily obtained.

Athletes are considered a high-risk group because some start taking the drugs in their early teenage years and continue for years. The number of teens taking anabolic steroids is thought to be small in comparison with the number using marijuana, amphetamines, and other illegal drugs. However, the number is also thought to be increasing, and long-term effects may be as bad as the effects that occur with use of other illegal drugs. Although steroids have a reputation for being dangerous to adult athletes, such as bodybuilders and football players, they are considered even more dangerous for teens because teens are still growing. Anabolic steroids can stop bone growth and damage the heart, kidneys, and liver of adolescents. In addition to those who take steroids to enhance athletic performance, some males take the drugs to produce a more muscular appearance and impress females. Steroid abusers usually take massive doses and often take several drugs or combine injectable and oral drugs for maximum effects. The large doses produce potentially serious adverse effects in several body tissues:

■ **Cardiovascular disorders** include hypertension, decreased high-density lipoprotein (HDL) and increased low density lipoprotein (LDL) cholesterol, all of which promote heart attacks and strokes.
■ **Liver disorders** include benign and malignant neoplasms, cholestatic hepatitis and jaundice, and peliosis hepatis, a disorder in which blood-filled cysts develop in the liver and may lead to hemorrhage or liver failure.
■ **Central nervous system disorders** include aggression, hostility, combativeness, and dependence charac-

## AT THE FOUNDATION: *Effects of Testosterone on Body Tissues*

### Fetal Development

The placenta produces large amounts of chorionic gonadotropin during pregnancy. Chorionic gonadotropin is similar to luteinizing hormone (LH) from the anterior pituitary gland. It promotes development of the interstitial or Leydig's cells in fetal testes, which then secrete testosterone. Testosterone production begins the second month of fetal life. When present, testosterone promotes development of male sexual characteristics (eg, penis, scrotum, prostate gland, seminal vesicles, and seminiferous tubules) and suppresses development of female sexual characteristics. In the absence of testosterone, the fetus develops female sexual characteristics.

Testosterone also provides the stimulus for the descent of the testes into the scrotum. This normally occurs after the seventh month of pregnancy, when the fetal testes are secreting relatively large amounts of testosterone. If the testes do not descend before birth, administration of testosterone or gonadotropic hormone, which stimulates testosterone secretion, produces descent in most cases.

### Adult Development

Little testosterone is secreted in boys until 11 to 13 years of age. At the onset of puberty, testosterone secretion increases rapidly and remains at a relatively high level until about 50 years of age, after which it gradually declines.

• The testosterone secreted at puberty acts as a growth hormone to produce enlargement of the penis, testes, and scrotum until about 20 years of age. The prostate gland, seminal vesicles, seminiferous tubules, and vas deferens also increase in size and functional ability. Under the combined influence of testosterone and follicle-stimulating hormone (FSH) from the anterior pituitary gland, sperm production is initiated and maintained throughout the man's reproductive life.

• **Skin.** Testosterone increases skin thickness and activity of the sebaceous glands. Acne in the male adolescent is attributed to the increased production of testosterone.

• **Voice.** The larynx enlarges and deepens the voice of the adult man.

• **Hair.** Testosterone produces the distribution of hair growth on the face, limbs, and trunk typical of the adult man. In men with a genetic trait toward baldness, large amounts of testosterone cause alopecia (baldness) of the scalp.

• **Skeletal muscles.** Testosterone is largely responsible for the larger, more powerful muscles of men. The effects of testosterone on protein metabolism cause this characteristic. Testosterone helps the body retain nitrogen, form new amino acids, and build new muscle protein. At the same time, it slows the loss of nitrogen and amino acids formed by the constant breakdown of body tissues. Overall, testosterone increases protein anabolism (buildup) and decreases protein catabolism (breakdown).

• **Bone.** Testosterone makes bones thicker and longer. After puberty, more protein and calcium are deposited and retained in bone matrix. This causes a rapid rate of bone growth. The height of a male adolescent increases rapidly for a time, then stops as epiphyseal closure occurs. This happens when the cartilage at the end of the long bones in the arms and legs becomes bone. Further lengthening of the bones is then prevented.

### Anterior Pituitary Function

High blood levels of testosterone decrease secretion of FSH and LH from the anterior pituitary gland. This, in turn, decreases testosterone production.

---

ized by preoccupation with drug use, inability to stop taking the drugs, and withdrawal symptoms similar to those that occur with alcohol, cocaine, and narcotics. In some cases, psychosis may develop.

■ **Reproductive system disorders** include decreased testicular function (eg, decreased secretion of endogenous testosterone and decreased formation of sperm), testicular atrophy, and erectile dysfunction in men and amenorrhea in women.

■ **Metabolic disorders** include atherosclerosis-promoting changes in cholesterol metabolism and retention of fluids, with edema and other imbalances. Fluid and electrolyte retention contribute to the increased weight associated with drug use.

■ **Dermatologic disorders** include moderate to severe acne in both sexes, depending on drug dosage.

Many of these adverse effects persist several months after the drugs are stopped and may be irreversible.

Names of anabolic steroids include nandrolone (Deca-Durabolin), oxandrolone (Oxandrin), oxymetholone (Anadrol-50), and stanozolol (Winstrol).

## ANDROGENS AND ANABOLIC STEROIDS USED AS DRUGS

■ When male sex hormones or androgens are given from exogenous sources for therapeutic purposes, they produce the same effects as the naturally occurring hormones. These effects include inhibition of endogenous sex hormones and sperm formation through negative feedback of pituitary LH and follicle-stimulating hormone (FSH).

■ Male sex hormones given to women antagonize or reduce the effects of female sex hormones. Thus, administration of androgenic or anabolic steroids to women suppresses menstruation and causes atrophy of the endometrial lining of the uterus.

■ Several dosage forms of androgens are available; they differ mainly in route of administration and pharmacokinetics.

■ Naturally occurring androgens are given by injection because, if given orally, the liver metabolizes them rapidly. Some esters of testosterone have been modified to slow the rate of metabolism and thus prolong action. For example, intramuscular (IM) testosterone cypionate and testosterone enanthate have slow onset of actions and last 2 to 4 weeks.

■ Oral testosterone is extensively metabolized in its first pass through the liver, so that nearly half of a dose is lost before it reaches the systemic circulation. As a result, doses as high as 400 mg/day may be needed to produce adequate blood levels for full replacement therapy. Methyltestosterone is a synthetic formulation that is less extensively metabolized by the liver and more suitable for oral administration.

■ Several transdermal formulations of testosterone are available. They have a rapid onset of action and last approximately 24 hours. A topical gel (a 10-g dose delivers 100 mg) produces normal serum testosterone levels within 4 hours after application, and absorption of testosterone into the blood continues for 24 hours. Steady-state serum concentrations occur by the second or third day of use. When the gel is discontinued, serum testosterone levels remain in the normal range for 24 to 48 hours, but decrease to pretreatment levels within about 5 days. With Testoderm, the serum testosterone concentration reaches a maximum level within 2 to 4 hours and declines within 2 hours after the skin patch is removed. Serum levels plateau at 3 to 4 weeks, with serum testosterone concentrations in the range for normal men. Testoderm must be applied to the scrotum to achieve adequate blood levels; scrotal skin is much more permeable to testosterone than other skin areas. Testoderm TTS is applied to skin on the arm, back, or buttocks. Androderm is also applied to nonscrotal skin, and testosterone is continuously absorbed for 24 hours, with normal blood levels achieved during the first day of drug use. Applying the patch at night produces serum testosterone levels similar to those in healthy young men (ie, higher concentrations in the morning and lower ones in the evening).

■ Like endogenous testosterone, drug molecules are highly bound (98%) to plasma proteins, and serum half-life varies (eg, 8 days for IM testosterone cypionate, 9 hours for oral fluoxymesterone). The drugs are inactivated primarily in the liver. About 90% of a dose is excreted in urine as conjugates of testosterone and its metabolites. About 6% of a dose is excreted in feces.

■ Danazol is a synthetic drug with weak androgenic activity. It is given orally, has a half-life of 4 to 5 hours, and is metabolized in the liver. Route of excretion is unknown.

■ All synthetic anabolic steroids are weak androgens. Consequently, giving these drugs for anabolic effects also produces masculinizing effects. This characteristic limits the clinical usefulness of these drugs in women and children. Profound changes in growth and sexual development may occur if these drugs are given to young children.

## Mechanism of Action

Like other steroid drugs, androgenic and anabolic drugs penetrate the cell membrane and bind to receptor proteins in the cell cytoplasm. The steroid–receptor complex is then transported to the nucleus, where it activates RNA and DNA production and stimulates cellular synthesis of protein.

## Indications for Use

With male sex hormones, the most clearcut indication for use is to treat androgen deficiency states (eg, hypogonadism, cryptorchidism, erectile dysfunction, oligospermia) in boys and men. Hypogonadism may result from hypothalamic–pituitary or testicular dysfunction. In prepubertal boys, administration of the drugs stimulates the development of masculine characteristics. In postpubertal men who become androgen deficient, the hormones reestablish and maintain masculine characteristics and functions.

In women, danazol (Danocrine) may be used to prevent or treat endometriosis or fibrocystic breast disease. Anabolic steroids are more often abused for bodybuilding purposes than used for therapeutic effects.

Although some drug literature still lists metastatic breast cancer and some types of anemia as indications for use, newer drugs have largely replaced androgens for these purposes. In breast cancer, for example, androgens are second-line hormonal agents, after anti-estrogens (eg, tamoxifen). In anemia associated with renal failure, synthetic erythropoietin is more effective and likely to be used.

## Management Considerations

### Duration of Therapy
Drug therapy with androgens may be short or long term, depending on the condition in question, the client's response to treatment, and the incidence of adverse reactions. If feasible, intermittent rather than continuous therapy is recommended.

### Effects of Androgens and Anabolic Steroids on Other Drugs
Androgens may increase effects of cyclosporine and warfarin, apparently by slowing their metabolism and

## CLIENT TEACHING GUIDELINES
### Androgens

#### General Considerations

✔ Take the drugs only if prescribed and as prescribed. Use by athletes for body building is inappropriate and, if not prescribed by a licensed physician, illegal.

✔ Continue medical supervision as long as the drugs are being taken.

✔ Weigh once or twice weekly and record the amount. An increase may indicate fluid retention and edema.

✔ Practice frequent and thorough skin cleansing to decrease acne, which is most likely to occur in women and children.

#### Self-administration

✔ Take oral preparations before or with meals, in divided doses.

✔ For buccal preparations:

✔ Take in divided doses.

✔ Place the tablet between the cheek and gum and allow to dissolve (do not swallow).

✔ Avoid eating, drinking, or smoking while the tablet is in place.

✔ With transdermal systems:

✔ Apply 2 Androderm systems nightly to clean, dry skin on back, abdomen, upper arm, or thigh. Do not apply to scrotum. Rotate sites, with 7 days between applications to a site. Press firmly into place for adherence.

✔ Apply 1 Testoderm system to clean, dry scrotal skin (shaved, for best adherence) once daily.

✔ Apply the prescribed amount of gel to clean, dry, intact skin of the shoulders and upper arms or the abdomen (do **not** apply to the genital area), once daily, preferably in the morning. Wash hands after application and allow sites to dry before dressing. After applications, wait at least 1 hour and preferably 4 to 6 hours before showering or swimming.

---

increasing their concentrations in the blood. These combinations should be avoided if possible. However, if required, serum creatinine and cyclosporine levels should be monitored with cyclosporine, and prothrombin time or international normalized ratio (INR) should be monitored with warfarin.

Androgens also increase effects of sulfonylurea antidiabetic drugs. Concurrent use should be avoided if possible. If required, smaller doses of sulfonylureas may be needed, blood glucose levels should be monitored closely, and clients should be assessed for signs of hypoglycemia. Danazol inhibits metabolism of carbamazepine and increases risks for toxicity. Concurrent use should be avoided.

## Contraindications to Use

Androgens and anabolic steroids are contraindicated during pregnancy (because of possible masculinizing effects on a female fetus), in clients with preexisting liver disease, and in men with prostate gland disorders. Men with enlarged prostates may have additional enlargement, and men with prostatic cancer may experience tumor growth. Although not contraindicated in children, these drugs must be used very cautiously, with x-rays taken approximately every 6 months to evaluate bone growth.

Androgens and anabolic steroids are contraindicated in clients with preexisting liver disease. Prolonged use of high doses may cause potentially life-threatening conditions such as peliosis hepatis, hepatic neoplasms, and hepatocellular carcinoma. In addition, androgen therapy should be discontinued if cholestatic hepatitis with jaundice occurs, or if liver function tests become abnormal.

Drug-induced jaundice is reversible when the medication is stopped.

## Individual Androgens

Clinical indications, routes, and dosage ranges are listed in Drugs at a Glance 25-1: Androgens.

## Herbal and Dietary Supplements

Androstenedione and DHEA, androgens produced by the adrenal cortex, are also available as over-the-counter (OTC) dietary supplements. They are marketed as safe, natural, alternative androgens for building muscles. These products, which have weak androgenic activity, act mainly as precursors for the production of sex hormones. Androstenedione, for example, may be converted to testosterone by way of an enzyme found in most body tissues. However, it may also be converted to estrogens, and the testosterone that is produced may be further converted to estrogen (estradiol). In one study, young men with normal serum testosterone levels were given an androstenedione supplement for 8 weeks. The researchers found little effect on serum testosterone levels or muscle development with resistance training. They also found increased serum levels of estrone and estradiol, which indicate that a significant proportion of the androstenedione was converted to estrogens. Thus, taking a supplement for masculinizing effects may produce feminizing effects instead.

DHEA is available alone as oral capsules or tablets and in a topical cream with vitamins and herbs. Most DHEA products of plant origin are produced in Europe and China. They are marketed with numerous claims for

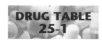

## Drugs at a Glance
**DRUG TABLE 25-1**
### Androgens

| Generic/Trade Name | Routes and Dosage Ranges | Comments |
|---|---|---|
| **Testosterone cypionate** (Depo-Testosterone) Pregnancy Category X | Hypogonadism: IM, 50–200 mg every 2–4 wk | Long duration of action of both cypionate and enanthate products make reversal of side effects difficult |
| **Testosterone enanthate** (Delatestryl) Pregnancy Category X | Hypogonadism: IM, 50–200 mg every 2–4 wk | Exogenous testosterone will result in premature epiphyseal closure and should be used with caution with young males Testosterone may cause serious liver toxicity |
| **Testosterone gel** (AndroGel 1%) Pregnancy Category X | Hypogonadism: 5 g (50 mg of drug) once daily to skin of shoulders and upper arms or abdomen | Skin should be clean and dry before application of product |
| **Testosterone pellets** Pregnancy Category X | Hypogonadism: Sub-Q, 150–450 mg every 3–6 mo Delayed puberty: Sub-Q, lower dosage range, for a limited duration (eg, every 3 mo for 2–3 doses) | Approximately ½ of the pellet is absorbed the first month; ⅓ the second; and ⅙ the third |
| **Testosterone transdermal systems** (Androderm, Testoderm) Pregnancy Category X | Hypogonadism: Apply two Androderm systems (dose of 5 mg) nightly to back, abdomen, upper arm or thigh; apply Testoderm (one 6-mg system) to scrotal sac daily | Skin should be clean and dry before application of product; patch can be removed and reapplied to bathe or swim Scrotum should be dry-shaved before application of patch |
| **Testolactone** (Teslac) Pregnancy Category X | Breast cancer: PO, 250 mg 4 times daily | Does not cause virilization |
| **Fluoxymesterone** (Halotestin) Pregnancy Category X | Hypogonadism: PO, 5–20 mg daily | Monitor serum glucose closely In children who have not reached puberty, hand and wrist x-rays should be taken |
| **Methyltestosterone** (Methitest, others) Pregnancy Category X | Cryptorchidism: PO, 30 mg daily; buccal tablets, 15 mg daily | May accelerate bone maturation without resultant linear bone growth |
| **Danazol** (Danocrine) Pregnancy Category X | Endometriosis: PO, 800 mg daily in two divided doses for 3–9 mo Fibrocystic breast disease: PO, 100–400 mg daily in two divided doses for 3–6 mo | Weak androgenic effect; for clients who have not tolerated or responded to other drug therapy |

health benefits, including inhibition of aging, atherosclerosis, cancer, diabetes mellitus, and osteoporosis. Most claims stem from laboratory and animal studies. A few small human studies have been done, most of which used a dose of 50 mg daily. Overall, there is no conclusive evidence that DHEA supplementation will prevent or treat such conditions. In addition, long-term effects in humans are unknown.

DHEA is contraindicated in men with prostate cancer or benign prostatic hypertrophy (BPH) and in women with estrogen-responsive breast or uterine cancer because DHEA may stimulate growth of these tissues. Clients older than 40 years of age should be aggressively screened for hormonally sensitive cancers before taking DHEA.

Adverse effects of DHEA include aggressiveness, hirsutism, insomnia, and irritability. Whether large doses of the OTC products can produce some of the serious side effects associated with standard anabolic steroids is unknown.

## ERECTILE DYSFUNCTION

Erectile dysfunction (ED), or impotence, is a condition whereby a male is persistently unable to achieve or sustain an erection adequate for satisfactory sexual performance. The condition affects nearly 30 million men, with an increased risk with advancing age and chronic illness.

Studies indicate that there is a reported prevalence of some degree of ED in 52% of males 40 to 70 years of age. Penile erection is a complex mechanism requiring functioning nervous, vascular, and hormonal systems. Additionally, the client must also be in the right mental state to respond to sensory sexual stimulation (see an attractive partner, smell a pleasant scent, hear a loving voice) to trigger an erection mediated by the central nervous system. Additionally, pharmacotherapy had been implicated as the cause of ED in roughly 10% to 25% of clients; these drugs are outlined in Table 25-1.

The multifactorial nature of ED makes management, including drug therapy, variable in its effect. Treatment of ED includes drug therapy, psychotherapy, mechanical devices, and surgical penile implantation. The focus of this section is on the pharmacologic treatment of the condition, predominately the use of the phosphodiesterase enzyme type 5 inhibitors.

## Mechanism of Action

The dorsal side of the penis contains two corpora cavernosa; the ventral side contains one corpus spongiosum. Blood flow through the corpora is through multiple interconnected sinuses that can fill with blood to produce an erection. When the penis is in a flaccid state, arterial flow into the corpora and venous flow outward are in a state of balance. During an erection (which is initiated by the action of nerves), arterial blood fills the sinuses, and the penis elongates and swells. Occlusion of venous outflow from the corpora sustains the erection.

The arterial flow into the corpora is improved by acetylcholine that acts along with other neurotransmitters through two different pathways. In the presence of sexual stimulation, acetylcholine works in one pathway to enhance the production of nitric oxide. Nitric oxide activates the activity of the enzyme, guanylate cyclase, leading to increased levels of cyclic guanosine monophosphate (cGMP), a vasodilatory neurotransmitter in the corporal tissue. With the resultant smooth muscle relaxation, inflow of blood increases, and an erection occurs.

In a second pathway, acetylcholine stimulates receptors to increase conversion of cyclic adenosine triphosphate (cATP) to cyclic adenosine monophosphate (cAMP), producing muscle relaxation and improved blood flow to the corpora. This also produces an erection.

The **phosphodiesterase enzyme type 5 inhibitors** are a class of drugs used for the management of ED. They cause decreased catabolism of cGMP; the class is highly selective for the phosphodiesterase enzyme type 5 found

---

### TABLE 25-1  Drugs Associated With Erectile Dysfunction

| Drug Class | Contributory Factor |
| --- | --- |
| Agents that decrease penile blood flow | Reduction of arteriolar flow to corpora |
|   Beta-adrenergic antagonists | |
|     Propranolol | |
|     Atenolol | |
|     Metoprolol | |
|   Central sympatholytic agents | |
|     Clonidine | |
|     Guanethidine | |
|     Methyldopa | |
|   Diuretics | |
| Anticholinergic agents | Anticholinergic effect |
|   Antihistamines | |
|   Antiparkinson agents | |
|   Tricyclic antidepressants | |
|   Phenothiazines | |
| Antiandrogens, estrogens | Suppression of testosterone-mediated stimulation of libido |
|   Cimetidine | |
|   Digoxin | |
|   Spironolactone | |
|   Ketoconazole | |
|   Luteinizing hormone–releasing hormone superantagonists | |
| Central nervous system depressants | Suppression of the perception of psychogenic stimuli |
|   Alcohol | |
|   Barbiturates | |
|   Benzodiazepines | |
| Dopamine agonists | Increased level of prolactin-inhibiting factor |
|   Metoclopramide | |
|   Phenothiazines | |

in genital tissue. Normally, cGMP is produced during sexual stimulation; therefore, the male must be stimulated after the drug is taken for an erection to occur. This enhances the effect of nitrous oxide, a chemical substance that relaxes the smooth muscles in the penis with sexual stimulation, increasing blood flow to the penis, and restoring the erectile response.

As previously described, **testosterone** is the principal endogenous androgen. Much of the testosterone that transfers to tissues undergoes intracellular conversion to dihydrotestosterone, especially in the prostate gland in the adult male. Almost all testosterone effects result from the increased formation of proteins throughout the body, especially in the cells of target organs and tissues responsible for development of male sexual characteristics. The use of testosterone replacement for ED may be indicated in an attempt to improve libido in clients with hypogonadism with decreased serum testosterone levels.

**Alprostadil** stimulates adenyl cyclase, which stimulates smooth muscle cell membrane receptors, increasing cAMP production. This results in an increase of arterial blood flow to the corpora.

## Indications for Use

The major clinical indication of drugs for ED is a history of inability to sustain an erection suitable for satisfactory sexual performance. The condition is associated with males with chronic illness, particularly hypertension, diabetes mellitus, and depression. Phosphodiesterase enzyme inhibitors are indicated for male clients experiencing ED.

The use of testosterone replacement may be indicated in clients with decreased libido and decreased serum testosterone levels. Testosterone replacement will not directly correct ED but will improve libido.

Alprostadil stimulates adenyl cyclase, which stimulates smooth muscle cell membrane receptors, increasing cAMP production. This results in an increase of arterial blood flow to the corpora.

The combination of papaverine plus phentolamine has been used to manage ED, but it is not described here because the drugs are not currently approved by the U.S. Food and Drug Administration (FDA) for this purpose.

## Goal of Treatment

Overall, the goal of treatment is to improve the quantity and quality of an erection suitable for satisfactory sexual performance with minimal or tolerable adverse drug effects. Ideally, the initial step in management is the identification and reversal of the underlying causes.

Drugs used for ED are self-administered at home. The home care nurse may encounter clients or family members taking one of the drugs when visiting the home for another purpose. Guidelines for strategies for ongoing

evaluation and intervention to aid the client in improving the quantity and quality of the sexual experience are addressed in Home Care Considerations. In addition, age-specific considerations are important in the management plan, particularly because this condition is commonly present in the older adult. Discussion of specific management considerations for older adults is found in Age-related Considerations.

## Contraindications to Use

Concurrent use of nitrates in any form or route of administration with phosphodiesterase enzyme inhibitors enhances severe hypotensive effects. This occurs because organic nitrates relax smooth muscle in blood vessel walls, decreasing blood pressure; nitrates also supply extra nitric oxide that can increase levels of cGMP. Therefore, nitrates are contraindicated within 24 hours of administration of phosphodiesterase enzyme inhibitors.

These drugs should be used with caution in individuals with conditions that may predispose them to priapism and in those with anatomic deformities of the penis, including cavernosal fibrosis, Peyronie's disease, or angulation.

## Home Care Considerations: Use of Drugs for Erectile Dysfunction

**ASSESS:** the client and family's knowledge of condition; the client for compliance with the prescribed regimen; for concurrent use with other drugs used for erectile dysfunction; and need for referral for treatment. Clients should be assessed for characteristics (eg, concurrent use of nitrates, older age group, renal or liver impairment, overuse of the drugs) that increase the risks for adverse effects.

**MONITOR:** the therapeutic and adverse effects of the drugs, satisfaction with quantity and quality of the sexual experience, and client's need for additional information, and provide that information.

**EDUCATE:** regarding importance of reading and following medication instructions, particularly timing of administration, not exceeding recommended dosages without consulting a health care provider, and interventions to minimize adverse effects, including avoiding the eating of grapefruit or drinking grapefruit juice with sildenafil or vardenafil. With alprostadil, emphasize importance of washing hands before drawing up medication and use of aseptic technique with administering, correct injection technique, and proper disposal of equipment after use. Reinforce that these drugs do not protect against sexually transmitted disease; use "safer sex" practices such as using latex condoms. Reinforce additional teaching points regarding specific drug preparations (see Client Teaching Guidelines: Androgens; Drugs for Erectile Dysfunction).

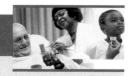

## Age-related Considerations:
## Use of Drugs That Affect Male Reproductive Health

### USE IN CHILDREN

The main indication for use of androgens is in boys with established deficiency states. Because the drugs cause epiphyseal closure, hands and wrists should be x-rayed every 6 months to detect bone maturation and prevent loss of adult height. Stimulation of skeletal growth continues for approximately 6 months after drug therapy is stopped. If premature puberty occurs (precocious sexual development, enlarged penis), the drug should be stopped. The drugs may cause or aggravate acne. Scrupulous skin care and other antiacne treatment may be needed, especially in adolescent boys.

### USE IN OLDER ADULTS

The main indication for use of androgens is a deficiency state in men. Older adults often have hypertension and other cardiovascular disorders that may be aggravated by the sodium and water retention associated with androgens and anabolic steroids. In men, the drugs may increase prostate size and interfere with urination, increase risk for prostatic cancer, and cause excessive sexual stimulation and priapism.

## Individual Drugs

The drugs that are used for ED include the phosphodiesterase enzyme inhibitors, testosterone, and alprostadil.

## Phosphodiesterase Enzyme Type 5 Inhibitors

Individual phosphodiesterase enzyme inhibitors are described below; routes and dosages ranges are listed in Drugs at a Glance 25-2: Drugs Used to Manage Erectile Dysfunction.

### Sildenafil

 **Sildenafil** (Viagra) was the first drug in this class to be approved for the treatment of ED and as such is considered the prototype (see Prototype Profile 25-1: Sildenafil). The drug is considered a first-line therapy, especially in younger clients, because of its convenient route of admin-

---

## ✔ CLIENT TEACHING GUIDELINES
## Drugs for Erectile Dysfunction

### General Considerations

✔ Take the drugs only if prescribed and as prescribed.

✔ Take as directed 30 minutes to 1 hour before sexual intercourse or as instructed.

✔ Report all drugs that are used to avoid the risk for untoward drug effect.

✔ Recognize that the drug does not protect against sexually transmitted disease; use "safer sex" practices such as latex condoms.

✔ Avoid concomitant use of other drug agents for erectile dysfunction.

✔ Do not share medications with others.

✔ If overdose is suspected, seek professional help at an emergency department immediately, or call the local poison control center.

### Self-administration

With sildenafil or vardenafil:

✔ Take oral preparations on an empty stomach because a high-fat meal may slow absorption.

✔ Do not use drug more than once a day or as instructed by a health care provider.

✔ Anticipate that sexual stimulation will be required for drug to be effective.

✔ Avoid eating grapefruit or drinking grapefruit juice because it may increase drug levels and therefore complications.

✔ Store medication at room temperature in a tightly closed container.

✔ Recognize that the drug could cause dizziness or vision changes; do not drive or operate machinery until the effects of the drug are known.

With alprostadil (Muse, Caverject, Edex):

✔ Use a ½-inch 27- to 30-gauge needle for injection; individuals with a needle phobia, or poor manual dexterity or vision, may be able to use an autoinjector.

✔ Inject into the dorsolateral area of the proximal third of the penis; hold pressure to injection site for at least 5 minutes to minimize risk for hematoma.

✔ Wash hands carefully before drawing up medication and use aseptic technique when administering.

✔ Dispose of vials, needles, and syringes in appropriate containers.

✔ Report to a health care provider any signs of infection, any fibrotic lumps in penis, pain in injected area, or priapism (a prolonged, painful erection lasting more than 1 hour).

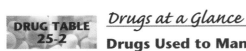

**DRUG TABLE 25-2**

*Drugs at a Glance*

## Drugs Used to Manage Erectile Dysfunction

| Generic/Trade Name | Routes and Dosage Ranges | Comments |
|---|---|---|
| Sildenafil (Viagra) | See Prototype Profile 25-1: Sildenafil | |
| Tadalafil (Cialis) Pregnancy Category B | 10 mg PO taken 30 min to 1 h before sexual intercourse; dosing range of 5–20 mg to be given as a single dose | Men who regularly consume grapefruit juice should not take more than 10 mg as a single dose or use more frequently than every 72 h, due to increased risk of toxicity |
| Vardenafil (Levitra) Pregnancy Category B | 10 mg PO taken 30 min to 1 h before sexual intercourse; dosing range of 5–20 mg to be given as a single dose | May take with or without food, although high-fat meals decrease absorption |
| Alprostadil (Muse, Caverject, Edex) Pregnancy Category X | Intracavernous: 2.5–60 mcg administered 5–10 min before sexual intercourse | Lowest effective dose should be used |
| | Intraurethral: 125–1000 mcg administered 5–10 min before sexual intercourse | The intraurethral inserts are marketed as Muse; the pellet is inserted with a urethral applicator |

## PROTOTYPE PROFILE 25-1
### ℗ Sildenafil (Sil DEN a fil)

**Drug Class**
*Chemical:* Phosphodiesterase enzyme type 5 inhibitor
*Functional:* Erectile dysfunction agent

**Trade Name**
Viagra

**Therapeutic Indications**
Treatment of erectile dysfunction

**Pharmacokinetics**
*Absorption*
Rapid

*Distribution*
Plasma protein binding: 96%

*Metabolism*
Hepatic

*Excretion*
Predominately feces; small amount in urine

**Pharmacodynamics**
*Onset of Action*
Approximately 60 min

*Duration*
2–4 h

**Contraindications/Precautions**
Concurrent use with nitrates, other drugs used to treat priapism, anatomic deformities of the penis (cavernosal fibrosis, Peyronie's disease, or angulation)

**Pregnancy Considerations**
Category B
Not indicated for use in women

**Dosage**
50 mg PO once daily; may decrease to 25 mg with hepatic or renal failure or in the older adult; increase to maximum of 100 mg as tolerated

**Adverse Effects**
Headache, dyspepsia, blurred or blue vision, sensitivity to light, flushing, dizziness, nasal congestion

**Drug Interactions**
*Increased Effects*
Hypotensive effects with nitrates, alpha blockers, and other antihypertensives
Serum levels of sildenafil with clarithromycin, erythromycin, digoxin, alcohol, ketoconazole, itraconazole, ritonavir, indinavir, or cimetidine
Risk for bleeding with concurrent use of heparin

*Decreased Effects*
Serum concentration of sildenafil with concurrent use of phenytoin, phenobarbital, rifampin, and carbamazepine

**Herbal Supplements and Dietary Considerations**
St. John's wort may decrease sildenafil levels
Absorption decreased with high-fat meal
Grapefruit juice may increase serum levels and risk for toxicity

istration, apparent efficacy, and low frequency of adverse effects. Sildenafil, in doses ranging from 25 to 100 mg, has been reported to produce an acceptable response in 56% to 82% of clients. The responses appear to be dose related. Dosage adjustment is necessary in clients with liver or renal disease, clients older than the age of 65 years, and clients currently taking drugs that are known to inhibit hepatic breakdown of sildenafil (eg, clarithromycin, erythromycin, ketoconazole, itraconazole, ritonavir, indinavir, and cimetidine).

Adverse effects are typically self-limiting and result from phosphodiesterase enzyme type 5 inhibition in tissue beyond the genital area. Common side effects include headache, nasal congestion, dyspepsia, and dizziness. The drug also enhances sensitivity to light, causing blurred vision or the loss of blue-green color discrimination, which is the "blue vision" reported with drug use.

Concurrent use of all forms and routes of nitrates with sildenafil enhance severe hypotensive effects. In 1998 when sildenafil was introduced, 123 deaths associated with the drug were reported. Approximately two thirds of users died as the result of a myocardial infarction or cardiac arrest; over one third of these clients developed cardiac symptoms within 5 hours of taking sildenafil. Of note, only one fifth of the clients had taken nitrates. Therefore, individuals with cardiac disease should undergo an overall cardiac workup and treadmill stress testing to determine risk category before beginning sildenafil therapy.

The drug should not be used in clients with normal erectile function or in combination with any other form of therapy for erectile dysfunction. The drug is not approved for use in women or children.

### Vardenafil

**Vardenafil** (Levitra) has recently been approved by the FDA for treatment of erectile dysfunction. The effectiveness of the drug and the expense of therapy are similar to those of sildenafil.

Adverse effects and warnings are indistinguishable from those with sildenafil. Vardenafil may not cause loss of blue-green color discrimination (and the same "blue vision" problem), but it is too soon to tell. The drug may be more effective in clients with diabetes or prostatectomy; however, both drugs in the class have been deemed effective, and no evidence currently indicates that one is superior.

### Tadalafil

**Tadalafil** (Cialis) is the most recent phosphodiesterase enzyme type 5 inhibitor approved by the FDA. Erectile function may be improved for up to 36 hours following a single dose, which may increase the drug's appeal. The same risk exists as with concurrent use of nitrates.

## Testosterone

Clinical indications, routes, and dosage ranges are listed in Drugs at a Glance: Androgens.

## Alprostadil

**Alprostadil** (Muse, Caverject, Edex) is also used to manage ED through direct injection into the corpus cavernosum or through pellets inserted in the urethra. The drug can increase arterial blood flow to the penis and reduce venous outflow. Dosages are based on an erection that is suitable for satisfactory sexual performance that does not last more than 1 hour. The drug should not be used by the intracavernous route more than once every 24 hours and not more than three times per week. The client should be instructed how to administer the injection with aseptic technique, to avoid visible veins, and to alternate sides of the penis for injection.

As an alternative, the drug can also be inserted directly as a pellet into the urethra using an applicator. The penis should be massaged after insertion to facilitate the absorption of the drug. An erection should develop in 5 to 10 minutes after administration and last up to 1 hour. The drug should not be used by the transurethral route more than twice in 24 hours.

Targeting the individual dose necessary for a satisfactory erection is completed in the health care provider's office. The client begins with the lowest dose. If no response occurs, the next highest dose is administered within the hour. Should no response be obtained, a one-day interval is recommended before titration is continued. Once a suitable erection is achieved, the client should remain in the health care provider's office until the erection completely subsides. The risk for hypotension and syncope may be enhanced when alprostadil is used with antihypertensive agents. The concomitant use of alcohol may produce a vasodilating effect.

Routes and dosage ranges are listed in Drugs at a Glance: Drugs Used to Manage Erectile Dysfunction.

## ℕURSING PROCESS

### Assessment

Before drug therapy is started, clients need a thorough history and physical examination. Periodic monitoring of the client's condition is needed throughout drug therapy.

- Assess for conditions in which androgens are used (eg, deficiency states).
- Assess for conditions that increase risks of adverse effects or are contraindications (eg, pregnancy, liver disease, prostatic hypertrophy).

*(continued)*

## NURSING PROCESS (Continued)

- Check laboratory reports of liver function tests (the drugs may cause cholestatic jaundice and liver damage), serum electrolytes (the drugs may cause sodium and water retention), and serum lipids (the drugs may increase levels and aggravate atherosclerosis).
- Assess weight and blood pressure regularly. These may be elevated by retention of sodium and water with resultant edema, especially in clients with congestive heart failure.
- For children, check x-ray reports of bone growth status initially and approximately every 6 months while the drugs are being taken.
- Assess the client's attitude toward taking male sex hormones.
- Assess the client's willingness to comply with instructions for taking the drugs and follow-up procedures.

### Nursing Diagnoses

- Disturbed Body Image related to masculinizing effects and menstrual irregularities
- Deficient Knowledge: Physiologic and psychological consequences of overuse and abuse of the drugs to enhance athletic performance
- Noncompliance: Overuse of drugs or dietary supplements
- Risk for Injury: Liver disease and other serious adverse drug effects

### Planning/Goals

*The client will:*
- Use the drugs for medical purposes only
- Receive or take the drugs as prescribed

- Avoid abuse of drugs or dietary supplements for body building
- Be counseled regarding effects of overuse and abuse if identified as being at risk (eg, athletes, especially weight lifters and football players)
- Avoid preventable adverse drug effects
- Comply with monitoring and follow-up procedures

### Interventions

- Assist clients to use the drug correctly.
- Assist clients to reduce sodium intake if edema develops.
- Record weight and blood pressure at regular intervals.
- Participate in school or community programs to inform children, parents, coaches, athletic trainers, and others of the risks of inappropriate use of androgens, anabolic steroids, and related dietary supplements.

### Evaluation

- Interview and observe for compliance with instructions for taking prescribed drugs.
- Interview and observe for therapeutic and adverse drug effects.
- Question athletes about illegal use of the drugs.
- Observe athletes for increased weight and behavioral changes that may indicate drug abuse.

---

## *Nursing Actions*
## Androgens and Anabolic Steroids

| Nursing Actions | Rationale/Explanation |
|---|---|
| 1. Administer accurately. | |
| a. Give intramuscular preparations of testosterone, other androgens and anabolic steroids deeply, preferably in the gluteal muscle. | |
| b. Give oral preparations before or with meals, in divided doses. | To decrease gastrointestinal disturbances |
| c. For buccal preparations: | |
| (1) Give in divided doses. | |
| (2) Place the tablet between the cheek and gum. | Buccal preparations must be absorbed through the mucous membranes. |
| (3) Instruct the client not to swallow the tablet and not to drink, chew, or smoke until the tablet is completely absorbed. | |
| d. With transdermal systems: | |
| (1) Apply 2 Androderm systems nightly to clean, dry skin on back, abdomen, upper arm, or thigh. Do *not* apply to scrotum. Rotate sites, with 7 days between applications to a site. Press firmly into place for adherence. | Correct site selection and application are necessary for therapeutic effects. Scrotal skin is more permeable to testosterone than other skin areas. |

*(continued)*

*Nursing Actions*

## Androgens and Anabolic Steroids (Continued)

| Nursing Actions | Rationale/Explanation |
|---|---|
| (2) Apply 1 Testoderm system to clean, dry scrotal skin (shaved, for best adherence) once daily. | |
| (3) Apply Androgel 1% to shoulders and upper arms or abdomen, once daily, preferably in the morning. | Manufacturer's recommendation. Clients may prefer self-application. Skin should be clean, dry, and intact; hands should be washed after application; and showering and swimming should be avoided for at least 1 hour and preferably 4 to 6 hours after application. |
| e. Inject testosterone pellets (Testopel) subcutaneously. | Manufacturer's recommendation |
| **2. Observe for therapeutic effects.** | |
| a. When the drug is given for hypogonadism, observe for masculinizing effects, such as growth of sexual organs, deepening of voice, growth of body hair, and acne. | |
| b. When the drug is given for anabolic effects, observe for increased appetite, euphoria, or statements of feeling better. | |
| **3. Observe for adverse reactions.** | |
| a. Virilism or masculinizing effects: | |
| (1) In adult men with adequate secretion of testosterone—priapism, increased sexual desire, reduced sperm count, and prostate enlargement | |
| (2) In prepubertal boys—premature development of sex organs and secondary sexual characteristics, such as enlargement of the penis, priapism, pubic hair | |
| (3) In women—masculinizing effects include hirsutism, deepening of the voice, menstrual irregularities | |
| b. Jaundice—dark urine, yellow skin and sclera, itching | |
| c. Edema | More likely in clients who are elderly or who have heart or kidney disease |
| d. Hypercalcemia | More likely in women with advanced breast cancer |
| e. Difficulty voiding due to prostate enlargement | More likely in middle-aged or elderly men |
| f. Inadequate growth in height of children | |
| **4. Observe for drug interactions.** | |
| a. Drugs that *decrease* effects of androgens | |
| (1) Barbiturates | Increase enzyme induction and rate of metabolism |
| (2) Calcitonin | Decreases calcium retention and thus antagonizes calcium-retaining effects of androgens |

## Herbal and Dietary Supplements

**Yohimbine** is widely touted as an aphrodisiac to improve sexual performance. The drug is derived from tree bark and is thought to possess alpha-adrenergic blocking effects in the central nervous system. Yohimbine increases catecholamines and enhances mood. Although controversial, it is thought that the drug reduces peripheral alpha-adrenergic blocking effects, creating a predominant cholinergic effect and a vasodilatory response.

The usual dose is 5.4 mg three times a day. The American Urological Association has cautioned against the use of yohimbine because of findings of a metaanalysis of published studies on the use of yohimbine in high doses that indicated that the drug was no more effective than a placebo. Common adverse effects include hypertension, tachycardia, anxiety, and insomnia.

## Critical Thinking Exercises

1. The most clearcut therapeutic indication for use of male sex hormones is:
   a. To treat androgen deficiency states in boys and men
   b. For bodybuilding purposes
   c. To treat metastatic breast cancer
   d. To treat anemia associated with renal failure

**2.** Androgens may increase effects of all of the following except:

   a. Cyclosporine

   b. Warfarin

   c. Sulfonylureas

   d. Heparin

**3.** What percentage of testosterone secreted by the testes binds to plasma albumin or to sex hormone–binding globulin and circulates in the blood?

   a. 26%

   b. 49%

   c. 78%

   d. 97%

**4.** Concurrent use of nitrates in any form or route of administration with phosphodiesterase enzyme inhibitors produces:

   a. Enhanced erectile potential

   b. Significant tachycardia

   c. Severe hypotensive effects

   d. Mild bronchodilation

**5.** Yohimbine is widely touted as an aphrodisiac to improve sexual performance. Findings of a metaanalysis of published studies on the use of yohimbine in high doses indicated that the drug was:

   a. Equal to sildenafil in therapeutic benefit

   b. More effective than testosterone

   c. Useful for erectile dysfunction because it produced no side effects

   d. No more effective than a placebo

## SELECTED REFERENCES

DiPiro, J. T., Talbert, R. L., Yee, G. C., Matzke, G. R., Wells, B. G., & Posey, L. M. (2002). *Pharmacotherapy: A pathophysiologic approach* (5th ed.). New York: McGraw-Hill.

*Drug facts and comparisons.* (Updated monthly). St. Louis: Facts and Comparisons.

Guyton, A. C., & Hall, J. E. (2000). *Textbook of medical physiology* (10th ed.). Philadelphia: W. B. Saunders.

Lacy, C. F., Armstrong, L. L., Goldman, M. P., & Lance, L. L. (2003). *Lexi-Comp's drug information handbook* (11th ed.). Hudson, OH: American Pharmaceutical Association.

Porth, C. M. (2002). *Pathophysiology: Concepts of altered health states* (6th ed.). Philadelphia: Lippincott Williams & Wilkins.

Snyder, P. J. (2000). Disorders of gonadal function in men. In H. D. Humes (Ed.), *Kelley's textbook of internal medicine* (4th ed., pp. 2743–2750). Philadelphia: Lippincott Williams & Wilkins.

# Nutrients and Weight Control

26

# Nutritional Support Products

## OBJECTIVES

*After studying this chapter, the student will be able to:*

1. Assess clients for risk factors and manifestations of fluid imbalances and undernutrition.

2. Evaluate the types and amounts of nutrients provided in commercial products for oral and tube feedings.

3. Collaborate with nutritionists and health care providers in designing and implementing nutritional support measures for undernourished or malnourished clients.

4. Minimize complications of enteral and parenteral nutrition.

5. Monitor laboratory reports that indicate nutritional status.

## CRITICAL THINKING SCENARIO

*M*ichelle, 2 months of age, had a gastrostomy tube placed after surgical repair of her esophagus. She is being sent home with her parents to receive tube feedings for a period of 6 to 8 weeks.

✔ What questions and anxieties might the parents have?

✔ What is the potential impact of tube feeding on infant–parent bonding?

✔ Compare and contrast how tube feedings are the same and different for an infant and adult.

✔ Review priority teaching needs for Michelle's parents before discharge.

# OVERVIEW

Water, carbohydrates, proteins, fats, vitamins, and minerals are required for human nutrition, to promote or maintain health, to prevent illness, and to promote recovery from illness or injury. The first four nutrients are discussed in this chapter and are highlighted in At the Foundation: Nutrient Requirements; vitamins and minerals are discussed in Appendix E.

Although recommended amounts of these nutrients can be used as rough estimates of clients' nutritional needs, actual requirements vary widely, depending on age, sex, size, illness, and other factors. Thus, nutritional care should be individualized. Although health care providers typically order diets, and nutritionists advise about dietary matters, it is often the nurse who must coordinate others to implement nutritional care. Consequently, this chapter discusses the use of products to improve nutritional status in clients with deficiency states and special needs.

# NUTRITIONAL DEFICIENCY STATES

Nutritional deficiencies result from inadequate amounts of water, carbohydrates, proteins, or fats. Treatment of deficiency states may lead to excess states. Causes and symptoms of water imbalances are listed in Table 26-1; those of protein-calorie imbalances are listed in Table 26-2.

Nurses encounter many clients who are unable to ingest adequate fluid and food because of illness. Debilitating illnesses such as cancer, acquired immunodeficiency syndrome, and chronic lung, kidney, or cardiovascular disorders often interfere with appetite and gastrointestinal (GI) function. Therapeutic drugs often cause anorexia, nausea, vomiting, diarrhea, or constipation. Nutritional deficiencies may impair the function of essentially every body organ, impair wound healing, and increase risks for infection. The nurse is involved with nutritional matters in almost any home care setting. Because nutrition is so important to health, the nurse should take advantage of any opportunity for health promotion in this area. Health promotion may involve assessing the nutritional status of all members of a household, especially children,

older adults, and those with obvious deficiencies or excesses, and providing counseling or other assistance to improve nutritional status. Guidelines for ongoing evaluation and intervention specific for age and in the home are addressed in Age-related Considerations and Home Care Considerations, respectively.

## TABLE 26-1    Water Imbalances

### Water Deficit

| Causes | Signs and Symptoms |
|---|---|
| 1. Inadequate fluid intake, most likely to occur in people who are comatose, unable to swallow, or otherwise incapacitated | 1. Thirst |
| | 2. Oliguria and concentrated urine |
| | 3. Weakness |
| | 4. Dry tongue and oral mucous membranes |
| 2. Excessive fluid loss due to vomiting, diarrhea, fever, diuretic drug therapy, high environmental temperatures, strenuous physical activity, or excessive sweating | 5. Flushed skin |
| | 6. Weight loss |
| | 7. Fever |
| | 8. Increased hematocrit |
| | 9. Mental disturbances ranging from mild confusion to delirium, convulsions, and coma |
| 3. A combination of 1 and 2 | 10. Hypovolemic shock if the deficiency is severe or develops rapidly |

### Water Excess

| Causes | Signs and Symptoms |
|---|---|
| 1. Excessive intake, most likely to occur with excessive amounts or rapid infusion of intravenous fluids | 1. Drowsiness |
| | 2. Weakness and lethargy |
| | 3. Weight gain |
| | 4. Edema |
| 2. Impaired excretion of fluids due to endocrine, renal, cardiovascular, or central nervous system disorders | 5. Low serum sodium and hematocrit |
| | 6. Disorientation |
| | 7. Circulatory overload and pulmonary edema if water excess is severe or develops rapidly |

## AT THE FOUNDATION: *Nutrient Requirements*

Water, carbohydrates, proteins, and fats are necessary for life. Water is required for cellular metabolism and excretion of metabolic waste products; 2000 to 3000 mL is needed daily. Proteins are basic anatomic and physiologic components of all body cells and tissues; the recommended amount for adults is 50 to 60 g daily. Carbohydrates and fats serve primarily as sources of energy for cellular metabolism. Energy is measured in kilocalories (kcal) per gram of food oxidized in the body. Carbohydrates and proteins supply 4 kcal/g; fats supply 9 kcal/g.

## TABLE 26-2 Carbohydrate, Protein, and Fat Imbalances

### Protein-Calorie Deficit

| Causes | Signs and Symptoms |
|---|---|
| 1. Inadequate intake of protein, carbohydrate, and fat | 1. Weight loss with eventual loss of subcutaneous fat and muscle mass |
| 2. Impaired ability to digest, absorb, or use nutrients | 2. Increased susceptibility to infection |
| 3. Excessive losses | 3. Weakness and fatigability |
| | 4. Dry, scaly skin |
| | 5. Impaired healing |
| | 6. Impaired growth and development in children |
| | 7. Edema |
| | 8. Decreased hemoglobin |
| | 9. Acidosis |
| | 10. Disordered brain function |
| | 11. Coma |
| | 12. Starvation |

### Protein-Calorie Excess

| Causes | Signs and Symptoms |
|---|---|
| 1. Excessive intake, especially of carbohydrates and fats | 1. Weight gain |
| | 2. Obesity |

# NUTRITIONAL SUPPORT PRODUCTS

Numerous products are available to supplement or substitute for dietary intake in clients who cannot ingest, digest, absorb, or use nutrients. For example, liquid enteral formulas are available for oral or tube feedings. Many are nutritionally complete, except for water, when given in sufficient amounts. Additional water must be given to meet fluid needs. Some products contain extra protein, fiber, calories, or other nutrients. Most oral products are available in a variety of flavors and contain 1 kcal/mL; some contain 1.5 or 2 kcal/mL. Some products are formulated for clients with particular organ impairments (eg, renal insufficiency) or disease processes (eg, diabetes mellitus), and some are contraindicated for clients with particular organ impairments or disease processes. Clients and caregivers who purchase over-the-counter products should read labels carefully or consult a nutritionist.

Intravenous (IV) fluids are also available. Most are nutritionally incomplete and are designed for short-term use when oral or tube feedings are contraindicated. They are most useful in meeting fluid and electrolyte needs. When nutrients must be provided parenterally for more than a few days, a special formula can be given. Parenteral nutritional formulas can be designed to meet all nutritional needs or to supplement other feeding methods.

## Age-related Considerations: Use of Nutritional Support Products

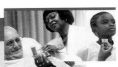

### USE IN CHILDREN

Children need increased amounts of water, protein, carbohydrate, and fat in proportion to their size to support growth and increased physical activity. Therefore, the goal of nutritional support is to meet needs without promoting obesity.

With tube feedings, to prevent nausea and regurgitation, the recommended rate of administration is no more than 5 mL every 5 to 10 minutes for premature and small infants and 10 mL/minute for older infants and children. Preparation of formulas, positioning of children, and administration are the same as for adults to prevent aspiration, diarrhea, and infection.

Parenteral nutrition may be indicated in infants and children who cannot eat or be fed enterally. In newborns, especially preterm and low-birth-weight infants, parenteral nutrition is needed within approximately 3 days of birth because they have little nutritional reserve. However, lipid emulsions should be given cautiously in preterm infants because deaths have been attributed to increased serum levels of lipids and free fatty acids. In other infants and children, parenteral nutrition may be used during medical illnesses or perioperative conditions to improve or maintain nutritional status. Overall, benefits include weight gain, increased height, increased liver synthesis of plasma proteins, and improved healing and recovery.

### USE IN OLDER ADULTS

Older adults are at risk for development of deficits and excesses in fluid volume. Inadequate intake is common and may result from numerous causes (eg, impaired thirst mechanism, impaired ability to obtain and drink fluids, inadequate water with tube feedings). Increased losses also occur with diuretic drugs, which are commonly prescribed for older adults. Fluid volume excess is most likely to occur with large amounts or rapid administration of IV fluids, especially in older adults with impaired cardiovascular function.

Older adults are also at risk for undernutrition in terms of protein, carbohydrate, and fat intake. Inadequate intake may result from the inability to obtain and prepare food as well as disease processes that interfere with the ability to digest and use nutrients. When alternative feeding methods (tube feedings, IV fluids) are used, careful assessment of nutritional status is required to avoid deficits or excesses.

### Home Care Considerations: Use of Nutritional Support Products

*ASSESS:* immediate and long-term care needs, safety risks and quality-of-life issues, use of resources, and ability to coordinate activities among IV therapy personnel and other health care providers.

*MONITOR:* compliance with the prescribed regimen; client responses and therapeutic and adverse effects; and that client is keeping appointments for lab work and follow-up care.

*EDUCATE:* with tube feeding, about the goals of treatment, administration, preparation or storage of solutions, equipment (eg, obtaining, cleaning), and monitoring responses (eg, weight, urine output); with parenteral nutrition, provide initial setup and ongoing client care management regarding solutions, infusion pumps, and other equipment that are often obtained from a pharmacy, home health agency, or independent company. Reinforce additional teaching points (see Client Teaching Guidelines: Nutritional Supplements and Tube Feedings).

Fat emulsions are usually included to supply additional calories and essential fatty acids.

Intravenous fluids and representative enteral products for infants, children, and adults are listed in Tables 26-3 and 26-4, respectively. For nutritional deficiencies due to malabsorption of carbohydrates, protein, and fat, pancreatic enzymes may be given.

**Pancreatin** and **pancrelipase** are commercial preparations of pancreatic enzymes (eg, lipase, protease, and amylase). The preparations are used to aid digestion and absorption of dietary carbohydrate, protein, and fat in conditions characterized by pancreatic enzyme deficiency. These conditions include cystic fibrosis, chronic pancreatitis, pancreatectomy, and pancreatic obstruction. No enzyme is recognized as a prototype, and dosages of the enzymes are listed in Drugs at a Glance 26-1: Pancreatic Enzymes.

## ■ DRUG USE IN SPECIFIC SITUATIONS

## Managing Fluid Disorders

### Fluid Deficiency

Treatment of fluid deficiency is aimed toward increasing intake or decreasing loss, depending on causative factors. The safest and most effective way of replacing body fluids is to give oral fluids when possible. Water is probably best, at least initially. Fluids containing large amounts of carbohydrate, fat, or protein are hypertonic and may increase fluid volume deficit if taken without sufficient water. If the client cannot take oral food or fluids for a few days or can take only limited amounts, IV fluids can

be used to provide complete or supplemental amounts of fluids. Frequently used solutions include 5% dextrose in water or sodium chloride.

To meet fluid needs over a longer period, a nasogastric or other GI tube may be used to administer fluids. Fluid needs must be assessed carefully for the client receiving food and fluid only by tube. Additional water is needed after or between tube feedings. Another way of meeting long-term fluid needs when the GI tract cannot be used is parenteral nutrition. These IV solutions provide other nutrients as well as fluids.

Optimal amounts of fluid may vary greatly. For most clients, 2000 to 3000 mL daily is adequate. A person with severe heart failure or oliguric kidney disease needs smaller amounts, but someone with fever or extra losses (eg, vomiting, diarrhea) needs more.

### Fluid Excess

Treatment of fluid excess is aimed toward decreasing intake and increasing loss. In acute circulatory overload or pulmonary edema, the usual treatment is to stop fluid intake (if the client is receiving IV fluids, slow the rate but keep the vein open for medication) and administer an IV diuretic. Because fluid excess may be a life-threatening emergency, prevention is better than treatment.

## Managing Nutritional Deficiencies

Undernutrition impairs the function of essentially every body organ, impairs wound healing, and increases risks for infection. The goal of treatment is to provide an adequate quantity and quality of nutrients to meet tissue needs. Requirements for nutrients vary with age, level of activity, level of health or illness, and other factors that must be considered when designing appropriate therapy.

### Enteral Nutrition: Oral Feedings

The safest and most effective way of increasing nutritional intake is by oral feedings, when feasible. High-protein, high-calorie foods can be included in many diets and given as between-meal or bedtime snacks. If the client cannot ingest enough food and fluid, many of the commercial nutritional preparations can be given as between-meal supplements to increase intake of protein and calories. These preparations vary in taste and acceptability. Measures to improve taste may include chilling, serving over ice, freezing, or mixing with fruit juice or another beverage. Specific methods depend on the client's taste preferences and the available formulas. Refer to instructions, usually on the labels, for appropriate diluting and mixing of beverages. Pudding formulations of several oral supplements are available and may be preferred by some clients.

### Enteral Nutrition: Tube Feedings

When oral feeding is contraindicated but the GI tract is functioning, tube feeding is usually preferred over IV flu-

## TABLE 26-3    Intravenous Fluids

| | Type/Characteristics | Uses | Comments |
|---|---|---|---|
| **Dextrose Injection** | | | |
| | Available in preparations containing 2.5%, 5%, 10%, 20%, 25%, 30%, 40%, 50%, 60%, and 70% dextrose<br>The most frequently used concentration is 5% dextrose in water ($D_5W$) or sodium chloride injection.<br>5% dextrose in water is isotonic with blood. It provides water and 170 kcal/L.<br>10% dextrose solution provides twice the calories in the same volume of fluid but is hypertonic and therefore may cause phlebitis.<br>Except for 25% or 50% solutions sometimes used to treat hypoglycemia, the higher concentrations are used in parenteral nutrition. They are hypertonic and must be given through a central or subclavian catheter. | To provide water and calories<br>Treat hypoglycemia (eg, insulin overdose)<br>As a component of parenteral nutritional mixtures | The dextrose in $D_5W$ is rapidly used, leaving "free" water for excreting waste products, maintaining renal function, and maintaining urine output.<br><br>Coinfusion of 10% dextrose solutions with lipid emulsions in peripheral parenteral nutrition may prevent or decrease phlebitis. |
| **Dextrose and Sodium Chloride Injection** | | | |
| | Available in several concentrations<br>Frequently used are 5% dextrose in 0.225% (also called $D_5\frac{1}{4}$ normal saline) and 5% dextrose in 0.45% sodium chloride ($D_5\frac{1}{2}$ normal saline)<br>These provide approximately 170 kcal/L, water, sodium, and chloride. | Maintenance fluids, usually with added potassium chloride, in clients who cannot eat or drink<br>Replacement fluids when large amounts are lost<br>To keep IV lines open<br>Administration of IV medications | |
| **Crystalline Amino Acid Solutions (Aminosyn, Freamine)** | | | |
| | Contain essential and nonessential amino acids | As a component of peripheral or central IV parenteral nutrition, with concentrated dextrose solutions | Special formulations are available for use in patients with renal or hepatic failure. |
| **Fat Emulsions (Intralipid, Liposyn)** | | | |
| | Provide concentrated calories and essential fatty acids<br>Available in 10% and 20% emulsions<br>500 mL of 10% emulsion provides 550 calories. | As a component of peripheral or central total parenteral nutrition | More calories can be supplied with a fat emulsion than with dextrose-protein solutions alone. |

ids, especially for long-term use. First, tube feeding is usually safer, more convenient, and more economical. Second, it helps to prevent GI atrophy, maintain GI function, and maintain immune system function. Third, several tubes and placement sites are available. For example, a nasogastric tube may be used for approximately 4 weeks. For long-term feedings, a gastrostomy tube may be placed percutaneously (called *percutaneous endoscopic gastrostomy*) or surgically. Nasointestinal tubes are recom-

*(text continues on page 454)*

## TABLE 26-4    Representative Enteral Formulas for Infants, Children, and Adults

| Name/Characteristics | Uses | Comments |
|---|---|---|
| *Infants and Children* | | |
| **Enfamil, Enfamil Premature**<br>Complete nutritional formulas | Alone for bottle-fed infants; as a supplement for breast-fed infants<br>Alone for bottle-fed or tube-fed premature infants | Formulas are similar to human breast milk<br>Nutritional needs of preterm infants differ from those of full-term infants. |
| **Lofenalac**<br>Contains less phenylalanine than other products | For infants and children with phenylketonuria (a metabolic disorder in which phenylalanine cannot be metabolized normally) | Inadequate for complete nutrition and growth. It is recommended that 85% of a child's protein needs be supplied with Lofenalac and the remaining with foods containing phenylalanine, which is an essential amino acid. |
| **Nursoy, ProSobee, Soyalac**<br>Hypoallergenic, milk-free formulas<br>Contain soy protein<br>Provide 20 calories/oz when mixed as directed | As milk substitutes for infants who are allergic to milk | Provide all other essential nutrients for normal growth and development |
| **Nutramigen**<br>Nutritionally complete, hypoallergenic formula containing predigested protein | Infants and children who are allergic to ordinary food proteins or have diarrhea or other GI problems | |
| **PediaSure**<br>Nutritionally complete, for oral use | Children 1–6 years of age | Amounts should be individualized |
| **Precision diets**<br>Nutritionally complete, high-nitrogen, low-residue formulas for oral or tube feedings | These formulas can be given to children if the amount is calculated to provide recommended amounts of nutrients for the particular age group. | These preparations are ingested or given by tube slowly over 4 hours.<br>Contraindicated in children with diabetes mellitus because the carbohydrate may produce hyperglycemia |
| **Pregestimil**<br>Contains easily digested protein, fat, and carbohydrate | For infants with severe malabsorption disorders | |
| **Vivonex**<br>Nutritionally complete diet, for oral or tube feedings<br>Requires little digestion and leaves little fecal residue | For children with GI disorders | Individualize the amount, concentration, and rate of administration to meet nutritional needs and tolerance. |
| *Adults* | | |
| **Amin-Aid**<br>Provides amino acids, carbohydrates, and a few electrolytes | As a source of protein for clients with acute or chronic renal failure | |
| **Ensure, Isocal, Osmolite**<br>Nutritionally complete<br>May be given orally or by tube feeding | As the sole source of nutrients or a supplement when food intake is decreased or does not meet nutritional needs | 2000 mL daily meets basic nutritional needs for adults. |
| **MCT Oil**<br>A preparation of medium-chain triglycerides, which are easier to digest than the long-chain triglycerides found in most foods<br>Can be mixed with fruit juices, used with salads or vegetables, or used in cooking and baking | Clients with fat malabsorption syndromes | Limit use in clients with severe hepatic cirrhosis because it may precipitate encephalopathy and coma.<br>Although useful as a caloric substitute for dietary fat (1 tbsp provides 115 kcal), it does not promote absorption of fat-soluble vitamins or provide essential fatty acids as the long-chain triglycerides do. |

*(continued)*

## TABLE 26-4    Representative Enteral Formulas for Infants, Children, and Adults (Continued)

| Name/Characteristics | Uses | Comments |
|---|---|---|
| **Polycose**<br>An oral supplement derived from carbohydrate<br>Available in liquid and powder<br>May be mixed with water or other beverages and with foods | Increase caloric intake in clients on protein-, electrolyte-, or fat-restricted diets | Individualize amounts by calories needed and tolerance. |
| **Portagen**<br>Nutritionally complete formula that contains medium-chain triglycerides, an easily digested form of fat | For clients with fat malabsorption problems, as the complete diet, as a beverage with meals, or as an addition to various recipes | May induce coma in clients with severe hepatic cirrhosis |
| **Precision diets**<br>Nutritionally complete, high nitrogen, low-residue formulas for oral or tube feedings | For supplemental or total nutrition | These preparations are ingested or given by tube slowly over 4 hours. The carbohydrate content may produce hyperglycemia; therefore, they should not be used in clients with diabetes mellitus. |
| **Pulmocare, Nutrivent**<br>These products are high in fat and low in carbohydrates because fat metabolism produces less carbon dioxide than carbohydrate metabolism. | Clients with chronic obstructive pulmonary disease or respiratory insufficiency | Clients with impaired breathing have difficulty eliminating carbon dioxide, a waste product of carbohydrate metabolism. When carbon dioxide accumulates in the body, it may produce respiratory acidosis and respiratory failure. |
| **Sustacal**<br>Nutritionally complete<br>May be given orally or by tube feeding | As the complete diet or to supplement other sources of nutrients | |
| **TraumaCal, Vivonex**<br>Nutritionally complete, high-protein formulas with easily assimilated amino acids and other nutrients<br>Can be used for oral or tube feedings | Clients with hypermetabolic states (eg, severe burns, trauma, or sepsis), to help meet nutritional needs and promote healing | The amount, concentration, and rate of administration can be adjusted to meet nutritional needs and tolerance. |

## *Drugs at a Glance*

**DRUG TABLE 26-1**

### Pancreatic Enzymes

| Generic/Trade Name | Route and Dosage Ranges | Comments |
|---|---|---|
| **Pancreatin** (Creon, others)<br>Pregnancy Category C | *Adults:* PO, 1 or 2 capsules or tablets with meals or snacks<br>*Children:* PO, 1 or 2 capsules or tablets with each meal initially, increased in amount or frequency if necessary and if adverse effects do not occur <6 mo. Dosage not established | Pancreatic lipase irreversibly inactivated at a pH ≤4<br>As with all enzymes, advise clients to not change brands without consulting health care provider or chew or crush enteric coated forms of drug |
| **Pancrelipase** (Viokase, others)<br>Pregnancy Category C | *Adults:* PO, 1 to 3 capsules or tablets before or with meals or snacks; or 1 or 2 packets of powder with meals or snacks | Overdose may cause diarrhea or temporary intestinal distress |

mended for clients at risk for aspiration from gastric feedings or with gastric disorders. Except for gastrostomy tubes, the tubes should be soft and small bore to decrease trauma.

When tube feedings are the client's only source of nutrients, they should be nutritionally complete and given in amounts calculated to provide adequate water, protein, calories, vitamins, and minerals. Although tube-feeding formulas vary in the volume needed for adequate intake

# Ⓝ URSING PROCESS

## Assessment

Assess each client for current or potential nutritional disorders. Some specific assessment factors include the following:

- What are usual drinking and eating patterns? Does fluid intake seem adequate? Does food intake seem adequate in terms of normal nutrition? Is the client financially able to purchase sufficient food? What are fluid and food likes and dislikes?
- Does the client know the basic foods for normal nutrition? Does the client view nutrition as important in maintaining health?
- Does the client appear underweight? Has there been a recent change in weight (eg, unintended weight loss)? If the client is underweight, assess for contributing factors (eg, appetite; ability to obtain, cook, or chew food). If a BMI is calculated, a BMI less than 18.5 kg/m² indicates undernutrition.
- Does the client have symptoms, disease processes, treatments, medications, or diagnostic tests that are likely to interfere with nutrition? For example, many illnesses and oral medications cause anorexia, nausea, vomiting, and diarrhea.
- Are any conditions present that increase or decrease nutritional requirements?
- Check available reports of laboratory tests, such as serum albumin, complete blood count, and blood glucose. Nutritional disorders, as well as many other disorders, may cause abnormal values.

## Nursing Diagnoses

- Imbalanced Nutrition:  Less Than Body Requirements related to inadequate intake or impaired ability to digest nutrients
- Deficient Fluid Volume related to inadequate intake
- Excess Fluid Volume related to excessive intake
- Diarrhea related to enteral nutrition
- Feeding Self Care Deficit

## Planning/Goals

**The client will:**
- Improve nutritional status in relation to body needs
- Maintain fluid and electrolyte balance

- Avoid complications of enteral nutrition, including aspiration, diarrhea, deficient or excess fluid volume, and infection
- Avoid complications of parenteral nutrition, including deficient or excess fluid volume and infection
- Identify the types and amounts of foods to meet nutritional needs

## Interventions

Implement measures to prevent nutritional disorders by promoting a well-balanced diet for all clients. Depending on the client's condition, diet orders, food preferences, knowledge and attitudes about nutrition, and other factors, specific activities may include the following:

- Provide food and fluid the client is willing and able to take, at preferred times when possible.
- Assist the client to a sitting position, cut meat, open containers, feed the client, and perform other actions if indicated.
- Treat symptoms or disorders that are likely to interfere with nutrition, such as pain, nausea, vomiting, or diarrhea.
- Consult with the physician or dietitian when needed, especially when special diets are ordered. Compliance is improved when the ordered diet differs as little as possible from the usual diet. Also, preferred foods often may be substituted for disliked ones.
- Promote exercise and activity. For undernourished clients, this may increase appetite, improve digestion, and aid bowel elimination.
- Minimize the use of sedative-type drugs when appropriate. Although no one should be denied pain relief, strong analgesics and other sedatives may cause drowsiness and decreased desire or ability to eat and drink as well as constipation and a feeling of fullness.
- Weigh clients at regular intervals.
- Use available resources to individualize nutritional care according to the client's clinical status and needs. For example, in hospitalized clients who are able to eat, consult a nutritionist about providing foods the client is able and willing to take. In hospitalized or outpatient clients who need a nutritional supplement, consult a nutritionist about choices, amounts, and costs.

*(continued)*

## NURSING PROCESS (Continued)

- For clients receiving parenteral nutrition, monitor weight, fluid intake, urine output, vital signs, blood glucose, serum electrolytes, and complete blood count daily or weekly, according to the client's status and whether hospitalized or at home.

### Evaluation

- Observe undernourished clients for quantity and quality of nutrient intake, weight gain, and improvement in labora-

tory tests of nutritional status (eg, serum proteins, blood sugar, electrolytes).
- Observe children for quantity and quality of food intake and appropriate increases in height and weight.
- Interview and observe for signs and symptoms of complications of enteral and parenteral nutrition.

---

## CLIENT TEACHING GUIDELINES
## Nutritional Supplements and Tube Feedings

### General Considerations

✔ Nutrition is extremely important in promoting health and recovery from illness. For people who are unable to take in enough nutrients because of poor appetite or illness, nutritional supplements can be very beneficial in improving their nutritional status. For example, supplemental feedings can slow or stop weight loss, increase energy and feelings of well-being, and increase resistance to infection.

✔ With oral supplements, choose one or more that the client is able and willing to take. Many are available, some in different flavors, and trying several different ones may be helpful. If a health care provider recommends one that the client does not like, ask for the names of others with comparable nutritional value.

✔ With feedings by a tube inserted into the stomach or intestinal tract, taste is not a consideration. However, there may be other factors that make a formula more or less acceptable, such as the occurrence of nausea or diarrhea.

### Self-administration or Caregiver Administration

✔ For oral supplemental feedings:
 ✔ Take or give at the preferred time and temperature, when possible. Chilling may improve taste.
 ✔ Mix powders or concentrated liquid preparations in preferred beverages, when possible. Some can be mixed with fruit juice, milk, tea, or coffee, which may improve taste and acceptability.
 ✔ Provide a variety of flavors, when possible, to improve acceptability.

✔ For tube feedings:
 ✔ Use or give with the client in a sitting position, if possible, to decrease risks of strangling and pulling formula into the lungs.
 ✔ Be sure the tube is placed correctly before each feeding. Ask a health care provider the best way of checking placement for your type of tube.

✔ Be sure the solution is room temperature. Cold formulas may cause abdominal cramping.
✔ Do not take or give more than 1 pint (500 mL) per feeding, including 2 to 3 oz of water for rinsing the tube. This helps to avoid overfilling the stomach and possible vomiting.
✔ Take or give slowly, over approximately 30 to 60 minutes. Rapid administration may cause nausea and vomiting.
✔ With continuous feedings, change containers and tubing daily. With intermittent feedings, rinse all equipment after each use, and change at least every 24 hours. Most tube feeding formulas are milk based and infection may occur if formulas become contaminated or equipment is not kept clean.
✔ Ask a health care provider about the amount of water to take or give. Most people receiving 1.5 to 2 quarts (1500 to 2000 mL) of tube feeding daily need approximately 1 quart (1000 mL) or more of water daily. However, clients' needs vary. Water can be mixed with the tube feeding formula, given after the tube feeding, or given between feedings. Be sure to include the amount of water used for rinsing the tube in the total daily amount.

✔ For giving medications by tube:
 ✔ Give liquid preparations when available. When not available, some tablets may be crushed and some capsules may be emptied and mixed with 1 to 2 tablespoons of water. Ask a health care provider which medications can safely be crushed or altered, because some (eg, long-acting or enteric-coated) can be harmful if crushed.
 ✔ Do not mix medications with the tube feeding formula because some medications may not be absorbed.
 ✔ Do not mix medications; give each one separately.
 ✔ Rinse the tube with water before and after each medication to get the medication through the tube and to keep the tube open.

of nutrients, any of the complete formulas can be used effectively. Other guidelines include the following:

- Once the kind and amount of formula are chosen, the method of feeding is selected. For feedings that enter the stomach, an intermittent schedule of administration every 4 to 6 hours, over 30 to 60 minutes, is usually recommended. For feedings that enter the duodenum or jejunum, a continuous drip method is required because the small bowel cannot tolerate the larger volumes of intermittent feedings. Continuous feedings require an infusion pump for accurate control of the flow rate. When used at home, enteral feedings are often given overnight to allow daytime oral feedings and more activity, if feasible, for the client.
- A common practice has been to initiate feedings with small amounts of diluted solution (ie, half strength), then increase to larger amounts and full strength. The rationale is to decrease the diarrhea and dehydration that may ensue when hypertonic solutions are given and water is drawn into the GI tract. Some authorities question the value of this regimen and prefer starting with small amounts of full-strength formulas. Isocal and Osmolite are isotonic and should be given full strength. Most formulas provide 1 kcal/mL so that caloric intake can be quickly calculated. Water can be given with, after, or between regular feedings and with medications, according to the client's fluid needs.
- Other than problems resulting from hypertonic solutions and inadequate fluid intake (diarrhea, fluid volume deficit, hypernatremia), a major complication of tube feeding is aspiration of the formula into the lungs. This is more likely to occur with unconscious clients and can be prevented by correctly positioning clients, verifying tube placement (before every intermittent feeding and approximately every 4 hours with continuous feedings), and giving feedings slowly.

### Parenteral Nutrition: Intravenous Feedings

Parenteral feedings are indicated when the GI tract is nonfunctioning, when enteral feedings would aggravate conditions such as inflammatory bowel diseases or pancreatitis, and when nutritional needs cannot be met by enteral feedings. For short-term use (eg, 3 to 5 days) of IV fluids, the goal is to provide adequate amounts of fluids and electrolytes and enough carbohydrate to minimize oxidation of body protein and fat for energy. The choice of specific solution depends on individual needs, but it should contain at least 5% dextrose. A frequently used solution is 5% dextrose in 0.22% sodium chloride, 2000 to 3000 mL per 24 hours. Potassium chloride is often added, and vitamins may be added. These solutions are nutritionally inadequate.

For long-term IV feedings (weeks to months), the goal is to provide all nutrients required for normal body functioning, including tissue growth and repair. Basic nutritional solutions provide water, carbohydrate, protein, vitamins, and minerals. Calories are usually supplied by

dilution of concentrated glucose solutions. Hypertonic solutions are given in a central vein so that they can be diluted rapidly. Central parenteral nutrition requires special techniques to increase safety and decrease complications. For example, a physician must insert the central IV catheter, and placement must be verified by a chest x-ray. Complications include air embolism and pneumothorax. Peripheral nutrition solutions are less hypertonic because they contain 5% or 10% dextrose. They can be given alone or in combination with oral or enteral feedings to increase nutrient intake.

Intravenous fat emulsions provide calories and essential fatty acids. These solutions are isotonic and may be given centrally or peripherally. When given peripherally, they are co-infused with the nutrition solution. The fat emulsion is thought to protect the vein and decrease phlebitis.

Guidelines for administration of central and peripheral parenteral nutrition include the following:

- Administer with an infusion pump to control the flow rate accurately. The solution must be given at a consistent rate so that nutrients can be used and complications prevented. The initial flow rate is usually 50 mL/hour; flow rate is then increased as tolerated to meet nutritional requirements (approximately 1500 to 3000 mL/day). With home administration, the entire daily amount may be infused overnight.
- To prevent infection, several measures are indicated. First, the IV catheter must be inserted with aseptic technique. Second, all solutions must be prepared aseptically in a pharmacy under a laminar-flow hood. Third, use an appropriate in-line filter. Fourth, change solution containers, administration sets, and dressings at the venipuncture site on a regular schedule, according to agency policies. Protocols for dressing changes usually include cleansing around the catheter with povidone-iodine solution (Betadine), applying povidone-iodine ointment, and reapplying an occlusive dressing. Sterile technique is used throughout.
- "Piggyback" fat emulsions into the IV line beyond the filter.

## Use in Renal Impairment

Because the kidneys excrete water and waste products of food metabolism, clients with renal impairment often have accumulation of water and urea nitrogen. As a result, these clients have special needs in relation to nutritional support. The needs differ with acute renal failure (ARF) and chronic renal failure (CRF).

With ARF, clients usually have major physiologic stress (eg, serious illness, sepsis, major surgery) that leads to metabolic disorders. These disorders include glucose intolerance (hyperglycemia and peripheral insulin resistance); accumulation of urea nitrogen, the end product of protein metabolism; and increased serum triglyceride levels from disordered fat metabolism. With CRF, clients are not usually as stressed as those with ARF. However, they often have multiple metabolic and fluid and electrolyte disorders. Those on dialysis have impaired host defense mechanisms and increased risk of infection. Undernourished clients have increased morbidity and mortality. Some considerations in nutritional support of clients with ARF and CRF are listed in the following sections.

### Acute Renal Failure

- In early ARF, dietary protein is usually restricted to 20 to 30 g/day to minimize urea nitrogen production.
- In oliguric ARF, small volumes of concentrated nutrients with minimal sodium are needed.
- In nonoliguric ARF, large amounts of sodium may be lost in urine, and sodium replacement may be needed.
- Enteral nutrition is preferred if possible. However, most clients are unable to tolerate enteral feedings because they are critically ill.
- Parenteral nutrition formulas should be carefully calculated according to nutritional status and metabolic disorders. Several amino acid solutions are formulated for clients with renal failure (eg, Aminosyn-RF, Aminess, NephrAmine, RenAmin). In addition, clients with ARF often have hyperkalemia, hyperphosphatemia, and hypermagnesemia, so that potassium, phosphorus, and magnesium should be omitted until serum levels return to normal.
- Intravenous fat emulsions should not be given to clients with ARF if serum triglyceride levels exceed 300 mg/dL.

### Chronic Renal Failure

- Enteral nutritional support is usually indicated because the GI tract is functional. Normal amounts of protein (eg, 1 g/kg/day) may be given. The former recommendation that protein restriction delayed progression of renal failure and the need for dialysis is not supported by newer data.
- High-calorie, low-electrolyte enteral formulations are usually indicated. Nepro is a formulation for clients receiving dialysis; Suplena, which is lower in protein and some electrolytes than Nepro, may be used in clients who are not receiving dialysis.
- If parenteral nutrition is needed, solutions should be carefully formulated according to nutritional status, the extent of metabolic disorders, and whether the client is receiving dialysis. Several amino acid solutions are formulated for clients with renal failure (eg, Aminosyn-RF, Aminess, NephrAmine, RenAmin).
- Serum triglyceride levels should be measured before IV fat emulsions are given. Many clients with CRF have hypertriglyceridemia, which would be worsened by fat emulsions, possibly leading to pancreatitis.

## Use in Hepatic Impairment

The liver is extremely important in digestion and metabolism of carbohydrates, proteins, and fat as well as storage of nutrients. Thus, clients with impaired hepatic function are often undernourished, with impaired metabolism of foodstuffs, vitamin deficiencies, and fluid and electrolyte imbalances. Depending on the disease process and the extent of liver impairment, these clients have special needs in relation to nutritional support.

- Clients with alcoholic hepatitis or cirrhosis have a high rate of metabolism and therefore need foods to supply extra energy. However, metabolic disorders interfere with the liver's ability to process and use foodstuffs.
- Disorders of glucose metabolism are common. Clients with cirrhosis often have hyperglycemia. Clients with severe hepatitis often have hypoglycemia because of impaired hepatic production of glucose and possibly impaired hepatic metabolism of insulin.
- Protein restriction is usually needed in clients with cirrhosis to prevent or treat hepatic encephalopathy, which is caused by excessive protein or excessive production of ammonia (from protein breakdown in the GI tract). For clients able to tolerate enteral feedings (usually by GI tube), Hepatic-Aid II is formulated for clients with liver failure. When peripheral or central parenteral nutrition is necessary for clients with hepatic failure and hepatic encephalopathy, HepatAmine, a special formulation of amino acids, may be used. Other amino acid preparations are contraindicated in clients with hepatic encephalopathy and coma.
- Enteral and parenteral fat preparations must be used cautiously. Medium-chain triglycerides (eg, MCT oil), which are used to provide calories in other malnourished clients, may lead to coma in clients with advanced cirrhosis. Clients who require parenteral nutrition may develop high serum triglyceride levels and pancreatitis if given usual amounts of IV fat emulsions. If serum triglyceride levels exceed 300 mg/dL, fat emulsions should be used only to prevent a deficiency of essential fatty acids.
- Sodium and fluid restrictions are often needed to decrease edema.

## Use in Pulmonary Impairment

- In clients with chronic obstructive pulmonary disease (COPD), major concerns are weight loss and decreasing the work of breathing. Weight loss is attributed mainly to hyperactive metabolism. However, increasing caloric intake in these clients must be done cautiously because overfeeding leads to increased carbon dioxide production, increased work of breathing, and perhaps respiratory acidosis. Thus, excessive carbohydrate in enteral or parenteral feedings may cause respiratory failure.
- Enteral nutrition is preferred if the GI tract is functional and accessible. Nutrivent and Pulmocare are enteral products for clients with COPD or respiratory failure and mechanical ventilation. They contain less carbohydrate and more fat than other products.
- Clients need adequate amounts of protein, but too much can increase the work of breathing and lead to muscle fatigue and respiratory failure. Moderate

amounts (1 to 1.5 g/kg/day) are recommended for clients with stable COPD. Clients with sepsis and respiratory failure who require mechanical ventilation usually need higher amounts of protein.

- Enteral formulas with more concentrated calories (eg, 2 kcal/mL) may be useful for clients with adult respiratory distress syndrome (ARDS), pulmonary edema, or other conditions requiring fluid restriction.
- Parenteral nutrition is often needed because clients with pulmonary failure from severe pneumonia or septicemia may have a prolonged ileus and be unable to tolerate enteral feedings. As with enteral feedings, excessive carbohydrate must be avoided.
- Intravenous fat emulsions should be infused slowly, over 24 hours. Rapid infusion may lead to pulmonary vasoconstriction.
- Excessive amounts of sodium and fluids should be avoided with both enteral and parenteral nutrition because they may worsen impaired pulmonary function.

## Use in Cardiac Impairment

- Undernutrition may lead to decreased cardiac output and stroke volume, with resultant hypotension and bradycardia.
- Excessive amounts of nutrients or fluids may worsen heart failure by increasing cardiac workload.
- Restricting sodium and fluid intake and increasing serum albumin may decrease edema and prevent or treat congestive heart failure, which commonly occurs in clients with impaired cardiac function. Also, loop diuretics are often given to increase excretion of sodium and water.
- With enteral nutrition, concentrated products (eg, 1.5 to 2 kcal/mL) provide more calories and help with fluid restrictions.
- Parenteral nutrition is usually needed only when a superimposed illness prevents use of the GI tract. Excessive amounts of sodium and fluid or rapid administration may precipitate or worsen heart failure and

should be avoided. If IV fat emulsions are used, they should be given over 24 hours because faster infusion may depress myocardial function.

## Use in Multiple Organ Dysfunction Syndrome

- Clients with multiple organ dysfunction syndrome (MODS), who are usually in critical care units, require nutritional support because they have high rates of metabolism and tissue breakdown (catabolism). However, nutritional support is complex because a client may have a combination of renal, hepatic, pulmonary, and cardiac impairments. Thus, it must be individualized according to the type and extent of organ impairment.
- Clients often have an ileus and GI dysfunction so that they require parenteral nutrition.
- Usual amounts of glucose are usually recommended. Clients with oliguric ARF or ARDS as part of their MODS need concentrated nutrients because fluid intake must be limited.
- During the severe physiologic stress of MODS, clients need higher than usual amounts of protein (eg, 1.5 to 2.5 g/kg/day) for growth, tissue maintenance and repair, and enzyme and hormone production. However, many clients may not be able to tolerate this amount because of organ impairments. For example, clients with ARF and dialysis or severe hepatic failure usually have protein intake restricted.
- Intravenous fat emulsions, a readily used source of energy, should provide 20% to 30% of calories. They also provide essential fatty acids. Some clients with MODS already have high serum triglyceride levels and are at risk for development of acute pancreatitis and further organ impairment. In these clients, IV fat emulsions are usually avoided until serum triglyceride levels are less than 300 mg/dL. In clients with MODS who receive IV fat emulsions, serum triglyceride levels should be monitored at least weekly.

## Nursing Actions
### Nutritional Products

| Nursing Actions | Rationale/Explanation |
|---|---|
| 1. Administer accurately.<br>  a. For oral supplemental feedings:<br>    (1) Chill liquids or pour over ice and give through a straw, from a closed container, between meals. | Chilling (or freezing) may improve formula taste and decrease formula odor. A straw directs the formula toward the back of the throat and decreases its contact with taste buds. A closed container also decreases odor. Giving between meals may have less effect on appetite at mealtimes. |
|     (2) Mix powders or concentrated liquid preparations in preferred beverages if not contraindicated. | Some can be mixed with fruit juice, milk, tea, or coffee, which may improve taste and acceptability. |

*(continued)*

## Nursing Actions

### Nutritional Products (Continued)

| Nursing Actions | Rationale/Explanation |
|---|---|

b. For intravenous (IV) feedings:

(1) Administer fluids at the prescribed flow rate. Use an infusion control device for hyperalimentation solutions.

> To administer sufficient fluids without a rapid flow rate. Rapid flow rates or large amounts of IV fluids can cause circulatory overload and pulmonary edema. In addition, hyperglycemia and osmotic diuresis may occur with hyperalimentation solutions.

(2) With IV fat emulsions, connect to the primary IV line beyond the filter; start slowly (0.5–1 mL/min) for approximately 30 minutes. If no adverse effects occur, increase rate to a maximum of 125 mL/h for the 10% solution or 60 mL/h for a 20% solution.

> Lipid emulsions should not be filtered.

(3) Use sterile technique when changing containers, tubings, or dressings.

> To prevent infection

(4) When adding drugs, use sterile technique, and add only those drugs known to be compatible with the IV solution.

> To avoid physical or chemical incompatibility

(5) Do not administer antibiotics or other drugs through central venous catheters.

> To avoid incompatibilities and possible precipitation or inactivation of the drug or fluid components

c. For tube feedings:

(1) Have the client sitting, if possible.

> To decrease risks of aspirating formula into lungs

(2) Check tube placement before each feeding by aspirating stomach contents or instilling air into the tube while listening over the stomach with a stethoscope.

> To prevent aspiration or accidental instillation of feedings into lungs

(3) Give the solution at room temperature.

> Cold formulas may cause abdominal cramping.

(4) If giving by intermittent instillation, do not give more than 500 mL per feeding, including water for rinsing the tube.

> To avoid gastric distention, possible vomiting, and aspiration into lungs

(5) Give by gravity flow (over 30–60 minutes) or infusion pump.

> Rapid administration may cause nausea, vomiting, and other symptoms.

(6) With continuous feedings, change containers and tubing daily. With intermittent bolus feedings, rinse all equipment after each use, and change at least every 24 hours.

> Most tube feeding formulas are milk based and provide a good culture medium for bacterial growth. Clean technique, not sterile technique, is required.

(7) Give an adequate amount of water, based on assessment of fluid needs. This may be done by mixing water with the tube feeding formula, giving it after the tube feeding, or giving it between feedings.

> To avoid dehydration and promote fluid balance. Most clients receiving 1500 to 2000 mL of tube feeding formula daily will need 1000 mL or more of water daily.

(8) Rinse nasogastric tubes with at least 50 to 100 mL water after each bolus feeding or administration of medications through the tube.

> To keep the tube patent and functioning. This water is included in calculation of fluid intake.

(9) When medications are ordered by tube, liquid preparations are preferred over crushed tablets or powders emptied from capsules.

> Tablets or powders may stick in the tube lumen. This may mean the full dose of the medication does not reach the stomach. Also, the tube is likely to become obstructed.

d. With pancreatic enzymes, give before or with meals or food.

> To obtain therapeutic effects, these agents must be in the small intestine when food is present.

2. **Observe for therapeutic effects.**

a. With water and other fluids, observe for fluid balance (amber-colored urine, approximately 1500 mL daily; moist mucous membranes in the oral cavity; adequate skin turgor).

b. With nutritional formulas given orally or by tube feeding, observe for weight gain and increased serum albumin. For infants and children receiving milk substitutes, observe for decreased diarrhea and weight gain.

> Therapeutic effects depend on the reason for use (ie, prevention or treatment of undernutrition).

*(continued)*

## *Nursing Actions*

## Nutritional Products (Continued)

| *Nursing Actions* | *Rationale/Explanation* |
|---|---|
| c. With parenteral hyperalimentation, observe for weight maintenance or gain and normal serum levels of glucose, electrolytes, and protein. | These are indications of improved metabolism, nitrogen balance, and nutritional status. When parenteral hyperalimentation is used for gastrointestinal malabsorption syndromes, diarrhea and other symptoms are usually relieved when oral feedings are stopped. |
| d. With pancreatic enzymes, observe for decreased diarrhea and steatorrhea. | The pancreatic enzymes function the same way as endogenous enzymes to aid digestion of carbohydrate, protein, and fat. |
| 3. Observe for adverse effects. | |
| a. With fluids, observe for peripheral edema, circulatory overload, and pulmonary edema (severe dyspnea, crackles). | Fluid excess is most likely to occur with rapid administration or large amounts of IV fluids, especially in people who are elderly or have congestive heart failure. |
| b. With commercial nutritional formulas (except Osmolite and Isocal), observe for hypotension, tachycardia, increased urine output, dehydration, nausea, vomiting, or diarrhea. | These adverse reactions are usually attributed to the hyperosmolality or hypertonicity of the preparations. They can be prevented or minimized by starting with small amounts of formula, given slowly. |
| c. With parenteral hyperalimentation, observe for elevated blood and urine glucose levels, signs of infection (fever, inflammation at the venipuncture site), concentrated urine or high specific gravity ($\geq$1.035), hypertension, dyspnea. | These signs and symptoms indicate complications of therapy. Except for infection, they are likely to occur when the solution is given in a concentration or at a rate that delivers more glucose than can be used. This produces hyperglycemia, which in turn causes excessive amounts of fluid to be excreted in the urine (osmotic diuresis). Hyperglycemic, hyperosmolar, nonketotic coma also may occur. |
| d. With IV fat emulsions, observe for signs of fat embolism (dyspnea, fever, chills, pain in the chest and back), phlebitis from vein irritation, and sepsis from contamination. Hyperlipidemia and hepatomegaly also may occur. | Thrombophlebitis and sepsis are the most frequent adverse effects. |
| 4. Observe for drug interactions. | |
| a. Drugs that *decrease* effects of anorexiants: | |
| (1) Antacids with calcium carbonate or magnesium hydroxide | May prevent action of enzymes; do not give at the same time. |

## Critical Thinking Exercises

1. A complication of enteral therapy that causes the greatest risk to the client is:
   a. Abdominal cramping
   b. Diarrhea
   c. Increased urine output
   d. Aspiration pneumonia

2. A client is receiving an intermittent bolus of tube feeding. After ascertaining proper tube placement, the nurse initially flushes the tube with 50 mL of water and administers 8 ounces of tube feeding. The nurse then follows the tube feeding with 100 mL of water. How much total intake should be recorded on the intake and output (I/O) record for that feeding?

   a. 240 mL
   b. 340 mL
   c. 390 mL
   d. 440 mL

3. A client receives an enteric-coated aspirin daily following his myocardial infarction. The nurse is administering the medication through the client's nasogastric tube. Before administration, the nurse should:

   a. Crush the medication
   b. Attempt to administer the medication orally
   c. Call the health care provider to clarify the medical order
   d. Hold the medication and ask the health care provider when he or she makes rounds in the morning

4. The nurse is supervising a student nurse while she is administering IV fat emulsions. The nurse should intervene if the student nurse:

   a. Uses sterile technique when changing the container
   b. Uses a separate in-line filter with the fat emulsions
   c. Starts the infusion slowly (0.5 to 1 mL/min), then increases the rate if no adverse effects are observed
   d. Uses an infusion control device while administering the fat emulsions

5. A client receiving parenteral nutrition at 100 mL/hour for several days has a blood glucose level of 420 mg/100 mL and a urine specific gravity of 1.016. Her urine output over the past 24 hours has been 3600 mL with and intake of 1500 mL. The nurse should suspect that the client:

   a. Is responding appropriately to the dextrose in the parenteral solution
   b. Has developed renal insufficiency from the parenteral solution
   c. Is getting too much parenteral solution, and the rate should be reduced to 50 mL/hour
   d. Has developed glucose intolerance

## SELECTED REFERENCES

Brown, R. O. (2000). Parenteral and enteral nutrition in adult patients. In E. T. Herfindal & D. R. Gourley (Eds.), *Textbook of therapeutics: Drug and disease management* (7th ed., pp. 193–211). Philadelphia: Lippincott Williams & Wilkins.

Coulston, A. M., Rock, C. L., & Monsen, E. R. (Eds.). (2001). *Nutrition in the prevention and treatment of disease.* San Diego: Academic Press.

DerMarderosian, A. (Ed.). (2000). *The review of natural products.* St. Louis: Facts and Comparisons.

*Drug facts and comparisons.* (Updated monthly). St. Louis: Facts and Comparisons.

Favreau, J. T., Ryu, M. L., Braunstein, G., Orshansky, G., Park, S. S., Coody, G. L., et al. (2002). Severe hepatotoxicity associated with the dietary supplement LipoKinetix. *Annals of Internal Medicine, 136*(8), 590–595.

Fetrow, C. W., & Avila, J. R. (1999). *Professional's handbook of complementary and alternative medicines.* Springhouse, PA: Springhouse Corporation.

Kim, R. B. (Ed.). (2001). *Handbook of adverse drug interactions.* New Rochelle, NY: The Medical Letter.

Lacy, C. F., Armstrong, L. L., Goldman, M. P., & Lance, L. L. (2003). *Lexi-Comp's drug information handbook* (11th ed.). Hudson, OH: American Pharmaceutical Association.

Pleuss, J. (2002). Alterations in nutritional status. In C. M. Porth (Ed.), *Pathophysiology: Concepts of altered health states* (6th ed., pp. 209–229). Philadelphia: Lippincott Williams & Wilkins.

Voss, A. C., & Mayer, K. E. (2001). Role of liquid dietary supplements. In A. M. Coulston, C. L. Rock, & E. R. Monsen (Eds.), *Nutrition in the prevention and treatment of disease* (pp. 229–243). San Diego: Academic Press.

Wallace, J. I., & Schwartz, R. S. (2000). Geriatric clinical nutrition, including malnutrition, obesity, and weight loss. In H. D. Humes (Ed.), *Kelley's textbook of internal medicine* (4th ed., pp. 3107–3114). Philadelphia: Lippincott Williams & Wilkins.

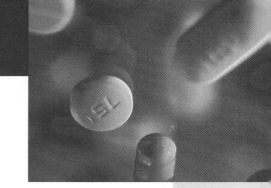

# 27

# Drugs for Weight Management

## OBJECTIVES

*After studying this chapter, the student will be able to:*

1 Assess clients for risk factors and manifestations of obesity.

2 Review health consequences of obesity.

3 Outline the management of obesity, including lifestyle changes and drugs to aid weight loss.

4 Identify the adverse effects of drugs used for obesity, including herbal and dietary supplements.

5 Assist clients who are overweight or obese to develop and maintain a safe and realistic weight loss program.

## CRITICAL THINKING SCENARIO

*C*ora Barker, a 48-year-old accountant, tells you that she had dieted on and off for the past 30 years, losing weight then gaining more weight than she lost. She has a body mass index (BMI) of 32 kg/m², tells you that she does not have time to exercise, and asks you about the new drugs on the market. She wants to get "jump started" on her weight loss program by taking medication until she can lose enough weight to get motivated.

✔ What advice would you have for Mrs. Barker?

✔ What are the goals of a successful weight loss program?

✔ What priority teaching needs are important to implement for this client?

# OVERVIEW

It is estimated that 97 million adults are overweight and obese in the United States, and reports of childhood obesity and inadequate exercise abound and are steadily increasing. Obesity and being overweight are considered major public health problems because of their association with high rates of morbidity and mortality. This chapter discusses obesity and pharmacologic therapy to aid weight loss.

# OBESITY

*Overweight* is defined as a body mass index (BMI) of 25 to 29.9 kg/m²; *obesity* is defined as a BMI of 30 kg/m² or more. The BMI reflects weight in relation to height and is a better indicator than weight alone. The desirable range for BMI is 18.5 to 24.9 kg/m², with any values below 18.5 indicating underweight and any values of 25 or above indicating excessive weight.

Obesity may occur in any group but is more likely to occur in women, minority groups, and poor people. It results from consistent ingestion of more calories than are used, and it substantially increases risks for development of cardiovascular disease (eg, hypertension, angina pectoris, myocardial infarction, stroke), diabetes mellitus, dyslipidemias (eg, increased triglycerides and low-density-lipoprotein [LDL] cholesterol; decreased high-density-lipoprotein [HDL] cholesterol, some types of cancer (eg, breast, prostate, endometrium, and colon), gallbladder disease, sleep apnea, and osteoarthritis of the knees. These disorders are attributed mainly to the multiple metabolic abnormalities associated with obesity. Abdominal fat out of proportion to total body fat (also called *central obesity*), which often occurs in men, is considered a greater risk factor for disease and death than lower body obesity. Many people consider obesity a chronic disease.

Overweight and obesity are common and increasing among children, especially those with overweight parents. Overweight is defined as a BMI above the 85th percentile for the age group. Studies indicate that obesity in childhood and adolescence is predictive of obesity and increased health risks in adulthood. In addition, more children are developing type 2 diabetes, which was formerly thought to occur only in adults. The increase in obesity and type 2 diabetes is mainly attributed to poor eating habits and too little exercise. Therefore, the goal of nutritional support is to meet needs without promoting obesity. Overweight and obesity are also common among older adults. Although caloric needs are usually decreased, primarily because of slowed metabolism and decreased physical activity, most people continue usual eating patterns. Discussion of obesity as it relates to age is summarized in Age Related Considerations. A nurse is involved with nutritional matters in almost any home care setting. Because obesity is a national health concern, the home care nurse should take advantage of any opportunity for health promotion in this area. Home Care Considerations outlines assessment, monitoring, and education concerns with these clients.

The general goals of weight management are to assist clients to prevent further weight gain, to lose weight, and to maintain a lower body weight more conducive to health. People who want to lose a few pounds should be encouraged to decrease caloric intake and increase exercise. For people with a BMI of 27 kg/m², treatment is recommended for those with two or more risk factors (eg, hypertension, dyslipidemia, diabetes) or a high waist circumference (central obesity) (Table 27-1). For people with a BMI of 30 kg/m² or above, treatment is recommended. Considerations for an effective weight loss program are included in At the Foundation: Principles of Weight Loss Management. The evidence report from the National Heart, Lung, and Blood Institute of the National Institutes of Health (Publication No. 98-4083): Clinical Guidelines on the Identification, Evaluation, and Treatment of Overweight and Obesity in Adults (September, 1998), can be found at www.nhlbi.nih.gov/guidelines/obesity/ob_gdlns.htm.

## Age-related Considerations: Obesity

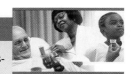

### USE IN CHILDREN

Treatment of childhood obesity should focus on normalizing food intake, especially fat intake, and increasing physical activity. One study indicates more success when caregivers work with the parents rather than the children themselves. None of the available weight loss drugs are indicated for use in children.

Emphasis is being placed on prevention of obesity, especially in children, adolescents, and young adults. The main elements are a more active lifestyle, a low-fat diet, regular meals, avoidance of snacking, drinking water instead of calorie-containing beverages, and decreasing the time spent watching television.

### USE IN OLDER ADULTS

With the high incidence of atherosclerosis and cardiovascular disease in older adults, it is especially important that fat intake be reduced. Anorexiant drugs should be used very cautiously, if at all, because older adults often have cardiovascular, renal, or hepatic impairments that increase risks for adverse drug effects. The use of orlistat in older adults has not been studied.

## Home Care Considerations: Supporting the Client With Obesity

*ASSESS:* the client and family's knowledge of condition and ability to implement a lifestyle that is conducive to safe, sustained weight loss; the client for compliance with the prescribed regimen, quality of life; and need for referral for treatment.

*MONITOR:* the therapeutic and adverse effects of the drugs, for signs and symptoms of a successful weight loss program, and client's need for additional information, and provide that information.

*EDUCATE:* regarding importance of reading and following dosing instructions, not exceeding recommended dosages without consulting a health care provider, and including a lifestyle program that incorporates a reduced-calorie diet and physical activity. Reinforce additional teaching points (see Client Teaching Guidelines: Drugs That Aid Weight Loss).

## Drugs for Obesity

Pharmacologic therapy for obesity (see Drugs at a Glance 27-1: Drugs for Obesity) has a problematic history because available drugs had potentially serious adverse effects and were recommended only for short-term use, and weight was rapidly regained when the drugs were stopped. No drug serves as the prototype. Two widely used drugs, fenfluramine and dexfenfluramine, were taken off the market in 1997 because of their association with diseased heart valves and pulmonary hypertension. More recently, phenylpropanolamine (PPA) was taken off the market because of its association with hypertension and

### TABLE 27-1  Heights and Weights Indicating Overweight and Obesity

| Height (ft/in) | Weight (lb) Indicating Overweight (BMI 25) | Weight (lb) Indicating Obesity (BMI 30) |
|---|---|---|
| 5'2" (62 in) | 135 | 165 |
| 5'3" | 140 | 170 |
| 5'4" | 145 | 175 |
| 5'5" | 150 | 180 |
| 5'6" | 155 | 185 |
| 5'7" | 160 | 190 |
| 5'8" | 165 | 195 |
| 5'9" | 170 | 200 |
| 5'10" | 175 | 205 |
| 5'11" | 180 | 210 |
| 6'0" | 185 | 220 |
| 6'1" | 190 | 225 |
| 6'2" (74 in) | 195 | 230 |

hemorrhagic strokes. PPA was the active ingredient in some over-the-counter diet aids (eg, Dexatrim, Acutrim) as well as the nasal decongestant component of many multisymptom cold remedies.

Older drugs include amphetamines and similar drugs. Amphetamines (see Chap. 15) are not recommended because they are controlled substances (Schedule II) with a high potential for abuse and dependence. Benzphetamine, diethylpropion, phendimetrazine, and phentermine are adrenergic drugs (see Chap. 16) that stimulate the release of norepinephrine and dopamine in the brain. This action in nerve terminals of the hypothalamic feeding center suppresses appetite. Other drug actions that may contribute to decreased appetite and weight loss include increasing energy and decreasing gastric secretion.

These drugs are central nervous system (CNS) and cardiovascular stimulants and are contraindicated in cardiovascular disease, hyperthyroidism, glaucoma, and agitated states. In addition, they are promoted for short-term use (8 to 12 weeks), weight is usually rapidly regained when the drugs are stopped, and they are controlled substances. Overall, their use as appetite suppressants is not recommended.

**Phentermine** (Ionamin, others) is the most frequently prescribed adrenergic anorexiant. Its use should be limited to clients with a BMI higher than 30 kg/m², or higher than 27 kg/m² if the client also has risk factors or other health problems that are aggravated by excessive weight. Its use is contraindicated in clients with hypertension or other cardiovascular disease and in those with a history of drug abuse. Clients with diabetes may experience altered insulin or oral hypoglycemic dosage requirements. Phentermine is pharmacologically and chemically similar to amphetamines; physical and psychological dependence may occur. The drug should also be used cautiously in clients with anxiety or agitation because of powerful CNS stimulant effects. The most commonly reported adverse effects are nervousness, dry mouth, constipation, and hypertension. Most individuals experience weight gain after discontinuing use.

**Sibutramine** (Meridia) was approved by the U.S. Food and Drug Administration (FDA) in late 1997 and became the most commonly prescribed antiobesity drug. This drug inhibits the reuptake of serotonin and norepinephrine in the brain, thereby increasing the amounts of these neurotransmitters. Clinical effects include increased satiety, decreased food intake, and a faster metabolism rate. Sibutramine is approved by the FDA for long-term use, but effects are mostly unknown beyond 1 year. The drug increases blood pressure and heart rate and is contraindicated in cardiovascular disorders (eg, hypertension, dysrhythmias). It should be used cautiously in clients who take other medications that increase blood pressure and pulse rate. It should also be used cautiously in clients with impaired hepatic function, narrow-angle glaucoma (may cause mydriasis), or a history of substance abuse or dependency.

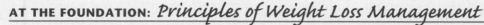

## AT THE FOUNDATION: *Principles of Weight Loss Management*

- Any weight reduction program needs to include a reduced-calorie diet and physical activity. Diets should consist of nutritionally sound foods in balanced meals. "Fad" diets are potentially hazardous to health and should be avoided. Exercise increases use of calories and helps preserve lean body mass during weight loss. It may also help to prevent the decreased metabolic rate that usually occurs with low-calorie diets.
- Emphasize health benefits of weight reduction. There is strong evidence that weight loss reduces risk factors for cardiovascular disease, including blood pressure, serum triglycerides, and total and LDL cholesterol. It also increases HDL cholesterol. In addition, in overweight and obese people without diabetes, weight loss reduces blood glucose levels and the risk for development of type 2 diabetes. For people who already have type 2 diabetes, weight loss reduces blood levels of glucose and glycosylated hemoglobin. These effects make the diabetes easier to manage, reduce complications of diabetes, and may allow smaller doses of antidiabetic medications. In general, modest weight losses of only 5 to 10 lb lower blood pressure and blood lipids and improve insulin resistance and glucose tolerance.
- Clients in a weight loss regimen should have regular measurements of body weight, BMI, blood pressure, blood lipids, and other factors as indicated.

- Provide psychological support and positive reinforcement for efforts toward weight management.
- There is increasing consensus that obesity is a chronic disease and that obese people should take weight loss medications on a long-term basis. Usually, however, the medications are recommended only in clients whose health is significantly endangered by obesity.
- When drug therapy is indicated, a single drug in the lowest effective dose is recommended. As with most other drugs, low doses decrease risks for adverse drug effects.
- A client taking an appetite suppressant who has not lost 4 lb during the first month of treatment is unlikely to benefit from longer use of the drug.
- Maximum weight loss usually occurs during the first 6 months of drug therapy. With most available drugs, use for this long is an unlabeled use of the drug.
- After a weight loss regimen of a few months, some experts recommend letting the body adjust to the lower weight before attempting additional losses. Thus, a weight maintenance program, possibly with continued drug therapy, is indicated.
- The National Institutes of Health do not recommend combining weight loss medications except in the context of clinical trials. This recommendation may change with orlistat, which works in the intestines and is not systemically absorbed.

Oral sibutramine is rapidly absorbed from the intestine and undergoes first-pass metabolism, during which active metabolites are formed. Peak plasma levels of the active metabolites occur within 3 to 4 hours, and drug half-life is 14 to 16 hours. The drug is highly bound to plasma proteins and rapidly distributed to most body tissues, with the highest concentrations in the liver and kidneys. It is metabolized in the liver, mainly by the cytochrome P450 3A4 enzymes. The active metabolites produced by first-pass metabolism are further metabolized to inactive metabolites, which are then excreted in urine and feces.

Common adverse effects include dry mouth, headache, insomnia, nervousness, and constipation; cardiovascular effects include hypertension, tachycardia, and palpitations. Potentially serious drug interactions may occur if sibutramine is taken with other cardiovascular stimulants (increased risk for hypertension and dysrhythmias), CNS stimulants (increased anxiety and insomnia), and serotonergic drugs (serotonin syndrome). Other drugs that increase serotonin include the selective serotonin reuptake inhibitors (eg, fluoxetine [Prozac] and related drugs), the triptan antimigraine drugs (eg, sumatriptan [Imitrex]), dextromethorphan (a common ingredient in cough syrups), and lithium. The combination of sibutramine with any of these drugs may cause serotonin syndrome, a condition characterized by agitation, confusion, hypomania, impaired coordination, loss of consciousness, nausea, tachycardia, and other symptoms.

In March 2002, a consumer group petitioned the FDA to take sibutramine off the market, saying the drug's risks outweigh its benefits. At the time, the FDA had received reports of 25 deaths, worldwide, of people who were taking the drug. It was unknown whether the deaths were related to the use of sibutramine. Most of the deaths (16) were related to cardiac problems. The

### ? How Can You Avoid This Medication Error?

Mr. Thompson, who is 46 years old, is admitted to the emergency department complaining of a migraine headache. He is currently successfully taking sibutramine as part of his weight loss program. The health care provider orders sumatriptan (Imitrex), and the nurse administers sumatriptan, 6 mg subcutaneously, and reduces the lighting in the room to allow the client to rest. The nurse checks on Mr. Thompson in 1 hour, and he is agitated, confused, tachycardic, and nauseated. Identify the error and how it could be prevented.

**DRUG TABLE 27-1**

## *Drugs at a Glance*
## Drugs for Obesity

| Generic/Trade Name | Routes and Dosage Ranges (Adults) | Comments |
|---|---|---|
| *Appetite Suppressants* | | |
| **Benzphetamine** (Didrex) Pregnancy Category X | PO, 25–50 once daily initially, increased up to three times daily if indicated | Controlled Substance: Schedule III Because it is a CNS stimulant, a single dose is preferably given in the mid-morning or mid-afternoon |
| **Diethylpropion** (Tenuate) Pregnancy Category B | Immediate release tablets, PO, 25 mg three times daily Controlled release tablets, PO, 75 mg once daily in midmorning | Controlled Substance: Schedule IV Take before meals or with food |
| **Phendimetrazine** (Bontril) Pregnancy Category C | Immediate release tablets, PO, 35 mg two or three times daily, 1 h before meals Sustained release capsules, PO, 105 mg once daily, 30–60 min before the first morning meal | Controlled Substance: Schedule III |
| **Phentermine hydrochloride** (Adipex) Pregnancy Category C | PO, 8 mg three times daily or 15–37.5 mg daily in the morning | Controlled Substance: Schedule IV |
| **Phentermine resin** (Ionamin) Pregnancy Category C | PO, 15–30 mg once daily in the morning | |
| **Sibutramine** (Meridia) Pregnancy Category C | PO, 10–15 mg once daily, in the morning, with or without food | Controlled Substance: Schedule IV |
| *Fat Blocker* | | |
| **Orlistat** (Xenical) Pregnancy Category B | PO, 1 capsule with each main meal, up to 3 capsules daily | A multivitamin containing the fat-soluble vitamins (A, D, E, K) should be taken 2 h before orlistat |

manufacturer reported knowledge of 32 deaths of people taking sibutramine, but stated there was no evidence that the drug was to blame.

**Orlistat** (Xenical) differs from other antiobesity drugs because it decreases absorption of dietary fat from the intestine (by inhibiting gastric and pancreatic lipase enzymes that normally break down fat into absorbable triglycerides). The drug blocks absorption of approximately 30% of the fat ingested in a meal. Decreased fat absorption leads to decreased caloric intake, resulting in weight loss and improved serum cholesterol values (eg, decreases total and low-density lipoprotein [LDL] cholesterol levels). The improvement in cholesterol is thought to be independent of weight loss effects.

Orlistat is not absorbed systemically, and its action occurs in the gastrointestinal (GI) tract. Consequently, it does not cause systemic adverse effects or drug interactions, as do phentermine and sibutramine. Its main disadvantages are frequent administration (three times daily) and GI symptoms (abdominal pain, oily spotting, fecal urgency, flatulence with discharge, fatty stools, fecal incontinence, and increased defecation). Adverse GI effects occur in almost all orlistat users but usually sub-

side after about 4 weeks. In addition, the drug prevents absorption of the fat-soluble vitamins, A, D, E, and K. As a result, people taking orlistat should also take a daily multivitamin containing these vitamins. The multivitamin should be taken 2 hours before or after the orlistat dose. If taken at the same time, the orlistat prevents absorption of the fat-soluble vitamins.

Orlistat is intended for people who are clinically obese, not those wanting to lose a few pounds. In addition, high-fat foods still need to be decreased because total caloric intake is a major determinant of weight, and adverse effects (eg, diarrhea and fatty, malodorous stools) worsen with high fat consumption. Long-term effects of orlistat are unknown, although one study reported safe and effective use for 2 years. In addition to weight loss and reduced cholesterol levels, clinical trials found a reduction in other risk factors associated with obesity, such as hypertension, hyperglycemia, and excessive waist circumference.

## Herbal and Dietary Supplements

Many people use herbal or dietary supplements for weight loss, even though reliable evidence of both safety and effectiveness are generally lacking. Some herbal products claim to decrease appetite and increase the rate at which the body burns calories. However, their effectiveness varies, and in most cases, there is no scientific evidence that they work at all. Most supplements for weight loss contain cardiovascular and CNS stimulants that may cause serious, even life-threatening, adverse effects. The manufacturing and labeling of these products are not strictly regulated by FDA.

In one survey of college students, researchers asked about the use of nonvitamin, nonmineral dietary supplements. Almost half (48.5%) of the 272 respondents reported they took such a product during the previous year. Although echinacea, ginseng, and St. John's wort were more frequently used, 27 students took weight loss products. Of these, 81.5% had a BMI in the acceptable range, and 11 of the 19 participants who reported an adverse reaction continued to take the products.

In general, many consumers do not seem to appreciate the benefits of proven weight management techniques (ie, appropriate diet and exercise) or the potential risks of taking weight loss products. Selected products are described below.

**Chromium** is a trace element in the hexavalent form and is an essential nutrient. In animals, it has been demonstrated that chromium is an insulin cofactor involved in carbohydrate, fat, and protein metabolism. In humans, a few cases of severe chromium deficiency in long-term total parenteral nutrition have been reported in patients with insulin resistance. No reliable assessment measures are available to identify the total body chromium level and thus chromium deficiency. Sources of chromium include wheat germ, brewer's yeast, calves liver, and American cheese. One study failed to demonstrate the effectiveness of chromium picolinate as a supplement to aerobic activity in a weight loss program.

**Ephedra** (ma huang) is an herb in many weight loss products (eg, Metabolife, Herbalife, others). It is not recommended for use by anyone, particularly individuals with hypertension, other cardiovascular disease, and diabetes, because it is a strong cardiovascular and CNS stimulant that increases risks for heart attack, seizure, stroke, and sudden death. Many ephedra-containing products also contain caffeine, which can further increase cardiovascular and CNS stimulation. The amount of ephedra varies among products, and there is a lack of consistency in labeling of the actual product content.

**Glucomannan** expands on contact with body fluids. It is included in weight loss regimens because of its supposed ability to produce feelings of stomach fullness, causing a person to eat less. It also has a laxative effect. There is little evidence to support its use as a weight loss aid. Products containing glucomannan should not be used by people with diabetes; it may cause hypoglycemia and increases hypoglycemic effects of antidiabetic medications.

**Guarana,** a major source of commercial caffeine, is found in weight loss products as well as caffeine-containing soft drinks, bodybuilding supplements, smoking cessation products, vitamin supplements, candies, and chewing gums. Caffeine is the active ingredient; the amount varies among products, and caffeine content of any particular product cannot be accurately predicted. Guarana is promoted to decrease appetite and increase energy and mental alertness. It is contraindicated in clients with dysrhythmias and may aggravate gastroesophageal reflux disease (GERD) and peptic ulcer disease.

Adverse effects include diuresis, cardiovascular symptoms (premature ventricular contractions, tachycardia), CNS symptoms (agitation, anxiety, insomnia, seizures, tremors), and GI symptoms (nausea, vomiting, diarrhea). Such effects are more likely to occur with higher doses or concomitant use of guarana and other sources of caffeine. Adverse drug–drug interactions include additive CNS and cardiovascular stimulation with beta-adrenergic agonists (eg, epinephrine, albuterol and related drugs, pseudoephedrine) and theophylline. In addition, concurrent use of cimetidine, fluoroquinolones, or oral contraceptives may increase or prolong serum caffeine levels and subsequent adverse effects.

**Guar gum** is a dietary fiber included in weight loss products because it is bulk forming, produces feelings of fullness, and may decrease appetite. It may cause esophageal or intestinal obstruction if not taken with an adequate amount of water and may interfere with the absorption of other drugs if taken at the same time. Adverse effects include nausea, diarrhea, flatulence, and abdominal discomfort.

**Hydroxycitric acid** (HCA, found in CitriMax) apparently suppresses appetite in animals, but there are no reliable studies that indicate its effectiveness in humans.

**Laxative and diuretic herbs** (eg, aloe, rhubarb root, buckthorn, cascara, senna, parsley, juniper, and dandelion leaves) are found in several products such as Super Dieter's Tea, Trim-Maxx Tea, and Water Pill. These products cause a significant loss of body fluids, not fat. Adverse effects may include low serum potassium levels, with subsequent cardiac dysrhythmias and other heart problems. In addition, long-term use of laxatives may lead to loss of normal bowel function and the necessity for continued use (ie, laxative dependency).

**LipoKinetix,** a combination dietary supplement, was recently associated with severe hepatotoxicity in seven previously healthy individuals (ages 20 to 32 years), who developed acute hepatitis. Of the four women and three men, five Japanese clients were diagnosed in 1 month or less; two white bodybuilders were diagnosed within 3 months. Three people were taking only LipoKinetix; four were also taking other supplements, which they resumed later without recurrence of hepatitis. All reported taking LipoKinetix according to the manufacturer's instructions; all recovered after the product was discontinued.

LipoKinetix contains norephedrine, caffeine, sodium usniate, 3,5-diiodothyronine, and yohimbe. The ingredients responsible for the hepatotoxicity were unknown. The reactions were considered idiosyncratic, and no other cause of the hepatitis was found.

With the observation that the five Japanese developed hepatotoxicity more rapidly than the two white bodybuilders, there is a possibility that Asians are less able to metabolize and excrete this product. As discussed in the early chapters of this text, smaller doses of several prescription drugs are needed in this population because of genetic or ethnic differences in metabolism. This princi-

ple may also apply to some herbal and dietary supplements and should be considered in teaching clients of Asian descent.

**St. John's wort** has been used as a weight-loss supplement based on thoughts that the herbal supplement inhibits monoamine oxidase (MAO), which would increase synaptic concentrations of serotonin and norepinephrine. There is no scientific evidence that the supplement has a role in the management of obesity, and its safety and efficacy are uncertain.

---

# NURSING PROCESS

## Assessment

Assess each client for current or potential nutritional issues leading to obesity. Some specific assessment factors include the following:

- What are usual drinking and eating patterns? Does food intake seem adequate in terms of normal nutrition? What are food likes and dislikes?
- Does the client know the basic foods for normal nutrition? Does the client view nutrition as important in maintaining health?
- Has there been a recent change in weight?
- Does the client appear overweight? If so, calculate the BMI or use the information in Table 27-5 to estimate the BMI. If the BMI is 25 kg/m² or above, ask the client if there are concerns about weight, if there are health problems caused or aggravated by excessive weight, if there is interest in a weight-management program to improve health, and what methods, over-the-counter products, or herbal or dietary supplements, if any, have been used to reduce weight. The nurse must be very tactful in eliciting information and assessing whether a client would like assistance with weight management. If the nurse–client contact stems from a health problem caused or aggravated by excessive weight, the client may be more motivated to lose weight and improve health.

## Nursing Diagnoses

- Disturbed Body Image related to weight gain

- Deficient Knowledge: Nutritional needs and weight management

## Planning/Goals

*The client will:*
- Avoid overuse of anorexiant drugs
- Avoid unproven weight loss dietary supplements

## Interventions

Implement measures to prevent nutritional disorders by promoting a well-balanced diet for all clients. Depending on the client's condition, diet orders, food preferences, knowledge and attitudes about nutrition, and other factors, specific activities may include the following:

- Promote exercise and activity. For overweight and obese clients, exercise may decrease appetite and distract from eating behaviors as well as increase calorie expenditure.
- Weigh clients at regular intervals. Calculate or estimate the BMI when indicated.
- Use available resources to individualize nutritional care according to the client's clinical status and needs.

## Evaluation

- Observe overweight or obese clients for food intake, weight loss, and appropriate use of exercise and anorexiant drugs.
- Observe children for quantity and quality of food intake and appropriate increases in height and weight.

---

## CLIENT TEACHING GUIDELINES
### Drugs That Aid Weight Loss

### General Considerations

✔ In addition to feeling better, health benefits of weight loss may include reduced blood pressure, reduced blood fats, less likelihood of having a heart attack or stroke, and less risk for development of diabetes mellitus.

✔ Any weight loss program should include a nutritionally adequate diet with decreased calories and increased exercise. The recommended rate of weight loss is approximately 2 lb weekly.

✔ Regular physical examinations and follow-up care are needed during weight loss programs.

✔ Diet and exercise are recommended for people who want to lose a few pounds. Medications to aid weight loss are usually recommended only for people whose health is endangered (ie, those who are overweight and have other risk factors for heart disease and those who are obese).

*(continued)*

## CLIENT TEACHING GUIDELINES
### Drugs That Aid Weight Loss (Continued)

✔ Read package inserts and other available information about the drug being taken, who should not take the drug, instructions and precautions for safe usage, and so forth. Keep the material for later reference if questions arise. If unclear about any aspect of the information, consult a health care provider before taking the drug.

✔ Appetite-suppressant drugs must be used correctly to avoid potentially serious adverse effects. Because these drugs stimulate the heart and the brain, adverse effects may include increased blood pressure, fast heart beat, irregular heart beat, heart attack, stroke, dizziness, nervousness, insomnia (if taken late in the day), and mental confusion. In addition, prolonged use of prescription drugs may lead to psychological dependence.

✔ Avoid over-the-counter decongestants, allergy, asthma, and cold remedies and weight loss herbal or dietary supplements when taking a prescription appetite suppressant. The combination can cause serious adverse effects from excessive heart and brain stimulation.

✔ Inform health care providers when taking an appetite suppressant, mainly to avoid other drugs with similar effects.

✔ Orlistat (Xenical) is not an appetite suppressant and does not cause heart or brain stimulation. It works in the intestines to prevent the fats in foods from being absorbed. It should be taken with a low-fat diet. Adverse effects include fatty stools and bloating.

**Self-administration**

✔ Take appetite suppressants in the morning to decrease appetite during the day and avoid interference with sleep at night.

✔ Do not crush or chew sustained-release products.

✔ With sibutramine (Meridia):

✔ Take once daily, with or without food.

✔ Have blood pressure and heart rate checked at regular intervals (the drug increases them).

✔ Notify a health care provider if a skin rash, hives, or other allergic reaction occurs.

✔ With orlistat:

✔ Take one capsule with each main meal or up to 1 hour after a meal, up to 3 capsules daily. If you miss a meal or eat a non-fat meal, you may omit a dose of orlistat.

✔ Take a multivitamin containing fat-soluble vitamins (A,D,E, and K) daily, at least 2 hours before or after taking orlistat. Orlistat prevents absorption of fat-soluble vitamins from food or multivitamin preparations if taken at the same time.

## *Nursing Actions*
## Drugs for Obesity

| Nursing Actions | Rationale/Explanation |
|---|---|
| 1. Administer accurately. | |
| a. With adrenergic anorexiants: | |
| (1) Give single-dose drugs in the early morning. | For maximum appetite-suppressant effects during the day |
| (2) Give multiple-dose preparations 30–60 minutes before meals and the last dose of the day about 6 h before bedtime. | For maximum appetite-suppressant effects at mealtime and to avoid interference with sleep from the drug's stimulating effects on the central nervous system (CNS) |
| b. With sibutramine, give once daily, in the morning | |
| c. With orlistat, give 1 capsule with each main meal or up to 1 h after a meal, up to 3 capsules daily. If a meal is missed or contains no fat, the dose can be omitted. | The drug needs to be in the gastrointestinal tract when fat-containing foods are eaten to prevent fat absorption. |
| 2. Observe for therapeutic effects. | |
| a. With anorexiant drugs and orlistat, observe for decreased caloric intake and weight loss. | The recommended rate of weight loss is approximately 2 to 3 lb weekly. |
| 3. Observe for adverse effects. | |
| a. With anorexiant drugs, observe for: | |
| (1) Nervousness, insomnia, hyperactivity | These adverse effects are caused by excessive stimulation of the CNS. They are more likely to occur with large doses or too frequent administration. |
| (2) Hypertension | Anorexiant drugs stimulate the sympathetic nervous system and may cause or aggravate hypertension. |

*(continued)*

## *Nursing Actions*
## Drugs for Obesity (Continued)

| *Nursing Actions* | *Rationale/Explanation* |
|---|---|
| (3) Development of tolerance to appetite-suppressant effects | This usually occurs within 4 to 6 weeks and is an indication for discontinuing drug administration. Continued administration does not maintain appetite-suppressant effects but increases incidence of adverse effects. In addition, taking large doses of the drug does not restore appetite-suppressant effects. |
| (4) Signs of psychological drug dependence | More likely with large doses or long-term use |
| b. With orlistat, observe for abdominal cramping, gas pains, diarrhea, and fatty stools. | These effects commonly occur and worsen with a high intake of dietary fat. The drug should not be used as an excuse for eating large amounts of fatty foods. |
| **4. Observe for drug interactions with weight loss drugs.** | |
| a. Drugs that *increase* effects of anorexiants: | |
| (1) Antidepressants, tricyclic | May increase hypertensive effects |
| (2) Other CNS stimulants | Additive stimulant effects |
| (3) Other sympathomimetic drugs (eg, epinephrine) | Additive hypertensive and other cardiovascular effects |
| b. Drugs that *decrease* effects of anorexiants: | |
| (1) Antihypertensive drugs | Decrease blood pressure raising effects of anorexiants |
| (2) CNS depressants (eg, alcohol) | Antagonize or decrease effects |
| c. Drugs that *increase* effects of sibutramine: | |
| (1) Adrenergics (eg, epinephrine, pseudoephedrine) | Additive increases in blood pressure |
| (2) Antidepressants (tricyclics [TCAs; eg, amitriptyline], selective serotonin reuptake inhibitors [SSRIs; eg, fluoxetine]) | TCAs and sibutramine increase levels of norepinephrine and serotonin in the brain; SSRIs increase serotonin levels. Concurrent use of these drugs may cause excessive CNS stimulation, hypertension, and serotonin syndrome and should be avoided. |
| (3) Antifungals (eg, itraconazole, ketoconazole) | Decrease metabolism and may increase adverse effects and toxicity of sibutramine. |
| (4) Antimigraine triptans (eg, sumatriptan) | Additive serotonin effects |
| (5) Lithium | Additive serotonin effect |

### How Can You Avoid This Medication Error?

**Answer:** Actually, there are two errors in this situation. A nurse should be more diligent in her assessment and not leave a client alone for 1 hour after administering a medication in the emergency department. Additionally, in this situation, a potentially serious drug interaction may have occurred when sibutramine was taken with a triptan antimigraine drug, such as sumatriptan (Imitrex). Other drugs, such as dextromethorphan (a common ingredient in cough syrups), lithium, fluoxetine (Prozac), and other CNS and cardiovascular stimulants, may also produce adverse effects with concomitant use. The combination of sibutramine with any of these drugs may cause serotonin syndrome, a condition characterized by agitation, confusion, hypomania, impaired coordination, loss of consciousness, nausea, tachycardia, and other symptoms.

### Critical Thinking Exercises

1. The antiobesity drug that decreases absorption of dietary fat from the intestine by inhibiting gastric and pancreatic lipase enzymes that normally break down fat into absorbable triglycerides is:
   a. Sibutramine (Meridia)
   b. Phentermine (Ionamin)
   c. Hydroxycitric acid (HCA)
   d. Orlistat (Xenical)

2. A multivitamin containing the fat-soluble vitamins (A, D, E, K) should be taken 2 hours before administration of which drug used for the treatment of obesity?
   a. Phentermine resin (Ionamin)
   b. Orlistat (Xenical)
   c. Sibutramine (Meridia)
   d. Phendimetrazine (Bontril)

**3.** The adrenergic anorexiant that is pharmacologically and chemically similar to amphetamines and may cause physical and psychological dependence is:

   a. Sibutramine (Meridia)

   b. Phentermine (Ionamin)

   c. Hydroxycitric acid (HCA)

   d. Orlistat (Xenical)

**4.** A client is calculated to have a BMI of 30.5 kg/m². This value would indicate that the client is:

   a. Underweight

   b. Within normal weight range

   c. Overweight

   d. Obese

**5.** The nurse is completing discharge teaching for a client taking oralist (Xenical). The nurse recognizes that the client needs additional discharge teaching if the client makes which of the following comments?

   a. "I need make sure that I take a multivitamin daily that contains the fat-soluble vitamins."

   b. "I should increase my dietary fat content if I develop any side effects."

   c. "Common side effects I should look for are abdominal pain, increased flatulence with discharge, fatty stools, diarrhea, and incontinence with my stools."

   d. "I should take my orlistat 2 hours before or after taking my multivitamin."

## SELECTED REFERENCES

Campbell, M. L., & Mathys, M. L. (2001). Pharmacologic options for the treatment of obesity. *American Journal of Health-System Pharmacy, 58*(14), 1301–1308.

Davidson, M. H., Hauptman, J., DiGirolamo, M., Foreyt, J. P., Halsted, C. H., Heber, D., et al. (1999). Weight control and risk factor reduction in obese subjects treated for 2 years with orlistat: A randomized controlled trial. *Journal of the American Medical Association, 281*(3), 235–242.

DerMarderosian, A. (Ed.) (2000). *The review of natural products.* St. Louis: Facts and Comparisons.

*Drug facts and comparisons.* (Updated monthly). St. Louis: Facts and Comparisons.

Expert Panel. (1998). Clinical guidelines on the identification, evaluation, and treatment of overweight and obesity in adults: Executive summary. *American Journal of Clinical Nutrition, 68,* 899–917.

Golan, M., Weizman, A., Apter, A., & Fainara, M. (1998). Parents as the exclusive agents of change in the treatment of childhood obesity. *American Journal of Clinical Nutrition, 67,* 1130–1135.

Gunnell, D. J., Frankel, S. J., Nanchahal, K., Peters, T. J., & Smith, G. D. (1998). Childhood obesity and adult cardiovascular mortality. *American Journal of Clinical Nutrition, 67,* 1111–1118.

Kim, R. B. (Ed.). (2001). *Handbook of adverse drug interactions.* New Rochelle, NY: The Medical Letter.

Lacy, C. F., Armstrong, L. L., Goldman, M. P., & Lance, L. L. (2003). *Lexi-Comp's drug information handbook* (11th ed.). Hudson, OH: American Pharmaceutical Association.

Mandl, E. L., & Iltz, J. L. (2000). Obesity and eating disorders. In E. T. Herfindal & D. R. Gourley (Eds.), *Textbook of therapeutics: Drug and disease management* (7th ed., pp. 1271–1288). Philadelphia: Lippincott Williams & Wilkins.

National Institutes of Health. (1998). Clinical guidelines on the identification, evaluation, and treatment of overweight and obesity in adults: The evidence report. [On-line.] Available: www.nhlbi.nih.gov/guidelines/obesity/ob_gdlns.htm. Accessed December 25, 2003.

Pinkowish, M. D. (1998). Obesity: A chronic disease. *Patient Care, 32*(16), 29–50.

Pleuss, J. (2002). Alterations in nutritional status. In C. M. Porth (Ed.), *Pathophysiology: Concepts of altered health states* (6th ed., pp. 209–229). Philadelphia: Lippincott Williams & Wilkins.

St. Peter, J. V., & Khan, M. A. (2002). Obesity. In J. T. DiPiro, R. L. Talbert, G. C. Yee, G. R. Matzke, B. G. Wells, & L. M. Posey (Eds.), *Pharmacotherapy: A pathophysiologic approach* (5th ed., pp. 219–250). New York: McGraw-Hill.

Stunkard, A. J., & Wadden, T. A., (2000). Obesity. In H. D. Humes (Ed.), *Kelley's textbook of internal medicine* (4th ed., pp. 233–244). Philadelphia: Lippincott Williams & Wilkins.

Wallace, J. I., & Schwartz, R. S. (2000). Geriatric clinical nutrition, including malnutrition, obesity, and weight loss. In H. D. Humes (Ed.), *Kelley's textbook of internal medicine* (4th ed., pp. 3107–3114). Philadelphia: Lippincott Williams & Wilkins.

Williamson, D. F. (1999). Pharmacotherapy for obesity (Editorial). *Journal of the American Medical Association, 281,* 278–280.

Yanovski, S. Z., & Yanovski, J. A. (2002). Obesity. *New England Journal of Medicine, 346*(8), 591–601.

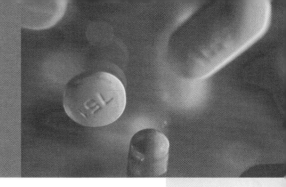

# Drugs Used to Treat Infections

## 28

# General Characteristics of Antimicrobial Drugs

**OBJECTIVES**

*After studying this chapter, the student will be able to:*

1 Identify populations who are at increased risk for development of infections.

2 Discuss common pathogens and methods of infection control.

3 Assess clients for local and systemic signs of infection.

4 Discuss common and potentially serious adverse effects of antimicrobial drugs.

5 Identify clients at increased risk for adverse drug reactions.

6 Discuss ways to increase benefits and decrease hazards of antimicrobial drug therapy.

7 Describe ways to minimize emergence of drug-resistant microorganisms.

8 State appropriate nursing implications for a client receiving an antimicrobial drug.

9 Discuss important elements of using antimicrobial drugs in children, older adults, those with renal or hepatic impairment, and those with critical illness.

## OVERVIEW

Antimicrobial drugs are used to prevent or treat infections caused by pathogenic (disease-producing) microorganisms. The human body and the environment contain many microorganisms, most of which live in a state of balance with the human host and do not cause disease. When the balance is upset and infection occurs, characteristics of the infecting microorganisms and the adequacy of host defense mechanisms are major factors in the severity of the infection and the person's ability to recover. Individuals who are very young or aged are at greater risk for developing infections. General principles of pediatric and geriatric drug therapy apply (see Chap. 4). Other guidelines regarding antimicrobial drug therapy in children and older adults are outlined in Age-related Considerations.

Conditions that impair defense mechanisms increase the incidence and severity of infections and impede recovery. In addition, use of antimicrobial drugs may lead to serious infections caused by drug-resistant microorganisms.

## MICROORGANISMS AND INFECTIONS

Infections are among the most common illnesses in all age groups, and they are often treated by antibiotic therapy at home, with medications administered by the client or a family member caregiver. Guidelines for ongoing evaluation and intervention are addressed in Home Care Considerations.

To help prevent infectious diseases and participate effectively in antimicrobial drug therapy, the nurse must

---

### Age-related Considerations: Use of Antimicrobial Drugs

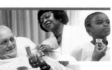

#### USE IN CHILDREN

1. **Penicillins and cephalosporins** are considered safe for most age groups. However, they are eliminated more slowly in neonates because of immature renal function and must be used cautiously and dosed appropriately for age. As with other classes of drugs, many penicillins and cephalosporins have not been FDA approved for use in children (usually younger than the age of 12 years). However, pediatric specialty references reflect the growing body of experience in using these drugs in younger children.

2. **Erythromycin**, oral azithromycin (Zithromax), and clarithromycin (Biaxin) are considered safe. Dirithromycin (Dynabac) has not been FDA approved for use in children younger than 12 years of age.

3. **Aminoglycosides** (eg, gentamicin) may cause nephrotoxicity and ototoxicity in any client population. Neonates are at high risk because of immature renal function.

4. **Tetracyclines** are contraindicated in children younger than 8 years of age because of drug effects on teeth and bone (see Chap. 31).

5. When **clindamycin** (Cleocin) is given to neonates and infants, liver and kidney function should be monitored.

6. **Fluoroquinolones** (eg, ciprofloxacin [Cipro]) are contraindicated for use in children (younger than the age of 18 years) because weight-bearing joints have been impaired in young animals given the drugs. However, if fluoroquinolones are the only therapeutic option for a resistant pathogen, the prescriber may decide to use a fluoroquinolone in children.

7. **Trimethoprim-sulfamethoxazole** (Bactrim) can be used for urinary tract infections and acute otitis media. However, its utility as a first-line drug has decreased during the past several years owing to increased bacterial resistance.

#### USE IN OLDER ADULTS

1. **Penicillins** are usually safe. However, hyperkalemia may occur with large IV doses of penicillin G potassium (1.7 mEq potassium per 1 million units), and hypernatremia may occur with ticarcillin (Ticar), which contains 5.6 mEq sodium per gram. Hyperkalemia and hypernatremia are more likely to occur with impaired renal function.

2. **Cephalosporins** (eg, cefazolin) are considered safe but may cause or aggravate renal impairment, especially when other nephrotoxic drugs are used concurrently. Dosage of most cephalosporins should be reduced in the presence of renal impairment (see Chap. 29).

3. **Macrolides** (eg, erythromycin) are usually safe. Dosage of clarithromycin should be reduced with severe renal impairment.

4. **Aminoglycosides** (eg, gentamicin) are contraindicated in the presence of impaired renal function if less toxic drugs are effective against causative microorganisms. Older adults are at high risk for nephrotoxicity and ototoxicity from these drugs. Interventions to decrease adverse drug effects are described in Chapter 30.

5. **Clindamycin** may cause diarrhea and should be used with caution in the presence of GI disease, especially colitis.

6. **Trimethoprim-sulfamethoxazole** (Bactrim, Septra) may be associated with an increased risk for severe adverse effects in older adults, especially those with impaired liver or kidney function. Severe skin reactions and bone marrow depression are the most frequently reported severe reactions.

7. **Tetracyclines** (except doxycycline) and nitrofurantoin (Macrodantin) are contraindicated in the presence of impaired renal function if less toxic drugs are effective against causative organisms.

## Home Care Considerations: Use of Antimicrobial Drug

*ASSESS:* client and family's ability and willingness to manage some aspects of therapy, prepare and use IV infusion pumps, maintain compliance with the prescribed regimen; therapeutic and adverse drug effects; and that client is keeping appointments for serum drug levels (if indicated) and follow-up care

*MONITOR:* general infection control practices, including frequent and thorough handwashing, use of gloves when indicated, and appropriate handling and disposal of body substances (eg, blood, urine, feces, sputum, vomitus, wound drainage); coordination of arrangements for procuring equipment, supplies, and medication. Also monitor for therapeutic and adverse effects of drugs and client's need for additional information, and provide that information

*EDUCATE:* family members how to administer antibiotics (eg, teaching a parent how to store and measure a liquid antibiotic), care for the person with an infection, how to protect other people in the environment from the infection, and that completion of antibiotic regimen is important to prevent resistant organisms. Reinforce additional teaching points (see Client Teaching Guidelines: Antimicrobial Drugs).

be knowledgeable about microorganisms, host responses to microorganisms, and antimicrobial drugs. This information is outlined in At the Foundation: Microorganisms and Infections. Classification, normal microbial flora, and common pathogenic microorganisms are described in the following sections.

## Classification

*Bacteria* are subclassified according to whether they are aerobic (require oxygen) or anaerobic (cannot live in the presence of oxygen), their reaction to Gram's stain (gram positive or gram negative), and their shape (eg, cocci, bacilli).

*Viruses* are intracellular parasites that survive only in living tissues. They are officially classified according to their structures but are more commonly described according to origin and the disorders or symptoms they produce. Human pathogens include adenoviruses, herpesviruses, and retroviruses (see Chap. 33).

*Fungi* are plantlike organisms that live as parasites on living tissue or as saprophytes on decaying organic matter. Approximately 50 species are pathogenic in humans (see Chap. 33).

## Normal Microbial Flora

Normal flora protects the human host by occupying space and consuming nutrients. This interferes with the ability of potential pathogens to establish residence and proliferate. Microorganisms that are part of the normal flora and nonpathogenic in one area of the body may be pathogenic in other parts of the body; for example, *Escherichia coli* often cause urinary tract infections.

If the normal flora is suppressed by antimicrobial drug therapy, potential pathogens may thrive. Much of the normal flora can cause disease under certain conditions, especially in elderly, debilitated, or immunosuppressed people. Normal bowel flora also synthesizes vitamin K and vitamin B complex.

## Infectious Diseases

Colonization involves the presence of normal microbial flora or transient environmental organisms that do not harm the host. Infectious disease involves the presence of a pathogen plus clinical signs and symptoms indicative of an infection. Accurate assessment and documentation of symptoms can aid diagnosis of infectious diseases.

### Laboratory Identification of Pathogens
Laboratory tests of infected fluids or tissues can identify probable pathogens. Bacteria can be identified based on Gram's stain and culture. *Gram's stain* identifies microscopic appearance, including shape and color of the organisms. *Culture* involves growing a microorganism in the laboratory. Growth on selective culture media will

## AT THE FOUNDATION: *Microorganisms and Infections*

In an infection, microorganisms initially attach to host cell receptors (ie, proteins, carbohydrates, lipids). Most microorganisms preferentially attach themselves to particular body tissues, invade the tissues, multiply, and produce infection. A major characteristic of microorganisms is their ability to survive in various environments. Bacteria survive in a variety of environments and adapt to protect themselves from normal body defense mechanisms and antimicrobial drugs. Drug-resistant bacterial strains can be produced in the presence of antimicrobial drugs.

Symptoms of infection are the result of the immune system's response to the presence of potential threats. Fever, for instance, results from the body's natural defense mechanism; higher temperatures reduce the ability of viruses and bacteria to replicate. Overall, the body's immune system is usually successful in preventing serious injury from infections.

characterize color, shape, and texture of the growing colonies. Identification of other microorganisms (eg, intracellular pathogens such as chlamydiae and viruses) may require different techniques. *Serology* identifies infectious agents indirectly by measuring the antibody level (titer) in the serum of a diseased host. A tentative diagnosis can be made if the antibody level against a specific pathogen rises during the acute phase of the disease and falls during convalescence. *Detection of antigens* uses features of culture and serology but reduces the time required for diagnosis. Another technique to identify an organism involves polymerase chain reaction (PCR), which can detect whether DNA for a specific organism is present in a sample.

## Common Human Pathogens

Common human pathogens are viruses, gram-positive enterococci, streptococci and staphylococci, and gram-negative intestinal organisms (*E. coli, Bacteroides, Klebsiella, Proteus, Pseudomonas* species, and others; Box 28-1). These microorganisms are usually spread by direct contact with an infected person or contaminated hands, food, water, or objects.

"Opportunistic" microorganisms are usually normal endogenous or environmental flora and nonpathogenic. They become pathogens, however, in hosts whose defense mechanisms are impaired. Opportunistic infections are likely to occur in people with severe burns, cancer, indwelling intravenous (IV) or urinary catheters, and antibiotic or corticosteroid drug therapy. Opportunistic bacterial infections, often caused by drug-resistant microorganisms, are usually serious and may be life threatening.

## Community–acquired Versus Nosocomial Infections

Infections are often categorized as community acquired or hospital acquired (nosocomial). Because the microbial environments differ, the two types of infections often have different etiologies and require different antimicrobial drugs. As a general rule, community-acquired infections are less severe and easier to treat. Nosocomial infections may be more severe and difficult to manage because they often result from drug-resistant microorganisms and occur in people whose resistance to disease is impaired. Drug-resistant strains of staphylococci, *Pseudomonas*, and *Proteus* are common causes of nosocomial infections.

## Antibiotic–resistant Microorganisms

The increasing prevalence of bacteria resistant to the effects of antibiotics, in both community-acquired and nosocomial infections, is a major public health concern (Box 28-2). Antibiotic resistance occurs in most human pathogens. Infections caused by drug-resistant organisms often require more toxic and expensive drugs, lead to prolonged illness or hospitalization, and increase mortality rates.

Resistant microorganisms grow and multiply when susceptible organisms (eg, normal flora) are suppressed by antimicrobial drugs or when immunosuppressive disorders or drugs impair normal body defenses. They may emerge during or after antimicrobial drug therapy. Contributing factors include (1) widespread use of antimicrobial drugs, especially broad-spectrum agents; (2) interrupted or inadequate antimicrobial treatment of infections; (3) type of bacteria; (4) type of infection; (5) clinical condition of the host; and (6) location or environmental setting where host resides.

### Mechanisms of Resistance

Antibiotics damage bacteria by disrupting essential functions of their life cycle. For example, penicillins and cephalosporins inhibit cell wall formation, fluoroquinolones interfere with DNA replication, and macrolides and clindamycin prevent protein synthesis. Regrettably, bacteria have adapted to overcome these disruptions. The mechanisms that lead to antibiotic resistance are diverse, but they can be classified into categories. In general, bacteria demonstrate resistance to antibiotics through five major mechanisms:

1. **Generating enzymes that inactivate the antibiotic.** For example, beta-lactamase enzymes change the chemical structure of penicillins and cephalosporins by opening the beta-lactam ring and preventing the antibiotic from binding with its target site (called penicillin-binding proteins) in the bacterial cell wall, thereby inactivating the drug.
2. **Changing the structure of the target site.** This mechanism generally involves structural changes in the amino acid sequence of the target site. The genetic mutations change antibiotic target sites or change the genetic code to produce new targets. These changes decrease bacterial susceptibility to an antibiotic, largely by altering binding sites. This mechanism is significant in the resistance to beta-lactam antibiotics, chloramphenicol, and aminoglycosides.
3. **Preventing cellular accumulation of the antibiotic.** This can occur by varying the membrane's permeability to the antibiotic by:
   - **Altering outer membrane proteins** (porin expression). Outer membrane porin proteins normally act as molecular sieves, allowing the movement of molecules into the cell according to charge and size. This mechanism is vital in the development of resistance to beta-lactam antibiotics, fluoroquinolones, and aminoglycosides.
   - **Introducing efflux pumps that regularly pump the antibiotic out of the cell.** Efflux pumps present on the surface of epithelial cells acquire the ability to pump drug molecules out of the cell using the cell's energy to achieve efficient protection against chemical invasion. Effective antibiotic transport has been recognized for many classes of drug efflux pumps, including tetracyclines and fluoroquinolones.

*(text continues on page 480)*

## BOX 28-1    Common Bacterial Pathogens

### Gram-positive Bacteria

*Staphylococci*

*Staphylococcus aureus* organisms are part of the normal microbial flora of the skin and upper respiratory tract and also are common pathogens. Some people carry (are colonized with) the organism in the anterior nares. The organisms are spread mainly by direct contact with people who are infected or who are carriers. The hands of health care workers are considered a major source of indirect spread and nosocomial infections. The organisms also survive on inanimate surfaces for long periods of time.

*S. aureus* organisms cause boils, carbuncles, burn and surgical wound infections, and internal abscesses. Burns or surgical wounds often become infected from clients' own nasal carriage or from health care personnel. The organisms cannot penetrate intact skin or mucous membranes. However, they can penetrate damaged tissues and produce endotoxins that destroy erythrocytes, leukocytes, platelets, fibroblasts, and other human cells. Also, many strains produce enterotoxins that cause food poisoning when ingested. The enterotoxins survive heating at temperatures high enough to kill the organisms, so reheating foods does not prevent food poisoning.

High-risk groups for staphylococcal infections include newborns, the elderly, and those who are malnourished, diabetic, or obese. In children, staphylococcal infections of the respiratory tract are most common in those younger than 2 years of age. In adults, staphylococcal pneumonia often occurs in people with chronic lung disease or as a secondary bacterial infection after influenza. The influenza virus destroys the ciliated epithelium of the respiratory tract and thereby aids bacterial invasion.

Staphylococcus species, non-aureus (SSNA), describes a group of organisms that are also part of the normal microbial flora of the skin and mucosal surfaces and are increasingly common pathogens. The most common member of this group involved in infections is *Staphylococcus epidermidis*. However, not all laboratories routinely further identify the specific organism when SSNA is identified, and microbiology laboratory reports may just report SSNA. For this discussion, we will use the term SSNA unless a specific reference needs to be made to *Staphylococcus epidermidis*.

Infections due to SSNA are associated with the use of treatment devices such as intravascular catheters, prosthetic heart valves, cardiac pacemakers, orthopedic prostheses, cerebrospinal fluid shunts, and peritoneal catheters. SSNA infections include endocarditis, bacteremia, and other serious infections and are especially hazardous to neutropenic and immunocompromised clients. Treatment usually requires removal of any infected medical device as well as appropriate antibiotic therapy.

*Streptococci*

Certain streptococci are part of the normal microbial flora of the throat and nasopharynx in many healthy people. Infections are usually spread by inhalation of droplets from the upper respiratory tracts of carriers or people with infections. However, these organisms do not cause disease unless the mucosal barrier is damaged by trauma, previous infection, or

surgical manipulation. Such damage allows the organisms to enter the bloodstream and gain access to other parts of the body. For example, the organisms may cause endocarditis if they reach damaged heart valves.

*S. pneumoniae* organisms, often called pneumococci, are common bacterial pathogens. They cause pneumonia, sinusitis, otitis media, and meningitis. Pneumococcal pneumonia usually develops when the mechanisms that normally expel organisms inhaled into the lower airway (ie, the mucociliary blanket and cough reflex) are impaired by viral infection, smoking, immobility, or other insults. When *S. pneumoniae* reach the alveoli, they proliferate, cause acute inflammation, and spread rapidly to involve one or more lobes. Alveoli fill with proteinaceous fluid, neutrophils, and bacteria. When the pneumonia resolves, there is usually no residual damage to the pulmonary parenchyma. Elderly adults have high rates of illness and death from pneumococcal pneumonia, which can often be prevented by pneumococcal vaccine. Pneumococcal vaccine (see Chap. 34) contains 23 strains of the pneumococci that cause most of the serious infections.

Pneumococcal sinusitis and otitis media usually follow a viral illness, such as the common cold. The viral infection injures the protective ciliated epithelium and fills the air spaces with nutrient-rich tissue fluid, in which the pneumococci thrive. *S. pneumoniae* cause approximately 35% of cases of bacterial sinusitis. In young children, upper respiratory tract infections may be complicated by acute sinusitis. With otitis media, most children have repeated episodes by 6 years of age and the pneumococcus causes approximately half of these cases. Recurrent otitis media during early childhood may result in reduced hearing acuity. Otitis media rarely occurs in adults.

Pneumococcal meningitis may develop from sinus or middle ear infections or an injury that allows organisms from the nasopharynx to enter the meninges. *S. pneumoniae* are a common cause of bacterial meningitis in adults. Other potential secondary complications include septicemia, endocarditis, pericarditis, and empyema.

Susceptible pneumococcal infections may be treated with penicillin G. For people who are allergic to penicillin, a cephalosporin or a macrolide may be effective.

*S. pneumoniae* organisms are developing resistance such that empiric treatment must be based on the likelihood of drug-resistant *S. pneumoniae* (DRSP). Rates of DRSP vary by locale; if high, the organisms will be resistant to penicillin and also cross-resistant to other alternatives such as second- and third-generation cephalosporins and possibly macrolides. Alternatives include fluoroquinolones, vancomycin, and chloramphenicol. Empiric treatment of meningitis where *S. pneumoniae* is known or suspected should include a third-generation cephalosporin (ceftriaxone or cefotaxime) plus vancomycin. Empiric treatment for pneumonia should include a fluoroquinolone or a macrolide in those areas with high penicillin and cephalosporin resistance rates.

*S. pyogenes* (beta-hemolytic streptococcus) are often part of the normal flora of the skin and oropharynx. The organisms spread from person to person by direct contact with oral or

*(continued)*

## BOX 28-1    Common Bacterial Pathogens (Continued)

respiratory secretions. They cause severe pharyngitis ("strep throat"), scarlet fever, rheumatic fever, and endocarditis. With streptococcal pharyngitis, people remain infected with the organism for weeks after symptoms resolve and thus serve as a reservoir for infection.

### Enterococci

Enterococci are normal flora in the human intestine but are also found in soil, food, water, and animals. Although the genus *Enterococcus* contains approximately 12 species, the main pathogens are *E. faecalis* and *E. faecium.* Most enterococcal infections occur in hospitalized patients, especially those in critical care units. Risk factors for nosocomial infections include serious underlying disease, prior surgery, renal impairment, and the presence of urinary or vascular catheters. These organisms, especially *E. faecalis,* are usually secondary invaders in urinary tract or wound infections. Enterococci may also cause endocarditis. This serious infection occurs most often in people with underlying heart disease, such as an injured valve. When the organisms reach a heart valve, they multiply and release emboli of foreign particles into the bloodstream. Symptoms of endocarditis include fever, heart murmurs, enlarged spleen, and anemia. This infection is diagnosed by isolating enterococci from blood cultures. If not treated promptly and appropriately, often with ampicillin and gentamicin, enterococcal endocarditis may be fatal.

### Gram-negative Bacteria

#### Bacteroides

*Bacteroides* are anaerobic bacteria normally found in the digestive, respiratory, and genital tracts. They are the most common bacteria in the colon, where they greatly outnumber *Escherichia coli. B. fragilis,* the major human pathogen, causes intra-abdominal and pelvic abscesses (eg, after surgery or trauma that allows fecal contamination of these tissues), brain abscesses (eg, from bacteremia or spread from a middle ear or sinus infection), and bacteremia, which may spread the organisms throughout the body.

#### Escherichia coli

*E. coli* inhabit the intestinal tract of humans and animals. They are normally nonpathogenic in the intestinal tract but common pathogens in other parts of the body. They may be beneficial by synthesizing vitamins and by competitively discouraging growth of potential pathogens.

*E. coli* cause most urinary tract infections. They also cause pneumonia and sepsis in immunocompromised hosts and meningitis and sepsis in newborns. *E. coli* pneumonia often occurs in debilitated patients after colonization of the oropharynx with organisms from their endogenous microbial flora. In healthy people, the normal gram-positive organisms of oral cavities attach to material that coats the surface of oral mucosa and prevents transient *E. coli* from establishing residence. Debilitated or severely ill people produce an enzyme that destroys the material that allows gram-positive flora to adhere to oral mucosa. This allows *E. coli* (and other gram-negative enteric bacteria) to compete successfully with the normal gram-positive flora and colonize the oropharynx. Then, droplets of the oral flora

are aspirated into the respiratory tract, where impaired protective mechanisms allow survival of the aspirated organisms.

*E. coli* also cause enteric gram-negative sepsis, which is acquired from the normal enteric bacterial flora. When *E. coli* and other enteric organisms reach the bloodstream of healthy people, host defenses eliminate the organisms. When the organisms reach the bloodstream of people with severe illnesses and conditions such as neutropenia, the host is unable to mount adequate defenses and sepsis occurs. In neonates, *E. coli* are the most common gram-negative organisms causing nosocomial septic shock and meningitis.

In addition, *E. coli* often cause diarrhea and dysentery. One strain, called O157:H7, causes hemorrhagic colitis, a disease characterized by severe abdominal cramps, copious bloody diarrhea, and hemolytic-uremic syndrome (hemolytic anemia, thrombocytopenia, and acute renal failure). Hemolytic-uremic syndrome occurs most often in children. The main reservoir of this strain is the intestinal tract of animals, especially cattle, and several epidemics have been associated with ingestion of undercooked ground beef. Other sources include contaminated water and milk and person-to-person spread. Because it cannot survive in nature, the presence of *E. coli* in milk or water indicates fecal contamination.

#### Klebsiella

*Klebsiella* organisms, which are normal bowel flora, may infect the respiratory tract, urinary tract, bloodstream, burn wounds, and meninges, most often as opportunistic infections in debilitated persons. *K. pneumoniae* are a common cause of pneumonia, especially in people with pulmonary disease, bacteremia, and sepsis.

#### Proteus

*Proteus* organisms are normally found in the intestinal tract and in decaying matter. They most often cause urinary tract and wound infections but may infect any tissue, especially in debilitated people. Infection usually occurs with antibiotic therapy, which decreases drug-sensitive bacteria and allows drug-resistant bacteria to proliferate.

#### Pseudomonas

*Pseudomonas* organisms are found in water, soil, skin, and intestines. They are found in the stools of some healthy people and possibly 50% of hospital patients. *P. aeruginosa,* the species most often associated with human disease, can cause infections of the respiratory tract, urinary tract, wounds, burns, meninges, eyes, and ears. Because of its resistance to many antibiotics, it can cause severe infections in people receiving antibiotic therapy for burns, wounds, and cystic fibrosis. *P. aeruginosa* colonizes the respiratory tract of most clients with cystic fibrosis and infects approximately 25% of burn patients. Infection is more likely to occur in hosts who are very young or very old or who have impaired immune systems. Sources of infection include catheterization of the urinary tract, trauma or procedures involving the brain or spinal cord, and contamination of respiratory ventilators.

*P. cepacia* infections are increasing, especially in patients with burns, cystic fibrosis, debilitation, or immunosuppression.

*(continued)*

BOX
28-1 **Common Bacterial Pathogens** (Continued)

These infections are especially difficult to treat because the organism is resistant to many of the antibiotics used to treat other gram-negative infections.

*Serratia*
S. marcescens organisms are found in infected people, water, milk, feces, and soil. They cause serious nosocomial infections of the urinary tract, respiratory tract, skin, burn wounds, and bloodstream. They also may cause hospital epidemics and produce drug-resistant strains. High-risk patients include newborns, the debilitated, and the immunosuppressed.

*Salmonella*
Approximately 1400 species have been identified; several are pathogenic to humans. The organisms cause gastroenteritis, typhoid fever, septicemia, and a severe, sometimes fatal type of food poisoning. The primary reservoir is the intestinal tract of many animals. Humans become infected through ingestion of contaminated water or food. Water becomes polluted by introduction of feces from any animal excreting salmonellae. Infection by food usually results from ingestion of contaminated meat or by hands transferring organisms from an infected source. In the United States, undercooked poultry and eggs are common sources.

Salmonella enterocolitis is a common cause of food-borne outbreaks of gastroenteritis. Diarrhea usually begins several hours after ingesting contaminated food and may continue for several days, along with nausea, vomiting, headache, and abdominal pain.

*Shigella*
Shigella species cause gastrointestinal problems ranging from mild diarrhea to severe bacillary dysentery. Humans, who seem to be the only natural hosts, become infected after ingestion of contaminated food or water. Effects of shigellosis are attributed to the loss of fluids, electrolytes, and nutrients and to the ulceration that occurs in the colon wall.

BOX
28-2 **Antibiotic-Resistant Staphylococci, Streptococci, and Enterococci**

### Methicillin-resistant *Staphylococcus* Species
Penicillin-resistant staphylococci developed in the early days of penicillin use because the organisms produced beta-lactamase enzymes (penicillinases) that destroyed penicillin. Methicillin was one of five drugs developed to resist the action of beta-lactamase enzymes and thus be effective in treating staphylococcal infections. Eventually, strains of S. aureus became resistant to these drugs as well. The mechanism of resistance in methicillin-resistant S. aureus (MRSA) is alteration of penicillin-binding proteins (PBPs). PBPs, the target sites of penicillins and other beta-lactam antibiotics, are proteins required for maintaining integrity of bacterial cell walls. Susceptible S. aureus have five PBPs called 1, 2, 3, 3a or 3', and 4. Beta-lactam antibiotics bind to these enzymes and produce defective bacterial cell walls, which kill the organisms. MRSA have an additional PBP called 2a or 2'. Methicillin cannot bind effectively to the PBPs and inhibit bacteria cell wall synthesis except with very high drug concentrations. Consequently, minimum inhibitory concentrations (MICs) of methicillin increased to high levels that were difficult to achieve.

The term MRSA is commonly used but misleading because the organisms are widely resistant to penicillins (including all of the antistaphylococcal penicillins, not just methicillin) and cephalosporins. Many strains of MRSA are also resistant to erythromycin, clindamycin, tetracycline, and the aminoglycosides. MRSA frequently colonize nasal passages of health care workers and are increasing as a cause of nosocomial infections, especially in critical care units. In addition, the incidence of methicillin-resistant S. epidermidis (MRSE, often reported as methicillin-resistant SSNA) isolates is increasing.

A major reason for concern about infections caused by MRSA and MRSE is that vancomycin is the drug of choice for treatment. However, vancomycin has been used extensively to treat infections caused by S. epidermidis and enterococci, and vancomycin resistance is increasing in those species. Because resistance genes from the other organisms can be transferred to S. aureus, vancomycin-resistant S. aureus may develop. Vancomycin-resistant enterococci (VRE) are discussed later.

### Penicillin-Resistant *Streptococcus pneumoniae* (Pneumococci)
Penicillin has long been the drug of choice for treating pneumococcal infections (eg, community-acquired pneumonia, bacteremia, meningitis, and otitis media in children). However, penicillin-resistant strains and multidrug-resistant strains are being identified with increasing frequency. Risk factors for the development of resistant strains include frequent antibiotic use and prophylactic antibiotics. Once developed, resistant strains spread to other people, especially in children's day care centers and in hospital settings. Children in day care centers are often colonized or infected with antibiotic-resistant S. pneumoniae. This is attributed to a high incidence of otitis media, which is often treated with a penicillin or cephalosporin. Resistant strains in adults and elderly clients are often associated with previous use of a penicillin or cephalosporin and hospitalization.

S. pneumoniae are thought to develop resistance to penicillin by decreasing the ability of their PBPs to bind with penicillin (and other beta-lactam antibiotics). Organisms displaying high-level penicillin resistance may be cross-resistant to second- and third-generation cephalosporins, amoxicillin/clavulanate, and the macrolides azithromycin and clarithromycin. In pneumococcal infections resistant to penicillins and cephalosporins, vancomycin, quinolones, and macrolides are drugs of choice.

*(continued)*

**BOX 28-2    Antibiotic-Resistant Staphylococci, Streptococci, and Enterococci** (Continued)

To decrease spread of resistant *S. pneumoniae,* the Centers for Disease Control and Prevention (CDC) have proposed:

- Improved surveillance to delineate prevalence by geographic area and assist clinicians in choosing appropriate antimicrobial therapy.
- Rational use of antimicrobials to reduce exposures to drug-resistant pneumococci. For example, prophylactic antibiotic therapy for otitis media may increase colonization and infection of young children with resistant organisms.
- Pneumococcal vaccination for people older than 2 years of age with increased risk of pneumococcal infection, and for all people older than 65 years of age.

### Vancomycin-resistant Enterococci

Enterococci have intrinsic and acquired resistance to many antibacterial drugs. For example, penicillins and cephalosporins inhibit rather than kill the organisms at achievable concentrations, and aminoglycosides are ineffective if used alone. As a result, standard treatment of an enterococcal infection outside of the urinary tract has involved a combination of ampicillin and gentamicin or streptomycin. This combination is often successful because the ampicillin damages the bacterial cell wall and allows the aminoglycoside to penetrate the bacterial cell. For ampicillin-allergic clients, vancomycin is given with an aminoglycoside.

This treatment is becoming less effective because some strains of enterococci have developed resistance to ampicillin, gentamicin, and vancomycin. The incidence of multidrug-resistant enterococci and VRE has increased in recent years. Two major types (Van A and Van B) of VRE have been described, with different patterns of antimicrobial susceptibility. Van B is susceptible to teicoplanin; Van A is resistant to teicoplanin but may be susceptible to minocycline, ciprofloxacin, or quinupristin/dalfopristin (Synercid).

A major contributing factor to VRE is increased use of vancomycin to prevent or treat other infections such as staphylococcal (MRSA and MRSE) infections and antibiotic-associated (pseudomembranous) colitis (caused by toxins released by *Clostridium difficile* organisms). Therefore, to decrease the spread of VRE, the CDC recommends limiting the use of vancomycin. Specific recommendations include avoiding or minimizing use in routine surgical prophylaxis, empiric therapy for febrile patients with neutropenia (unless the prevalence of MRSA or MRSE is high), systemic or local prophylaxis for intravascular catheter infection or colonization, selective decontamination of the gastrointestinal tract, eradication of MRSA colonization, primary treatment of antibiotic-associated colitis, and routine prophylaxis for very low birth weight infants or patients on continuous ambulatory peritoneal dialysis. Thorough handwashing and environmental cleaning are also important because VRE can survive for long periods on hands, gloves, stethoscopes, and environmental surfaces. Personnel should remove or change gloves after contact with clients known to be colonized or infected with VRE. Stethoscopes should be used only with an infected patient or cleaned thoroughly between patients if used for both VRE-infected and uninfected patients.

---

4. **Changing the metabolic pathway that is being blocked.** Antibiotics that seek a specific metabolic event become ineffective if the bacterium can carry out the reaction by another pathway. As an illustration, trimethoprim-sulfamethoxazole (Bactrim) normally inhibits folic acid synthesis, but resistance has developed in gram-negative organisms, which acquire their resistance from enzymes that allow them to bypass the metabolic step under attack by the antibiotic.

5. **Titration.** This involves the overproduction of the target enzyme to overpower the effects of the antibiotic, resulting in resistance. For instance, some bacteria have become resistant to trimethoprim by extracting excessive quantities of the antibiotic's target enzyme.

A few bacteria are naturally resistant to specific antibiotics because of their structure. For instance:

- Gram-negative bacteria possess an outer membrane and a cytoplasmic membrane, and larger antibiotics are unable to pass their narrow porins.
- Mycoplasma lacks a cell wall, making it impervious to penicillins.
- Sulfonamides have no impact on bacteria that obtain their folic acid from the environment.

## HOST DEFENSE MECHANISMS

Although the numbers and virulence of microorganisms help to determine whether a person acquires an infection, another major factor is the host's ability to defend itself against the would-be invaders.

Major defense mechanisms of the human body are intact skin and mucous membranes, various anti-infective secretions, mechanical movements, phagocytic cells, and the immune and inflammatory processes. Many factors impair host defense mechanisms and predispose to infection by disease-producing microorganisms:

- Breaks in the skin and mucous membranes related to trauma, inflammation, open lesions, or insertion of prosthetic devices, tubes, and catheters for diagnostic or therapeutic purposes
- Impaired blood supply
- Neutropenia and other blood disorders
- Malnutrition
- Poor personal hygiene
- Suppression of normal bacterial flora by antimicrobial drugs

- Suppression of the immune system and the inflammatory response by immunosuppressive drugs, cytotoxic antineoplastic drugs, and adrenal corticosteroids
- Diabetes mellitus and other chronic diseases
- Advanced age

## CHARACTERISTICS OF ANTI-INFECTIVE DRUGS

### Terms and Concepts

Several terms are used to describe these drugs. *Anti-infective* and *antimicrobial* include antibacterial, antiviral, and antifungal drugs; *antibacterial* and *antibiotic* usually refer only to drugs used in bacterial infections. Most of the drugs in this section are antibacterials. Antiviral and antifungal drugs are discussed in Chapter 33.

Additional terms for antibacterial drugs include *broad spectrum*, for those effective against several groups of microorganisms, and *narrow spectrum*, for those effective against a few groups. The action of an antibacterial drug is usually described as *bactericidal* (kills the microorganism) or *bacteriostatic* (inhibits growth of the microorganism). Whether a drug is bactericidal or bacteriostatic often depends on its concentration at the infection site and the susceptibility of the microorganism to the drug. Successful treatment with bacteriostatic antibiotics depends on the ability of the host's immune system to eliminate the inhibited bacteria and an adequate duration of drug therapy. Stopping an antibiotic prematurely can result in rapid resumption of bacterial growth. Bactericidal drugs are preferred in serious infections, especially in people with impaired immune function.

### Mechanisms of Action

Most antibiotics act on a specific target in the bacterial cell (Fig. 28-1). Almost any structure unique to bacteria, such as proteins or nucleic acids, can be a target for antibiotics. Specific mechanisms include the following:

1. Inhibition of bacterial cell wall synthesis or activation of enzymes that disrupt bacterial cell walls (eg, penicillins, cephalosporins, vancomycin)
2. Inhibition of protein synthesis by bacteria or production of abnormal bacterial proteins (eg, aminoglycosides, clindamycin, erythromycin, tetracyclines). These drugs bind irreversibly to bacterial ribosomes, intracellular structures that synthesize proteins. When antimicrobial drugs are bound to the ribosomes, bacteria cannot synthesize the proteins necessary for cell walls and other structures.
3. Disruption of microbial cell membranes (eg, antifungals)
4. Inhibition of organism reproduction by interfering with nucleic acid synthesis (eg, fluoroquinolones,

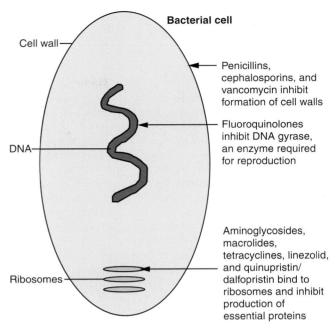

**FIGURE 28–1** Actions of antibacterial drugs on bacterial cells.

rifampin, anti–acquired immunodeficiency syndrome antivirals)

5. Inhibition of cell metabolism and growth (eg, sulfonamides, trimethoprim)

### Indications for Use

Antimicrobial drugs are used to treat and prevent infections. Empiric therapy against the most likely pathogens is often begun until organisms are identified when more specific therapy is instituted. Prophylactic therapy is recommended to prevent:

1. Group A streptococcal infections and possibly rheumatic fever, rheumatic heart disease, and glomerulonephritis. Penicillin is commonly used.
2. Bacterial endocarditis in clients with cardiac valvular disease who are having dental, surgical, or other invasive procedures
3. Tuberculosis. Isoniazid (see Chap. 32) is used.
4. Perioperative infections in high-risk clients (eg, those whose resistance to infection is lowered because of age, poor nutrition, disease, or drugs) and for high-risk surgical procedures (eg, cardiac or GI surgery, certain orthopedic procedures, organ transplantations)
5. Sexually transmitted diseases (eg, gonorrhea, syphilis, chlamydial infections) after exposure has occurred
6. Recurrent urinary tract infections in premenopausal, sexually active women. A single dose of trimethoprim-sulfamethoxazole, cinoxacin, or cephalexin, taken after sexual intercourse, is often effective.

*(text continues on page 484)*

# Nursing Process

## Assessment

Assess for current or potential infection:

- General signs and symptoms of infection are the same as those of inflammation, although the terms are not synonymous. Inflammation is the normal response to any injury; infection requires the presence of a microorganism. The two often occur together. Inflammation may weaken tissue, allowing microorganisms to invade and cause infection. Infection (tissue injury by microorganisms) arouses inflammation. Local signs include redness, heat, edema, and pain; systemic signs include fever and leukocytosis. Specific manifestations depend on the site of infection. Common sites are the respiratory tract, surgical or other wounds, and the genitourinary tract.
- Assess each client for the presence of factors that increase risks of infection (see the section on Host Defense Mechanisms, earlier).
- Assess culture reports for causative organisms.
- Assess susceptibility reports for appropriate antibacterial drug therapy.
- Assess clients for drug allergies. If present, ask about specific signs and symptoms.
- Assess baseline data about renal and hepatic function and other factors that aid monitoring for therapeutic and adverse drug effects.
- Assess for characteristics that increase risks of adverse drug effects.

## Nursing Diagnoses

- Fatigue related to infection
- Activity Intolerance related to fatigue
- Diarrhea related to antimicrobial therapy
- Imbalanced Nutrition: Less Than Body Requirements related to anorexia, nausea, and vomiting associated with antimicrobial therapy
- Risk for Injury related to infection or adverse drug effects
- Risk for Infection related to emergence of drug-resistant microorganisms
- Deficient Knowledge: Methods of preventing infections

## Planning/Goals

*The client will:*

- Receive antimicrobial drugs accurately when given by health care providers or caregivers
- Take drugs as prescribed and for the length of time prescribed when self-administered as an outpatient
- Experience decreased fever, white blood cell (WBC) count, and other signs and symptoms of infection
- Be monitored regularly for therapeutic and adverse drug effects
- Receive prompt recognition and treatment of potentially serious adverse effects
- Verbalize and practice measures to prevent future infections
- Be safeguarded against nosocomial infections by health care providers

## Interventions

- Use measures to prevent and minimize the spread of infection.
- Wash hands thoroughly and often. This is probably the most effective method of preventing infections.
- Support natural defense mechanisms by promoting general health measures (eg, nutrition, adequate fluid intake, rest, exercise).
- Keep the client's skin clean and dry, especially the hands, underarms, groin, and perineum, because these areas harbor large numbers of microorganisms. Also, take care to prevent trauma to the skin and mucous membrane. Damaged tissues are susceptible to infection.
- Treat all body fluids (eg, blood, aspirates from abdomen or chest) and body substances (eg, sputum, feces, urine, wound drainage) as infectious. Major elements of standard precautions to prevent transmission of hepatitis B, human immunodeficiency virus, and other pathogens include wearing gloves when likely to be exposed to any of these materials and thorough handwashing when the gloves are removed. Rigorous and consistent use of the recommended precautions helps to protect health care providers and clients.
- Implement isolation procedures appropriately.
- To prevent spread of respiratory infections, have clients wash hands after coughing, sneezing, or contact with infected people; cover mouth and nose with tissues when sneezing or coughing and dispose of tissues by placing them in a paper bag and burning it; expectorate sputum (swallowing may cause reinfection); avoid crowds when possible, especially during influenza season (approximately November through February); and recommend annual influenza vaccine to high-risk populations (eg, people with chronic diseases such as diabetes and heart, lung, or renal problems; older adults; and health care personnel who are likely to be exposed). Pneumococcal vaccine (see Chap. 34) is recommended as a single dose for the same populations.
- Assist or instruct clients at risk about pulmonary hygiene measures to prevent accumulation or promote removal of respiratory secretions. These measures include ambulating, turning, coughing and deep-breathing exercises, and incentive spirometry. Retained secretions are good culture media for bacterial growth.
- Use sterile technique when changing any dressing. If a wound is not infected, sterile technique helps prevent infection; if the wound is already infected, sterile technique avoids introducing new bacteria. For all but the smallest of dressings without drainage, remove the dressing with clean gloves, discard it in a moisture-proof bag, and wash hands before putting on sterile gloves to apply the new dressing.
- To minimize spread of staphylococcal infections, infected personnel with skin lesions should not work until lesions are healed; infected clients should be isolated. Personnel

*(continued)*

## NURSING PROCESS (Continued)

with skin lesions probably spread more staphylococci than clients because personnel are more mobile.

- For clients with infections, monitor temperature for increased or decreased fever, and monitor WBC count for decrease.
- For clients receiving antimicrobial therapy, maintain a total fluid intake of approximately 3000 mL/24 hours, if not contraindicated by the client's condition. An adequate intake and avoidance of fluid volume deficit may help to decrease drug toxicity, especially with aminoglycoside antibiotics. On the other hand, a client receiving IV antibiotics, with 50 to 100 mL of fluid per dose, may be at risk for development of fluid volume overload.

- Assist clients with handwashing, maintaining nutrition and fluid balance, getting adequate rest, and handling secretions correctly. These measures help the body to fight the infection, prevent further infection, and enhance the effectiveness of anti-infective drugs.
- Assist clients in using antimicrobial drugs safely and effectively.

### Evaluation
- Interview and observe for compliance with instructions for using antimicrobial drugs.
- Observe for adverse drug effects.
- Interview and observe for practices to prevent infection.

## CLIENT TEACHING GUIDELINES
## Antimicrobial Drugs

### General Considerations
✔ Wash hands often and thoroughly, especially before preparing food or eating and after exposure to any body secretions (eg, urine, feces, sputum, nasal secretions). This is probably the most effective way to prevent infection and to avoid spreading an infection to others.

✔ A balanced diet and adequate fluid intake, rest, and exercise also help the body to fight infection, prevent further infection, and increase the effectiveness of antimicrobial drugs.

✔ Take all prescribed doses of an antimicrobial; do not stop when symptoms are relieved. If medication is stopped too soon, symptoms of the current infection may recur and new infections that are caused by antibiotic-resistant organisms and harder to treat may develop.

✔ If problems occur with taking an antimicrobial drug, report them to a health care provider rather than stopping the drug.

✔ Do not take antimicrobials left over from a previous illness or prescribed for someone else. Even if infection is present, the likelihood of having the appropriate drug on hand, and in adequate amounts, is extremely small. Thus, taking drugs not prescribed for the particular illness tends to maximize risks and minimize benefits. Also, if the infection is viral, antibacterial drugs are ineffective and should not be used.

✔ Report any other drugs being taken to the prescribing physician. Drug interactions may occur, and changes in drug therapy may be indicated.

✔ Report any drug allergies to all health care providers and wear a medical identification emblem that lists allergens.

✔ Some antibiotics (eg, ampicillin, nitrofurantoin, penicillin V, sulfonamides, tetracyclines) decrease the effectiveness of estrogens and oral contraceptives. Women taking these drugs should use another method of contraception. Inadequate blood levels of estrogen may be indicated by breakthrough bleeding.

### Self-administration
✔ Unless instructed otherwise, take antimicrobial drugs at evenly spaced intervals around the clock. This helps maintain beneficial blood levels of most drugs.

✔ Take most oral antimicrobials on an empty stomach, approximately 1 hour before or 2 hours after meals. Food may decrease absorption and effectiveness. If the medication causes intolerable nausea or vomiting, a few bites of food may be taken.

✔ Store most liquid preparations in the refrigerator, check expiration dates, and discard them when indicated. These preparations are stable and effective for a limited time.

✔ Take the medications with a full glass of water. This helps tablets and capsules to dissolve better in the stomach and decreases stomach irritation.

✔ Report nausea, vomiting, diarrhea, skin rash, recurrence of symptoms for which the antimicrobial drug was prescribed, or signs of new infection (eg, fever, cough, sore mouth, drainage). These problems may indicate adverse effects of the drug, lack of therapeutic response to the drug, or another infection. Any of these requires evaluation and may indicate changes in drug therapy.

## ▨ MANAGEMENT CONSIDERATIONS

### Treating Infection

The goal of treatment is to eradicate the causative microorganism and return the host to full physiologic functioning. This differs from the goal of most drug therapy, which is to relieve signs and symptoms rather than cure the underlying disorder.

### Rational Use of Antimicrobial Drugs

Antimicrobials are among the most frequently used drugs worldwide. Their success in saving lives and decreasing severity and duration of infectious diseases has encouraged their extensive use. Authorities believe that much antibiotic use involves overuse, misuse, or abuse of the drugs. That is, an antibiotic is not indicated at all, or the wrong drug, dose, route, or duration is prescribed. Inappropriate use of antibiotics increases adverse drug effects, infections with drug-resistant microorganisms, and health care costs. In addition, it decreases the number of effective drugs for serious or antibiotic-resistant infections.

Guidelines to promote more appropriate use of the drugs include:

1. Avoid the use of broad-spectrum antibacterial drugs to treat viral or trivial bacterial infections; use narrow-spectrum agents when likely to be effective.
2. Give antibacterial drugs only when a significant bacterial infection is diagnosed or strongly suspected or when there is an established indication for prophylaxis. These drugs are ineffective and should not be used to treat viral infections. The Centers for Disease Control and Prevention (CDC) estimate that one third of all outpatient prescriptions for antibiotics are unnecessary.
3. Minimize antimicrobial drug therapy for fever unless other clinical manifestations or laboratory data indicate infection.
4. Use the drugs along with other interventions to decrease microbial proliferation, such as universal precautions, medical isolation techniques, frequent and thorough handwashing, and preoperative skin and bowel cleansing.
5. Follow recommendations of the CDC for prevention and treatment of infections, especially those caused by drug-resistant organisms (eg, gonorrhea, penicillin-resistant streptococcal infections, methicillin-resistant staphylococcal infections, vancomycin-resistant enterococcal (VRE) infections, and multidrug-resistant tuberculosis [MDR-TB]).
6. Finish an antibiotic prescription and take exactly as directed even if symptoms have resolved. Not completing the full course may allow some resistant bacteria to survive. These surviving resistant bacteria multiply as a resistant strain, or group, and are more complicated to treat. The drug-resistant bacteria can also spread from one individual to another.
7. Consult infectious disease physicians, infection control nurses, and infectious disease pharmacists about local patterns of drug-resistant organisms and treatment of complicated infections.

### Collection of Specimens

Collect specimens for culture and Gram's stain before giving the first dose of an antibiotic. For best results, specimens must be collected accurately and taken directly to the laboratory. If analysis is delayed, contaminants may overgrow pathogenic microorganisms.

### Drug Selection

Once an infection requiring treatment is diagnosed, numerous factors influence the choice of an antimicrobial drug or combination of drugs.

**Initial empiric therapy.** Because most laboratory tests to identify definitively the causative organisms and to determine susceptibility to antibiotics require 48 to 72 hours (except Gram's stain and a rapid test for group A streptococci), the health care provider usually prescribes for immediate administration a drug that is likely to be effective. This empiric therapy is based on an informed estimate of the most likely pathogen, given the client's signs and symptoms and apparent site of infection. A single broad-spectrum antibiotic or a combination of drugs is often chosen.

**Culture and susceptibility studies** allow the therapist to "match the drug to the bug." Culture identifies the causative organism; susceptibility tests determine which drugs are likely to be effective against the organism. Culture and susceptibility studies are especially important with suspected gram-negative infections because of the high incidence of drug-resistant microorganisms. However, drug-resistant gram-positive organisms are being identified with increasing frequency.

When a specific organism is identified by a laboratory culture, tests can be performed to measure the organism's susceptibility to particular antibiotics. Laboratory reports indicate whether the organism is susceptible (S) or resistant (R) to the tested drugs. One indication of susceptibility is the minimum inhibitory concentration (MIC). The MIC is the lowest concentration of an antibiotic that prevents visible growth of microorganisms. Some laboratories report MIC instead of, or in addition to, susceptible (S) or resistant (R). *Susceptible organisms* have low or moderate MICs that can be attained by giving usual doses of an antimicrobial agent. For the drug to be effective, serum and tissue concentrations should usually exceed the MIC of an organism for a period of time. How much and how long drug concentrations need to exceed the MIC depend on the drug class and the bacterial species. *Resistant organisms* have high MICs and may require higher concentrations of drug than can be achieved in the body, even with large doses. In some cases, the minimum bactericidal concentration (MBC) is reported, indicating no growth of the organism in the presence of a particular antibiotic. The MBC is especially desirable for infected hosts with impaired immune functions.

Clients' responses to antimicrobial therapy cannot always be correlated with the MIC of an infecting pathogen. Thus, reports of drug susceptibility testing must be applied in the context of the site of infection, the characteristics of the drug, and the clinical status of the client.

**Knowledge of antibiotic resistance patterns in the community and agency.** Because these patterns change, continuing efforts must be made. *Pseudomonas aeruginosa* is resistant to many antibiotics. Those strains resistant to gentamicin may be susceptible to amikacin, ceftazidime, imipenem, or aztreonam. Some gram-negative organisms have become increasingly resistant to aminoglycosides, third-generation cephalosporins, and aztreonam, but may be susceptible to imipenem.

**Knowledge of the organisms most likely to infect particular body tissues.** For example, urinary tract infections are often caused by *E. coli*, and a drug effective against this organism is indicated.

**A drug's ability to penetrate infected tissues.** Several antimicrobials are effective in urinary tract infections because they are excreted in the urine. However, the choice of an effective antimicrobial drug may be limited in infections of the brain, eyes, gallbladder, or prostate gland because many drugs are unable to reach therapeutic concentrations in these tissues.

**A drug's toxicity and the risk-to-benefit ratio.** In general, the least toxic drug should always be used. However, for serious infections, more toxic drugs may be necessary.

**Drug costs.** If an older, less expensive drug meets the criteria for rational drug selection and is likely to be effective against a given infection, it should be used as opposed to a more expensive agent. For hospitals and nursing homes, personnel costs in relation to preparation and administration should be considered as well as purchasing costs.

## Antibiotic Combination Therapy

Antimicrobial drugs are often used in combination. Indications for combination therapy may include:

■ Infections caused by multiple microorganisms (eg, abdominal and pelvic infections)
■ Nosocomial infections, which may be caused by many different organisms
■ Serious infections in which a combination is synergistic (eg, an aminoglycoside and an antipseudomonal penicillin for pseudomonal infections)
■ Likely emergence of drug-resistant organisms if a single drug is used (eg, tuberculosis). Although drug combi-

nations to prevent resistance are widely used, the only clearly effective use is for treatment of tuberculosis.
■ Fever or other signs of infection in clients whose immune systems are suppressed. Combinations of antibacterial plus antiviral drugs, antifungal drugs, or both may be needed.

## Dosage

Dosage (amount and frequency of administration) should be individualized according to characteristics of the causative organism, the chosen drug, and the client's size and condition (eg, type and severity of infection, ability to use and excrete the chosen drug). For example, dosage may need to be increased for more resistant organisms such as *Pseudomonas* species and for infections in which antibiotics have difficulty penetrating to the site of infection (eg, meningitis). Antimicrobial drug therapy requires close monitoring in clients with renal impairment. Many drugs are excreted primarily by the kidneys; some are nephrotoxic and may further damage the kidneys. In the presence of renal impairment, drugs may accumulate and produce toxic effects. Thus, dosages often must be reduced if the client has renal impairment or other disorders that delay drug elimination. In clients with renal failure who are receiving hemodialysis or peritoneal dialysis, some drugs are removed by dialysis, and an extra dose may be needed during or after dialysis. Reference texts or scientific articles should be consulted to determine appropriate doses of antibiotics in these clients.

Antimicrobial therapy in clients with liver impairment is not well defined. Some drugs are metabolized by the liver (eg, cefoperazone, chloramphenicol, clindamycin, erythromycin), and dosage must be reduced in clients with severe liver impairment. Some are associated with elevations of liver enzymes or hepatotoxicity (eg, certain fluoroquinolones, tetracyclines, isoniazid, rifampin). Laboratory monitoring may be helpful in high-risk populations.

## Route of Administration

Most antimicrobial drugs are given orally or intravenously for systemic infections. The route of administration depends on the client's condition (eg, location and severity of the infection, ability to take oral drugs) and the available drug dosage forms. In serious infections, the IV route is preferred for most drugs.

## Duration of Therapy

Duration of therapy varies from a single dose to years, depending on the reason for use. For most acute infections, the average duration is approximately 7 to 10 days or until the recipient has been afebrile and asymptomatic for 48 to 72 hours.

## Perioperative Use

When used to prevent infections associated with surgery, a single dose of an antimicrobial is usually given within 2 hours before the first incision. This provides effective tissue concentration during the procedure. If contamination occurs, the client should be treated for an infection. The choice of drug depends on the pathogens most likely to colonize the operative area. For most surgeries involving an incision through the skin, a first-generation cephalosporin with activity against *Staphylococcus aureus* or *Streptococcus* species, such as cefazolin (Kefzol), is commonly used. Repeated doses may be given during surgery for procedures of long duration, procedures involving insertion of prosthetic materials, and contaminated or infected operative sites. Postoperative antimicrobials are indicated with contaminated surgeries, traumatic wounds, or ruptured viscera.

## Nursing Actions
## Antimicrobial Drugs

| Nursing Actions | Rationale/Explanation |
|---|---|
| 1. Administer accurately. | |
| a. Schedule at evenly spaced intervals around the clock. | To maintain therapeutic blood levels |
| b. Give most oral antimicrobials on an empty stomach, approximately 1 h before or 2 h after meals. | To decrease binding to foods and inactivation by gastric acid |
| c. For oral and parenteral solutions from powder forms, follow label instructions for mixing and storing. Check expiration dates. | Several antimicrobial drugs are marketed in powder forms because they are unstable in solution. When mixed, measured amounts of diluent must be added for drug dissolution and the appropriate concentration. Parenteral solutions are usually prepared in the pharmacy. Most solutions require refrigeration to prolong stability. None of the solutions should be used after the expiration date because drug decomposition is likely. |
| d. Give parenteral antimicrobial solutions alone; do not mix with any other drug in a syringe or intravenous (IV) solution. | To avoid chemical and physical incompatibilities that may cause drug precipitation or inactivation |
| e. Give intramuscular (IM) antimicrobials deeply into large muscle masses (preferably gluteal muscles), and rotate injection sites. | To decrease tissue irritation |
| f. For IV administration, use dilute solutions, give direct injections slowly and intermittent infusions over 30 to 60 min. After infusions, flush the IV tubing with at least 10 mL of IV solution. For children, check references about individual drugs to avoid excessive concentrations and excessive fluids. | Most antimicrobials that are given IV can be given by intermittent infusion. Although instructions vary with specific drugs, most reconstituted drugs can be further diluted with 50 to 100 mL of IV fluid ($D_5W$, NS, $D_5$-$\frac{1}{4}$% or $D_5$-$\frac{1}{2}$% NaCl). Dilution and slow administration minimize vascular irritation and phlebitis. Flushing ensures that the entire dose is given and prevents contact between drugs in the tubing. |
| 2. Observe for therapeutic effects. | |
| a. With local infections, observe for decreased redness, edema, heat, and pain. | Signs and symptoms of inflammation and infection usually subside within approximately 48 h after antimicrobial therapy is begun. Although systemic manifestations of infection are similar regardless of the cause, local manifestations vary with the type or location of the infection. |
| b. With systemic infections, observe for decreased fever and white blood cell count, increased appetite, and reports of feeling better. | |
| c. With wound infections, observe for decreased signs of local inflammation and decreased drainage. Drainage also may change from purulent to serous. | |
| d. With respiratory infections, observe for decreased dyspnea, coughing, and secretions. Secretions may change from thick and colored to thin and white. | |
| e. With urinary tract infections, observe for decreased urgency, frequency, and dysuria. If urinalysis is done, check the laboratory report for decreased bacteria and white blood cells. | |
| f. Absence of signs and symptoms of infection when given prophylactically. | |

*(continued)*

## Nursing Actions

### Antimicrobial Drugs (Continued)

| Nursing Actions | Rationale/Explanation |
|---|---|
| 3. Observe for adverse effects. | |
| a. Hypersensitivity | Reactions are more likely to occur in those with previous hypersensitivity reactions and those with a history of allergy, asthma, or hay fever. |
| (1) Anaphylaxis—hypotension, respiratory distress, urticaria, angioedema, vomiting, diarrhea | Hypersensitivity may occur with most antimicrobial drugs but is more common with penicillins. Anaphylaxis may occur with oral administration but is more likely with parenteral administration and may occur within 5 to 30 min of injection. Hypotension results from vasodilation and circulatory collapse. Respiratory distress results from bronchospasm or laryngeal edema. |
| (2) Serum sickness—chills, fever, vasculitis, generalized lymphadenopathy, joint edema and inflammation, bronchospasm, urticaria | This is a delayed allergic reaction, occurring 1 wk or more after the drug is started. Signs and symptoms are caused by inflammation. |
| (3) Acute interstitial nephritis (AIN), hematuria, oliguria, proteinuria, pyuria | AIN is considered a hypersensitivity reaction that may occur with many antimicrobials, including penicillins, cephalosporins, aminoglycosides, sulfonamides, tetracyclines, and others. It is usually reversible if the causative agent is promptly stopped. |
| b. Superinfection | Superinfection is a new or secondary infection that occurs during antimicrobial therapy of a primary infection. Super-infections are common and potentially serious because responsible microorganisms are often drug-resistant staphylococci, gram-negative organisms (eg, *Pseudomonas aeruginosa*), or fungi (eg, *Candida*). |
| (1) Recurrence of systemic signs and symptoms (eg, fever, malaise) | |
| (2) New localized signs and symptoms—redness, heat, edema, pain, drainage, cough | |
| (3) Stomatitis or "thrush"—sore mouth; white patches on oral mucosa; black, furry tongue | From overgrowth of fungi |
| (4) Pseudomembranous colitis—severe diarrhea characterized by blood, pus, and mucus in stools | May occur with most antibiotics, but is most often associated with ampicillin, the cephalosporins, and clindamycin. These and other antibiotics suppress normal bacterial flora and allow the overgrowth of *Clostridium difficile*. The organism produces a toxin that kills mucosal cells and produces superficial ulcerations that are visible with sigmoidoscopy. Discontinuing the drug and giving metronidazole or oral vancomycin are curative measures. However, relapses may occur. |
| (5) Monilial vaginitis—rash in perineal area, itching, vaginal discharge | From overgrowth of yeast organisms |
| c. Phlebitis at IV sites; pain at IM sites | Many antimicrobial parenteral solutions are irritating to body tissues. |
| d. Nausea and vomiting | These often occur with oral antimicrobials, probably from irritation of gastric mucosa. |
| e. Diarrhea | Commonly occurs, caused by irritation of gastrointestinal mucosa and changes in intestinal bacterial flora; and may range from mild to severe. Pseudomembranous colitis is one type of severe diarrhea. |
| f. Nephrotoxicity | |
| (1) See AIN, earlier | More likely to occur in clients who are elderly or who have impaired renal function. |

*(continued)*

## Nursing Actions
### Antimicrobial Drugs (Continued)

| Nursing Actions | Rationale/Explanation |
|---|---|
| (2) Acute tubular necrosis (ATN)—increased blood urea nitrogen and serum creatinine, decreased creatinine clearance, fluid and electrolyte imbalances | Aminoglycosides are the antimicrobial agents most often associated with ATN. |
| g. Neurotoxicity—confusion, hallucinations, neuromuscular irritability, convulsive seizures | More likely with large IV doses of penicillins or cephalosporins, especially in clients with impaired renal function. |
| h. Bleeding—hypoprothrombinemia, platelet dysfunction | Most often associated with penicillins and cephalosporins. |
| 4. Observe for drug interactions. | See following chapters. The most significant interactions are those that alter effectiveness or increase drug toxicity. |

## Critical Thinking Exercises

1. The incidence of multidrug-resistant enterococci and VRE has increased in recent years. Two major types (Van A and Van B) of VRE have been described, with different patterns of antimicrobial susceptibility. Van B is susceptible to:
   a. Teicoplanin
   b. Minocycline
   c. Ciprofloxacin
   d. Quinupristin-dalfopristin (Synercid)

2. The term antibiotic usually refers only to drugs used to treat infections caused by:
   a. Viruses and fungus
   b. Bacteria and viruses
   c. Viruses only
   d. Bacteria only

3. A client is diagnosed with an opportunistic infection. Which of the following is most likely correct?
   a. The client has acquired the infection in a health care facility
   b. The client is infected by a virulent microorganism
   c. The client has acquired the infection in the community
   d. The client's defense mechanisms are impaired

4. Which of the following terms refers to the ability of bacteria to produce disease in an individual?
   a. Latency
   b. Virulence
   c. Pathogenicity
   d. Colonization

5. When teaching a client about a prescribed antibiotic, a common instruction is to take all the medicine and not to stop prematurely. Why is this information important?
   a. An iatrogenic infection may develop
   b. Phagocytosis is enhanced
   c. The ability of the organism is reduced
   d. Risk for development of resistant organisms increases

## SELECTED REFERENCES

Abate, B. J., & Barriere, S. L. (2002). Antimicrobial regimen selection. In J. T. DiPiro, R. L. Talbert, G. C. Yee, G. R. Matzke, B. G. Wells, & L. M. Posey (Eds.), *Pharmacotherapy: A pathophysiologic approach* (5th ed., pp. 1817–1829). New York: McGraw-Hill.

Ambrose, P. G., Owens, R. C., Quintiliani, R., Yeston, N., Crowe, H. M., Cunha, B. A., et al. (1998). Antibiotic use in the critical care unit. *Critical Care Clinics, 14*(2), 283–308.

Chambers, H. F. (2001). Antimicrobial agents: General considerations. In J. G. Hardman & L. E. Limbird (Eds.), *Goodman & Gilman's the pharmacological basis of therapeutics* (10th ed., pp. 1143–1170). New York: McGraw-Hill.

*Drug facts and comparisons.* (Updated monthly). St. Louis: Facts and Comparisons.

Gill, V. J., Fedorko, D. P., and Witebsky, F. G. (2000). The clinician and the microbiology laboratory. In G. L. Mandell, J. E. Bennett, & R. Dolin (Eds.), *Principles and practice of infectious diseases* (5th ed., pp. 184–221). New York: Churchill Livingstone.

Harwell, J. L., & Brown, R. B. (2000). The drug-resistant pneumococcus: Clinical relevance, therapy, and prevention. *Chest, 117*(2), 530–541.

Lacy, C. F., Armstrong, L. L., Goldman, M. P., & Lance, L. L. (2003). *Lexi-Comp's drug information handbook* (11th ed.). Hudson, OH: American Pharmaceutical Association.

Mangram, A. J., Horan, T. C., Pearson, M. L., Silver, L. C., Jarvis, W. R., and the Hospital Infection Control Practices Advisory

Committee. (1999). Guideline for the prevention of surgical site infection. *Infection Control and Hospital Epidemiology, 20*(4), 247–278.

Moellering, R. C. (2000). Principles of anti-infective therapy. In G. L. Mandell, J. E. Bennett, & R. Dolin (Eds.), *Principles and practice of infectious diseases* (5th ed., pp. 223–233). Philadelphia: Churchill Livingstone.

Murthy, R. (2001). Hospital-acquired infections: Realities of risks and resistance. *Chest, 119*(2), 405S–411S.

Nolin, T. D., Abraham, P. A., & Matzke, G. R. (2002). Drug-induced renal disease. In J. T. DiPiro, R. L. Talbert, G. C. Yee, G. R. Matzke, B. G. Wells, & L. M. Posey (Eds.), *Pharmacotherapy: A pathophysiologic approach* (5th ed., pp. 889–909). New York: McGraw-Hill.

Rybak, M. J., & Aeschlimann, J. R. (2002). Laboratory tests to direct antimicrobial pharmacotherapy. In J. T. DiPiro, R. L. Talbert, G. C. Yee, G. R. Matzke, B. G. Wells, & L. M. Posey (Eds.), *Pharmacotherapy: A pathophysiologic approach* (5th ed., pp. 1797–1815). New York: McGraw-Hill.

Weber, D. J., Raasch, R., and Rutala, W. R. (1999). Nosocomial infections in the ICU: The growing importance of antibiotic-resistant pathogens. *Chest, 115*, 34S–41S.

# 29

# Beta-Lactam Antibacterials: Penicillins, Cephalosporins, and Others

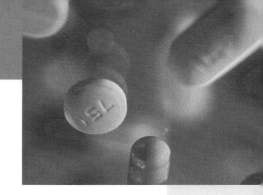

## OBJECTIVES

*After studying this chapter, the student will be able to:*

1 Describe general characteristics of beta-lactam antibiotics.

2 Discuss penicillins in relation to effectiveness, safety, spectrum of antimicrobial activity, mechanism of action, indications for use, administration, observation of client response, and teaching of clients.

3 Differentiate among extended-spectrum penicillins.

4 Question clients about allergies before the initial dose of a penicillin.

5 Describe characteristics of beta-lactamase inhibitor drugs.

6 State the rationale for combining a penicillin and a beta-lactamase inhibitor drug.

7 Discuss similarities and differences between cephalosporins and penicillins.

8 Differentiate cephalosporins in relation to antimicrobial spectrum, indications for use, and adverse effects.

9 Give major characteristics of carbapenems and monobactam drugs.

10 Apply principles of using beta-lactam antimicrobials in selected client situations.

## CRITICAL THINKING SCENARIO

*B*rad, 5 months of age, is brought to the urgent care center at 4:00 AM. He has had a cold for 3 days and started to run a high temperature (over 39°C) last evening. His parents are visibly upset and worried. He has been crying continuously for the last 8 hours and appears to be in pain. The physician examines him and tells the parents Brad has a middle ear infection, for which the doctor prescribes amoxicillin, 200 mg every 8 hours for 10 days.

✔ What factors contribute to the increased incidence of ear infections in this age group?

✔ Why is amoxicillin is a good choice for treatment (hint: think of the spectrum of coverage)?

✔ What teaching is necessary for the parents to limit the potential for antimicrobial resistance?

✔ Describe factors in the situation that may make learning difficult for the parents and how you will individualize teaching.

# OVERVIEW

Beta-lactam antibacterials, which include penicillins and cephalosporins, have been among the most effective of all antibiotics, but overuse and misuse have jeopardized their effectiveness. The penicillin structure is derived from 6-aminopenicillanic acid (6-APA); the cephalosporin ring structure is derived from 7-aminocephalosporanic acid (7-ACA). The drugs derive their name from the beta-lactam ring that is part of their chemical structure; the cephalosporin structure has different side chains that allow for variation in the spectrum of activity and duration of action. An intact beta-lactam ring is essential for antibacterial activity. Several gram-positive and gram-negative bacteria produce beta-lactamase enzymes that disrupt the beta-lactam ring and inactivate the drugs, allowing bacterial infection to develop unchecked. This is a major mechanism by which microorganisms acquire resistance to beta-lactam antibiotics. Penicillinase and cephalosporinase are beta-lactamase enzymes that act on penicillins and cephalosporins, respectively.

Despite the common element of a beta-lactam ring, characteristics of beta-lactam antibiotics differ widely because of variations in their chemical structures. The drugs may differ in antimicrobial spectrum of activity, routes of administration, susceptibility to beta-lactamase enzymes, and adverse effects. Beta-lactam antibiotics include penicillins, cephalosporins, carbapenems, and monobactams, which are described in the following sections. Pharmacokinetic characteristics of selected drugs are listed in Table 29-1, and routes and dosage ranges are listed later in the Drugs at a Glance tables. At the foundation of beta-lactam antibiotic therapy is general management of infection and characteristics of antimicrobial drugs addressed in Chapter 28.

## Mechanism of Action

Beta-lactam antibacterial drugs inhibit synthesis of bacterial cell walls by binding to proteins (penicillin-binding proteins) in bacterial cell membranes. This binding produces a defective cell wall that allows intracellular contents to leak out, destroying the microorganism. In subbactericidal concentrations, the drugs may inhibit growth, decrease viability, and alter the shape and structure of organisms. The latter characteristic may help to explain the development of mutant strains of microorganisms exposed to the drugs. Beta-lactam antibiotics are most effective when bacterial cells are dividing.

# PENICILLINS

The penicillins are effective, safe, and widely used antimicrobial agents. The group includes natural extracts from the *Penicillium* mold and several semisynthetic derivatives. When **P** penicillin G, the prototype, was introduced, it was effective against streptococci, staphylococci, gonococci, meningococci, *Treponema pallidum*, and other organisms. It had to be given parenterally because it was destroyed by gastric acid, and injections were painful. With extensive use, strains of drug-resistant staphylococci appeared. Later, penicillins were developed to increase gastric acid stability, beta-lactamase stability, and antimicrobial spectrum of activity, especially against gram-negative microorganisms. Semisynthetic derivatives are formed by adding side chains to the penicillin nucleus.

After absorption, penicillins are widely distributed and achieve therapeutic concentrations in most body fluids, including joint, pleural, and pericardial fluids and bile. Therapeutic levels are not usually obtained in intraocular fluid and cerebrospinal fluid (CSF) unless inflammation is present because normal cell membranes act as barriers to drug penetration. Penicillins are rapidly excreted by the kidneys and produce high drug concentrations in the urine (an exception is nafcillin, which is excreted by the liver).

The most serious, and potentially fatal, adverse effect of the penicillins is hypersensitivity. Seizures, interstitial nephritis, and nephropathy may also occur.

## Indications for Use

Clinical indications for use of penicillins include bacterial infections caused by susceptible microorganisms. As a class, penicillins usually are more effective in infections caused by gram-positive bacteria than those caused by gram-negative bacteria. However, their clinical uses vary significantly according to the subgroup or individual drug and microbial patterns of resistance. The drugs are often useful in skin, soft tissue, respiratory, gastrointestinal, and genitourinary infections. However, the incidence of resistance among streptococci, staphylococci, and other microorganisms continues to grow.

## Contraindications to Use

Contraindications include hypersensitivity or allergic reactions to any penicillin preparation. An allergic reaction to one penicillin means the client is allergic to all members of the penicillin class. The potential for cross-allergenicity with cephalosporins and carbapenems exists; thus, other alternatives should be selected in penicillin-allergic clients when possible.

## Management Considerations

### Drug Selection

Choice of a beta-lactam antibacterial depends on the organism causing the infection, severity of the infection, and other factors. With penicillins, penicillin G or amoxicillin is the drug of choice in many infections; an anti-

**TABLE 29-1    Pharmacokinetics of Selected Beta-Lactam Drugs**

| Group/ Drug Name | Route of Administration | Protein Binding (%) | Half-Life (Minutes) With Normal Renal Function | Main Route of Elimination | Action Onset | Peak | Duration |
|---|---|---|---|---|---|---|---|
| *Penicillins* | | | | | | | |
| Penicillin G (aqueous) | IM, IV | 60 | 30–60 | Renal | Rapid | 30 min | 4–6 h |
| Penicillin V | PO | 80 | 30–60 | Renal | Varies | 60 min | 4–6 h |
| Amoxicillin | PO | 20 | 60–90 | Renal | 30–60 min | 1–2 h | 6–8 h |
| Dicloxacillin | PO | 98 | 30–60 | Hepatic/renal | Varies | 30–60 min | 4–6 h |
| Nafcillin | PO, IM, IV | 87–90 | 60 | Hepatic/renal | PO varies | 60 min | 4 h |
| | | | | | IV immediate | 15 min | 4 h |
| Piperacillin | IM, IV | 16 | 60 | Renal | Rapid | 30–60 min | |
| Ticarcillin | IM, IV | 45 | 60 | Renal | Rapid | 30–75 min | |
| *Cephalosporins* | | | | | | | |
| Cefaclor | PO | 25 | 35–54 | Renal | | 30–60 min | 8–10 h |
| Cefazolin | IM, IV | 80–86 | 90–120 | Renal | IM 30 min | 1.5–2 h | 6–8 h |
| | | | | | IV immediate | 5 min | 6–8 h |
| Cefepime | IM, IV | 20 | 102–138 | Renal | IM 30 min | 1.5–2 h | 10–12 h |
| | | | | | IV immediate | 5 min | 10–12 h |
| Cefixime | PO | 65 | 180–240 | Renal | | 2–6 h | |
| Cefoperazone | IM, IV | 82–93 | 120 | Biliary | IM 1 h | 1–2 h | 6–12 h |
| | | | | | IV 5–10 min | 15–20 min | 6–12 h |
| Cefotetan | IM, IV | 88–90 | 180–276 | Renal | IM 30–60 min | 1.5–3 h | 18–24 h |
| | | | | | IV 15–20 min | 30 min | 18–24 h |
| Ceftazidime | IM, IV | <10 | 114–120 | Renal | IM 30 min | 1 h | 24–28 h |
| | | | | | IV rapid | 1h | 24–28 h |
| Ceftriaxone | IM, IV | 85–95 | 348–522 | Hepatic | IM 30 min | 1.5–4 h | 15–18 h |
| | | | | | IV rapid | Immediate | 15–18 h |
| Cefuroxime | PO, IM, IV | 50 | 80 | Renal | PO varies | 2 h | 18–24 h |
| | | | | | IM 20 min | 30 min | 18–24 h |
| | | | | | IV rapid | Immediate | 18–24 h |
| Cephalexin | PO | 10 | 50–80 | Renal | | 60 min | 8–10 h |
| Cephradine | PO, IM, IV | 8–17 | 48–80 | Renal | PO varies | 1 h | 6–8 h |
| | | | | | IM 20 min | 1–2 h | 6–8 h |
| | | | | | IV rapid | 5 min | 6–8 h |
| *Carbapenem* | | | | | | | |
| Imipenem-Cilastatin | IM, IV | 20/40 | 60 (for each component) | Renal | Varies | 2 h | 6–8 h |
| *Monobactam* | | | | | | | |
| Aztreonam | IM, IV | | 90–120 | Renal | IV rapid | 30 min | 6–8 h |
| | | | | | IM varies | 60–90 min | 6–8 h |

pseudomonal penicillin is indicated in most *Pseudomonas* infections; and an antistaphylococcal penicillin is indicated in staphylococcal infections. Antistaphylococcal drugs of choice are nafcillin for intravenous (IV) use and dicloxacillin for oral use.

Many beta-lactam antibiotics are given in the home setting. Guidelines for ongoing evaluation and intervention are addressed in Home Care Considerations. In addition, age-specific considerations are important in the management of individuals requiring antibiotic therapy of any kind. Discussion of the management significance of penicillins and other beta-lactam antibacterials in children and older adults is found in Age-related Considerations.

## Route of Administration and Dosage

Choice of route and dosage depends largely on the seriousness of the infection being treated. For serious infections, beta-lactam antibacterials are usually given in large IV doses. With penicillins, most must be given every 4 to 6 hours to maintain therapeutic blood levels because the

## Home Care Considerations: Use of Beta-Lactam Drugs

**ASSESS:** client for compliance with the prescribed regimen; therapeutic and adverse drug effects, especially with changes in drugs or dosages; that client is keeping appointments for serum drug levels and follow-up care.

**MONITOR:** for therapeutic and adverse effects of drugs and client's need for additional information, and provide that information.

**EDUCATE:** about importance of completion of antibiotic therapy to prevent resistant organisms; that with liquid suspensions for children, shaking to resuspend medication and measuring with a measuring spoon or calibrated device are required for safe dosing. Household spoons should *not* be used because they vary widely in capacity. General guidelines for IV therapy are discussed in Chapter 28; specific guidelines depend on the drug being given.

kidneys rapidly excrete them. The oral route is often used, especially for less serious infections and for long-term prophylaxis of rheumatic fever; the intramuscular (IM) route is rarely used in hospitalized clients but may be used in ambulatory settings.

### Guidelines Related to Hypersensitivity to Penicillins

1. Before giving the initial dose of any penicillin preparation, ask the client if he or she has ever taken penicillin, and if so, whether an allergic reaction occurred. Penicillin is the most common cause of drug-induced anaphylaxis, a life-threatening hypersensitivity reaction, and a person known to be hypersensitive should be given another type of antibiotic.

2. In the rare instance in which penicillin is considered essential, a skin test may be helpful in assessing hypersensitivity. Benzylpenicilloyl polylysine (Pre-Pen) or a dilute solution of the penicillin to be administered (10,000 units/mL) may be applied topically to a skin scratch made with a sterile needle. If the scratch test is negative (no urticaria, erythema, or pruritus), the preparation may be injected intradermally. Allergic reactions, including fatal anaphylactic shock, have occurred with skin tests and after negative skin tests. If the scratch test is positive, desensitization can be accomplished by giving gradually increasing doses of penicillin.

3. Because anaphylactic shock may occur with administration of the penicillins, especially by parenteral routes, emergency drugs and equipment must be readily available. Treatment may require parenteral epinephrine, oxygen, and insertion of an endotracheal or tracheostomy tube if laryngeal edema occurs.

## Subgroups and Individual Penicillins

Characteristics of penicillins are outlined in Drugs at a Glance 29-1: Penicillins.

### Penicillins G and V

**Penicillin G,** the prototype, remains widely used because of its effectiveness and minimal toxicity (see Prototype Profile 29-1: Penicillin G Benzathine). Many strains of staphylococci and gonococci have acquired resistance to penicillin G, preventing its use for treatment of infections caused by these organisms. Some strains of streptococci have acquired resistance to penicillin G, although the drug is still effective in many streptococcal infections. Thus, it is often the drug of choice for the treatment of streptococcal pharyngitis; for prevention of rheumatic fever, a complication of streptococcal pharyngitis; and for prevention of bacterial endocarditis in people with diseased heart valves who undergo dental or some surgical procedures.

*(text continues on page 497)*

## Age-related Considerations: Use of Beta-Lactam Antibacterials

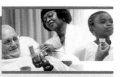

### USE IN CHILDREN

Penicillins and cephalosporins are widely used to treat infections in children and are generally safe. They should be used cautiously in neonates because immature kidney function slows their elimination. Dosages should be based on age, weight, severity of the infection being treated, and renal function. Specialized pediatric dosing references can provide guidance to dosing of most beta-lactams based on the child's age and weight.

### USE IN OLDER ADULTS

Beta-lactam antibacterials are relatively safe, although decreased renal function, other disease processes, and con-

current drug therapies increase the risks for adverse effects in older adults. With penicillins, hyperkalemia may occur with large IV doses of penicillin G potassium, and hypernatremia may occur with ticarcillin (Ticar). Hypernatremia is less likely with other antipseudomonal penicillins such as mezlocillin and piperacillin. Cephalosporins may aggravate renal impairment, especially when other nephrotoxic drugs are used concurrently. Dosage of most cephalosporins must be reduced in the presence of renal impairment, depending on creatinine clearance.

With aztreonam, imipenem-cilastatin, and meropenem, dose and frequency of administration are determined by renal status as indicated by creatinine clearance.

### CLIENT TEACHING GUIDELINES
## Oral Penicillins

### General Considerations

✔ Do not take any penicillin if you have ever had an allergic reaction to penicillin with which you had difficulty breathing, swelling, or skin rash. However, some people call a minor stomach upset an allergic reaction and are not given penicillin when that is the best antibiotic in a given situation.

✔ Complete the full course of drug treatment for greater effectiveness and prevention of secondary infection with drug-resistant bacteria.

✔ Follow instructions carefully about the dose and how often it is taken. Drug effectiveness depends on maintaining adequate blood levels.

✔ Penicillins often need more frequent administration than some other antibiotics, because they are rapidly excreted by the kidneys.

### Self-administration or Caregiver Administration

✔ Take most penicillins on an empty stomach, 1 hour before or 2 hours after a meal. Penicillin V, amoxicillin, and Augmentin can be taken without regard to meals.

✔ Take each dose with a full glass of water; do not take with orange juice or with other acidic fluids (they may destroy the drug).

✔ Take at even intervals, preferably around the clock.

✔ Shake liquid penicillins well, to mix thoroughly and measure the dose accurately.

✔ Discard liquid penicillin after 1 week if stored at room temperature or after 2 weeks if refrigerated. Liquid forms deteriorate and should not be taken after their expiration dates.

✔ Report skin rash, hives, itching, severe diarrhea, shortness of breath, fever, sore throat, black tongue, or any unusual bleeding. These symptoms may indicate a need to stop the penicillin.

---

### DRUG TABLE 29-1
## *Drugs at a Glance*
## Penicillins

| Generic/Trade Name | Routes and Dosage Ranges | Comments |
|---|---|---|
| **Penicillins G and V** | | |
| **Penicillin G potassium and sodium** (Pfizerpen) Pregnancy Category B | *Adults:* IM, 300,000–8 million U daily IV, 6–20 million U daily by continuous or intermittent infusion q2–4h. Up to 60 million U daily have been given in certain serious infections. *Children:* IM, IV, 50,000–300,000 U/kg/d in divided doses q4h | Modify dose in renal insufficiency; reconstituted solution stable for 7 days when refrigerated |
| **Penicillin G benzathine** (Bicillin) Pregnancy Category B | See Prototype Profile 29-1: Penicillin G Benzathine | |
| **Penicillin G procaine** (Wycillin) Pregnancy Category B | *Adults:* IM, 600,000–2.4 million U daily in one or two doses *Children:* IM, 300,000 U/day in divided doses q12h | Do not inject into gluteal muscle in children < 2 yr |
| **Penicillin V** (Veetids) Pregnancy Category B | *Adults:* PO, 125–500 mg q4–6h *Children:* Same as adults *Infants:* PO, 15–50 mg/kg/d in 3–6 divided doses | Administer around-the-clock to minimize variation in peak and trough serum levels |

*(continued)*

**DRUG TABLE 29-1**

*Drugs at a Glance*

## Penicillins (Continued)

| Generic/Trade Name | Routes and Dosage Ranges | Comments |
|---|---|---|
| **Penicillinase-Resistant (Antistaphylococcal) Penicillins** | | |
| **Dicloxacillin** Pregnancy Category B | *Adults:* PO, 250 mg q6h *Children:* Weight ≥ 40 kg: Same as adults Weight < 40 kg: 25 mg/kg/d in four divided doses q6h | Administer around-the-clock |
| **Nafcillin** Pregnancy Category B | *Adults:* IM, 500 mg q4–6h IV, 500 mg–2 g in 15–30 mL sodium chloride injection, infused over 5–10 min, q4h; maximal daily dose, 18 g for serious infections *Children:* IM, IV, 50–200 mg/kg/d in four to six divided doses q4–6h | Not dialyzable by hemodialysis |
| **Oxacillin** Pregnancy Category B | *Adults:* PO, IM, IV 500 mg–1 g q4–6h. For direct IV injection, the dose should be well diluted and given over 10–15 min. *Children:* Weight > 40 kg: Same as adults Weight ≤ 40 kg: PO, IM, IV 50–100 mg/kg/d in four divided doses q6h | Administer around-the-clock |
| ***Ampicillins*** | | |
| **Ampicillin** (Principen) Pregnancy Category B | *Adults:* PO, IM, IV 250–500 mg q6h. In severe infections, doses up to 2 g q4h may be given IV. *Children:* Weight > 20 kg: Same as adults Weight ≤ 20 kg: PO, IM, IV 50–200 mg/kg/d in divided doses q6h | To increase absorption, administer on an empty stomach |
| **Amoxicillin** (Amoxil) Pregnancy Category B | *Adults:* PO, 250–500 mg q8h *Children:* Weight > 20 kg: Same as adults Weight ≤ 20 kg: 20–40 mg/kg/d in divided doses q8h | May be taken with food |
| **Extended-Spectrum (Antipseudomonal) Penicillins** | | |
| **Carbenicillin indanyl sodium** (Geocillin) Pregnancy Category B | *Adults:* PO, 382–764 mg four times daily *Children:* PO, 30–50 mg/kg/d in divided doses q6h | Administer around-the-clock Tablets have bitter taste; take on empty stomach with full glass of water (sodium content: 382 mg tablet has 23 mg [1mEq]) |
| **Ticarcillin** (Ticar) Pregnancy Category B | *Adults:* IM, IV, 1–3 g q6h. IM injections should not exceed 2 g/injection. *Children:* Weight < 40 kg: 100–300 mg/kg/d q6–8h | Obtain culture and sensitivity samples before administering first dose, if possible |
| **Piperacillin** (Pipracil) Pregnancy Category B | *Adults:* IV, IM, 200–300 mg/kg/d in divided doses q4–6h. Usual adult dosage, 3–4 g q4–6h; maximal daily dose, 24 g *Children:* Age < 12 y: Dosage not established | Dosage adjustment required in renal insufficiency |
| **Penicillin/Beta-Lactamase Inhibitor Combinations** | | |
| **Ampicillin/sulbactam** (Unasyn) Pregnancy Category B | *Adults:* IM, IV, 1.5–3 g q6h *Children:* Weight ≥ 40 kg: same as adults Weight < 40 kg: 300 mg/kg/d in divided doses q6h | Each 3g vial contains ampicillin, 2 g, and sulbactam, 1g |

*(continued)*

**DRUG TABLE 29-1**

## Drugs at a Glance

## Penicillins (Continued)

| Generic/Trade Name | Routes and Dosage Ranges | Comments |
|---|---|---|
| **Amoxicillin clavulanate** (Augmentin) Pregnancy Category B | *Adults:* PO, 250–500 mg q8h or 875 mg q12h *Children:* Weight < 40 kg: 20–40 mg/ kg/d in divided doses q8h Weight ≥ 40 kg: same as adults | Product-specific considerations available through pharmacist |
| **Piperacillin-tazobactam** (Zosyn) Pregnancy Category B | *Adults:* IV, 2.25–4.5 g q6–8h *Children:* IV, 100–300 mg/kg/d in divided doses q4–6h | Vials have an 8:1 ratio of piperacillin sodium to tazobactam sodium; sodium content: piperacillin sodium 2 g and tazobactam sodium 0.25 g |
| **Ticarcillin-clavulanate** (Timentin) Pregnancy Category B | *Adults:* IV, 3.1 g q4-6h *Children:* Weight < 60 kg: 200–300 mg/ kg/d in divided doses q4–6h | Obtain culture and sensitivity samples before administering first dose, if possible |

## PROTOTYPE PROFILE 29-1

### P Penicillin G (pen I SIL in jee) Benzathine

**Drug Class**
*Chemical:* Beta-lactam antibiotic
*Functional:* Antibiotic, penicillin

**Trade Names**
Bicillin LA, Isoject, Permapen

**Therapeutic Indications**
For treatment of streptococcal pharyngitis; for prevention of rheumatic fever; for prevention of bacterial endocarditis in people with diseased heart valves who undergo dental or surgical procedures; and for treatment of syphilis

**Pharmacokinetics**
*Absorption*
Slow

*Distribution*
Plasma protein binding: 60%

*Metabolism*
Excreted largely unchanged

*Excretion*
Urine

**Pharmacodynamics**
*Onset of Action*
Rapid

*Duration*
1–4 wk

**Contraindications/Precautions**
Hypersensitivity to penicillin, use with caution in impaired renal function or seizure disorder

**Pregnancy Considerations**
Category B
Enters breast milk; compatible

**Dosage**
*Adults:* Group A strep: URI: IM, 25,000 to 50,000 mcg/kg as a single dose; maximum, 1.2 million units
Rheumatic fever prophylaxis: 25,000 to 50,000 mcg/kg every 3–4 wk; maximum, 1.2 million units/dose
Early syphilis: 50,000 mcg/kg as a single dose; divided into two injection sites
Syphilis >1 y duration: 2.4 million units divided into two injection sites weekly for three doses
*Children:* Group A strep: URI: 25,000 to 50,000 mcg/kg as a single dose; maximum, 1.2 million units
Rheumatic fever prophylaxis: 25,000–50,000 mcg/kg every 3–4 wk; maximum 1.2 million units/dose
Early syphilis: 50,000 mcg/kg as a single dose; divided into two injection sites
Syphilis >1 y duration: 50,000 mcg/kg every 3–4 wk; maximum, 2.4 million units/dose

**Adverse Effects**
Convulsions, confusion, electrolyte imbalance, hemolytic anemia, anaphylaxis

**Drug Interactions**
*Increased Effects*
Penicillin levels with probenecid
Synergistic activity with aminoglycosides

*Decreased Effects*
Penicillin effectiveness with tetracycline

**Herbal Supplements and Dietary Considerations**
None noted

Several preparations of penicillin G are available for IV and IM administration. They cannot be used interchangeably. Only aqueous preparations can be given intravenously. Preparations containing benzathine or procaine can be given only intramuscularly. Long-acting repository forms have additives that decrease their solubility in tissue fluids and delay their absorption.

**Penicillin V** is derived from penicillin G and has the same antibacterial spectrum. It is not destroyed by gastric acid and is given only by the oral route. It is well absorbed and produces therapeutic blood levels.

### Penicillinase-resistant (Antistaphylococcal) Penicillins

This group includes four drugs (**cloxacillin, dicloxacillin, nafcillin,** and **oxacillin**) that are effective in some infections caused by staphylococci resistant to penicillin G. An older member of this group, methicillin, is no longer marketed for clinical use. However, susceptibility of bacteria to the antistaphylococcal penicillins is determined by exposing the bacteria to methicillin (methicillin susceptible or resistant) or oxacillin (oxacillin susceptible or resistant) in bacteriology laboratories.

These drugs are formulated to resist the penicillinases that inactivate other penicillins. They are recommended for use in known or suspected staphylococcal infections, except for methicillin-resistant *Staphylococcus aureus* (MRSA) infections. Although called methicillin resistant, these staphylococcal microorganisms are also resistant to other antistaphylococcal penicillins.

### Aminopenicillins

**Ampicillin** is a broad-spectrum, semisynthetic penicillin that is bactericidal for several types of gram-positive and gram-negative bacteria. It has been effective against enterococci, *Proteus mirabilis, Salmonella, Shigella,* and *Escherichia coli,* but resistant forms of these organisms are increasing. It is ineffective against penicillinase-producing staphylococci and gonococci.

Ampicillin is excreted mainly by the kidneys; thus, it is useful in urinary tract infections (UTIs). Because some is excreted in bile, it is useful in biliary tract infections not caused by biliary obstruction. It is used in the treatment of bronchitis, sinusitis, and otitis media.

**Amoxicillin** is similar to ampicillin except it is only available orally. It is better absorbed and produces therapeutic blood levels more rapidly than oral ampicillin. It also causes less gastrointestinal distress.

### Extended-Spectrum (Antipseudomonal) Penicillins

The drugs in this group (**carbenicillin, ticarcillin, mezlocillin,** and **piperacillin**) have a broad spectrum of antimicrobial activity, especially against gram-negative organisms such as *Pseudomonas* and *Proteus* species and *E. coli.* For pseudomonal infections, one of these drugs is usually given concomitantly with an aminoglycoside or a fluoroquinolone (see Chap. 30). Carbenicillin is available as an oral formulation for UTI or prostatitis caused by susceptible pathogens. The other drugs are usually given by intermittent IV infusion, although most can be given intramuscularly.

### Penicillin and Beta-Lactamase Inhibitor Combinations

To overcome bacterial resistance to beta-lactams, current drugs combine a beta-lactam antibiotic and a beta-lactamase inhibitor. Beta-lactamase inhibitors are proteins designed to inhibit or destroy the effectiveness of beta-lactamase enzymes. Inhibitors generally have little antibacterial activity themselves and so are combined with a beta-lactam antibiotic. These inhibitors function by binding and inactivating the beta-lactamase enzymes produced by many bacteria (eg, *E. coli, Klebsiella, Enterobacter,* and *Bacteroides* species, and *S. aureus*). When combined with a penicillin, the beta-lactamase inhibitor protects the penicillin from destruction by the enzymes and extends the penicillin's spectrum of antimicrobial activity. Thus, the combination drug may be effective in infections caused by bacteria that are resistant to a beta-lactam antibiotic alone. Clavulanate, sulbactam, and tazobactam are the beta-lactamase inhibitors available in combinations with penicillins.

**Unasyn** is a combination of ampicillin and sulbactam available in vials with 1 g of ampicillin and 0.5 g of sulbactam or 2 g of ampicillin and 1 g of sulbactam. **Augmentin** contains amoxicillin and clavulanate. It is available in 250-, 500-, and 875-mg tablets, each of which contains 125 mg of clavulanate. Thus, two 250-mg tablets are not equivalent to one 500-mg tablet. **Timentin** is a combination of ticarcillin and clavulanate in an IV formulation containing 3 g ticarcillin and 100 mg clavulanate. **Zosyn** is a combination of piperacillin and tazobactam in an IV formulation. Three dosage strengths are available, with 2 g piperacillin and 0.25 g tazobactam, 3 g piperacillin and 0.375 g tazobactam, or 4 g piperacillin and 0.5 g tazobactam.

## ◼ CEPHALOSPORINS

Cephalosporins are a widely used group of drugs that are derived from a fungus. Although technically cefoxitin and cefotetan (cephamycins derived from a different fungus) and loracarbef (a carbacephem) are not cephalosporins, they are categorized with the cephalosporins because of their similarities to the group. Cephalosporins are broad-spectrum agents with activity against both gram-positive and gram-negative bacteria. Compared with penicillins, they are less active against gram-positive organisms but more active against gram-negative ones.

Once absorbed, cephalosporins are widely distributed into most body fluids and tissues, with maximum concentrations in the liver and kidneys. Many cephalosporins do not reach therapeutic levels in CSF; exceptions are cefuroxime, a second-generation drug, and the third-generation agents. These drugs reach therapeutic levels when meninges are inflamed. Most cephalosporins are excreted through the kidneys. Exceptions include cefoperazone, which is excreted in bile, and ceftriaxone, which undergoes dual elimination through the biliary tract and kidneys. Cefotaxime is primarily metabolized in the liver to an active metabolite, desacetyl cefotaxime, which is eliminated by the kidneys.

## First-Generation Cephalosporins

The first cephalosporin, cephalothin, is no longer available for clinical use. However, it is used for determining susceptibility to first-generation cephalosporins, which have essentially the same spectrum of antimicrobial activity. They are effective against streptococci, staphylococci (except MRSA), *Neisseria, Salmonella, Shigella, Escherichia, Klebsiella,* and *Bacillus* species, *Corynebacterium diphtheriae, Proteus mirabilis,* and *Bacteroides* species (except *Bacteroides fragilis*). They are not effective against *Enterobacter, Pseudomonas,* and *Serratia* species.

## Second-Generation Cephalosporins

Second-generation cephalosporins are more active against some gram-negative organisms than the first-generation drugs. Thus, they may be effective in infections resistant to other antibiotics, including infections caused by *Haemophilus influenzae, Klebsiella* species, *E. coli,* and some strains of *Proteus.* Because each of these drugs has a different antimicrobial spectrum, susceptibility tests must be performed for each drug rather than for the entire group, as may be done with first-generation drugs. Cefoxitin (Mefoxin), for example, is active against *B. fragilis,* an anaerobic organism resistant to most drugs.

## Third-Generation Cephalosporins

Third-generation cephalosporins further extend the spectrum of activity against gram-negative organisms. In addition to activity against the usual enteric pathogens (eg, *E. coli, Proteus* and *Klebsiella* species), they are also active against several strains resistant to other antibiotics and to first- and second-generation cephalosporins. Thus, they may be useful in infections caused by unusual strains of enteric organisms such as *Citrobacter, Serratia,* and *Providencia.* Another difference is that third-generation cephalosporins penetrate inflamed meninges to reach therapeutic concentrations in CSF. Thus, they may be useful in meningeal infections caused by common pathogens, including *H. influenzae, Neisseria meningitidis,* and *Streptococcus pneumoniae.* Although some of the drugs are active against *Pseudomonas* organisms, drug-resistant strains may emerge when a cephalosporin is used alone for treatment of pseudomonal infection.

Overall, cephalosporins gain gram-negative activity and lose gram-positive activity as they move from the first to the third generation. The second- and third-generation drugs are more active against gram-negative organisms because they are more resistant to the beta-lactamase enzymes (cephalosporinases) produced by some bacteria to inactivate cephalosporins.

## Fourth-Generation Cephalosporins

Fourth-generation cephalosporins have a greater spectrum of antimicrobial activity and greater stability against breakdown by beta-lactamase enzymes compared with third-generation drugs. Cefepime is the first fourth-generation cephalosporin to be developed. It is active against both gram-positive and gram-negative organisms. With gram-positive organisms, it is active against streptococci and staphylococci (except for methicillin-resistant staphylococci). With gram-negative organisms, its activity against *Pseudomonas aeruginosa* is similar to that of ceftazidime, and its activity against Enterobacteriaceae is greater than that of third-generation cephalosporins. Moreover, cefepime retains activity against strains of Enterobacteriaceae and *P. aeruginosa* that have acquired resistance to third-generation agents.

## Indications for Use

Clinical indications for the use of cephalosporins include surgical prophylaxis and treatment of infections of the respiratory tract, skin and soft tissues, bones and joints, urinary tract, brain and spinal cord, and bloodstream (septicemia). In most infections with streptococci and staphylococci, penicillins are more effective and less expensive. In infections caused by MRSA, cephalosporins are not clinically effective even if *in vitro* testing indicates susceptibility. Infections caused by *Neisseria gonorrhoeae,* once susceptible to penicillin, are now preferentially treated with a third-generation cephalosporin such as ceftriaxone. Cefepime is indicated for use in severe infections of the lower respiratory and urinary tracts, skin and soft tissue, and female reproductive tract, as well as in febrile neutropenic clients. It may be used as monotherapy for all infections caused by susceptible organisms except *P. aeruginosa;* a combination of drugs should be used for serious pseudomonal infections.

## Contraindications to Use

A major contraindication to the use of a cephalosporin is a previous severe anaphylactic reaction to a penicillin. Because cephalosporins are chemically similar to penicillins, there is a risk for cross-sensitivity. However, incidence of cross-sensitivity is low, especially in clients who have had delayed reactions (eg, skin rash) to penicillins. Another contraindication is cephalosporin allergy. Immediate allergic reactions with anaphylaxis, bronchospasm, and urticaria occur less often than delayed reactions with skin rash, drug fever, and eosinophilia.

## Management Considerations

### Drug Selection

With cephalosporins, *first-generation* drugs are often used for surgical prophylaxis, especially with prosthetic implants, because gram-positive organisms such as staphylococci cause most postimplant infections. They may also be used alone for treatment of infections caused by susceptible organisms in body sites where drug penetration and host defenses are adequate. Cefazolin (Kefzol) is a frequently used parenteral agent. It reaches a higher serum concentration, is more protein bound, and has a slower rate of elimination than other first-generation drugs. These factors prolong serum half-life, so that cefazolin can be given less frequently. Cefazolin may also be administered intramuscularly.

*Second-generation* cephalosporins are also often used for surgical prophylaxis, especially for gynecologic and colorectal surgery. They are also used for treatment of intraabdominal infections such as pelvic inflammatory disease, diverticulitis, penetrating wounds of the abdomen, and other infections caused by organisms inhabiting pelvic and colorectal areas.

*Third-generation* cephalosporins are recommended for serious infections caused by susceptible organisms that are resistant to first- and second-generation cephalosporins. They are often used in the treatment of infections caused by *E. coli*, *Proteus*, *Klebsiella*, and *Serratia* species, and other Enterobacteriaceae, especially when the infections occur in body sites not readily reached by other drugs (eg, CSF, bone) and in clients with immunosuppression. Although effective against many *Pseudomonas* strains, these drugs should not be used alone in treating pseudomonal infections because drug resistance develops.

*Fourth-generation* drugs are most useful in serious gram-negative infections, especially infections caused by organisms resistant to third-generation drugs. Cefepime has the same indications for use as ceftazidime, a third-generation drug.

### Route of Administration

With cephalosporins, a few are sufficiently absorbed for oral administration; these are most often used in mild infections and UTI. Although some cephalosporins can be given intramuscularly, the injections cause pain and induration. Cefazolin is preferred for IM administration because it is less irritating to tissues (see Drugs at a Glance 29-2: Oral Cephalosporins and Drugs at a Glance 29-3: Parenteral Cephalosporins for characteristics of specific drugs).

## ■ CARBAPENEMS

Carbapenems are broad-spectrum, bactericidal, beta-lactam antimicrobials. Like other beta-lactam drugs, they inhibit synthesis of bacterial cell walls by binding with

*(text continues on page 502)*

---

**DRUG TABLE 29-2**

## *Drugs at a Glance*
## Oral Cephalosporins

| Generic/Trade Name | Routes and Dosage Ranges | Comments/Uses |
|---|---|---|
| ***First Generation*** | | |
| **Cefadroxil** (Duricef, Ultracef) Pregnancy Category B | *Adults:* PO, 1–2 g twice daily *Children:* 30 mg/kg/d in two doses q12h | A derivative of cephalexin that has a longer half-life and can be given less often |
| **Cephalexin** (Keflex) Pregnancy Category B | *Adults:* PO, 250–500 mg q6h, increased to 4 g q6h if necessary in severe infections *Children:* PO, 25–50 mg/kg/d in divided doses q6h | First oral cephalosporin; still used extensively |
| **Cephradine** (Anspor, Velosef) Pregnancy Category B | *Adults:* PO, 250–500 mg q6h, up to 4 g daily in severe infections *Children:* PO, 25–50 mg/kg/d in divided doses q6h. In severe infections, up to 100 mg/kg/d may be given. | Essentially the same as cephalexin, except it also can be given parenterally |
| ***Second Generation*** | | |
| **Cefaclor** (Ceclor) Pregnancy Category B | *Adults:* PO, 250–500 mg q8h *Children:* PO, 20–40 mg/kg/d in three divided doses q8h | More active against *H. influenzae* and *E. coli* than first-generation drugs |

*(continued)*

## DRUG TABLE 29-2

### *Drugs at a Glance*

### Oral Cephalosporins (Continued)

| Generic/Trade Name | Routes and Dosage Ranges | Comments/Uses |
|---|---|---|
| **Cefprozil** (Cefzil) Pregnancy Category B | *Adults:* PO, 250–500 mg q12–24h *Children:* PO, 15 mg/kg q12h | Similar to cefaclor |
| **Cefuroxime** (Ceftin) Pregnancy Category B | *Adults:* PO, 250 mg q12h; severe infections, 500 mg q12h; urinary tract infection, 125 mg q12h *Children:* >12 y, same as adults; <12 y, 125 mg q12h Otitis media, >2 y, 250 mg q12h, <2 y, 125 mg q12h | 1. Can also be given parenterally 2. Available only in tablet form 3. The tablet may be crushed and added to a food (eg, applesauce), but the crushed tablet leaves a strong, bitter, persistent aftertaste. |
| **Loracarbef** (Lorabid) Pregnancy Category B | *Adults:* PO, 200–400 mg q12h *Children:* PO, 15–30 mg/kg/d in divided doses q12h | A synthetic drug similar to cefaclor |
| ***Third Generation*** | | |
| **Cefdinir** (Omnicef) Pregnancy Category B | *Adults:* PO, 300 mg q12h or 600 mg q24h for 10 d *Children:* ≥13 y: PO Same as adults 6 mo–12 y: PO 7 mg/kg q12h or 14 mg/kg q24h for 10 d | Indicated for bronchitis, pharyngitis, and otitis media caused by streptococci or *H. influenzae* |
| **Cefditoren pivoxil** (Spectracef) Pregnancy Category B | *Adults:* Bronchitis or pharyngitis, PO, 400 mg twice daily (q12h) for 10 days Skin infections, PO 200 mg twice daily for 10 days Renal impairment: CrCl 30–49 mL/min, PO 200 mg twice daily CrCl <30 mL/min, PO 200 mg once daily *Children:* ≥12 y: Same as adults | Indicated for pharyngitis, bacterial exacerbations of chronic bronchitis, and skin/skin structure infections |
| **Cefixime** (Suprax) Pregnancy Category B | *Adults:* PO, 200 mg q12h or 400 mg q24h *Children:* PO, 4 mg/kg q12h or 8 mg/kg q24h; give adult dose to children 50 kg of weight or ≥12 y | First oral third-generation drug |
| **Cefpodoxime** (Vantin) Pregnancy Category B | *Adults:* PO, 200–400 mg q12h *Children:* PO, 5 mg/kg q12h Give 10 mg/kg (400 mg or adult dose) to children ≥13 y with skin and soft-tissue infections | Similar to cefixime except has some activity against staphylococci (except methicillin-resistant *S. aureus*) |
| **Ceftibuten** (Cedax) Pregnancy Category B | *Adults:* PO, 400 mg daily for 10 d Renal impairment: CrCl 30–49 mL/min, 200 mg q24h CrCl 5–29 mL/min, 100 mg q24h *Children:* Oral suspension with 90 mg/5 mL *10 kg:* 5 mL daily *20 kg:* 10 mL daily *40 kg:* 20 mL daily *Above 45 kg:* Same as adults Oral suspension with 180 mg/5 mL *10 kg:* 2.5 mL daily *20 kg:* 5 mL daily *40 kg:* 10 mL daily *Above 45 kg:* Same as adults | 1. Indicated for bronchitis, otitis media, pharyngitis, or tonsillitis caused by streptococci or *H. Influenzae.* 2. Can be given once daily 3. Available in a capsule for oral use and an oral pediatric suspension that comes in two concentrations (90 mg/5 mL and 180 mg/5 mL). |

| DRUG TABLE 29-3 | Drugs at a Glance |
|---|---|

## Parenteral Cephalosporins

| Generic/Trade Name | Routes and Dosage Ranges | Comments/Uses |
|---|---|---|
| **First Generation** | | |
| **Cefazolin** (Kefzol, Ancef) Pregnancy Category B | *Adults:* IM, IV, 250 mg–1 g q6–8h *Children:* IM, IV, 50–100 mg/kg/d in 3–4 divided doses | Active against streptococci, staphylococci, *Neisseria, Salmonella, Shigella, Escherichia, Klebsiella, Listeria, Bacillus, Hemophilus influenzae, Corynebacterium diphtheriae, Proteus mirabilis,* and *Bacteroides* (except *B. fragilis*) |
| **Cephapirin** (Cefadyl) Pregnancy Category B | *Adults:* IV, IM, 500 mg–1 g q4–6h, up to 12 g daily, IV, in serious infections *Children:* IV, IM, 40–80 mg/kg/d in 4 divided doses (q6h) | No significant differences from cefazolin |
| **Cephradine** (Anspor, Velosef) Pregnancy Category B | *Adults:* IV, IM, 500 mg–1 g 2–4 times daily, depending on severity of infection *Children:* IV, IM, 75–125 mg/kg/d in divided doses q6h | No significant differences from cefazolin except it also can be given orally |
| **Second Generation** | | |
| **Cefotetan** (Cefotan) Pregnancy Category B | *Adults:* IV, IM, 1–2 g q12h for 5–10 d; maximum dose, 3 g q12h in life-threatening infections Perioperative prophylaxis, IV 1–2 g 30–60 min before surgery | 1. Effective against most organisms except *Pseudomonas* 2. Highly resistant to beta-lactamase enzymes |
| **Cefoxitin** (Mefoxin) Pregnancy Category B | *Adults:* IV, 1–2 g q4–6h Surgical prophylaxis, IV 1 or 2 g 30–90 min before surgery *Children:* IV, 80–160 mg/kg/d in divided doses q4–6h. Do not exceed 12 g/d. | 1. The first cephamycin (derived from a different fungus than cephalosporins) 2. A major clinical use may stem from increased activity against *B. fragilis,* an organism resistant to most other antimicrobial drugs. |
| **Cefuroxime** (Ceftin, Kefurox, Zinacef) Pregnancy Category B | *Adults:* IV, IM, 750 mg–1.5 g q8h Surgical prophylaxis, IV 1.5 g 30–60 min before initial skin incision *Children:* >3 mo: IV, IM, 50–100 mg/kg/d in divided doses q6–8h Bacterial meningitis, IV 200–240 mg/kg/d in divided doses q6–8h, reduced to 100 mg/kg/d on clinical improvement | 1. Similar to other second-generation cephalosporins 2. Penetrates cerebrospinal fluid in presence of inflamed meninges |
| **Third Generation** | | |
| **Cefoperazone** (Cefobid) Pregnancy Category B | *Adults:* IV, IM, 2–4 g/d in divided doses q8–12h *Children:* Dosage not established | 1. Active against gram-negative and gram-positive organisms, including gram-negative organisms resistant to earlier cephalosporins 2. Excreted primarily in bile; half-life prolonged in hepatic failure |
| **Cefotaxime** (Claforan) Pregnancy Category B | *Adults:* IV, IM, 1 g q6–8h; maximum dose, 12 g/24h *Children:* Weight > 50 kg: same as adults Weight < 50 kg and age > 1 mo: IV, IM 50–180 mg/kg/d, in divided doses q4–6h Neonates: ≤1 wk, IV 50 mg/kg q12h; 1–4 wk, IV 50 mg/kg q8h | 1. Antibacterial activity against most gram-positive and gram-negative bacteria, including several strains resistant to other antibiotics. 2. Recommended for serious infections caused by susceptible microorganisms |

*(continued)*

**DRUG TABLE 29-3**

*Drugs at a Glance*

**Parenteral Cephalosporins** (Continued)

| Generic/Trade Name | Routes and Dosage Ranges | Comments/Uses |
|---|---|---|
| **Ceftazidime** (Fortaz) Pregnancy Category B | *Adults:* IV, IM, 1 g q8–12h *Children:* 1 mo to 12 y: IV 30–50 mg/kg q8h, not to exceed 6 g/d <1 mo: IV 30 mg/kg q12h | 1. Active against gram-positive and gram-negative organisms 2. Especially effective against gram-negative organisms, including *P. aeruginosa* and other bacterial strains resistant to aminoglycosides 3. Indicated for serious infections caused by susceptible organisms |
| **Ceftizoxime** (Cefizox) Pregnancy Category B | *Adults:* IV, IM, 1–2 g q8–12h *Children:* >6 mo: IV, IM 50 mg/kg q6–8h, increased to a total daily dose of 200 mg/kg if necessary | 1. Broader gram-negative and anaerobic activity, especially against *B. fragilis* 2. More active against Enterobacteriaceae than cefoperazone 3. Dosage must be reduced with even mild renal insufficiency (CrCl < 80 mL/min) |
| **Ceftriaxone** (Rocephin) Pregnancy Category B | *Adults:* IV, IM, 1–2 g once daily (q24h) *Children:* IV, IM, 50–75 mg/kg/d, not to exceed 2 g daily, in divided doses q12h Meningitis, IV, IM 100 mg/kg/d, not to exceed 4 g daily, in divided doses q12h | 1. First third-generation cephalosporin approved for once-daily dosing 2. Antibacterial activity against most gram-positive and gram-negative bacteria, including several strains resistant to other antibiotics |
| ***Fourth Generation*** | | |
| **Cefepime** (Maxipime) Pregnancy Category B | *Adults:* IV, 0.5–2 g q12h IM, 0.5–1 g q12h Renal impairment: CrCl 30–60 mL/min, 0.5–2 g q24h; CrCl 11–29 mL/min, 0.5–1 g q24h; CrCl ≤ 10 mL/min, 250–500 mg q24h *Children:* ≤ 40 kg: 50–150 mg/kg/d in 2–3 divided doses not to exceed recommended adult dose | 1. Indicated for urinary tract infections caused by *Escherichia coli* or *Klebsiella pneumoniae*; skin and soft tissue infections caused by susceptible streptococci or staphylococci; pneumonia caused by *Streptococcus pneumoniae* or *Pseudomonas aeruginosa*; complicated intra-abdominal infection and empiric therapy of febrile, neutropenic clients 2. Dosage must be reduced with renal impairment. |

CrCl, creatinine clearance

penicillin-binding proteins. Drugs at a Glance 29-4: Carbapenems and Monobactams describes specific drugs. The group consists of three drugs.

**Imipenem-cilastatin** (Primaxin) is given parenterally and distributed in most body fluids. Imipenem is rapidly broken down by an enzyme (dehydropeptidase) in renal tubules and therefore reaches only low concentrations in urine. Cilastatin was synthesized to inhibit the enzyme and reduce potential renal toxicity of the antibacterial agent. Recommended doses indicate the amount of imipenem; the solution contains an equivalent amount of cilastatin.

The drug is effective in infections caused by a wide range of bacteria, including penicillinase-producing staphylococci, *E. coli*, *Proteus*, *Enterobacter*, *Klebsiella*, and *Serratia* species, *P. aeruginosa*, and *Enterococcus faecalis*. Its main indication for use is treatment of infections caused by

organisms resistant to other drugs. Adverse effects are similar to those of other beta-lactam antibiotics, including the risk for cross-sensitivity in clients with penicillin hypersensitivity. Central nervous system toxicity, including seizures, has been reported. Seizures are more likely in clients with a seizure disorder or when recommended doses are exceeded; however, they have occurred in other clients as well. To prepare the solution for IM injection, lidocaine, a local anesthetic, is added to decrease pain. This solution is contraindicated in people allergic to this type of local anesthetic and in those who have severe shock or heart block.

**Meropenem** (Merrem) has a broad spectrum of antibacterial activity and may be used as a single drug for empiric therapy before causative microorganisms are identified. It is effective against penicillin-susceptible staphy-

## CLIENT TEACHING GUIDELINES
## Oral Cephalosporins

### General Considerations

✔ Inform your physician if you have ever had a severe allergic reaction to penicillin in which you had difficulty breathing, swelling, or skin rash. A small number of people are allergic to both penicillins and cephalosporins because the drugs are somewhat similar in their chemical structures.

✔ Also inform your physician if you have had a previous allergic reaction to a cephalosporin (eg, Ceclor, Keflex). If not sure whether a new prescription is a cephalosporin, ask the pharmacist before having the prescription filled.

✔ Complete the full course of drug treatment for greater effectiveness and prevention of secondary infection with drug-resistant bacteria.

✔ Follow instructions about dosing frequency; effectiveness depends on maintaining adequate blood levels.

### Self-administration or Caregiver Administration

✔ Take most oral drugs with food or milk to prevent stomach upset.

✔ Take cefpodoxime (Vantin) and cefuroxime (Ceftin, Kefurox, Zinacef) with food to increase absorption.

✔ Do not take cefditoren (Spectracef) with antacids containing aluminum or magnesium (eg, Maalox, Mylanta) or Pepcid, Tagamet, or Zantac. These drugs decrease absorption of Spectracef and make it less effective. If necessary to take one of the drugs, take it 2 hours before or 2 hours after a dose of Spectracef.

✔ Shake liquid preparations well to mix thoroughly and measure the dose accurately.

✔ Report the occurrence of diarrhea, especially if it is severe or contains blood, pus, or mucus. Cephalosporins can cause antibiotic-associated colitis and the drug may need to be stopped.

✔ Inform the prescribing physician if you are breast-feeding. These drugs enter breast milk.

**DRUG TABLE 29-4**

### *Drugs at a Glance*
### Carbapenems and Monobactams

| Generic/Trade Name | Routes and Dosage Ranges | Comments/Uses |
|---|---|---|
| **Carbapenems** | | |
| **Ertapenem** (Invanz) Pregnancy Category B | *Adults:* IM, 1 g once daily IV 1 g once daily over 15 to 30 min *Children:* Dosage not established | Lidocaine added to reduce pain with IM administration; do not use lidocaine with epinephrine; assess for allergy to drug; do not use with diluents containing dextrose |
| **Imipenem-cilastatin** (Primaxin) Pregnancy Category C | *Adults:* IV, 250–1000 mg q6–8h Maximum dose, 4 g/d IM, 500–750 mg q12h *Children:* >40 kg weight, same as adults <40 kg weight: IV, up to 10 mg/kg/d in divided doses. Maximum dose, 2 g/d | Lidocaine added to reduce pain with IM administration; do not use lidocaine with epinephrine; assess for allergy to drug |
| **Meropenem** (Merrem) Pregnancy Category B | *Adults:* IV, 1 g q8h, as a bolus injection over 3–5 min or infusion over 15–30 min *Children:* 3 mo and older: IV, 20–40 mg/ kg q8h | Potentially subtherapeutic serum levels of valproic acid may be reported with meropenem therapy |
| **Monobactam** | | |
| **Aztreonam** (Azactam) Pregnancy Category B | *Adults:* UTI, IM, IV 0.5–1.0 g q8–12h Moderate systemic infection, 1–2 g q8–12h Severe systemic infection, 2 g q6–8h *Children:* IM, IV, 30 mg/kg q6–8h | Drug has nearly pure gram-negative aerobic activity; should not be used for gram-positive infections |

UTI, urinary tract infection

lococci and *S. pneumoniae*, most gram-negative aerobes (eg, *E. coli*, *H. influenzae*, *Klebsiella pneumoniae*, *P. aeruginosa*), and some anaerobes, including *B. fragilis*. It is indicated for use in intraabdominal infections and bacterial meningitis caused by susceptible organisms. Compared with imipenem, meropenem costs more and seems to offer no clinical advantages. Adverse effects are similar to those of imipenem.

**Ertapenem** (Invanz) also has a broad spectrum of antibacterial activity, although more limited than imipenem and meropenem. It is approved for complicated intraabdominal, skin and skin structure, acute pelvic, and urinary tract infections. It can be used to treat community-acquired pneumonia caused by penicillin-susceptible *S. pneumoniae*. Unlike imipenem and meropenem, ertapenem does not have *in vitro* activity against *P. aeruginosa* and *Acinetobacter baumannii*.

Ertapenem shares the adverse effect profile of the other carbapenems. Lidocaine is also used in preparation of the solution for IM injection, and the same cautions should be used as with imipenem.

## MONOBACTAM

**Aztreonam** (Azactam) is active against gram-negative bacteria, including Enterobacteriaceae and *P. aeruginosa*, and many strains that are resistant to multiple antibiotics. Activity against gram-negative bacteria is similar to that of the aminoglycosides, but the drug does not cause kidney damage or hearing loss. Aztreonam is stable in the presence of beta-lactamase enzymes. Because gram-positive and anaerobic bacteria are resistant to aztreonam, the drug's ability to preserve normal gram-positive and anaerobic flora may be an advantage over most other antimicrobial agents.

Indications for use include infections of the urinary tract, lower respiratory tract, and skin and skin structures, as well as intraabdominal and gynecologic infections and septicemia. Adverse effects are similar to those of penicillin, including possible hypersensitivity reactions.

Drugs at a Glance 29-4 describes specific carbapenems and monobactams.

## USE OF PENICILLINS IN SPECIFIC SITUATIONS

### Streptococcal Infections

Clinicians need to perform culture and susceptibility studies and know local patterns of streptococcal susceptibility or resistance before prescribing penicillins for streptococcal infections. When used, penicillins should

---

## NURSING PROCESS

General aspects of the nursing process in antimicrobial drug therapy, as described in Chapter 28, apply to the client receiving penicillins, cephalosporins, aztreonam, and carbapenems. In this chapter, only those aspects related specifically to these drugs are included.

### Assessment

With penicillins, ask clients whether they have ever taken a penicillin and, if so, whether they ever had a skin rash, hives, swelling, or difficulty breathing associated with the drug. With cephalosporins, ask clients if they have ever taken one of the drugs, as far as they know, and whether they ever had a severe reaction to penicillin. Naming a few cephalosporins (eg, Ceclor, Keflex, Rocephin, Suprax) may help the client identify previous usage.

### Nursing Diagnoses

- Risk for Injury: Hypersensitivity reactions with penicillins or cephalosporins
- Risk for Injury: Renal impairment with cephalosporins
- Deficient Knowledge: Correct home care administration and usage of oral beta-lactams

### Planning/Goals

*The client will:*

- Take oral beta-lactam antibacterials as directed
- Receive parenteral beta-lactam drugs by appropriate techniques to minimize tissue irritation
- Receive prompt and appropriate treatment if hypersensitivity reactions occur

### Interventions

- After giving a penicillin parenterally in an outpatient setting, keep the client in the area for at least 30 minutes. Anaphylactic reactions are more likely to occur with parenteral than oral use and within a few minutes after injection.
- In any client care setting, keep emergency equipment and supplies readily available.
- Monitor client response to beta-lactam drugs.
- Monitor dosages of beta-lactam drugs for clients with impaired renal function.

### Evaluation

- Observe for improvement in signs of infection.
- Interview and observe for adverse drug effects.

be given for the full prescribed course to prevent complications such as rheumatic fever, endocarditis, and glomerulonephritis.

## With Probenecid

Probenecid (Benemid) can be given concurrently with penicillins to increase serum drug levels. Probenecid acts by blocking renal excretion of the penicillins. This action may be useful when high serum levels are needed with oral penicillins or when a single large dose is given intramuscularly for prevention or treatment of syphilis.

## With an Aminoglycoside

A penicillin is often given concomitantly with an aminoglycoside for serious infections, such as those caused by *P. aeruginosa*. The drugs should not be admixed in a syringe or an IV solution because the penicillin inactivates the aminoglycoside.

## Use in Renal Impairment

Beta-lactam antimicrobials are excreted mainly by the kidneys and may accumulate in the presence of renal impairment. Dosage of many beta-lactams must be decreased according to creatinine clearance (CrCl) levels. In addition, some of the drugs are nephrotoxic. References should be consulted to determine dosages recommended for various levels of creatinine clearance. Additional considerations are included in the following sections.

- Dosage of penicillin G, bacampicillin, carbenicillin, mezlocillin, piperacillin, piperacillin-tazobactam, and ticarcillin should be reduced.
- Clients on hemodialysis usually need an additional dose after treatment because hemodialysis removes substantial amounts and produces subtherapeutic serum drug levels.
- Carbenicillin, which is used to treat UTIs, does not reach therapeutic levels in urine in clients with severe renal impairment (CrCl <10 mL/minute).
- Nephropathy, such as interstitial nephritis, although infrequent, has occurred with all penicillins. It is most often associated with high doses of parenteral penicillins and is attributed to hypersensitivity reactions. Manifestations include fever, skin rash, eosinophilia, and possibly increased levels of blood urea nitrogen and serum creatinine.
- Electrolyte imbalances, mainly hypernatremia and hyperkalemia, may occur. Hypernatremia is most likely to occur when ticarcillin (5.6 mEq sodium/g) is given to clients with renal impairment or congestive heart failure. Hypokalemic metabolic acidosis may also occur with ticarcillin because potassium loss is enhanced by high sodium intake. Hyperkalemia may occur with large IV doses of penicillin G potassium (1.7 mEq/ 1 million units).

## Use in Hepatic Impairment

A few beta-lactam antibiotics may cause or aggravate hepatic impairment. Amoxicillin-clavulanate (Augmentin) should be used with caution in clients with hepatic impairment. It is contraindicated in clients who have had cholestatic jaundice and hepatic dysfunction with previous use of the drug. Cholestatic liver impairment usually subsides when the drug is stopped. Hepatotoxicity is attributed to the clavulanate component and has also occurred with ticarcillin-clavulanate (Timentin).

## ■ USE OF CEPHALOSPORINS IN SPECIFIC SITUATIONS

### Perioperative Use

Some cephalosporins are used in surgical prophylaxis. The particular drug depends largely on the type of organism likely to be encountered in the operative area. First-generation drugs, mainly cefazolin, are used for procedures associated with gram-positive postoperative infections, such as prosthetic implant surgery. Second-generation cephalosporins (mainly cefotetan and cefoxitin) are often used for abdominal procedures, especially gynecologic and colorectal surgery, in which enteric gram-negative postoperative infections may occur. Third-generation drugs should not be used for surgical prophylaxis because they are less active against staphylococci than cefazolin, the gram-negative organisms they are most useful against are rarely encountered in elective surgery, widespread use for prophylaxis promotes emergence of drug-resistant organisms, and they are very expensive.

When used perioperatively, a cephalosporin should be given within 2 hours before the first skin incision is made so that the drug has time to reach therapeutic serum and tissue concentrations. A single dose is usually sufficient, although clients undergoing a surgical procedure exceeding 3 hours should receive additional doses at 3-hour intervals. Postoperative doses are rarely necessary but, if used, should generally not exceed 24 hours.

### Use in Renal Impairment

- Reduce dosage because usual doses may produce high and prolonged serum drug levels. In renal failure (CrCl <20 to 30 mL/minute), dosage of all cephalosporins except cefoperazone should be reduced. Cefoperazone is excreted primarily through the bile and therefore does not accumulate with renal failure.
- Cefotaxime is converted to active metabolites that are normally eliminated by the kidneys. These metabolites accumulate and may cause toxicity in clients with renal impairment.

## Use in Hepatic Impairment

Cefoperazone is excreted mainly in bile, and its serum half-life increases in clients with hepatic impairment or biliary obstruction. Adverse effects include cholestasis, jaundice, and hepatitis. Serum drug levels should be monitored if high doses are given (>4 g).

## ■ USE OF AZTREONAM IN SPECIFIC SITUATIONS

### Use in Renal Failure

- After an initial loading dose of aztreonam, reduce dosage by 50% or more in clients with CrCl levels of 30 mL/minute or less. Give at the usual intervals of 6, 8, or 12 hours.
- For serious or life-threatening infections in clients on hemodialysis, give 12.5% of the initial dose after each hemodialysis session, in addition to maintenance doses.

### Use in Hepatic Impairment

Aztreonam, imipenem, meropenem, and ertapenem may cause abnormalities in liver function test results (ie, elevated aspartate and alanine aminotransferase and alkaline phosphatase), but hepatitis and jaundice rarely occur.

## ■ USE OF CARBAPENEMS IN SPECIFIC SITUATIONS

### Use in Renal Failure

- Dosage of imipenem should be reduced in most clients with renal impairment, and the drug is contraindicated in clients with severe renal impairment (CrCl ≤5 mL/minute) unless hemodialysis is started within 48 hours. For clients already on hemodialysis, the drug may cause seizures and should be used very cautiously, if at all.
- Dosage of meropenem should be reduced with renal impairment (CrCl <50 mL/minute).
- Dosage of ertapenem should be reduced to 500 mg daily with renal impairment (CrCl <30 mL/minute). For clients on hemodialysis, administer the daily dose after dialysis.

### Use in Hepatic Impairment

Dosages of imipenem, meropenem, and ertapenem do not require reduction in most clients with hepatic impairment because the drugs are excreted through the kidneys.

---

*Nursing Actions*

## Beta-Lactam Antibacterials

| Nursing Actions | Rationale/Explanation |
|---|---|
| 1. Administer accurately. | |
| a. With penicillins: | |
| (1) Give most oral penicillins on an empty stomach, approximately 1 h before or 2 h after a meal. Penicillin V, amoxicillin, and amoxicillin/clavulanate may be given without regard to meals. | To decrease binding to foods and inactivation by gastric acid. The latter three drugs are not significantly affected by food. |
| (2) Give oral drugs with a full glass of water, preferably; do not give with orange juice or other acidic fluids. | To promote absorption and decrease inactivation, which may occur in an acidic environment |
| (3) Give intramuscular (IM) penicillins deeply into a large muscle mass. | To decrease tissue irritation |
| (4) For intravenous (IV) administration, usually dilute reconstituted penicillins in 50 to 100 mL of 5% dextrose or 0.9% sodium chloride injection and infuse over 30 to 60 min. | To minimize vascular irritation and phlebitis |
| (5) Give reconstituted ampicillin IV or IM within 1 h. | The drug is stable in solution for a limited time, after which effectiveness is lost. |
| b. With cephalosporins: | |
| (1) Give most oral drugs with food or milk. | To decrease nausea and vomiting. Food delays absorption but does not affect the amount of drug absorbed. An exception is the pediatric suspension of ceftibuten, which must be given at least 2 h before or 1 h after a meal. |

*(continued)*

## *Nursing Actions*

### Beta-Lactam Antibacterials (Continued)

| Nursing Actions | Rationale/Explanation |
|---|---|
| (2) Give IM drugs deeply into a large muscle mass. | The drugs are irritating to tissues and cause pain, induration, and possibly sterile abscess. The IM route is rarely used. |
| (3) For IV administration, usually dilute reconstituted drugs in 50 to 100 mL of 5% dextrose or 0.9% sodium chloride injection and infuse over 30 min. | These drugs are irritating to veins and cause thrombophlebitis. This can be minimized by using small IV catheters, large veins, adequate dilution, slow infusion rates, and changing venipuncture sites. Thrombophlebitis is more likely to occur with doses of more than 6 g/d for longer than 3 d. |
| c. With carbapenems: | |
| (1) For IV imipenem/cilastatin, mix reconstituted solution in 100 mL of 0.9% NaCl or 5% dextrose injection. Give 250- to 500-mg doses over 20 to 30 min; give 1-g doses over 40 to 60 min. | Manufacturer's recommendations |
| (2) For IM imipenem, inject deeply into a large muscle mass with a 21-gauge, 2-inch needle. | |
| (3) For IV meropenem, give as an injection (5–20 mL) over 3 to 5 min or as an infusion over 15 to 30 min. | |
| (4) For IV ertapenem, infuse over 30 min. | |
| d. With aztreonam: | |
| (1) For IM administration, add 3 mL diluent per gram of drug, and inject into a large muscle mass. | |
| (2) For IV injection, add 6 to 10 mL sterile water, and inject into vein or IV tubing over 3 to 5 min. | |
| (3) For IV infusion, mix in at least 50 mL of 0.9% NaCl or 5% dextrose injection per gram of drug and give over 20 to 60 min. | |
| 2. Observe for therapeutic effects. | See Chapter 28. |
| a. Decreased signs of local and systemic infection | |
| b. Decreased signs and symptoms of the infection for which the drug is given | |
| c. Absence of signs and symptoms of infection when given prophylactically | |
| 3. Observe for adverse effects. | |
| a. Hypersensitivity—anaphylaxis, serum sickness, skin rash, urticaria | See Nursing Actions in Chapter 28 for signs and symptoms. Reactions are more likely to occur in those with previous hypersensitivity reactions and those with a history of allergy, asthma, or hay fever. Anaphylaxis is more likely with parenteral administration and may occur within 5 to 30 min of injection. |
| b. Phlebitis at IV sites and pain at IM sites | Parenteral solutions are irritating to body tissue. |
| c. Superinfection | See Chapter 28 for signs and symptoms. |
| d. Nausea and vomiting | May occur with all beta-lactam drugs, especially with high oral doses |
| e. Diarrhea, colitis, pseudomembranous colitis | Diarrhea commonly occurs with beta-lactam drugs and may range from mild to severe. The most severe form is pseudomembranous colitis, which is more often associated with ampicillin and the cephalosporins than other beta-lactams. |
| f. Nephrotoxicity | |
| (1) Acute interstitial nephritis (AIN)—hematuria, oliguria, proteinuria, pyuria | AIN may occur with any of the beta-lactams, especially with high parenteral doses of penicillins. |
| (2) Increased blood urea nitrogen and serum creatinine; casts in urine | More likely with cephalosporins, especially in clients who are elderly or have impaired renal function, unless dosage is reduced |

*(continued)*

## Nursing Actions

### Beta-Lactam Antibacterials (Continued)

| Nursing Actions | Rationale/Explanation |
|---|---|
| g. Neurotoxicity—confusion, hallucinations, neuromuscular irritability, convulsive seizures | More likely with large IV doses of penicillins or cephalosporins, especially in clients with impaired renal function |
| h. Coagulation disorders and bleeding from hypoprothrombinemia or platelet dysfunction | Ticarcillin may cause decreased platelet aggregation. Cefmetazole, cefoperazone, cefotetan, and ceftriaxone may cause hypoprothrombinemia (by killing intestinal bacteria that normally produce vitamin K or a chemical structure that prevents activation of prothrombin) or platelet dysfunction. Bleeding can be treated by giving vitamin K. Vitamin K does not restore normal platelet function or normal bacterial flora in the intestines. |
| **4. Observe for drug interactions.** | |
| a. Drugs that *increase* effects of penicillins: | |
| (1) Gentamicin and other aminoglycosides | Synergistic activity against *Pseudomonas* organisms when given concomitantly with extended-spectrum (antipseudomonal) penicillins |
| | Synergistic activity against enterococci that cause subacute bacterial endocarditis, brain abscess, meningitis, or urinary tract infection |
| | Synergistic activity against *S. aureus* when used with nafcillin |
| (2) Probenecid (Benemid) | Decreases renal excretion of penicillins, thus elevates and prolongs penicillin blood levels |
| b. Drugs that *decrease* effects of penicillins: | |
| (1) Acidifying agents (ascorbic acid, cranberry juice, orange juice) | Most oral penicillins are destroyed by acids, including gastric acid. Amoxicillin and penicillin V are acid stable. |
| (2) Erythromycin | Erythromycin inhibits the bactericidal activity of penicillins against most organisms but potentiates activity against resistant strains of *S. aureus*. |
| (3) Tetracyclines | These bacteriostatic antibiotics slow multiplication of bacteria and thereby inhibit the penicillins, which act against rapidly multiplying bacteria. |
| c. Drugs that *increase* effects of cephalosporins: | |
| (1) Loop diuretics (furosemide, ethacrynic acid) | Increased renal toxicity |
| (2) Gentamicin and other aminoglycoside antibiotics | Additive renal toxicity especially in older clients, those with renal impairment, those receiving high dosages, and those receiving probenecid |
| (3) Probenecid | Increases blood levels by decreasing renal excretion of the cephalosporins. This may be a desirable interaction to increase blood levels and therapeutic effectiveness or allow smaller doses. |
| d. Drugs that *decrease* effects of cephalosporins: | |
| (1) Tetracyclines | Tetracyclines are bacteriostatic and slow the rate of bacterial reproduction. Cephalosporins are bactericidal and are most effective against rapidly multiplying bacteria. Thus, tetracyclines should not be given concurrently with cephalosporins. |
| (2) Antacids containing aluminum or magnesium (eg, Mylanta) and histamine $H_2$ antagonists (eg, cimetidine, ranitidine) | These drugs decrease absorption of cefditoren (Spectracef). Give the drugs at least 2 hours apart. |
| e. Drugs that *increase* effects of carbapenems | |
| (1) Probenecid | Probenecid minimally increases serum drug levels of carbapenems, but it is not recommended for concomitant use with any of the drugs. |
| (2) Cyclosporine | May increase central nervous system (CNS) adverse effects of imipenem |
| f. Drugs that *alter* effects of aztreonam | Few documented, clinically significant interactions reported, but potential interactions are those that occur with other beta-lactam antibiotics. |

## How Can You Avoid This Medication Error?

**Answer:** You have just administered the wrong medication to this patient. Although the names are similar (many cephalosporin names sound and look alike), these are two different drugs. Cefuroxime is a second-generation cephalosporin and ceftizoxime is a third-generation cephalosporin, meaning their bacterial coverage and pharmacokinetics are different. When the dispensed medication is not identical to the prescribed medication, check with the pharmacist to see if the substitution is appropriate or if it is a mistake.

## Critical Thinking Exercises

1. The only penicillin that is excreted by the liver is:
   a. Nafcillin
   b. Cloxacillin
   c. Piperacillin
   d. Penicillin G

2. The health care provider orders Augmentin, 500 mg PO. No 500-mg tablets are available, but the nurse has in stock 250-mg tablets. The nurse should:
   a. Administer 2 of the 250 mg tablets
   b. Call the health care provider to clarify the order
   c. Request a 500-mg tablet from the pharmacy
   d. Substitute with available amoxicillin, 500 mg

3. When combined with a penicillin, the beta-lactamase inhibitor protects the penicillin from destruction by enzymes produced by many bacteria, resulting in:
   a. An extended spectrum of antimicrobial activity
   b. Increased drug resistance
   c. Reduced enzyme availability
   d. Limited adverse effects

4. Imipenem-cilastatin (Primaxin) is given parenterally. Because of the way the solution is prepared for IM injection, this drug should only be administered to which of the following individuals?
   a. An individual allergic to lidocaine
   b. A client with infections caused by organisms resistant to other beta-lactams
   c. A client with heart block
   d. An individual who has severe shock

5. A client being treated for a serious respiratory infection has an allergy to penicillin G. The nurse can anticipate that the client will be started on which group of antibiotics?
   a. Cephalosporins
   b. Carbapenems
   c. Penicillin and beta-lactamase inhibitor combinations
   d. Macrolides

## SELECTED REFERENCES

Bush, L. M., & Johnson, C. C. (2000). Antibacterial therapy: Ureidopenicillins and beta-lactam/beta-lactamase inhibitor combinations. *Infectious Disease Clinics of North America, 14*(2), 409–433.

Dancer, S. J. (2001). The problem with cephalosporins. *Journal of Antimicrobial Chemotherapy, 48*, 463–478.

*Drug facts and comparisons.* (Updated monthly). St. Louis: Facts and Comparisons.

Lacy, C. F., Armstrong, L. L., Goldman, M. P., & Lance, L. L. (2003). *Lexi-Comp's drug information handbook* (11th ed.). Hudson, OH: American Pharmaceutical Association.

Limauro, D. L., Chan-Tompkins, N. H., Carter, R. W., Brodmerkel, G. J., Jr., & Agrawal, R. M. (1999). Amoxicillin/clavulanate associated hepatic failure with progression to Stevens-Johnson syndrome. *Annals of Pharmacotherapy, 33*, 560–564.

Petri, W. A., Jr. (2001). Antimicrobial agents: Penicillins, cephalosporins, and other beta-lactam antibiotics. In J. G. Hardman, & L. E. Limbird (Eds.), *Goodman & Gilman's the pharmacological basis of therapeutics* (10th ed., pp. 1189–1218). New York: McGraw-Hill.

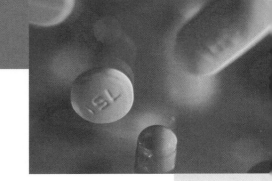

# 30

# Aminoglycosides, Fluoroquinolones, Macrolides, and Miscellaneous Antibacterials

## OBJECTIVES

*After studying this chapter, the student will be able to:*

1 Give characteristics of aminoglycosides in relation to effectiveness, safety, spectrum of antimicrobial activity, indications for use, administration, and observation of client responses.

2 List factors influencing selection and dosage of aminoglycosides.

3 Discuss the importance of serum drug levels during aminoglycoside therapy.

4 Describe measures to decrease nephrotoxicity and ototoxicity with aminoglycosides.

5 Identify characteristics, uses, adverse effects, and nursing process implications of fluoroquinolones.

6 Discuss characteristics and specific uses of macrolide antibacterials.

7 Compare and contrast macrolides with other commonly used antibacterial drugs.

8 Apply principles of using macrolides in selected client situations.

9 Discuss characteristics and clinical indications for using chloramphenicol, clindamycin, linezolid, metronidazole, quinupristin-dalfopristin, and vancomycin.

## CRITICAL THINKING SCENARIO

*Y*ou are an infection control nurse who will be providing long-term care nurses with an update on methicillin-resistant *Staphylococcus aureus* (MRSA). Because MRSA has been a significant problem during the past decade, especially in long-term care facilities, your goal is to increase knowledge about the development of drug resistance and appropriate measures to prevent spread of this organism.

✔ What factors promote resistance to antibiotics?

✔ Why may vancomycin be the drug of choice for MRSA?

✔ What risks are involved when vancomycin is used consistently to treat MRSA?

✔ What infection control practices are necessary to limit the spread of MRSA and other resistant organisms?

# OVERVIEW

The drugs described in this chapter are heterogeneous in their antimicrobial spectra, characteristics, and clinical uses. Some are used often; some are used only in specific circumstances. Parenteral administration of these drugs is typically done in a hospital setting, depending on the severity of the health condition, although the frequency of intravenous (IV) administration in the home is increasing. Oral medications are often self-administered at home. Guidelines for ongoing evaluation and intervention are addressed in Home Care Considerations. In addition, age-specific considerations are important in the management of individuals requiring antibiotic therapy of any kind. Discussion of management significance in children and older adults is found in Age-related Considerations.

The aminoglycosides have been widely used to treat serious gram-negative infections for many years. The quinolones are also older drugs originally used only for treatment of urinary tract infections (see Chap. 31). The fluoroquinolones are synthesized by adding a fluorine molecule to the quinolone structure. This addition increases drug activity against gram-negative microorganisms, broadens the antimicrobial spectrum to include several other microorganisms, and allows use of the drugs in treating systemic infections. The macrolides have similar antibacterial spectra and mechanisms of action and may be bacteriostatic or bactericidal, depending on drug concentration in infected tissues. General characteristics, mechanisms of action, indications for and contraindications to use, nursing process implications, and management considerations for these drugs are described in this chapter. At the foundation of antibiotic therapy is general management of infection and characteristics of antimicrobial drugs addressed in Chapter 28.

# AMINOGLYCOSIDES

Aminoglycosides are bactericidal agents with similar pharmacologic, antimicrobial, and toxicologic characteristics. They are used to treat infections caused by gram-negative microorganisms such as *Pseudomonas* and *Proteus* species, *Escherichia coli*, and *Klebsiella*, *Enterobacter*, and *Serratia* species. Individual drugs, with routes of administration and dosage ranges, are listed in the Drugs at a Glance 30-1: Aminoglycosides.

These drugs are poorly absorbed from the gastrointestinal (GI) tract. Thus, when given orally, they exert local effects in the GI tract. They are well absorbed from intramuscular injection sites and reach peak effects in 30 to 90 minutes with adequate circulation. After IV administration, peak effects occur within 30 to 60 minutes. Plasma half-life is 2 to 4 hours with normal renal function.

After parenteral administration, aminoglycosides are widely distributed in extracellular fluid and reach therapeutic levels in blood, urine, bone, inflamed joints, and pleural and ascitic fluids. They accumulate in high concentrations in the kidney and inner ear. They are poorly distributed to the central nervous system, intraocular fluids, and respiratory tract secretions.

Injected drugs are not metabolized; they are excreted unchanged in the urine, primarily by glomerular filtration. Oral drugs are excreted in feces.

## Mechanism of Action

Aminoglycosides penetrate the cell walls of susceptible bacteria and bind irreversibly to 30S ribosomes, intracellular structures that synthesize proteins. As a result, the bacteria cannot synthesize the proteins necessary for their function and replication.

## Indications for Use

The major clinical use of parenteral aminoglycosides is to treat serious systemic infections caused by susceptible aerobic gram-negative organisms. Gram-negative organisms cause many hospital-acquired infections. These infections have become more common with control of other types of infections, widespread use of antimicrobial drugs, and diseases (eg, acquired immunodeficiency syndrome [AIDS]) or treatments (eg, radical surgery and therapy with antineoplastic or immunosuppressive drugs) that lower host resistance. Although they can occur anywhere, infections due to gram-negative organisms commonly involve the respiratory and genitourinary tracts, skin, wounds, bowel, and bloodstream. Any infection with gram-negative organisms may be serious and potentially life threatening. Management is difficult

**Home Care Considerations:
Use of Aminoglycosides,
Fluoroquinolones, Macrolides,
and Miscellaneous Antibacterials**

**ASSESS:** client for compliance with the prescribed regimen; therapeutic and adverse drug effects, especially with changes in drugs or dosages; that client is keeping appointments for serum drug levels and follow-up care.

**MONITOR:** for therapeutic and adverse drug effects and client's need for additional information, and provide that information.

**EDUCATE:** that completion of antibiotic therapy is important to prevent resistant organisms; that with liquid suspensions for children, shaking to resuspend medication and measuring with a measuring spoon or calibrated device are required for safe dosing. Household spoons should *not* be used because they vary widely in capacity. General guidelines for IV therapy are discussed in Chapter 28; specific guidelines depend on the drug being given. Reinforce additional teaching points (see Client Teaching Guidelines: Oral Fluoroquinolones; Macrolides).

## Age-related Considerations: Use of Aminoglycosides, Fluoroquinolones, Macrolides, and Miscellaneous Antibacterials

### USE IN CHILDREN

Aminoglycosides must be used cautiously in children as with adults. Dosage must be accurately calculated according to weight and renal function. Serum drug concentrations must be monitored and dosage adjusted as indicated to avoid toxicity. Neonates may have increased risk for nephrotoxicity and ototoxicity because of their immature renal function. Neomycin is not recommended for use in infants and children. Fluoroquinolones are not recommended for use in children if other alternatives are available because they have been associated with permanent damage in cartilage and joints in some animal studies.

Erythromycin is usually considered safe for treatment of infections caused by susceptible organisms. Azithromycin and clarithromycin are used in young children for some infections (eg, pharyngitis, tonsillitis, and acute otitis media). Safety and effectiveness of dirithromycin have not been established for children younger than 12 years of age.

Dosage of chloramphenicol must be reduced in premature infants and in full-term infants younger than 2 weeks of age because impaired metabolism may lead to accumulation and adverse effects. Clindamycin should be given to neonates and infants only if clearly indicated, and then liver and kidney function must be monitored. Diarrhea and pseudomembranous colitis may occur with topical clindamycin for treatment of acne. The safety and efficacy of metronidazole have been established in children only for the treatment of amebiasis. Vancomycin is often used in children, including preterm and full-term neonates, for the same indications as in adults. Monitoring serum drug levels is recommended with IV vancomycin.

With the newer drugs, linezolid and quinupristin-dalfopristin, there has been little experience with their use in children and pediatric dosages have not been identified.

### USE IN OLDER ADULTS

With aminoglycosides, advanced age is considered a major risk factor for development of toxicity. Because of impaired renal function, other disease processes (eg, diabetes), and multiple-drug therapy, older adults are at high risk for development of aminoglycoside-induced nephrotoxicity and ototoxicity. However, the drugs are commonly used in older adults for infections caused by organisms resistant to other antibacterials. Aminoglycosides should not be given to older adults with impaired renal function if less toxic drugs are effective against causative organisms. When the drugs are given, extreme caution is required. Interventions to decrease the incidence and severity of adverse drug effects are listed in the section on Guidelines for Reducing Toxicity of Aminoglycosides. These interventions are important for any client receiving an aminoglycoside, but are especially important for older adults. In addition, prolonged therapy (>1 week) increases risk for toxicity and should be avoided when possible.

Fluoroquinolones are commonly used in older adults for the same indications as in younger adults. In older adults with normal renal function, the drugs should be accompanied by an adequate fluid intake and urine output to prevent drug crystals from forming in the urinary tract. In addition, urinary alkalinizing agents, such as calcium-containing antacids, should be avoided because drug crystals form more readily in alkaline urine. In those with impaired renal function, a common condition in older adults, the drugs should be used cautiously and in reduced dosages.

Erythromycin is generally considered safe. Because it is metabolized in the liver and excreted in bile, it may be useful in clients with impaired renal function. Dosage reductions are not indicated with azithromycin and dirithromycin, but may be needed if clarithromycin is given to older adults with severe renal impairment. Dosage of vancomycin should be adjusted for impaired renal function in older adults as in other age groups.

Quinupristin-dalfopristin and linezolid do not require dosage adjustment in older adults. The miscellaneous drugs are used in older adults for the same indications as in younger adults.

---

because the organisms are in general less susceptible to antibacterial drugs, and drug-resistant strains develop rapidly. In pseudomonal infections, an aminoglycoside is often given concurrently with an antipseudomonal penicillin (eg, piperacillin) for synergistic therapeutic effects. The penicillin-induced breakdown of the bacterial cell wall makes it easier for the aminoglycoside to reach its site of action inside the bacterial cell. However, the drugs are chemically and physically incompatible. Therefore, they should not be mixed in a syringe or an IV fluid because the aminoglycoside will be deactivated.

A second clinical use is for treatment of tuberculosis. Streptomycin was often used before the development of isoniazid and rifampin. Now, it may be used for treatment of tuberculosis resistant to other antitubercular drugs. Multidrug-resistant strains of the tuberculosis organism, including strains resistant to both isoniazid and rifampin, are being identified with increasing frequency. This development is leading some authorities to recommend an aminoglycoside as part of a four- to six-drug regimen (see Chap. 32).

A third clinical use is for synergistic action when combined with ampicillin, penicillin G, or vancomycin in the treatment of enterococcal infections. Regimens for enterococcal infections, particularly meningitis or endocarditis, should include **P** **gentamicin,** the prototype, in divided doses rather than once-daily dosing (see Prototype Profile 30-1: Gentamicin). Some enterococcal strains are resistant to gentamicin, however, and microbiology results should be reviewed for each client.

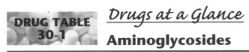

## Drugs at a Glance
**Aminoglycosides**

**DRUG TABLE 30-1**

| Generic/Trade Name | Routes and Dosage Ranges | Comments |
|---|---|---|
| **Amikacin** (Amikin)<br>Pregnancy Category C | *Adults:* IM, IV, 15 mg/kg q24h, 7.5 mg/kg q12h, or 5 mg/kg q8h<br>*Children: Older children:* Same as adults<br>*Neonates:* IM, IV, 10 mg/kg initially, then 7.5 mg/kg q12h | Retains a broader spectrum of antibacterial activity than other aminoglycosides because it resists degradation by most enzymes that inactivate gentamicin and tobramycin<br>Major clinical use is in infections caused by organisms resistant to other aminoglycosides (eg, *Pseudomonas, Proteus, Escherichia coli, Klebsiella, Enterobacter, Serratia*), whether community or hospital acquired |
| **Gentamicin** (Garamycin, Gentak, Gentacidin)<br>Pregnancy Category C | See Prototype Profile 30-1: Gentamicin | |
| **Kanamycin** (Kantrex)<br>Pregnancy Category D | *Adults:* IV, IM, 15 mg/kg/d, in two or three divided doses<br>Suppression of intestinal bacteria PO 1 g every hour for four doses, then 1 g q6h for 36 to 72 h<br>Hepatic coma PO 8–12 g daily in divided doses<br>*Children:* IV, IM same as adults | Occasionally used to decrease bowel organisms before surgery, treat hepatic coma, or to treat multidrug-resistant tuberculosis |
| **Neomycin** (Neo-Fradin; Neo-Rx)<br>Pregnancy Category C | *Adults:* Suppression of intestinal bacteria (with erythromycin 1 g) PO 1 g at 19, 18, and 9 h before surgery (three doses)<br>Hepatic coma PO 4–12 g daily in divided doses | Given orally or topically only because too toxic for systemic use<br>Although poorly absorbed from GI tract, toxic levels may accumulate in presence of renal failure.<br>Used topically, often in combination with other drugs, to treat infections of the eye, ear, and skin (burns, wounds, ulcers, dermatoses)<br>When used for wound or bladder irrigations, systemic absorption may occur if the area is large or if drug concentration exceeds 0.1%. |
| **Paromomycin** (Humatin)<br>Pregnancy Category C | *Adults:* Intestinal amebiasis: PO, 25–35 mg/kg/d, in three divided doses, with meals, for 5–10 d. Repeat after 2 wk, if necessary.<br>Hepatic coma: PO, 4 g/d in divided doses for 5–6 d<br>*Children:* Intestinal amebiasis, same as adults | Acts against bacteria and amebae in the intestinal lumen<br>Used to treat hepatic coma and intestinal amebiasis. It is not effective in amebic infections outside the intestine.<br>Usually not absorbed from GI tract and unlikely to cause ototoxicity and nephrotoxicity associated with systemically absorbed aminoglycosides. However, systemic absorption may occur in the presence of inflammatory or ulcerative bowel disease. |
| **Streptomycin**<br>Pregnancy Category D | *Adults:* IM, 15 mg/kg/d (maximum 1 g) or 25–30 mg/kg two or three times weekly (maximum 1.5 g per dose)<br>*Children:* IM 20–40 mg/kg/d in two divided doses, q12h (maximum dose, 1 g/d) | May be used in a four- to six-drug regimen for treatment of multidrug-resistant tuberculosis |

*(continued)*

**DRUG TABLE 30-1**

## Drugs at a Glance
### Aminoglycosides (Continued)

| Generic/Trade Name | Routes and Dosage Ranges | Comments |
|---|---|---|
| **Tobramycin** (Nebcin; Tobrex, Tobi) <br> Pregnancy Category D (injection, inhalation) <br> Pregnancy Category B (ophthalmic) | *Adults:* IV, IM, 3–5 mg/kg q24h, 1.5–2.5 mg/kg q12h, or 1–1.7 mg/kg q8h <br> *Children:* Same as adults <br> *Neonates (≤1 wk):* IM, IV, up to 4 mg/kg/d in two divided doses, q12h | Similar to gentamicin in antibacterial spectrum, but may be more active against *Pseudomonas* organisms <br> Often used with other antibiotics for septicemia and infections of burn wounds, other soft tissues, bone, the urinary tract, and the central nervous system |

A final clinical use is oral administration to suppress intestinal bacteria. Neomycin and kanamycin may be given before bowel surgery and to treat hepatic coma. In hepatic coma, intestinal bacteria produce ammonia, which enters the bloodstream and causes encephalopathy. Drug therapy to suppress intestinal bacteria decreases ammonia production. Paromomycin is used mainly in the treatment of intestinal amebiasis.

---

## PROTOTYPE PROFILE 30-1
### P Gentamicin (jen ta MYE sin)

**Drug Class**
*Chemical:* Aminoglycoside
*Functional:* Antibiotic

**Trade Names**
Garamycin, Genoptic, Gentak, Gentacidin

**Therapeutic Indications**
Treatment of susceptible infections, normally gram-negative organisms

**Pharmacokinetics**

*Absorption*
PO: none; crosses placenta; relative diffusion into CSF from blood minimal

*Distribution*
Plasma protein binding: <30%

*Metabolism*
Varies with age and renal function

*Excretion*
Urine

**Pharmacodynamics**
*Onset of Action*
Time to peak: IM, 30–90 min; IV, 30 min after 30-min infusions

*Duration*
Directly related to renal function

**Contraindications/Precautions**
Hypersensitivity to gentamicin or other aminoglycosides; with caution in renal insufficiency, myasthenia gravis, hypocalcemia, cochlear or vestibular impairment
Risk of nephrotoxicity and ototoxicity with long-term use

**Pregnancy Considerations**
Category C
Enters breast milk in small amounts; compatible

**Dosage**
Use of ideal body weight appears to be more accurate than total body weight; peak and trough levels should guide dosing
*Adults:* IV, IM, 3 to 7 mg/kg q 24h, 1.5–2.5 mg/kg q12h, or 1–1.7 mg/kg q8h
*Children:* IV, IM, 6–7.5 mg/kg/d in 3 divided doses, q8h
*Infants and neonates:* IV, IM, 7.5 mg/kg/d in 3 divided doses, q8h
*Premature infants and neonates < 1 wk:* 5 mg/kg/d in 2 divided doses, q 12h

**Adverse Effects**
Dizziness, drowsiness, gait instability, ototoxicity, nephrotoxicity, impaired creatinine clearance

**Drug Interactions**
*Increased Effects*
Nephrotoxic potential with penicillins, cephalosporins, amphotericin B, or loop diuretics
Neuromuscular blocking effects with aminoglycosides

*Decreased Effects*
None recognized

**Herbal Supplements and Dietary Considerations**
Calcium, potassium, and magnesium intake should be adequate because renal wasting may cause low serum levels of these electrolytes

A few aminoglycosides are administered topically to the skin or to the eye. These are discussed in Appendices F and G, respectively.

## Contraindications to Use

Aminoglycosides are contraindicated in infections for which less toxic drugs are effective. The drugs are nephrotoxic and ototoxic and must be used very cautiously in the presence of renal impairment. Dosages are adjusted according to serum drug levels and creatinine clearance. The drugs must also be used cautiously in clients with myasthenia gravis and other neuromuscular disorders because muscle weakness may be increased.

## Management Considerations

### Choice of Drug

The choice of aminoglycoside depends on local susceptibility patterns and specific organisms causing an infection. Gentamicin is often given for systemic infections if resistant microorganisms have not developed in the clinical setting. If gentamicin-resistant organisms have developed, amikacin or tobramycin may be given because they are usually less susceptible to drug-destroying enzymes. In terms of toxicity, the aminoglycosides cause similar effects.

### Dosage of Aminoglycosides

Dosage of aminoglycosides must be carefully regulated because therapeutic doses are close to toxic doses. Two major dosing schedules are used, one involving multiple daily doses and one involving a single daily dose. The multiple-dose regimen has been used traditionally, and guidelines are well defined. The single-dose regimen is being used increasingly, and guidelines are still evolving as studies and clinical experience accumulate. These two regimens are described in the following sections.

### *Multiple Daily Dosing*

1. An *initial loading dose*, based on client weight and the desired peak serum concentration, is given to achieve therapeutic serum concentrations rapidly. If the client is obese, lean or ideal body weight should be used because aminoglycosides are not significantly distributed in body fat. In clients with normal renal function, the recommended loading dose for gentamicin, tobramycin, and netilmicin is 1.5 to 2 mg/kg of body weight; for amikacin, the loading dose is 5 to 7.5 mg/kg.
2. *Maintenance doses* are based on serum drug concentrations. Peak serum concentrations should be assessed 30 to 60 minutes after drug administration (5 to 8 mcg/mL for gentamicin and tobramycin, 20 to 30 mcg/mL for amikacin, 4 to 12 mcg/mL for netilmicin). Measurement of both peak and trough levels helps to main-

tain therapeutic serum levels without excessive toxicity. For gentamicin and tobramycin, peak levels above 10 to 12 mcg/mL and trough levels above 2 mcg/mL for prolonged periods have been associated with nephrotoxicity. For accuracy, blood samples must be drawn at the correct times, and the timing of drug administration and blood sampling must be accurately documented.

3. *With impaired renal function*, dosage of aminoglycosides must be reduced. Methods of adjusting dosage include lengthening the time between doses or reducing doses. References should be consulted for specific recommendations on adjusting aminoglycoside doses for renal impairment.
4. *In urinary tract infections*, smaller doses can be used than in systemic infections because the aminoglycosides reach high concentrations in the urine.

### *Single Daily Dosing*

The use of once-daily (or extended-interval) aminoglycoside dosing is increasing. This dosing method uses high doses (7 mg/kg) to produce high initial drug concentrations, but a repeat dose is not administered until the serum concentration is quite low. Most clients can be successfully managed with one daily dose using this approach. However, certain populations require more than one daily dose, but still require fewer daily doses than are necessary in multiple dosing strategies (thus extended-interval dosing).

This practice evolved from increased knowledge about the concentration-dependent bactericidal effects and postantibiotic effects of aminoglycosides. Concentration-dependent bactericidal effects mean that the drugs kill more microorganisms with a large dose and high peak serum concentrations. Postantibiotic effects mean that aminoglycosides continue killing microorganisms even with low serum concentrations. These characteristics allow administration of high doses to achieve high peak serum concentrations and optimal killing of microorganisms. The longer interval until the next dose allows the client to eliminate the drug to very low serum concentrations for approximately 6 hours. During this low-drug period, the postantibiotic effect is active while there is minimal drug

> **? How Can You Avoid This Medication Error?**
>
> Your client has vancomycin 1 g IV ordered for 0900. The pharmacy sends up a 250-mL IV bag with 1 g of vancomycin, to infuse over 1 hour. Your IV drip rate is 10 drops/mL. You calculate and regulate the IV rate at 42 drops per minute. When you return in 30 minutes, the entire 250 mL has infused into the client and he appears very flushed and complains of feeling hot.

accumulation in body tissues. Reported advantages of this regimen include increased bactericidal effects, less nephrotoxicity, reduced need for serum drug concentration data, and reduced nursing time for administration.

## FLUOROQUINOLONES

Fluoroquinolones are synthetic bactericidal drugs with activity against gram-negative and gram-positive organisms. They may allow oral ambulatory treatment of infections that previously required parenteral therapy and hospitalization. Most are given orally, after which they are well absorbed, achieve therapeutic concentra-

tions in most body fluids, and are metabolized to some extent in the liver. The kidneys are the main route of elimination, with approximately 30% to 60% of an oral dose excreted unchanged in the urine. Dosage should be reduced in renal impairment. Individual drugs, with routes of administration and dosage ranges, are listed in the Drugs at a Glance 30-2: Fluoroquinolones.

## Mechanism of Action

The drugs act by interfering with deoxyribonucleic acid (DNA) gyrase, an enzyme required for synthesis of bacterial DNA and therefore required for bacterial growth and replication.

**DRUG TABLE 30-2**

### Drugs at a Glance
### Fluoroquinolones

| Generic/Trade Name | Routes and Dosage Ranges | Comments/Uses |
|---|---|---|
| **Cinoxacin** (Cinobac) Pregnancy Category C | *Adults:* PO, 1 g daily in two to four divided doses for 7–14 d | 1. Used only for UTI 2. Effective against most gram-negative bacteria that commonly cause UTI (*Escherichia coli, Klebsiella, Enterobacter, Proteus*) |
| **Ciprofloxacin** (Cipro) Pregnancy Category C | *Adults:* PO, 250–750 mg q12h IV, 200–400 mg q8–12h | 1. Effective in respiratory, urinary tract, gastrointestinal tract, and skin and soft tissue infections as well as sexually transmitted diseases caused by chlamydiae and gonorrhea organisms 2. Used as one of four to six drugs in treatment of multidrug-resistant tuberculosis |
| **Gatifloxacin** (Tequin, Zymar) Pregnancy Category C | *Adults:* PO, IV, infusion 400 mg once daily Give IV dose over 60 minutes; avoid rapid administration | Indicated for pneumonia, bronchitis, sinusitis, skin and soft tissue infections, urinary infections, pyelonephritis, and gonorrhea |
| **Levofloxacin** (Levaquin) Pregnancy Category C | *Adults:* PO, IV, 250–750 mg once daily. Infuse IV dose slowly over 60 min | A broad-spectrum agent effective for treatment of bronchitis, cystitis, pneumonia, sinusitis, skin and skin structure infections, and pyelonephritis |
| **Lomefloxacin** (Maxaquin) Pregnancy Category C | *Adults:* PO, 400 mg once daily Preoperatively, PO 400 mg as a single dose, 1–6 h before surgery | Approved for bronchitis, urinary infections, and transurethral surgical procedures |
| **Moxifloxacin** (Avelox, Vigamox) Pregnancy Category C | *Adults:* PO, IV, 400 mg once daily. Infuse IV dose slowly over 60 min | Indicated for pneumonia, sinusitis, bronchitis, skin and soft tissue infections |
| **Norfloxacin** (Noroxin) Pregnancy Category C | *Adults:* PO, 400 mg twice daily | Used only for UTI and uncomplicated gonorrhea |
| **Ofloxacin** (Floxin, Ocuflox) Pregnancy Category C | *Adults:* PO, IV, 200–400 mg q12h for 3–10 d Gonorrhea, PO 400 mg as a single dose | 1. Effective in respiratory, urinary tract, gastrointestinal tract, and skin and soft tissue infections as well as sexually transmitted disease caused by chlamydiae and gonorrhea organisms |

*(continued)*

**DRUG TABLE 30-2**

*Drugs at a Glance*

**Fluoroquinolones** (Continued)

| Generic/Trade Name | Routes and Dosage Ranges | Comments/Uses |
|---|---|---|
| | | 2. Used as one of four to six drugs in treatment of multidrug-resistant tuberculosis |
| **Sparfloxacin** (Zagam) Pregnancy Category C | *Adults:* PO, 400 mg as loading dose, then 200 mg once daily for 10 d Renal impairment (creatinine clearance <50 mL/min), PO 400 mg as loading dose, then 200 mg q48h for a total of 9 d of therapy | Indicated for community-acquired pneumonia caused by *Chlamydia pneumoniae*, *Streptococcus pneumoniae*, or *Haemophilus influenzae* and acute bacterial exacerbations of chronic bronchitis caused by above organisms, *Klebsiella pneumoniae*, or *Staphylococcus aureus* |

UTI, urinary tract infection.

## Indications for Use

Fluoroquinolones are indicated for various infections caused by aerobic gram-negative and other microorganisms. Thus, they may be used to treat infections of the respiratory, genitourinary, and GI tracts as well as infections of bones, joints, skin, and soft tissues. Additional uses include treatment of gonorrhea, multidrug-resistant tuberculosis (see Chap. 32), *Mycobacterium avium* complex (MAC) infections in clients with AIDS, and fever in neutropenic cancer clients. Indications vary with individual drugs and are listed in Drugs at a Glance 30-2: Fluoroquinolones.

## Management Considerations

### Choice of Drug

Local susceptibility patterns and specific organisms also determine the choice of fluoroquinolone because individual drugs differ somewhat in their antimicrobial spectra. The drugs cause similar adverse effects.

### Dosage of Fluoroquinolones

Recommended dosages of fluoroquinolones should not be exceeded in any clients, and dosages should be reduced in the presence of renal impairment.

## Contraindications to Use

Fluoroquinolones are contraindicated in clients who have experienced a hypersensitivity reaction and in children younger than 18 years of age, if other alternatives are available. Limited data are available on the safety of fluoroquinolones in pregnant or lactating women; they should not be used unless the benefits outweigh the potential risks.

## **N**URSING PROCESS

General aspects of the nursing process as described in Chapter 28 apply to the client receiving aminoglycosides, fluoroquinolones, macrolides, and miscellaneous antibiotics. In this chapter, only those aspects related specifically to these drugs are included.

### Assessment

With aminoglycosides, assess for the presence of factors that predispose to nephrotoxicity or ototoxicity:

- Check laboratory reports of renal function (eg, serum creatinine, creatinine clearance, blood urea nitrogen [BUN]) for abnormal values.

- Assess for impairment of balance or hearing, including audiometry reports if available.
- Analyze current medications for drugs that interact with aminoglycosides to increase risks of nephrotoxicity or ototoxicity.

With fluoroquinolones, assess for the presence of factors that increase risks of adverse drug effects (eg, impaired renal function, inadequate fluid intake, frequent or prolonged exposure to sunlight in usual activities of daily living):

- Assess laboratory tests (eg, complete blood counts and tests of renal and hepatic function) for abnormal values.

*(continued)*

## NURSING PROCESS (Continued)

With macrolides and miscellaneous antibiotics.

- Assess for infections that macrolides and the designated miscellaneous drugs are used to prevent or treat.
- Assess each client for signs and symptoms of the specific current infection.
- Assess culture and susceptibility reports when available.
- Assess each client for risk factors that increase risks of infection (eg, immunosuppression) or risks of adverse drug reactions (eg, impaired renal or hepatic function).

### Nursing Diagnoses

- Deficient Knowledge related to type of infection and appropriate use of prescribed antimicrobial drugs
- Risk for Injury related to adverse drug effects
- Risk for Injury related to infection with antibiotic-resistant microorganisms

### Planning/Goals

*The client will:*

- Receive aminoglycoside dosages that are individualized by age, weight, renal function, and serum drug levels
- Have serum aminoglycoside levels monitored when indicated
- Have renal function tests performed regularly during aminoglycoside and fluoroquinolone therapy
- Be well hydrated during aminoglycoside and fluoroquinolone therapy
- Take or receive macrolides and miscellaneous antimicrobials accurately, for the prescribed length of time
- Experience decreased signs and symptoms of the infection being treated
- Be monitored regularly for therapeutic and adverse drug effects

- Verbalize and practice measures to prevent recurrent infection

### Interventions

- With aminoglycosides, weigh clients accurately (dosage is based on weight), monitor laboratory reports of BUN, serum creatinine, serum drug levels, and urinalysis for abnormal values.
- Force fluids to at least 2000 to 3000 mL daily if not contraindicated. Keeping the client well hydrated reduces risks of nephrotoxicity with aminoglycosides and crystalluria with fluoroquinolones.
- Encourage fluid intake to decrease fever and maintain good urinary tract function.
- Provide foods and fluids with adequate nutrients to maintain or improve nutritional status, especially if febrile and hypermetabolic.
- Avoid concurrent use of other nephrotoxic drugs when possible.
- Use measures to prevent and minimize the spread of infection (see Chap. 28).
- Monitor for fever and other signs and symptoms of infection.
- Monitor laboratory reports for indications of the client's response to drug therapy (eg, white blood cells [WBC], tests of renal function).
- Assist clients to prevent or minimize infections with streptococci, staphylococci, and enterococci organisms.

### Evaluation

- Interview and observe for improvement in the infection being treated.
- Interview and observe for adverse drug effects.

---

## CLIENT TEACHING GUIDELINES
## Oral Fluoroquinolones

### General Considerations

✔ Avoid exposure to sunlight during and for several days after taking one of these drugs. Stop taking the drug and notify the prescribing physician if skin burning, redness, swelling, rash, or itching occurs. Sunscreen lotions do not prevent photosensitivity reactions.

✔ Be very careful if driving or doing other tasks requiring alertness or physical coordination. These drugs may cause dizziness or lightheadedness.

### Self-administration

✔ Take norfloxacin (Noroxin) and enoxacin (Penetrex) 1 hour before or 2 hours after meals. Do not take ofloxacin with food. Ciprofloxacin (Cipro), gatifloxacin (Tequin), lomefloxacin (Maxaquin), moxifloxacin (Avelox), and sparfloxacin (Zagam) can be taken without regard to meals.

✔ Drink 2 to 3 quarts of fluid daily if able. This helps to prevent kidney problems.

✔ Do not take antacids containing magnesium or aluminum (eg, Mylanta or Maalox) or any products containing iron or zinc at the same time, within 4 hours before, or within 2 hours after a dose of the antibiotic.

# MACROLIDES

The macrolides, which include erythromycin, azithromycin (Zithromax), clarithromycin (Biaxin), and dirithromycin (Dynabac), have similar antibacterial spectra and mechanisms of action. They are widely distributed into body tissues and fluids and may be bacteriostatic or bactericidal, depending on drug concentration in infected tissues. They are effective against gram-positive cocci, including group A streptococci, pneumococci, and most staphylococci. They are also effective against species of *Corynebacterium*, *Treponema*, *Neisseria*, and *Mycoplasma* and against some anaerobic organisms such as *Bacteroides* and *Clostridia*. Azithromycin and clarithromycin also are active against the atypical mycobacteria that cause *Mycobacterium avium* complex (MAC) disease. MAC disease is an opportunistic infection that occurs mainly in people with advanced human immunodeficiency virus (HIV) infection. Individual drugs, with routes of administration and dosage ranges, are listed in the Drugs at a Glance 30-3: Macrolides.

**DRUG TABLE 30-3** *Drugs at a Glance*
## Macrolides

| Generic/Trade Name | Routes and Dosage Ranges | Comments |
|---|---|---|
| **Azithromycin** (Zithromax) Pregnancy Category B | *Adults:* Respiratory and skin infections, PO, 500 mg as a single dose on the first day, then 250 mg once daily for 4 d. Nongonococcal urethritis and cervicitis caused by *Chlamydia trachomatis*, give 1 g as a single dose. *Children: 6 mo and older:* Acute otitis media PO, 10 mg/kg as a single dose (not to exceed 500 mg) on the first day, then 5 mg/kg (not to exceed 250 mg) once daily for 4 d *2 y and older:* Pharyngitis/tonsillitis, PO, 12 mg/kg (not to exceed 500 mg) once daily for 5 d | Do not administer concurrently with magnesium or aluminum antacids |
| **Clarithromycin** (Biaxin, Biaxin XL) Pregnancy Category C | *Adults:* PO, 250–500 mg q12h for 7 to 14 d. Prevention or treatment of MAC, PO, 500 mg q12h Extended release, bronchitis and community-acquired pneumonia, PO, 1000 mg (two 500-mg tablets) once daily for 7 d Acute maxillary sinusitis, PO 1000 mg once daily for 14 d *Children:* PO, 7.5 mg/kg q12h, not to exceed 500 mg q12h *Prevention or treatment of MAC:* same as above | May be used to prevent bacterial endocarditis in clients with a penicillin allergy |
| **Dirithromycin** (Dynabac) Pregnancy Category C | *Adults:* Bronchitis caused by *Streptococcus pneumoniae* or *Moraxella catarrhalis* and skin infections caused by methicillin-susceptible *Staphylococcus aureus*, PO 500 mg once daily for 7 d Pharyngitis/tonsillitis caused by *Streptococcus pyogenes*, PO 500 mg once daily for 10 d Community-acquired pneumonia caused by *Legionella pneumophila*, *Mycoplasma pneumoniae*, or *S. pneumoniae*, PO 500 mg once daily for 14 d *Children: 12 y and older:* same as adults | Do not crush tablets May cause insomnia |

*(continued)*

**DRUG TABLE 30-3**

## *Drugs at a Glance*
### Macrolides (Continued)

| Generic/Trade Name | Routes and Dosage Ranges | Comments |
|---|---|---|
| **Erythromycin base** (E-mycin) Pregnancy Category B | See Prototype Profile: Erythromycin | |
| **Erythromycin estolate** (Ilosone) Pregnancy Category B | *Adults:* PO, 250 mg q6h; maximal daily dose, 4 g<br>*Children:* Weight >25 kg, PO same as adults<br>Weight 10–25 kg, PO 30–50 mg/kg/d in divided doses<br>Weight <10 kg, PO 10 mg/kg/d in divided doses q6–12h<br>Dosages may be doubled in severe infections. | Do not crush enteric coated products. GI upset with all erythromycins is common |
| **Erythromycin ethylsuccinate** (E.E.S.) Pregnancy Category B | *Adults:* PO, 400 mg four times daily; severe infections, up to 4 g or more daily in divided doses<br>*Children:* PO, 30–50 mg/kg/d in four divided doses q6–12h. Severe infections, 60–100 mg/kg/d in divided doses | |
| **Erythromycin lactobionate** Pregnancy Category B | *Adults:* IV, 15–20 mg/kg/d in divided doses; severe infections, up to 4 g daily<br>*Children:* IV same as adults | |
| **Erythromycin stearate** (Erythrocin stearate) Pregnancy Category B | *Adults:* PO 250 mg q6h or 500 mg q12h; severe infections, up to 4 g daily<br>*Children:* PO, 30–50 mg/kg/d in four divided doses q6h; severe infections, 60–100 mg/kg/d | |

**℗  Erythromycin,** the prototype, is now used less often because of microbial resistance, numerous drug interactions, and the development of newer macrolides. Erythromycin is outlined in Prototype Profile 30-2: Erythromycin. Depending on the specific salt formulation used, food can have a variable effect on the absorption of oral erythromycin. Compared with erythromycin, the newer drugs require less frequent administration and cause less nausea, vomiting, and diarrhea. Azithromycin and dirithromycin are excreted mainly in bile, and clarithromycin is metabolized to an active metabolite in the liver, which is then excreted in urine.

Erythromycin is available in several preparations. Topical and ophthalmic preparations are discussed in Appendices F and G, respectively.

A relative of the macrolides, telithromycin (Ketek), is the first of a new class of antibiotics, named the ketolides. Telithromycin and a similar drug have not yet received U.S. Food and Drug Administration (FDA) approval for marketing. These drugs are expected to offer better activity against multidrug-resistant strains of *Streptococcus pneumoniae,* an increasingly common cause of infections in children and adults.

## Mechanism of Action

The macrolides enter microbial cells and attach to 50S ribosomes, thereby inhibiting microbial protein synthesis.

## Indications for Use

The macrolides are widely used for treatment of respiratory tract and skin and soft tissue infections caused by streptococci and staphylococci. Erythromycin is also used as a penicillin substitute in clients who are allergic to penicillin; for prevention of rheumatic fever, gonorrhea, syphilis, pertussis, and chlamydial conjunctivitis in newborns (ophthalmic ointment); and to treat other infections (eg, Legionnaires disease, genitourinary infections caused by *Chlamydia trachomatis,* intestinal amebiasis caused by *Entamoeba histolytica*).

In addition, azithromycin is approved for treatment of urethritis and cervicitis caused by *C. trachomatis* organisms and is being used for the prevention and treatment of MAC disease. Clarithromycin is approved for prevention and treatment of MAC disease. For prevention, clarithromycin may be used alone; for treatment, it is combined with one

## PROTOTYPE PROFILE 30-2

### P Erythromycin (eh rith roe MYE cin)

**Drug Class**
*Chemical:* Macrolide
*Functional:* Antibiotic

**Trade Name**
E-mycin

**Therapeutic Indications**
Treatment of susceptible infections

**Pharmacokinetics**

*Absorption*
PO, variable but better with salt form than with base formulation

*Distribution*
Plasma protein binding: 75%–90%; crosses placenta

*Metabolism*
Liver

*Excretion*
Mainly in bile; approximately 20% is excreted in urine.

**Pharmacodynamics**

*Onset of Action*
Time to peak: Base, 4 h; ethylsuccinate: 0.5–2.5 h; food delays absorption

*Duration*
Peak half-life elimination: 1.5–2 h

**Contraindications/Precautions**
Sensitivity to erythromycin, hepatic impairment; lactobionate formulation contains benzyl alcohol that has been associated with toxicity in neonates

**Pregnancy Considerations**
Category B
Enters breast milk; compatible

**Dosage**
*Adults:* PO (base, estolate, sterate), 250 mg q6h; (ethylsuccinate), 400 mg q6 or 800 mg q12h
IV (gluceptate and lactobionate), 25–500 mg (up to 1 g) q6h
*Children:* 7.5–12.5 mg/kg q6h or 12.5 to 25 mg/kg q12h (up to 100 mg/kg/d)
IV (gluceptate and lactobionate) 3.75–5 mg/kg q6h

**Adverse Effects**
Nausea, vomiting, diarrhea, abdominal pain, ventricular dysrhythmias, headache, mouth sores

**Drug Interactions**

*Increased Effects*
Risk for dysrhythmias with thioridazine, astemizole, gatifloxacin, cisapride, pimozide
Serum concentrations of alfentanil, diazepam, buspirone, calcium channel blockers, benzodiazepines, clozapine, cyclosporine, digoxin, dihydropyridine, cilostazol, sildenafil, vinblastine, tacrolimus, theophylline, methylprednisolone, disopyramide, ergot alkaloids, loratadine, and zopiclone with concurrent use

*Decreased Effects*
Erythromycin may antagonize the therapeutic effects of lincomycin and clindamycin.

**Herbal Supplements and Dietary Considerations**
Do not give with milk or acidic beverages; may take with food to decrease GI complaints; depending on the specific salt formulation used, food can have a variable effect on the absorption of oral erythromycin; avoid alcohol

---

or two other drugs (eg, ethambutol or rifabutin) to prevent the emergence of drug-resistant organisms. Clarithromycin is also used to treat *Helicobacter pylori* infections associated with peptic ulcer disease.

## Management Considerations

### Effects of Macrolides on Other Drugs

Erythromycin interferes with the elimination of several drugs, especially those metabolized by the cytochrome P450 enzymes in the liver. As a result, the affected drugs are eliminated more slowly, their serum levels are increased, and they are more likely to cause adverse effects and toxicity unless dosage is reduced. Interacting drugs include alfentanil (Alfenta), bromocriptine (Parlodel), carbamazepine (Tegretol), cyclosporine (Sandimmune), digoxin (Lanoxin), disopyramide (Norpace), methyl-

prednisolone (Medrol), theophylline (Theo-Dur), triazolam (Halcion), and warfarin (Coumadin). These drugs represent a variety of drug classes. Erythromycin is contraindicated in clients who are receiving fluoroquinolone antibacterials (eg, ciprofloxacin) because serious ventricular dysrhythmias and fatalities have been reported.

The newer macrolides have fewer effects on other drugs, but some differences are apparent. Clarithromycin, for example, increases carbamazepine levels, but azithromycin does not.

## Contraindications to Use

Macrolides are contraindicated in people who have had hypersensitivity reactions. They are also contraindicated or must be used with caution in clients with preexisting liver disease.

## CLIENT TEACHING GUIDELINES
### Macrolides

**General Considerations**

✔ Complete the full course of drug therapy. The fastest and most complete relief of infections occurs with accurate usage of antibiotics. Moreover, inaccurate use may cause other, potentially more severe infections.

✔ These drugs are often given for infections of the respiratory tract or skin (eg, bronchitis, pneumonia, cellulitis). Good handwashing can help prevent the development and spread of these infections.

✔ Report symptoms of infection that recur or develop during antibiotic therapy. Such symptoms can indicate recurrence of the original infection (ie, the antibiotic is not effective because it is the wrong drug or wrong dosage for the infection or it is not being taken accurately) or a new infection with antibiotic-resistant bacteria or fungi.

✔ Report nausea, vomiting, diarrhea, abdominal cramping or pain, yellow discoloration of the skin or eyes (jaundice), dark urine, pale stools, or unusual tiredness. These symptoms may indicate liver damage, which sometimes occurs with these drugs.

**Self-administration**

✔ Take each dose with 6 to 8 oz of water, at evenly spaced time intervals, preferably around the clock.

✔ With erythromycin, ask a health care provider if not instructed when to take the drug in relation to food. Erythromycin is available in several preparations. Some should be taken on an empty stomach (at least 1 h before or 2 h after meals) or may be taken with a small amount of food if gastrointestinal upset occurs. Some preparations may be taken without regard to meals.

✔ Take azithromycin (Zithromax) oral solution on an empty stomach, 1 h before or 2 h after a meal; take tablets without regard to meals. Do not take with an antacid.

✔ Take clarithromycin (Biaxin) regular tablets and the oral suspension without regard to meals. Take extended-release tablets (Biaxin XL) with food. With the oral suspension, do not refrigerate and shake well before measuring the dose.

✔ Take dirithromycin (Dynabac) with food or within 1 h of having eaten. Do not cut, chew, or crush the tablets.

## MISCELLANEOUS ANTIBACTERIAL DRUGS

Individual drugs are discussed in Drugs at a Glance 30-4: Miscellaneous Antibacterials.

**Chloramphenicol** (Chloromycetin) is a broad-spectrum, bacteriostatic antibiotic that is active against most gram-positive and gram-negative bacteria, rickettsiae, chlamydiae, and treponemes. It acts by interfering with microbial protein synthesis. It is well absorbed and diffuses well into body tissues and fluids, including cerebrospinal fluid (CSF), but low drug levels are obtained in urine. It is metabolized in the liver and excreted in the urine.

Chloramphenicol is rarely used in infections caused by gram-positive organisms because of the effectiveness and low toxicity of penicillins, cephalosporins, and macrolides. Each of the alternate classes of antibiotics has a more favorable safety profile and should be considered first, before chloramphenicol. It is indicated for use in serious infections for which no adequate substitute drug is available. Specific infections include meningococcal, pneumococcal, or *Haemophilus* meningitis in penicillin-allergic clients; anaerobic brain abscess; *Bacteroides fragilis* infections; rickettsial infections and brucellosis when tetracyclines are contraindicated; and *Klebsiella* and *Haemophilus* infections that are resistant to other drugs.

**Clindamycin** (Cleocin) is similar to the macrolides in its mechanism of action and antimicrobial spectrum. It is bacteriostatic in usual doses. It is effective against gram-positive cocci, including group A streptococci, pneumococci, most staphylococci, and some anaerobes such as *Bacteroides* and *Clostridia*. Clindamycin enters microbial cells and attaches to 50S ribosomes, thereby inhibiting microbial protein synthesis.

Clindamycin is often used to treat infections caused by *B. fragilis*. Because these bacteria are usually mixed with gram-negative organisms from the gynecologic or GI tracts, clindamycin is usually given with another drug, such as gentamicin, to treat mixed infections. The drug may be useful as a penicillin substitute in clients who are allergic to penicillin and who have serious streptococcal, staphylococcal, or pneumococcal infections in which the causative organism is susceptible to clindamycin. A topical solution is used in the treatment of acne, and a vaginal cream is available. Clindamycin does not reach therapeutic concentrations in the central nervous system (CNS) and should not be used for treating meningitis.

Clindamycin is well absorbed with oral administration and reaches peak plasma levels within 1 hour after a dose. It is widely distributed in body tissues and fluids, except CSF, and crosses the placenta. It is highly bound (90%) to plasma proteins. It is metabolized in the liver, and the metabolites are excreted in bile and urine. Dosage may need to be reduced in clients with severe hepatic failure to prevent accumulation and toxic effects.

**Linezolid** (Zyvox) is a member of the oxalodinone class, a newer class of antibiotics. It is active against aerobic gram-positive bacteria, in which it acts by inhibiting protein synthesis. The drug is well absorbed orally, distributes widely, and undergoes hepatic elimination. Its effects in pregnancy and in children are largely unknown.

## DRUG TABLE 30-4 — *Drugs at a Glance*
### Miscellaneous Antibacterials

| Generic/Trade Name | Routes and Dosage Ranges | Comments |
|---|---|---|
| **Chloramphenicol** (Chloromycetin) Pregnancy Category C | *Adults:* PO, IV, 50–100 mg/kg/d, in four divided doses, q6h *Children and full-term infants >2 wk:* PO, 50 mg/kg/d, in three or four divided doses, q6–8h | Do not administer IM; draw peak level 2 h after oral dose or 90 min after the end of the infusion |
| **Clindamycin hydrochloride** (Cleocin) Pregnancy Category B | *Adults:* PO, 150–300 mg q6h; up to 450 mg q6h for severe infections *Children:* PO, 8–16 mg/kg/d in three or four divided doses, q6–8h; up to 20 mg/kg/d in severe infections | Food may delay peak concentration; avoid St. John's wort because it may decrease drug levels |
| **Clindamycin phosphate** (Cleocin phosphate) Pregnancy Category B | *Adults:* IM, 600 mg–2.7 g/d in two to four divided doses, q6–12h IV, 600 mg–2.7 g/d in two to four divided doses; up to 4.8 g/d in life-threatening infections *Children:* IM, IV, 15–40 mg/kg/d in three or four divided doses, q6–8h; up to 40 mg/kg/d in severe infections | Food may delay peak concentration; avoid St. John's wort because it may decrease drug levels |
| **Clindamycin palmitate** (Cleocin Pediatric—75 mg/mL) Pregnancy Category B | *Children:* PO, 8–12 mg/kg/d in three or four divided doses; up to 25 mg/kg/d in very severe infections. For children weighing 10 kg or less, the minimum dose is 37.5 mg, three times per day. | Refrigeration of reconstituted oral solution will cause thickening; will be stable at room temperature for 16 d |
| **Linezolid** (Zyvox) Pregnancy Category C | *Adults:* PO, 400–600 mg q12h IV, 600 mg over 30–120 min q12h (for serious infections) *Children:* Dosage not established | Myelosuppression has been reported with drug; weekly CBC monitoring is recommended |
| **Metronidazole** (Flagyl) Pregnancy Category B; may be contraindicated in first trimester | *Adults:* Anaerobic bacterial infection, IV 15 mg/kg (about 1 g for a 70-kg adult) as a loading dose, infused over 1 h, followed by 7.5 mg/kg (about 500 mg for a 70-kg adult) q6h as a maintenance dose, infused over 1 h. Duration usually 7–10 d; maximum dose 4 g/d *Surgical prophylaxis,* colorectal surgery: IV, 15 mg/kg, infused over 30–60 min, infusion to be completed about 1 h before surgery, followed by 7.5 mg/kg, infused over 30–60 min, at 6 h and 12 h after the initial dose *C. difficile* colitis: PO, 1–2 g daily for 7–10 d *Children:* Dosage not established | Recommended that breast-feeding be discontinued for 12–24 h following single dose therapy to allow for excretion Alcohol ingestion may cause a disulfiram-like response |
| **Quinupristin-dalfopristin** (Synercid) Pregnancy Category B | *Adults:* IV, 7.5 mg/kg over 60 min q12h for skin and skin structure infections, and q8h for VREF bacteremia *Children:* Dosage not established | Incompatible with saline for infusion |
| **Spectinomycin** (Trobicin) Pregnancy Category B | *Adults:* IM, 2 g in a single dose *Children:* Dosage not established | For IM use only |

*(continued)*

**DRUG TABLE 30-4**

## *Drugs at a Glance*
## Miscellaneous Antibacterials (Continued)

| Generic/Trade Name | Routes and Dosage Ranges | Comments |
|---|---|---|
| **Vancomycin** (Vancocin) Pregnancy Category C | *Adults:* PO, 500 mg q6h or 1 g q12h; maximum dose, 4 g/d IV, 2 g/d in two to four divided doses, q6–12h *Children:* PO, IV, 40 mg/kg/d in divided doses *Infants and Neonates:* IV, 15 mg/kg initially, then 10 mg/kg q12h for neonates up to 7 d of age, then q8h up to 1 mo of age | Drug levels should be obtained after the third dose unless otherwise directed; peaks are drawn 1 h after infusion; troughs obtained before next dose |

Linezolid is indicated for septicemia, pneumonia (both community acquired and nosocomial) and skin and skin structure infections. The drug is bacteriostatic against enterococci (including faecalis and faecium) and staphylococci (including methicillin-resistant strains), and bactericidal for most streptococci.

Myelosuppression (eg, anemia, leukopenia, pancytopenia, thrombocytopenia) is a serious adverse effect. The client's complete blood count should be monitored; if myelosuppression occurs, linezolid should be discontinued. Myelosuppression usually improves with drug discontinuation. Pseudomembranous colitis may also occur. Mild cases usually resolve with drug discontinuation; moderate or severe cases may require fluid and electrolyte replacement and an antibacterial drug that is effective against *Clostridium difficile* organisms. Hypertension may occur with the concomitant ingestion of linezolid and adrenergic drugs or large amounts of tyramine-containing foods (eg, aged cheeses, tap beers, red wines, sauerkraut, soy sauce).

**Metronidazole** (Flagyl) is effective against anaerobic bacteria, including gram-negative bacilli such as *Bacteroides,* gram-positive bacilli such as *Clostridia,* and some gram-positive cocci. It is also effective against protozoa that cause amebiasis, giardiasis, and trichomoniasis (see Chap. 33).

Clinical indications for use include prevention or treatment of anaerobic bacterial infections (eg, in colorectal surgery and intraabdominal infections) and treatment of *Clostridium difficile* infections associated with pseudomembranous colitis. It is contraindicated during the first trimester of pregnancy and must be used with caution in clients with CNS or blood disorders.

Metronidazole is carcinogenic in rodents, if given in high doses for prolonged periods, but there is no evidence that people treated with therapeutic doses have increased risks for development of cancer. The drug is widely distributed in body fluids and tissues, metabo-

lized in the liver, and excreted mostly (60% to 80%) in urine, with a small amount excreted in feces.

**Quinupristin-dalfopristin** (Synercid) belongs to a class of antimicrobials referred to as streptogramins. Both components are active antimicrobials that affect bacterial ribosomes to decrease protein synthesis. The combination is bacteriostatic against *Enterococcus faecium* (including vancomycin-resistant strains) and bactericidal against both methicillin-susceptible and methicillin-resistant strains of staphylococci. It is not active against *Enterococcus faecalis.* The combination undergoes biliary excretion and fecal elimination.

Quinupristin-dalfopristin is indicated for skin and skin structure infections caused by *S. aureus* or group A streptococcus. It is also used for treatment of clients with serious or life-threatening infections associated with vancomycin-resistant *Enterococcus faecium* (VREF) bacteremia.

Quinupristin-dalfopristin is a strong inhibitor of cytochrome P450 3A4 enzymes and therefore interferes with the metabolism of drugs such as cyclosporine, antiretrovirals, carbamazepine, and many others. Toxicity may occur with the inhibited drugs.

**Spectinomycin** (Trobicin) is used for treatment of gonococcal exposure or infection in people who are allergic to or unable to take preferred drugs (the cephalosporins ceftriaxone or cefixime, or the fluoroquinolones ciprofloxacin or ofloxacin). It may be used during pregnancy when clients cannot tolerate cephalosporins and when fluoroquinolones are contraindicated. Spectinomycin has no activity against infections caused by *Chlamydia* organisms, which often accompany gonorrhea.

**Vancomycin** is active only against gram-positive microorganisms. It acts by inhibiting cell wall synthesis. Vancomycin is indicated only for the treatment of severe infections. Parenteral vancomycin has been used extensively to treat infections caused by MRSA and methicillin-resistant staphylococcal species non-aureus (SSNA, including *Staphylococcus epidermidis*) and endocarditis caused by *Streptococcus viridans* (in clients allergic to or with infections resistant to penicillins and cephalosporins) or *Enterococcus faecalis* (with an aminoglycoside). *S. pneumoniae* remain susceptible to vancomycin, although vancomycin-tolerant strains have been identified. The drug has also been widely used for prophylaxis of gram-positive infections in clients who are at high risk for developing MRSA infections (eg, those with diabetes, previous hospitalization, or MRSA in their nasal passages) and who require placement of long-term intravascular catheters and other invasive treatment or monitoring devices. Oral vancomycin has been used extensively to treat staphylococcal enterocolitis and pseudomembranous colitis caused by *C. difficile.*

Partly because of this widespread use, vancomycin-resistant enterococci (VRE) are being encountered more often, especially in critical care units, and treatment options for infections caused by these organisms are very limited. To decrease the spread of VRE, the Centers for Disease Control and Prevention recommends limiting the use of vancomycin. Specific recommendations include avoiding or minimizing use in empiric treatment of febrile clients with neutropenia (unless the prevalence of MRSA or SSNA is high); initial treatment for *C. difficile* colitis (metronidazole is preferred); and prophylaxis for surgery, low-birthweight infants, intravascular catheter colonization or infection, and peritoneal dialysis.

For systemic infections, vancomycin is given intravenously and reaches therapeutic plasma levels within 1 hour after infusion. It is very important to give IV infusions slowly, over 1 to 2 hours, to avoid an adverse reaction characterized by hypotension and flushing and skin rash. This reaction, sometimes called *red man syndrome,* is attributed to histamine release. Vancomycin is excreted through the kidneys; dosage should be reduced in the presence of renal impairment. For bacterial colitis, vancomycin is given orally because it is not absorbed from the GI tract and acts within the bowel lumen. Large amounts of vancomycin are excreted in the feces after oral administration.

Culture and susceptibility reports and local susceptibility patterns should be reviewed to determine whether an antibiotic-resistant pathogen is present in the client. This is particularly important before starting vancomycin, quinupristin-dalfopristin, or linezolid. These drugs have relatively narrow spectra of activity, and appropriate indications for their use should be observed to decrease the likelihood of resistance.

## Management Considerations

### Preventing Toxicity with Chloramphenicol

Blood dyscrasias (potentially serious and life-threatening) have occurred in clients taking chloramphenicol. Irreversible bone marrow depression may appear weeks or months after therapy. A dose-related reversible bone marrow depression usually responds to discontinuation of the drug. Clients should be monitored with a complete blood count, platelet count, reticulocyte count, and serum iron level every 2 days. In addition, periodic measurements of serum drug levels are recommended. Therapeutic levels are 10 to 20 mcg/mL.

### Preventing Toxicity With Clindamycin

If diarrhea develops in a client receiving clindamycin, the drug should be stopped. If the diarrhea is severe and persistent, stools should be checked for white blood cells, blood, mucus, and the presence of *C. difficile* toxin. Proctoscopy can be done to determine more definitively whether the client has pseudomembranous colitis, a potentially fatal adverse reaction. If lesions are seen on proctoscopy, the drug should be stopped immediately. Although pseudomembranous colitis may occur with any antibiotic, it has often been associated with clindamycin therapy.

## Use of Aminoglycosides in Specific Situations

### Guidelines for Reducing Toxicity of Aminoglycosides

In addition to the preceding recommendations, guidelines to decrease the incidence and severity of adverse effects include the following:

1. Identify clients at high risk for adverse effects (eg, neonates, older adults, clients with renal impairment, clients with disease processes or drug therapies that impair blood circulation and renal function).
2. Keep clients well hydrated to decrease drug concentration in serum and body tissues. The drugs reach higher concentrations in the kidneys and inner ears than in other body tissues. This is a major factor in nephrotoxicity and ototoxicity. The goal of an adequate fluid intake is to decrease the incidence and severity of these adverse effects.
3. Use caution with concurrent administration of diuretics. Diuretics may increase the risk for nephrotoxicity by decreasing fluid volume, thereby increasing drug concentration in serum and tissues. Dehydration is most likely to occur with loop diuretics such as furosemide.
4. Give the drug for no longer than 10 days unless necessary for treatment of certain infections. Clients are most at risk when high doses are given for prolonged periods.
5. Detect adverse effects early and reduce dosage or discontinue the drug. Changes in renal function tests that indicate nephrotoxicity may not occur until the client has received an aminoglycoside for several days. If nephrotoxicity occurs, it is usually reversible if the drug is stopped. Early ototoxicity is detectable only with audiometry and is generally not reversible.

### Use in Renal Impairment

Aminoglycosides are nephrotoxic and must be used very cautiously in clients with renal impairment; they require dosage adjustments in renal impairment. Dosage guidelines have been established according to creatinine clearance and often involve lower dosages and prolonged intervals between doses (eg, 36 to 72 hours). Guidelines for reducing nephrotoxicity of aminoglycosides are as listed previously.

### Use in Hepatic Impairment

With aminoglycosides, hepatic impairment is not a significant factor because the drugs are excreted through the kidneys.

## Use of Fluoroquinolones in Specific Situations

### Use in Renal Impairment

Fluoroquinolones are nephrotoxic and must be used very cautiously and require dosage adjustments in clients with renal impairment. Dosage guidelines have been established according to creatinine clearance and often involve lower dosages and prolonged intervals between doses (eg, 36 to 72 hours).

With fluoroquinolones, reported renal effects include azotemia, crystalluria, hematuria, interstitial nephritis, nephropathy, and renal failure. Nephrotoxicity occurs less often than with aminoglycosides, and most cases of acute renal failure have occurred in older adults. It is unknown whether renal failure is caused by hypersensitivity or a direct toxic effect. Crystalluria rarely occurs in acidic urine but may occur in alkaline urine. Guidelines for reducing nephrotoxicity include lower dosages, longer intervals between doses, adequate hydration, and avoiding substances that alkalinize the urine.

Oral fluoroquinolones are often self-administered at home. Individuals with renal or hepatic failure are at greater risk for complications associated with therapy and should often be monitored in the home.

### Use in Hepatic Impairment

With fluoroquinolones, hepatotoxicity has been observed with some of the drugs. Clinical manifestations range from abnormalities in liver enzyme test results to hepatitis, liver necrosis, or hepatic failure. Because of serious hepatotoxicity with trovafloxacin, the FDA issued a public health advisory to use the drug only for serious infections, give initial doses in an inpatient setting, administer no longer than 14 days, and discontinue the drug if liver dysfunction occurs.

## Use of Macrolides and Miscellaneous Drugs in Specific Situations

### Use in Renal Impairment

With the macrolides, dosage of erythromycin does not need reduction because erythromycin is excreted mainly by the liver. With the newer drugs, there are no data about azithromycin dosage in renal impairment, and no dosage reduction is recommended for dirithromycin. However, clarithromycin dosage should be halved or the dosing interval doubled in clients with severe renal impairment (creatinine clearance [CrCl] <30 mL/minute). In addition, the combination of clarithromycin and ranitidine bismuth citrate therapy (Tritec; used to treat peptic ulcers associated with *H. pylori* infection) is not recommended in clients with severe renal impairment (CrCl <25 mL/minute).

Dosage of clindamycin does not need reduction in renal impairment because clindamycin is excreted primarily by the liver. Dosage of vancomycin should be reduced because vancomycin is excreted mainly by the kidneys and accumulates in renal impairment. In addition, vancomycin may be nephrotoxic with IV administration, high serum concentrations, prolonged therapy, use in elderly or neonates, and concomitant use of other nephrotoxic drugs. Thus, in addition to reduced dosage, renal function and serum drug levels should be monitored (therapeutic levels are 10 to 25 mcg/mL). Dosages of quinupristin-dalfopristin and linezolid do not need to be reduced in clients with renal failure.

### Use in Hepatic Impairment

Erythromycin should be used cautiously, if at all, in clients with hepatic impairment. It is metabolized in the liver to an active metabolite that is excreted in the bile. Avoiding the drug or dosage reduction may be needed in liver failure. It has also been associated with cholestatic hepatitis, most often with the estolate formulation (eg, Ilosone). Symptoms, which may include nausea, vomiting, fever, and jaundice, usually occur after 1 to 2 weeks of drug administration and subside when the drug is stopped.

Other macrolides vary in their hepatic effects. Azithromycin is mainly eliminated unchanged in bile and could accumulate with impaired liver function. It should be used with caution. Clarithromycin is metabolized in the liver to an active metabolite that is then excreted through the kidneys. Dosage reduction is not recommended for clients with hepatic impairment and normal renal function but is required with severe renal impairment (see earlier). Dirithromycin is metabolized in the liver to an active metabolite that is then excreted in bile and feces. No dosage reduction is recommended for mild hepatic impairment. Because effects in moderate to severe hepatic impairment have not been studied, the drug should be used only if absolutely necessary.

Clindamycin, chloramphenicol, and metronidazole should be used cautiously, if at all, in the presence of liver disease. Because these drugs are eliminated through the liver, they may accumulate and cause toxic effects. When feasible, other drugs should be substituted. If no effective substitutes are available, dosage should be reduced. With quinupristin-dalfopristin and linezolid, there are currently no recommendations to alter dosage in hepatic impairment.

*(text continues on page 531)*

## Nursing Actions

## Aminoglycosides, Fluoroquinolones, Macrolides, and Miscellaneous Antibacterials

| Nursing Actions | Rationale/Explanation |
|---|---|
| 1. Administer accurately. | |
| a. With aminoglycosides: | |
| (1) For intravenous (IV) administration, dilute the drug in 50 to 100 mL of 5% dextrose or 0.9% sodium chloride injection and infuse over 30 to 60 min. The concentration of gentamicin solution should not exceed 1 mg/mL. | To achieve therapeutic blood levels |
| (2) Give intramuscular aminoglycosides in a large muscle mass, and rotate sites. | To avoid local tissue irritation. This is less likely to occur with aminoglycosides than with most other antibiotics. |
| b. With fluoroquinolones: | |
| (1) Give norfloxacin and enoxacin 1 h before or 2 h after a meal. Do not give ofloxacin with food. Ciprofloxacin, lomefloxacin, and sparfloxacin may be given without regard to food intake. | To promote therapeutic plasma drug levels. Food in the gastrointestinal (GI) tract interferes with absorption of most oral fluoroquinolones. |
| (2) Give IV infusions over 60 min. | To decrease vein irritation and phlebitis |
| (3) When giving ciprofloxacin IV into a primary IV line (eg, using piggyback or Y connector), stop the primary solution until ciprofloxacin is infused. | To avoid physical or chemical incompatibilities |
| c. With macrolides: | |
| (1) Give oral erythromycin preparations according to manufacturers' instructions, with 6 to 8 oz of water, at evenly spaced intervals, around the clock. | Some should be taken on an empty stomach; some can be taken without regard to meals. Adequate water aids absorption; regular intervals help to maintain therapeutic blood levels. |
| (2) With azithromycin, give the oral suspension on an empty stomach, 1 h before or 2 h after a meal. Give tablets without regard to meals. Do not give oral azithromycin with aluminum- or magnesium-containing antacids. | Food decreases absorption of the suspension; antacids decrease absorption of tablets and the suspension |
| (3) With clarithromycin, give regular tablets and the oral suspension with or without food. Give the extended-release tablets (Biaxin XL) with food. Shake the suspension well before measuring the dose. | Manufacturer's recommendations. All suspensions should be mixed well to measure accurately. |
| (4) With dirithromycin, give with food or within 1 h after a meal. | |
| (5) For IV erythromycin, consult the manufacturer's instructions for dissolving, diluting, and administering the drug. Infuse continuously or intermittently (eg, q6h over 30–60 min). | The IV formulation has limited stability in solution, and instructions must be followed carefully to achieve therapeutic effects. Also, instructions differ for intermittent and continuous infusions. IV erythromycin is the treatment of choice for Legionnaires disease. Otherwise, it is rarely used. |
| d. With chloramphenicol: | |
| (1) Give oral drug 1 h before or 2 h after meals, q6h around the clock. If GI upset occurs, give with food. | To increase absorption and maintain therapeutic blood levels |
| (2) Mix IV chloramphenicol in 50–100 mL of 5% dextrose in water and infuse over 15–30 min. | |
| e. With clindamycin: | |
| (1) Give capsules with a full glass of water. | To avoid esophageal irritation |
| (2) Do not refrigerate reconstituted oral solution. | Refrigeration is not required for drug stability and may thicken the solution, making it difficult to measure and pour accurately. |

(continued)

## Nursing Actions

## Aminoglycosides, Fluoroquinolones, Macrolides, and Miscellaneous Antibacterials (Continued)

| Nursing Actions | Rationale/Explanation |
|---|---|
| (3) Give IM injections deeply, and rotate sites. Do not give more than 600 mg in a single injection. | To decrease pain, induration, and abscess formation |
| (4) For IV administration, dilute 300 mg in 50 mL of IV fluid and give over 10 min, or dilute 600 mg in 100 mL and give over 20 min. **Do not** give clindamycin undiluted or by direct injection. | Dilution decreases risks for phlebitis. Cardiac arrest has been reported with bolus injections of clindamycin. |
| f. With linezolid: | |
| (1) Give oral tablets and suspension without regard to meals. | Manufacturer's recommendations. |
| (2) For IV administration, the drug is compatible with 5% dextrose, 0.9% sodium chloride, and lactated Ringer's solutions. | |
| (3) Infuse the drug over 30 to 120 minutes. If other drugs are being given through the same IV line, flush the line with one of the above solutions before and after linezolid administration. | |
| g. With IV metronidazole, check the manufacturer's instructions. | The drug requires specific techniques for preparation and administration. |
| h. With quinupristin-dalfopristin: | |
| (1) Give IV, mixed in a minimum of 250 mL of 5% dextrose solution and infused over 60 minutes. | Dilution in at least 250 mL of IV solution decreases venous irritation. A central venous catheter may also be used for drug administration, to decrease irritation. |
| (2) Do *not* mix the drug or flush the IV line with saline- or heparin-containing solutions. | The drug is incompatible with saline- and heparin-containing solutions. |
| i. With vancomycin, dilute 500-mg doses in 100 mL and 1-g doses in 200 mL of 0.9% NaCl or 5% dextrose injection and infuse over at least 60 min. | To decrease hypotension and flushing (ie, "red man syndrome") that may occur with more rapid IV administration. This reaction is attributed to histamine release and may be prevented by prior administration of diphenhydramine, an antihistamine. Dilution also decreases pain and phlebitis at the injection site. |
| 2. **Observe for therapeutic effects.** | See Chapter 28. |
| a. Decreased local and systemic signs of infection | |
| b. Decreased signs and symptoms of the specific infection for which the drug is being given | |
| 3. **Observe for adverse effects.** | Adverse effects are more likely to occur with parenteral administration of large doses for prolonged periods. However, they may occur with oral administration in the presence of renal impairment and with usual therapeutic doses. |
| a. With aminoglycosides, observe for: | |
| (1) Nephrotoxicity—casts, albumin, red or white blood cells in urine, decreased creatinine clearance, increased serum creatinine, increased blood urea nitrogen. | Renal damage is most likely to occur in clients who are elderly, receive high doses or prolonged therapy, have prior renal damage, or receive other nephrotoxic drugs. This is the most serious adverse reaction. Risks of kidney damage can be minimized by using the drugs appropriately, detecting early signs of renal impairment, and keeping clients well hydrated. |
| (2) Ototoxicity—deafness or decreased hearing, tinnitus, dizziness, ataxia | This results from damage to the eighth cranial nerve. Incidence of ototoxicity is increased in older clients and those with previous auditory damage, high doses or prolonged duration, and concurrent use of other ototoxic drugs. |

*(continued)*

## Nursing Actions

### Aminoglycosides, Fluoroquinolones, Macrolides, and Miscellaneous Antibacterials (Continued)

| Nursing Actions | Rationale/Explanation |
|---|---|
| (3) Neurotoxicity—respiratory paralysis and apnea | This is caused by neuromuscular blockade and is more likely to occur after rapid IV injection, administration to a client with myasthenia gravis, or concomitant administration of general anesthetics or neuromuscular blocking agents (eg, succinylcholine, tubocurarine). This effect also may occur if an aminoglycoside is administered shortly after surgery, owing to the residual effects of anesthetics or neuromuscular blockers. Neostigmine or calcium may be given to counteract apnea. |
| (4) Hypersensitivity—skin rash, urticaria | This is an uncommon reaction except with topical neomycin, which may cause sensitization in as many as 10% of recipients. |
| (5) Nausea, vomiting, diarrhea, peripheral neuritis, paresthesias | Uncommon with parenteral aminoglycosides. Diarrhea often occurs with oral administration. |
| b. With fluoroquinolones, observe for: | The drugs are usually well tolerated. |
| (1) Hepatotoxicity (abnormal liver enzyme tests, hepatitis, hepatic failure) | Hepatotoxicity has been observed with most of the drugs. Trovafloxacin use is restricted because of liver damage and failure. |
| (2) Allergic reactions (anaphylaxis, urticaria) | Uncommon, but some fatalities have been reported. |
| (3) Nausea, vomiting, diarrhea, pseudomembranous colitis | Nausea is the most common GI symptom. |
| (4) Headache, dizziness | |
| (5) Crystalluria | Uncommon, but may occur with an inadequate fluid intake |
| (6) Photosensitivity (skin redness, rash, itching) | May occur with most fluoroquinolones with exposure to sunlight |
| (7) Other | Adverse effects involving most body systems have been reported with one or more of the fluoroquinolones. Most have a low incidence (<1%) of occurrence. |
| c. With macrolides: | |
| (1) Nausea, vomiting, diarrhea | These are the most frequent adverse reactions, reportedly less common with azithromycin and clarithromycin than with erythromycin. |
| (2) With IV erythromycin, phlebitis at the IV infusion site | The drug is very irritating to body tissues. Phlebitis can be minimized by diluting the drug well, infusing it slowly, and not using the same vein more than 48–72 h, if possible. |
| (3) Hepatotoxicity—nausea, vomiting, abdominal cramps, fever, leukocytosis, abnormal liver function, cholestatic jaundice | More likely to occur with the estolate formulation of erythromycin; less likely to occur with the newer macrolides than with erythromycin. |
| (4) Allergic reactions (anaphylaxis, skin rash, urticaria) | Potentially serious but infrequent |
| d. With chloramphenicol: | |
| (1) Bone marrow depression (anemia, leukopenia, thrombocytopenia) | Blood dyscrasias are the most serious adverse reaction to chloramphenicol. |
| (2) Clinical signs of infection or bleeding | |
| e. With clindamycin: | |
| (1) Nausea, vomiting, diarrhea | These are the most frequent adverse effects and may be severe enough to require stopping the drug. |
| (2) Pseudomembranous colitis (also called antibiotic-associated colitis)—severe diarrhea, fever, stools containing neutrophils and shreds of mucous membrane | May occur with most antibiotics but is more common with oral clindamycin. It is caused by *Clostridium difficile*. The organism produces a toxin that kills mucosal cells and produces superficial ulcerations that are visible with sigmoidoscopy. Discontinuing the drug and giving oral metronidazole are curative measures. |

*(continued)*

## Nursing Actions

### Aminoglycosides, Fluoroquinolones, Macrolides, and Miscellaneous Antibacterials (Continued)

| Nursing Actions | Rationale/Explanation |
|---|---|
| f. With linezolid: | |
| (1) Nausea, vomiting, diarrhea | These are common effects. |
| (2) Bone marrow depression (anemia, leukopenia, thrombocytopenia) | Complete blood cell counts (CBCs) are recommended weekly to monitor for myelosupression. If it occurs, the drug should be discontinued. |
| (3) Pseudomembranous colitis (PMC) | May occur with linezolid as with other antibiotics. If it occurs, the drug should be discontinued. |
| g. With metronidazole: | |
| (1) Central nervous system effects—convulsive seizures, peripheral paresthesias, ataxia, confusion, dizziness, headache | Convulsions and peripheral neuropathy may be serious effects; GI effects are most common. |
| (2) GI effects—nausea, vomiting, diarrhea | |
| (3) Dermatologic effects—skin rash, pruritus, thrombophlebitis at infusion sites | |
| h. With quinupristin-dalfopristin: | |
| (1) IV infusion site reactions (pain, edema, inflammation) | The most common adverse effects during clinical trials. Moderate to severe venous irritation can occur with administration through peripheral veins. This can be prevented by infusion through a central venous IV line. |
| (2) Nausea, vomiting, diarrhea | These effects occurred in 2.7% to 4.6% of subjects in clinical trials. Most other adverse effects occurred in fewer than 1%. |
| i. With vancomycin: | |
| (1) Nephrotoxicity—oliguria, increased blood urea nitrogen and serum creatinine | Uncommon. Most likely to occur with large doses, concomitant administration of an aminoglycoside antibiotic, or pre-existing renal impairment. Usually resolves when vancomycin is discontinued. |
| (2) Ototoxicity—hearing loss, tinnitus | Most likely to occur in people with renal impairment or a preexisting hearing loss |
| (3) Red man syndrome—hypotension, skin flushing | Occurs with rapid infusion of IV vancomycin. Can be prevented by adequate dilution and infusing over 1–2 h or premedicating with diphenhydramine (an antihistamine). |
| 4. Observe for drug interactions. | |
| a. Drugs that *increase* effects of aminoglycosides: | The listed drugs increase toxicity. |
| (1) Amphotericin B, cephalosporins, cisplatin, cyclosporine, enflurane, vancomycin | These drugs are nephrotoxic alone and may increase nephrotoxicity of aminoglycosides. |
| (2) Loop diuretics (furosemide, bumetanide) | Increased ototoxicity |
| (3) Neuromuscular blocking agents (eg, pancuronium, vecuronium) | Increased neuromuscular blockade with possible paralysis of respiratory muscles and apnea |
| b. Drugs that *increase* effects of fluoroquinolones: Cimetidine, probenecid | Cimetidine inhibits hepatic metabolism and probenecid inhibits renal excretion of fluoroquinolones. These actions may increase serum drug levels. |
| c. Drugs that *increase* effects of erythromycin: | |
| (1) Chloramphenicol | The combination is effective against some strains of resistant *Staphylococcus aureus.* |
| (2) Streptomycin | The combination is effective against the enterococcus in bacteremia, brain abscess, endocarditis, meningitis, and urinary tract infection |
| d. Drugs that *increase* effects of clarithromycin: | |
| (1) Fluconazole | Probably inhibits metabolism of clarithromycin |
| e. Drugs that *increase* effects of dirithyromycin: | |
| (1) Antacids, histamine-2 ($H_2$) receptor antagonists | These agents raise gastric pH and slightly increase absorption of dirithromycin. |
| f. Drug that *increases* effects of metronidazole: | Inhibits hepatic metabolism of metronidazole |
| (1) Cimetidine | |

*(continued)*

## Nursing Actions

### Aminoglycosides, Fluoroquinolones, Macrolides, and Miscellaneous Antibacterials (Continued)

| Nursing Actions | Rationale/Explanation |
|---|---|
| g. Drugs that *decrease* effects of fluoroquinolones: | |
| (1) Antacids, iron preparations, sucralfate, zinc preparations | These drugs interfere with absorption of fluoroquinolones from the GI tract. |
| (2) Antineoplastic drugs | These drugs may decrease serum levels of fluoroquinolones. |
| (3) Bismuth subsalicylate (eg, Pepto-Bismol) decreases enoxacin absorption if given with or within 1 h after enoxacin. | These drugs should not be taken together or within 1 h of each other. |
| (4) Nitrofurantoin may decrease the antibacterial effect of norfloxacin in the urinary tract | |
| h. Drugs that *decrease* effects of azithromycin: | |
| (1) Antacids | Antacids decrease peak serum levels |
| i. Drugs that *decrease* effects of chloramphenicol: | |
| (1) Enzyme inducers (eg, rifampin) | Reduce serum levels, probably by accelerating liver metabolism of chloramphenicol |
| j. Drugs that *decrease* effects of clindamycin: | |
| (1) Erythromycin | Delays absorption |
| (2) Kaolin-pectin | |
| k. Drugs that *decrease* effects of metronidazole: | |
| (1) Enzyme inducers (phenobarbital, phenytoin, prednisone, rifampin) | These drugs induce hepatic enzymes and decrease effects of metronidazole by accelerating its rate of hepatic metabolism. |

## ? How Can You Avoid This Medication Error?

**Answer:** This error occurred because the drug infused too rapidly. Although the IV rate was calculated correctly, the IV could have been positional, which could have caused the sudden infusing of medication. When giving a medication such as this, it is best to use an IV controller pump to regulate the infusion rate. The rapid infusion of vancomycin caused the flushing, which is sometimes referred to as the "red man effect." This is not an allergic reaction, but is caused by histamine release and vasodilation when infusion is too fast. This reaction can be limited by slowing the infusion or premedication with an antihistamine.

## Critical Thinking Exercises

1. Erythromycin interferes with the elimination of several drugs, especially those:
   a. Excreted by the kidneys
   b. Metabolized by the cytochrome P450 enzymes in the liver
   c. That have significant first-pass effect in the liver
   d. With prolonged half-life following oral administration

2. Although an aminoglycoside and an antipseudomonal penicillin are administered together for synergistic therapeutic effects, they should not be combined in a syringe or IV fluid for administration because the aminoglycoside will:
   a. Be deactivated
   b. Cause a hypersensitivity reaction
   c. Reach toxic levels
   d. Cause ototoxicity

3. In urinary tract infections, smaller doses of aminoglycosides can be used than in systemic infections because the aminoglycosides:
   a. Are broken down in the liver
   b. Reach high concentrations in the urine
   c. Have minimal side effects
   d. Have local susceptibility patterns

4. Measurement of both peak and trough levels helps to maintain therapeutic serum levels without excessive toxicity. When should peak serum concentrations be assessed?
   a. 15 to 30 minutes before drug administration
   b. 30 to 60 minutes before drug administration
   c. 15 to 30 minutes after drug administration
   d. 30 to 60 minutes after drug administration

**5.** Early ototoxicity with an aminoglycoside is:
   a. Generally not reversible
   b. Usually reversible
   c. Unlikely with intravenous administration
   d. Readily detectible in normal conversations

## SELECTED REFERENCES

Chambers, H. F. (2001). Antimicrobial agents: Protein synthesis inhibitors and miscellaneous antibacterial agents; Antimicrobial agents: The aminoglycosides. In J. G. Hardman & L. E. Limbird (Eds.), *Goodman & Gilman's the pharmacological basis of therapeutics* (10th ed., pp. 1219–1271). New York: McGraw-Hill.

*Drug facts and comparisons.* (Updated monthly). St. Louis: Facts and Comparisons.

Fisman, D. N., and Kaye, K. M. (2000). Antibacterial therapy: Once-daily dosing of aminoglycoside antibiotics. *Infectious Disease Clinics of North America, 14*(2), 475–487.

Harwell, J. I., & Brown, R. B. (2000). The drug-resistant pneumococcus: Clinical relevance, therapy, and prevention. *Chest, 117*(2), 530–541.

Hooper, D. C. (1998). Expanding uses of fluoroquinolones: Opportunities and challenges. *Annals of Internal Medicine, 129*, 908–911.

Hospital Infection Control Practices Advisory Committee (HICPAC) (1995). Recommendations for preventing the spread of vancomycin resistance: Recommendations of the Hospital Infection Control Practices Advisory Committee (HICPAC). *Morbidity & Mortality Weekly, 44*(RR12), 1–13.

Lacy, C. F., Armstrong, L. L., Goldman, M. P., & Lance, L. L. (2003). *Lexi-Comp's drug information handbook* (11th ed.). Hudson, OH: American Pharmaceutical Association.

Lipsky, B. A., & Baker, C. A. (1999). Fluoroquinolone toxicity profiles: A review focusing on newer agents. *Clinical Infectious Diseases, 28*, 352–364.

Moellering, R. C. (1998). Vancomycin-resistant enterococci. *Clinical Infectious Diseases, 26*, 1196–1199.

Paterson, D. L., Robson, J. M. B., & Wagener, M. M. (1998). Risk factors for toxicity in elderly clients given aminoglycosides once daily. *Journal of General Internal Medicine, 13*, 735–739.

Petri, W. A., Jr. (2001). Antimicrobial agents: Sulfonamides, trimethoprim-sulfamethoxazole, quinolones, and agents for urinary tract infections. In J. G. Hardman & L. E. Limbird (Eds.), *Goodman & Gilman's the pharmacological basis of therapeutics* (10th ed., pp. 1171–1188). New York: McGraw-Hill.

Steigbigel, N. H. (2000). Macrolides and clindamycin. In G. L. Mandell, J. E. Bennett, & R. Dolin (Eds.), *Principles and practice of infectious diseases* (5th ed., pp 367–382). Philadelphia: Churchill Livingstone.

U.S. Food and Drug Administration. (1999). *Public health advisory: Trovan (trovafloxacin)*. Washington, DC: Author.

Zuckerman, J. M. (2000). The newer macrolides: Azithromycin and clarithromycin. *Infectious Disease Clinics of North America, 14*(2), 449–462.

# 31

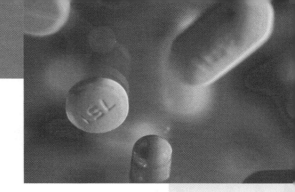

# Tetracyclines, Sulfonamides, and Urinary Agents

## OBJECTIVES

*After studying this chapter, the student will be able to:*

1 Discuss major characteristics and clinical uses of tetracyclines.

2 Recognize doxycycline as the tetracycline of choice for use in clients with renal failure.

3 Give characteristics, clinical uses, adverse effects, and nursing implications of selected sulfonamides.

4 Recognize trimethoprim-sulfamethoxazole as a combination drug that is commonly used for urinary tract and systemic infections.

5 Describe the use of urinary antiseptics in the treatment of urinary tract infections.

6 Teach clients strategies for preventing, recognizing, and treating urinary tract infections.

## CRITICAL THINKING SCENARIO

*F*aye Sullivan, 15 years of age, comes to the walk-in clinic with symptoms of urgency, frequency, and dysuria. A routine urinalysis indicates the presence of infection. The urinary tract infection (UTI) is treated with Bactrim for 10 days.

✔ What factors increase the incidence of UTI in adolescent girls?

✔ What important information should be included when teaching Faye about Bactrim therapy?

✔ Describe strategies to prevent future UTIs.

✔ List the data you need to collect to determine whether Faye's UTI is responding to treatment.

## PROTOTYPE PROFILE

tetracycline, (Achromycin, others) p. 539

# OVERVIEW

Tetracyclines and sulfonamides are older, broad-spectrum, bacteriostatic drugs that are rarely used for systemic infections because of microbial resistance and the development of more effective or less toxic drugs. However, the drugs are useful in selected infections. Urinary antiseptics are used only in urinary tract infections (UTIs). These drugs are described later in this chapter and listed later in Drugs at a Glance 31-1, 31-2, and 31-3.

The tetracyclines are similar in pharmacologic properties and antimicrobial activity. They are effective against a wide range of gram-positive and gram-negative organisms, although they are usually not drugs of choice. Bacterial infections caused by *Brucella* species and *Vibrio cholerae* are still treated by tetracyclines. The drugs also remain effective against rickettsiae, chlamydia, mycoplasma, some protozoa, spirochetes, and others. They are widely distributed into most body tissues and fluids. The older tetracyclines are excreted mainly in urine; doxycycline is eliminated in urine and feces, and minocycline is eliminated mainly by the liver. Individual tetracyclines are discussed in Drugs at a Glance 31-1: Tetracyclines.

Sulfonamides are bacteriostatic against a wide range of gram-positive and gram-negative bacteria, although increasing resistance is making them less useful. Susceptibility should be documented, but sulfonamides may be active against *Streptococcus pyogenes,* some staphylococcal strains, *Haemophilus influenzae, Nocardia* species, *Chlamydia trachomatis,* and toxoplasmosis. The combination of trimethoprim-sulfamethoxazole is useful in urinary tract infections due to Enterobacteriaceae, bronchitis, and *Pneumocystis carinii* infection (in high doses). Individual drugs vary in extent of systemic absorption and clinical indications. Some are well absorbed and can be used in systemic infections; others are poorly absorbed and exert more local effects. Sulfonamides are discussed in Drugs at a Glance 31-2: Sulfonamide Preparations.

**DRUG TABLE 31-1**

## *Drugs at a Glance*
## Tetracyclines

| Generic/Trade Name | Routes and Dosage Ranges | Comments/Uses |
|---|---|---|
| **Tetracycline** (Achromycin, others) Pregnancy Category D | See Prototype Profile 31-1: Tetracycline | |
| **Demeclocycline** (Declomycin) Pregnancy Category D | *Adults:* PO, 150 mg q6h or 300 mg q12h Gonorrhea in penicillin-sensitive clients, PO 600 mg initially, followed by 300 mg q12h for 4 d *Children:* Age>8 y: PO, 6–12 mg/kg/d in two to four divided doses | 1. The tetracycline most likely to cause photosensitivity 2. Primarily used to treat inappropriate secretion of antidiuretic hormone |
| **Doxycycline** (Vibramycin) Pregnancy Category D | *Adults:* PO, 100 mg q12h for two doses, then 100 mg once daily or in divided doses; severe infections, 100 mg q12h IV, 200 mg the first day, then 100–200 mg daily in one or divided doses; give over 1–4 hours *Children:* Age > 8 y: PO, IV weight ≥ 45 kg: same as adults Weight <45 kg: PO, 4.4 mg/kg/d divided q12h for two doses, then 2.2 mg/kg/d in a single dose; severe infections, 4.4 mg/kg/d in divided doses q12h IV 4.4 mg/kg/d in one or two doses for 1 d, then 2.2–4.4 mg/kg/d as 1 or 2 infusions Give over 1–4 hours | 1. Well absorbed from the gastrointestinal tract. Oral administration yields serum drug levels equivalent to those obtained by parenteral administration. 2. Highly lipid soluble; therefore, reaches therapeutic levels in CSF, the eye, and the prostate gland 3. Can be given in smaller doses and less frequently than other tetracyclines because of long serum half-life (approximately 18 h) 4. Excreted by kidneys to a lesser extent than other tetracyclines and is considered safe for clients with impaired renal function |
| **Minocycline** (Minocin) Pregnancy Category D | *Adults:* PO, IV 200 mg initially, then 100 mg q12h *Children:* >8 y: PO, IV 4 mg/kg initially, then 2 mg/kg, q12h | 1. Well absorbed after oral administration 2. Like doxycycline, readily penetrates CSF, the eye, and the prostate 3. Metabolized more than other tetracyclines, and smaller amounts are excreted in urine and feces |

**DRUG TABLE 31-2**

*Drugs at a Glance*

## Sulfonamide Preparations

| Generic/Trade Name | Routes and Dosage Ranges | Comments/Uses |
|---|---|---|
| **Single Agents** | | |
| **Sulfadiazine**<br>Pregnancy Category B;<br>  D at term | *Adults:* PO, 2–8 gm daily<br>*Children:* >2 mo: PO, 75 mg/kg initially, then 150 mg/kg/d in four to six divided doses; maximal daily dose, 6 g | A short-acting, rapidly absorbed, rapidly excreted agent for systemic infections<br>The addition of folinic acid may be recommended<br>For treatment of<br>  Nocardiosis<br>  Toxoplasmosis |
| **Sulfamethizole**<br>  (Thiosulfil)<br>Pregnancy Category C;<br>  D at term by expert analysis | *Adults:* PO, 500 mg–1 g three or four times daily<br>*Children:* >2 mo: PO 30–45 mg/kg/d in 4 divided doses | A highly soluble, rapidly absorbed, and rapidly excreted agent that is similar to sulfisoxazole in actions and uses |
| **Sulfamethoxazole**<br>  (Gantanol)<br>Pregnancy Category C;<br>  D at term by expert analysis | *Adults:* PO, 2 g initially, then 1–2 g two or three times daily<br>*Children:* >2 mo: PO 50–60 mg/kg initially, then 30 mg/kg q12h; maximal daily dose, 75 mg/kg | For treatment of urinary tract infections<br>Similar to sulfisoxazole in therapeutic effects but absorbed and excreted more slowly. More likely to produce excessive blood levels and crystalluria than sulfisoxazole.<br>An ingredient in mixtures with trimethoprim (see Combination Agent, below)<br>For treatment of<br>  Systemic infections<br>  Urinary tract infections |
| **Sulfasalazine**<br>  (Azulfidine)<br>Pregnancy Category B;<br>  D at term | *Adults:* Ulcerative colitis, PO 3–4 g daily in divided doses initially; 2 g daily in four doses for maintenance; maximal daily dose, 8 g<br>Rheumatoid arthritis, PO 2 g daily in divided doses<br>*Children:* PO 40–60 mg/kg/d in three to six divided doses initially, followed by 30 mg/kg/d in four divided doses | Poorly absorbed<br>Does not alter normal bacterial flora in the intestine. Effectiveness in ulcerative colitis may be due to antibacterial (sulfapyridine) and anti-inflammatory (aminosalicylic acid) metabolites.<br>For treatment of<br>  Ulcerative colitis<br>  Rheumatoid arthritis |
| **Sulfisoxazole**<br>Pregnancy Category B;<br>  D at term | *Adults:* PO, 2–4 g initially, then 4–8 g daily in four to six divided doses<br>Intravaginally, 2.5–5 g of vaginal cream (10%) twice daily<br>*Children:* >2 mo: PO, 75 mg/kg of body weight initially, then 150 mg/kg/d in four to six divided doses; maximal daily dose, 6 g | Rapidly absorbed, rapidly excreted:<br>Highly soluble and less likely to cause crystalluria than most other sulfonamides<br>Used for prevention of bacterial colonization and infection of severe burn wounds |
| **Combination Agent** | | |
| **Trimethoprim-sulfamethoxazole**<br>  (Bactrim, Septra, others)<br>Pregnancy Category C;<br>  D at term by expert analysis | *Adults:* Urinary tract infections, trimethoprim 160 mg and sulfamethoxazole 800 mg PO q12h for 10–14 d<br>Shigellosis, same dose as above for 5 d<br>Severe urinary tract infections, PO, 8–10 mg (trimethoprim component) per kg/d in two to four divided doses, up to 14 d | May exhibit synergistic effectiveness against many organisms (verify susceptibility first), including streptococci (*S. viridans*); staphylococci (*S. epidermidis, S. aureus*); *Escherichia coli; Salmonella; Shigella; Serratia; Klebsiella; Nocardia;* and others. Most strains of *Pseudomonas* are resistant.<br>*(continued)* |

## *Drugs at a Glance*

## Sulfonamide Preparations (Continued)

| Generic/Trade Name | Routes and Dosage Ranges | Comments/Uses |
|---|---|---|
| | *P. carinii* pneumonia, IV, 15–20 mg (trimethoprim component) per kg/d in three or four divided doses, q6–8h up to 14 d<br><br>*Children:* Urinary tract infections, otitis media, and shigellosis, PO, 8 mg/kg trimethoprim and 40 mg/kg sulfamethoxazole in two divided doses q12h for 10 d<br>Severe urinary tract infections, IV, 8–10 mg (trimethoprim component)/kg in two to four divided doses q6–8h or q12h up to 14 d<br>*P. carinii* pneumonia, IV, 15–20 mg (trimethoprim component) per kg/d in three or four divided doses, q6–8h up to 14 d | The two drugs have additive antibacterial effects because they interfere with different steps in bacterial synthesis and activation of folic acid, an essential nutrient.<br>The combination is less likely to produce resistant bacteria than either agent alone.<br>Oral preparations contain different amounts of the two drugs, as follows:<br>a. "Regular" tablets contain trimethoprim 80 mg and sulfamethoxazole 400 mg.<br>b. Double-strength tablets (eg, Bactrim D.S., Septra D.S.) contain trimethoprim 160 mg and sulfamethoxazole 800 mg.<br>c. The oral suspension contains trimethoprim 40 mg and sulfamethoxazole 200 mg in each 5 mL.<br>The IV preparation contains trimethoprim 80 mg and sulfamethoxazole 400 mg in 5 mL.<br>Dosage must be reduced in renal insufficiency.<br>The preparation is contraindicated if creatinine clearance is less than 15 mL/min.<br>The agent is used for acute and chronic urinary tract infections; acute exacerbations of chronic bronchitis; acute otitis media caused by susceptible strains of *Haemophillus influenzae* and *S. pneumoniae;* shigellosis; infection by *Pneumocystis carinii* (prevention and treatment); intravenous preparation indicated for *P. carinii* pneumonia, severe urinary tract infections, and shigellosis. |
| **Topical Sulfonamides**<br><br>**Mafenide**<br>(Sulfamylon)<br>Pregnancy Category C | *Adults:* Topical application to burned area, once or twice daily, in a thin layer<br>*Children:* Same as adults | Effective against most gram-negative and gram-positive organisms, especially *Pseudomonas*<br>Application causes pain and burning.<br>Mafenide is absorbed systemically and may produce metabolic acidosis.<br>Prevention of bacterial colonization and infection of severe burn wounds |

*(continued)*

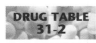

**DRUG TABLE 31-2**

## *Drugs at a Glance*

### Sulfonamide Preparations (Continued)

| Generic/Trade Name | Routes and Dosage Ranges | Comments/Uses |
|---|---|---|
| **Silver sulfadiazine** (Silvadene) Pregnancy Category B | *Adults:* Same as mafenide. Usually the preferred drug. Topical application to burned area once or twice daily in a thin layer *Children:* Same as adults | Effective against most *Pseudomonas* species, the most common pathogen in severe burn sepsis, *E. coli, Klebsiella, Proteus,* staphylococci, and streptococci Application is painless. Does not cause electrolyte or acid–base imbalances Significant amounts may be absorbed systemically with large burned areas and prolonged use. |

UTI, urinary tract infection.

Urinary antiseptics may be bactericidal for sensitive organisms in the urinary tract because they are concentrated in renal tubules and reach high levels in urine. They are not used in systemic infections because they do not attain therapeutic plasma levels. An additional drug, phenazopyridine, is given to relieve pain associated with UTI. It has no antibacterial activity. The general management of infection and common characteristics of antimicrobial drugs are addressed in Chapter 28. Drugs for treatment of UTIs are discussed in Drugs at a Glance 31-3: Miscellaneous Drugs for Urinary Tract Infections. The tetracyclines, sulfonamides, and urinary agents are often self-administered at home. Guidelines for evaluation and intervention are addressed in Home Care Considerations. A discussion of management significance in children and older adults is found in Age-related Considerations.

## Mechanisms of Action

Tetracyclines penetrate microbial cells by passive diffusion and an active transport system. Intracellularly, they bind to 30S ribosomes, like the aminoglycosides, and inhibit microbial protein synthesis. Sulfonamides act as antimetabolites of paraaminobenzoic acid (PABA), which microorganisms require to produce folic acid; folic acid, in turn, is required for the production of bacterial intracellular proteins. Sulfonamides enter into the reaction instead of PABA, compete for the enzyme involved, and cause formation of nonfunctional derivatives of folic acid. Thus, sulfonamides halt multiplication of new bacteria but do not kill mature, fully formed bacteria. With the exception of the topical sulfonamides used in burn therapy, the presence of pus, serum, or necrotic tissue interferes with sulfonamide action because these materials contain PABA. Some bacteria can change

their metabolic pathways to use precursors or other forms of folic acid and thereby develop resistance to the antibacterial action of sulfonamides. Once resistance to one sulfonamide develops, cross-resistance to others is common.

## Indications for Use

A ℗ **tetracycline** is the drug of choice or alternate (sometimes as part of combination therapy) in a few infections (eg, brucellosis, chancroid, cholera, granuloma inguinale, psittacosis, Rocky Mountain spotted fever, syphilis, trachoma, typhus, gastroenteritis due to *V. cholerae* or *Helicobacter pylori*). Tetracycline is discussed in Prototype Profile 31-1: Tetracycline. The drugs are also useful in some animal bites and Lyme disease. Other drugs (eg, penicillins) are usually preferred in gram-positive infections, and most gram-negative organisms are resistant to tetracyclines. However, a tetracycline may be used if bacterial susceptibility is confirmed. Specific clinical indications for tetracyclines include the following:

1. Treatment of uncomplicated urethral, endocervical, or rectal infections caused by *Chlamydia* organisms.
2. Adjunctive treatment, with other antimicrobials, in the treatment of pelvic inflammatory disease and sexually transmitted diseases.
3. Long-term treatment of acne. Tetracyclines interfere with the production of free fatty acids and decrease *Corynebacterium* species in sebum. These actions decrease the inflammatory, pustular lesions associated with severe acne.
4. As a substitute for penicillin in penicillin-allergic clients. Tetracyclines may be effective in treating syphilis when penicillin cannot be given. They should

**DRUG TABLE 31-3**

*Drugs at a Glance*

## Miscellaneous Drugs for Urinary Tract Infections

| Generic/Trade Name | Routes and Dosage Ranges | Comments |
|---|---|---|
| **Fosfomycin** (Monurol) Pregnancy Category B | *Adults:* PO, 3 g in a single dose, taken with or without food. Powder should be mixed with one-half cup of water and drunk immediately. *Children:* Dosage not established | Broad-spectrum, long-acting agent Most common adverse effects are diarrhea and headache. |
| **Methenamine mandelate** (Mandelamine; Dehydral) Pregnancy Category C | *Adults:* PO, 1 g four times daily *Children:* Age 6–12 y: PO, 500 mg four times daily Age <6 y: PO, 50 mg/kg/d, in 3 divided doses | Antibacterial activity only at a urine pH <5.5. In acidic urine, the drug forms formaldehyde, which is the antibacterial component. Acidification of urine (eg, with ascorbic acid) is usually needed. Formaldehyde is active against several gram-positive and gram-negative organisms, including *Escherichia coli*. It is most useful for long-term suppression of bacteria in chronic, recurrent infections. It is not indicated in acute infections. Contraindicated in renal failure |
| **Methenamine-hippurate** (Hiprex) Pregnancy Category C | *Adults:* PO, 1 g twice daily *Children:* PO, 500 mg–1 g twice daily | See methenamine mandelate, above |
| **Nalidixic acid** (NegGram) Pregnancy Category B | *Adults:* PO, 4 g daily in four divided doses for 1–2 wk, then 2 g/d if long-term treatment is required *Children:* PO, 55 mg/kg/d in four divided doses, reduced to 33 mg/kg/d for long-term use in children <12 y. Contraindicated in infants <3 mo. >3 mo: PO 5–7 mg/kg/d, in four divided doses | Active against most gram-negative organisms that cause UTI, but rarely used because organisms develop resistance rapidly and other effective drugs are available. |
| **Nitrofurantoin** (Furadantin, Macrodantin) Pregnancy Category B | *Adults:* PO, 50–100 mg four times daily Prophylaxis of recurrent UTI in women, PO 50–100 mg at bedtime | Antibacterial activity against *E. coli* and most other organisms that cause UTI. Used for short-term treatment of UTI or long-term suppression of bacteria in chronic, recurrent UTI. Bacterial resistance develops slowly and to a limited degree. Contraindicated in severe renal disease |
| **Phenazopyridine** (Pyridium) Pregnancy Category B | *Adults:* PO, 200 mg three times daily after meals *Children:* 6–12 y: PO, 12 mg/kg/d, in three divided doses | An azo dye that acts as a urinary tract analgesic and relieves symptoms of dysuria, burning, and frequency and urgency of urination, which occur with UTI. It has no anti-infective action. It turns urine orange-red, which may be mistaken for blood. It is contraindicated in renal insufficiency and severe hepatitis. |

## PROTOTYPE PROFILE 31-1

### P Tetracycline (tet ra SYE kleen)

**Drug Class**
*Chemical:* Tetracycline
*Functional:* Antibiotic

**Trade Names**
Sumycin, Wesmycin

**Therapeutic Indications**
Treatment of susceptible bacterial infections of both gram-negative and gram-positive organisms

**Pharmacokinetics**
*Absorption*
PO, 75%

*Distribution*
Small amount appears in bile
Relative diffusion into CSF from blood significant only with inflammation

*Metabolism*
Plasma protein binding: 65%

*Excretion*
Urine (60% unchanged drug); feces (as active form)

**Pharmacodynamics**
*Onset of Action*
PO: 1–2 h; time to peak: 2–4 h

*Duration*
Half-life elimination: with normal renal function: 8–11 h; with end-stage renal disease 57–108 h

**Contraindications/Precautions**
Hypersensitivity to tetracycline; pregnancy; children younger than 8 years of age
Use with caution with renal or hepatic disease

**Pregnancy Considerations**
Category D
Crosses placenta; may cause permanent discoloration of teeth in fetus if used during last half of pregnancy
Enters breast milk; potential to stain unerupted teeth of infant

**Dosage**
*Adults:* Systemic infection: 250–500 mg q6h
*Helicobacter pylori* eradication: 500 mg 2–4 times/d as combination therapy
*Children >8 years of age:* Systemic infection: 25–50 mg/kg/d PO in divided doses q6h

**Adverse Effects**
Pericarditis, photosensitivity, nausea, vomiting, diarrhea, headache, superinfection; intracranial hypertension

**Drug Interactions**
*Increased Effects*
Anticoagulation with concomitant use of warfarin
Fatal nephrotoxicity when used with methoxyflurane anesthesia

*Decreased Effects*
Absorption of tetracycline with calcium, aluminum, or magnesium containing antacids, zinc, iron, sucralfate, didanosine, quinapril, or sodium bicarbonate
Possible decreased efficacy of oral contraceptives has been refuted

**Herbal Supplements and Dietary Considerations**
Avoid dong quai, St. John's wort (may also cause photosensitivity)
Taking with dairy products may decrease serum concentration of drug
Administer on an empty stomach

---

not be substituted for penicillin in treating streptococcal pharyngitis because microbial resistance is common, and tetracyclines do not prevent rheumatic fever. In addition, they should not be substituted for penicillin in any serious staphylococcal infection because microbial resistance commonly occurs.

5. Doxycycline may be used to prevent traveler's diarrhea due to enterotoxic strains of *E. coli.*

6. Demeclocycline may be used to inhibit antidiuretic hormone in the management of chronic inappropriate antidiuretic hormone secretion.

Sulfonamides are commonly used to treat UTI (eg, acute and chronic cystitis, asymptomatic bacteriuria) caused by *E. coli* and *Proteus* or *Klebsiella* species organisms. In acute pyelonephritis, other agents are preferred.

Additional uses include ulcerative colitis and uncommon infections such as chancroid, lymphogranuloma venereum, nocardiosis, toxoplasmosis, and trachoma. Topical sulfonamides are used in prevention of burn wound infections and in treatment of ocular, vaginal, and other soft tissue infections. For specific clinical indications of individual drugs, see Drugs at a Glance 31-2: Sulfonamide Preparations.

Urinary antiseptics are used only for UTI.

## Contraindications to Use

Both tetracyclines and sulfonamides are contraindicated in clients with renal failure. Tetracyclines are also contraindicated in pregnant women and in children up to 8 years of age. In the fetus and young child, tetracyclines are deposited in bones and teeth along with calcium. If given during active mineralization of these tissues, tetracyclines can cause permanent brown coloring (mottling) of tooth enamel and can depress bone growth. With the exception of doxycycline, they should not be used in renal failure because accumulation may increase the likelihood of liver toxicity. Increased photosensitivity is a common side effect, and clients should be warned to take precaution to prevent sunburn while on these drugs. Sulfonamides are also contraindicated in late pregnancy, lactation, children younger than 2 months of age (except for treatment of congenital toxoplasmosis), and people who have had hypersensitivity reactions to them or to chemically related drugs (eg, thiazide diuretics or antidiabetic sulfonylureas). Sulfasalazine (Azulfidine) is contraindicated in people who are allergic to salicylates and in people with intestinal or urinary tract obstruction.

## Management Considerations

### Tetracyclines

1. Culture and susceptibility studies are needed before tetracycline therapy is started because many strains of organisms are either resistant or vary greatly in drug susceptibility. Cross-sensitivity and cross-resistance are common among tetracyclines.

### How Can You Avoid This Medication Error?

Trimethoprim-sulfamethoxazole (Bactrim) DS bid is ordered for a client after urologic surgery. He takes no medications and reports an allergy to eggs, nuts, sulfa, and morphine. The unit dose provided from the pharmacy is a tablet containing 160 mg of trimethoprim and 800 mg of sulfamethoxazole. You give him one tablet at 0900 for his morning dose.

2. The oral route of administration is usually effective and preferred. Intravenous therapy is used when oral administration is contraindicated or for initial treatment of severe infections.

3. Tetracyclines decompose with age, exposure to light, and extreme heat and humidity. Because the breakdown products may be toxic, it is very important to store these drugs correctly. Also, the manufacturer's expiration dates on containers should be noted, and outdated drugs should be discarded.

### Sulfonamides and Urinary Antiseptics

1. With systemically absorbed sulfonamides, an initial loading dose may be given to produce therapeutic blood levels (12 to 15 mg/100 mL) more rapidly. The amount is usually twice the maintenance dose.

2. Urine pH is important in drug therapy with sulfonamides and urinary antiseptics.

   a. With sulfonamide therapy, alkaline urine increases drug solubility and helps prevent crystalluria. It also increases the rate of sulfonamide excretion and the concentration of sulfonamide in the urine. The urine can be alkalinized by giving sodium bicarbonate. Alkalinization is not needed with sulfisoxazole (because the drug is highly soluble) or sulfonamides used to treat intestinal infections or burn wounds (because there is little systemic absorption).

   b. With methenamine mandelate (Mandelamine) therapy, urine pH must be acidic (<5.5) for the drug to be effective. At a higher pH, Mandelamine does not hydrolyze to formaldehyde, the antibacterial component. Urine can be acidified by concomitant administration of ascorbic acid.

3. Urine cultures and sensitivity tests are indicated in suspected UTI because of wide variability in possible pathogens and their susceptibility to antibacterial drugs. The best results are obtained with drug therapy indicated by the microorganisms isolated from each client.

---

## ✔ CLIENT TEACHING GUIDELINES
## Oral Tetracyclines

### General Considerations

✔ Because tetracyclines inhibit rather than kill bacteria, they must be taken correctly to achieve desired effects.

✔ These drugs increase sensitivity to sunlight and risks of sunburn. Avoid sunlamps, tanning beds, and intense or prolonged exposure to sunlight; if unable to avoid exposure, wear protective clothing and a sunblock preparation.

✔ Report severe nausea, vomiting, diarrhea, skin rash, or perineal itching. These symptoms may indicate a need for changing or stopping the tetracycline.

### Self-administration

✔ Take most tetracyclines on an empty stomach, at least 1 hour before or 2 hours after meals. Doxycycline and minocycline may be taken with food (except dairy products).

✔ Do not take with or within 2 hours of dairy products, antacids, or iron supplements. If an antacid must be taken, take at least 2 hours before or after tetracycline.

✔ Take each dose with at least 8 oz of water.

## CLIENT TEACHING GUIDELINES
## Oral Sulfonamides

### General Considerations

✔ Sulfonamides inhibit rather than kill bacteria. Thus, it is especially important to take them as prescribed, for the length of time prescribed.

✔ These drugs increase sensitivity to sunlight and risks of sunburn. Avoid sunlamps, tanning beds, and intense or prolonged exposure to sunlight; if unable to avoid exposure, wear protective clothing and a sunblock preparation.

✔ Notify the prescribing physician if you have blood in urine, skin rash, difficulty in breathing, fever, or sore throat. These symptoms may indicate adverse drug effects and the need to change or stop the drug.

### Self-administration

✔ Take oral sulfonamides on an empty stomach with at least 8 oz of water.

✔ With oral suspensions, shake well, refrigerate after opening, and discard the unused portion after 14 days.

✔ Drink 2 to 3 quarts of fluid daily, if able. A good fluid intake helps the drugs to be more effective, especially in urinary tract infections, and decreases the likelihood of damaging the kidneys.

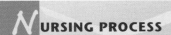

## NURSING PROCESS

General aspects of the nursing process in antimicrobial drug therapy, as described in Chapter 28, apply to the client receiving tetracyclines, sulfonamides, and urinary antiseptics. In this chapter, only those aspects related specifically to these drugs are included.

### Assessment

With tetracyclines, assess for conditions in which the drugs must be used cautiously or are contraindicated, such as impaired renal or hepatic function.

With sulfonamides, assess for signs and symptoms of disorders for which the drugs are used:

- For *UTI,* assess urinalysis reports for white blood cells and bacteria, urine culture reports for type of bacteria, and symptoms of dysuria, frequency, and urgency of urination.
- For *burns,* assess the size of the wound, amount and type of drainage, presence of edema, and amount of eschar.
- Ask clients specifically if they have ever taken a sulfonamide and, if so, whether they had an allergic reaction.

With urinary antiseptics, assess for signs and symptoms of UTI.

### Nursing Diagnoses

- Risk for Injury: Hypersensitivity reaction, kidney, liver, or blood disorders with sulfonamides
- Deficient Knowledge: Correct administration and use of tetracyclines, sulfonamides, and urinary antiseptics

### Planning/Goals

*The client will:*
- Receive or self-administer the drugs as directed
- Receive prompt and appropriate treatment if adverse effects occur

### Interventions

- During tetracycline therapy for systemic infections, monitor laboratory tests of renal function for abnormal values.

- During sulfonamide therapy, encourage sufficient fluids to produce a urine output of at least 1200 to 1500 mL daily. A high fluid intake decreases the risk of crystalluria (precipitation of drug crystals in the urine).
- Avoid urinary catheterization when possible. If catheterization is necessary, use sterile technique. The urinary tract is normally sterile except for the lower third of the urethra. Introduction of any bacteria into the bladder may cause infection.
- A single catheterization may cause infection. With indwelling catheters, bacteria colonize the bladder and produce infection within 2 to 3 weeks, even with meticulous care.
- When indwelling catheters must be used, measures to decrease UTI include using a closed drainage system; keeping the perineal area clean; forcing fluids, if not contraindicated, to maintain a dilute urine; and removing the catheter as soon as possible. Do not disconnect the system and irrigate the catheter unless obstruction is suspected. *Never* raise the urinary drainage bag above bladder level.
- Force fluids in anyone with a UTI unless contraindicated. Bacteria do not multiply as rapidly in dilute urine. In addition, emptying the bladder frequently allows it to refill with uninfected urine. This decreases the bacterial population of the bladder.
- Teach women to cleanse themselves from the urethral area toward the rectum after voiding or defecating to avoid contamination of the urethral area with bacteria from the vagina and rectum. Also, voiding after sexual intercourse helps cleanse the lower urethra and prevent UTI.

### Evaluation

- Observe for improvement in signs of the infection for which drug therapy was given.
- Interview and observe for adverse drug effects.

## Age-related Considerations: Use of Tetracyclines, Sulfonamides, and Urinary Agents

### USE IN CHILDREN

Tetracyclines should not be used in children younger than 8 years of age because of their effects on teeth and bones. In teeth, the drugs interfere with enamel development and may cause a permanent yellow, gray, or brown discoloration. In bone, the drugs form a stable compound in bone-forming tissue and may interfere with bone growth.

Systemic sulfonamides are contraindicated during late pregnancy, lactation, and in children younger than 2 months. If a fetus or young infant receives a sulfonamide by placental transfer, in breast milk, or by direct administration, the drug displaces bilirubin from binding sites on albumin. As a result, bilirubin may accumulate in the bloodstream (hyperbilirubinemia) and central nervous system (kernicterus) and cause life-threatening toxicity.

Sulfonamides are often used to treat UTIs in children older than 2 months. Few data are available regarding the effects of long-term or recurrent use of sulfamethoxazole in children younger than 6 years of age with chronic renal disease. **Sulfamethoxazole** is often given in combination with trimethoprim (Bactrim, Septra), although trimethoprim has not been established as safe and effective in children younger than 12 years of age.

Some clinicians recommend that asymptomatic bacteriuria be treated in children younger than 5 years of age to decrease risks for long-term renal damage. Treatment is the same as for symptomatic UTI.

### USE IN OLDER ADULTS

A major concern with the use of tetracyclines and sulfonamides in older adults is renal impairment, which commonly occurs in this population. Except for doxycycline and minocycline, tetracyclines are contraindicated in clients with renal impairment. Sulfonamides may cause additional renal impairment. As with younger adults, a fluid intake of about 2 L daily is needed to reduce formation of crystals and stones in the urinary tract.

With the combination of sulfamethoxazole and trimethoprim (Bactrim, Septra), older adults are at increased risk for severe adverse effects. Severe skin reactions and bone marrow depression are most often reported. Folic acid deficiency may also occur because both of the drugs interfere with folic acid metabolism.

## ■ DRUG USE IN SPECIFIC SITUATIONS

### Use in Renal Impairment

As discussed previously, most tetracyclines are contraindicated in clients with renal impairment. High concentrations of tetracyclines inhibit protein synthesis in human cells. This antianabolic effect increases tissue breakdown (catabolism) and the amount of waste products to be excreted by the kidneys. The increased workload can be handled by normally functioning kidneys, but waste products are retained when renal function is impaired. This leads to azotemia, increased blood urea nitrogen, hyperphosphatemia, hyperkalemia, and acidosis. If a tetracycline is necessary because of an organism's sensitivity or the host's inability to take other antimicrobial drugs, doxycycline or minocycline may be given.

Systemic sulfonamides should probably be avoided in clients with renal impairment, if other effective drugs are available. Acute renal failure (ARF) has occurred when the drugs or their metabolites precipitated in renal tubules and caused obstruction. ARF is rarely associated with newer sulfonamides, which are more soluble than older ones, but has increased with the use of sulfadiazine to treat toxoplasmosis in clients with acquired immunodeficiency syndrome (AIDS). Preventive measures include a fluid intake of 2 to 3 L daily.

### Use in Hepatic Impairment

Tetracyclines are contraindicated in pregnant women because they may cause fatal hepatic necrosis in the

## Home Care Considerations: Use of Tetracyclines, Sulfonamides, and Urinary Agents

**ASSESS:** adverse drug effects should be reviewed with clients, and clients should be assessed for characteristics (eg, prolonged exposure to sunlight, renal impairment, failing to take full course of antibiotic) that increase the risks for adverse effects.

**MONITOR:** client for compliance with the prescribed regimen; therapeutic and adverse drug effects; signs of superinfection (oral ulcers, genital or anal discharge); that client is keeping appointments for follow-up care.

**EDUCATE:** how to use, store out of extreme heat or light; parents about need to avoid use in children younger than 8 years of age because it can discolor permanent teeth. Stress the importance of completing entire course of treatment and for women to consult with health care provider if contemplating pregnancy (possible teratogenic effect). Reinforce additional teaching points (see Client Teaching Guidelines: Oral Tetracyclines; Oral Sulfonamides).

mother. They must be used cautiously in the presence of liver or kidney impairment. Because tetracyclines are metabolized in the liver, hepatic impairment or biliary obstruction slows drug elimination. In clients with renal impairment, high intravenous (IV) doses (>2 g/day) have been associated with death from liver failure. If necessary in clients with known or suspected renal and hepatic impairment, renal and liver function test results should be monitored. In addition, serum tetracycline levels should not exceed 15 mcg/mL, and other hepatotoxic drugs should be avoided.

Sulfonamides cause cholestatic jaundice in a small percentage of clients and should be used with caution in clients with hepatic impairment.

## Nursing Actions

## Tetracyclines, Sulfonamides, and Urinary Agents

| Nursing Actions | Rationale/Explanation |
|---|---|
| **1. Administer accurately**<br>a. With tetracyclines:<br>(1) Give oral drugs with food that does not contain dairy products; do not give with or within 2 h of dairy products, antacids, or iron supplements.<br>(2) For intravenous (IV) administration, dilute with an appropriate type and amount of IV solution, and infuse over 1–4 h. | To decrease nausea and other gastrointestinal (GI) symptoms. Tetracyclines combine with metallic ions (eg, aluminum, calcium, iron, magnesium) and are not absorbed.<br>Rapid administration should be avoided. IV doses are usually mixed in hospital pharmacies. |
| b. With sulfonamides:<br>(1) Give oral drugs before or after meals, with a full glass of water.<br>(2) Infuse IV trimethoprim-sulfamethoxazole (diluted in 125 mL of 5% dextrose in water) over 60–90 min. Do not mix with other drugs or solutions and flush IV lines to remove any residual drug.<br>(3) For topical sulfonamides to burn wounds, apply a thin layer with a sterile gloved hand after the surface has been cleansed of previously applied medication. | Absorption is better when taken on an empty stomach; however, taking with food decreases GI upset.<br>Manufacturer's recommendations<br><br><br>Burn wounds may be cleansed by whirlpool, shower, or spot cleansing with sterile saline, gauze pads, and gloves. |
| c. Give nitrofurantoin with or after meals. | Food decreases nausea, vomiting, and diarrhea. |
| **2. Observe for therapeutic effects** | Therapeutic effects depend on the reason for use. |
| a. With tetracyclines, observe for decreased signs and symptoms of the infection for which the drug is being given. | |
| b. With sulfonamides, observe for decreased symptoms of urinary tract infection (UTI), decreased diarrhea when given for ulcerative colitis or bacillary dysentery, lack of fever, and wound drainage and evidence of healing in burn wounds. | Topical sulfonamides for burns are used to prevent rather than treat infection. |
| c. With urinary antiseptics, observe for decreased symptoms of UTI. | |
| **3. Observe for adverse effects**<br>a. Nausea, vomiting, diarrhea | Commonly occur with tetracyclines, sulfonamides, and urinary antiseptics, probably from local irritation of GI mucosa. After several days of an oral tetracycline, diarrhea may be caused by superinfection. |
| b. Hematologic disorders—anemia, neutropenia, thrombocytopenia<br>c. Hypersensitivity—anaphylaxis, skin rash, urticaria, serum sickness<br>d. Photosensitivity—sunburn reaction | This can be prevented or minimized by avoiding exposure to sunlight or other sources of ultraviolet light, wearing protective clothing and using sunscreen lotions. |

*(continued)*

## Nursing Actions

## Tetracyclines, Sulfonamides, and Urinary Agents (Continued)

| Nursing Actions | Rationale/Explanation |
|---|---|
| e. Thrombophlebitis at IV infusion sites | These drugs are irritating to tissues. Irritation can be decreased by diluting the drugs and infusing them at the recommended rates. |
| f. Nephrotoxicity—increased blood urea nitrogen and serum creatinine, hematuria, proteinuria, crystalluria | Nephrotoxicity is more likely to occur in people who already have impaired renal function. Keeping clients well hydrated may help prevent renal damage. |
| g. Hepatotoxicity—elevated aspartate aminotransferase and other enzymes | Hepatitis, cholestasis, and other serious liver disorders rarely occur with these drugs. |
| h. Superinfection—sore mouth, white patches on oral mucosa, black, furry tongue, diarrhea, skin rash, itching in the perineal area, pseudomembranous colitis | Superinfection may occur with tetracyclines because of their broad spectrum of antimicrobial activity. Signs and symptoms usually indicate monilial infection. Meticulous oral and perineal hygiene helps prevent these problems. The drug should be stopped if severe diarrhea occurs, with blood, mucus, or pus in stools. |
| 4. Observe for drug interactions<br>  a. Drugs that *decrease* effects of tetracyclines:<br>    (1) Aluminum, calcium, iron, or magnesium preparations (eg, antacids, ferrous sulfate) | These metals combine with oral tetracyclines to produce insoluble, nonabsorbable compounds that are excreted in feces. |
|     (2) Cathartics | Decrease absorption |
|     (3) Barbiturates, carbamazepine, phenytoin, rifampin | These drugs induce drug-metabolizing enzymes in the liver and may speed up metabolism of doxycycline. |
|   b. Drugs that *increase* effects of sulfonamides:<br>    (1) Alkalinizing agents (eg, sodium bicarbonate) | Increase rate of urinary excretion, thereby raising levels of sulfonamides in the urinary tract and increasing effectiveness in UTIs |
|     (2) Methenamine compounds, urinary acidifiers (eg, ascorbic acid) | These drugs increase the risk of nephrotoxicity and should not be used with sulfonamides. They may cause precipitation of sulfonamide with resultant blockage of renal tubules. |
|     (3) Salicylates (eg, aspirin), nonsteroidal anti-inflammatory drugs (eg, ibuprofen), oral anticoagulants, phenytoin, methotrexate | Increase toxicity by displacing sulfonamides from plasma protein-binding sites, thereby increasing plasma levels of free drug |
|   c. Drugs that alter effects of nitrofurantoin:<br>    (1) Antacids | May decrease absorption |
|     (2) Acidifying agents | Increase antibacterial activity of nitrofurantoin by decreasing renal excretion. Nitrofurantoin is most active against organisms causing UTI when urine pH is 5.5 or less. |

## ? How Can You Avoid This Medication Error?

**Answer:** Bactrim should not be given to this client because he has an allergy to sulfa, and the sulfamethoxazole component is a sulfonamide. You might want to ask him what type of reaction he experienced when he previously took sulfa. If he reports nausea, this is an adverse side effect rather than an allergic response. An allergic response is a histamine-mediated reaction with symptoms such as hives, rash, pruritus, or, in severe cases, bronchospasm and cardiovascular collapse. If any allergic symptoms occurred, hold the medication and call the physician. If the client is not allergic to sulfa, giving one tablet would provide an accurate double-strength (DS) dose.

## Critical Thinking Exercises

1. Which of the tetracyclines is eliminated mainly by the liver?
   a. Doxycycline
   b. Minocycline
   c. Demeclocycline
   d. Tetracycline

2. Tetracyclines are contraindicated in children up to 8 years of age because they are associated with:
   a. Depression of bone growth
   b. Increased risks for long-term renal damage
   c. Displacement of bilirubin from binding sites on albumin
   d. Drug-induced anaphylaxis

**3.** Long-term, low-dose administration of a tetracycline is prescribed for the treatment of acne. The rationale for this treatment includes all of the following except the:

a. Interference with the production of free fatty acids
b. Decrease of *Corynebacterium* species in sebum
c. Decrease in inflammatory pustular lesions
d. Increase in drug resistance

**4.** Sulfasalazine (Azulfidine) is contraindicated in people who are allergic to:

a. Salicylates
b. Penicillin
c. Sulfonylureas
d. Clindamycin hydrochloride

**5.** With the combination of sulfamethoxazole and trimethoprim (Bactrim, Septra), older adults are at increased risk for severe adverse effects. Which of the following potential adverse effects is unlikely the result of therapy with this drug combination?

a. Severe skin reactions
b. Bone marrow depression
c. Folic acid deficiency
d. Tinnitus

## SELECTED REFERENCES

Chambers, H. F. (2001). Antimicrobial agents: Protein synthesis inhibitors and miscellaneous antibacterial agents. In J. G. Hardman & L. E. Limbird (Eds.), *Goodman & Gilman's the pharmacological basis of therapeutics* (10th ed., pp. 1239–1271). New York: McGraw-Hill.

*Drug facts and comparisons.* (Updated monthly). St. Louis: Facts and Comparisons.

Lacy, C. F., Armstrong, L. L., Goldman, M. P., & Lance, L. L. (2003). *Lexi-Comp's drug information handbook* (11th ed.). Hudson, OH: American Pharmaceutical Association.

Marchiondo, K. (1998). A new look at urinary tract infection. *American Journal of Nursing 98*(3), 34–38.

Petri, W. A., Jr. (2001). Antimicrobial agents: Sulfonamides, trimethoprim-sulfamethoxazole, quinolones, and agents for urinary tract infections. In J. G. Hardman & L. E. Limbird (Eds.), *Goodman & Gilman's the pharmacological basis of therapeutics* (10th ed., pp. 1171–1188). New York: McGraw-Hill.

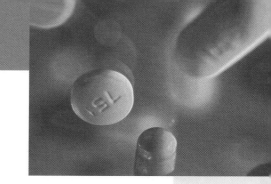

# 32

# Drugs for Tuberculosis and Mycobacterium avium Complex (MAC) Disease

## OBJECTIVES

*After studying this chapter, the student will be able to:*

1 Describe characteristics of latent, active, and drug-resistant tuberculosis infections.

2 Identify populations at high risk for developing tuberculosis.

3 List characteristics, uses, effects, and nursing implications of using primary antitubercular drugs.

4 Give the rationale for multiple drug therapy in treatment of tuberculosis.

5 Discuss ways to increase adherence to antitubercular drug therapy regimens.

6 Differentiate the advantages and disadvantages of directly observed therapy (DOT).

7 Describe factors affecting the use of primary, secondary, and other drugs in the treatment of multidrug-resistant tuberculosis (MDR-TB).

8 Discuss *Mycobacterium avium* complex disease and the drugs used to prevent or treat it.

## CRITICAL THINKING SCENARIO

*J*ohn Phillips, a homeless person with a history of drug and alcohol abuse, comes to the emergency department with a productive cough, complaints of night sweats, and fatigue. The health care provider suspects tuberculosis (TB) and orders a purified protein derivative (PPD) skin test, chest x-ray, and sputum for acid-fast bacilli.

✔ Describe the necessary infection control measures to use before TB is confirmed or ruled out.

✔ Why would multidrug treatment be important if TB were confirmed?

✔ What factors affect compliance with drug treatment for Mr. Phillips? Develop a plan to improve and monitor compliance.

✔ How long will Mr. Phillips require drug treatment, and how you can evaluate when the TB is cured?

### PROTOTYPE PROFILE

isoniazid (Nydrazid), p. 555

# OVERVIEW

Tuberculosis (TB) is an infectious disease that usually affects the lungs (>80% of cases) but may involve most parts of the body, including lymph nodes, pleurae, bones, joints, kidneys, and gastrointestinal (GI) tract. It is caused by *Mycobacterium tuberculosis*, the tubercle bacillus. In general, these bacilli multiply slowly; they may lie dormant in the body for many years; they resist phagocytosis and survive in phagocytic cells; and they develop resistance to antitubercular drugs.

Tuberculosis commonly occurs in many parts of the world and causes many deaths annually. In the United States, active disease has waned to a historically low level. However, there are now large numbers of people with inactive or latent tuberculosis infection (LTBI). Contributing factors include increased exposure during a resurgence of active disease between 1985 and 1992, immigration from countries where the disease is common, and increasing numbers of people with conditions or medications that depress the immune system. The epidemiology of the disease is discussed in At the Foundation: Epidemiology of Tuberculosis.

# DRUG-RESISTANT TUBERCULOSIS

In addition to LTBI, a major concern among public health and infectious disease experts is an increase in drug-resistant infections. A major factor in drug-resistant infections is poor client adherence to prescribed antitubercular drug therapy.

Drug-resistant mutants of *M. tuberculosis* microorganisms are present in any infected person. When infected people receive antitubercular drugs, drug-resistant mutants continue to appear and reproduce in the presence of the drugs. These strains may become predominant as the drugs eliminate susceptible strains and provide more space and nutrients for resistant strains. Most drug-resistant strains develop when previously infected clients do not take the drugs and doses prescribed for the length of time prescribed. However, drug-resistant strains can also be spread from one person to another and cause new infections, especially in people whose immune systems are suppressed.

Multidrug-resistant tuberculosis (MDR-TB) indicates organisms that are resistant to isoniazid (INH) and rifampin, the most effective drugs available, with or without resistance to other antitubercular drugs. MDR-TB is associated with rapid progression, with 4 to 16 weeks from diagnosis to death, and with high death rates (50% to 80%). It is also very difficult and expensive to treat.

# PREVENTING THE DEVELOPMENT AND SPREAD OF TUBERCULOSIS

Recommendations for tuberculosis control have changed considerably in recent years. Current recommendations from the Centers for Disease Control and Prevention

---

**AT THE FOUNDATION:** *Epidemiology of Tuberculosis*

There are four distinct phases in the initiation and progression of tuberculosis:

1. **Transmission** occurs when an uninfected person inhales infected airborne particles that are exhaled by an infected person (Fig. 32-1). Major factors affecting transmission are the number of bacteria expelled by the infected person and the closeness and duration of the contact between the infected and the uninfected person.
2. **Primary infection.** It is estimated that 30% of persons exposed to tuberculosis bacilli become infected and develop a mild, pneumonia-like illness that is often undiagnosed. About 6 to 8 weeks after exposure, those infected have positive reactions to tuberculin skin tests. Within approximately 6 months of exposure, spontaneous healing occurs as the bacilli are encapsulated in calcified tubercles.
3. **Latent tuberculosis infection (LTBI).** In most people who become infected with TB bacteria, the immune system is able to stop bacterial growth. The bacteria become inactive, but they remain alive in the body and can become active later. People with inactive or latent TB infection have no symptoms, do not feel sick, do not spread TB to others, usually have a positive skin test reaction, and can develop

active TB disease years later if the latent infection is not effectively treated. In many people with LTBI, the infection remains inactive throughout their lives. In others, the TB bacteria become active and cause tuberculosis, usually when a person's immune system becomes weak as a result of disease, immunosuppressive drugs, or aging.

4. **Active tuberculosis** usually results from reactivation of latent infection, although new infection can also occur. Both reactivated and new infections are more likely to occur in people whose immune systems are depressed by disease (eg, human immunodeficiency virus [HIV] infection, diabetes mellitus, cancer) or drug therapy (eg, for cancer or organ transplantation). Among people with LTBI, signs and symptoms of active disease (eg, cough that is persistent and often productive of sputum, chest pain, chills, fever, hemoptysis, night sweats, weight loss, weakness, lack of appetite, a positive skin test, abnormal chest radiograph, and/or positive sputum smear or culture) are estimated to develop in 5% within 2 years and in another 5% after 2 years. Among people with both LTBI and HIV infection, LTBI progresses to active disease more rapidly (approximately 10% each year), is more severe, and often involves extrapulmonary sites.

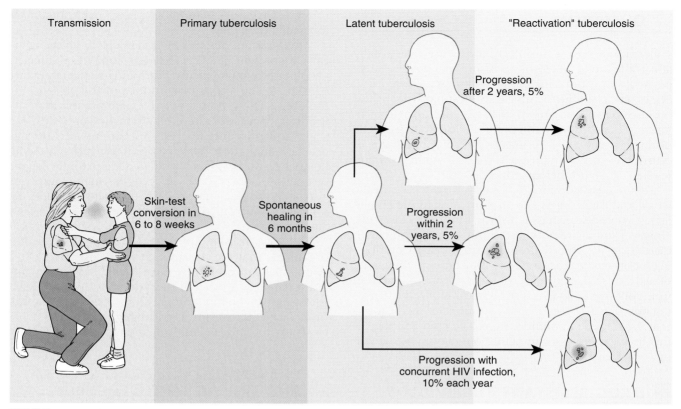

| Transmission | Primary tuberculosis | Latent tuberculosis | "Reactivation" tuberculosis |

Progression after 2 years, 5%

Skin-test conversion in 6 to 8 weeks

Spontaneous healing in 6 months

Progression within 2 years, 5%

Progression with concurrent HIV infection, 10% each year

**FIGURE 32–1** Transmission of tuberculosis and progression from latent infection to reactivated disease. Among persons who are seronegative for the human immunodeficiency virus (HIV), approximately 30 percent of heavily exposed persons will become infected. In 5% of persons with latent infection, active disease will develop within two years, and in an additional 5%, progression to active disease will occur later. The rate of progression to active disease is dramatically increased among persons who are coinfected with HIV. (Adapted from Small, P.M. and Fujiwara, P.I. [2001]. Management of tuberculosis in the United States. *New England Journal of Medicine, 345*(3), 189–200.)

(CDC), the American Thoracic Society (ATS), and the Infectious Diseases Society of America (IDSA) emphasize continued treatment of active disease and expanded efforts to identify and treat latent infection (LTBI). For identification, tuberculin skin testing is recommended only for high-risk groups (Box 32-1). When LTBI is found in these groups, it should be treated, to eradicate this reservoir of infection (Box 32-2).

Recommendations for treatment are also changing, as authorities strive to design more effective regimens and overcome barriers to their effective implementation. One major change is increasing use of short-course regimens. Numerous studies indicate that these regimens are effective for many people. In addition, clients are more likely to complete a shorter course of therapy, which reduces the occurrence of drug-resistant TB.

Although local health departments are largely responsible for TB control programs, some authorities urge increased testing and treatment in primary care settings and settings where high-risk groups are found (eg, homeless shelters). In addition, they urge recognition and effective management of language, social, economic, transportation, and other barriers that limit access to health care and inhibit diagnosis and treatment.

Nurses have important roles to play in TB control. Some of the roles include performing and reading tuberculin skin tests; managing TB clinics; tracking contacts of clients with active disease; assessing clients, homes, and other settings for risk factors; educating clients and families about the tuberculosis infection and its treatment; administering or directing the administration of antitubercular drugs (eg, directly observed therapy [DOT]); and maintaining records (eg, skin tests performed, positive results, clients starting or completing drug therapy, and adherence or lack of adherence to prescribed treatment regimens). Most children are infected in their homes. Children in close contact with a case of tuberculosis should receive skin testing, a physical examination, and a chest x-ray. General issues to be considered regarding clients in the home setting and specific issues regarding children and older adults are outlined in Home Care Considerations and Age-related Considerations, respectively.

Numerous strategies have been proposed to increase adherence, including:

1. **Client, family, and contact education.** This may be especially important with treatment of LTBI. Most people are more motivated to take medications and

*(text continues on page 552)*

## BOX 32-1    Targeted Tuberculin Testing for Latent Tuberculosis Infection (LTBI)

### Purpose

To identify people with latent tuberculosis infection (LTBI) who are at high risk for developing active tuberculosis and who would benefit by treatment of LTBI, if detected.

### Who Should Be Tested?

Numerous high-risk groups have been identified, including persons with the following circumstances or conditions:

- Recent infection with *Mycobacterium tuberculosis* organisms
- Close contact with someone diagnosed with infectious pulmonary TB
- Immigration from areas of the world with high rates of TB. For about 5 years, immigrants have incidence rates similar to those of their countries of origin and are thought to have become infected in their native countries. After 5 years, rates become similar to those of the general U.S. population.
- Belonging to younger age groups. Young children (eg, <5 years) with a positive skin test are at high risk for progression to active disease. The risk is also increased in adolescents and young adults.
- Belonging to older age groups, especially if also living or working in institutions with high-risk populations (eg, hospitals, homeless shelters, correctional facilities, nursing homes, residential homes for patients with AIDS)
- Being homeless
- Being an injection drug user
- Having HIV infection or AIDS. HIV infection greatly increases the risk for progression of LTBI to active TB.
- Having chest radiographs that show fibrotic lesions in the lungs. Such lesions are likely to stem from prior, untreated, healed TB.
- Being underweight, especially if more than 10% to 15% under ideal weight.
- Having silicosis (a pulmonary disorder caused by inhalation of dust particles from mining or stonecutting). People with silicosis and a positive tuberculin test are about 30 times more likely to develop active disease than the general population.
- Having chronic renal failure and being on hemodialysis. These people are 10 to 25 times more likely to develop active disease than the general population.
- Having diabetes mellitus. These people are 2 to 4 times more likely to develop active TB than those without diabetes, and the risk is probably greater in those with insulin-dependent or poorly controlled diabetes.
- Having a history of gastrectomy (which is often accompanied by weight loss and malabsorption), jejunoileal bypass, renal or cardiac transplantation, carcinoma of the head or neck, lung cancer, lymphoma, or leukemia.
- Receiving high-dose corticosteroid therapy (eg, prednisone >15 mg/d or equivalent amounts of other drugs for several weeks). These people may be at risk for reactivation of TB, but the exact risk is unknown. Lower doses and intermittent administration of corticosteroids are not associated with TB.

### Where Should Testing Be Done?

Traditionally, local health departments have been responsible for testing, interpreting, and providing follow-up care; some institutions have tested residents and employees, and some large businesses have tested employees. More recently, the Centers for Disease Control (CDC) and other authorities have recommended that more testing be done in primary care settings and any other locations where high risk individuals are. Such testing sites include neighborhood health centers, jails, homeless shelters, inner-city sites, methadone clinics, syringe and needle-exchange programs, and other community-based social service organizations. In the latter situations, local health departments are urged to assist local providers in developing, implementing, and evaluating TB screening programs appropriate for their communities.

### Test Interpretation

Positive reactions differ according to the amount of induration (a nodule or area of hardened tissue, not to be confused with the area of redness, which may be larger than the area of induration) and characteristics of the group being tested, as follows:

- **Induration of 5 mm or more.** Persons at highest risk (eg, close contacts of someone with active, infectious TB; those with HIV infection or risk factors for HIV infection; and those with chest radiographs that are consistent with previous TB)
- **Induration of 10 mm or more.** Persons at high risk (eg, those with conditions or characteristics such as diabetes mellitus; silicosis; immunosuppressive drug therapy; leukemia, lymphoma, head or neck cancer; chronic renal failure; gastrectomy; jejunoileal bypass; low body weight; injecting drug users known to be seronegative for HIV infection; recent immigrants from countries that have high TB rates; residents and employees of prisons, long-term care institutions, and other congregate settings for high-risk populations; low-income groups; high-risk racial and ethnic groups; migrant farm workers; and infants, children, and adolescents exposed to adults in high-risk categories).
- **Induration of 15 mm or more.** Persons who are at low risk for developing TB and do not meet the criteria listed for the above groups. Routine testing is not recommended for low-risk groups.
- **False-positive reactions.** These may occur with infections caused by nontuberculous strains of mycobacteria or a previous intradermal injection of Bacille Calmette-Guérin (BCG), a live attenuated strain derived from *Mycobacterium bovis.* In many parts of the world, BCG is used as a vaccine against tuberculosis, especially in children. There is currently no reliable way to differentiate tuberculin reactions caused by vaccination with BCG from those caused by infection with *M. tuberculosis.* However, large areas of induration (>20 mm) are unlikely to result from BCG.
- **False-negative reactions.** These may occur with HIV infection or other conditions that suppress the immune system and inhibit the ability to react to the tuberculin antigen. Thus, a negative skin test may occur in the presence of tuberculosis infection.

## BOX 32-2    Treatment of Latent Tuberculosis Infection (LTBI)

### Recommended Regimens for Adults

**Isoniazid (INH) daily or twice weekly for 9 months** is the preferred regimen, including persons with HIV infection or radiographic evidence of prior TB.

**Isoniazid daily or twice weekly for 6 months.** The main advantage of this regimen over the 9-month schedule is greater adherence because of the shorter length. It is also less costly. This regimen may be used for HIV-negative adults with normal chest radiographs; it is *not* recommended for HIV-positive persons, those <18 years of age, or those with fibrotic lesions on chest radiographs.

**Rifampin and pyrazinamide (RIF-PZA) daily or twice weekly for 2 months.** This regimen may be used for contacts of patients with INH-resistant TB and for those who are unlikely to complete a longer course of treatment. Rifampin is contraindicated in HIV-positive patients who are receiving protease inhibitors or nonnucleoside reverse transcriptase inhibitors, because rifampin greatly stimulates metabolism and decreases the effectiveness of the antiviral drugs. Rifabutin, which causes less enzyme induction than rifampin, may be substituted in some cases. Pyrazinamide is contraindicated during pregnancy.

This regimen was revised in 2001 because of several reports of liver failure and death. To reduce the risks of liver injury, the American Thoracic Society and the CDC, with the endorsement of the Infectious Diseases Society of America, issued new recommendations for choosing patients and for more intensive clinical and laboratory monitoring, as follows:

1. The RIF-PZA regimen is not recommended for persons who have underlying liver disease or who have had INH-associated liver injury. It should be used with caution in patients who take other hepatotoxic medications or use alcohol, even if alcohol use is stopped during treatment. Persons being considered for treatment with this regimen should be informed about potential hepatotoxicity and asked whether they have had liver disease or adverse effects from INH.
2. The RIF-PZA regimen is recommended mainly for clients who are unlikely to complete longer courses of treatment and who can be monitored closely. (For other adults not infected with HIV, the 9-month daily regimen of INH is preferred, with 4 months of daily RIF as an acceptable alternative.)
3. The RIF-PZA regimen does increase risks of hepatotoxicity in clients with HIV infection. Still, INH daily for 9 months is the treatment of choice for HIV-infected persons with LTBI when completion of treatment can be assured.
4. Increase safety by limiting the pyrazinamide dose to <20 mg/kg/d and a maximum of 2 g/d; giving no more than a 2-week supply of rifampin and pyrazinamide at a time; and assessing patients at 2, 4, and 6 weeks of treatment for adherence, tolerance, and adverse effects, and at 8 weeks to document treatment completion. For non-English-speaking clients, health care providers who speak the clients' language should instruct them to stop taking the drugs immediately and seek medical care if abdominal pain, emesis, jaundice, or other symptoms

of hepatitis develop. Provider continuity is recommended for monitoring.

5. Perform liver function tests (eg, serum aspartate and alanine aminotransferases [AST and ALT] and bilirubin) at baseline and at 2, 4, and 6 weeks. RIF-PZA treatment should be stopped and not resumed if enzyme levels are higher than five times the upper limit of normal in an asymptomatic person, are higher than normal range if symptoms of hepatitis are present, or if a serum bilirubin is above normal range.

**Rifampin daily for 4 months.** This regimen is used mainly for clients who cannot tolerate INH or pyrazinamide.

### Special Populations

1. Pregnant women. The preferred regimen for treatment of LTBI is INH, administered daily or twice weekly for 9 or 6 months. Pregnant women taking INH should also take pyridoxine supplementation. For HIV-positive women with higher risks of progression to active TB, treatment should not be delayed; for those with lower risks, some experts recommend waiting until after delivery to start treatment. In general, INH, rifampin, and ethambutol have good safety records in pregnancy. Pyrazinamide and streptomycin are contraindicated during pregnancy.
2. Children and adolescents. INH daily or twice weekly for 9 months is recommended. Infants and children under 5 years of age with LTBI are at high risk for progression to disease. They are also more likely than older children and adults to develop life-threatening forms of TB, including meningeal and disseminated disease. INH therapy appears to be more effective for children than adults, and the risk for INH-related hepatitis is minimal in infants, children, and adolescents, who generally tolerate the drug better than adults. Routine administration of pyridoxine is not recommended for children taking INH, but should be given to breast-feeding infants, children and adolescents with pyridoxine-deficient diets, and children who experience paresthesias when taking INH.

   Although few studies have been done in infants, children, and adolescents, rifampin alone, rifampin with INH, and rifampin with pyrazinamide have been used to treat LTBI with effectiveness. Although the optimal length of rifampin therapy in children with LTBI is unknown, the American Academy of Pediatrics recommends 6 months.

   There have been no reported studies of any regimen for treatment for LTBI in HIV-infected children. The American Academy of Pediatrics recommends INH for 9 months; most experts recommend routine monitoring of serum liver enzyme concentrations and pyridoxine administration.
3. Contacts of patients with drug-susceptible TB and positive skin-test reactions (>5 mm) should be treated with one of the recommended regimens described above, regardless of age.
4. Contacts of patients with INH-resistant, rifampin-susceptible TB should generally be given rifampin and pyrazinamide for 2 months. For patients with intolerance to pyrazinamide, rifampin alone for 4 months is recommended. If rifampin cannot be used, rifabutin can be substituted.

*(continued)*

## BOX 32-2    Treatment of Latent Tuberculosis Infection (LTBI) (Continued)

5. Contacts of patients with multidrug-resistant (MDR)-TB who are at high risk for developing active TB are generally given pyrazinamide and ethambutol or pyrazinamide and a fluoroquinolone (levofloxacin, ofloxacin, or sparfloxacin) for 6 to 12 months. Immunocompetent contacts may be observed without treatment or treated for 6 months; immunocompromised contacts (eg, HIV-infected persons) should be treated for 12 months.

   For children exposed to MDR-TB, pyrazinamide and ethambutol are recommended for 9 to 12 months if the isolate is susceptible to both drugs. If these drugs cannot be used, two other drugs to which the infecting organism is likely susceptible should be given. Fluoroquinolones are contraindicated in children.

6. HIV-infected persons. With INH, the 9-month regimen is recommended. With rifampin, the drug is contraindicated or should be used with caution in persons who are taking protease inhibitors or nonnucleoside reverse transcriptase inhibitors (NNRTIs). Rifabutin can be substituted for rifampin in some circumstances, but it should not be used with hard-gel saquinavir or delavirdine and must be used cautiously with soft-gel saquinavir and nevirapine because data are limited. Dosage of rifabutin needs to be reduced to one half the usual daily dose (ie, from 300 mg/d to 150 mg/d) with indinavir, nelfinavir, or amprenavir and to one fourth the usual dose (ie, 150 mg every other day or 3 times a week) with ritonavir. Usual dosage (300 mg/d) can be given with nevirapine and 450 mg or 600 mg/d are needed with efavirenz. Rifapentine is not recommended as a substitute for rifampin because its safety, effectiveness, and interactions with anti-HIV medication have not been established.

7. BCG-vaccinated persons. A history of Bacille Calmette-Guérin (BCG) vaccination should not influence the decision to treat LTBI.

### Additional Recommendations

1. Before beginning treatment for LTBI, active TB should be ruled out by history, physical examination, chest radiography, and bacteriologic studies, if indicated.

2. Allow patients to participate in choosing a treatment regimen, when feasible, by discussing options and characteristics of each (eg, the length and complexity, possible adverse effects, and potential drug interactions).

3. Directly observed therapy (DOT) should be used consistently with intermittent regimens (eg, twice weekly) and when possible with 2-month regimens and in certain settings (eg, institutional settings, community outreach programs, and for persons living in households with patients who are receiving home-based DOT for active TB).

4. Try to ensure completion of treatment. This is determined by the total number of doses administered as well as the duration of therapy. For daily INH, the 9-month regimen should include at least 270 doses in 12 months and the 6-month regimen should include at least 180 doses in 9 months. For twice-weekly INH, the 9-month regimen should include at least 76 doses in 12 months and the 6-month regimen should include at least 52 doses in 9 months. For the 2-month regimen of daily rifampin (or rifabutin) and pyrazinamide, at least 60 doses should be given in 3 months. For the 4-month regimen of daily rifampin alone, at least 120 doses should be given in 6 months.

   These schedules allow minor interruptions in therapy although, ideally, patients should receive medication on a regular schedule until the course of therapy is completed. When doses are missed, the duration of therapy should be lengthened. When restarting therapy after interruptions, the original regimen may be continued as long as needed to complete the recommended duration of the particular regimen or a new regimen may be needed if interruptions were frequent or prolonged. If treatment is interrupted for longer than 2 months, the client should be reassessed for active TB before restarting drug therapy.

## Home Care Considerations: Drugs to Treat Tuberculosis

***ASSESS:*** the client and family's knowledge of tuberculosis and how to prevent spread of infection; the client for compliance with the prescribed regimen; the client for signs of peripheral neuropathy, visual disturbances, or ototoxicity (with streptomycin administration), need for referral for treatment.

***MONITOR:*** the therapeutic and adverse effects of the drugs; that client is continuing prescribed drug regimen even when feeling better, keeping appointments for sputum, blood testing, and chest x-rays, and follow-up care.

***EDUCATE:*** on safe use of the drugs (eg, avoidance of alcohol to reduce risk for liver damage, use of pyridoxine with

isoniazid to prevent peripheral neuropathy); on ways to minimize adverse effects (eg, not taking isoniazid with meals or using antacids to enhance absorption); about the importance of taking the drugs and the possible consequences of not taking them (ie, more severe disease, longer treatment regimens with more toxic drugs, spreading the disease to others). Women of childbearing age should use an alternate form of contraception than birth control pills while taking rifampin and should notify a health care provider when contemplating pregnancy if taking ethambutol and rifampin. Reinforce additional teaching points (see Client Teaching Guidelines: Isoniazid, Rifampin, and Pyrazinamide).

## Age-related Considerations: Use of Drugs for Tuberculosis and MAC Disease

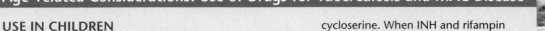

### USE IN CHILDREN

Tuberculosis occurs in children of all ages. Infants and preschool-aged children are especially in need of early recognition and treatment because they can rapidly progress from primary infection to active pulmonary disease and perhaps to extrapulmonary involvement. Tuberculosis is usually discovered during examination of a sick child or investigation of the contacts of someone with newly diagnosed active tuberculosis.

For treatment of latent infection, only one of the four regimens currently recommended for adults (INH for 9 months) is recommended for those younger than 18 years of age. For treatment of active disease, the prescribed regimens are similar to those used for adults. That is, the same primary drugs are used and may be given daily, twice weekly, or 3 times weekly with child-appropriate reductions in dosage. If the drug-susceptibility patterns of the *Mycobacterium tuberculosis* strain causing the index case are known, the child is treated with those drugs; if this information is not available, the pattern of drug resistance in the community where the child likely became infected should be the guide for selecting the drug therapy regimen. As in adults, drug-susceptible tuberculosis is treated with INH, rifampin, and pyrazinamide for 2 months. Then, pyrazinamide is stopped, and the INH and rifampin are continued for 4 more months. If drug-resistant organisms have been identified in the community, a fourth drug, ethambutol or streptomycin, should be given until the client's culture and susceptibility reports become available. If pyrazinamide is not given, INH and rifampin are recommended for 9 months. When INH or rifampin cannot be used, therapy should continue for 12 to 24 months.

Drug-resistant tuberculosis in children is usually acquired from an adult family member or other close contact with active, drug-resistant disease. For children exposed to MDR-TB, there is no proven preventive therapy. Several regimens are used empirically, including ethambutol and pyrazinamide or ethionamide and

cycloserine. When INH and rifampin cannot be given because of MDR-TB, drug therapy should continue for 24 months after sputum smears or cultures become negative. Fluoroquinolones (eg, levofloxacin, ofloxacin) are used for treatment of MDR-TB in adults, but are not recommended for use in children. Clients with MDR-TB may require months of treatment before sputum smears become negative, and they are infectious during this period. To guide dosage and minimize adverse drug effects, serum drug levels should be measured periodically, especially in clients with GI, renal, or hepatic disease or with advanced HIV infection.

In children with HIV infection, the American Academy of Pediatrics recommends three drugs for at least 12 months. If drug-resistant or extrapulmonary disease is suspected, four drugs are indicated.

Overall, as with adults, drug therapy regimens vary with particular circumstances and continue to evolve. Health care providers need to follow current recommendations of pediatric infectious disease specialists.

### USE IN OLDER ADULTS

Although INH is the drug of choice for treatment of latent infection, its use is controversial in older adults. Because risks for drug-induced hepatotoxicity are higher in this population, some clinicians believe those with positive skin tests should have additional risk factors (eg, recent skin test conversion, immunosuppression, or previous gastrectomy) before receiving INH. When INH is given, people who drink alcoholic beverages daily are most likely to sustain serious liver impairment.

For treatment of active disease caused by drug-susceptible organisms, INH, rifampin, and pyrazinamide are given, as in younger adults. Because all three drugs may cause hepatotoxicity, liver function tests should be monitored and the drugs discontinued if signs and symptoms of hepatotoxicity occur. For treatment of suspected or known MDR-TB, four to six drugs are used.

schedule follow-up care when they have symptoms than when they feel well and have no symptoms. The importance of treatment for the future health of the individual, significant others, and the community must be emphasized. In addition, clients should be informed about common and potential adverse effects of drug therapy and what to do if they occur.

2. **Providing support services and resources.** These require substantial financial resources and may include more workers to provide DOT at the client's location; flexible clinic hours; reducing waiting times for clients; and assisting clients with child care, transportation, or other social service needs that encourage them to initiate and continue treatment. Lack of these services

(eg, clinics far from clients' homes, with inconvenient hours, long waiting times, and unsupportive staff) may deter clients from being evaluated for a positive skin test, initiating treatment, or completing the prescribed treatment and follow-up care.

3. **Individualizing treatment regimens,** when possible, to increase client convenience and minimize disruption of usual activities of daily living. Short-course regimens, intermittent dosing (eg, 2 or 3 times weekly rather than daily), and fixed-dose combinations of drugs (eg, Rifater or Rifamate) reduce the number of pills and the duration of therapy.

4. **Promoting communication and continuity of care.** With clients for whom English is not their primary

language, it is very desirable to have a health care worker who speaks their language or who belongs to their ethnic group. This worker may be able to teach clients and others more effectively, elicit cooperation with treatment, administer DOT, and be a consistent support person.

## Monitoring Antitubercular Drug Therapy

There are two main methods of monitoring client responses to treatment: clinical and laboratory. The current trend seems to be increasing clinical monitoring and decreasing laboratory monitoring.

1. **Clinical monitoring** is indicated for all clients. It includes teaching clients about signs and symptoms of adverse drug effects and which effects require stopping drug therapy and obtaining medical care (eg, hepatotoxicity). It also includes regular assessment by a health care provider. Clinical monitoring should be repeated at each monthly visit. Clients should be assessed for signs of liver disease (eg, loss of appetite, nausea, vomiting, dark urine, jaundice, numbness or tingling of the hands and feet, fatigue, abdominal tenderness, easy bruising or bleeding) at least monthly if receiving INH alone or rifampin alone and at 2, 4, and 8 weeks if receiving rifampin and pyrazinamide. In addition to detecting adverse effects, these ongoing contacts are opportunities to reinforce teaching, assess adherence with therapy since the last visit, and observe for drug interactions. A standardized interview form may be helpful in eliciting appropriate information.

2. **Laboratory monitoring** mainly involves liver function tests (serum alanine and aspartate aminotransferases [ALT and AST] and bilirubin). Baseline measurements are indicated for clients with possible liver disorders, those infected with human immunodeficiency virus (HIV), women who are pregnant or early postpartum (within 3 months of delivery), those with a history of liver disease (eg, hepatitis B or C, alcoholic hepatitis or cirrhosis), those who use alcohol regularly, and those with risk factors for liver disease. Monitoring during therapy is indicated in clients who have abnormal baseline values or other risk factors for liver disease and those who develop symptoms of liver damage. Some clinicians recommend that INH be stopped for transaminase levels more than 3 times the upper limit of normal if associated with symptoms and 5 times the upper limit of normal if the client is asymptomatic.

## ■ ANTITUBERCULAR DRUGS

Antitubercular drugs are divided into primary and secondary agents. The main primary drugs (eg, isoniazid, rifampin, and pyrazinamide) are used to treat latent, active, and drug-resistant tuberculosis infection when possible. Ethambutol and streptomycin are also considered primary drugs. Because of their varied characteristics, the primary drugs are described individually below and their dosages are listed in Drugs at a Glance 32-1: Primary Antitubercular Drugs. Most antitubercular drugs are metabolized in the liver and several (eg, INH, rifampin, and pyrazinamide) are hepatotoxic. Moreover, they are often used concomitantly, which increases risks for hepatotoxicity. To detect hepatotoxicity as early as possible, clients should be thoroughly instructed to report any signs of liver damage, and health care providers who administer DOT or have any client contact should observe for and ask about symptoms. For clients at risk for developing hepatotoxicity, ALT and AST should be measured before starting and periodically during drug therapy. If hepatitis occurs, these enzymes usually increase before other signs and symptoms develop.

Secondary drugs are used only for clients who are unable to tolerate primary drugs and for clients who are infected with organisms that are resistant to primary drugs. In general, they are less effective, more toxic, or both.

## Primary Antitubercular Drugs

**Isoniazid** (INH), the most commonly used antitubercular drug, is bactericidal, relatively inexpensive, and nontoxic, and it can be given orally or by injection. Although it can be used alone for treatment of LTBI, it must be used with other antitubercular drugs for treatment of active disease. It is considered the prototype of the group of drugs and is highlighted in Prototype Profile 32-1: Isoniazid.

INH penetrates body cells and mycobacteria, kills actively growing intracellular and extracellular organisms, and inhibits the growth of dormant organisms in macrophages and tuberculous lesions. Its mechanism of action is inhibiting formation of cell walls in mycobacteria. Metabolism of INH is genetically determined; some people are "slow acetylators," and others are "rapid acetylators." A person's rate of acetylation may be significant in determining response to INH. Slow acetylators have less *N*-acetyltransferase, the acetylating enzyme, in their livers. In these clients, INH is more likely to accumulate to toxic concentrations, and the development of peripheral neuropathy is more likely. However, there is no significant difference in the clinical effectiveness of INH. Rapid acetylators may require unusually high doses of INH. They also may be more susceptible to serious liver injury because of rapid formation of hepatotoxic metabolites.

Potentially serious adverse effects include hepatotoxicity and peripheral neuropathy. Hepatotoxicity may be manifested by symptoms of hepatitis (eg, anorexia, nausea, fatigue, malaise, and jaundice) or elevated liver enzymes. The drug should be stopped if hepatitis develops or liver enzymes (eg, ALT and AST) are more than 5 times the normal values. Hepatitis is more likely to

## DRUG TABLE 32-1
### Drugs at a Glance
### Primary Antitubercular Drugs

| Name/Route | Adults Daily | Adults 2×/wk | Children Daily | Children 2×/wk | Comments |
|---|---|---|---|---|---|
| **Isoniazid** (INH) PO or IM Pregnancy Category C | See Prototype Profile 32-1: Isoniazid | | | | |
| **Rifampin** (Rifadin) PO or IV infusion Pregnancy Category C | 10 mg/kg (600 mg) | 10 mg/kg (600 mg) | 10–20 mg/kg (600 mg) | 10–20 mg/kg (600 mg) | LTBI: Given 4 mo alone or 2 mo with pyrazinamide Active TB: Given for 6 mo, with other drugs |
| **Pyrazinamide** PO Pregnancy Category C | 15–30 mg/kg (2 g) | 50–70 mg/kg (4 g) | 15–30 mg/kg (2 g) | 50–70 mg/kg (4 g) | LTBI: Given 2 mo with rifampin Active TB: Given for 2 mo with INH and rifampin |
| **Streptomycin** IM Pregnancy Category D | 15 mg/kg (1 g) | 25–30 mg/kg (1.5 g) | 20–40 mg/kg (1 g) | 25–30 mg/kg (1.5 g) | Used for active TB, with other drugs |
| **Ethambutol** (Myambutol) PO Pregnancy Category C | 15–25 mg/kg (2.5 g) | 50 mg/kg (2.5 g) | 15–25 mg/kg (2.5 g) | 50 mg/kg (2.5 g) | Used for active TB, with other drugs, and MAC disease |
| **Rifabutin** (Mycobutin) PO Pregnancy Category B | 300 mg | | Not established | | Used to treat MAC disease and to substitute for rifampin in clients taking certain anti-HIV medications |
| **Rifapentine** (Priftin) PO Pregnancy Category C | | 150 mg 2×/wk for 2 mo, then 1×/wk for 4 mo | Not established | | May be used instead of rifampin, with other drugs |

LTBI, latent tuberculosis infection

occur during the first 8 weeks of INH therapy and in people who use alcohol. Clients receiving INH should be monitored monthly for signs and symptoms of hepatitis. Because of the risk for hepatotoxicity, INH should be used very cautiously in clients with preexisting liver disease. Peripheral neuropathy may be manifested by numbness and tingling in the hands and feet. It is most likely to occur in clients who are malnourished or elderly, or who have alcoholism, diabetes mellitus, or uremia. Pyridoxine, 25 to 50 mg daily, is usually given with INH to minimize peripheral neuropathy.

**Rifampin** is a rifamycin drug that is bactericidal for both intracellular and extracellular tuberculosis organisms. It kills mycobacteria by inhibiting synthesis of RNA and thereby causing defective, nonfunctional proteins to be produced. Its ability to penetrate intact cells contributes to its effectiveness in tuberculosis because mycobacteria are harbored in host cells. Rifampin and INH are synergistic in combination, and they eliminate tuberculosis bacilli from sputum and produce clinical improvement faster than any other drug regimen, unless organisms resistant to one or both drugs are causing the disease.

## PROTOTYPE PROFILE 32-1

### *P* Isoniazid (eye soe NYE a zid)

**Drug Class**
*Chemical:* Antitubercular agent
*Functional:* Antitubercular agent

**Trade Name**
Nydrazid

**Therapeutic Indications**
Treatment of susceptible tuberculosis infection; prophylaxis in individuals exposed to tuberculosis

**Pharmacokinetics**
*Absorption*
PO, rapid

*Distribution*
Well distributed to all body tissues including CSF; penetrates and reaches therapeutic concentrations in essentially all body fluids and cavities

*Metabolism*
Hepatic; acetylation phenotype determines decay rate

*Excretion*
Kidneys

**Pharmacodynamics**
*Onset of Action*
Time to peak: 1–2 h

*Duration*
Fast acetylators: 3–100 min half-life elimination; slow acetylators: 2–5 h half-life elimination

**Contraindications/Precautions**
Hypersensitivity to isoniazid; acute liver disease
With caution in patients with renal impairment, chronic liver disease

**Pregnancy Considerations**
Category C
Enters breast milk/compatible

**Dosage**
*Adults:* Prophylaxis: 300 mg/d PO for 6 mo (without HIV infection) or for 12 mo (with HIV infection)
Treatment: 5 mg/kg/d PO given daily
Directly observed therapy: 2 to 3 times per week, 15 mg/kg PO (maximum 900 mg)
*Children:* Prophylaxis: 10 mg/kg/d PO in 1–2 divided doses (maximum of 300 mg/d) for 6 mo (without HIV infection) or for 12 mo (with HIV infection)
Treatment: 10–20 mg/kg/d in 1–2 divided doses (maximum, 300 mg/d)
Directly observed therapy: 3 times per week, 20–30 mg/kg (maximum, 900 mg)

**Adverse Effects**
Nausea, vomiting, dizziness, blurred vision, slurred speech; peripheral neuropathy

**Drug Interactions**
*Increased Effects*
Levels of hydantoins, carbamazepines, cycloserine, oral anticoagulants, benzodiazepines (those that are metabolized in liver)

*Decreased Effects*
Effectiveness of INH with aluminum salts

**Herbal Supplements and Dietary Considerations**
Take on empty stomach 1 h before or 2 h after meals
Avoid alcohol and tyramine-containing foods
Should increase dietary intake of magnesium, niacin, and folate

---

Rifampin is well absorbed with oral administration and diffuses well into body tissues and fluids, with highest concentrations in the liver, lungs, gallbladder, and kidneys. Peak serum concentration occurs in 1 to 3 hours with oral administration and immediately with intravenous administration. It is metabolized in the liver and excreted primarily in bile; a small amount is excreted in urine. Its elimination half-life is about 3 hours with a 300-mg dose and about 5 hours with a 600-mg dose. Because it is a strong inducer of drug-metabolizing enzymes, its half-life becomes shorter with continued use. The drug causes a harmless red-orange discoloration of body secretions, including urine, tears, saliva, sputum, perspiration, and feces. It may permanently stain soft contact lenses.

Adverse effects include gastrointestinal upset, skin rashes, and hepatitis, and it has many interactions with other drugs. It induces hepatic microsomal enzymes and accelerates the metabolism of numerous other drugs, thereby decreasing their serum concentrations, half-lives, and therapeutic effects. Affected drugs include acetaminophen, anti–acquired immunodeficiency syndrome (anti-AIDS) drugs (protease inhibitors and nonnucleoside reverse transcriptase inhibitors; see Chap. 33), benzodiazepines, corticosteroids, cyclosporine, estrogens, fluconazole, ketoconazole, mexiletine, methadone, metoprolol, phenytoin, propranolol, quinidine, oral contraceptives, oral sulfonylureas, theophylline, verapamil, and warfarin. With warfarin, decreased anticoagulant effect occurs approximately 5 to 8 days after rifampin is started and lasts for 5 to 7 days after rifampin is stopped. With methadone, concurrent administration with rifampin may precipitate signs and symptoms of opiate withdrawal unless methadone dosage is increased.

**Rifabutin** (Mycobutin) is another rifamycin that is active against mycobacteria. Its mechanism of action is the same as that of rifampin, so that most rifampin-resistant strains are also resistant to rifabutin. Its two main uses are in clients with HIV infection, to treat *Mycobacterium avium* complex (MAC) disease, and to substitute for rifampin in clients who need both antitubercular and certain antiviral drugs. The major advantages of rifabutin over rifampin are a longer serum half-life (45 hours, on average) and reduced hepatic induction of microsomal metabolism. Rifabutin has no advantage over rifampin in treatment of tuberculosis but may be given concurrently with INH to clients who need prophylaxis against both *M. tuberculosis* and *M. avium.*

Rifabutin is well absorbed from the GI tract; a dose of 300 mg produces peak serum concentration in about 23 hours. It is extensively metabolized in the liver (and to a lesser extent in the intestinal wall); it is excreted in urine and bile.

Like rifampin, rifabutin and its metabolites may cause a harmless red-orange discoloration of urine, feces, saliva, sputum, perspiration, and tears. Soft contact lenses may be permanently stained. Adverse effects include GI upset (nausea, vomiting, diarrhea), hepatitis, muscular aches, neutropenia, skin rash, and uveitis (an eye disorder characterized by inflammation, pain, and impaired vision). Hepatotoxicity is rare. Adverse effects increase when rifabutin is administered with a drug that inhibits cytochrome P4503A4 enzymes (eg, clarithromycin) and inhibits rifabutin metabolism. Safety and effectiveness in children have not been established.

Also similar to rifampin, but to a lesser extent, rifabutin induces drug-metabolizing enzymes in the liver and accelerates the metabolism of numerous drugs. This action decreases concentration and clinical efficacy of beta-blockers, corticosteroids, cyclosporine, digoxin, hormonal contraceptives, itraconazole and ketoconazole, methadone, nonnucleoside reverse transcriptase inhibitors, oral hypoglycemic agents, phenytoin, protease inhibitors, theophylline, warfarin, and zidovudine. If these drugs are administered with rifabutin, their dosage may need to be increased.

**Rifapentine** (Priftin) is similar to rifampin in effectiveness, adverse effects, and enzyme induction activity. It is indicated for use in the treatment of pulmonary tuberculosis and must be used with at least one other drug to which the causative organisms are susceptible. The main advantage over rifampin is less frequent administration (once or twice weekly). Its action has a slow onset and peaks in 5 to 6 hours. It is metabolized in the liver and excreted in urine and feces. It has a half-life of 14 hours.

**Ethambutol** (Myambutol) is a tuberculostatic drug that inhibits synthesis of RNA and thus interferes with mycobacterial protein metabolism. It may be a component in a four-drug regimen for initial treatment of active tuberculosis that may be caused by drug-resistant organisms. When culture and susceptibility reports become available (usually several weeks), ethambutol may be stopped if the causative organisms are susceptible to INH and rifampin or continued if the organisms are resistant to INH or rifampin and susceptible to ethambutol. Ethambutol is not recommended for young children (eg, <5 years of age) whose visual acuity cannot be monitored, but it may be considered for children of any age when organisms are susceptible to ethambutol and resistant to other drugs. Mycobacterial resistance to ethambutol develops slowly.

Ethambutol is well absorbed from the GI tract, even when given with food. Dosage is determined by body weight and should be changed during treatment if significant changes in weight occur.

To obtain therapeutic serum levels, the total daily dose is given at one time. Drug action has a rapid onset, peaks in 2 to 4 hours and lasts 20 to 24 hours. The drug has a half-life of 3 to 4 hours, is metabolized in the liver, and is excreted primarily by the kidneys, either unchanged or as metabolites. Dosage must be reduced with impaired renal function.

A major adverse effect is optic neuritis, an inflammatory, demyelinating disorder of the optic nerve, which decreases visual acuity and ability to differentiate red from green. Tests of visual acuity and red–green discrimination are recommended before starting ethambutol and periodically during therapy. If optic neuritis develops, the drug should be promptly stopped. Recovery usually occurs when ethambutol is discontinued.

**Pyrazinamide** is used with INH and rifampin for the first 2 months of treating active tuberculosis treatment and with rifampin alone for treatment of latent infection. It is bactericidal against actively growing mycobacteria in macrophages, but its exact mechanism of action is unknown. It is well absorbed from the GI tract and penetrates most body fluids and tissues, including macrophages containing TB organisms. Its action has a rapid onset and peaks in 2 hours. It is metabolized in the liver and excreted mainly through the kidneys. Its half-life is 9 to 10 hours.

The most common adverse effect is GI upset; the most severe adverse effect is hepatotoxicity, and the drug should not be given to a client with preexisting liver impairment unless it is considered essential. Clients without liver impairment should be assessed for symptoms of liver dysfunction every 2 weeks during the usual 8 weeks of therapy. If symptoms occur, liver enzymes (ALT and AST) should be measured. If significant liver damage is indicated, pyrazinamide should be stopped.

Pyrazinamide inhibits urate excretion. This characteristic causes hyperuricemia in most clients and may cause acute attacks of gout, but these are uncommon.

**Streptomycin,** an aminoglycoside antibiotic (see Chap. 30), acts only against extracellular organisms; it does not penetrate macrophages and tuberculous lesions. It may be used in a regimen of four drugs to treat active TB when the susceptibility of the causative organism is unknown or in a regimen of four to six drugs in the treatment of tuberculosis suspected or known to be resistant to INH, rifampin, or both. It may be discontinued when cultures become negative or after a few months of therapy.

## Combination Primary Drugs

Rifamate and Rifater are combination products developed to increase convenience to clients and promote adherence to the prescribed drug therapy regimen (for drug-susceptible tuberculosis). Each Rifamate tablet contains INH 150 mg and rifampin 300 mg, and two tablets daily provide the recommended doses for a 6-month, short-course treatment regimen. Rifater contains INH 50 mg, rifampin 120 mg, and pyrazinamide 300 mg and is approved for the first 2 months of a 6-month, short-course treatment regimen. Dosage depends on weight, with 4 tablets daily for clients weighing 44 kg or less, 5 tablets daily for those weighing 45 to 54 kg, and 6 tablets daily for those weighing 55 kg or more.

## Secondary Antitubercular Drugs

Paraaminosalicylic acid (PAS), capreomycin (Capastat), cycloserine (Seromycin), and ethionamide (Trecator SC) are diverse drugs that share tuberculostatic properties. They are indicated for use only when other agents are contraindicated or in disease caused by drug-resistant organisms. They must be given concurrently with other drugs to inhibit emergence of resistant mycobacteria. PAS is available only by special order from the manufacturer.

## Other Drugs Used in Multidrug-resistant Tuberculosis

Amikacin and kanamycin are aminoglycoside antibiotics with activity against mycobacteria. Although they are not usually considered antitubercular drugs, one may be a component of a four- to six-drug regimen to treat suspected or known MDR-TB. Similarly, the fluoroquinolones (eg, levofloxacin, ofloxacin, sparfloxacin) have antimycobacterial activity and may be used to treat MDR-TB.

## ■ TREATMENT OF ACTIVE TUBERCULOSIS

Adequate drug therapy of clients with active disease usually produces improvement within 2 to 3 weeks, with decreased fever and cough, weight gain and improved well-being, and improved chest x-rays. Treatment should generally be continued at least 6 months, or 3 months after cultures become negative. Most clients have negative sputum cultures within 3 to 6 months. If the client is symptomatic or the culture is positive after 3 months, noncompliance or drug resistance must be considered. Cultures that are positive after 6 months often include drug-resistant organisms, and an alternative drug therapy regimen is needed. With the increasing prevalence of MDR-TB, guidelines for treatment have changed and continue to evolve in the attempt to promote client adherence to treatment and to manage MDR-TB, two of the major problems in drug therapy of tuberculosis.

■ The most commonly used regimen consists of INH, rifampin, and pyrazinamide daily for 2 months, followed by INH and rifampin (daily, 2 times weekly, or

3 times weekly) for 4 additional months. If 4% or more of the tuberculosis isolates in the community are INH-resistant organisms, ethambutol or streptomycin should also be given until susceptibility reports become available. If the causative strain of *M. tuberculosis* is susceptible to INH, rifampin, and pyrazinamide, the regimen is continued as with the three-drug regimen described previously, and the fourth drug (ethambutol or streptomycin) is discontinued. If rifampin is not used, an 18-month course of therapy is considered the minimum. In the absence of drug resistance, INH and rifampin in a 9-month regimen are effective; adding pyrazinamide for the initial 2 months of therapy allows the regimen to be shortened to 6 months.

■ For INH-resistant TB, the recommended regimen is rifampin, pyrazinamide, and ethambutol for 6 months. For rifampin-resistant TB, recommended regimens are INH and ethambutol for 18 months or INH, pyrazinamide, and streptomycin for 9 months. For MDR-TB, a 5- or 6-drug regimen, individualized according to susceptibility reports and containing at least three drugs to which the organism is susceptible, should be instituted. Such regimens include primary and secondary antitubercular drugs as well as other drugs with activity against *M. tuberculosis*, such as amikacin, kanamycin, levofloxacin, ofloxacin, or sparfloxacin. Some clinicians include at least one injectable agent. The drugs should be given for 1 to 2 years after cultures become negative, preferably with direct observation. Intermittent administration is not recommended for MDR-TB.

■ In the intermittent schedules, health care providers (or other responsible adults) either administer the drugs or observe the client taking them (ie, DOT). This method was developed for clients unable or unwilling to self-administer the drugs independently. DOT increases adherence to and completion of prescribed courses of treatment. It is considered desirable for all treatment regimens and mandatory for intermittent regimens (eg, 2 or 3 times weekly) and regimens for MDR-TB.

■ During pregnancy, a three-drug regimen of INH, rifampin, and ethambutol is usually used, with close monitoring of liver function tests. Pyrazinamide and streptomycin should not be used during pregnancy.

## ■ *MYCOBACTERIUM AVIUM* COMPLEX DISEASE

*Mycobacterium avium* and *Mycobacterium intracellulare* are different types of mycobacteria that resemble each other so closely they are usually grouped together as MAC. These atypical mycobacteria are found in water and soil throughout the United States. The organisms are thought to be transmitted by inhalation of droplets of contaminated water; there is no evidence of spread to humans from animals or other humans.

*M. avium* complex rarely causes significant disease in immunocompetent people but causes an opportunistic pulmonary infection in approximately 50% of clients with advanced HIV infection. Symptoms include a productive cough, weight loss, hemoptysis, and fever. As the disease becomes disseminated through the body, chronic lung disease develops, and the organism is found in the blood, bone marrow, liver, lymph nodes, and other body tissues.

The main drugs used in prevention of MAC disease are the macrolides, azithromycin and clarithromycin (see Chap. 30), and rifabutin (described earlier). Lifelong prophylactic drug therapy is recommended. For treatment, a three-drug regimen of a macrolide (azithromycin, 250 mg daily, or clarithromycin, 1000 mg daily), rifabutin (300 mg daily), and ethambutol (25 mg/kg per day for 2 months, then 15 mg/kg per day) is often used. The drugs may also be given 2 or 3 times weekly. Drug dosages are the same for intermittent regimens, except that the larger dose of ethambutol is continued throughout. Streptomycin, 500 to 1000 mg twice weekly, is usually added for the initial 3 months of treatment when extensive MAC disease is present.

## NURSING PROCESS

### Assessment

Assess for latent or active tuberculosis infection:

- For latent infection, identify high-risk clients (ie, people who are close contacts of someone with active tuberculosis; are elderly or undernourished; have diabetes mellitus, silicosis, Hodgkin's disease, leukemia, or AIDS; are alcoholics; are receiving immunosuppressive drugs; or are immigrants from Southeast Asia and other parts of the world where the disease is endemic).
- For active disease, clinical manifestations include fatigue, weight loss, anorexia, malaise, fever, and a productive cough. In early phases, however, there may be no symptoms. If available, check diagnostic test reports for indications of tuberculosis (chest x-ray, tuberculin skin test, and sputum smear and culture).
- In children, initial signs and symptoms may occur within a few weeks after exposure, before skin tests become positive, and resemble those of bacterial pneumonia. In addition, indications of disease in lymph nodes, GI and urinary tracts, bone marrow, and meninges may be present.
- In older adults, signs and symptoms of tuberculosis are often less prominent than in younger adults, or similar to those in other respiratory disorders. Thus, an older adult is less likely to have fever, a positive skin test, significant sputum production, hemoptysis, or night sweats. However, mental status changes and mortality rates are higher in older than in younger adults.
- In clients with HIV infection, skin tests showing 5 mm of induration are considered positive. In addition, disease manifestations in clients with AIDS differ from those of people with undamaged immune systems. For example, malaise, weight loss, weakness, and fever are prominent. Other symptoms often resemble those of bacterial pneumonia, involve multiple lobes of the lungs, and involve extrapulmonary sites of infection.
- Assess candidates for antitubercular drug therapy for previous exposure and reaction to the primary drugs and for the current use of drugs that interact with the primary drugs.
- Assess for signs and symptoms of MAC disease, especially in clients with advanced HIV infection who have a CD4+ cell count of 100/mm³ or less.

### Nursing Diagnoses

- Anxiety or Fear related to chronic illness and long-term drug therapy

- Deficient Knowledge: Disease process and need for treatment
- Noncompliance related to adverse drug effects and need for long-term treatment
- Deficient Knowledge: Consequences of noncompliance with the drug therapy regimen
- Risk for Injury: Adverse drug effects

### Planning/Goals

*The client will:*
- Take drugs as prescribed
- Keep appointments for follow-up care
- Report adverse drug effects
- Act to prevent spread of tuberculosis

### Interventions

Assist clients to understand the disease process and the necessity for long-term treatment and follow-up. This is extremely important for the client and the community, because lack of knowledge and failure to comply with the therapeutic regimen lead to disease progression and spread. The American Lung Association publishes many helpful pamphlets, written for the general public, that can be obtained from a local chapter and given to clients and their families. Do not use these as a substitute for personal contact, however.

Use measures to prevent the spread of tuberculosis:

- Isolate suspected or newly diagnosed hospitalized clients in a private room for 2 or 3 weeks, until drug therapy has rendered them noninfectious.
- Wear masks with close contact, and wash hands thoroughly afterward.
- Have clients wear masks when out of the room for diagnostic tests.
- Assist clients to take antitubercular drugs as prescribed, for the length of time prescribed.

### Evaluation

- Observe for improvement in signs and symptoms of tuberculosis and MAC disease.
- Interview and observe for adverse drug effects; check laboratory reports of hepatic and renal function, when available.
- Question regarding compliance with instructions for taking antitubercular and anti-MAC drugs.

## CLIENT TEACHING GUIDELINES
## Isoniazid, Rifampin, and Pyrazinamide

✔ Isoniazid (also called INH) is one of the most commonly used medications for tuberculosis infection. It is given to people with positive skin tests to prevent development of active disease. Vitamin B₆ (pyridoxine) is usually given along with the INH to prevent leg numbness and tingling. Take INH and pyridoxine in a single dose once daily. Take on an empty stomach if possible; if stomach upset occurs, the drugs may be taken with food.

✔ For treatment of active disease, INH, rifampin, and pyrazinamide are usually given daily or twice weekly for 2 months; then the pyrazinamide is stopped and the others are continued for an additional 4 months.

✔ For treatment of inactive or latent tuberculosis infection, various regimens of INH alone, rifampin and pyrazinamide, or rifampin alone may be used. Any one of these regimens can be effective in preventing active disease if the drugs are taken correctly and for the time prescribed.

✔ INH, rifampin, and pyrazinamide can all cause liver damage. As a result, you should avoid alcoholic beverages and watch for signs and symptoms of hepatitis (eg, nausea, yellowing of skin or eyes, dark urine, light-colored stools). If such symptoms occur, you should stop taking the drugs and report the symptoms to the nurse or physician managing the tuberculosis infection immediately. Blood tests of liver function will also be ordered. In some cases, liver failure has occurred, most often when clients continued to take the medications for a week or longer after symptoms of liver damage occurred.

✔ Rifampin should be taken in a single dose, once daily or twice weekly, on an empty stomach, 1 hour before or 2 hours after a meal.

✔ Rifampin causes a reddish discoloration of urine, tears, saliva, and other body secretions. This is harmless, except that soft contact lenses may be permanently stained.

✔ Use all available resources to learn about tuberculosis and the medications used to prevent or treat the infection. This is extremely important because the information can help you understand the reasons long-term treatment and follow-up care are needed. In addition to personal benefit, taking medications as prescribed can help your family and community by helping to prevent spread of tuberculosis. The American Lung Association publishes many helpful pamphlets that are available from local health departments and health care providers. Additional information is available on the Internet. Some sites that provide reliable information include the Centers for Disease Control and Prevention (CDC) Division of Tuberculosis Elimination (DTBE) at http://www.cdc.gov/nchstp/tb/dtbe/html; and the National Tuberculosis Center at http://www.nationaltbcenter.edu/resource.html.

✔ Learn how to prevent spread of tuberculosis:

✔ Cover mouth and nose when coughing or sneezing. This prevents expelling tuberculosis germs into the surrounding air, where they can be inhaled by and infect others.

✔ Cough and expectorate sputum into at least two layers of tissue. Place the used tissues in a waterproof bag, and dispose of the bag, preferably by burning.

✔ Wash hands after coughing or sneezing.

✔ A nourishing diet and adequate rest help healing of infection.

✔ Periodic visits to a health care provider are needed for follow-up care and to monitor medications.

✔ The importance of taking medications as prescribed cannot be overemphasized. If not taken in the doses and for the length of time needed, there is a high likelihood for development of tuberculosis infection that is resistant to the most effective antituberculosis drugs. If this happens, treatment is much longer, very expensive, and requires strong drugs that cause more adverse effects. In addition, this very serious infection can be spread to family members and other close contacts. Thus, avoiding drug-resistant tuberculosis should be a strong incentive to complete the full course of treatment.

✔ Rifampin decreases the effectiveness of oral contraceptive tablets; a different type of contraception should be used during rifampin therapy.

## ▪ DRUG USE IN SPECIFIC SITUATIONS

### Effects of Antitubercular Drugs on Other Drugs

Isoniazid (INH) increases risks for toxicity with several drugs, apparently by inhibiting their metabolism and increasing their blood levels. These include acetaminophen, carbamazepine, haloperidol, ketoconazole, phenytoin (effects of rifampin are opposite to those of INH and tend to predominate if both drugs are given with phenytoin), and vincristine. INH increases the risk for hepatotoxicity with most of these drugs; concurrent use should be avoided when possible, or blood levels of the inhibited drug should be monitored. With vincristine, INH may increase peripheral neuropathy.

The rifamycins (rifampin, rifabutin, rifapentine) induce cytochrome P450 drug-metabolizing enzymes and therefore accelerate the metabolism and decrease the effectiveness of many drugs. Rifampin is the strongest inducer and may decrease the effects of angiotensin-converting enzyme (ACE) inhibitors, anticoagulants, antidysrhythmics, some antifungals (eg, fluconazole), anti-HIV protease inhibitors (eg, amprenavir, indinavir, nelfinavir, ritonavir), anti-HIV nonnucleoside reverse transcriptase inhibitors (NNRTIs; delavirdine, efavirenz, nevirapine), benzodiazepines, beta blockers, corticosteroids, cyclosporine, digoxin, diltiazem, doxycycline, estrogens and oral contraceptives, fexofenadine, fluoroquinolones, fluvastatin, haloperidol, lamotrigine, losartan, macrolide antibiotics, narcotic analgesics (eg, methadone, morphine), nifedipine, ondansetron, phenytoin, propafenone, rofecoxib, sertraline, sirolimus, sulfonylureas (eg, glyburide), tacrolimus, tamoxifen, theophylline, thyroid hormones, toremifene, tricyclic antidepressants, verapamil, zaleplon, zidovudine, and zolpidem.

Rifabutin is reportedly a weaker enzyme inducer and may be substituted for rifampin in some cases. It is probably substituted most often for clients who require anti-HIV medications.

Pyrazinamide may decrease effects of allopurinol and cyclosporine.

## Use in Human Immunodeficiency Virus Infection

Tuberculosis is a common opportunistic infection in people with advanced HIV infection and may develop from an initial infection or reactivation of an old infection. For treatment of latent infection (LTBI) in clients with positive skin tests, 9 months of INH or 2 months of rifampin and pyrazinamide are effective. Both regimens may be given daily or twice weekly. Several cases of serious liver damage, and a few deaths have been reported with the rifampin-pyrazinamide combination. Monitoring of liver function is recommended at weeks 2, 4, and 8 of the combination.

Treatment of active disease is similar to that of persons who do not have HIV infection. Those with HIV infection who adhere to standard treatment regimens do not have an increased risk for treatment failure or relapse. Thus, these clients are usually treated with antitubercular drugs for 6 months, as are HIV seronegative clients. The regimen may be longer if the bacteriologic (eg, negative cultures) or clinical response (eg, improvement in symptoms) is slow or inadequate.

A major difficulty with treatment of TB in clients with HIV infection is that rifampin interacts with many protease inhibitors (PIs) and nonnucleoside reverse transcriptase inhibitors (NNRTIs). If the drugs are given concurrently, rifampin decreases blood levels and therapeutic effects of the anti-HIV drugs. Rifabutin has fewer interactions and may be substituted for rifampin. The PIs indinavir and nelfinavir and most of the NNRTIs can be used with rifabutin. Ritonavir (PI) and delavirdine (NNRTI) should not be used with rifabutin. Also, amprenavir and indinavir increase risks for rifabutin toxicity. Dosage of rifabutin should be decreased if given with one of these drugs.

## Nursing Actions

### Antitubercular Drugs

| Nursing Actions | Rationale/Explanation |
|---|---|
| 1. Administer accurately. | |
| a. Give isoniazid (INH), ethambutol, and rifampin in a single dose once daily, twice a week, or 3 times a week. | A single dose with the resulting higher blood levels is more effective. Also, less frequent administration is more convenient for clients and more likely to be completed. |
| b. Give INH and rifampin on an empty stomach, 1 h before or 2 h after a meal, with a full glass of water. INH may be given with food if GI upset occurs. | Food delays absorption. |
| c. Give parenteral INH by deep IM injection into a large muscle mass, and rotate injection sites. | To decrease local pain and tissue irritation. Used only when clients are unable to take the medication orally. |
| d. Give IV rifampin by infusion, over 1 to 3 h, depending on dose and volume of IV solution. | For a 600-mg dose, reconstitute with 10 mL sterile water for injection; withdraw the entire amount and add it to 500 mL 5% Dextrose or 0.9% Sodium chloride solution; infuse over 3 h. |
| e. Give rifabutin 300 mg once daily; if GI upset occurs, may give 150 mg twice daily. | Manufacturer's recommendation |
| f. Give rifapentine on an empty stomach when possible; may give with food if GI upset occurs. | Usually given twice weekly for 2 mo, with 72 h between doses, then once weekly for 4 mo, along with other anti-TB drugs, for treatment of active TB. |
| g. Give secondary anti-TB drugs daily. See drug literature for specific instructions. | These drugs are used only to treat TB infection caused by organisms that are resistant to the primary anti-TB drugs. |

*(continued)*

## *Nursing Actions*

## Antitubercular Drugs (Continued)

| Nursing Actions | Rationale/Explanation |
|---|---|
| 2. Observe for therapeutic effects. | Therapeutic effects are usually apparent within the first 2 or 3 wk of drug therapy for active disease. |
| a. With latent infection, observe for the absence of signs and symptoms. | |
| b. With active disease, observe for clinical improvement (eg, decreased cough, sputum, fever, night sweats, and fatigue; increased appetite, weight, and feeling of well-being; negative sputum smear and culture; improvement in chest radiographs). | |
| 3. Observe for adverse effects. | |
| a. Nausea, vomiting, diarrhea | These symptoms are likely to occur with any of the oral antitubercular drugs. |
| b. Neurotoxicity: | |
| (1) Eighth cranial nerve damage—vertigo, tinnitus, hearing loss | A major adverse reaction to aminoglycoside antibiotics |
| (2) Optic nerve damage—decreased vision and color discrimination | The major adverse reaction to ethambutol |
| (3) Peripheral neuritis—tingling, numbness, paresthesias | Often occurs with INH but can be prevented by administering pyridoxine (vitamin $B_6$). Also may occur with ethambutol. |
| (4) Central nervous system changes—confusion, convulsions, depression | More often associated with INH, but similar changes may occur with ethambutol |
| c. Hepatotoxicity—increased serum ALT, AST, and bilirubin; jaundice; and other symptoms of hepatitis (eg, anorexia, nausea, vomiting, abdominal pain) | May occur with INH, rifampin, and pyrazinamide, especially if the client already has liver damage. Report these symptoms to the prescribing physician immediately, to prevent possible liver failure and death. |
| d. Nephrotoxicity—increased blood urea nitrogen and serum creatinine, cells in urine, oliguria | A major adverse reaction to aminoglycosides |
| e. Hypersensitivity—fever, tachycardia, anorexia, and malaise are early symptoms. If the drug is not discontinued, exfoliative dermatitis, hepatitis, renal abnormalities, and blood dyscrasias may occur. | Hypersensitivity reactions are more likely to occur between the third and eighth weeks of drug therapy. Early detection and drug discontinuation are necessary to prevent progressive worsening of the client's condition. Severe reactions can be fatal. |
| f. Miscellaneous—rifampin, rifabutin, and rifapentine can cause: | The color change is harmless, but clients should avoid wearing soft contact lenses during therapy. |
| (1) a red-orange discoloration of body fluids, including urine and tears | |
| (2) permanent staining of soft contact lenses | |
| (3) increased sensitivity to sunlight | |
| (4) unplanned pregnancy, most often associated with rifampin, which makes hormonal birth control pills and implants less effective | Women who take rifampin should use a different form of birth control. |
| 4. Observe for drug interactions. | |
| a. Drugs that *increase* effects of antitubercular drugs: | |
| (1) Other antitubercular drugs | Potentiate antitubercular effects and risks of hepatotoxicity. These drugs are always used in combinations of two or more for treatment of active tuberculosis. |
| b. Drugs that *increase* effects of INH: | |
| (1) Alcohol | Increases risk of hepatotoxicity, even if use is stopped during INH therapy |
| (2) Carbamazepine | Accelerates metabolism of INH to hepatotoxic metabolites and increases risk of hepatotoxicity |
| (3) Stavudine | Increases risk of peripheral neuropathy; avoid the combination if possible |
| c. Drug that *decreases* effects of INH: | Decreases risk of peripheral neuritis |
| (1) Pyridoxine (vitamin $B_6$) | |
| d. Drug that *decreases* effects of rifampin: | |
| (1) Ketoconazole | May decrease absorption |

## Critical Thinking Exercises

**1.** An intermittent administration schedule that is designed to increase adherence and completion of prescribed course of treatment is:

   **a.** Directly observed therapy
   **b.** Short-term therapy
   **c.** Mandatory intermittent regimen
   **d.** Sporadic management

**2.** Isoniazid (INH) increases risks for toxicity with several drugs, apparently by inhibiting their metabolism and increasing their blood levels. There is concern for all of the following drugs except:

   **a.** Acetaminophen
   **b.** Rifampin
   **c.** Carbamazepine
   **d.** Phenytoin

**3.** Pyrazinamide inhibits urate excretion. This characteristic causes what condition in most clients?

   **a.** Elevated cholesterol levels
   **b.** Pruritus
   **c.** Urinary tract infection
   **d.** Hyperuricemia

**4.** Rifamate differs from isoniazid (INH) in that Rifamate:

   **a.** Is a combination product containing INH and rifampin
   **b.** Is considered an aminoglycoside
   **c.** Must be administered intramuscularly
   **d.** Requires a longer course of administration

**5.** A tuberculin skin test in persons considered at highest risk is considered a positive reaction with an area of:

   **a.** Induration of 5 mm or more
   **b.** Induration of 10 mm or more
   **c.** Redness of 5 mm or more
   **d.** Redness of 10 mm or more

## SELECTED REFERENCES

Al-Dossary, F. S., Ong, L. T., Correa, A. G., & Starke, J. R. (2002). Treatment of childhood tuberculosis with a six month directly observed regimen of only two weeks of daily therapy. *Pediatric Infectious Diseases Journal, 21*(2), 91–96.

American Thoracic Society, Centers for Disease Control and Prevention. (2000). Diagnostic standards and classification of tuberculosis in adults and children. *American Journal of Respiratory and Critical Care Medicine, 161,* 1376–1395.

American Thoracic Society, Centers for Disease Control and Prevention (2000). Targeted tuberculin testing and treatment of latent tuberculosis infection. *American Journal of Respiratory and Critical Care Medicine, 161,* S221—S247.

Centers for Disease Control and Prevention. (2001). Fatal and severe liver injuries associated with rifampin and pyrazinamide for latent tuberculosis infection and revisions in American Thoracic Society/CDC recommendations. *Morbidity and Mortality Weekly Report, 50*(34), 733–735 (August 31, 2001).

Daley, C. L. (2000). Pulmonary tuberculosis. In H. D. Humes (Ed.), *Kelley's textbook of internal medicine* (4th ed., pp. 2454–2460). Philadelphia: Lippincott Williams & Wilkins.

Fitzpatrick, L. K., & Braden, C. (2000). Tuberculosis. In H. D. Humes (Ed.), *Kelley's textbook of internal medicine* (4th ed., pp. 2055–2065). Philadelphia: Lippincott Williams & Wilkins.

Kamholz, S. L. (2001). Current trends in multidrug-resistant tuberculosis. Presented at the 67th Annual Scientific Assembly of the American College of Chest Physicians, November 4, 2001.

Kim, R. B. (Ed.) (2001). *Handbook of adverse drug interactions.* New Rochelle, NY: The Medical Letter.

Lacy, C. F., Armstrong, L. L., Goldman, M. P., & Lance, L. L. (2003). *Lexi-Comp's drug information handbook* (11th ed.). Hudson, OH: American Pharmaceutical Association.

Porth, C. M. (Ed.). (2002). *Pathophysiology: Concepts of altered health states* (6th ed., pp. 615–619). Philadelphia: Lippincott Williams & Wilkins.

Small, P. M., & Fujiwara, P. I. (2001). Management of tuberculosis in the United States. *New England Journal of Medicine, 345*(3), 189–200.

Starke, J. R. (2002). Tuberculosis. In H. B. Jenson & R. S. Baltimore (Eds.), *Pediatric infectious diseases: Principles and practice* (2nd ed., pp. 396–419). Philadelphia: W. B. Saunders.

Zeind, C. S., Gourley, G. K., & Chandler-Toufieli, D. M. (2000). Tuberculosis. In E. T. Herfindal & D. R. Gourley, (Eds.), *Textbook of therapeutics: Drug and disease management* (7th ed., pp. 1427–1450). Philadelphia: Lippincott Williams & Wilkins.

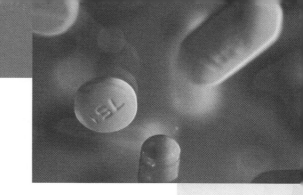

# 33

# Antiviral, Antifungal, and Antiparasitic Drugs

## OBJECTIVES

*After studying this chapter, the student will be able to:*

1 Identify characteristics of viruses.

2 Differentiate types of antiviral drugs used for herpes infections, human immunodeficiency virus (HIV) infections, influenza A, and respiratory syncytial virus infections.

3 Describe commonly used antiviral drugs in terms of indications for use, adverse effects, and nursing process implications.

4 Give the rationale for using combinations of drugs in treating HIV infection.

5 Provide guidelines for using antiviral drugs in special populations.

6 Discuss the drugs used to treat *Pneumocystis carinii* pneumonia in clients with acquired immunodeficiency syndrome (AIDS).

7 Discuss antibacterial drug therapy and immunosuppression as risk factors for development of fungal infections.

8 Describe commonly used antifungal drugs in terms of indications for use, adverse effects, and nursing process implications.

9 Give environmental and other major factors in prevention and recognition of selected parasitic diseases.

10 Discuss assessment and treatment of pinworm infestations and pediculosis in school-aged children.

11 Teach clients techniques to prevent viral, fungal, and selected parasitic infections.

## CRITICAL THINKING SCENARIO

$\mathcal{M}$ark O'Malley, a 32-year-old man, was recently diagnosed with HIV infection with a CD4+ cell count of less than 200. He is started on aggressive drug therapy with Combivir, a reverse transcriptase inhibitor combination, and nelfinavir, a protease inhibitor. Each day, he takes 12 pills at a cost of approximately $450.00 per week.

✔ What is the expected outcome of antiviral therapy in a person infected with HIV?

✔ Does Mr. O'Malley have AIDS?

✔ Is the HIV-infected person still able to spread the infection to others while on antiviral treatment?

✔ Who should be responsible for the cost of treatment if private insurance lapses when Mr. O'Malley is no longer able to work?

## PROTOTYPE PROFILE

zidovudine (AZT, ZVD, Retrovir), p. 575

# OVERVIEW

This chapter focuses on a variety of organisms that can produce disease. Viruses, fungi, and parasites and their related drug therapy are outlined. At the foundation of drug therapy to treat these organisms is general management of infection and characteristics of antimicrobial drugs addressed in Chapter 28.

Most drugs in these classes are self-administered or dosed by caregivers in the home setting. Precautions to prevent infections from occurring or spreading are important because of the close contacts among members of a household. Discussions of age-dependent factors and additional issues in the home are addressed in Age-related Considerations and Home Care Considerations, respectively.

## Viruses

Viruses produce many diseases, including AIDS, hepatitis, pneumonia, and other disorders that affect almost every body system. Many potentially pathogenic viral strains exist. Viruses can be spread by secretions from infected people, ingestion of contaminated food or water, breaks in skin or mucous membrane, blood transfusions, sexual contact, pregnancy, breast-feeding, and organ transplantation. Severe infections are more common when disease or drugs impair host defense mechanisms.

1. Viruses are intracellular parasites that can live and reproduce only while inside other living cells. They gain entry to human host cells by binding to receptors on cell membranes.

## Age-related Considerations: Use of Antiviral, Antifungal, and Antiparasitic Drugs

### USE IN CHILDREN

#### Antiviral Drugs

The use of systemic antiviral drugs may be difficult in children because several of the available agents have not been tested in this group, are not available in pediatric formulations, or do not have pediatric dosages.

Amantadine may be given to prevent or treat influenza A in children 1 year of age or older, and rimantadine is given only for prevention in children. The optimal dose and duration of amantadine or rimantadine therapy have not yet been established.

Cidofovir is highly nephrotoxic and should probably not be used in children because of long-term risks for carcinogenicity and reproductive toxicity.

#### HIV Drugs

Consistent with most other viral infections, few guidelines exist regarding the use of anti-HIV drugs in children. Most HIV infections in children result from perinatal transmission, and HIV testing should be a part of routine perinatal care. HIV-seropositive females should receive zidovudine to prevent perinatal transmission. At 14 to 34 weeks of gestation, zidovudine should be administered at a dose of 100 mg PO five times a day until delivery. At delivery, a loading dose of 2 mg/kg should be administered, followed by 1 mg/kg per hour until birth. The infant is then administered zidovudine, 2 mg/kg every 6 hours for the first 6 weeks of life. If perinatal infection occurs, the infant usually develops symptoms (eg, an opportunistic infection or failure to thrive) within the first 3 to 8 months of life. Zidovudine, which is approved for treatment of HIV infection in children, is usually the drug of choice. As in adults, anemia and neutropenia are common adverse effects of zidovudine.

Abacavir can be used in clients 3 months to 13 years of age; amprenavir can be used in children 4 to 16 years of age; didanosine is an alternative for children who do not respond to zidovudine; nelfinavir may be used in children 2 years of age and older; and delavirdine and zalcitabine may be used in adolescents. Safety and effectiveness of several drugs have not been established (eg, famciclovir, indinavir, and stavudine for any age group; ritonavir for those younger than 12 years of age; and saquinavir for those younger than 16 years). Kaletra can be used for children 6 months or older.

#### Antifungal Drugs

Guidelines for the use of topical antifungal drugs in children are generally the same as those for adults. With most oral and parenteral agents, safety, effectiveness, and guidelines for use have not been established. In addition, some agents have no established dosages, and others have age restrictions. Despite these limitations, most oral and parenteral drugs have been used successfully to treat children with serious fungal infections, without unusual or severe adverse effects. These include conventional and lipid formulations of amphotericin B, fluconazole, itraconazole, and ketoconazole. As in other populations receiving these drugs, children should receive the lowest effective dosage and be monitored closely for adverse effects. The safety and efficacy of caspofungin in children have not been established.

#### Antiparasitic Drugs

Children often receive an antiparasitic drug for head lice or worm infestations. These products should be used exactly as directed and with appropriate precautions to prevent reinfection. Malaria is usually more severe in children than in adults, and children should be protected from exposure when possible. When chemoprophylaxis or treatment for malaria is indicated, the same drugs are used for children as for adults, with appropriate dosage adjustments. An exception is that tetracyclines should not be given to children younger than 8 years of age.

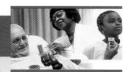

## Age–related Considerations: Use of Antiviral, Antifungal, and Antiparasitic Drugs (Continued)

### USE IN OLDER ADULTS
#### Antiviral Drugs

Selection and dosing should proceed cautiously in the elderly, who often have impaired organ function, concomitant diseases, or other drug therapy. Most systemic antiviral drugs are excreted by the kidneys, and renal impairment is common in older adults. Therefore, greater risk for toxicity exists. These risks may be minimized by dose reduction when indicated by decreased creatinine clearance (CrCl). When amantadine is given to prevent or treat influenza A, dosage should be reduced with renal impairment, and older adults should be closely monitored for CNS (eg, hallucinations, depression, confusion) and cardiovascular (eg, congestive heart failure, orthostatic hypotension) effects.

#### HIV Drugs

There is little information regarding the effects of anti-HIV medications in older adults. As potent antiretroviral therapy continues to extend the lifespan of HIV-seropositive clients, clinicians can expect to encounter greater numbers of older adults on these medications. As a general rule, renal impairment may necessitate adjustment of NRTI and NNRTI doses, whereas hepatic impairment will affect dosing of protease inhibitors.

#### Antifungal Drugs

Specific guidelines for the use of antifungal drugs have not been established. The main concern is with oral or parenteral drugs because topical agents produce few adverse effects.

Virtually all adults receiving IV amphotericin B experience adverse effects. With the impaired renal and cardiovascular functions that usually accompany aging, older adults are especially vulnerable to serious adverse effects. They must be monitored closely to reduce the incidence and severity of nephrotoxicity, hypokalemia, and other adverse drug reactions. Lipid formulations are less nephrotoxic than the conventional deoxycholate formulation and may be preferred for older adults. Azole drugs should probably be stopped if hypertension, edema, or hypokalemia occurs. In addition, itraconazole has been associated with heart failure, a common condition in older adults.

#### Antiparasitic Drugs

Older adults are more likely to experience adverse effects of antiparasitic drugs because they often have impaired renal and hepatic function.

---

2. Once inside host cells, viruses use cellular metabolic activities for their own survival and replication. Viral replication involves dissolution of the protein coating and exposure of the genetic material (DNA or RNA). With DNA viruses, the viral DNA enters the host cell's nucleus, incorporates into the host cell's chromosomal DNA, coding the host cell genes to produce new viruses. In addition, the viral DNA is transmitted to the host's daughter cells during host cell mitosis and becomes part of the inherited genetic information of the host cell and its progeny. With RNA viruses (eg, HIV), viral RNA must be converted to DNA by an enzyme called *reverse transcriptase* before replication can occur.

---

## Home Care Considerations: Use of Antiviral, Antifungal, and Antiparasitic Drugs

***ASSESS:*** willingness to persist with the long-term treatment usually required; managing symptoms of infection or adverse drug effects, and preventing or minimizing opportunistic infections. Because many of these clients' immune functions are often severely suppressed, be prepared to triage and refer client to hospitalization or other resources as indicated.

***MONITOR:*** for therapeutic and adverse effects; ability of client and family to coordinate medical and social services, manage the environment, administer the drugs. When children have parasitic infestations, the home care nurse may need to collaborate with daycare centers and schools to prevent or control outbreaks.

***EDUCATE:*** about personal and environmental hygiene measures and protective interventions, such as frequent and thorough handwashing by clients, all members of the household, and visitors; safe food preparation and storage; removing potted plants and fresh flowers; and avoiding activities that generate dust in the patient's environment. In addition, air-conditioning and air-filtering systems should be kept meticulously clean, and any plans for renovations should be postponed or canceled. Reinforce additional teaching points related to specific infections (see Client Teaching Guidelines: Antiretroviral Drugs; Oral and Topical Antifungal Drugs; Antiparasitic Drugs).

3. Viruses induce antibodies and immunity. The protein coat of the virus allows the immune system of the host to recognize the virus as a "foreign invader" and to produce antibodies against it. The exception is the influenza A virus, which can alter its protein covering so efficiently that the immune system does not recognize it as foreign. Thus, last year's antibody cannot recognize and neutralize this year's virus.

Once the virus has penetrated the cell, it is protected from antibody action, and the host depends on cell-mediated immunity (lymphocytes and macrophages) to eradicate the virus along with the cell harboring it.

## Fungi

Fungi are molds and yeasts that are widely dispersed in the environment. Molds are multicellular organisms that form a fuzzy coating on various surfaces (eg, the mold that forms on spoiled food and the mildew that forms on clothing in damp environments). Yeasts are unicellular organisms. Fungi that are pathogenic in humans exist in soil, decaying plants, and other environmental habitats or as part of the endogenous human flora. For example, *Candida albicans* organisms are part of the normal microbial flora of the skin, mouth, gastrointestinal (GI) tract, and vagina. Growth of *Candida* organisms is normally restrained by intact immune mechanisms and bacterial competition for nutrients. With suppression of the immune system or antibacterial drug therapy, fungal overgrowth and opportunistic infection can occur. In addition, some fungi have characteristics that enhance their ability to cause disease. *Cryptococcus neoformans* organisms, for example, can become encapsulated, which allows them to evade the normal immune defense mechanism of phagocytosis. *Aspergillus* species organisms produce protease, an enzyme that allows them to destroy structural proteins and penetrate body tissues.

## Parasites

A parasite is a living organism that survives at the expense of another organism, called the *host*. Parasitic infestations are common human ailments worldwide. The effects of parasitic diseases on human hosts vary from minor to major and life threatening. Parasitic diseases in this chapter are those caused by protozoa, helminths (worms), scabies, and pediculi (lice). Protozoa and helminths can infect the digestive tract and other body tissues; scabies and pediculi affect the skin.

## NURSING PROCESS

### Assessment

#### Viral

- Assessment varies with the type of viral infection and may include signs and symptoms of influenza or other viral infections of the respiratory tract, genital herpes, viral infections of the eye, or other conditions.
- Assess renal function and adequacy of fluid intake.
- With HIV infection, assess baseline data to assist in monitoring response to drug therapy. Baseline data may include vital signs, weight and nutritional status, signs and symptoms of the disease, signs and symptoms of opportunistic infections associated with the disease and immunosuppression, and available reports of laboratory tests (eg, complete blood count, CD4+ lymphocyte counts, plasma levels of viral RNA, blood urea nitrogen and serum creatinine, liver function tests).

#### Fungal

Assess for fungal infections. Specific signs and symptoms vary with location and type of infection as well as the immune state of the client.

- Superficial lesions of skin, hair, and nails are usually characterized by pain, burning, and itching. Some lesions are moist; others are dry and scaling. They also may appear inflamed or discolored.
- Candidiasis occurs in warm, moist areas of the body. Skin lesions are likely to occur in perineal and intertriginous areas. They are usually moist, inflamed, pruritic areas with papules, vesicles, and pustules. Oral lesions are white patches that adhere to the buccal mucosa. Vaginal infection causes a cheesy vaginal discharge, burning, and itching. Intestinal infection causes diarrhea. Systemic infection causes chills and fever, myalgia, arthralgia, and prostration.
- Blastomycosis, coccidioidomycosis, and histoplasmosis may be asymptomatic or mimic influenza, pneumonia, or tuberculosis, with cough, fever, malaise, and other pulmonary manifestations. Severe histoplasmosis may also cause fever, anemia, enlarged spleen and liver, leukopenia, and gastrointestinal tract ulcers.
- Cryptococcosis may involve the lungs, skin, and other body organs. In clients with AIDS or other immunosuppressant disorders, it often involves the central nervous system (CNS) and produces mental status changes, headache, dizziness, and neck stiffness.
- Sporotrichosis involves the skin and lymph nodes. It usually produces small nodules that look like insect bites initially and ulcerations later. Nodules and ulcers also may develop in local lymphatic channels and nodes. The infection can spread to other parts of the body in immunocompromised clients.
- Systemic mycoses produce severe symptoms and may be life-threatening. They are confirmed by recovery of organisms from specimens of body tissues or fluids.

## NURSING PROCESS (Continued)

### Parasitic

Assess for conditions in which antiparasitic drugs are used.

- Assess for exposure to parasites. Exposure is influenced by many variables (eg, geographic location, personal hygiene, environmental sanitation).
- Assess for signs and symptoms. These vary greatly, depending on the type and extent of parasitic infestation.
  - **Amebiasis.** The person may be asymptomatic, have nausea, vomiting, diarrhea, abdominal cramping, and weakness, or experience symptoms from ulcerations of the colon or abscesses of the liver (amebic hepatitis) if the disease is severe, prolonged, and untreated. Amebiasis is diagnosed by identifying cysts or trophozoites of *E. histolytica* in stool specimens.
  - **Malaria.** Initial symptoms may resemble those produced by influenza (eg, headache, myalgia). Characteristic paroxysms of chills, fever, and copious perspiration may not be present in early malaria. During acute malarial attacks, the cycles occur every 36 to 72 hours. Additional symptoms include nausea and vomiting, splenomegaly, hepatomegaly, anemia, leukopenia, thrombocytopenia, and hyperbilirubinemia. Malaria is diagnosed by identifying the plasmodial parasite in peripheral blood smears (by microscopic examination).
  - **Trichomoniasis.** Women usually have vaginal burning, itching, and yellowish discharge; men may be asymptomatic or have symptoms of urethritis. The condition is diagnosed by finding *T. vaginalis* organisms in a wet smear of vaginal exudate, semen, prostatic fluid, or urinary sediment (by microscopic examination). Cultures may be necessary.
  - **Helminthiasis.** Light infestations may be asymptomatic. Heavy infestations produce symptoms according to the particular parasitic worm. Hookworm, roundworm, and threadworm larvae migrate through the lungs and may cause symptoms of pulmonary congestion. The hookworm may cause anemia by feeding on blood from the intestinal mucosa; the fish tapeworm may cause megaloblastic or pernicious anemia by absorbing folic acid and vitamin $B_{12}$. Large masses of roundworms or tapeworms may cause intestinal obstruction. The major symptom usually associated with pinworms is intense itching in the perianal area (pruritus ani). Helminthiasis is diagnosed by microscopic identification of parasites or ova in stool specimens. Pinworm infestation is diagnosed by identifying ova on anal swabs, obtained by touching the sticky side of cellophane tape to the anal area. (Early-morning swabs are best because the female pinworm deposits eggs during sleeping hours.)
  - **Scabies and pediculosis.** Pruritus is usually the primary symptom. Secondary symptoms result from scratching and often include skin excoriation and infection (ie, vesicles, pustules, and crusts). Pediculosis is diagnosed by visual identification of lice or ova (nits) on the client's body or clothing.

### Nursing Diagnoses

#### Viral

- Anxiety related to a medical diagnosis of HIV infection, genital herpes, or CMV retinitis
- Altered Sexuality Patterns related to sexually transmitted viral infections (HIV infection, genital herpes)
- Disturbed Body Image related to sexually transmitted infection
- Social Isolation related to a medical diagnosis of HIV infection or genital herpes
- Deficient Knowledge: Disease process and methods of spread; availability of vaccines and other prophylactic interventions
- Risk for Injury: Recurrent infection; adverse drug effects or interactions; infections and other problems associated with compromised immune systems in HIV infection

#### Fungal

- Risk for Injury related to fungal infection
- Deficient Knowledge: Prevention of fungal infection; accurate drug usage
- Noncompliance related to the need for long-term therapy
- Risk for Injury: Adverse drug effects with systemic antifungal drugs

#### Parasitic

- Deficient Knowledge: Management of disease process and prevention of recurrence
- Deficient Knowledge: Accurate drug administration
- Imbalanced Nutrition: Less Than Body Requirements related to parasitic disease or drug therapy
- Self-Esteem Disturbance related to a medical diagnosis of parasitic infestation
- Noncompliance related to need for hygienic and other measures to prevent and treat parasitic infestations

### Planning/Goals

**The client will:**

#### Viral

- Receive or take antiviral drugs as prescribed
- Be safeguarded against new or recurrent infection
- Act to prevent spread of viral infection to others and recurrence in self
- Avoid preventable adverse drug effects
- Receive emotional support and counseling to assist in coping with HIV infection or genital herpes

#### Fungal

- Take or receive systemic antifungal drugs as prescribed
- Apply topical drugs accurately
- Act to prevent recurrence of fungal infection
- Avoid preventable adverse effects from systemic drugs

#### Parasitic

- Experience relief of symptoms for which antiparasitic drugs were taken
- Self-administer drugs accurately

*(continued)*

## NURSING PROCESS (Continued)

- Avoid preventable adverse effects
- Act to prevent recurrent infestation
- Keep appointments for follow-up care

### Interventions

#### Viral

- Follow recommended policies and procedures for preventing spread of viral infections.
- Assist clients in learning ways to control spread and recurrence of viral infection.
- Assist clients to maintain immunizations against viral infections.
- For clients receiving systemic antiviral drugs, monitor serum creatinine and other tests of renal function, complete blood count, and fluid balance.
- Spend time with the client when indicated to reduce anxiety and support usual coping mechanisms.
- For clients with HIV infection, monitor for changes in baseline data during each contact; prevent opportunistic infections (eg, CMV retinitis, herpes infections) when possible; and manage signs and symptoms, disease complications, and adverse effects of drug therapy to promote quality of life.

#### Fungal

- Use measures to prevent spread of fungal infections:
  - Observe universal precautions while assessing or providing care to clients with skin lesions. Superficial infections (eg, ringworm) are highly contagious and can be spread by sharing towels and hairbrushes. Systemic mycoses are not usually considered contagious.
  - Decrease client exposure to environmental fungi. For inpatients who are neutropenic or otherwise immunocompromised, do not allow soil-containing plants in the room and request regular cleaning and inspection of air-conditioning systems. Aspergillosis has occurred after inhalation of airborne mold spores from air-conditioning units and hospital water supplies. For outpatients, assist to identify and avoid areas of potential exposure (eg, soil contaminated by chicken, bird, or bat droppings; areas where buildings are being razed, constructed, or renovated). If exposure is unavoidable, instruct to spray areas with water to minimize airborne spores and to wear disposable clothing and a face mask. For clients at risk of exposure to sporotrichosis (eg, those who garden or work in plant nurseries), assist to identify risk factors and preventive measures (eg, wearing gloves and long sleeves).
- For obese clients with skin candidiasis, apply dry padding to intertriginous areas to help prevent irritation and candidal growth.
- For clients with oropharyngeal ulcerations, provide soothing oral hygiene, nonacidic fluids, and soft, bland foods.
- For clients with systemic fungal infections, monitor respiratory, cardiovascular, and neurologic status at least every 8 hours. Provide comfort measures and medications (eg, analgesics, antihistamines, antipyretics, antiemetics) for clients receiving IV amphotericin B.

#### Parasitic

Use measures to avoid exposure to or prevent transmission of parasitic diseases.

- Environmental health measures include the following:
  - Sanitary sewers to prevent deposition of feces on surface soil and the resultant exposure to helminths
  - Monitoring of community water supplies, food-handling establishments, and food-handling personnel
  - Follow-up examination and possibly treatment of household and other close contacts of people with helminthiasis, amebiasis, trichomoniasis, scabies, and pediculosis
  - Mosquito control in malarious areas and prophylactic drug therapy for travelers to malarious areas. In addition, teach travelers to decrease exposure to mosquito bites (eg, wear long-sleeved, dark clothing; use an effective insect repellent such as DEET; and sleep in well-screened rooms or under mosquito netting). These measures are especially needed at dusk and dawn, the maximal feeding times for mosquitoes.
- Personal and other health measures include the following:
  - Maintain personal hygiene (ie, regular bathing and shampooing, handwashing before eating or handling food and after defecation or urination).
  - Avoid raw fish and undercooked meat. This is especially important for anyone with immunosuppression.
  - Avoid contaminating streams or other water sources with feces.
  - Control flies and avoid foods exposed to flies.
  - With scabies and pediculosis infestations, drug therapy must be accompanied by adjunctive measures to avoid reinfection or transmission to others. For example, close contacts should be examined carefully and treated if indicated. Clothes, bed linens, and towels should be washed and dried on hot cycles. Clothes that cannot be washed should be dry cleaned. With head lice, combs and brushes should be cleaned and disinfected; carpets and upholstered furniture should be vacuumed.
  - With pinworms, clothing, bed linens, and towels should be washed daily on hot cycles. Toilet seats should be disinfected daily.
  - Ensure follow-up measures, such as stool specimens, vaginal examinations, anal swabs, smears, and cultures.
  - With vaginal infections, avoid sexual intercourse, or have the male partner use a condom.

### Evaluation

#### Viral

- Observe for improvement in signs and symptoms of the viral infection for which a drug is given.
- Interview outpatients regarding their compliance with instructions for taking antiviral drugs.
- Interview and observe for use of infection control measures.
- Interview and observe for adverse drug effects.

## NURSING PROCESS (Continued)

- Observe the extent and severity of any symptoms in clients with HIV infection.

### Fungal

- Observe for relief of symptoms for which an antifungal drug was prescribed.
- Interview outpatients regarding their compliance with instructions for using antifungal drugs.
- Interview and observe for adverse drug effects with systemic antifungal agents.

### Parasitic

- Interview and observe for relief of symptoms.
- Interview outpatients regarding compliance with instructions for taking antiparasitic drugs and measures to prevent recurrence of infestation.
- Interview and observe for adverse drug effects.
- Interview and observe regarding food intake or changes in weight.

## ANTIVIRAL DRUGS

Few antiviral drugs were available before the AIDS epidemic. Since then, numerous drugs have been developed to treat HIV infection and opportunistic viral infections that occur in hosts whose immune systems are suppressed by AIDS or immunosuppressant drugs given to organ transplant recipients. Drug therapy for viral infections is still limited, however, because drug development is difficult. Viruses use the metabolic and reproductive mechanisms of host cells for their own vital functions, and few drugs inhibit viruses without being excessively toxic to host tissues. Most of these agents inhibit viral reproduction but do not eliminate viruses from tissues. Available drugs are expensive, relatively toxic, and effective in a limited number of infections. Some may be useful in treating an established infection if given promptly and in chemoprophylaxis if given before or soon after exposure. Protection conferred by chemoprophylaxis is immediate but lasts only while the drug is being taken. Antiviral drugs should be used cautiously in clients with impaired renal function because some are nephrotoxic, most are eliminated by the kidneys, and many require dosage reductions because their elimination may be decreased. The antiviral drugs of most concern in hepatic impairment are the anti-HIV agents, especially the protease inhibitors. Although most antiretroviral drugs have not been studied in clients with hepatic impairment, several are primarily metabolized in the liver and may produce high blood levels and cause adverse effects in the presence of liver dysfunction. Subgroups of antiviral drugs are described in the following sections; additional characteristics and dosage ranges are listed in the Drugs at a Glance 33-1: Drugs for Prevention or Treatment of Selected Viral Infections and Drugs at a Glance 33-2: Drugs for Human Immunodeficiency Virus Infection and Acquired Immunodeficiency Syndrome.

## Viral Vaccines

Viral vaccines are used to produce active immunity in clients before exposure or to control epidemics of viral disease in a community. Vaccines for prevention of polio-myelitis, measles, rubella, mumps, smallpox, chickenpox, and yellow fever and for protection against influenza and rabies are available (see Chap. 34). Live attenuated viral vaccines are generally safe and nontoxic. However, they should not be used in clients who are pregnant or immunodeficient, or who are receiving corticosteroids, antineoplastic or immunosuppressive drugs, or irradiation. Influenza vaccines prevent infection in most clients. If infection does occur, less virus is shed in respiratory secretions. Thus, vaccination reduces transmission of influenza by decreasing the number of susceptible people and by decreasing transmission by immunized people who still become infected. The multiplicity of rhinoviruses (common cold), enteroviruses, and respiratory viruses hinders development of practical, specific vaccines for these common diseases.

## Drugs for Herpesvirus Infections

**Acyclovir, famciclovir,** and **valacyclovir** penetrate virus-infected cells, become activated by an enzyme, and inhibit viral DNA reproduction. They are used in the treatment of herpes simplex and herpes zoster infections. Acyclovir is used to treat genital herpes, in which it decreases viral shedding and the duration of skin lesions and pain. It does not eliminate inactive virus in the body and thus does not prevent recurrence of the disease unless oral drug therapy is continued. Acyclovir is also used for treatment of herpes simplex infections in immunocompromised clients. Prolonged or repeated courses of acyclovir therapy may result in the emergence of acyclovir-resistant viral strains, especially in immunocompromised clients. Acyclovir can be given orally or intravenously, or applied topically to lesions. Intravenous (IV) use is recommended for severe genital herpes in nonimmunocompromised clients and any herpes infections in immunocompromised clients. Oral and IV acyclovir are excreted mainly in urine, and dosage should be decreased in clients who are elderly or have renal impairment.

Famciclovir and valacyclovir are oral drugs for herpes zoster and recurrent genital herpes. Famciclovir is

**DRUG TABLE 33-1**

*Drugs at a Glance*

## Drugs for Prevention or Treatment of Selected Viral Infections

| Generic/Trade Name | Routes and Dosage Ranges | Comments/Uses |
|---|---|---|
| **Herpes Virus Infections** | | |
| **Acyclovir** (Zovirax) Pregnancy Category B | *Adults:* Genital herpes, PO, 200 mg q4h, five times daily for 10 d for initial infection; 400 mg two times daily to prevent recurrence of chronic infection; 200 mg q4h five times daily for 5 d to treat recurrence Herpes zoster, PO, 800 mg q4h five times daily for 7–10 d Chickenpox, PO, 20 mg/kg (maximum dose 800 mg) four times daily for 5 d Mucosal and cutaneous herpes simplex virus (HSV) infections in immunocompromised hosts (ICH), IV 5 mg/kg infused at constant rate over 1 h, q8h for 7 d Varicella-zoster infections in ICH, IV 10 mg/kg, infused as above, q8h for 7 d HSV encephalitis, IV 10 mg/kg infused as above, q8h for 10 d *Children:* <12 y: IV 250 mg/m² q8h for 7 d | For treatment of oral mucocutaneous lesions (eg, cold sores, fever blisters) Genital herpes Herpes simplex encephalitis Varicella (chickenpox) in immunocompromised hosts Herpes zoster (shingles) in normal and immunocompromised hosts |
| **Cidofovir** (Vistide) Pregnancy Category C | *Adults:* Topically to lesions q3h, six times daily for 7 d IV infusion, 5 mg/kg over 1 h, every 2 wk *Children:* Dosage not established | As treatment of CMV retinitis in persons with AIDS |
| **Famciclovir** (Famvir) Pregnancy Category B | *Adults:* Herpes zoster, PO, 500 mg q8h for 7 d Genital herpes, PO, 125 mg twice daily for 5 d *Children:* Dosage not established | Used to treat: Acute herpes zoster Genital herpes, recurrent episodes |
| **Foscarnet** (Foscavir) Pregnancy Category C | *Adults:* CMV retinitis, IV, 60 mg/kg q8h for 2–3 wk, depending on clinical response, then 90–120 mg/kg/d for maintenance HSV infections, IV, 40 mg/kg q8–12h for 2–3 wk or until lesions are healed Reduce dosage with impaired renal function | For treatment of CMV retinitis in persons with AIDS Treatment of acyclovir-resistant mucocutaneous HSV infections in immunocompromised clients |
| **Ganciclovir** (Cytovene) Pregnancy Category C | *Adults:* CMV retinitis, IV, 5 mg/kg q12h for 14–21 d, then 5 mg/kg once daily for 7 d/wk or 6 mg/kg once daily for 5 d/wk or PO 1000 mg three times daily for maintenance Prevention in transplant recipients, IV 5 mg/kg once daily 7 d/wk or 6 mg/kg once daily 5 d/wk Prevention in clients with HIV infection, PO 1000 mg three times daily | Used to treat: CMV retinitis in immunocompromised clients Prevention of CMV disease in clients with organ transplants or advanced HIV infection |

*(continued)*

**DRUG TABLE 33-1**

*Drugs at a Glance*

## Drugs for Prevention or Treatment of Selected Viral Infections (Continued)

| Generic/Trade Name | Routes and Dosage Ranges | Comments/Uses |
|---|---|---|
| **Trifluridine**<br>(Viroptic)<br>Pregnancy Category C | *Adults:* Topically to eye, 1% ophthalmic solution, 1 drop q2h while awake (maximum 9 drops/d) until re-epithelialization of corneal ulcer occurs; then 1 drop q4h (maximum 5 drops/d) for 7 d | For keratoconjunctivitis caused by herpes viruses |
| **Valacyclovir**<br>(Valtrex)<br>Pregnancy Category B | *Adults:* Herpes zoster, PO, 1 g q8h for 7 d<br>Recurrent genital herpes, PO 500 mg q12h daily for 5 d<br>Reduce dosage with renal impairment (creatinine clearance <50 mL/min) | For herpes zoster and recurrent genital herpes in immunocompetent clients |
| **Vidarabine**<br>(Vira-A)<br>Pregnancy Category C | *Adults:* IV, 15 mg/kg/d dissolved in 2500 mL of fluid and given over 12–24 h daily for 10 d<br>Topically to eye, 3% ophthalmic ointment, applied q3h until re-epithelialization, then twice daily for 7 d | Keratoconjunctivitis caused by herpes viruses |
| ***Influenza Virus Infection*** | | |
| **Amantadine**<br>(Symmetrel)<br>Pregnancy Category C | *Adults:* PO, 200 mg once daily or 100 mg twice daily<br>Reduce dosage with renal impairment (creatinine clearance <50 mL/min)<br>*Children: 9 to 12 y:* PO, 100 mg twice daily<br>*1 to 9 y:* PO, 4.4 to 8.8 mg/kg/d given in one single dose or two divided doses, not to exceed 150 mg/d | Prevention or treatment of influenza A infection |
| **Oseltamivir**<br>(Tamiflu)<br>Pregnancy Category C | *Adults:* PO, 75 mg twice daily for 5 d<br>*Children:* Dosage not established | Treatment of influenza |
| **Rimantadine**<br>(Flumadine)<br>Pregnancy Category C | *Adults:* PO, 100 mg twice daily<br>*Children: <10 y:* 5 mg/kg once daily, not exceeding 150 mg<br>*>10 y:* Same as adults | Prevention or treatment of influenza A infection in adults<br>Prophylaxis of influenza A in children |
| **Zanamivir**<br>(Relenza)<br>Pregnancy Category C | *Adults:* Oral inhalation, 1 Rotadisk twice daily for 5 days<br>*Children: ≥12 y:* Same as adults | Treatment of influenza A or B infection |
| ***Respiratory Syncytial Virus Infection*** | | |
| **Ribavirin**<br>(Virazole)<br>Pregnancy Category X | *Children:* Inhalation; diluted to a concentration of 20 mg/mL for 12 to 18 h/d for 3 to 7 d | Treatment of hospitalized infants and young children with severe lower respiratory tract infections |

AIDS, acquired immunodeficiency syndrome; CMV, cytomegalovirus.

metabolized to penciclovir, its active form, and excreted mainly in the urine. Valacyclovir is metabolized to acyclovir by enzymes in the liver and intestine and is eventually excreted in the urine. As with acyclovir, dosage of these drugs must be reduced in the presence of renal impairment.

**Cidofovir, foscarnet, ganciclovir,** and **valganciclovir** also inhibit viral reproduction after activation by a viral enzyme found in virus-infected cells. The drugs are used to treat cytomegalovirus (CMV) retinitis most commonly in clients with AIDS. In addition, foscarnet is used to treat *(text continues on page 574)*

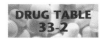

*Drugs at a Glance*

## Drugs for Human Immunodeficiency Virus Infection and Acquired Immunodeficiency Syndrome

| Generic/Trade Name | Routes and Dosage Ranges | Comments/Uses |
|---|---|---|
| *Nucleoside Reverse Transcriptase Inhibitors (NRTIs)* | | |
| **Zidovudine** (AZT, ZVD, Retrovir) Pregnancy Category C | | See Prototype Profile: Zidovudine |
| **Abacavir** (Ziagen) Pregnancy Category C | *Adults:* PO 300 mg twice daily *Children:* >3 mo: PO 8 mg/kg twice daily (maximum dose, 300 mg twice daily) | Well absorbed with oral administration Approximately 50% bound to plasma proteins Metabolized to inactive metabolites that are excreted in urine and feces May cause serious hypersensitivity reactions |
| **Didanosine** (ddI, Videx, Videx EC) Pregnancy Category B | *Adults:* PO 200 mg twice daily or 400 mg (enteric coated) once daily *Children:* <0.4 m² BSA: PO 25 mg q12h 0.5–0.7 m² BSA: PO 50 mg q12h 0.8–1 m² BSA: PO 75 mg q12h 1.1–1.4 m² BSA: PO 100 mg q12h | Used for patients who do not respond to or cannot tolerate zidovudine |
| **Lamivudine** (Epivir) Pregnancy Category C | *Adults:* PO 150 mg twice daily Weight <50 kg (110 lbs): PO 2 mg/kg twice daily *Children:* 3 mo to 12 y: PO 4 mg/kg twice daily 12–16 y: PO same as adults | Used to treat advanced HIV infection and chronic hepatitis B Well absorbed with oral administration and mainly eliminated unchanged in urine Dosage should be reduced with renal impairment |
| **Stavudine** (Zerit) Pregnancy Category C | *Adults:* Weight ≥60 kg, PO 40 mg q12h Weight <60 kg, PO 30 mg q12h *Children:* Dosage not established | Used to treat adults who do not improve with or do not tolerate other anti-HIV medications May be useful against zidovudine-resistant strains of HIV Approximately 40% is eliminated through the kidneys, and dosage should be reduced with renal impairment May cause peripheral neuropathy |
| **Zalcitabine** (Hivid) Pregnancy Category C | *Adults:* PO 0.75 mg q8h (2.25 mg/d) with zidovudine 200 mg q8h (600 mg/d) *Children:* Dosage not established | Used with zidovudine to treat advanced HIV infection in adults whose condition continues to deteriorate while receiving zidovudine May cause peripheral neuropathy |
| **Zidovudine and lamivudine** (Combivir) Pregnancy Category C | *Adults:* One capsule twice daily *Children:* Dosage not established | Combination product to reduce pill burden |
| **Zidovudine, Lamivudine, and Abacavir** (Trizivir) Pregnancy Category C | *Adults:* One capsule twice daily *Children:* Dosage not established | Combination product to reduce pill burden |

*(continued)*

DRUG TABLE
33-2

*Drugs at a Glance*

## Drugs for Human Immunodeficiency Virus Infection and Acquired Immunodeficiency Syndrome (Continued)

| Generic/Trade Name | Routes and Dosage Ranges | Comments/Uses |
|---|---|---|
| *Nucleotide Reverse Transcriptase Inhibitors* | | |
| **Tenofovir DF** (Viread) Pregnancy Category B | *Adults:* 300 mg once daily *Children:* Dosage not established | Used for salvage therapy after multiple drug failures Efficacious against hepatitis B |
| *Non-nucleoside Reverse Transcriptase Inhibitors (NNRTIs)* | | |
| **Delavirdine** (Rescriptor) Pregnancy Category C | *Adults:* PO 400 mg (four 100-mg tablets) three times daily *Children:* Dosage not established | Used with NRTIs and protease inhibitors Well absorbed with oral administration and metabolized in the liver Induces drug-metabolizing enzymes in the liver and increases metabolism of itself and other drugs Common adverse effects are nausea and skin rash. |
| **Efavirenz** (Sustiva) Pregnancy Category C | *Adults:* PO, 600 mg at bedtime *Children:* ≥3 y and weight 10–40 kg (22–88 lbs): PO 200–400 mg, depending on weight *Weight >40 kg:* PO same as adults | May cause CNS side effects |
| **Nevirapine** (Viramune) Pregnancy Category C | *Adults:* PO, 200 mg once daily for 2 wk, then 200 mg twice daily *Children:* Dosage not established | Well absorbed with oral administration and metabolized in the liver Induces drug-metabolizing enzymes in the liver and increases metabolism of itself and other drugs Adverse effects include severe skin reactions and hepatotoxicity. |
| *Protease Inhibitors* | | |
| **Amprenavir** (Agenerase) Pregnancy Category C | *Adults:* PO, 1200 mg (eight 150-mg capsules) twice daily *Children: 13–16 y and weight ≥50 kg:* PO same as adults *4–12 y, or 13–16 y and weight <50 kg:* PO 20/mg/kg twice daily or 15 mg/kg three times daily (maximum daily dose, 2400 mg); Oral solution, 22.5 mg/kg twice daily or 17 mg/kg three times daily (maximum daily dose, 2800 mg) | Well absorbed after oral administration Oral solution less bioavailable than capsules, thus the two dosage forms are not equivalent on a milligram basis Highly bound to plasma proteins Metabolized in liver; small amount of unchanged drug excreted in urine and feces May cause serious skin reactions |
| **Indinavir** (Crixivan) Pregnancy Category C | *Adults:* PO, 800 mg (two 400-mg capsules) q8h *Children:* Dosage not established | Well absorbed and approximately 60% bound to plasma proteins Metabolized in the liver and excreted mainly in feces May cause GI upset and kidney stones |
| **Lopinavir and Ritonavir** (Kaletra) Pregnancy Category C | *Adults:* 3 capsules twice daily *Children: 7–15 kg:* 12/3 mg/kg twice daily *15–40 kg:* 10/2.5 mg/kg twice daily | Combination product composed of two protease inhibitors Ritonavir boosts lopinavir levels many fold |
| **Nelfinavir** (Viracept) Pregnancy Category B | *Adults:* 1250 mg twice daily *Children: 2–13 y:* PO 20–30 mg/kg/dose, three times daily | Metabolized in the liver Most common adverse effect is diarrhea, which can be controlled with over-the-counter drugs such as loperamide. |

*(continued)*

**DRUG TABLE 33-2**

*Drugs at a Glance*

## Drugs for Human Immunodeficiency Virus Infection and Acquired Immunodeficiency Syndrome (Continued)

| Generic/Trade Name | Routes and Dosage Ranges | Comments |
|---|---|---|
| **Ritonavir** (Norvir) Pregnancy Category B | *Adults:* PO, 600 mg twice daily *Children:* PO, 400 mg/m² daily | Metabolized in the liver May cause GI upset |
| **Saquinavir** (Fortovase) Pregnancy Category B | *Adults:* PO, 1200 mg (six 200-mg tablets) three times daily *Children:* Dosage not established | Not well absorbed, undergoes first-pass metabolism in the liver, and is highly bound to plasma proteins Metabolized in the liver and excreted mainly in feces May cause GI upset May produce fewer drug interactions than indinavir and ritonavir |

BSA, body surface area.

acyclovir-resistant mucocutaneous herpes simplex infections in people with impaired immune functions. Valganciclovir and ganciclovir are used to prevent CMV disease, mainly in clients with organ transplants or HIV infection. Dosage of these drugs must be reduced with renal impairment. Ganciclovir causes granulocytopenia and thrombocytopenia in approximately 20% to 40% of recipients. These hematologic effects often occur during the first 2 weeks of therapy but may occur at any time. If severe bone marrow depression occurs, ganciclovir should be discontinued. Recovery usually occurs within a week of stopping the drug. Foscarnet and cidofovir should be used cautiously in clients with renal disease.

**Trifluridine** and **vidarabine** are applied topically to treat keratoconjunctivitis and corneal ulcers caused by the herpes simplex virus (herpetic keratitis). Trifluridine should not be used longer than 21 days because of possible ocular toxicity. Vidarabine also is given intravenously to treat herpes zoster infections in clients whose immune systems are impaired and to treat encephalitis caused by herpes simplex viruses. IV dosage must be reduced with impaired renal function.

## Drugs for HIV Infection and AIDS (Antiretrovirals)

Four classes of drugs currently exist for the management of HIV infection: nucleoside reverse transcriptase inhibitors (NRTIs), nucleotide reverse transcriptase inhibitors, non-nucleoside reverse transcriptase inhibitors (NNRTIs), and protease inhibitors. Each class inhibits enzymes required for viral replication in human host cells (Fig. 33-1). To increase effectiveness and decrease viral mutations and emergence of drug-resistant viral strains, the drugs are used in combination. All of the drugs can cause serious adverse effects and require intensive monitoring. In addition, clients with HIV infection may have concomitant liver disease that further impairs hepatic metabolism and elimina-

tion of the drugs. Although few guidelines are available, dosages should be individualized according to the severity of hepatic impairment and HIV infection, other drug therapies (for HIV infection, opportunistic infections, or other conditions), additional risk factors for drug toxicity, and the potential for drug interactions. In addition, all clients with hepatic impairment should be monitored closely for abnormal liver function tests (LFTs) and drug-related toxicity. Updated treatment guidelines are readily available on the Internet at www.hivatis.org.

### Nucleoside Reverse Transcriptase Inhibitors

The NRTIs are structurally similar to specific DNA components (adenosine, cytosine, guanosine, or thymidine) and thus easily enter human cells and viruses in human cells. For example, **ℙ zidovudine,** the prototype, is able to substitute for thymidine. In infected cells, these drugs inhibit reverse transcriptase, an enzyme required by retroviruses to convert RNA to DNA and allow replication. The drugs are more active in preventing acute infection than in treating chronically infected cells. Thus, they slow progression but do not cure HIV infection or prevent transmission of the virus through sexual contact or blood contamination.

Zidovudine, the first NRTI to be developed, is still widely used and is described in Prototype Profile 33-1: Zidovudine. However, zidovudine-resistant viral strains are common. Other NRTIs are usually given in combination with zidovudine or as a substitute for zidovudine in clients who are unable to take or do not respond to zidovudine.

### Nucleotide Reverse Transcriptase Inhibitors

This class of antiretroviral drugs is the newest and currently includes one agent. These drugs, like the NRTIs, inhibit the reverse transcriptase enzyme. However, they differ structurally from the NRTIs, and this difference helps them to circumvent acquired drug resistance. The drugs are partially activated and begin inhibiting HIV

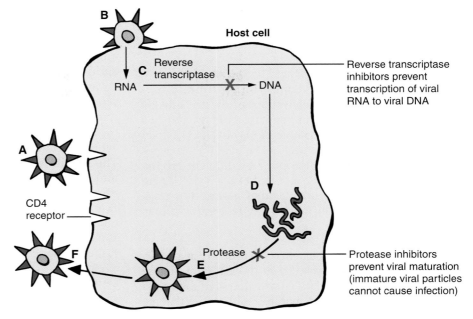

**FIGURE 33-1** HIV replication and actions of anti-HIV drugs. **(A)** The virus attaches to receptors (eg, CD4 molecules) on the host cell membrane and fuses to the cell membrane. **(B)** The virus becomes uncoated and releases its RNA into the host cell. **(C)** The enzyme reverse transcriptase converts RNA to DNA, which is necessary for viral replication. **(D)** The DNA codes for protein synthesis, which produces immature viral particles. **(E)** The enzyme protease assembles the immature viral particles into mature viruses. **(F)** Mature viruses are released from the host cell.

---

## PROTOTYPE PROFILE 33-1

### *P* Zidovudine (zye DOE vue deen)

**Drug Class**
*Chemical:* Nucleoside reverse transcriptase inhibitor
*Functional:* Antiretroviral

**Trade Names**
AZT, ZVD, Retrovir

**Therapeutic Indications**
Management of HIV infection typically in combination with other retrovirals
Reduction of maternal–fetal transmission of HIV

**Pharmacokinetics**
*Absorption*
Well absorbed PO

*Distribution*
Widely distributed; enters the CNS

*Metabolism*
Hepatic

*Excretion*
Renal

**Pharmacodynamics**
*Onset of Action*
PO: unknown; IV rapid

*Duration*
PO, IV; 4 h

**Contraindications/Precautions**
Hypersensitivity to drug, lactation, severe hepatic or renal disease, bone marrow suppression, IV additive incompatibility with blood products and protein solutions

**Pregnancy Considerations**
Category C
Crosses the placenta

**Dosage**
Management of HIV:
*Adults:* PO, 100 mg q4h while awake or 200 mg tid
IV, 1 mg/kg over 1 h q4h
*Children:* <12 y: PO, 90–100 mg/m² q6h (not to exceed 200 mg q6h)
IV, 120 mg/m² q6h (not to exceed 160 mg q6h)
Prevention of maternal–fetal transmission:
*Adults:* >14 wk pregnant: 100 mg five times a day until labor; during labor: 2 mg/kg over 1 h and then 1 mg/kg/h until cord is clamped
*Neonate:* IV, 1.5 mg/kg q6h until able to take PO; 2 mg/k q6h started within 6 h of birth and continued for 6 wk

**Adverse Effects**
Weakness, headache, dizziness, mental depression, seizures, gastrointestinal effects, granulocytopenia, anemia, tremor

**Drug Interactions**
*Increased Effects*
Additive retroviral toxicity with probenecid and fluconazole
Additive bone marrow suppression with ganciclovir, antineoplastics, or radiation therapy
Neurotoxicity with acyclovir
Concurrent use with phenytoin may alter phenytoin level and decreases clearance of retroviral by 30%

*Decreased Effects*
Reduced retroviral activity with clarithromycin
Concurrent use with phenytoin decreases clearance of retroviral by 30%.

**Herbal Supplements and Dietary Considerations**
Take PO without regard to food

replication soon after ingestion. Tenofovir is the first available drug from this class; it can be dosed once daily. Tenofovir has also demonstrated efficacy in the treatment of hepatitis B.

### Non-nucleoside Reverse Transcriptase Inhibitors

The NNRTIs inhibit viral replication in infected cells by directly binding to reverse transcriptase and preventing its function. They are used in combination with NRTIs to treat clients with advanced HIV infection. Because the two types of drug inhibit reverse transcriptase by different mechanisms, they have synergistic antiviral effects. NNRTIs are also used with other antiretroviral drugs because drug-resistant strains emerge rapidly when the drugs are used alone.

### Protease Inhibitors

Protease inhibitors exert their effects against HIV at a different phase of its life cycle than reverse transcriptase inhibitors. Protease is an HIV enzyme required to process viral protein precursors into mature viral particles that are capable of infecting other cells. The drugs inhibit the enzyme by binding to the protease-active site. This inhibition causes the production of immature, noninfectious viral particles. These drugs are active in both acutely and chronically infected cells because they block viral maturation.

Most protease inhibitors are metabolized in the liver by the cytochrome P450 enzyme system and should be used cautiously in clients with impaired liver function. They should be used cautiously in pregnant women because few data exist. It is unknown whether the drugs are excreted in breast milk, but this may be irrelevant because the Centers for Disease Control and Prevention (CDC) advises women with HIV infection to avoid breast-feeding because HIV may be transmitted to an uninfected infant. Safety and efficacy of protease inhibitors in children have not been established.

Indinavir, ritonavir, and saquinavir are the oldest and best-known protease inhibitors, but their long-term effects are unknown. Two major concerns are viral resistance and drug interactions. Viral resistance develops fairly rapidly, with resistant strains developing in approximately half of the recipients within a year of drug therapy. In relation to drug interactions, protease inhibitors interfere with metabolism, increase plasma concentrations, and increase risks for toxicity of numerous other drugs metabolized by the cytochrome P450 (CYP450) enzymes in the liver.

Ritonavir is the most potent CYP450 inhibitor among the protease inhibitor class. It may increase plasma concentrations of amiodarone, bepridil, bupropion, clozapine, flecainide, meperidine, piroxicam, propafenone, propoxyphene, quinidine, and rifabutin. None of these drugs should be given concomitantly with ritonavir because high plasma concentrations may cause cardiac dysrhythmias, hematologic abnormalities, seizures, and other potentially serious adverse effects. In addition, ritonavir may increase sedation and respiratory depression when used concurrently with benzodiazepines (eg, alprazolam, diazepam) and zolpidem.

Indinavir increases plasma concentrations of several of the same drugs listed previously and should not be given concomitantly with them because of potential cardiac arrhythmias or prolonged sedation. Saquinavir may produce fewer interactions because it inhibits the CYP450 enzyme system to a lesser extent than indinavir and ritonavir. However, if saquinavir is given with clindamycin, quinidine, triazolam, or a calcium channel blocker, clients should be monitored closely for increased plasma levels and adverse drug effects.

Amprenavir is a sulfonamide and should be used with caution in clients known to be allergic to sulfonamides. The likelihood of cross-sensitivity reactions between amprenavir and other sulfonamides is unknown. The drug formulation contains high concentrations of vitamin E, and clients using this drug should be cautioned against taking any additional vitamin E supplements. Amprenavir should be discontinued with the occurrence of severe skin rashes or moderate rashes with systemic symptoms.

### Combination Drugs

In HIV infection, as in many other conditions, the use of combination drugs is increasing. Antiretroviral drug regimens are complex and involve the ingestion of many pills daily. Adherence to the regimens is difficult but critical in preventing the development of drug resistance. Combination products decrease the "pill burden" and promote adherence. Combivir (lamivudine and zidovudine), Trizivir (abacavir, lamivudine, and zidovudine), and Kaletra (lopinavir and ritonavir) are currently available. Kaletra is a combination of two protease inhibitors in which ritonavir is added to increase serum concentrations of lopinavir. Lopinavir is not available as a single agent.

## Drugs for Influenza A

**Amantadine** and **rimantadine** inhibit replication of the influenza A virus and are used to prevent or treat influenza A infections. Postexposure prophylaxis with either drug protects contacts of people with influenza A infections. Seasonal prophylaxis may be used in high-risk clients if the influenza vaccine cannot be given or may be ineffective. In epidemics, one of the drugs is recommended for clients at high risk who have not been vaccinated. The high-risk population includes older adults, those who have chronic lung disease, and those who have immunodeficiency disorders. During an epidemic, amantadine or rimantadine may be given for approximately 2 weeks if the client is vaccinated at the beginning of drug therapy or for approximately 4 to 8 weeks if the client is not vaccinated. Protection is lost within a few days after drug therapy is stopped. For treatment of influenza A infection, either drug may shorten the illness if started soon after onset and continued for 5 days. The drugs may also decrease viral shedding and spread.

Amantadine and rimantadine accumulate in the body of elderly adults and others with impaired renal function, and dosage therefore should be reduced in these groups. The most common adverse effects of the drugs are GI (anorexia, nausea) and central nervous system (CNS; nervousness, lightheadedness, difficulty concentrating) symptoms. Amantadine has also been associated with exacerbations of preexisting seizure disorders and psychiatric symptoms. Amantadine is teratogenic in animals, and neither drug has been established as safe for pregnant women.

Amantadine is also used in the treatment of Parkinson's disease and for extrapyramidal symptoms associated with the use of certain antipsychotic drugs (see Chap. 9).

**Oseltamivir** (Tamiflu) and **zanamivir** (Relenza) are approved for treatment of influenza A or B in clients with symptoms for 2 days or less. They are used for 5 days. Oseltamivir is an oral drug; zanamivir is a powder form for oral inhalation with a device called a Diskhaler. Zanamivir may cause bronchospasm in clients with asthma or chronic obstructive pulmonary disease.

## Drug for Respiratory Syncytial Virus Respiratory Tract Infections

**Ribavirin** is used for the treatment of bronchiolitis or pneumonia caused by the respiratory syncytial virus (RSV). It is used in hospitalized infants and young children and given by inhalation with the Viratek Small Particle Aerosol Generator. The drug is not recommended for clients on ventilators because it precipitates and may block breathing tubes, including endotracheal tubes. Deterioration of pulmonary function is a common adverse effect. The drug is absorbed systemically after administration by aerosol. Most infants and children with RSV infections have mild, self-limited disease that does not involve the lower respiratory tract and therefore does not require hospitalization or ribavirin therapy.

## ▨ FUNGAL INFECTIONS

Fungal infections (mycoses) may be mild and superficial or life threatening and systemic. Dermatophytes cause superficial infections of the skin, hair, and nails. They obtain nourishment from keratin, a protein in skin, hair, and nails. Dermatophytic infections include tinea pedis (athlete's foot) and tinea capitis (ringworm of the scalp) (see Appendix F).

Most fungal infections occur in healthy people but are more severe and invasive in immunocompromised hosts. For example, *C. albicans* organisms often cause superficial mucosal infections (eg, oral, intestinal, or vaginal candidiasis) with antibacterial drug therapy. In immunocompromised hosts, candidal infections are more likely to be deep, widespread, and caused by non-*albicans* species. Other fungi that cause serious infections are not part of the body's normal flora. Instead, they grow in soil and decaying organic matter. Most invasive fungal infections are acquired by inhalation of airborne spores from contaminated soil, and severity of disease increases with intensity of exposure. Infections such as histoplasmosis, coccidioidomycosis, and blastomycosis usually occur as pulmonary disease but may be systemic. Other serious systemic infections include aspergillosis, cryptococcosis, and sporotrichosis.

Serious systemic fungal infections commonly occur and are increasing in incidence, largely because of HIV infections, the use of immunosuppressant drugs to treat clients with cancer or organ transplants, the use of indwelling IV catheters for prolonged drug therapy or parenteral nutrition, implantation of prosthetic devices, and widespread use of broad-spectrum antibacterial drugs. Characteristics of selected fungal infections are described in Box 33-1.

## Antifungal Drugs

Development of drugs that are effective against fungal cells without being excessively toxic to human cells has been limited because fungal cells are very similar to human cells. Available antifungal drugs, which differ in their chemical structures and mechanisms of action, produce their therapeutic effects by disrupting the structure and function of various fungal cell components (Fig. 33-2).

Polyenes (eg, amphotericin B) and azoles (eg, fluconazole) act on ergosterol to disrupt fungal cell membranes. Amphotericin B (and nystatin) binds to ergosterol and forms holes in the membrane, causing leakage of the fungal cell contents and lysis of the cell. The azole drugs bind to a CYP450 enzyme (14-alpha-demethylase) that is required for synthesis of ergosterol from lanosterol, a precursor. This action causes production of a defective cell membrane, which also allows leakage of intracellular contents and destruction of the cell. Both types of drugs also affect cholesterol in human cell membranes, and this characteristic is considered primarily responsible for the drugs' toxicity.

Echinocandins or glucan synthesis inhibitors (eg, caspofungin) are a new class of antifungal drugs that disrupt fungal cell walls rather than fungal cell membranes. They act by inhibiting beta-(1,3)-D-glucan synthetase, an enzyme required for synthesis of glucan. Glucan is an essential polysaccharide in the fungal cell wall; its depletion leads to leakage of cellular contents and cell death. Because human cells do not contain cell walls, these drugs are less toxic than the polyene and azole antifungals.

Drugs for superficial fungal infections of skin and mucous membranes are usually applied topically. Numerous preparations are available, many without a prescription. Drugs for systemic infections are given intravenously or orally. Patients with HIV infection need aggressive treatment of primary fungal infections and prolonged or lifelong secondary prophylaxis. Patients with prolonged or severe neutropenia secondary to treatment with cytotoxic cancer drugs also require aggressive treatment of fungal infections because they are at high risk for acute, life-threatening, systemic mycoses such as candidiasis and aspergillosis. Selected antifungal drugs are further described in the following sections. In addition, pharmacokinetic characteristics of selected drugs are listed in Table 33-1; clinical indications for use and dosage ranges are listed in Drugs at a Glance 33-3: Selected Antifungal Drugs.

### Polyenes

**Amphotericin B** is active against most types of pathogenic fungi, including those that cause aspergillosis,

## CLIENT TEACHING GUIDELINES
### Antiretroviral Drugs

**General Considerations**

✔ Prevention is better than treatment, partly because medications used to treat viral infections may cause serious adverse effects. Thus, whenever possible, techniques to prevent viral infections should be employed.

✔ Frequent and thorough handwashing helps prevent most infections.

✔ Maintain immunizations against viral infections as indicated.

✔ Always practice safer sex by using a condom.

✔ In cases of IV drug abuse, use or promote the use of clean needles.

✔ Drugs may relieve symptoms but do not cure HIV infection, prevent transmission of the virus, or prevent other illnesses associated with advanced HIV infection.

✔ Effective treatment of HIV infection requires close adherence to drug therapy regimens involving several drugs and daily doses. Missing as few as one or two doses can decrease blood levels of antiretroviral drugs and result in increased HIV replication and selection for drug-resistant viral strains.

✔ It is generally recommended that herbal products not be used with antiretroviral medications. The protease inhibitors are particularly sensitive to the effects of herbal remedies, and the use of these products may result in decreased serum levels. In controlled clinical trials, St. John's wort and garlic reduced serum levels of specific protease inhibitors. Echinacea should also be avoided because it may stimulate viral replication.

✔ Request information about adverse effects associated with the specific drugs you are taking and what you should do if they occur. Adverse effects vary among the drugs; some are potentially serious.

✔ Have regular blood tests including viral load, CD4+ cell count, complete blood count, and others as indicated (eg, tests of kidney and liver function).

✔ Keep your health care providers informed about all medications being taken; do not take any other drugs (including drugs of abuse, herbal preparations, vitamin/mineral supplements, nonprescription drugs) without consulting a health care provider. These preparations may make anti-HIV medications less effective or more toxic.

✔ If amprenavir is prescribed:

✔ Tell the prescriber if you are allergic to sulfa drugs (eg, Bactrim). Amprenavir is a sulfonamide; it is unknown whether people allergic to sulfa drugs are allergic to amprenavir.

✔ Women who take hormonal contraceptives may need to use a second form of contraception.

✔ Do not take vitamin E supplements because amprenavir capsules and oral solution contain more than the recommended daily amount of vitamin E.

✔ With nelfinavir, women using oral contraceptives may need to use a second form of contraception.

**Self-administration**

✔ Take the medications exactly as prescribed. Do not change doses or stop the medications without consulting a health care provider. If a dose is missed, do not double the next dose. The drugs must be taken consistently to suppress HIV infection and minimize adverse drug effects.

✔ These medications vary in their interactions with food and should be taken appropriately for optimal benefit. Unless otherwise instructed, take the drugs as follows:

✔ **Abacavir, amprenavir, Combivir, delavirdine, efavirenz, famciclovir, lamivudine, nevirapine, stavudine, tenofovir,** and **valacyclovir** may be taken with or without food. However, do not take abacavir, amprenavir, or efavirenz with a high-fat meal. Also, if taking an antacid or didanosine, take **amprenavir** at least 1 hour before or after a dose of antacid or didanosine.

✔ Take **didanosine** and **indinavir** on an empty stomach. This usually means 1 hour before or 2 hours after a meal. Although indinavir is best absorbed if taken on an empty stomach, with water, it may also be taken with skim milk, juice, coffee, tea, or a light meal (eg, toast, cereal). If you are taking indinavir and didanosine, the drugs should be taken at least 1 hour apart on an empty stomach.

✔ Take **ganciclovir, Kaletra, nelfinavir,** and **ritonavir** with food. The oral solution of ritonavir may be mixed with chocolate milk to improve the taste.

✔ Take **saquinavir** within 2 hours after a meal.

✔ **Delavirdine** tablets may be mixed in water by adding four tablets to at least 3 oz of water, waiting a few minutes, and then stirring. Drink the mixture promptly, rinse the glass, and swallow the rinse to be sure the entire dose is taken.

✔ To give **nelfinavir** to infants and young children, the oral powder can be mixed with a small amount of water, milk, or formula. Once mixed, the entire amount must be taken to obtain the full dose. Acidic foods or juices (eg, apple sauce, orange juice, apple juice) should not be used because they produce a bitter taste.

---

blastomycosis, candidiasis, coccidioidomycosis, cryptococcosis, histoplasmosis, and sporotrichosis. The drug is fungicidal or fungistatic depending on the concentration in body fluids and on the susceptibility of the causative fungus. Amphotericin B is highly toxic to humans and

is therefore recommended only for serious, potentially fatal fungal infections, in which it is usually the initial drug of choice. The drug is usually given for 4 to 12 weeks but may be needed longer by some clients.

*(text continues on page 584)*

## Nursing Actions
### Antiviral Drugs

| Nursing Actions | Rationale/Explanation |
|---|---|
| 1. Administer accurately. | |
| a. Give oral drugs as recommended in relation to meals: | Manufacturers' recommendations to promote absorption and bioavailability |
| (1) Give abacavir, amprenavir, delavirdine, efavirenz, famciclovir, lamivudine, nevirapine, stavudine, tenofovir, and valacyclovir with or without food. However, do not give abacavir, amprenavir, or efavirenz with a high-fat meal. Also, if the patient is taking an antacid or didanosine, give amprenavir at least 1 h before or after a dose of antacid or didanosine. | |
| (2) Give didanosine and indinavir on an empty stomach, 1 h before or 2 h after a meal. Although indinavir is best absorbed if taken on an empty stomach, with water, it may also be taken with skim milk, juice, coffee, tea, or a light meal (eg, toast, cereal). If the patient is taking indinavir and didanosine, the drugs should be given at least 1 h apart on an empty stomach. | |
| (3) Give ganciclovir, nelfinavir, Kaletra, and ritonavir with food. The oral solution of ritonavir may be mixed with chocolate milk to improve the taste. | |
| (4) Give saquinavir within 2 h after a meal. | |
| b. Delavirdine tablets may be mixed in water by adding four tablets to at least 3 oz of water, waiting a few minutes, and then stirring. Have the client drink the mixture promptly, rinse the glass, and swallow the rinse to be sure the entire dose is taken. | |
| c. To give nelfinavir to infants and young children, the oral powder can be mixed with a small amount of water, milk, or formula. Once mixed, the entire amount must be taken to obtain the full dose. | Acidic foods or juices (eg, orange juice, apple juice, apple sauce) should not be used because they produce a bitter taste. |
| d. Give intravenous (IV) acyclovir, cidofovir, foscarnet, and ganciclovir over 1 h. | To decrease tissue irritation and increased toxicity from high plasma levels |
| e. With cidofovir therapy, give probenecid 2 g 3 h before cidofovir, 1 g 2 h before cidofovir, and 1 g 8 h after completion of the cidofovir infusion | To slow renal excretion of cidofovir and decrease nephrotoxic effects |
| f. When applying topical acyclovir, wear a glove to apply. | |
| g. When administering ribavirin, follow the manufacturer's instructions. | |
| 2. Observe for therapeutic effects. | |
| a. With acyclovir for genital herpes, observe for fewer recurrences when given for prophylaxis; observe for healing of lesions and decreased pain and itching when given for treatment. | |
| b. With amantadine, observe for absence of symptoms when given for prophylaxis of influenza A and decreased fever, cough, muscle aches, and malaise when given for treatment. | |
| c. With cidofovir, ganciclovir, or foscarnet for cytomegalovirus retinitis, observe for improved vision. | |
| d. With ophthalmic drugs, observe for decreased signs of eye infection. | |
| e. With antiretroviral drugs, observe for improved clinical status (fewer signs and symptoms) and improved laboratory markers (eg, decreased viral load, increased CD4+ cell count) | |

*(continued)*

## Nursing Actions

## Antiviral Drugs (Continued)

| Nursing Actions | Rationale/Explanation |
|---|---|
| 3. Observe for adverse effects. | |
| a. General effects—anorexia, nausea, vomiting, diarrhea, fever, headache | These effects occur with most systemic antiviral drugs and may range from mild to severe. |
| b. With IV acyclovir—phlebitis at injection site, skin rash, urticaria, increased blood urea nitrogen or serum creatinine, encephalopathy manifested by confusion, coma, lethargy, seizures, tremors | Encephalopathy is rare but potentially serious; other effects commonly occur. |
| c. With topical acyclovir—burning or stinging and pruritus | These effects are usually transient. |
| d. With amantadine and rimantadine—central nervous system (CNS) effects with anxiety, ataxia, dizziness, hyperexcitability, insomnia, mental confusion, hallucinations, slurred speech | CNS symptoms are reportedly more likely with zalcitabine and amantadine than with rimantadine and may be similar to those caused by atropine and CNS stimulants. Adverse reactions are more likely to occur in older adults and those with renal impairment. |
| e. With didanosine, zalcitabine, and zidovudine—peripheral neuropathy (numbness, burning, pain in hands and feet), pancreatitis (abdominal pain, severe nausea and vomiting, elevated serum amylase) | Peripheral neuropathy is more likely with zalcitibine and the drug should be discontinued if symptoms occur. Pancreatitis may be more likely with didanosine, especially in those with previous episodes, alcohol consumption, elevated serum triglycerides, or advanced HIV infection. Didanosine should be stopped promptly if symptoms of pancreatitis occur. Renal impairment may be more likely to occur with foscarnet. |
| f. With ganciclovir and foscarnet—bone marrow depression (anemia, leukopenia, neutropenia, thrombocytopenia), renal impairment (increased serum creatinine and decreased creatinine clearance), neuropathy | |
| g. With indinavir, ritonavir, and saquinavir—circumoral and peripheral paresthesias, debilitation, fatigue | The most frequent adverse effects are the general ones listed above. Most are relatively mild. |
| h. With lamivudine and stavudine—peripheral neuropathy, flu-like syndrome (fever, malaise, muscle and joint aches or pain), dizziness, insomnia, depression | |
| i. With abacavir—anaphylactic–like symptoms—if skin rash or shortness of breath develops, immediately discontinue the drug and do not readminister. | |
| j. With ribavirin—increased respiratory distress | Pulmonary function may deteriorate. |
| k. With zidovudine—bone marrow depression (BMD; anemia, leukopenia, granulocytopenia, thrombocytopenia); anemia and neutropenia in newborn infants | Anemia may occur within 2–4 wk of starting the drug; granulocytopenia is more likely after 6–8 wk. A complete blood count should be performed every 2 wk. Colony-stimulating factors have been used to aid recovery of bone marrow function. Blood transfusions may be given for anemia. The hematologic effects on newborn infants may occur when the mothers received zidovudine during pregnancy. |
| l. With ophthalmic antiviral drugs—pain, itching, edema, or inflammation of the eyelids | These symptoms result from tissue irritation or hypersensitivity reactions. |
| 4. Observe for drug interactions. | Antiviral drugs are often given concomitantly with each other and with many other drugs, especially those used to treat opportunistic infections and other illnesses associated with HIV infection and organ transplantation. In general, combinations of drugs that cause similar, potentially serious adverse effects (eg, bone marrow depression, peripheral neuropathy) should be avoided, when possible. |
| a. Drugs that *increase* effects of acyclovir: | |
| (1) Probenecid | May increase blood levels of acyclovir by slowing its renal excretion |
| (2) Zidovudine | Severe drowsiness and lethargy may occur. |

*(continued)*

## Nursing Actions

## Antiviral Drugs (Continued)

| Nursing Actions | Rationale/Explanation |
|---|---|
| b. Drugs that *increase* effects of amantadine and rimantadine:<br>(1) Anticholinergics—atropine, first-generation antihistamines, antipsychotics, tricyclic antidepressants<br><br>(2) CNS stimulants | These drugs add to the anticholinergic effects (eg, blurred vision, mouth dryness, urine retention, constipation, tachycardia) of the antiviral agents.<br>These drugs add to the CNS-stimulating effects (eg, confusion, insomnia, nervousness, hyperexcitability) of the antiviral agents. |
| c. Drugs that *increase* effects of cidofovir and foscarnet:<br>(1) Aminoglycoside antibiotics, amphotericin B, didanosine, IV pentamidine | These drugs are nephrotoxic and increase risks of nephrotoxicity. |
| d. Drugs that *increase* effects of ganciclovir:<br>(1) Imipenem/cilastatin<br>(2) Nephrotoxic drugs (eg, amphotericin B, cyclosporine)<br><br>(3) Probenecid | Increased risk of seizures; avoid the combination if possible.<br>Increased serum creatinine and potential nephrotoxicity<br><br>May increase blood levels of ganciclovir by decreasing its renal excretion |
| e. Drugs that *increase* effects of indinavir:<br>(1) Clarithromycin, ketoconazole, quinidine, zidovudine. | Increase blood levels of indinavir, probably by decreasing its metabolism and elimination |
| f. Drugs that *decrease* effects of indinavir:<br>(1) Didanosine<br><br><br><br>(2) Fluconazole<br>(3) Rifampin, rifabutin | Didanosine increases gastric pH and decreases absorption of indinavir. If the two drugs are given concurrently, give at least 1 h apart, on an empty stomach.<br>Decreases blood levels of indinavir<br>These drugs speed up metabolism of indinavir by inducing hepatic drug-metabolizing enzymes. |
| g. Drug that *increases* the effects of lamivudine:<br>(1) Trimethoprim/sulfamethoxazole | Decreases elimination of lamivudine |
| h. Drugs that *increase* the effects of ritonavir:<br>(1) Clarithromycin, fluconazole, fluoxetine: | Increase blood levels, probably by slowing metabolism of ritonavir |
| i. Drug that *decreases* the effects of ritonavir:<br>(1) Rifampin | Accelerates metabolism of ritonavir by inducing drug-metabolizing enzymes in the liver |
| j. Drug that *increases* the effects of saquinavir:<br>(1) Ketoconazole | Increases blood levels of saquinavir |
| k. Drugs that *decrease* the effects of saquinavir:<br>(1) Rifampin, rifabutin | Accelerate metabolism of ritonavir by inducing drug-metabolizing enzymes in the liver |
| l. Drugs that *increase* the effects of zalcitabine:<br>(1) Chloramphenicol, cisplatin, didanosine, ethionamide, isoniazid, metronidazole, nitrofurantoin, phenytoin, ribavirin, vincristine<br>(2) Cimetidine, probenecid<br><br>(3) Pentamidine (IV) | Zalcitabine and these drugs are associated with peripheral neuropathy; concomitant use increases risks of this adverse effect.<br>Increase blood levels of zalcitabine by decreasing its elimination<br>Increased risk of pancreatitis. If IV pentamidine is used to treat *Pneumocystis carinii* pneumonia, zalcitabine should be interrupted. |
| m. Drugs that *decrease* effects of zalcitabine:<br>(1) Antacids, metoclopramide | Decrease absorption. Do not give antacids at the same time as zalcitabine. |

*(continued)*

## Nursing Actions

### Antiviral Drugs (Continued)

| Nursing Actions | Rationale/Explanation |
|---|---|
| n. Drugs that *increase* effects of zidovudine: | |
| (1) Doxorubicin, vincristine, vinblastine | Increased bone marrow depression, including neutropenia |
| (2) Amphotericin B, flucytosine | Increased nephrotoxicity |
| (3) Ganciclovir and pentamidine | Increased neutropenia |
| (4) Probenecid, trimethoprim | May increase blood levels of zidovudine, probably by decreasing renal excretion |
| o. Drugs that *decrease* effects of zidovudine: | |
| (1) Rifampin, rifabutin | Accelerate metabolism of zidovudine |
| p. Drugs that *decrease* effects of Kaletra: | |
| (1) Efavirenz | Dosage of Kaletra may need to be increased if it is given concomitantly with one of these drugs. |
| (2) Nevirapine | |

### BOX 33-1    Selected Fungal Infections

**Aspergillosis,** the most common invasive mold infection worldwide, occurs in debilitated and immunocompromised people, including those with leukemia, lymphoma, or acquired immunodeficiency syndrome (AIDS), and those with neutropenia from a disease process or drug therapy. Invasive aspergillosis is characterized by inflammatory granulomatous lesions, which may develop in the bronchi, lungs, ear canal, skin, or mucous membranes of the eye, nose, or urethra. It may extend into blood vessels, which leads to infection of the brain, heart, kidneys, and other organs. Invasive aspergillosis is a serious illness associated with thrombosis, ischemic infarction of involved tissues, and progressive disease. It is often fatal.

Allergic bronchopulmonary aspergillosis, an allergic reaction to inhaled aspergillus spores, may develop in people with asthma and cause bronchoconstriction, wheezing, dyspnea, cough, muscle aches, and fever. The condition is aggravated if the spores germinate and grow in the airways, thereby producing chronic exposure to the antigen and permanent fibrotic damage.

*Aspergillus* mold may be found in soil, decaying plant matter, cellars, potted plants, peppers and spices, showerheads, hot water faucets, public buildings, and private homes. It is estimated to comprise about 40% of the fungal flora in homes and hospitals. It has also been found in library books, on soft contact lenses, and in food. In neutropenic patients, ingestion of cereals, powdered milk, tea, and soy sauce has been linked to aspergillosis. A few cases in immunocompromised patients have been associated with marijuana smoking and the organism can infest peanuts, cashews, and coffee beans. Large numbers of spores are released into the air during soil excavations (eg, for construction or renovation of buildings) or handling of decaying organic matter and carried into most human environments. There are several species that cause invasive disease in humans but *A. fumigatus* is the most common (about 90% of cases). *A. fumigatus* reproduces by releasing spores, which are small enough to reach the alveoli when inhaled. Most aspergillus

organisms (80% to 90%) enter the body through the respiratory system, and pulmonary aspergillosis is acquired by inhalation of the spores. Other potential entry sites include damaged skin (eg, burn wounds, intravenous catheter insertion sites), operative wounds, the cornea, and the ear.

Aspergillosis in hospitalized patients has long been attributed to entry of outside air containing aspergillus spores into hospital ventilation systems. Consequently, preventive measures have focused on removing aspergillus spores from the air and preventing exposure by using high efficiency particle air (HEPA) filtration, laminar air flow, and positive pressure systems in rooms used by high-risk patients (eg, those with bone marrow or organ transplants). Specific recommendations are to place HEPA filters where outside air enters patient rooms; position air intake and exhaust ports so that room air enters from one side of the room, flows across the room, and exits on the opposite side; and maintain room air pressure above that of the corridor so that corridor air cannot enter the room. In addition, monitor filtration systems (eg, regular preventive maintenance and checking of pressures and airflow) and construct windows, doors, and air entry and exit ports to seal patients' rooms and prevent air leaks. Doors to patients' rooms should be kept closed as much as possible.

Despite the use of the above measures, the incidence of aspergillosis continued to increase and researchers began looking for other sources of infection. One recent study identified a hospital water system as a source of exposure. More airborne particles containing aspergillus were found in bathrooms than in patient rooms and hallways and *A. fumigatus* organisms isolated from a patient with aspergillosis were identical to those recovered from the shower wall in the patient's room. The researchers concluded that the hospital water supply can be a source of nosocomial aspergillosis. Another study investigated the spread of invasive aspergillosis in an intensive care unit for liver transplant patients. The index case developed a wound infection 11 days after liver

*(continued)*

BOX
33-1    Selected Fungal Infections (Continued)

transplantation. Two other patients in the unit developed invasive pulmonary aspergillosis. The researchers concluded that *Aspergillus* organisms can form spores in infected wounds and that debriding and dressing those wounds may result in aerosolization of spores and airborne person-to-person transmission. With these organisms, inhalation of spores and direct inoculation of tissues by spores are common routes of infection. Health care providers, especially those who work with immunocompromised patients, should be aware of this potential risk. Hospitalized patients with wound or skin infections caused by *Aspergillus* species should have their lesions covered with a clean dressing and disruptions minimized. If this is not feasible, the patient should be placed in a private room with monitored negative room air pressure and HEPA filtration of the room air, if available. These recommendations may also be helpful with lung transplant recipients who develop tracheobronchial aspergillosis and may potentially be a source of airborne *Aspergillus* organisms.

**Blastomycosis** is initiated by inhalation of spores from a fungus that grows in soil and decaying organic matter. The organism is widespread in the southeastern United States, Minnesota, Wisconsin, Michigan, and New York. Sporadic cases most often occur in adult males who have extensive exposure to woods and streams with vocational or recreational activities. The infection may be asymptomatic or produce pulmonary symptoms resembling pneumonia, tuberculosis, or lung cancer. It may also be systemic and involve other organs, especially the skin and bone. Skin lesions (eg, pustules, ulcerations, abscesses) may progress over a period of years and eventually involve large areas of the body. Bone invasion, with arthritis and bone destruction, occurs in 25% to 50% of clients.

Blastomycosis can occur in healthy people with sufficient exposure but is usually more severe and more likely to involve multiple organ involvement and CNS disease in immunocompromised clients. However, it infrequently occurs in patients with HIV infection.

**Candidiasis** is a yeast infection that often occurs in clients with malignant lymphomas, diabetes mellitus, or AIDS and in clients receiving antibiotic, antineoplastic, corticosteroid, and immunosuppressant drug therapy. *Candida* organisms are found in soil, on inanimate objects, in hospital environments, and in food. In the human body, they are found on diseased skin and along the entire gastrointestinal (GI) tract, in sputum, along the female genital tract, and in the urine of patients with indwelling bladder catheters. Most infections arise from the normal endogenous organisms, often from the GI tract or skin, and are caused by *Candida albicans*. Oral, intestinal, vaginal, and systemic candidiasis can occur. Early recognition and treatment of local infections may prevent systemic candidiasis.

- **Oral candidiasis** (thrush) is characterized by painless white plaques on oral and pharyngeal mucosa. It often occurs in newborn infants who become infected during passage through an infected or colonized vagina. In older children and adults, thrush may occur as a complication of diabetes mellitus, as a result of poor oral hygiene, or after taking antibiotics or corticosteroids. It may also occur as an early manifestation of AIDS.

- **Gastrointestinal candidiasis** most often occurs after prolonged broad-spectrum antibacterial therapy, which destroys a large part of the normal flora of the intestine. The main symptom is diarrhea.
- **Vaginal candidiasis** commonly occurs in women who are pregnant, have diabetes mellitus, or take oral contraceptives or antibacterial drugs. The main symptom is a yellowish vaginal discharge. The infection may produce inflammation of the perineal area and spread to the buttocks and thighs. The organism is difficult to eradicate, and many women have recurrent infections.
- **Skin candidiasis** usually occurs in people with continuously moist skinfolds or moist surgical dressings. The organism also may cause diaper rash and perineal rashes. Skin lesions are red and macerated.
- **Systemic** or **invasive candidiasis** occurs when the organism gets into the bloodstream and is circulated throughout the body, with the brain, heart, kidneys, and eyes as the most common sites of infection. It often occurs as a nosocomial infection in clients with serious illnesses or drug therapies that suppress their immune systems and may be fatal. Invasive infections may be present in any organ and may produce such disorders as urinary tract infection, endocarditis, and meningitis. It is usually diagnosed by positive cultures of blood or tissue. Signs and symptoms depend on the severity of the infection and the organs affected.

The incidence of severe candidal infections has increased in recent years, in part because of increased numbers of neutropenic and immunodeficient patients. In addition, the frequent use of strong, broad-spectrum antibiotics leads to extensive candidal colonization in debilitated patients and the widespread use of medical devices (eg, intravascular catheters, monitoring equipment, endotracheal tubes, and urinary catheters) allows the organisms to reach sites that are normally sterile. People who use intravenous drugs also develop invasive candidiasis because the injections inoculate the fungi directly into the bloodstream.

The incidence of invasive infections caused by non-albicans *Candida* species also seems to be increasing. These infections are probably related to the widespread use of antifungal drugs such as fluconazole. In general, non-albicans candidal infections are less susceptible to azole antifungal drugs (eg, fluconazole, itraconazole) and are more difficult to treat effectively with the currently available agents.

**Coccidioidomycosis** is caused by an organism that grows as a mold in soil and decaying organic matter and is commonly found in the southwestern United States and northern Mexico. Infection results from inhalation of spores that convert to yeasts in the warm environment of the body and often cause asymptomatic or mild respiratory infection. However, the organism may cause acute pulmonary infection with fever, chest pain, cough, headache, and loss of appetite. Radiographs may show small nodules in the lung like those seen in tuberculosis. In some cases, chronic disease develops in which the organisms remain localized and cause large, organism-

*(continued)*

## BOX 33-1 Selected Fungal Infections (Continued)

filled cavities in the lung. These cavities may become fibrotic and eventually require surgical excision. In a few cases, severe, disseminated disease occurs, either soon after the primary infection or after years of chronic pulmonary disease. Disseminated coccidioidomycosis may produce an acute or chronic meningitis or a generalized disease with lesions in many internal organs. Skin lesions appear as granulomas that may eventually heal or become ulcerations. Most clients with primary infection recover without treatment; clients with disseminated disease require prolonged chemotherapy.

Coccidioidomycosis may occur in healthy or immuno-compromised people but is more severe and more likely to become systemic in immunocompromised clients. For example, clients with AIDS who live in endemic areas are highly susceptible to this infection. The severity of the disease also increases with intensity of exposure.

**Cryptococcosis** is caused by inhalation of spores of *Cryptococcus neoformans,* an organism found worldwide. *C. neoformans* organisms grow most abundantly in bird excreta, especially pigeon droppings. They have also been isolated from nonavian sources such as fruits, vegetables, and dairy products.

When cryptococcosis occurs in healthy people, the primary infection is localized in the lungs, is asymptomatic or produces mild symptoms, and heals without treatment. However, pneumonia may occur and lead to spread of the organisms by the bloodstream. When cryptococcosis occurs in immunocompromised people, it is likely to be more severe and to become disseminated to the CNS, skin, and other body organs. People with AIDS are highly susceptible and cryptococcosis is the fourth most frequent opportunistic infection in this population. Infection most often affects the lungs and CNS. Cryptococcal pneumonia in patients with AIDS has a mortality rate of 40% or more. Cryptococcal meningitis, the most common manifestation of disseminated disease, often produces abscesses in the brain. Clinical manifestations include headache, dizziness, and neck stiffness, and the condition is often mistaken for brain tumor. Later symptoms include coma, respiratory failure, and death if the meningitis is not treated effectively.

**Histoplasmosis** is a common fungal infection that occurs worldwide, especially in the central and mideastern United States. The causative fungus is found in soil and organic debris around chicken houses, bird roosts, and caves inhabited by bats. Exposure to spores may result from activities such as demolishing or remodeling old buildings, clearing brush from urban parks, or cleaning chicken coops. Spores can be picked up by the wind and spread over large areas. Histoplasmosis develops when the spores are inhaled into the lungs, where

they rapidly develop into the tissue-invasive yeast cells that reach the bloodstream and become distributed throughout the body. In most cases, the organisms are destroyed or encapsulated by the host's immune system. The lung lesions heal by fibrosis and calcification and resemble the lesions of tuberculosis.

Clinical manifestations may vary widely. In people with normal immune responses, manifestations can be correlated with the extent of exposure. Most infections are asymptomatic or produce minimal symptoms for which treatment is not sought. When symptoms occur, they usually resemble an acute, influenza-like respiratory infection and improve within a few weeks. However, people exposed to large amounts of spores may have a high fever and severe pneumonia, which usually resolves with a low mortality rate. Some people, most often adult men with underlying emphysema or other lung disease, develop chronic pulmonary histoplasmosis with recurrent episodes of cough, fever, and weakness. Some people (10% or fewer) also develop inflammatory complications such as arthritis, arthralgia, or pericarditis. These disorders are usually managed with anti-inflammatory drugs rather than antifungal drug therapy. Some people also develop histoplasmosis years after the primary infection, probably from reactivation of a latent infection. This is likely to occur in clients with AIDS. Histoplasmosis is the most frequent endemic fungal infection occurring in patients with HIV infection and has been recognized as an AIDS-defining illness since 1987.

In addition, histoplasmosis occasionally infects the liver, spleen, and other organs and is rapidly fatal if not treated effectively. As with many other infections, the severe, disseminated form usually occurs in patients whose immune systems are suppressed by diseases or drugs.

**Sporotrichosis** occurs when contaminated soil or plant material is inoculated into the skin through small wounds (eg, thorn pricks) on the fingers, hands, or arms. It is most likely to occur among people who handle sphagnum moss, roses, or baled hay. Thus, infection is a hazard for gardeners and greenhouse workers. It can occur in both healthy and immunocompromised people, but is usually more severe and disseminated in the immunocompromised host.

Initial lesions, usually small, painless bumps resembling insect bites, occur 1 week to 6 months after inoculation. The subcutaneous nodule develops into a necrotic ulcer, which heals slowly as new ulcers appear in adjacent areas. Local lymphatic channels and lymph nodes also develop abscesses, nodules, and ulcers that may persist for years if the disease is not treated effectively. In immunocompromised people, sporotrichosis may spread to various tissues, including the meninges.

Lipid formulations were developed to decrease adverse effects, especially nephrotoxicity. Compared with the original deoxycholate formulation (Fungizone), these mixtures of amphotericin B with lipids penetrate and reach higher concentrations in diseased tissues (eg, those infected or inflamed). This increases therapeutic effects. At the same time, lipid formulations do not penetrate normal tissues well and therefore reach lower concentrations in normal tissues. This decreases adverse effects and also allows higher doses to be given. Although these products cause much less nephrotoxicity, chills, and fever, they are much more expensive than the deoxycholate formulation. As a result, they are usually recommended for use only in clients who cannot tolerate the older formulation or who

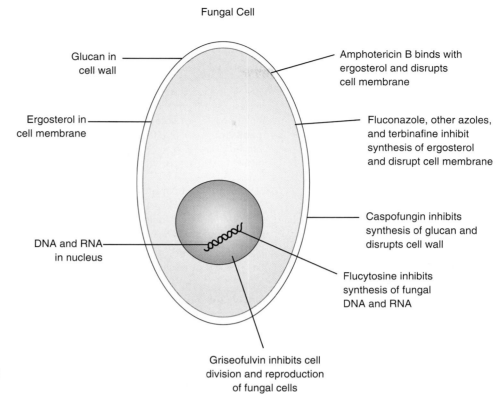

Fungal Cell

Glucan in cell wall

Ergosterol in cell membrane

DNA and RNA in nucleus

Amphotericin B binds with ergosterol and disrupts cell membrane

Fluconazole, other azoles, and terbinafine inhibit synthesis of ergosterol and disrupt cell membrane

Caspofungin inhibits synthesis of glucan and disrupts cell wall

Flucytosine inhibits synthesis of fungal DNA and RNA

Griseofulvin inhibits cell division and reproduction of fungal cells

**FIGURE 33-2** Actions of antifungal drugs on fungal cells.

are at risk for developing nephrotoxicity. The various lipid preparations differ in their characteristics and cannot be used interchangeably.

Amphotericin B is not well absorbed orally and must be given intravenously for systemic infections. After infusion, the liver and other organs rapidly take up the drug. It is then slowly released back into the bloodstream. Despite its long-term use, little is known about its distribution and metabolic pathways. Drug concentrations in most body fluids (eg, pleural, peritoneal, synovial, aqueous and vitreous humors) are higher in the presence of inflammation (about two thirds of serum levels). Concentrations in cerebrospinal fluid (CSF) are low with or without inflammation. The drug has an initial serum half-life of 24 hours, which represents redistribution from

*(text continues on page 589)*

**TABLE 33-1  Pharmacokinetics of Systemic Antifungal Drugs**

| Generic/ Trade Name | Protein Binding (%) | Half-life | Metabolism/Excretion | Action | | |
|---|---|---|---|---|---|---|
| | | | | *Onset* | *Peak* | *Duration* |
| **Amphotericin B deoxycholate** (Fungizone) | >90 | 24 h, then 15 d | Tissues/urine | IV 20–30 min | 1–2 h | 20–24 h |
| **Fluconazole** (Diflucan) | 11–12 | 30 h | 80% eliminated as unchanged drug in urine | PO slow IV rapid | 1–2 h 1 h | 2–4 d 2–4 d |
| **Flucytosine** (Ancobon) | Minimal | 2–4 h | Mainly eliminated in urine as unchanged drug | PO varies | 2 h | 10–12 h |
| **Itraconazole** (Sporanox) | 99 | 21 h, then 64 h | Hepatic/urine | PO slow IV rapid | 4 h | 4–6 d End of infusion |
| **Ketoconazole** (Nizoral) | 99 | 8 h | Hepatic/bile | Varies | 1–4 h | 8 h |
| **Terbinafine** (Lamisil) | 99 | 36 h | Hepatic/urine | Topical slow | 1–2 h | 200–400 h (oral) |

**DRUG TABLE 33-3**

*Drugs at a Glance*

## Selected Antifungal Drugs

| Generic/Trade Name | Routes and Dosage Ranges | Comments/Uses |
|---|---|---|
| **Amphotericin B deoxycholate** (Fungizone) Pregnancy Category B | *Adults:* IV, individualized according to disease severity and client tolerance. Initial dose often 0.25 mg/kg/d, gradually increased to 0.5–1 mg/kg/d, infused over 2–6 h. Topically to skin lesions two to four times daily for 1–4 wk Oral suspension (100 mg/mL), 1 mL "swish and swallow" 4 times daily *Children:* Same as for adults for IV, skin preparations, and oral suspension | For treatment of serious, systemic fungal infections (eg, candidiasis, histoplasmosis) Cutaneous candidiasis Oral candidiasis |
| **Amphotericin B lipid complex** (Abelcet) Pregnancy Category B | *Adults:* IV, 5 mg/kg/d *Children:* Same as adults | For systemic infections in clients who do not tolerate Fungizone |
| **Liposomal amphotericin B** (AmBisome) Pregnancy Category B | *Adults:* IV, 3–5 mg/kg/d *Children:* Same as adults | For systemic infections in clients who do not tolerate Fungizone Empiric treatment of presumed fungal infections in febrile, neutropenic clients |
| **Amphotericin B cholesteryl** (Amphotec) Pregnancy Category B | *Adults:* IV, 3–4 mg/kg/d *Children:* Same as adults | For systemic infections in clients who do not tolerate Fungizone |
| **Butenafine** (Mentax) Pregnancy Category B | *Adults:* Topically to skin lesions 1–2 times daily for 1–4 wk *Children:* Safety and efficacy not established for children <12 y | Used for tinea infections |
| **Butoconazole** (Femstat, Gynazole) Pregnancy Category C; use only in second and third trimesters | *Adults:* Intravaginally, once daily for 3 d | Used for vaginal candidiasis |
| **Caspofungin** (Cancidas) Pregnancy Category C | *Adults:* IV infusion over 1 h, 70 mg initially, then 50 mg daily Hepatic impairment, 70 mg initially, then 35 mg daily *Children:* Safety and efficacy not established | Used to treat invasive aspergillosis |
| **Ciclopirox** (Loprox) Pregnancy Category B | *Adults:* Topically to skin lesions, twice daily for 2–4 wk | For tinea infections, cutaneous candidiasis |
| **Clotrimazole** (Lotrimin, Mycelex, Gyne-Lotrimin) Pregnancy Category B (topical); C (troches) | *Adults:* PO, 1 troche dissolved in mouth five times daily Topically to skin daily for 2–4 wk Intravaginally, once daily for 3–7 d *Children:* Same as adults | For cutaneous dermatophytosis; oral, cutaneous, and vaginal candidiasis |
| **Econazole** (Spectazole) Pregnancy Category C | *Adults:* Topically to skin lesions, once or twice daily for 2–4 wk *Children:* Dosage not established | For treatment of tinea infections, cutaneous candidiasis |
| **Fluconazole** (Diflucan) Pregnancy Category C | *Adults:* Oropharyngeal candidiasis, PO, IV 200 mg first day, then 100 mg daily for 2 wk *Children:* Oropharyngeal candidiasis, PO, IV 6 mg/kg first day, then 3 mg/kg/d for at least 2 wk | To treat oropharyngeal, esophageal, vaginal, and systemic candidiasis Prevention of candidiasis after bone marrow transplantation Cryptococcal meningitis |

*(continued)*

**DRUG TABLE
33-3**

*Drugs at a Glance*

## Selected Antifungal Drugs (Continued)

| Generic/Trade Name | Routes and Dosage Ranges | Comments/Uses |
|---|---|---|
| | *Adults:* Esophageal candidiasis, PO, IV, 200 mg first day, then 100 mg daily for at least 3 wk<br>*Children:* Esophageal candidiasis, PO, IV, 6 mg/kg first day, then 3 mg/kg/d for at least 3 wk<br>*Adults:* Vaginal candidiasis, PO, 150 mg as a single dose<br>*Adults:* Systemic candidiasis, PO, IV, 400 mg first day, then 200 mg daily for at least 4 wk<br>*Children:* Systemic candidiasis, PO, IV 6–12 mg/kg/d<br>*Adults:* Prophylaxis, PO, IV, 400 mg once daily<br>Cryptococcal meningitis, PO, IV, 400 mg first day, then 200–400 mg/d for 10–12 wk<br>*Children:* Cryptococcal meningitis, PO, IV 12 mg/kg first day, then 6 mg/kg/d for 10–12 wk | |
| **Flucytosine** (Ancobon)<br>Pregnancy Category C | *Adults:* PO, 50–150 mg/kg/d in divided doses q6h<br>Dosage must be decreased with impaired liver function.<br>*Children:* Safety and efficacy not established | For systemic mycoses due to *Candida* species or *Cryptococcus neoformans* |
| **Griseofulvin** (Fulvicin)<br>Pregnancy Category C | *Adults:* Microsize, PO, 500 mg–1 g daily in divided doses q6h<br>Ultramicrosize, PO 250–500 mg daily<br>*Children:* Microsize, PO, 10–20 mg/kg in divided doses, q6h<br>Ultramicrosize, PO, 5–10 mg/kg/d | For dermatophytosis (skin, hair, nails) |
| **Haloprogin** (Halotex) | *Adults:* Topically to skin, 1% cream or solution twice daily for 2–4 wk<br>*Children:* Dosage not established | For dermatophytosis, mainly tinea pedis (athlete's foot), cutaneous candidiasis |
| **Itraconazole** (Sporanox)<br>Pregnancy Category C | *Adults:* Systemic infection, PO, 200 mg once or twice daily for 3 mo<br>Blastomycosis, histoplasmosis, aspergillosis, IV, 200 mg twice daily for 4 doses, then 200 mg/d<br>Fingernail onychomycosis, PO, 200 mg twice daily for 1 wk, no drug for 3 wk, then repeat dosage for 1 wk<br>Oral solution, 100–200 mg daily (10–20 mL), swish and swallow 3 times daily for 3–5 d<br>Tinea infections, PO, 100–200 mg daily for 1–4 wk<br>*Children:* Safety and efficacy not established. 3–16-y-old patients have been treated with 100 mg daily for systemic infections and patients 6 mo–12 y have been treated with 5 mg/kg once daily for 2 wk without serious or unusual adverse effects. | For systemic fungal infections, including aspergillosis, in neutropenic and immunocompromised hosts<br>Onychomycosis<br>Tinea infections |

*(continued)*

*Drugs at a Glance*

**DRUG TABLE 33-3**

### Selected Antifungal Drugs (Continued)

| Generic/Trade Name | Routes and Dosage Ranges | Comments/Uses |
|---|---|---|
| **Ketoconazole** (Nizoral)<br>Pregnancy Category C | *Adults:* PO, 200 mg once daily, increased to 400 mg once daily if necessary in severe infections<br>Topically, once daily for 2–6 wk<br>*Children:* 2 y and older: PO 3.3–6.6 mg/kg/d as a single dose | To treat candidiasis, histoplasmosis, coccidioidomycosis<br>Cutaneous candidiasis<br>Tinea infections |
| **Miconazole** (Monistat)<br>Pregnancy Category C | *Adults:* Topically, twice daily for 2–4 wk<br>Intravaginally, vaginal cream, once daily at bedtime for 3–7 d; vaginal suppository, once daily at bedtime (1 d for 1200 mg; 3 d for 200 mg; 7 d for 100 mg) | For dermatophytosis, cutaneous and vulvovaginal candidiasis |
| **Naftifine** (Naftin)<br>Pregnancy Category B | *Adults:* Topically, once daily (cream) or twice daily (gel)<br>*Children:* Safety and efficacy not established | Used for tinea infections (athlete's foot, jock itch, ringworm) |
| **Natamycin** (Natacyn)<br>Pregnancy Category C | *Adults:* Topically, 1 drop q1–2h for 3–4 d, then 1 drop 6–8 times daily for 14–24 d<br>*Children:* Safety and efficacy not established | For fungal infections of the eye |
| **Nystatin** (Mycostatin)<br>Pregnancy Category B/C (oral) | *Adults:* Oral or intestinal infection, PO tablets 1–2 (500,000–1,000,000 units) 3 times daily; oral suspension, 4–6 mL (400,000–600,000 units) 4 times daily; oral troches 1–2 (200,000–400,000 units) 4–5 times daily<br>*Children:* >1 y: PO oral suspension, same as adults; infants, 2 mL (200,000 units) 4 times daily<br>Oral troches, same as adults for children old enough to suck on the lozenge until it dissolves<br>Topically to skin lesions, 2–3 times daily<br>Intravaginally, 1 vaginal tablet once daily for 14 d | For candidiasis of skin, mucous membrane, and intestinal tract |
| **Oxiconazole** (Oxistat)<br>Pregnancy Category B | *Adults:* Topically to skin lesions, once or twice daily for 2–4 wk<br>*Children:* Safety and efficacy not established | To treat tinea infections |
| **Sulconazole** (Exelderm)<br>Pregnancy Category C | *Adults:* Topically to skin lesions, once or twice daily for 3–4 wk<br>*Children:* Safety and efficacy not established for children <12 y | To treat tinea infections |
| **Terbinafine** (Lamisil)<br>Pregnancy Category B | *Adults:* Tinea infections, topically to skin, once or twice daily for at least 1 wk and no longer than 4 wk<br>Fingernail infections, PO, 250 mg daily for 6 wk<br>Toenail infections, PO, 250 mg daily for 12 wk | For tinea infections<br>Onychomycosis of fingernails or toenails |

*(continued)*

## DRUG TABLE 33-3
### *Drugs at a Glance*
### Selected Antifungal Drugs (Continued)

| Generic/Trade Name | Routes and Dosage Ranges | Comments/Uses |
|---|---|---|
| **Terconazole** (Terazol) Pregnancy Category C | *Adults:* Intravaginally, 1 applicator once daily at bedtime for 7 doses (0.4% cream) or 3 doses (0.8% cream) Vaginal suppository, 1 daily at bedtime for 3 d | Used for vaginal candidiasis |
| **Tioconazole** (Vagistat) Pregnancy Category C | *Adults:* Intravaginally, 1 applicator at bedtime | Used for vaginal candidiasis |
| **Tolnaftate** (Tinactin) Pregnancy Category C | *Adults:* Topically to skin lesions, twice daily for 2–6 wk | For cutaneous mycoses (dermatophytosis) |
| **Triacetin** (Fungoid) Pregnancy Category C | *Adults:* Topically to skin lesions, 3 times daily | For dermatophytosis (eg, athlete's foot), cutaneous candidiasis |
| **Zinc undecylenate** (Desenex) Pregnancy Category B | *Adults:* Topically to skin twice daily for 2–4 wk *Children:* Same as for adults | For dermatophytosis |

the bloodstream to tissues. This is followed by a second elimination phase, with a half-life of approximately 15 days, which represents elimination from tissue storage sites. Most of the drug is thought to be metabolized in the tissues; about 5% of the active drug is excreted daily in the urine. After administration is stopped, amphotericin B can be detected in the urine for several weeks.

Adverse effects include an infusion reaction characterized by fever, chills, and tachypnea. This reaction does not represent drug hypersensitivity. It is usually managed by premedication with acetaminophen, diphenhydramine (an antihistamine), or the addition of hydrocortisone to the IV infusion fluids. Chills, which occur despite premedication, can be treated with meperidine. Nephrotoxicity is the most common and the most serious long-term adverse effect. The drug apparently damages the kidneys by constricting afferent renal arterioles and reducing blood flow to the kidneys. Several measures may decrease nephrotoxicity, such as keeping the client well hydrated, giving sodium chloride 0.9% IV solution before drug administration, and avoiding the concomitant administration of other nephrotoxic drugs (eg, aminoglycoside antibiotics) or diuretics. Increasing the dosing interval to every other day has also been proposed, but this lessens nephrotoxicity only if the total dose of the drug is reduced. Hypokalemia and hypomagnesemia also occur and may require oral or IV replacement. Additional adverse effects include anorexia, nausea, vomiting, anemia, and phlebitis or thrombophlebitis at peripheral infusion sites. A central vein is preferred for administration.

**Nystatin** has the same mechanism of action as amphotericin B. However, it is used only for topical therapy of oral, intestinal, and vaginal candidiasis because it is too toxic for systemic use. Although given orally for oral or intestinal infections, the drug is not absorbed systemically, and it is excreted in the feces after oral use. With oral use, adverse effects include nausea, vomiting, and diarrhea; with vaginal application, adverse effects include local irritation and burning.

### Azoles

The azoles comprise the largest group of commonly used antifungal agents. Many of these are used topically, and some are available without a prescription for dermatologic (see Appendix F) or vaginal use (eg, butoconazole, clotrimazole, miconazole, terconazole, tioconazole). The ones discussed in this chapter are used systemically or both topically and systemically. In serious, invasive fungal infections, these drugs are often used long-term following initial treatment with amphotericin B. However, their use as initial treatment for some systemic infections is increasing. Ketoconazole, the first azole, is chemically an imidazole;

### ? How Can You Avoid This Medication Error?

Amphotericin B is ordered for Harry Little, who has aspergillosis. You collect the following information before administering the medication: blood pressure 110/68, pulse 92, respiratory rate 18, temperature 37.8°C. Laboratory test results include K⁺ 3.2 mEq/L, Na⁺ 140 mEq/L, hemoglobin 14 g/dL, hematocrit 43%, blood urea nitrogen (BUN) 48 mg/dL, and creatinine 3.5 mg/dL. You have an order to premedicate Mr. Little with meperidine and diphenhydramine IV, which you do. He has a central line and the IV amphotericin is diluted in 500 cc, to run over 2 hours. You set the IV infusion pump for 250 cc/hour after you check the site and see that there is no redness.

fluconazole and itraconazole are triazoles. The triazoles have replaced ketoconazole for most uses because they have a broader spectrum of antifungal activity, better absorption, better drug distribution in body tissues, fewer adverse effects, and fewer drug interactions. Several newer triazoles are being developed. All azoles are contraindicated during pregnancy. Teratogenicity has occurred in animals, and fetal malformations have been reported in women who took fluconazole during pregnancy.

**Ketoconazole** (Nizoral) was an important antifungal agent when it was first introduced. It had several advantages over amphotericin B in that it could be given orally, on an outpatient basis, and was somewhat less toxic. Little absorption occurs with topical use. Adverse effects include nausea, vomiting, hypersensitivity reactions (including anaphylaxis), pruritus with oral use, and irritation, stinging, and itching with local application. A major disadvantage that evolved during several years of use includes many interactions with other drugs whereby ketoconazole decreases the metabolism and increases the risks for toxicity with affected drugs. The drug also requires gastric acid for tablet dissolution and drug absorption. Consequently, administration is problematic for patients with achlorhydria and those receiving drugs that decrease gastric acidity (eg, antacids, histamine-2 blocking agents, proton pump inhibitors). These drugs must be given at least 2 hours after ketoconazole. In addition, the drug has been associated with hepatotoxicity. As a result of these difficulties and the development of the triazole drugs, ketoconazole has largely been replaced by fluconazole and itraconazole for systemic fungal infections. It is still used in some patients who require long-term therapy because it is much less expensive than fluconazole or itraconazole. It may also be used with cyclosporine and tacrolimus because it increases blood levels of these immunosuppressant drugs and allows smaller dosages in patients with organ transplants.

**Fluconazole** (Diflucan) is a synthetic, broad-spectrum agent that is effective for candidiasis, cryptococcosis, and coccidioidomycosis and may be used as first-line or second-line (after amphotericin B) therapy. It is also used for long-term maintenance therapy of cryptococcal meningitis in clients with AIDS, after initial use of amphotericin B. It is very effective in treatment of candidal infections. A single oral dose of 150 mg is given for vaginal candidiasis. However, more infections with resistant strains of *Candida* organisms are being seen with the extensive use of fluconazole during recent years. Aspergillosis does not respond to fluconazole therapy, and fluconazole has less activity against blastomycosis and histoplasmosis than itraconazole.

Fluconazole can be given orally or intravenously and, except for a more rapid onset with IV use, pharmacokinetics and dosage are similar with the two routes. Oral drug does not require gastric acid for absorption, and the drug reaches therapeutic levels in most body fluids and tissues, including normal and inflamed meninges. With a one-time loading dose of twice the usual daily dose, steady-state blood levels are reached in about 2 days; without a loading dose, 5 to 10 days are required. Once-daily dosing may be effective in some clients with normal renal function. Most of the drug is excreted as unchanged drug in urine; dosage may need to be reduced in clients with impaired renal function.

Fluconazole is usually well tolerated. Adverse effects, including nausea, vomiting, diarrhea, abdominal pain, headache, and skin rash, have been reported in fewer than 3% of patients. In addition, elevation of liver enzymes and hepatic necrosis have been reported, and alopecia often occurs in clients receiving prolonged, high-dose treatment.

Fluconazole increases the effects of several drugs, including cyclosporine, phenytoin, oral sulfonylureas, and warfarin, but apparently has fewer interactions than ketoconazole and itraconazole.

**Itraconazole** (Sporanox) is a synthetic, broad-spectrum agent similar to fluconazole. It is a drug of choice for blastomycosis, histoplasmosis, and sporotrichosis and is useful in treating aspergillosis. It may be most useful for long-term suppression of disseminated histoplasmosis in patients with AIDS and for nonmeningeal, non–life-threatening blastomycosis. It is probably the drug of choice for all forms of sporotrichosis except meningitis. It may also be used to treat vaginal candidiasis, tinea infections, dermatophytic infections, and onychomycosis. It is contraindicated for the treatment of dermatophytic infections and onychomycosis in patients with congestive heart failure.

Itraconazole can be given orally or intravenously. However, both the oral capsule and suspension require a low gastric pH for drug dissolution and absorption. The suspension is better absorbed than the capsule. Drug absorption is especially problematic in patients with HIV infection who have achlorhydria and in those receiving a concurrent antacid, histamine-2 antagonist, or proton pump inhibitor. Serum levels should be measured to ensure adequate absorption. Drug concentrations are higher in visceral organs than in serum; little drug appears in urine or CSF.

The drug is well tolerated in usual doses but may cause nausea and gastric distress. Higher doses may cause impotence, hypokalemia, hypertension, edema, and congestive heart failure. Itraconazole has significant interactions with several commonly prescribed drugs. Drugs that increase the pH of gastric acid (eg, antacids, histamine-2 blockers, proton pump inhibitors) decrease absorption of itraconazole and should be given at least 2 hours after itraconazole. Drugs that induce drug-metabolizing enzymes (eg, carbamazepine, phenytoin, rifampin) decrease serum levels and therapeutic effectiveness of itraconazole. Itraconazole increases serum levels of cyclosporine, digoxin, oral sulfonylureas, and warfarin. It decreases serum levels of carbamazepine, phenytoin, and rifampin.

## Miscellaneous Antifungal Drugs

**Caspofungin** (Cancidas) is the first echinocandin antifungal drug; others are being developed. These drugs are usually fungicidal, but they do not act as rapidly as amphotericin B. They are active against *Candida* organisms, including azole-resistant strains, *Aspergillus* organisms, and the organisms that cause blastomycosis and histoplasmosis. They lack activity against *Cryptococcus* species. These drugs inhibit beta-(1,3)-D-glucan synthase, the enzyme responsible for incorporation of glucose into the glucan fibrils that compose the walls of most fungi. Depletion of glucan in the fungal cell wall leads to leakage of cellular contents and cell death. Because human cells do not have cell walls or contain beta-glucan, these drugs are less toxic than other systemic antifungal drugs. At present, caspofungin is indicated for treatment of invasive aspergillosis in clients who cannot take or do not respond to amphotericin B or itraconazole. It has not been studied for initial treatment of invasive aspergillosis.

Caspofungin is given intravenously and is highly bound to plasma albumin. After a single 1-hour infusion, plasma levels decline in three main phases. A short alpha phase occurs immediately after infusion; an intermediate beta phase has a half-life of 8 to 11 hours; and a longer gamma phase has a half-life of 40 to 50 hours. There is minimal biotransformation or excretion during the first 30 hours after infusion; the drug is then metabolized slowly and excreted in feces and urine.

Caspofungin is usually well tolerated with doses of 50 mg/day. Adverse effects occur in fewer than 3% of recipients and include nausea, vomiting, and infusion site complications. With doses of 50 to 70 mg daily, adverse effects include fever, headache, nausea, phlebitis or thrombophlebitis at infusion sites, and abnormal laboratory reports (eg, decreased white blood cells, hemoglobin and hematocrit; increased serum potassium and liver aminotransferase enzymes). Dosage must be reduced with moderate hepatic impairment (eg, after a 70-mg loading dose, a 35-mg daily dose is recommended rather than the 50-mg daily dose recommended for clients with normal liver function). The drug has not been studied in clients with severe hepatic impairment. No dosage adjustment is needed for renal impairment.

Cyclosporine increases effects of caspofungin, including potential liver damage. Concomitant use is not recommended unless potential benefits outweigh potential risks. Drugs that decrease effects include anti-HIV drugs (eg, efavirenz, nelfinavir, nevirapine), anticonvulsants (eg, carbamazepine, phenytoin), dexamethasone, and rifampin. Concurrent administration may significantly reduce caspofungin blood levels and therapeutic effectiveness unless dosage is increased (eg, from the usual 50 mg to 70 mg daily).

**Flucytosine** is a nucleoside analog that is converted to 5-fluorouracil inside the fungal cell. The 5-fluorouracil is then metabolized to products that interfere with the synthesis of fungal RNA and DNA. Flucytosine has little activity against molds or dimorphic fungi and is mainly used for yeast infections. It has significant activity against *Candida* species and *C. neoformans*. Flucytosine is not used alone because drug resistance develops. It is most often used in combination with amphotericin B to treat systemic candidiasis and cryptococcal meningitis. The combination allows smaller doses of amphotericin B and prevents emergence of flucytosine resistance. If high doses of amphotericin B are used, flucytosine adds no additional benefit.

Flucytosine is well absorbed with oral use and widely distributed into most body fluids, including urine, aqueous humor, bronchial secretions, and CSF. Levels in CSF reach 60% to 80% of serum levels. More than 90% of each dose is excreted unchanged in urine. Dosage must be reduced and serum drug levels monitored in the presence of impaired renal function.

Flucytosine causes fewer adverse effects than amphotericin B and the azole antifungals, but it may be associated with GI upset (nausea, vomiting, diarrhea) and bone marrow depression (eg, leukopenia, thrombocytopenia), especially when given concurrently with amphotericin B. AIDS patients with systemic fungal infections do not tolerate flucytosine well because of their baseline leukopenia. Adverse effects are attributed to conversion of flucytosine to toxic metabolites in human cells.

**Griseofulvin** (Fulvicin) has long been used orally for dermatophyte infections of the scalp and nails and for skin eruptions that were too extensive to be treated with topical agents alone. The drug acts by interfering with cell division and reproduction in actively growing fungal cells. In infections of keratinized tissues, the drug binds to keratin (a protein in hair, nails, and the epidermis of the skin). Over time, the infected tissues are shed and replaced by uninfected tissues. Dermatophytic infections (eg, ringworm) of skin usually improve in 3 to 8 weeks. A year or more may be needed to eliminate onychomycosis of toenails. As a result, griseofulvin is being used less often, and itraconazole, which is effective with shorter courses of therapy, is being used more often. Griseofulvin is contraindicated in patients with liver disease.

Oral griseofulvin is poorly absorbed; absorption is improved by reducing the particle size (microsize or ultramicrosize formulations are available) and by taking the drug with fatty meals. Doses are about 30% lower with the ultramicrosized formulation because it is better absorbed than the microsized formulation.

Griseofulvin is usually well tolerated. Common adverse effects include GI upset (eg, nausea, vomiting, diarrhea), fatigue, headache, insomnia, and skin rash. Hepatotoxicity may also occur. Griseofulvin may decrease the effects of cyclosporine, oral contraceptives, salicylates, and warfarin. Warfarin doses may need to be increased, and an alternative method of contraception may be needed during griseofulvin therapy.

**Terbinafine** (Lamisil) is a synthetic allylamine with a broad spectrum of antifungal activity. It inhibits an enzyme (squalene epoxidase) needed for synthesis of ergosterol, a structural component of fungal cell membranes. Terbinafine has fungicidal activity against dermatophytes and has been used primarily for topical treatment of ringworm infections and oral treatment of onychomycosis (fungal infection of nails). Therapeutic effects may not be evident until months after drug therapy is stopped, because of the time required for growth of healthy nail. Because of its activity against *Candida, Aspergillus,* and possibly other fungal organisms, terbinafine is being evaluated for possible use in invasive mycoses.

Oral terbinafine is about 70% absorbed, but first-pass metabolism reduces bioavailability to approximately 40%. The drug is extensively metabolized to inactive metabolites and excreted in the urine.

Adverse effects with topical terbinafine are minimal. Common effects with oral use are headache, diarrhea, and abdominal discomfort. Oral drug may also cause skin reactions and liver failure with long-term therapy of onychomycosis. Hepatotoxicity is uncommon but has occurred in people with and without preexisting liver disease and has led to liver transplantation or death. Terbinafine is not recommended for patients with chronic or active liver disease, and serum alanine aminotransferase (ALT) and aspartate transaminase (AST) should be checked before starting the drug.

## ■ PROTOZOAL INFECTIONS

The protozoal infections include amebiasis, giardiasis, malaria, pneumocystosis, toxoplasmosis, and trichomoniasis. An overview of these infections is provided next.

*(text continues on page 595)*

---

### CLIENT TEACHING GUIDELINES
### Oral and Topical Antifungal Drugs

**General Considerations**

✔ If you have a condition or take a medicine that suppresses your immune system (eg, bone marrow or organ transplant, leukemia, lymphoma, diabetes mellitus, HIV infection, cancer chemotherapy, corticosteroid therapy), you need to avoid exposure to molds and fungi when possible. For example, aspergillus organisms, which can be in the air, dust, soil, and other environments, can cause serious illness and death. To minimize exposure, you should avoid areas of building construction or renovation, avoid cleaning carpets or potentially moldy areas, and avoid potted plants and live flowers.

✔ With skin lesions, wash hands often and do not share towels, hairbrushes, or other personal items.

✔ With vaginal yeast infections, do not use over-the-counter medications repeatedly without consulting a physician or other health care provider. Recurrent infections may indicate inadequate treatment, reinfection, or a bacterial infection (for which an antifungal drug is not effective), and a different treatment may be needed.

✔ With histoplasmosis and other potentially serious fungal infections, avoid or minimize future exposure to chicken, pigeon, and bat excreta.

✔ For people who work with plants (eg, roses, sphagnum moss) or baled hay, sporotrichosis can be prevented by wearing gloves and long sleeves and avoiding injuries that cause breaks in the skin.

**Self-administration**

✔ Use antifungal drugs as prescribed.

✔ With topical skin preparations, wash and dry the area before each application of medication.

✔ With vaginal antifungal preparations:

✔ Read instructions carefully, with prescribed and over-the-counter drugs.

✔ Insert high into the vagina (except during pregnancy).

✔ Continue use through menstruation.

✔ Wear a minipad to avoid staining clothing; do not use a tampon.

✔ Wash applicator with mild soap and rinse thoroughly after each use.

✔ Avoid sexual intercourse while using the drug.

✔ With flucytosine, take capsules a few at a time over 15 minutes to decrease nausea and vomiting.

✔ With oral ketoconazole, take with food to decrease gastrointestinal upset. However, do not take with antacids or drugs such as ranitidine (Zantac) or omeprazole (Prilosec). If one of these drugs is required, take it approximately 2 hours after a dose of ketoconazole.

✔ With itraconazole capsules, take after a full meal for best absorption. With the oral suspension, take on an empty stomach, usually by swishing in the mouth and then swallowing it.

✔ With nystatin suspension for mouth lesions (thrush), swish the medication around in the mouth for a few minutes (to increase drug contact with the lesions), then swallow the medication.

✔ With oral fluconazole (Diflucan), itraconazole (Sporanox), ketoconazole (Nizoral), or terbinafine (Lamisil), notify a health care provider of unusual fatigue, loss of appetite, nausea, vomiting, jaundice, dark urine, pale stools, fever, abdominal pain, or diarrhea. These may be signs of liver damage or other adverse drug effects. Drug therapy may need to be discontinued.

✔ With griseofulvin, avoid prolonged exposure to sunlight or sunlamps; the drug may cause photosensitivity.

## Nursing Actions

## Antifungal Drugs

| Nursing Actions | Rationale/Explanation |
|---|---|
| **1. Administer accurately.** | |
| a. Give IV amphotericin B according to manufacturers' recommendations for each product: | Test doses and all other solutions should be prepared in the pharmacy. |
| (1) Follow recommendations for administration of test doses. | Preparation, concentration, and recommended infusion times vary among formulations. |
| (2) Use an infusion pump. | To regulate flow accurately |
| (3) Use a separate intravenous (IV) line if possible; if necessary to use an existing line, flush with 5% dextrose in water before and after each infusion. | |
| (4) Fungizone IV—give in 5% dextrose in water, over 2–6 h; use an in-line filter; do not mix with other IV medications. | Administration times can vary according to patient tolerance. |
| (5) Abelcet—give IV over approximately 2 h; if infusion time exceeds 2 h, shake the container q2h to mix contents; do not use an in-line filter. | |
| (6) AmBisome—infuse over 2 h or longer; may use an in-line filter. | |
| (7) Amphotec—refrigerate after reconstitution and use within 24 h; infuse over at least 2 h; do not use an in-line filter. | |
| (8) Apply cream or lotion liberally to skin lesions and rub in gently. | |
| b. Give azoles according to manufacturers' recommendations: | |
| (1) With IV fluconazole, follow instructions for preparation carefully; give as a continuous infusion at a maximum rate of 200 mg/h. | |
| (2) Shake the oral suspension of fluconazole thoroughly before measuring the dose. | To resuspend medication in the liquid vehicle and ensure accurate dosage |
| (3) Give itraconazole capsules after a full meal; give the oral solution on an empty stomach and ask the client to swish the medication around in the mouth, then swallow the medication. | To decrease GI upset and increase absorption. The oral solution is used to treat oropharyngeal and esophageal candidiasis, and correct administration enhances contact with mucosal lesions. |
| (4) Give ketoconazole tablets with food. However, do not give with antacids or other gastric acid suppressants. If such drugs are required, give them 2 h after a dose of ketoconazole. | Food decreases GI upset. Antacids and other drugs that suppress gastric acid decrease absorption because the drug is dissolved and absorbed only in an acidic environment. |
| c. With IV caspofungin, infuse over approximately 1 hour. Be sure it is added to 0.9% sodium chloride solutions only (dextrose solutions should be avoided). Do not mix or co-infuse with any other medications. | Caspofungin should be prepared in a pharmacy according to the manufacturer's instructions. The drug is available in single-dose vials of 50 mg or 70 mg. It must be reconstituted with 0.9% sodium chloride solution, then added to 250 mL of 0.9% sodium chloride solution. |
| d. With flucytosine, have the client take 1 or 2 capsules at a time over 15 min. | To decrease nausea and vomiting |
| **2. Observe for therapeutic effects.** | |
| a. Decreased fever and malaise with systemic mycoses | Most antifungal drug therapy is long-term, over weeks, months, or years. With skin infections, optimal therapeutic effects may occur 2–4 wks after drug therapy is stopped. With nail infections, optimal effects may occur 6–9 mo after drug therapy is stopped. |
| b. Healing of lesions on skin and mucous membranes | |
| c. Diminished diarrhea with intestinal candidiasis | |
| d. Decreased vaginal discharge and discomfort with vaginal candidiasis | |

*(continued)*

## *Nursing Actions*
## Antifungal Drugs (Continued)

| Nursing Actions | Rationale/Explanation |
|---|---|
| 3. Observe for adverse effects. | |
| a. With IV amphotericin B, observe for fever, chills, anorexia, nausea, vomiting, renal damage (elevated blood urea nitrogen and serum creatinine), hypokalemia, hypomagnesemia, headache, stupor, coma, convulsions, anemia from bone marrow depression, phlebitis at venipuncture sites, and anaphylaxis. | Amphotericin B is a highly toxic drug and most recipients develop adverse reactions, including some degree of renal damage. Antipyretic and antiemetic drugs may be given to help minimize adverse reactions and promote patient comfort. Adequate hydration and lipid formulations may decrease renal damage. Anaphylaxis is uncommon; however, appropriate treatment medications and supplies should be available during infusions. If severe respiratory distress occurs, the drug infusion should be stopped immediately and no additional doses should be given. |
| b. With fluconazole, itraconazole, or ketoconazole, observe for unusual fatigue, loss of appetite, nausea, vomiting, jaundice, dark urine, pale stools, fever, abdominal pain, or diarrhea. With ketoconazole, observe for nausea, vomiting, pruritus, and abdominal pain. | These may be signs of liver damage or other adverse effects. Drug therapy may need to be discontinued. With ketoconazole, GI upset occurs in about 20% of clients taking 200 mg daily and in 50% or more of clients taking 400 mg daily. |
| c. With caspofungin 50 mg daily, observe for nausea, vomiting, and phlebitis at infusion sites. With larger doses (50–70 mg daily), observe for the above plus fever, headache, and abnormal laboratory reports (eg, decreased white blood cells, hemoglobin, and hematocrit; increased serum potassium and liver aminotransferase enzymes). | The drug is usually well tolerated. |
| d. With flucytosine, observe for nausea, vomiting, and diarrhea. | These are common effects. Hepatic, renal, and hematologic functions also may be affected. |
| e. With griseofulvin, observe for GI symptoms, hypersensitivity (urticaria, photosensitivity, skin rashes, angioedema), headache, mental confusion, fatigue, dizziness, peripheral neuritis, and blood dyscrasias (leukopenia, neutropenia, granulocytopenia). | The incidence of serious reactions is very low. |
| f. With oral terbinafine, observe for diarrhea, dyspepsia, headache, skin rash or itching, and liver enzyme abnormalities. | Elevated liver enzymes (AST and ALT) may indicate liver damage and may occur in clients with or without pre-existing liver disease. |
| g. With topical drugs, observe for skin rash and irritation. | Adverse reactions are usually minimal with topical drugs, although hypersensitivity may occur. |
| 4. Observe for drug interactions. | |
| a. Drugs that *increase* effects of amphotericin B: | |
| (1) Antineoplastic drugs | May increase risks of nephrotoxicity, hypotension, and bronchospasm |
| (2) Corticosteroids | May potentiate hypokalemia and precipitate cardiac dysfunction. |
| (3) Zidovudine | Increases renal and hematologic adverse effects of the liposomal formulation of amphotericin B. Renal and hematologic functions should be monitored closely. |
| (4) Nephrotoxic drugs (eg, aminoglycoside antibiotics, cyclosporine) | Increase nephrotoxicity |
| b. Drug that *increases* effects of fluconazole: | |
| (1) Hydrochlorothiazide | Increases serum levels of fluconazole, attributed to decreased renal excretion |
| c. Drugs that *decrease* effects of fluconazole: | |
| (1) Cimetidine | Decreased absorption |
| (2) Rifampin | Accelerated metabolism from enzyme induction |

*(continued)*

## Nursing Actions

### Antifungal Drugs (Continued)

| Nursing Actions | Rationale/Explanation |
|---|---|
| d. Drugs that *decrease* effects of itraconazole and ketoconazole: | |
| (1) Antacids, histamine H₂ antagonists, proton pump inhibitors | These drugs decrease gastric acid, which inhibits absorption of itraconazole and ketoconazole. If one of these drugs is required, it should be given at least 2 h after the azole drug. |
| (2) Phenytoin, rifampin | Decrease serum levels, probably from accelerated metabolism |
| e. Drug that *increases* effects of caspofungin: | |
| (1) Cyclosporine | Increases serum levels |
| f. Drugs that *decrease* effects of caspofungin: | |
| (1) Enzyme inducers (efavirenz, nelfinavir, nevirapine, dexamethasone, carbamazepine, phenytoin, rifampin) | Decrease serum levels by accelerating caspofungin metabolism. The daily dose of caspofungin may need to be increased to 70 mg/d (instead of 50 mg/d) if given with one of these drugs. |
| g. Drugs that *decrease* effects of griseofulvin: | |
| (1) Enzyme inducers (eg, rifampin) | Enzyme inducers inhibit effects of griseofulvin by increasing its rate of metabolism. |
| h. Drug that *increases* effects of terbinafine: | |
| (1) Cimetidine | Slows metabolism and elimination of terbinafine so that serum levels are increased |
| i. Drug that *decreases* effects of terbinafine: | |
| (1) Rifampin | Causes rapid clearance of terbinafine |

## Amebiasis

Amebiasis is a common disease in Africa, Asia, and Latin America, but it can occur in any geographic region. In the United States, it is most likely to occur in residents of institutions for the mentally retarded, homosexual and bisexual men, and residents or travelers of countries with poor sanitation.

Drugs used to treat amebiasis (amebicides) are classified according to their site of action. For example, iodoquinol is an *intestinal amebicide* because it acts within the lumen of the bowel; chloroquine is a *tissue* or *extraintestinal amebicide* because it acts in the bowel wall, liver, and other tissues. Metronidazole (Flagyl) is effective in both intestinal and extraintestinal amebiasis. No amebicides are currently recommended for prophylaxis of amebiasis.

## Giardiasis

Giardiasis is caused by *Giardia lamblia,* a common intestinal parasite. It is spread by food or water contaminated with human feces containing encysted forms of the organism or by contact with infected people or animals. Person-to-person spread often occurs among children in day care centers, institutionalized people, and homosexual or bisexual men. The organism is also found in people who camp or hike in wilderness areas or who drink untreated well water in areas where sanitation is poor. Giardiasis may affect children more than adults and may cause community outbreaks of diarrhea.

Giardial infections occur 1 to 2 weeks after ingestion of the cysts and may be asymptomatic or produce diarrhea and abdominal cramping and distention. If untreated, giardiasis may resolve spontaneously or progress to a chronic disease with anorexia, nausea, malaise, weight loss, and continued diarrhea with large, foul-smelling, light-colored, fatty stools. Deficiencies of vitamin B₁₂ and fat-soluble vitamins may occur. Adults and children older than 8 years with symptomatic giardiasis should be treated with oral metronidazole.

## Malaria

Malaria is a common cause of morbidity and mortality in many parts of the world, especially in tropical regions. In the United States, malaria is rare and affects travelers or immigrants from malarious areas.

Malaria is caused by four species of protozoa of the genus *Plasmodium.* The human being is the only natural reservoir of these parasites. All types of malaria are transmitted only by *Anopheles* mosquitoes. *Plasmodium vivax, Plasmodium malariae,* and *Plasmodium ovale* cause recurrent malaria by forming reservoirs in the human host. In these types of malaria, signs and symptoms may occur months or years after the initial attack. *Plasmodium falciparum* causes the most life-threatening type of malaria but does not form a reservoir. This type of malaria may be cured and prevented from recurring.

Antimalarial drugs act at different stages in the life cycle of plasmodial parasites. Some drugs (eg, chloroquine) are effective against erythrocytic forms and are therefore useful in preventing or treating acute attacks of malaria. These drugs do not prevent infection with the parasite, but they do prevent clinical manifestations. Other drugs (eg, primaquine) act against exoerythrocytic or tissue forms of the parasite to prevent initial infection and recurrent attacks or to cure some types of malaria. Combination drug therapy, administered concomitantly or consecutively, is common with antimalarial drugs.

## Pneumocystosis

Pneumocystosis is caused by *Pneumocystis carinii*, a parasitic organism once considered a protozoan but now considered a fungus. Sources and routes of spread have not been clearly delineated. It is apparently widespread in the environment, and most people are exposed at an early age. Infections are mild or asymptomatic in immunocompetent people. However, the organism can form cysts in the lungs, persist for long periods, and become activated in immunocompromised hosts. Activation produces *Pneumocystis carinii* pneumonia (PCP), an acute, life-threatening respiratory infection characterized by cough, fever, dyspnea, and presence of the organism in sputum. Groups at risk include HIV-seropositive persons; those receiving corticosteroids or antineoplastics, and other immunosuppressive drugs; and caregivers of infected people. PCP is a common cause of death in people with AIDS.

## Toxoplasmosis

Toxoplasmosis is caused by *Toxoplasma gondii*, a parasite spread by ingesting undercooked meat or other food containing encysted forms of the organism, by contact with feces from infected cats, and by congenital spread from mothers with acute infection. Once infected, the organism may persist in tissue cysts for the life of the host. However, symptoms rarely occur unless the immune system is impaired or becomes impaired at a later time. Although symptomatic infection may occur in anyone with immunosuppression (eg, people with cancer or organ transplants), it is especially common and serious in people with AIDS, in whom it often causes encephalitis and death.

## Trichomoniasis

The most common form of trichomoniasis is a vaginal infection caused by *Trichomonas vaginalis*. The disease is usually spread by sexual intercourse. Antitrichomonal drugs may be administered systemically (ie, metronidazole) or applied locally as douche solutions or vaginal creams.

## HELMINTHIASIS

Helminthiasis, or infestation with parasitic worms, is a common finding in many parts of the world. Helminths are most often found in the GI tract. However, several types of parasitic worms penetrate body tissues or produce larvae that migrate to the blood, lymph channels, lungs, liver, and other body tissues.

Drugs used for treatment of helminthiasis are called *anthelmintics*. Most anthelmintics act locally to kill or cause expulsion of parasitic worms from the intestines; some anthelmintics act systemically against parasites that have penetrated various body tissues. The goal of anthelmintic therapy may be to eradicate the parasite completely or to decrease the magnitude of infestation ("worm burden").

## SCABIES AND PEDICULOSIS

Scabies and pediculosis are parasitic infestations of the skin. Scabies is caused by the itch mite (*Sarcoptes scabiei*), which burrows into the skin and lays eggs that hatch in 4 to 8 days. The burrows may produce visible skin lesions, most often between the fingers and on the wrists.

Pediculosis may be caused by one of three types of lice. Pediculosis capitis (head lice) is the most common type of pediculosis in the United States. It is diagnosed by finding louse eggs (nits) attached to hair shafts close to the scalp. Pediculosis corporis (body lice) is diagnosed by finding lice in clothing, especially in seams. Body lice can transmit typhus and other diseases. Pediculosis pubis (pubic or crab lice) is diagnosed by the presence of nits in the pubic and genital areas.

## ANTIPARASITIC DRUGS

Antiparasitic drugs include amebicides, antimalarials, other antiprotozoal agents, anthelmintics, scabicides, and pediculicides. These are briefly described below and listed in Drugs at a Glance 33-4: Antiparasitic Drugs.

## Amebicides

**Chloroquine** (Aralen) is used primarily for its antimalarial effects. When used as an amebicide, the drug is effective in extraintestinal amebiasis (ie, hepatic amebiasis) but usually ineffective in intestinal amebiasis. The phosphate salt is given orally. When the oral route is contraindicated, severe nausea and vomiting occur, or if the infection is severe, the hydrochloride salt can be given intramuscularly. Treatment is usually combined with an intestinal amebicide.

**Iodoquinol** (Yodoxin) is an iodine compound that acts against active amebae (trophozoites) in the intestinal lumen. Iodoquinol is ineffective in amebic hepatitis

*(text continues on page 601)*

**DRUG TABLE 33-4**

*Drugs at a Glance*

## Antiparasitic Drugs

| Generic/Trade Name | Routes and Dosage Ranges | Comments/Uses |
|---|---|---|
| *Amebicides* | | |
| **Chloroquine** (Aralen) Pregnancy Category C | *Adults:* Phosphate, PO, 1 g/d for 2 d, then 500 mg/d for 2 to 3 wk Hydrochloride, IM, 200 to 250 mg/d for 10 to 12 d *Children:* Phosphate, PO 20 mg/kg/d, in two divided doses, for 2 d, then 10 mg/kg/d for 2 to 3 wk Hydrochloride, IM, 15 mg/kg/d for 2 d, then 7.5 mg/kg/d for 2 to 3 wk | Used to treat extraintestinal amebiasis; may cause headache, visual changes, retinopathy, personality changes |
| **Iodoquinol** (Yodoxin) Pregnancy Category C | *Adults:* Asymptomatic carriers, PO, 650 mg/d Symptomatic intestinal amebiasis, PO, 650 mg three times daily after meals for 20 d; repeat after 2 to 3 wk if necessary *Children:* PO, 40 mg/kg/d in three divided doses for 20 d (maximum dose, 2 g/d); repeat after 2 to 3 wk if necessary | For treatment of intestinal amebiasis; should be taken after meals; optic neuritis or atrophy or peripheral neuropathy have occurred following long-term use |
| **Metronidazole** (Flagyl) Pregnancy Category B; may be contra-indicated during first trimester | *Adults:* Amebiasis, PO, 500 to 750 mg three times daily for 5–10 d Giardiasis, PO, 250 mg three times daily for 7 d Trichomoniasis, PO 250 mg three times daily for 7 d, 1 g twice daily for 1 d, or 2 g in a single dose. Repeat after 4 to 6 wk, if necessary. *Gardnerella vaginalis* vaginitis, PO 500 mg twice daily for 7 d *Children:* Amebiasis, PO, 35 to 50 mg/kg/d in three divided doses, for 10 d Giardiasis, PO, 15 mg/kg/d in three divided doses, for 7 d | Used for: Intestinal and extraintestinal amebiasis Giardiasis Trichomoniasis Avoid alcohol during therapy and 72 hrs after |
| **Tetracycline** (Sumycin) and **doxycycline** (Vibramycin) Pregnancy Category D | *Adults:* PO, 250–500 mg q6h, up to 14 d | See Prototype Profile 31-1: Tetracycline Used for intestinal amebiasis |
| *Antimalarial Agents* | | |
| **Chloroquine phosphate and chloroquine hydrochloride** (Aralen) Pregnancy Category C | *Adults:* Prophylaxis, PO, 5 mg/kg (chloroquine base) weekly (maximum of 300 mg weekly), starting 2 wk before entering a malarious area and continuing for 8 wk after return Treatment, PO, 1 g (600 mg of base) initially, then 500 mg (300 mg of base) after 6 to 8 h, then 500 mg daily for 2 d (total of 2.5 g in four doses) *Children:* Treatment, PO, 10 mg/kg (chloroquine base) initially, then 5 mg/kg after 6 h, then 5 mg/kg/d for 2 d (total of four doses) | For prevention and treatment of malaria |

*(continued)*

**DRUG TABLE 33-4**

*Drugs at a Glance*

## Antiparasitic Drugs (Continued)

| Generic/Trade Name | Routes and Dosage Ranges | Comments/Uses |
|---|---|---|
| | *Adults:* Treatment of malarial attacks, (hydrochloride) IM, 250 mg (equivalent to 200 mg of chloroquine base) initially, repeated q6h if necessary, to a maximal dose of 800 mg of chloroquine base in 24 h<br>*Children:* Treatment of malarial attacks, (hydrochloride) IM, 5 mg/kg chloroquine base initially, repeated after 6 h if necessary; maximal dose, 10 mg/kg/24 h | |
| **Hydroxychloroquine**<br>(Plaquenil)<br>Pregnancy Category C | *Adults:* Prophylaxis, PO, 5 mg/kg, not to exceed 310 mg (of hydroxychloroquine base), once weekly for 2 wk before entry to and 8 wk after return from malarious areas<br>*Children:* Prophylaxis, PO, 5 mg/kg (of hydroxychloroquine base) once weekly for 2 wk before entry to and 8 wk after return from malarious areas<br>*Adults:* Treatment of acute malarial attacks, PO, 620 mg initially, then 310 mg 6 h later, and 310 mg/d for 2 d (total of four doses)<br>*Children:* Treatment of acute malarial attacks, PO, 10 mg/kg initially, then 5 mg/kg 6 h later, and 5 mg/kg/d for two doses (total of four doses) | For treatment of erythrocytic malaria |
| **Chloroquine with primaquine**<br>Pregnancy Category C | *Adults:* PO, 1 tablet weekly for 2 wk before entering and 8 wk after leaving malarious areas<br>*Children:* PO, same as adults for children weighing >45 kg; 1/2 tablet for children weighing 25–45 kg. For younger children, a suspension is prepared (eg, 40 mg of chloroquine and 6 mg of primaquine in 5 mL). Dosages are then 2.5 mL for children weighing 5 to 7 kg, 5 mL for 8 to 11 kg, 7.5 mL for 12 to 15 kg, 10 mL for 16 to 20 kg, and 12.5 mL for 21 to 24 kg. Dosages are given weekly for 2 wk before entering and 8 wk after leaving malarious areas. | Used for prophylaxis of malaria |
| **Atovaquone-Proguanil**<br>(Malarone)<br>Pregnancy Category C | *Adults:* Prophylaxis, one tablet daily 1–2 days before and 7 d after travel.<br>Treatment, 4 tablets daily for 3 d.<br>*Children: 11–40 kg:* Prophylaxis, 1 to 3 pediatric tablets 1–2 d before and 7 d after travel.<br>Treatment, 1–4 adult tablets every day for 3 d | For prevention and treatment of malaria |

*(continued)*

**DRUG TABLE 33-4**

*Drugs at a Glance*

## Antiparasitic Drugs (Continued)

| Generic/Trade Name | Routes and Dosage Ranges | Comments/Uses |
|---|---|---|
| **Halofantrine** (Halfan)<br>Pregnancy Category C | *Adults:* PO, 500 mg q6h for three doses, repeat in 1 wk for clients without previous exposure to malaria (eg, travelers)<br>*Children: <40 kg:* PO, 8 mg/kg according to the schedule for adults | For treatment of malaria, including chloroquine- or multidrug-resistant strains. |
| **Mefloquine** (Lariam)<br>Pregnancy Category C | *Adults:* Prophylaxis, PO, 250 mg 1 wk before travel, then 250 mg weekly during travel and for 4 wk after leaving a malarious area<br>Treatment, 1250 mg (5 tablets) as a single dose<br>*Children:* Prophylaxis, PO, 1/4 tablet for 15–19 kg weight; 1/2 tablet for 20–30 kg; 3/4 tablet for 31–45 kg; and 1 tablet for >45 kg, according to the schedule for adults | Used for prevention and treatment of malaria |
| **Primaquine**<br>Pregnancy Category C | *Adults:* PO, 26.3 mg (equivalent to 15 mg of primaquine base) daily for 14 d, beginning immediately after leaving a malarious area, or 79 mg (45 mg of base) once a week for 8 wk. To prevent relapse, the same dose is given with chloroquine or a related drug daily for 14 d.<br>*Children:* PO, 0.3 mg of base/kg/d for 14 d, according to the schedule for adults, or 0.9 mg of base/kg/wk for 8 wk | For prevention of malaria |
| **Pyrimethamine** (Daraprim)<br>Pregnancy Category C | *Adults:* PO, 25 mg once weekly, starting 2 wk before entering and continuing for 8 wk after returning from malarious areas<br>*Children:* PO, 25 mg once weekly, as for adults, for children >10 y; 6.25–12.5 mg once weekly for children <10 y | For prevention of malaria |
| **Quinine** (Quinamm)<br>Pregnancy Category X | *Adults:* PO, 650 mg q8h for 10–14 d<br>*Children:* PO, 25 mg/kg/d in divided doses q8h for 10–14 d | Used for treatment of malaria |
| *Anti–Pneumocystis carinii Agents* | | |
| **Trimethoprim-sulfamethoxazole or TMP-SMX** (Bactrim, others)<br>Pregnancy Category C | *Adults:* Prophylaxis, PO, 1 double-strength tablet (160 mg TMP and 800 mg SMX) q24h<br>Treatment, IV, 15–20 mg/kg/d (based on trimethoprim) q6–8 h, for up to 14 d; PO 15–20 mg/kg TMP/100 mg/kg SMX per day, in divided doses, q6h, for 14–21 d<br>*Children:* Prophylaxis, PO, 150 mg/m² TMP/750 mg/m² SMX per d, in divided doses q12h, on 3 consecutive days per week. Maximum daily dose, 320 mg TMP/1600 mg SMX. | For prevention and treatment of *Pneumocystis carinii* pneumonia (PCP) |

*(continued)*

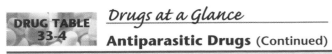

**DRUG TABLE
33-4**

*Drugs at a Glance*

## Antiparasitic Drugs (Continued)

| Generic/Trade Name | Routes and Dosage Ranges | Comments/Uses |
|---|---|---|
|  | Treatment, IV, 15–20 mg/kg/d (based on trimethoprim) q6–8 h, for up to 14 d; PO 15–20 mg/kg TMP/100 mg/kg SMX per day, in divided doses, q6h, for 14–21 d |  |
| **Atovaquone** (Mepron) Pregnancy Category C | *Adults:* Prevention, PO, 1500 mg once daily with a meal Treatment, PO 750 mg twice daily with food for 21 d *Children: 13–16 y:* Same as adults *<13 y:* Dosage not established | For prevention and treatment of PCP in people who are unable to take TMP-SMX |
| **Pentamidine** (Pentam 300, NebuPent) Pregnancy Category C | *Adults:* Treatment, IM, IV, 4 mg/kg once daily for 14 d Prophylaxis, inhalation, 300 mg every 4 wk *Children:* IM, IV, same as adults Inhalation, dosage not established | For prevention and treatment of PCP |
| **Dapsone** (Avlosulfon) Pregnancy Category C | *Adults:* PO, 100 mg daily *Children: >1 mo:* 2mg/kg/d maximum dose, 100 mg daily | For prevention of PCP |
| **Trimetrexate** (Neutrexin) Pregnancy Category D | *Adults:* IV infusion 45 mg/m² daily, over 60–90 min, for 21 d (with leucovorin, PO, IV, 20 mg/m² q6h for 24 d; give IV doses over 5–10 min) *Children:* Dosage not established | For treatment of PCP in immunocom-promised clients who are unable to take TMP-SMX |
| ***Anthelmintics*** |  |  |
| **Mebendazole** (Vermox) Pregnancy Category C | *Adults:* Most infections, PO, 100 mg morning and evening for 3 con-secutive d. For pinworms, a single 100-mg dose may be sufficient. A second course may be given in 3 wk, if necessary. *Children:* Same as adults | Treatment of hookworm, pinworm, roundworm, whipworm, and tape-worm infections |
| **Pyrantel** (Antiminth) Pregnancy Category C | *Adults:* Roundworms and pinworms, PO, 11 mg/kg (maximal dose, 1 g) as a single dose; for hookworms, the same dose is given daily for 3 con-secutive days. The course of therapy may be repeated in 1 mo, if necessary. *Children:* Same as adults | Treatment of roundworm, pinworm, and hookworm infections |
| **Thiabendazole** (Mintezol) Pregnancy Category C | *Adults:* PO, 22 mg/kg (maximal single dose, 3 g) twice daily after meals; 1 d for pinworms, repeated after 1–2 wk; 2 d for other infections, except trichinosis, which requires approximately 5 d *Children:* Same as adults | Treatment of threadworm, pinworm, hookworm, roundworm, and whip-worm infections |
| **Ivermectin** (Stromectol) Pregnancy Category C | *Adults:* 200 mcg/kg as a single dose *Children: ≥5 years:* 150 mcg/kg as a single dose | Treatment of strongyloidiasis |

*(continued)*

*Drugs at a Glance*

## Antiparasitic Drugs (Continued)

| Generic/Trade Name | Routes and Dosage Ranges | Comments/Uses |
|---|---|---|
| **Scabicides and Pediculicides** | | |
| **Permethrin** (Nix, Elimite)<br>Pregnancy Category B | *Adults:* Scabies, massage Elmite into the skin over the entire body except the face, leave on for 8–14 h, wash off. Pediculosis, apply Nix after shampooing, rinsing, and towel drying hair. Saturate hair and scalp, leave on for 10 min, rinse off with water.<br>*Children:* Same as adults | Pediculosis<br>Scabies |
| **Gamma benzene hexachloride** (Kwell, Lindane)<br>Pregnancy Category B | *Adults:* Scabies, apply topically to entire skin except the face, neck, and scalp, leave in place for 24 h, then remove by shower<br>*Children:* Same as adults<br>*Adults:* Pediculosis, rub cream or lotion into affected area, leave in place for 12 h, then wash or shampoo (rub into the affected area for 4 min and rinse thoroughly) | Pediculosis<br>Scabies |
| **Malathion** (Ovide)<br>Pregnancy Category B | *Adults:* Applied to hair, rubbed in well to wet hair, then hair dried without covering or using a hair dryer.<br>After 8–12 h, shampoo, rinse, and comb hair with a fine-toothed comb to remove dead lice and eggs. If necessary, treatment can be repeated in 7–9 d.<br>*Children:* Same as adults for children >2 y<br>Safety and effectiveness not established for children <2 y | Pediculosis (head lice) |

and abscess formation. Its use is contraindicated with iodine allergy and liver disease.

**Metronidazole** (Flagyl) is effective against protozoa that cause amebiasis, giardiasis, and trichomoniasis and against anaerobic bacilli, such as *Bacteroides* and *Clostridia* species. It is a drug of choice for all forms of amebiasis except asymptomatic intestinal amebiasis (in which amebic cysts are expelled in the feces). For trichomoniasis, metronidazole is the only systemic trichomonacide available, and it is more effective than any locally active agent. Because trichomoniasis is transmitted by sexual intercourse, partners should be treated simultaneously to prevent reinfection.

Metronidazole is usually contraindicated during the first trimester of pregnancy and must be used with caution in patients with CNS or blood disorders. Patients should also avoid all forms of ethanol while receiving this medication.

**Tetracycline** and **doxycycline** are antibacterial drugs (see Chap. 31) that act against amebae in the intestinal lumen by altering the bacterial flora required for amebic viability. One of these drugs may be used with other amebicides in the treatment of all forms of amebiasis except asymptomatic intestinal amebiasis.

## Antimalarial Agents

**Chloroquine** is a widely used antimalarial agent. It acts against erythrocytic forms of plasmodial parasites to prevent or treat malarial attacks. When used for prophylaxis, it is given before, during, and after travel or residence in endemic areas. When used for treatment of malaria caused by *P. vivax*, *P. malariae*, or *P. ovale*, chloroquine relieves symptoms of the acute attack. However, the drug does not prevent recurrence of malarial attacks because it does not act against the tissue (exoerythrocytic) forms of the parasite. When used for treatment of malaria caused by *P. falciparum*, chloroquine relieves symptoms of the acute attack and eliminates the parasite from the body because *P. falciparum* does not have tissue reservoirs. Concern about chloroquine-resistant strains of *P. falciparum* have developed in many areas.

Chloroquine is also used in protozoal infections other than malaria, including extraintestinal amebiasis and giardiasis. It should be used with caution in patients with hepatic disease or severe neurologic, GI, or blood disorders.

**Hydroxychloroquine** (Plaquenil) is a derivative of chloroquine with essentially the same actions, uses, and adverse effects as chloroquine. It has also been used to treat rheumatoid arthritis and lupus erythematosus.

**Chloroquine** with **primaquine** is a mixture available in tablets containing chloroquine phosphate, 500 mg (equivalent to 300 mg of chloroquine base), and primaquine phosphate, 79 mg (equivalent to 45 mg of primaquine base). This combination is effective for prophylaxis of malaria and may be more acceptable to clients. It also may be more convenient for use in children because no pediatric formulation of primaquine is available.

**Halofantrine** (Halfan) is indicated for treatment of malaria caused by *P. falciparum* or *P. vivax*, including chloroquine- or multidrug-resistant strains.

**Mefloquine** (Lariam) is used to prevent *P. falciparum* malaria, including chloroquine-resistant strains, and to treat acute malaria caused by *P. falciparum* or *P. vivax*.

**Primaquine** is used to prevent the initial occurrence of malaria; to prevent recurrent attacks of malaria caused by *P. vivax*, *P. malariae*, and *P. ovale*; and to achieve "radical cure" of these three types of malaria. (Radical cure involves eradicating the exoerythrocytic forms of the plasmodium and preventing the survival of the blood forms.) The clinical usefulness of primaquine stems primarily from its ability to destroy tissue (exoerythrocytic) forms of the malarial parasite. Primaquine is especially effective in *P. vivax* malaria. Thus far, plasmodial strains causing the three relapsing types of malaria have not developed resistance to primaquine. When used to prevent initial occurrence of malaria (causal prophylaxis), primaquine is given concurrently with a suppressive agent (eg, chloroquine or hydroxychloroquine) after the patient has returned from a malarious area. Primaquine is not effective for treatment of acute attacks of malaria.

**Pyrimethamine** (Daraprim) is a folic acid antagonist used to prevent malaria caused by susceptible strains of plasmodia. It is sometimes used with a sulfonamide and quinine to treat chloroquine-resistant strains of *P. falciparum*. Folic acid antagonists and sulfonamides act synergistically against plasmodia because they block different steps in the synthesis of folic acid, a nutrient required by the parasites.

**Quinine** (Quinamm) is derived from the bark of the cinchona tree. Quinine was the primary antimalarial drug for many years but has been largely replaced by synthetic agents that cause fewer adverse reactions. However, it may still be used in the treatment of chloroquine-resistant *P. falciparum* malaria, usually in conjunction with pyrimethamine and a sulfonamide. Quinine also relaxes skeletal muscles and has been used for prevention and treatment of nocturnal leg cramps.

**Malarone** is a new combination antimalarial medication containing 250 mg of atovaquone and 100 mg of proguanil per tablet. This product may be used for both the prevention and treatment of malarial infections, particularly those caused by *P. falciparum*. The drug also seems to be effective in chloroquine-resistant areas and is devoid of many of the side effects of mefloquine. Two drugs are combined to inhibit separate pathways involved in the synthesis of nucleic acids by the offending parasite. The drug should be taken daily with food or milk starting 1 or 2 days before entering an endemic area and for 7 days upon return.

## Anti–Pneumocystis carinii Agents

**Trimethoprim-sulfamethoxazole** (TMP-SMX, Bactrim, others; see Chap. 32) is the drug of choice for prevention and treatment of PCP. Prophylaxis is indicated for adults and adolescents with HIV infection and CD4$^+$ cell counts lower than 200; organ transplant recipients; patients with leukemia or lymphoma who are receiving cytotoxic chemotherapy; and patients receiving high doses of corticosteroids (equivalent to 20 mg or more daily of prednisone) for prolonged periods of time.

Common adverse effects include nausea, vomiting, and skin rash. These effects seem to be more common in patients who are HIV seropositive.

**Atovaquone** (Mepron) is used for both prophylaxis and treatment of PCP in people who are unable to take TMP-SMX. Adverse effects include nausea, vomiting, diarrhea, fever, insomnia, and elevated hepatic enzymes.

**Dapsone** (Avlosulfon) may be used for the prophylaxis of PCP infection in HIV-seropositive patients who are unable to tolerate TMP-SMX. Patients who are glucose-6-phosphate dehydrogenase (G6PD) deficient will develop hemolytic anemia; therefore, this laboratory parameter should be assessed before initiating therapy. Common side effects include nausea, vomiting, and rash.

**Trimetrexate** (Neutrexin) is a folate antagonist (which must be used with leucovorin rescue) approved only for treatment of moderate to severe PCP in immunocompromised patients, including those with advanced HIV infection, who are unable to take TMP-SMX. Hematologic toxicity is the main dose-limiting adverse effect. To minimize hematologic effects, leucovorin should be given daily during trimetrexate therapy and for 72 hours after the last trimetrexate dose. Dosage of trimetrexate must be reduced and dosage of leucovorin increased with significant neutropenia or thrombocytopenia.

**Pentamidine** (Pentam 300, NebuPent) may be used both for prophylaxis and treatment of PCP infection. Pentamidine interferes with production of ribonucleic acid and deoxyribonucleic acid by the organism. The drug is given parenterally for treatment of PCP and by inhalation for prophylaxis. It is excreted by the kidneys and accumulates in the presence of renal failure; therefore, dosage should be reduced in patients with renal impairment. Clinicians should also be aware that the intravenous form of pentamidine is particularly toxic to the pancreas. With parenteral pentamidine, appropriate tests should be performed before, during, and after treatment (eg, complete blood count, platelet count, serum creatinine, blood urea nitrogen, blood glucose, serum calcium, and electrocardiogram).

## Anthelmintics

**Mebendazole** (Vermox) is a broad-spectrum anthelmintic used in the treatment of parasitic infections by hookworms, pinworms, roundworms, and whipworms. It is also useful but less effective in tapeworm infection. Mebendazole kills helminths by preventing uptake of the glucose necessary for parasitic metabolism. The helminths become immobilized and die slowly; therefore, they may be expelled from the GI tract up to 3 days after drug therapy is completed. Mebendazole acts locally in the GI tract, and less than 10% of the drug is absorbed systemically.

Mebendazole is usually the drug of choice for single or mixed infections caused by the aforementioned parasitic worms. The drug is contraindicated during pregnancy because of teratogenic effects in rats; it is relatively contraindicated in children younger than 2 years of age because it has not been extensively investigated for use in this age group.

**Pyrantel** (Antiminth) is effective in infestations of roundworms, pinworms, and hookworms. The drug acts locally to paralyze worms in the intestinal tract. Pyrantel is poorly absorbed from the GI tract, and most of an administered dose may be recovered in feces. Pyrantel is contraindicated in pregnancy and is not recommended for children younger than 1 year of age.

**Thiabendazole** (Mintezol) is most effective against threadworms and pinworms. It is useful but less effective against hookworms, roundworms, and whipworms. Because of the broad spectrum of anthelmintic activity, thiabendazole may be especially useful in mixed parasitic infestations. In trichinosis, thiabendazole decreases symptoms and eosinophilia but does not eliminate larvae from muscle tissues. The mechanism of anthelmintic action is uncertain but probably involves interference with parasitic metabolism. The drug is relatively toxic compared with other anthelmintic agents.

Thiabendazole is a drug of choice for threadworm infestations. For other types of helminthiasis, it is usually considered an alternative drug. It is rapidly absorbed after oral administration, and most of the drug is excreted in urine within 24 hours. It should be used with caution in clients with liver or kidney disease.

**Ivermectin** (Stromectol) is used for numerous parasitic infections and is most active against strongyloidiasis. Ivermectin has also been used for the oral treatment of resistant lice. The drug has relatively few side effects but may cause some nausea and vomiting.

## Scabicides and Pediculicides

**Permethrin** is the drug of choice for both pediculosis and scabies. Although a single application eliminates parasites and ova, two applications are generally recommended. For pediculosis, permethrin is available as a 1% over-the-counter liquid (Nix). For scabies, a 5% permethrin cream (Elimite) is available by prescription. For scabies, a single application of 5% permethrin cream is considered curative. Permethrin is safer than other scabicides and pediculicides, especially for infants and children.

Permethrin is derived from a chrysanthemum plant, and people with a history of allergy to ragweed or chrysanthemum flowers should use it cautiously. The most frequent adverse effect is pruritus.

To avoid reinfection, close contacts should be treated simultaneously. With pediculosis, clothing and bedding should be sterilized by boiling or steaming and seams of clothes should be examined to verify that all lice are eliminated.

**Gamma benzene hexachloride** (Lindane) is a second-line drug for scabies and pediculosis. It may be used for people who have hypersensitivity reactions or resistance to treatment with permethrin. It is applied topically, and substantial amounts are absorbed through intact skin. CNS toxicity has been reported with excessive use, especially in infants and children. The drug is available in a 1% concentration in a cream, lotion, and shampoo.

**Malathion** (Ovide) is a pediculicide particularly used in the treatment of head lice, and **pyrethrin** preparations (eg, Barc, RID) are available over the counter as gels, shampoos, and liquid suspensions for treatment of pediculosis. **Crotamiton** (Eurax) is sometimes used as a 10% cream or lotion for scabies.

*(text continues on page 606)*

## CLIENT TEACHING GUIDELINES
### Antiparasitic Drugs

#### General Considerations
✔ Use measures to prevent parasitic infection or reinfection:

  ✔ Support public health measures to maintain a clean environment (ie, sanitary sewers, clean water, regulation of food-handling establishments and food-handling personnel).

✔ When traveling to wilderness areas or to tropical or underdeveloped countries, check with the local health department about precautions needed to avoid parasitic infections.

✔ Practice good handwashing and other personal hygiene practices.

*(continued)*

## CLIENT TEACHING GUIDELINES
### Antiparasitic Drugs (Continued)

✔ When a family member or other close contact contracts a parasitic infection, be sure appropriate treatment and follow-up care are completed.

✔ Avoid raw fish and undercooked meat.

✔ With vaginal infections, avoid sexual intercourse, or use a condom.

### Self-administration or Caregiver Administration

✔ Use antiparasitic drugs as prescribed; their effectiveness depends on accurate use.

✔ Take atovaquone, chloroquine and related drugs, iodoquinol, and oral metronidazole with or after meals. Food increases absorption of atovaquone and decreases gastrointestinal irritation of the other drugs.

✔ To use pentamidine by inhalation, dissolve the contents of one vial in 6 mL of sterile water, place the solution in the nebulizer chamber of a Respirgard II device, and deliver by way of oxygen or compressed air flow until the nebulizer chamber is empty (approximately 30 to 45 minutes).

✔ Take or give most anthelmintics without regard to mealtimes or food ingestion. Mebendazole tablets should be chewed or crushed and mixed with food; thiabendazole should be taken with food to decrease stomach upset. Chew chewable tablets thoroughly before swallowing.

✔ Use pediculicides and scabicides as directed on the label or product insert. Instructions vary among preparations.

## Nursing Actions
### Antiparasitics

| Nursing Actions | Rationale/Explanation |
|---|---|
| 1. Administer accurately. | |
| a. Give atovaquone, chloroquine and related drugs, iodoquinol, and oral metronidazole with or after meals. | Food improves absorption of atovaquone and decreases gastrointestinal (GI) irritation of the other drugs. |
| b. With pentamidine: (1) For intravenous administration, dissolve the calculated dose in 3–5 mL of sterile water or 5% dextrose in water. Dilute further with 50–250 mL of 5% dextrose solution and infuse over 60 min. | |
| c. Give anthelmintics without regard to mealtimes or food ingestion. Mebendazole tablets may be chewed, swallowed, or crushed and mixed with food. | Food in the GI tract does not decrease effectiveness of most anthelmintics. |
| d. For pediculicides and scabicides, follow the label or manufacturer's instructions. | Instructions vary among preparations. |
| 2. Observe for therapeutic effects. | |
| a. With chloroquine for acute malaria, observe for relief of symptoms and negative blood smears. | Fever and chills usually subside within 24–48 h, and blood smears are negative for plasmodia within 24–72 h. |
| b. With amebicides, observe for relief of symptoms and negative stool examinations. | Relief of symptoms does not indicate cure of amebiasis; laboratory evidence is required. Stool specimens should be examined for amebic cysts and trophozoites periodically for approximately 6 mo. |
| c. With anti–Pneumocystis carinii agents for prophylaxis, observe for absence of symptoms; when used for treatment, observe for decreased fever, cough, and respiratory distress. | |
| d. With anthelmintics, observe for relief of symptoms, absence of the parasite in blood or stool for three consecutive examinations, or a reduction in the number of parasitic ova in the feces. | The goal of anthelmintic drug therapy may be complete eradication of the parasite or reduction of the "worm burden." |
| e. With pediculicides, inspect affected areas for lice or nits. | For most clients, one treatment is effective. For others, a second treatment may be necessary. |

*(continued)*

## Nursing Actions

## Antiparasitics (Continued)

| Nursing Actions | Rationale/Explanation |
|---|---|
| 3. Observe for adverse effects. | |
| a. With amebicides, observe for anorexia, nausea, vomiting, epigastric burning, diarrhea. | GI effects may occur with all amebicides. |
| (1) With iodoquinol, observe for agitation, amnesia, peripheral neuropathy, and optic neuropathy. | These effects are most likely to occur with large doses or long-term drug administration. |
| b. With antimalarial agents, observe for nausea, vomiting, diarrhea, pruritus, skin rash, headache, central nervous system (CNS) stimulation. | These effects may occur with most antimalarial agents. However, adverse effects are usually mild because small doses are used for prophylaxis, and the larger doses required for treatment of acute malarial attacks are given only for short periods. |
| (1) With pyrimethamine, observe for anemia, thrombocytopenia, and leukopenia. | This drug interferes with folic acid metabolism. |
| (2) With quinine, observe for signs of cinchonism (headache, tinnitus, decreased auditory acuity, blurred vision). | These effects occur with usual therapeutic doses of quinine. They do not usually necessitate discontinuance of quinine therapy. |
| c. With metronidazole, observe for convulsions, peripheral paresthesias, nausea, diarrhea, unpleasant taste, vertigo, headache, and vaginal and urethral burning sensation. | CNS effects are most serious; GI effects are most common. |
| d. With parenteral pentamidine, observe for leukopenia, thrombocytopenia, hypoglycemia, hyperglycemia, hypocalcemia, hypokalemia, hypotension, acute renal failure. | Severe hypotension may occur after a single parenteral dose. Deaths from hypotension, hypoglycemia, and cardiac arrhythmias have been reported. |
| e. With aerosolized pentamidine, observe for fatigue, shortness of breath, bronchospasm, cough, dizziness, rash, anorexia, nausea, vomiting, chest pain. | These are the most common adverse effects. |
| f. With atovaquone, observe for nausea, vomiting, diarrhea, fever, headache, skin rash. | |
| g. With trimetrexate, observe for anemia, neutropenia, thrombocytopenia, increased bilirubin and liver enzymes (aspartate and alanine aminotransferases, alkaline phosphatase), fever, skin rash, pruritus, nausea, vomiting, hyponatremia, hypocalcemia. | |
| h. With topical antitrichomonal agents, observe for hypersensitivity reactions (eg, rash, inflammation), burning, and pruritus. | Hypersensitivity reactions are the major adverse effects. Other effects are minor and rarely require that drug therapy be discontinued. |
| i. With permethrin, observe for pruritus, burning, or tingling; with Lindane, observe for CNS stimulation (nervousness, tremors, insomnia, convulsions). | Antihistamines or topical corticosteroids may be used to decrease itching. CNS toxicity is more likely to occur with excessive use of Lindane (ie, increased amounts, leaving in place longer than prescribed, or applying more frequently than prescribed). |
| 4. Observe for drug interactions. | Few clinically significant drug interactions occur because many antiparasitic agents are administered for local effects in the GI tract or on the skin. Most of the drugs also are given for short periods. |
| a. Drugs that alter effects of chloroquine: | |
| (1) Acidifying agents (eg, ascorbic acid) | Inhibit chloroquine by increasing the rate of urinary excretion |
| (2) Alkalinizing agents (eg, sodium bicarbonate) | Potentiate chloroquine by decreasing the rate of urinary excretion |
| (3) Monoamine oxidase inhibitors | Increase risk of toxicity and retinal damage by inhibiting metabolism. |

*(continued)*

## Nursing Actions

### Antiparasitics (Continued)

| Nursing Actions | Rationale/Explanation |
| --- | --- |
| b. Drugs that alter effects of metronidazole:<br>(1) Phenobarbital, phenytoin<br><br>(2) Cimetidine<br><br>c. Drugs that *decrease* effects of atovaquone and trimetrexate: Rifampin and other drugs that induce CYP450 drug-metabolizing enzymes in the liver | These drugs induce hepatic enzymes and decrease effects of metronidazole by accelerating its rate of hepatic metabolism. May increase effects by inhibiting hepatic metabolism of metronidazole.<br>Although few interactions have been reported, any enzyme-inducing drug can potentially decrease effects of atovaquone and trimetrexate by accelerating their metabolism in the liver. |

### ? How Can You Avoid This Medication Error?

**Answer:** Amphotericin B is very nephrotoxic. You should not administer it to Mr. Little when his BUN is 48 mg/dL and his creatinine is 3.5 mg/dL because both values indicate renal impairment. Notify his physician of these laboratory data to see if he or she would like to decrease the dose.

## Critical Thinking Exercises

1. A client is started on acyclovir. What preexisting condition should the nurse recognize requires caution during this drug's use?
   a. Diabetes mellitus
   b. Asthma
   c. Renal impairment
   d. Liver disease

2. A client with advanced HIV infection was started on didanosine 1 month ago. He presents back to the clinic intoxicated, complaining of severe abdominal pain. The most likely cause of his symptoms associated with didanosine therapy is:
   a. Acute gastrointestinal bleeding
   b. Coronary artery disease
   c. Hepatitis
   d. Pancreatitis

3. Probenecid is administered with cidofovir therapy to:
   a. Increase renal excretion of cidofovir
   b. Decrease nephrotoxic effects
   c. Minimize gastrointestinal upset
   d. Decrease frequency of attacks of acute gout.

4. The nurse teaches the client about adverse reactions to stavudine. Which adverse reaction is most likely to occur?
   a. Peripheral neuropathy
   b. Acute tubular necrosis
   c. Pancreatitis
   d. Exacerbation of asthma

5. Indinavir belongs to which classification of drugs used to treat HIV infection and AIDS?
   a. Nucleoside reverse transcriptase inhibitors
   b. Nucleotide reverse transcriptase inhibitors
   c. Non-nucleoside reverse transcriptase inhibitors
   d. Protease inhibitors

## SELECTED REFERENCES

Acosta E. P., Kakuda T. N., Brundage R. C., Anderson, P. L., & Fletcher, C. V. (2000). Pharmacodynamics of HIV-1 protease inhibitors. *Clinical Infectious Diseases, 30,* 151S–159S.

Balfour, H. H. (1999). Antiviral drugs. *New England Journal of Medicine, 340,* 1255–1268.

Bartels, C. L., Peterson, K. E., & Taylor, K. L. (2001). Head lice resistance: Itching that just won't stop. *Annals of Pharmacotherapy, 35,* 109–112.

Burkhart, C. N., & Burkhart, C. G. (1999). Another look at ivermectin in the treatment of scabies and head lice. *International Journal of Dermatology, 38,* 235.

De Clerq, E. (2001). New developments in anti-HIV chemotherapy. *Current Medical Chemistry, 8,* 1529–1558.

Dodds, E. S., Drew, R. H., & Perfect, J. R. (2000). Antifungal pharmacodynamics: Review of the literature and clinical applications. *Pharmacotherapy, 20*(11), 1335–1355.

*Drug facts and comparisons.* (Updated monthly.) St. Louis: Facts and Comparisons.

Ernst, E. J. (2001). Investigational antifungal agents. *Pharmacotherapy, 21*(8 Pt. 2), 165S–174S.

Greenwood, B., & Mutabingwa, T. (2002, August 13). Malaria in 2002. *Nature, 415,* 670–672.

Panel on Clinical Practice for Treatment of HIV Infection convened by the Department of Health and Human Services (DHHS) and the Henry J. Kaiser Family Foundation. (2001). *Guidelines for the use of antiretroviral agents in HIV-infected adults and adolescents.* [On-line.] Available: http://www.hivatis.org.

Kaul, D. R., Cinti, S. K., Carver, P. L., & Kazanjian, P. H. (1999). HIV protease inhibitors: Advances in therapy and adverse reactions, including metabolic complications. *Pharmacotherapy, 19,* 281–298.

Lacy, C. F., Armstrong, L. L., Goldman, M. P., & Lance, L. L. (2003). *Lexi-Comp's drug information handbook* (11th ed.). Hudson, OH: American Pharmaceutical Association.

Lewis, R. E., & Kontoyiannis, D. P. (2001). Rationale for combination antifungal therapy. *Pharmacotherapy, 21*(8 Pt. 2), 149S–164S.

Morrison, C., & Lew, E. (2001). Aspergillosis. *American Journal of Nursing, 101*(8), 40–48.

Patterson, T. F. (2000). Infections caused by dimorphic fungi. In H. D. Humes (Ed.), *Kelley's textbook of internal medicine* (4th ed., pp. 2094–2099). Philadelphia: Lippincott Williams & Wilkins.

Pegues, D. A., Lasker, B. A., McNeil, M. M., Hamm, P. M., Lundal, J. L., & Kubak, B. M. (2002). Cluster of cases of invasive aspergillosis in a transplant intensive care unit: Evidence of person-to-person airborne transmission. *Clinical Infectious Diseases, 34*(3), 412–416.

Rana, K. Z., & Dudley, M. N. (1999). Human immunodeficiency virus protease inhibitors. *Pharmacotherapy 19*, 35–49.

Reed, M. D., & Blumer, J. L. (2002). Anti-infective therapy. In H. B. Jenson & R. S. Baltimore (Eds.), *Pediatric infectious diseases: Principles and practice* (2nd ed., pp. 147–215). Philadelphia: W. B. Saunders.

Rex, J. H. (2000). Approach to the treatment of systemic fungal infections. In H. D. Humes (Ed.), *Kelley's textbook of internal medicine* (4th ed., pp. 2279–2281). Philadelphia: Lippincott Williams & Wilkins.

Sepkowitz, K. A. (2002). Opportunistic infections in patients with and patients without acquired immunodeficiency syndrome. *Clinical Infectious Diseases, 34*, 1098–1107.

Winstanley, P. (2001). Modern chemotherapeutic options for malaria. *Lancet, 1*, 242–250.

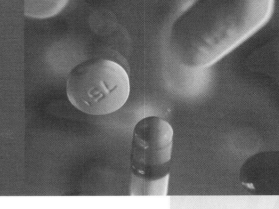

34

# Immunizing Agents

## OBJECTIVES

*After studying this chapter, the student will be able to:*

1 Give common characteristics of immunizations.

2 Discuss the importance of immunizations in promoting health and preventing disease.

3 List authoritative sources for immunization information.

4 Identify immunizations recommended for children.

5 Identify immunizations recommended for adults.

6 Discuss ways to promote immunization of all age groups.

7 Teach parents about recommended immunizations and record keeping.

## CRITICAL THINKING SCENARIO

*A* young couple, Jack and Diane Griffen, brings their 6-week-old infant, Sarah, to the clinic for a well-baby check and her required "shots." First, you examine Sarah and talk with the couple about how new parenthood is going. Both seem very motivated to be good parents. They have lots of questions and ask whether all those shots are really necessary. Mrs. Griffen admits that she has always been afraid of shots and just can't watch her baby be hurt.

✔ How can you acknowledge Mrs. Griffen's concerns without minimizing her feelings?

✔ What basic information will you provide the new parents regarding immunizations?

✔ What will you teach Mr. and Mrs. Griffen about appropriate symptom management and what to expect for 2 to 3 days after the injection?

✔ How will you convey to the parents the importance of keeping up-to-date immunization records?

## OVERVIEW

An abnormally functioning immune system causes numerous diseases. When the system is hypoactive, immunodeficiency disorders develop in which the person is highly susceptible to infectious and neoplastic diseases. When the system is hyperactive, it perceives ordinarily harmless environmental substances (eg, foods, plant pollens) as harmful and induces allergic reactions. When the system is inappropriately activated (it loses its ability to distinguish between self and nonself, so that an immune response is aroused against the host's own body tissues), the result is autoimmune disorders, such as systemic lupus erythematosus and rheumatoid arthritis.

Many antigens that activate the immune response are microorganisms that cause infectious diseases. Early scientists observed that people who contracted certain diseases were thereafter protected despite repeated exposure to the disease. As knowledge evolved, it was discovered that protection stemmed from body substances called *antibodies*, and that antibodies could also be induced by deliberate, controlled exposure to the antigen. Subsequently, immunization techniques were developed. To aid understanding of the concept of immunizations and the individual immunizing agents, more specific characteristics, processes, and functions of the immune system are described later in the chapter and in At the Foundation: Types of Immunity.

## IMMUNITY

Immunity indicates protection from a disease, and the major function of the immune system is to detect and eliminate foreign substances that may cause tissue injury or disease. Immunity is the third and last line of defense against infection (following anatomic barriers and the inflammatory response) and has three unique character-

---

**AT THE FOUNDATION:** *Types of Immunity*

**Innate or natural immunity** is not produced by the immune system and includes general protective mechanisms that protect an individual from infectious agents that cause illness in other species (species dependent) or through specific genetic characteristics in an individual (host dependent).

**Acquired immunity** develops during gestation or after birth and may be active or passive. *Active acquired immunity* is produced by the person's own immune system in response to a disease caused by a specific antigen or administration of an antigen (eg, a vaccine) from a source outside the body, usually by injection. The immune response stimulated by the antigen produces activated lymphocytes and antibodies against the antigen. When an antigen is present for the first time, production of antibodies requires several days. As a result, the serum concentration of antibodies does not reach protective levels for approximately 7 to 10 days, and the disease develops in the host. When the antigen is eliminated, the antibody concentration gradually decreases over several weeks.

The duration of active immunity may be brief (eg, to influenza viruses), or it may last for years or a lifetime. Long-term active immunity has a unique characteristic called *memory*. When the host is reexposed to the antigen, lymphocytes are activated, and antibodies are produced rapidly, and the host does not contract the disease. This characteristic allows "booster" doses of antigen to increase antibody levels and maintain active immunity against some diseases.

*Passive acquired immunity* occurs when antibodies are formed by the immune system of another person or animal and transferred to the host. For example, an infant is normally protected for several months by maternal antibodies received through the placenta during gestation. Also, antibodies previously formed by a donor can be transferred to the host by an injection of immune serum. These antibodies act against antigens immediately. Passive immunity is short term, lasting only a few weeks or months and is used in the treatment of clinical emergencies.

**Cellular and Humoral Immunity**
Types of acquired immunity have traditionally been separated into cellular immunity (mainly involving activated T lymphocytes in body tissues) and humoral immunity (mainly involving B lymphocytes and antibodies in the blood). However, it is now known that the two types are closely connected, that virtually all antigens elicit both cellular and humoral responses, and that most humoral (B cell) responses require cellular (T cell) stimulation.

Although most humoral immune responses occur when antibodies or B cells encounter antigens in blood, some occur when antibodies or B cells encounter antigens in other body fluids (eg, tears, sweat, saliva, mucus, and breast milk). The antibodies (mostly immunoglobulin A [IgA], some IgM and IgG) secreted at these sites act locally rather than systemically. This local protection combats foreign substances, especially pathogenic microorganisms that are inhaled, swallowed, or otherwise come in contact with external body surfaces. When the foreign substances bind to local antibodies, they are unable to attach to and invade mucosal tissue.

istics: specificity, memory, and inducibility to provide long-term protection against specific antigens. To perform this function, the immune system must be able to differentiate body tissues (self) from foreign substances (nonself). Self tissues are recognized by distinctive protein molecules on the surface membranes of body cells encoded by a group of genes called the major histocompatibility complex (MHC). Nonself or foreign antigens are also recognized by distinctive molecules, called *epitopes*, on their surfaces. Epitopes vary widely in type, number, and ability to elicit an immune response.

## ■ IMMUNIZATION

Immunization or vaccination involves administration of an antigen to induce antibody formation (for active immunity) or serum from immune people (for passive immunity). Preparations used for immunization are biologic products prepared by pharmaceutical companies and regulated by the U.S. Food and Drug Administration (FDA). No immunization product serves as a prototype.

Although immunizations against some diseases have long been used, the development of immunizing agents and recommendations for their use continue. Some recommendations and changes of recent years are summarized below:

■ The American Academy of Pediatrics (www.aap.org) recommends that only the inactivated polio vaccine (IPV) be used in the United States. The oral vaccine used for many years contained live virus and caused viral shedding and a few cases of polio. The main disadvantages of IPV are that it must be injected and is more expensive.
■ Hepatitis B virus (HBV) infection can cause serious liver diseases such as acute and chronic hepatitis, cirrhosis, and hepatocellular carcinoma. Chronic carriers of HBV may be asymptomatic reservoirs for viral transmission. Children who become infected are at high risk for chronic infection. Because of these circumstances, hepatitis B vaccine is now recommended for all newborns and for nonimmunized children before starting school as well as for other at-risk groups. Overall, the goal is to achieve universal immunization, decrease transmission, and eradicate the disease.
■ Everyone should be immunized against diphtheria and tetanus every 7 to 10 years for life.
■ Strategies to promote immunization continue to evolve. One strategy is to combine vaccines so that only one injection is required when the need and time for multiple vaccines coincide. In addition to the long used measles-mumps-rubella (MMR) and diphtheria-tetanus-pertussis (DTaP) combinations, available combinations include inactivated poliovirus vaccine with DTaP with hepatitis B (Pediarix), *Haemophilus b* (Hib)

with hepatitis B (Comvax), DTaP with *Haemophilus b* (DTaP-HIB; TriHIBit), and hepatitis A and hepatitis B (Twinrix). Another strategy is to give multiple vaccines (in separate syringes, at different sites) at one visit to a health care provider when feasible. For example, several vaccines are recommended to be given at the same time for routine immunization of infants and young children. In addition, influenza and pneumococcal vaccines can be administered concurrently, and at least one study indicates that varicella and MMR can be given at the same office visit.
■ Two vaccines were developed, marketed, and then withdrawn from the market. Rotavirus vaccine was withdrawn because of adverse effects, and Lyme disease vaccine was apparently withdrawn because of infrequent use.

## ■ AGENTS FOR ACTIVE IMMUNITY

The biologic products used for active immunity are vaccines and toxoids. *Vaccines* are suspensions of microorganisms or their antigenic products that have been killed or attenuated (weakened or reduced in virulence) so that they can induce antibody formation while preventing or causing very mild forms of the disease. Many vaccines produce long-lasting immunity. Attenuated live vaccines produce immunity, usually lifelong, that is similar to that produced by natural infection. However, there is a small risk for producing disease with live vaccines, especially in people with impaired immune function. Vaccines developed with recombinant DNA technology have a very low risk for causing active disease.

*Toxoids* are bacterial toxins or products that have been modified to destroy toxicity while retaining antigenic properties (ie, ability to induce antibody formation). Immunization with toxoids is not permanent; scheduled repeat doses (boosters) are required to maintain immunity.

Additional components of vaccines and toxoids may include aluminum phosphate, aluminum hydroxide, or calcium phosphate. Products containing aluminum should be given intramuscularly only because they cannot be given intravenously, and greater tissue irritation occurs with subcutaneous injections. These additives are used to delay absorption and increase antigenicity.

For maximum effectiveness, vaccines and toxoids must be given before exposure to the pathogenic microorganism. They should also be given by the recommended route, to ensure the desired immunologic response.

### Indications for Use

Clinical indications for use of vaccines and toxoids include the following:

1. Routine immunization of all children against diphtheria, *Haemophilus b* infection, hepatitis B, mumps, pertussis, pneumococcal infection, poliomyelitis,

rubella (German measles), rubeola (red measles), tetanus, and varicella.

2. Immunization of adolescents and adults against diphtheria and tetanus.

3. Immunization of prepubertal girls or women of childbearing age against rubella. Rubella during the first trimester of pregnancy is associated with a high incidence of birth defects in the newborn.

4. Immunization of people at high risk for serious morbidity or mortality from a particular disease. For example, hepatitis B, influenza, and pneumococcal vaccines are recommended for selected groups of people.

5. Immunization of adults and children at high risk for exposure to a particular disease. For example, some diseases (eg, yellow fever) rarely occur in most parts of the world. Thus, immunization is recommended only for people who live in or travel to geographic areas where the disease can be contracted.

## Contraindications to Use

Vaccines and toxoids are usually contraindicated during febrile illnesses; immunosuppressive drug therapy (see Chap. 36); immunodeficiency states; leukemia, lymphoma, or generalized malignancy; and pregnancy.

## ■ AGENTS FOR PASSIVE IMMUNITY

Immune serums are the biologic products used for passive immunity. They are used to provide temporary immunity in people exposed to or experiencing a particular disease. The goal of therapy is to prevent or modify the disease process (ie, decrease the incidence and severity of symptoms).

Immune globulin products are made from the serum of individuals with high concentrations of the specific antibody or immunoglobulin required. They may consist of whole serum or the immunoglobulin portion of serum in which the specific antibodies are concentrated. Immunoglobulin fractions are preferred over whole serum because they are more likely to be effective. Plasma used to prepare these products is negative for hepatitis B surface antigen (HBsAg). Hyperimmune serums are available for cytomegalovirus, hepatitis B, rabies, rubella, tetanus, varicella zoster (shingles), and respiratory syncytial virus infections.

## ■ INDIVIDUAL IMMUNIZING AGENTS

Individual vaccines, toxoids, and immune serums are listed in Drugs at a Glance 34-1: Vaccines and Toxoids for Active Acquired Immunity and in Drugs at a Glance 34-2: Immune Serums for Passive Acquired Immunity.

## ■ MANAGEMENT CONSIDERATIONS

### Keeping Up-to-Date with Immunization Recommendations

Recommendations regarding immunizations change periodically as additional information and new immunizing agents become available. Consequently, health care providers should update their knowledge at least annually. The best source of information regarding current recommendations is the Centers for Disease Control and Prevention (CDC), headquartered in Atlanta, Georgia (www.cdc.gov).

The main source of CDC recommendations is the Advisory Committee on Immunization Practices (ACIP, accessible at www.cdc.gov/nip/acip), which consists of 15 experts appointed by the Secretary of the U.S. Department of Health and Human Services (DHHS) to advise the Secretary, the Assistant Secretary for Health, and the CDC on strategies to prevent vaccine-preventable diseases. Other sources of information include the American Academy of Pediatrics (www.aap.org) and the American Academy of Family Physicians (www.aafp.org). Local health departments can also be consulted on routine immunizations and those required for foreign travel. These sources can also provide information on new vaccine release, vaccine supply, and statements on use of specific vaccines.

### Reporting of Vaccine-preventable Diseases

Health care providers who encounter cases of vaccine-preventable disease should report such cases to the local or state health department. This information is sent to the CDC to determine whether an outbreak is occurring and to help prevention and control strategies. The CDC can then determine the impact of the case on national policy and practice regarding immunizations.

### Reporting of Adverse Reactions

All health care providers must report any serious adverse reactions to the DHHS vaccine Adverse Reporting System (VAERS). The VAERS relies on health professionals, clients, or guardians to submit reports of adverse reactions following vaccination. All reports are entered into a computer database, and selected reports of serious events and all reports of fatalities are followed up individually by a health professional. General information and the VAERS form are available on the VAERS web site at www.fda.gov/cber/vaers.html.

### Storage of Vaccines

To maintain effectiveness of vaccines and other biologic preparations, the products must be stored properly. Most products require refrigeration at 2°C to 8°C (35.6°F to

(text continues on page 622)

**DRUG TABLE 34-1**

*Drugs at a Glance*

## Vaccines and Toxoids for Active Acquired Immunity

| Generic/Trade Name | Characteristics | Routes and Dosage Ranges | Comments/Uses |
|---|---|---|---|
| **Vaccines** | | | |
| **Haemophilus b (Hib) conjugate vaccine** (ActHIB, HibTITER, PedvaxHIB) Pregnancy Category C | Formed by conjugating a derivative of the organism with a protein. The protein increases antigenicity. | *Children:* HibTITER age 2–5 mo: IM, 0.5 mL every 2 mo for 3 doses; age 15 mo: 0.5 mL as a single booster dose<br>Age 7–11 mo: IM, 0.5 mL every 2 mo for two doses; age 15 mo: 0.5 mL as a single booster dose<br>Age 12–14 mo: IM, 0.5 mL as single dose; age 15 mo: 0.5 mL as a single booster dose, at least 2 mo after the first dose<br>Age 15–59 mo: IM, 0.5 mL as a single dose (no booster dose)<br>Pedvax HIB age 2–6 mo: IM, 0.5 mL every 2 mo for two doses; age 12 mo: 0.5 mL as a booster dose<br>Age 7–11 mo: IM, 0.5 mL every 2 mo for two doses; age 15 mo: 0.5 mL as booster dose<br>Age 12–14 mo: IM, 0.5 mL as single dose; age 15 mo: 0.5 mL as a single booster dose, at least 2 mo after the first dose<br>Age 15–59 mo: IM, 0.5 mL as a single dose (no booster dose)<br>ProHIBit age 15–59 mo: IM, 0.5 mL as a single dose (no booster dose) | Used to prevent infection with Hib, a common cause of serious bacterial infections, including meningitis, in children younger than 5 y |
| **Haemophilus b (Hib) conjugate vaccine with hepatitis B vaccine** (Comvax) Pregnancy Category C | May be given at the same time as DTaP, MMR, injected polio vaccine (IPV), but with separate syringes and in separate sites | *Children:* IM, 0.5 mL at 2, 4, and 12–15 mo | For routine immunization of children 6 wk to 15 mo born to HBsAg-negative mothers |
| **Hepatitis A vaccine** (Havrix, Vaqta) Pregnancy Category C | Inactivated whole virus<br>More than 90% effective<br>Duration of protection unknown<br>Contraindicated during febrile illness, immunosuppression<br>With Havrix, the adult formulation contains 1,440 units in 1 mL; the pediatric formulation contains 360 or 720 units in 0.5 mL<br>With Vaqta, the adult formulation contains 50 units/mL; the pediatric formulation contains 25 units/0.5 mL | *Adults:* Havrix, IM in deltoid, 1440 units initially and 6–12 mo later (total of 2 doses)<br>Vaqta, IM in deltoid, 50 units initially and 6–12 mo later (total of 2 doses)<br>*Children:* Havrix, 2–18 y, IM, 360 units initially, 1 mo later, and 6–12 mo later (total of 3 doses) or 720 units initially and 6–12 mo later (total of 2 doses)<br>Vaqta, IM 25 units initially and 6–18 mo later (total of 2 doses) | Indicated for workers in daycare centers, laboratories, food-handling establishments; homosexual men; intravenous drug users; military personnel; travelers to areas where hepatitis A is endemic; community residents during an outbreak; people with chronic liver disease (eg, hepatitis B or C, cirrhosis) |

*(continued)*

**DRUG TABLE 34-1**

*Drugs at a Glance*

## Vaccines and Toxoids for Active Acquired Immunity (Continued)

| Generic/Trade Name | Characteristics | Routes and Dosage Ranges | Comments/Uses |
|---|---|---|---|
| **Hepatitis B vaccine (recombinant)** (Recombivax HB, Engerix-B) Pregnancy Category C | Prepared by inserting the gene coding for production of HBsAg into yeast cells Contains no blood or blood products Approximately 96% effective in children and young adults; approximately 88% effective in adults >40 y Duration of protection unknown; can measure serum antibody levels periodically (protective levels approximately 10 million units/mL) | *Adults:* 20 y and older: Engerix, IM, 20 mcg (1 mL) initially and 1 mo and 6 mo later (3 doses) Predialysis and dialysis clients: IM, 40 mcg (2 mL) initially and 1, 2, and 6 mo later (4 doses) Recombivax: IM, 10 mcg (1 mL) initially and 1 mo and 6 mo later (3 doses) Predialysis and dialysis clients: IM, 40 mcg (1 mL) initially and 1 mo and 6 mo later (3 doses) *Children:* Neonates to 19 y: Engerix: IM, 10 mcg (0.5 mL), initially and 1 mo and 6 mo later (3 doses) Neonates to 19 y: Recombivax: IM, 5 mcg (0.5 mL) initially and 1 mo and 6 mo later (3 doses) Alternative for ages 11–15 y: IM, 10 mcg (1 mL) initially and at 4–6 mo (2 doses) | Indicated for preexposure immunization of high-risk groups, such as health care providers (nurses, physicians, dentists, laboratory workers); clients with cancer, organ transplants, hemodialysis, immunosuppressant drug therapy, or multiple infusions of blood or blood products; male homosexuals; intravenous drug abusers; household contacts of HBV carriers; residents and staff of institutions for mentally handicapped people Persons requiring postexposure vaccine include infants born to carrier mothers, people with accidental exposure of skin or mucous membrane to infected blood (eg, needle-stick injuries), and household contacts or sexual partners of persons with acute hepatitis B infection |
| **Hepatitis A, inactivated** and **hepatitis B, recombinant** (Twinrix) Pregnancy Category C | Contains 720 units of hepatitis A and 20 mcg of hepatitis B antigens per mL | IM, 1 mL initially, 1 and 6 mo later (total of 3 doses) | Used with adults exposed to hepatitis A or B (eg, medical personnel, staff in institutional settings such as daycare centers, prisons) Adults at risk for exposure, including travelers to areas of high incidence; people with chronic liver disease; laboratory workers, police, emergency medical personnel, sanitation workers |
| **Influenza vaccine** (Fluzone, FluShield, Fluvirin, FluMist) Pregnancy Category C | Inactivated strains of A and B influenza viruses, reformulated annually to include current strains Provides protective antibody concentrations for about 6 mo Grown in chick embryos; therefore, contraindicated in clients who are highly allergic to eggs | *Adults:* IM, 0.5 mL in a single dose *Children:* <3 y, IM 0.25 mL, 1 dose if previously vaccinated; 2 doses at least 1 mo apart if first vaccination 3–8 y, IM 0.5 mL, 1 dose if previously vaccinated; 2 doses at least 1 mo apart if first vaccination 9 y and older: IM, 0.5 mL in a single dose | Recommended annually for health care providers; all adults >65 y; and people in chronic care facilities or chronically ill with pulmonary, cardiovascular, or renal disorders, diabetes mellitus, or adrenocortical insufficiency Also recommended for pregnant women in their second or third trimester |

*(continued)*

**DRUG TABLE 34-1**

*Drugs at a Glance*

## Vaccines and Toxoids for Active Acquired Immunity (Continued)

| Generic/Trade Name | Characteristics | Routes and Dosage Ranges | Comments/Uses |
|---|---|---|---|
| | | Intranasal (FluMist):<br>*Adults:* 0.5 mL/dose (1 dose per season)<br>*Children:* >9 y: refer to adult dose<br>5–8 y previously not vaccinated with influenza vaccine: 0.5 mL/dose (2 doses per season given 60 d apart)<br>5–8 y, previously vaccinated with influenza vaccine: 0.5 mL/dose (1 dose per season) | Safety and efficacy of intranasal administration has not been established in children <5 y or adults ≥50 y |
| **Measles vaccine** (Attenuvax)<br>Pregnancy Category X | Preparation of live, attenuated measles (rubeola) virus<br>Protects approximately 95% of recipients for several years or lifetime<br>Usually given with mumps and rubella vaccines. A combination product containing all three antigens is available and preferred<br>Measles vaccine should not be given for 3 mo after administration of immune serum globulin, plasma, or whole blood | *Adults and children:* Sub-Q, 0.5 mL in a single dose | For routine immunization of children up to 1 y of age<br>Immunization of adults not previously immunized<br>Adults born before 1957 are generally considered immune. However, birth before 1957 is not acceptable evidence of immunity for women who could become pregnant |
| **Measles and rubella vaccine** (M-R-Vax II)<br>Pregnancy Category C | Mixture of live attenuated rubeola virus (Attenuvax) and rubella (German measles) virus | *Children:* Sub-Q, total volume of reconstituted vial | For immunization of 15-mo-old children against rubeola and rubella |
| **Measles, mumps, and rubella vaccine** (M-M-R II)<br>Pregnancy Category C | Mixture of rubeola, rubella, and mumps vaccines<br>Preferred over single immunizing agents | *Children:* Sub-Q, 0.5 mL | For immunization from age 15 mo to puberty |
| **Meningococcal polysaccharide vaccine** (Menomune-A/C Menomune-A/C/Y/W-135)<br>Pregnancy Category C | Suspension prepared from *Neisseria meningitidis*<br>Protective levels of antibody usually achieved 7–10 d after immunization | *Adults and children:* Sub-Q, 0.5 mL | Used for immunization of people at risk in epidemic or endemic areas<br>Type A only should be given to infants and children <2 y |
| **Mumps virus vaccine** (Mumpsvax)<br>Pregnancy Category X | Suspension of live, attenuated mumps virus<br>Provides immunity in about 97% of children and 93% of adults for at least 10 y<br>Most often given in combination with measles and rubella vaccines | *Adults:* Sub-Q, 0.5 mL in a single dose (reconstituted vaccine retains potency for 8 h if refrigerated; discard if not used within 8 h)<br>*Children:* >1 y, same as adults (vaccination not indicated in children <1 y) | For routine immunization of children 1 y and adults; adults born before 1957 are generally considered immune and need not be vaccinated<br>Trivalent measles-mumps-rubella vaccine is the preferred agent |

*(continued)*

## DRUG TABLE 34-1

*Drugs at a Glance*

## Vaccines and Toxoids for Active Acquired Immunity (Continued)

| Generic/Trade Name | Characteristics | Routes and Dosage Ranges | Comments/Uses |
|---|---|---|---|
| **Pneumococcal vaccine, polyvalent** (Pneumovax 23, Pnu-Imune 23) Pregnancy Category C | Consists of 23 strains of pneumococci, which cause approximately 85%–90% of the serious pneumococcal infections in the United States Protection begins about 3 wk after vaccination and lasts years Not recommended for children <2 y because they may be unable to produce adequate antibody levels | *Adults and children:* Sub-Q, IM, 0.5 mL as a single dose | For adults with chronic disorders associated with increased risk for pneumococcal infection (eg, cardiovascular or pulmonary disease, diabetes mellitus, Hodgkin's disease, multiple myeloma, cirrhosis, alcohol dependence, renal failure, immunosuppression) Adults 65 y and older who are otherwise healthy Children 2 y and older with chronic disease associated with increased risk for pneumococcal infection (eg, asplenia, nephrotic syndrome, immunosuppression) |
| **Pneumococcal 7-valent conjugate vaccine** (Prevnar) Pregnancy Category C | Contains 7 *Streptococcus pneumoniae* antigens conjugated to a protein to increase antigenicity | *Children:* Birth–6 mo: IM, 0.5 mL at 2, 4, and 6 mo and at 12–15 mo (4 doses) 7–11 mo: IM, 0.5 mL initially, at least 4 wk later, and after 1 y birthday (3 doses) 12–23 mo: IM, 0.5 mL initially and at least 2 mo later (2 doses) 24 mo–9 y: IM, 0.5 mL in a single dose | Active immunization to prevent invasive pneumococcal infections in young children |
| **Poliomyelitis vaccine, inactivated (IPV)** (IPOL) Pregnancy Category C | A suspension of inactivated poliovirus types I, II, and III | *Adults:* Sub-Q, 0.5 mL monthly for 2 doses, then a third dose 6–12 mo later *Children:* Sub-Q, 0.5 mL at 2, 4, 6–18 mo, and 4–6 y of age (4 doses) or at 2 and 4 mo (2 doses) | Routine immunization of infants Immunization of adults not previous immunized and at risk for exposure (eg, health care or laboratory workers) |
| **Rabies vaccine (human diploid cell rabies vaccine [HDCV])** (Imovax) Pregnancy Category C | An inactivated virus vaccine Immunity develops in 7–10 d and lasts 1 y or longer | *Adults and children:* Preexposure prophylaxis: IM, 1.0 mL for 3 doses. The second dose is given 1 wk after the first; the third dose is given 3–4 wk after the first. Then, booster doses (1 mL) every 2–5 y based on antibody titers Postexposure: IM, 1 mL for 5 doses. After the initial dose, other doses are given 3, 7, 14, and 28 d later. Rabies immunoglobulin is administered at the same time as the initial dose of HDCV vaccine | Preexposure immunization in people at high risk for exposure (veterinarians, animal handlers, laboratory personnel who work with rabies virus) Postexposure prophylaxis in people who have been bitten by potentially rabid animals or who have skin scratches or abrasions exposed to animal saliva (eg, animal licking of wound), urine, or blood *(continued)* |

**DRUG TABLE
34-1**

*Drugs at a Glance*

## Vaccines and Toxoids for Active Acquired Immunity (Continued)

| Generic/Trade Name | Characteristics | Routes and Dosage Ranges | Comments/Uses |
|---|---|---|---|
| **Rubella vaccine** (Meruvax II) Pregnancy Category C | Sterile suspension of live, attenuated rubella virus Protects about 95% of recipients at least 15 y, probably for lifetime Should not be given for 3 mo after receiving immune serum globulin, plasma, or whole blood Usually given with measles and mumps vaccines | *Adults and children:* Sub-Q, 0.5 mL in a single dose | Routine immunization of children 1 y and older Initial or repeat immunization of adolescent girls or women of childbearing age *if* serum antibody levels are low |
| **Tuberculosis vaccine** (bacillus Calmette-Guérin) (TICE BCG) Pregnancy Category C | Suspension of attenuated tubercle bacilli Converts negative tuberculin reactors to positive reactors. Therefore, precludes use of the tuberculin skin test for screening or early diagnosis of tuberculosis Contraindicated in clients with impaired immune responses | *Adults:* Percutaneous, by multiple puncture disk, 0.2–0.3 mL *Children:* Newborns, percutaneous, by multiple puncture disk, 0.1 mL >1 mo, same as adults | For use in people at high risk for exposure, including newborns of women with tuberculosis |
| **Typhoid vaccine** (Vivotif Berna, Typhim Vi) Pregnancy Category C | Suspension of attenuated or killed typhoid bacilli Protects >70% of recipients | *Adults:* Sub-Q, 0.5 mL for two doses at least 4 wk apart, then a booster dose of 0.5 mL (or 0.1 mL intradermal) at least every 3 y for repeated or continued exposure PO, 1 capsule every other day for four doses; repeat every 4 y as a booster dose with repeated or continued exposure *Children:* >10 y, Sub-Q, 0.5 mL for two doses at least 4 wk apart, then a booster dose of 0.5 mL at least every 3 y for repeated or continued exposure Age 6 mo–10 y: Sub-Q, 0.25 mL for two doses, at least 4 wk apart, then a booster dose of 0.25 mL (or 0.1 mL intradermal) every 3 y if indicated >6 y: PO, same as adults | For high-risk people (household contacts of typhoid carriers or people whose occupation or travel predisposes to exposure) |

*(continued)*

**DRUG TABLE 34-1**

*Drugs at a Glance*

## Vaccines and Toxoids for Active Acquired Immunity (Continued)

| Generic/Trade Name | Characteristics | Routes and Dosage Ranges | Comments/Uses |
|---|---|---|---|
| **Varicella virus vaccine** (Varivax) Pregnancy Category C | Contains live, attenuated varicella virus Contraindicated in people with hematologic or lymphatic malignancy, immunosuppression, febrile illness, or pregnancy | *Adults:* Sub-Q, 0.5 mL, followed by a second dose of 0.5 mL 4–8 wk after the first dose *Children:* 1–12 y: Sub-Q, 0.5 mL in a single dose *Adolescents:* 13 y and older: Sub-Q, 0.5 mL, followed by a second dose of 0.5 mL 4–8 wk after the first dose | Immunization of children 12 mo and older Immunization of adults |
| **Yellow fever vaccine** (YF-Vax) Pregnancy Category D | Suspension of live, attenuated yellow fever virus Protects about 95% of recipients for 10 y or longer | *Adults:* Sub-Q, 0.5 mL; booster dose of 0.5 mL every 10 y if in endemic areas *Children:* >6 mo: Sub-Q, same as adults | For laboratory personnel at risk for exposure Travel to endemic areas (Africa, South America) |
| ***Toxoids*** | | | |
| **Diphtheria and tetanus toxoids and acellular pertussis vaccine (DTaP)** (Tripedia, Certiva, Infanrix) Pregnancy Category C | The pertussis component is acellular bacterial particles, which decrease the adverse effects associated with the whole-cell vaccine used formerly | *Children:* IM, 0.5 mL at approximately 18 mo of age; repeat at 4–6 y of age | Active immunization of children aged 6 wk to 7 y |
| **Diphtheria and tetanus toxoids and acellular pertussis and *Haemophilus influenzae* type B conjugate vaccines (DTaP-HIB)** (TriHIBit) Pregnancy Category C | A combination product, to decrease the number of injections and increase compliance | *Children:* IM, 0.5 mL within 30 min or less after reconstitution | Active immunization of children 15–18 mo of age who have been previously immunized against diphtheria, tetanus, and pertussis |
| **Diphtheria and tetanus toxoids and acellular pertussis (DtaP), hepatitis B (recombinant), and inactivated poliovirus vaccine** (Pediarix) Pregnancy Category C | A combination vaccine product, to decrease the number of injections (from 9 to 3) and increase compliance with comparable protection | *Children:* IM, 0.5 mL at approximately 2, 4, and 6 months of age | Promotes active immunity to diphtheria, tetanus, pertussis, hepatitis B, and poliovirus types 1, 2, and 3. |
| **Diphtheria and tetanus toxoids adsorbed (pediatric type)** Pregnancy Category C | Also called DT Contains a larger amount of diphtheria antigen than tetanus and diphtheria toxoids, adult type (Td) | *Infants and children:* 6 y and younger: IM, 0.5 mL for two doses at least 4 wk apart, followed by a reinforcing dose 1 y later and at the time the child starts school | Routine immunization of infants and children 6 y and younger in whom pertussis vaccine is contraindicated (ie, those who have adverse reactions to initial doses of DTP) |
| **Tetanus toxoid, adsorbed** Pregnancy Category C | Preparation of detoxified products of *Clostridium tetani* Protects about 100% of recipients for 10 y or more | *Adults:* Primary immunization in adults not previously immunized: IM, 0.5 mL for 3 doses, initially, 4–8 wk later, then at 6–12 mo | Routine immunization of infants and young children Primary immunization of adults |

*(continued)*

| DRUG TABLE 34-1 | *Drugs at a Glance* |
|---|---|

## Vaccines and Toxoids for Active Acquired Immunity (Continued)

| Generic/Trade Name | Characteristics | Routes and Dosage Ranges | Comments/Uses |
|---|---|---|---|
| | Usually given in combination (eg, DTaP or DT) for primary immunization of infants and children 6 y of age or older<br>Usually given alone or combined with diphtheria toxoid (Td adult type) for primary immunization of adults | Then, 0.5 mL booster dose every 10 y<br>Prophylaxis: IM, 0.5 mL if wound severely contaminated and no booster dose received for 5 y; 0.5 mL if wound clean and no booster dose received for 10 y<br>*Children:* Primary immunization and prophylaxis, same as adults | Prevention of tetanus in previously immunized people who sustain a potentially contaminated wound |
| **Tetanus and diphtheria toxoids, adsorbed (adult type)**<br>Pregnancy Category C | Also called Td<br>Contains a smaller amount of diphtheria antigen than diphtheria and tetanus toxoids, pediatric type | IM, 0.5 mL for two doses, at least 4 wk apart, followed by a reinforcing dose 6–12 mo later and every 10 y thereafter<br>*Children:* >6 y: same as adults | Primary immunization or booster doses in adults and children >6 y of age |

| DRUG TABLE 34-2 | *Drugs at a Glance* |
|---|---|

## Immune Serums for Passive Acquired Immunity

| Generic/Trade Name | Characteristics | Routes and Dosage Ranges | Comments/Uses |
|---|---|---|---|
| **Cytomegalovirus immune globulin, IV, human (CMV-IGIV)** (CytoGam)<br>Pregnancy Category C | Contains antibodies against CMV | Posttransplantation: IV infusion, 150 mg/kg within 72 h, then 100–150 mg/kg at 2, 4, 6, and 8 wk, then 50–100 mg/kg at 12 and 16 wk | Treat CMV infection in renal, liver, and bone marrow transplant recipients |
| **Hepatitis B immune globulin, human** (H-BIG, BayHep B, Nabi-HB)<br>Pregnancy Category C | A solution of immunoglobulins that contains antibodies to HBsAg | *Adults and children:* IM, 0.06 mL/kg (usual adult dose is 3–5 mL) as soon as possible after exposure, preferably within 7 d. Repeat dose in 1 mo | To prevent hepatitis after exposure. Neonates born to HBsAg positive or unknown status mothers are given HBIG and the first dose of hepatitis B vaccine within 12 h of birth |
| **Immune globulin, human (IG; IGIM)** (BayGam)<br>Pregnancy Category C | Given IM only<br>Commonly called gamma globulin<br>Obtained from pooled plasma of normal donors<br>Consists primarily of IgG, which contains concentrated antibodies<br>Produces adequate serum levels of IgG in 2–5 d | *Adults and children:* Exposure to hepatitis A: IM, 0.02 mL/kg<br>Exposure to measles: IM, 0.25 mL/kg given within 6 d of exposure<br>Exposure to varicella: IM, 0.6–1.2 mL/kg<br>Exposure to rubella (pregnant women only): IM, 0.55 mL/kg<br>Immunoglobulin deficiency: IM, 1.3 mL/kg initially, then 0.6 mL/kg every 3–4 wk<br>Bacterial infections: IM, 0.5–3.5 mL/kg | To decrease the severity of hepatitis A, measles, and varicella after exposure<br>To treat immunoglobulin deficiency<br>Adjunct to antibiotics in severe bacterial infections and burns<br>To lessen possibility of fetal damage in pregnant women exposed to rubella virus (however, routine use in early pregnancy is not recommended) |

*(continued)*

**DRUG TABLE 34-2**

*Drugs at a Glance*

## Immune Serums for Passive Acquired Immunity (Continued)

| Generic/Trade Name | Characteristics | Routes and Dosage Ranges | Comments/Uses |
|---|---|---|---|
| **Immune globulin IV** (IGIV) (Gamimune N, Gammagard, Gammar-P IV, Iveegam, Polygam S/D, Panglobulin, Sandoglobulin, Venoglobulin-S) Pregnancy Category C | Given IV only Provides immediate antibodies Half-life about 3 wk Mechanism of action in idiopathic thrombocytopenic purpura (ITP) unknown **Warning:** IGIV products have been associated with renal dysfunction and failure and death. They should be used cautiously in clients with or at risk for developing renal impairment | Gamimune: IV, infusion, 100–200 mg/kg once a month May be given more often or increased to 400 mg/kg if clinical response or serum level of IgG is insufficient ITP: IV infusion, 400 mg/kg daily for 5 consecutive days Sandoglobulin: IV infusion, 200 mg/kg once a month. May be given more often or increased to 300 mg/kg if clinical response or level of IgG is inadequate. ITP: IV infusion, 400 mg/kg daily for 5 consecutive days Other products, see manufacturers' literature | Immunodeficiency syndrome ITP |
| **Rabies immune globulin,** human (BayRab, Imogam) Pregnancy Category C | Gamma globulin obtained from plasma of people hyperimmunized with rabies vaccine Not useful in treatment of clinical rabies infection | *Adults and children:* IM, 20 units/kg (half the dose may be infiltrated around the wound) as soon as possible after possible exposure (eg, animal bite) | Postexposure prevention of rabies, in conjunction with rabies vaccine |
| **Respiratory syncytial virus (RSV) immune globulin** IV, human (RSV-IGIV) (RespiGam) Pregnancy Category C | Reduces severity of RSV illness and the incidence and duration of hospitalization in high-risk infants May cause fluid overload Not established as safe and effective in children with congenital heart disease | *Children:* IV infusion via infusion pump, 1.5 mL/kg/h for 15 min, then 3 mL/kg/h for 15 min, then 6 mL/kg/h until the infusion is completed, then once monthly, if tolerated Maximum monthly dose, 750 mg/kg | Prevention of serious RSV infections in high-risk children <2 y (ie, those with bronchopulmonary dysplasia or history of premature birth [gestation of 35 wk or less]) Treatment of RSV lower respiratory tract infections in hospitalized infants and young children |
| **Rh₀(D) immune globulin,** human (Gamulin Rh, HypRho-D, RhoGAM) Pregnancy Category C | Prepared from fractionated human plasma A sterile concentrated solution of specific immunoglobulin (IgG) containing anti-Rh₀(D) | Obstetric use: Inject contents of 1 vial IM for every 15 mL fetal packed red cell volume within 72 h after delivery, miscarriage, or abortion Consult package instructions for blood typing and drug administration procedures. | To prevent sensitization in a subsequent pregnancy to the Rh₀(D) factor in an Rh-negative mother who has given birth to an Rh-positive infant by an Rh-positive father Also available in microdose form (MICRhoGAM) for the prevention of maternal Rh immunization after abortion or miscarriage up to 12 wk gestation |

*(continued)*

**DRUG TABLE 34-2**

*Drugs at a Glance*

## Immune Serums for Passive Acquired Immunity (Continued)

| Generic/Trade Name | Characteristics | Routes and Dosage Ranges | Comments/Uses |
|---|---|---|---|
| **Tetanus immune globulin,** human (Hyper-Tet) Pregnancy Category C | Solution of globulins from plasma of people hyper-immunized with tetanus toxoid Tetanus toxoid (Td) should also be given to initiate active immunization if minor wound and >10 y since Td, if major wound and >5 y since Td, or if Td primary immunization series was incomplete | *Adults and children:* Prophylaxis: IM, 250 units as a single dose Treatment of clinical disease: IM, 3000–6000 units in a single dose | To prevent tetanus in clients with wounds possibly contaminated with *Clostridium tetani* and whose immunization history is uncertain or incomplete Treatment of tetanus infection |
| **Varicella-zoster immune globulin,** human (VZIG) (Varicella-zoster immune globulin) Pregnancy Category C | The globulin fraction of human plasma Antibodies last 1 mo or longer | IM, 125 units/10 kg up to a maximum of 625 units within 48 h after exposure if possible; may be given up to 96 h after exposure. Minimal dose, 125 units | Postexposure to chickenpox or shingles, to prevent or decrease severity of infections in children <15 y of age who have not been immunized or who are immunodeficient because of illness or drug therapy Infants born to mothers who develop varicella 5 d before or 2 d after delivery and premature infants <28 wk gestation |

CMV, cytomegalovirus; IgG, immunoglobulin G; RSV, respiratory syncytial virus; HBsAg, hepatitis B surface antigen

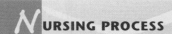

# NURSING PROCESS

## Assessment

Assess the client's immunization status by obtaining the following information:

- Determine the client's previous history of diseases for which immunizing agents are available (eg, measles, influenza).
- Ask if the client has had previous immunizations.
  - For which diseases were immunizations received?
  - Which immunizing agent was received?
  - Were any adverse effects experienced? If so, what symptoms occurred, and how long did they last?
  - Was tetanus toxoid given for any cuts or wounds?
  - Did any foreign travel require immunizations?
- Determine whether the client has any conditions that contraindicate administration of immunizing agents (eg, malignancy, pregnancy, immunosuppressive drug therapy).
- For pregnant women not known to be immunized against rubella, serum antibody titer should be measured to determine resistance or susceptibility to the disease.
- For clients with wounds, assess the type of wound and determine how, when, and where it was sustained. Such information may reveal whether tetanus immunization is needed.

- For clients exposed to infectious diseases, try to determine the extent of exposure (eg, household or brief, casual contact) and when it occurred.

## Nursing Diagnoses

- Deficient Knowledge: Importance of maintaining immunizations for both children and adults
- Risk for Fluid Volume Deficit related to inadequate intake and febrile reactions to immunizing agent
- Noncompliance in obtaining recommended immunizations related to fear of adverse effects
- Risk for Injury related to hypersensitivity, fever, and other adverse drug effects

## Planning/Goals

*The client will:*

- Avoid diseases for which immunizations are available and recommended
- Obtain recommended immunizations for children and self
- Keep appointments for immunizations

*(continued)*

## NURSING PROCESS (Continued)

### Interventions

Use measures to prevent infectious diseases, and provide information about the availability of immunizing agents. General measures include those to promote health and resistance to disease (eg, nutrition, rest, and exercise). Additional measures include the following:

- Education of the public, especially parents of young children, regarding the importance of immunizations to personal and public health. Include information about the diseases that can be prevented and where immunizations can be obtained.
- Assisting clients in developing a system to maintain immunization records for themselves and their children. This is important because immunizations are often obtained at different places and over a period of years. Written, accurate, up-to-date records help to prevent diseases and unnecessary immunizations.
- Prevention of disease transmission. The following are helpful measures:
  - Handwashing (probably the most effective method)
  - Avoiding contact with people who have known or suspected infectious diseases, when possible
  - Using isolation techniques when appropriate
  - Using medical and surgical aseptic techniques
- For someone exposed to rubeola, administration of measles vaccine within 48 hours to prevent the disease

- For someone with a puncture wound or a dirty wound, administration of tetanus immune globulin to prevent tetanus, a life-threatening disease
- For someone with an animal bite, washing the wound immediately with large amounts of soap and water. Health care should then be sought. Administration of rabies vaccine may be needed to prevent rabies, a life-threatening disease.
- Explaining to the client that contracting rubella or undergoing rubella immunization during pregnancy, especially during the first trimester, may cause severe birth defects in the infant. The goal of immunization is to prevent congenital rubella syndrome. Current recommendations are to immunize children against rubella at 12 to 15 months of age.

  It is recommended that previously unimmunized girls 11 to 13 years of age be immunized. Further, nonpregnant women of childbearing age should have rubella antibody tests. If antibody concentrations are low, the women should be immunized. Pregnancy should be avoided for 3 months after immunization.

### Evaluation

- Interview and observe for symptoms.
- Interview and observe for adverse drug effects.
- Check immunization records when indicated.

---

46.4°F); some (eg, MMR) require protection from light. Manufacturers' instructions for storage should be strictly followed.

## Vaccine Shortages

During 2000 to 2002, approximately, shortages of several vaccines occurred. Some shortages were localized; some were widespread. These shortages interrupted the recommended schedules for many immunizations, especially those for routine immunizations of children. Long-term consequences of altered immunization schedules are largely unknown.

During the shortages, public health officials regularly issued updates on availability and priorities for use among at-risk populations. One postulated reason for the shortages was the withdrawal of some manufacturers from vaccine production, probably because of relatively low profits and difficulties in complying with FDA regulations for manufacturing them. For example, a regulation requiring removal of thiomersal, a mercury-based preservative, resulted in the need for single-dose vials rather than multiple-dose vials and a smaller amount of marketable product from the same amount of vaccine. Mercury is toxic to humans, especially to infants. Also, preparations from previous seasons cannot be used, since each year the formulation is standardized according to the

U.S. Public Health Service. The introduction of intranasal influenza vaccine during the 2003–2004 influenza season increased the number of healthy individuals between the ages of 5 and 49 who were immunized.

## Use Throughout the Lifespan

Routine immunization of children has greatly reduced the prevalence of many common childhood diseases. However, many children are not being immunized appropriately, and diseases for which vaccines are available still occur. Standards of practice, aimed toward increasing immunizations, have been established and are supported by most pediatric provider groups (Box 34-1).

Guidelines for children whose immunizations begin in early infancy are given in Age-related Considerations. Different schedules are recommended for children 1 to 5 years of age and for those older than 6 years of age who are being immunized for the first time.

Adolescents who received all primary immunizations as infants and young children should have hepatitis B vaccine (if not received earlier) and a tetanus-diphtheria booster (adult type) at 14 to 16 years of age and every 10 years thereafter. Young adults who are health care workers, are sexually active, or belong to high-risk groups should have hepatitis B vaccine if not previously received; a tetanus-diphtheria booster every 10 years; MMR if not pregnant

## BOX 34-1  Standards for Pediatric Immunization Practices

The following standards are recommended for use by all health professionals in the public and private sector who administer vaccines to or manage immunization services for infants and children.

Standard 1: Immunization services are readily available.

Standard 2: There are no barriers or unnecessary prerequisites to the receipt of vaccines.

Standard 3: Immunization services are available free or for a minimal fee.

Standard 4: Providers use all clinical encounters to screen and, when indicated, immunize children.

Standard 5: Providers educate parents and guardians about pediatric immunizations in general terms.

Standard 6: Providers question parents or guardians about contraindications and, before immunizing a child, inform them in specific terms about the risks and benefits of the immunizations their child is to receive.

Standard 7: Providers follow only true contraindications.

Standard 8: Providers administer simultaneously all vaccine doses for which a child is eligible at the time of each visit.

Standard 9: Providers use accurate and complete recording procedures.

Standard 10: Providers coschedule immunization appointments in conjunction with appointments for other child health services.

Standard 11: Providers report adverse events after immunization promptly, accurately, and completely.

Standard 12: Providers operate a tracking system.

Standard 13: Providers adhere to appropriate procedures for vaccine management.

Standard 14: Providers conduct semiannual audits to assess immunization coverage levels and to review immunization records in the patient population they serve.

Standard 15: Providers maintain up-to-date, easily retrievable medical protocols at all locations where vaccines are administered.

Standard 16: Providers operate with patient-oriented and community-based approaches.

Standard 17: Vaccines are administered by properly trained individuals.

Standard 18: Providers receive ongoing education and training on current immunization recommendations.

---

and rubella titer is inadequate or proof of immunization is unavailable; and varicella. In addition, young adults who are health care providers should have influenza vaccine annually.

Middle-aged adults should maintain immunizations against tetanus; high-risk groups (eg, those with chronic illness) and health care providers should receive hepatitis B once (if not previously taken) and influenza vaccine annually. Age-related Considerations also discusses immunizations in the older adult.

The nurse can play an important role by clinical assessment of individuals receiving immunizations, interviewing the family about immunization records, and ensuring compliance with the prescribed regimen. Guidelines for strategies for ongoing evaluation and intervention are addressed in Home Care Considerations.

## ■ DRUG USE IN SPECIFIC SITUATIONS

### Use in Immunosuppression

Compared with healthy, immunocompetent individuals, the antibody response to immunization is usually adequate but reduced in immunosuppressed persons. With hepatitis A and B vaccines, larger doses may be required. Also, with hepatitis B vaccine, antibody concentrations should be measured and booster doses given if antibody concentrations fall.

Live bacterial (bacille Calmette-Guérin, oral typhoid) or viral (MMR, varicella, yellow fever) vaccines should generally not be given to people with human immunodeficiency virus (HIV) infection, other immune diseases, or impaired immune systems due to leukemia, lymphoma, systemic corticosteroid or anticancer drugs, or radiation therapy. The bacteria or viruses may be able to reproduce and cause active infection in these people. Persons with asymptomatic HIV infection should receive inactivated vaccines. If an immunosuppressed person is exposed to measles or varicella, immune globulin or varicella-zoster immune globulin may be given for passive immunization.

For children with HIV infection, the AAP and ACIP recommend administration of most routine immunizations (DTaP, IPV, MMR, Hib) regardless of symptoms and administration of influenza and pneumococcal vaccines if symptomatic. Varicella vaccine is not recommended.

### Use in Cancer

For clients with active malignant disease, live vaccines should not be given. Although killed vaccines and toxoids may be given, antibody production may be inadequate to provide immunity. When possible, clients should receive needed immunizations 2 weeks before or 3 months after immunosuppressive radiation or chemotherapy treatments. For example, clients with Hodgkin's lymphoma who are more than 2 years old should be immunized with pneumococcal and Hib vaccines 10 to 14 days before therapy is started. In addition, clients who have not received chemotherapy for 3 to 4 weeks may have an adequate antibody response to influenza vaccine.

## Age-related Considerations: Use of Immunizing Agents

### USE IN CHILDREN

Current recommendations for use of immunizing agents in children include:

1. Hepatitis B vaccine to all newborns with a second dose 4 weeks after the first dose, a third dose at least 8 weeks after the third dose or 16 weeks after the first dose. The last dose in the series (third or fourth dose) should not be given before 6 months of age. This schedule is for monovalent vaccine (hepatitis B vaccine only) and infants whose mothers were negative for hepatitis B surface antigen (HBsAg). If a combined hepatitis B, *Haemophilus influenzae* B vaccine is used (eg, the combination can be used for all but the first dose in newborns), the second dose should not be given before 6 weeks of age. Also, if the mother's HBsAg status is positive or unknown, newborns should be given hepatitis B vaccine within 12 hours of birth, along with a dose of hepatitis B immune globulin (HBIG).

   The annual Recommended Childhood Immunization Schedule of the American Academy of Pediatrics (AAP), the CDC Advisory Committee on Immunization Practices (ACIP), and the American Academy of Family Physicians (AAFP) is issued in January of each year. The 2002 schedule (*Pediatrics, 109*(1), 162) places more emphasis on giving hepatitis B vaccine to all infants before hospital discharge to "1) safeguard against maternal hepatitis B testing errors and test reporting failures; 2) protect neonates discharged to households in which hepatitis B chronic carriers other than the mother may reside; and 3) enhance the completion of the childhood immunization series."

2. DTaP (diphtheria and tetanus toxoids, acellular pertussis vaccine) at 2 months, 4 months, 6 months, 15 to 18 months, and 4 to 6 years of age.

3. *Haemophilus influenzae* type b vaccine (Hib) at 2, 4, 6, and 12 to 15 months of age. There are three Hib conjugate vaccines approved for use in infants. If PedvaxHIB or Comvax is given at 2 and 4 months of age, a dose at 6 months is not needed. DTaP/Hib combination products should not be used for primary immunization at 2, 4, or 6 months but can be used as boosters after any Hib vaccine.

4. Inactivated polio vaccine (IPV) injection at 2 and 4 months of age, at 6 to 18 months, and at 4 to 6 years of age. Oral polio vaccine (OPV) is no longer recommended for use in the United States.

5. MMR at 12 to 15 months of age, as a combined vaccine. These vaccines are given later than DTaP and IPV because sufficient antibodies may not be produced until passive immunity acquired from the mother dissipates (at 12 to 15 months of age).

6. Pneumococcal 7-valent conjugate vaccine (Prevnar) to all children at 2 to 23 months of age and pneumococcal polyvalent vaccine (Pneumovax 23 or Pnu-Imune 23) for children 2 years and older with chronic illnesses that increase their risk for developing serious pneumococcal infections.

7. Varicella at 12 to 18 months and again at approximately 12 years of age.

8. For children with chronic illnesses such as asthma, heart disease, diabetes, and others, influenza vaccine is recommended annually after 6 months of age.

9. For children with human immunodeficiency virus (HIV) infection, live viral and bacterial vaccines (MMR, varicella, bacillus Calmette-Guérin) are contraindicated because they may cause the disease rather than prevent it. However, immunizations with DTaP, IPV, and Hib are recommended even though they may be less effective than in children with competent immune systems. Also recommended is annual administration of influenza vaccine for children older than 6 months of age and one-time administration of pneumococcal vaccine for children older than 2 years of age.

### USE IN OLDER ADULTS

Annual influenza vaccine and one-time administration of pneumococcal vaccine at 65 years of age are recommended for healthy older adults and those with chronic respiratory, cardiovascular, and other diseases. As with younger adults, immunization for most other diseases is recommended for older adults at high risk for exposure.

---

## Home Care Considerations: Use of Immunizing Agents

***ASSESS:*** knowledge of immunization recommendations; the immunization record to evaluate immunization status; and need for additional information and provide that information.

***MONITOR:*** for compliance with the prescribed regimen, and for therapeutic and adverse drug effects.

***EDUCATE:*** regarding importance of immunization schedule and completing series as indicated; managing fever and pain, induration, and erythema at injection sites and importance of reporting severe or persistent reactions promptly. Stress the importance of women using effective contraception for 3 months following rubella immunizations to prevent rubella-induced abnormalities in the fetus. Reinforce additional teaching points (see Client Teaching Guidelines: Immunizations).

## CLIENT TEACHING GUIDELINES
### Immunizations

✔ Appropriate vaccinations should be maintained for adults as well as for children. Consult a health care provider periodically because recommendations and personal needs change fairly often.

✔ Maintain immunization records for yourself and your children. This is important because immunizations are often obtained at different places and over a period of years. Written, accurate, up-to-date records help to prevent diseases and unnecessary immunizations.

✔ If a physician recommends an immunization and you do not know whether you have had the immunization or the disease, it is probably safer to take the immunization than to risk having the disease. Immunization after a previous immunization or after having the disease usually is not harmful.

✔ To avoid rubella-induced abnormalities in fetal development, women of childbearing age who receive a rubella immunization must avoid becoming pregnant (ie, must use effective contraceptive methods) for 3 months.

✔ Women of childbearing age who receive a varicella immunization must avoid becoming pregnant (ie, must use effective contraceptive methods) for 3 months.

✔ Most vaccines cause fever and soreness at the site of injection. Acetaminophen (Tylenol) can be taken two to three times daily for 24 to 48 hours (by adults and children) to decrease fever and discomfort.

✔ After receiving varicella vaccine (to prevent chickenpox), avoid close contact with newborns, pregnant women, and anyone whose immune system is impaired. Also, use effective methods of contraception to avoid pregnancy for at least 3 months after immunization. Vaccinated people may transmit the vaccine virus to susceptible close contacts. Effects of the vaccine on the fetus are unknown, but fetal harm has occurred with natural varicella infection during pregnancy.

✔ After receiving a vaccine, stay in the area for approximately 30 minutes. If an allergic reaction is going to occur, it will usually do so within that time.

## Nursing Actions
### Immunizing Agents

| Nursing Actions | Rationale/Explanation |
|---|---|
| **1. Administer accurately.** | |
| a. Read the package insert, and check the expiration date on all biologic products (eg, vaccines, toxoids, and human immune serums). | Concentration, dosage, and administration of biologic products often vary with the products. Fresh products are preferred; avoid administration of expired products. Also, use reconstituted products within designated time limits because they are usually stable for only a few hours. |
| b. Check the child's temperature before giving diphtheria, tetanus, and pertussis (DTP) vaccine. | If the temperature is elevated, do not give the vaccine. |
| c. Give DTP in the lateral thigh muscle of the infant. | The vastus lateralis is the largest skeletal muscle mass in the infant and the preferred site for all intramuscular (IM) injections. |
| d. With measles, mumps, rubella (MMR) vaccine, use only the diluent provided by the manufacturer, and administer the vaccine subcutaneously (Sub-Q) within 8 h after reconstitution. | The reconstituted preparation is stable for approximately 8 h. If not used within 8 h, discard the solution. |
| e. Give hepatitis B vaccine IM in the anterolateral thigh of infants and young children and in the deltoid of older children and adults. Although the IM route is preferred, the drug can be given Sub-Q in people at high risk of bleeding from IM injections (eg, clients with hemophilia). | Higher blood levels of protective antibodies are produced when the vaccine is given in the thigh or deltoid than when it is given in the buttocks, probably because of injection into fatty tissue rather than gluteal muscles. |
| f. Give IM human immune serum globulin with an 18- to 20-gauge needle, preferably in gluteal muscles. If the dose is 5 mL or more, divide it and inject it into two or more IM sites. Follow manufacturer's instruction for preparation and administration of IV formulations. | To promote absorption and minimize tissue irritation and other adverse reactions |
| g. Aspirate carefully before IM or Sub-Q injection of any immunizing agent. | To avoid inadvertent IV administration and greatly increased risks of severe adverse effects |

*(continued)*

## Nursing Actions

## Immunizing Agents (Continued)

| Nursing Actions | Rationale/Explanation |
|---|---|
| h. Have aqueous epinephrine 1:1000 readily available before administering any vaccine. | For immediate treatment of allergic reactions |
| i. After administration of an immunizing agent in a clinic or office setting, have the client stay in the area for at least 30 min. | To observe for allergic reactions, which usually occur within 30 min |
| 2. Observe for therapeutic effects.<br>a. Absence of diseases for which immunized<br>b. Decreased incidence and severity of symptoms when given to modify disease processes | |
| 3. Observe for adverse effects. | Most adverse effects are mild and transient. However, serious reactions occasionally occur. The risk of serious adverse effects from immunization is usually much smaller than the risk of the disease immunized against.<br>Adverse effects may be caused by the immunizing agent or by foreign protein incorporated with the immunizing agent (eg, egg protein in viral vaccines grown in chick embryos). |
| a. General reactions<br>(1) Pain, tenderness, redness at injection sites | Local tissue irritation may occur with injected immunizing agents. |
| (2) Fever, malaise, muscle aches | These adverse effects commonly occur with vaccines and toxoids. They rarely occur with human immune serums given for passive immunity. |
| (3) Anaphylaxis (cardiovascular collapse, shock, laryngeal edema, urticaria, angioneurotic edema, severe respiratory distress) | Anaphylaxis occasionally occurs with immunizing agents. It is a medical emergency that requires immediate treatment with SC epinephrine (0.5 mL for adults; 0.01 mL/kg for children). Anaphylaxis is most likely to occur within 30 min after immunizing agents are injected. |
| (4) Serum sickness (urticaria, fever, arthralgia, enlarged lymph nodes) | Serum sickness is a delayed hypersensitivity reaction that occurs several days or weeks after an injection of serum. Treatment is symptomatic. Symptoms are usually relieved by acetaminophen, antihistamines, and corticosteroids. |
| b. With DtaP<br>(1) Soreness, erythema, edema at injection sites<br>(2) Anorexia, nausea | These effects are common |
| (3) Severe fever, encephalopathy, seizures | These are rare adverse reactions and less likely to occur with the acellular pertussis component now used. If they occur, they are thought to be caused by the pertussis antigen, and further administration of pertussis vaccine or DTP may be contraindicated. |
| c. With *Haemophilus influenzae* b vaccine—pain and erythema at injection sites | These effects occur in about 25% of recipients but are usually mild and resolve within 24 hours. |
| d. With hepatitis B vaccine<br>(1) Injection site soreness, erythema, induration<br>(2) Fever<br>(3) Anaphylaxis | Soreness and fever commonly occur and can be relieved by acetaminophen or ibuprofen. Anaphylaxis and other severe reactions rarely occur. |
| e. With influenza vaccine<br>(1) Pain, induration, and erythema at injection sites | Adverse effects can be minimized by administering acetaminophen at the time of immunization and at 4, 8, and 12 h later. |
| (2) Flu-like symptoms—chills, fever, malaise, muscle aches | Injection site reactions and flu-like symptoms may start within 12 h after vaccination. |
| (3) Febrile seizures | Febrile seizures have been reported in children, but are uncommon. |

(continued)

## Nursing Actions

### Immunizing Agents (Continued)

| Nursing Actions | Rationale/Explanation |
|---|---|
| f. With MMR vaccine | |
| (1) Mild symptoms of measles—cough, fever up to 39.4°C (102°F), headache, malaise, photophobia, skin rash, sore throat | These symptoms may occur 6–11 d after immunization. |
| (2) Febrile seizures | These are rare, but more likely to occur in children <2 years of age. |
| (3) Arthralgia (joint pain) | Joint pain has been reported in as many as 25% of adult females 2–6 wk after receiving rubella vaccine. |
| (4) Anaphylaxis in recipients who are allergic to eggs | The measles and mumps viruses used in MMR vaccine are grown in chick embryo cell cultures. Recipients who are allergic to eggs should be observed for 90 min after the vaccine is injected. MMR vaccine should be given only in a setting where personnel and equipment are available to treat anaphylaxis. |
| g. With pneumococcal vaccine | |
| (1) Local effects—soreness, induration, and erythema at injection sites | Local effects occur in 40–90% of recipients; systemic effects occur less frequently. |
| (2) Systemic effects—chills, fever, headache, muscle aches, nausea, photophobia, weakness | |
| h. With polio vaccine | Adverse effects are usually mild. Anaphylaxis rarely occurs. |
| (1) Soreness at injection sites | However, if it occurs within 24 h after administration of polio |
| (2) Fever | vaccine, no additional doses of the vaccine should be given. |
| (3) Anaphylaxis | |
| i. With varicella vaccine | |
| (1) Early effects—transient soreness or erythema at injection sites | Injection site reactions occur in 20%–35% of recipients; a skin rash develops in a few (about 8%) recipients within a month. Those who develop the rash from the vaccine have milder symptoms of shorter duration than those who develop varicella naturally. |
| (2) Late effect—a mild, maculopapular skin rash with a few lesions | |
| j. With immune globulin intravenous (IGIV)—chills, dizziness, dyspnea, fever, flushing, headache, nausea, urticaria, vomiting, tightness in chest, pain in chest, hip or back | These effects occur in as many as 10% of recipients and are related to the rate of infusion. If they occur, the infusion should be stopped until the symptoms subside and restarted at a slower rate. The symptoms can also be prevented or minimized by pre-infusion administration of acetaminophen and diphenhydramine or a corticosteroid. |
| **4. Observe for drug interactions.** | |
| a. Drugs that *decrease* effects of vaccines in general: immunosuppressants (eg, corticosteroids, antineoplastic drugs, phenytoin [Dilantin]) | Vaccines may be contraindicated in clients receiving immunosuppressive drugs. These clients cannot produce sufficient amounts of antibodies for immunity and may develop the illness produced by the particular organism contained in the vaccine. The disease is most likely to occur with the live virus vaccines (measles, mumps, rubella). Similar effects occur when the client is receiving irradiation and phenytoin, an anticonvulsant drug that suppresses both cellular and humoral immune responses |
| b. Drugs that *decrease* effects of measles and MMR vaccines | |
| (1) Immunosuppressants | May decrease effectiveness of immunization; patients may remain susceptible to measles despite immunization |
| (2) Immune globulins (eg, RIG, RSV-IGIV, VZIG, IGIV) | To avoid inactivation of the attenuated virus, give measles or MMR vaccine at least 14–30 d before or 6–8 wk after the immune globulin. Alternatively, may check antibody titers or repeat the measles vaccine dose 3 mo after immune globulin administration. |

*(continued)*

## Nursing Actions
### Immunizing Agents (Continued)

| Nursing Actions | Rationale/Explanation |
|---|---|
| (3) Interferon | May inhibit antibody response to the vaccine |
| c. Drugs that *decrease* effects of meningococcal vaccine | |
| (1) Measles vaccine | These vaccines should be given at least 1 mo apart. |
| d. With varicella vaccine, salicylates may *increase* risk of Reye's syndrome. | Aspirin and other salicylates should be avoided for 6 wk after vaccine administration because of potential Reye's syndrome, which has been reported with salicylate use after natural varicella infection. |

## Critical Thinking Exercises

1. At a follow-up postpartum visit, a new mother is offered and receives a rubella vaccine because her rubella titer was inadequate during pregnancy. The immunity she develops to subsequent rubella infections is an example of what type of immunity?

   a. Passive acquired immunity
   b. Active acquired immunity
   c. Natural immunity
   d. Both a and c

2. A 68-year-old client last received a tetanus immunization at age of 60 years. She asks the nurse if she needs to be reimmunized against tetanus. The nurse would be consistent with recommended guidelines if he stated:

   a. "You do not need a tetanus shot after the age of 65."
   b. "Everyone should be immunized against tetanus every 7 to 10 years for life."
   c. "You do not need a tetanus shot unless you have a break in the skin with a traumatic injury."
   d. "You should have a tetanus injection every 3 years for life."

3. While cleaning out the attic, a man sustains a bat bite and is exposed to rabies. The emergency department staff administers serum rabies immune globulin in conjunction with the rabies vaccine for postexposure prophylaxis. Administering the serum rabies immune globulin is an example of what type of immunity?

   a. Passive acquired immunity
   b. Active acquired immunity
   c. Natural immunity
   d. "Bat" luck

4. Which of the following children could receive the MMR immunization safely? A child:

   a. With an upper respiratory infection
   b. Taking phenytoin (Dilantin)
   c. Taking corticosteroids
   d. Receiving irradiation

5. Which of the following vaccines is no longer recommended?

   a. Diphtheria-tetanus-pertussis (DTaP) combination vaccine
   b. Oral polio vaccine (OPV)
   c. Hepatitis B vaccine
   d. Inactivated polio vaccine (IPV)

## SELECTED REFERENCES

Ad Hoc Working Group for the Development of Standards for Pediatric Immunization Practices. (1993). Standards for pediatric immunization practices. *Journal of the American Medical Association, 269,* 1817–1822.

American Academy of Pediatrics Committee on Infectious Diseases. (2002). Recommended childhood immunization schedule—United States, 2002. *Pediatrics, 109(1),* 162.

*Drug facts and comparisons.* (Updated monthly). St. Louis: Facts and Comparisons.

Eickhoff, T. C. (2000). Immunizations. In H. D. Humes (Ed.), *Kelley's textbook of internal medicine* (4th ed., pp. 169–174). Philadelphia: Lippincott Williams & Wilkins.

Hak, E. B., & McColl, M. P. (2000). Immunization therapy. In E. T. Herfindal & D. R. Gourley (Eds.), *Textbook of therapeutics: Drug and disease management* (7th ed., pp. 1363–1384). Philadelphia: Lippincott Williams & Wilkins.

Lacy, C. F., Armstrong, L. L., Goldman, M. P., & Lance, L. L. (2003). *Lexi-Comp's drug information handbook* (11th ed.). Hudson, OH: American Pharmaceutical Association.

Porth, C. M. (Ed.). (2002). *Pathophysiology: Concepts of altered health states* (6th ed.). Philadelphia: Lippincott Williams & Wilkins.

Shinefield, H. R., Black, S. B., Staehle, B. O., Matthews, H., Aldeman, T., Ensor, K. et al (2002). Vaccination with measles, mumps and rubella vaccine and varicella vaccine: Safety, tolerability, immunogenicity, persistence of antibody and duration of protection against varicella in healthy children. *Pediatric Infectious Diseases Journal 21(6),* 555–561.

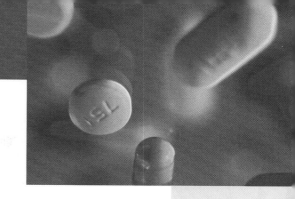

# 35

# Hematopoietic and Immunostimulant Drugs

## OBJECTIVES

*After studying this chapter, the student will be able to:*

1 Give the goals and methods of enhancing hematopoietic and immune functions.

2 Discuss the use of hematopoietic agents in the treatment of anemia and thrombocytopenia.

3 Describe the use of filgrastim and sargramostim in neutropenia and bone marrow transplantation.

4 Identify the adverse effects and nursing process implications of administering filgrastim and sargramostim.

5 Discuss interferons in terms of clinical uses, adverse effects, and nursing process implications.

## CRITICAL THINKING SCENARIO

Jean Reynolds, a 67-year-old client who has had chronic renal failure for the past 7 years, is severely anemic. Her health care provider prescribes epoetin alfa (Epogen) to stimulate red blood cell production. You are responsible for teaching her about the drug, including subcutaneous administration.

✔ Review why renal failure causes anemia and how Epogen works to increase red blood cell counts.

✔ What assessment data should you collect before teaching Mrs. Reynolds self-injection technique?

✔ How will you evaluate whether the Epogen is working? Consider decreased symptoms of anemia and expected changes in laboratory values.

## PROTOTYPE PROFILE

epoetin alfa (Epogen, Procrit), p. 635

# OVERVIEW

Enhancing a person's own body systems to fight infection and cancer is a concept that continues to evolve. Hematopoietic and immunostimulant drugs (also called *cytokines* or *biologic response modifiers*) are given to restore normal function or to increase the ability of the immune system to eliminate potentially harmful invaders. Those available for therapeutic use include colony-stimulating factors (CSF; eg, darbepoetin alfa, epoetin alfa, filgrastim, sargramostim), several interferons, and two interleukins. These drugs, which are the primary focus of this chapter, are described in the following sections and in Drugs at a Glance 35-1.

Bacillus Calmette-Guérin (BCG) vaccine, used in the treatment of bladder cancer, is also discussed. Other drugs with immunostimulant properties are discussed in other chapters. These include traditional immunizing agents (see Chap. 34); levamisole (Ergamisol), which restores functions of macrophages and T cells and is used with fluorouracil in the treatment of intestinal cancer; and antiviral drugs used in the treatment of acquired immunodeficiency syndrome (AIDS) (see Chap. 33). Levamisole and antiviral drugs are more accurately called *immunorestoratives* because they help a compromised immune system regain normal function rather than stimulating "supranormal" function. In AIDS, the human immunodeficiency virus (HIV) causes immune system malfunction; therefore, the antiviral drugs indirectly improve immunologic function.

# GENERAL CHARACTERISTICS OF HEMATOPOIETIC AND IMMUNOSTIMULANT DRUGS

1. Most hematopoietic and immunostimulant drugs are facsimiles of natural endogenous protein substances called *cytokines*. These endogenous cytokines control the reproduction, growth, and differentiation of stem cells and colony-forming units. Their role in cellular activity is described in At the Foundation: Hematopoietic Cytokines. Techniques of molecular biology are used to delineate the type and sequence of amino acids and to identify the genes responsible for producing the cytokines. These genes are then inserted into bacteria (usually *Escherichia coli*) or yeasts capa-

## AT THE FOUNDATION: *Hematopoietic Cytokines*

Cytokines are substances produced by bone marrow cells, activated helper T cells, activated macrophages, and other cells. They regulate many cellular activities by acting as chemical messengers among cells. Some cytokines are growth factors that induce proliferation and differentiation of blood cells. These cytokines comprise a large group of proteins that are structurally and functionally diverse. They were initially named and defined by their action on one type of blood cell, but some of them act on multiple types of blood cells. The term *cytokine* includes lymphokines secreted by lymphocytes and monokines secreted by monocytes and macrophages. The terms *lymphokines* and *monokines* are still used, but they are misleading because secretion of many lymphokines and monokines is not limited to lymphocytes and monocytes as these terms imply. In general, secretion of cytokines occurs after activation of a particular cell and lasts a few hours to a few days. Although a variety of cells can secrete cytokines, helper T cells and macrophages are the main producers.

Cytokines act by binding to receptors on the membranes of numerous types of target cells. A cytokine may bind to receptors on the membrane of the same cell that secreted it (autocrine action); it may bind to receptors on a target cell near the cell that produced it (paracrine action); and, occasionally, it may bind to target cells in distant parts of the body (endocrine or hormonal action). After binding, the cytokine–receptor complex triggers signal-transduction pathways that alter gene expression in the target cells. Overall, cytokines are involved in numerous physiologic responses, including hematopoiesis, cellular proliferation and differentiation, inflammation, wound healing, and cellular and humoral immunity.

Cytokine actions and functions are affected by several factors. First, although the immune response to an antigen may include the production of cytokines, cytokines do not act in response to specific antigens. Instead, they affect whatever cells they encounter that have cytokine receptors and are able to respond. Cytokine receptors are often expressed on a cell only after that cell has interacted with an antigen, so that cytokine activation is limited to antigen-activated lymphocytes. Second, the actions of most cytokines have been determined in laboratories by analysis of the effects of recombinant cytokines, often at nonphysiologic concentrations, and added individually to in vitro systems. Within the human body, however, cytokines rarely if ever act alone. Instead, a target cell is exposed to an environment containing a mixture of cytokines, which may have synergistic or antagonistic effects on each other. Third, cytokines often induce the synthesis of other cytokines. The resulting actions and interactions among cytokines may profoundly alter physiologic responses. Fourth, proteins that act as cytokine antagonists are found in the bloodstream and other extracellular fluids. These proteins may bind directly to a cytokine and inhibit its activity or bind to a cytokine receptor but fail to activate the cell.

ble of producing the substances exogenously. Cloning of the genes that encode interferons, for example, has made it possible to produce large amounts of these substances for research and clinical use. Some interferons (eg, interferon beta-1b) are synthetic versions of DNA recombinant products.

2. Despite extensive research efforts, relatively few cytokine-like drugs are available for clinical use. One of the difficulties in using cytokines is maintaining effective dose levels over treatment periods of weeks or months. During a natural immune response, interacting body cells produce adequate concentrations of cytokines around target cells. However, achieving adequate local concentrations from injected, exogenous cytokines is difficult.

   A second difficulty in using cytokines is that some of the drugs have a short half-life and require frequent administration. Some newer formulations (eg, darbepoetin alfa, pegfilgrastim, and peginterferon alfa-2b) can be given less often. An additional consideration is that the substances are very powerful biologic response modifiers and can cause unanticipated adverse effects.

3. Exogenous drug preparations have the same mechanisms of action as the endogenous products. Colony-stimulating factors bind to receptors on the cell surfaces of immature blood cells in the bone marrow and increase the number, maturity, and functional ability of the cells. Interferons, called alfa, beta, or gamma according to specific characteristics, also bind to specific cell surface receptors and alter intracellular activities. In viral infections, they induce enzymes that inhibit protein synthesis and degrade viral ribonucleic acid. As a result, viruses are less able to enter uninfected cells, reproduce, and release new viruses.

   In addition to their antiviral effects, interferons also have antiproliferative and immunoregulatory activities. They can increase expression of major histocompatibility complex (MHC) molecules, augment the activity of natural killer (NK) cells, increase the effectiveness of antigen-presenting cells in inducing the proliferation of cytotoxic T cells, aid the attachment of cytotoxic T cells to target cells, and inhibit angiogenesis. Because of these characteristics, the interferons are used mainly to treat viral infections and cancers. In chronic hepatitis C, interferon improves liver function in approximately 50% of clients, but relapse often occurs when drug therapy is stopped. In multiple sclerosis, the action of interferon beta is unknown. The drugs are being investigated for additional uses. Systemic interferons are usually well absorbed, widely distributed, and eliminated primarily by the kidneys.

4. In cancer, the exact mechanisms by which interferons and interleukins exert antineoplastic effects are unknown. However, their immunostimulant effects are thought to enhance activities of immune cells (ie, NK cells, T cells, B cells, and macrophages), induce tumor cell antigens (which make tumor cells more easily recognized by immune cells), or alter the expression of oncogenes (genes that can cause a normal cell to change to a cancer cell). BCG vaccine is thought to act against cancer of the urinary bladder by stimulating the immune system and eliciting a local inflammatory response, but its exact mechanism of action is unknown.

5. They are given by subcutaneous or intravenous (IV) injection because they are proteins that would be destroyed by digestive enzymes if given orally.

6. They may produce adverse effects, so that clients do not feel better when taking one of these drugs.

7. The combination of injections and adverse effects may lead to noncompliance in taking the drugs as prescribed.

8. All of the drugs are contraindicated for use in clients who have previously experienced hypersensitivity reactions to any component of the pharmaceutical preparations.

9. Darbepoetin alfa (Aranesp), epoetin alfa (Epogen), filgrastim (Neupogen, Neulasta), oprelvekin (Neumega), and the interferons are often self-administered or given by a caregiver to chronically ill clients. The home care nurse may need to provide assistance in obtaining appropriate laboratory tests (eg, complete blood count [CBC], platelet count, tests of renal or hepatic function) to monitor clients' responses to the medications. Other interventions depend on the drug being taken. General guidelines for strategies for ongoing evaluation and intervention specific for age and in the home are addressed in Age-related Considerations and Home Care Considerations, respectively.

## Characteristics of Individual Drugs

Individual drugs are described in Drugs at a Glance 35-1: Hematopoietic and Immunostimulant Agents.

## Hematopoietic Agents

**Darbepoetin alfa** and 🅟 **epoetin alfa** are drug formulations of erythropoietin, a hormone from the kidney that stimulates bone marrow production of red blood cells. They are used to prevent or treat anemia in several conditions; epoetin alfa serves as the prototype (see Prototype Profile 35-1: Epoetin Alfa). In chronic renal failure, epoetin has a serum half-life of 4 to 13 hours and produces detectable blood levels of erythropoietin within 24 hours with IV administration. With subcutaneous administration, peak serum levels occur within 5 to 24 hours and then decline slowly. Darbepoetin has a much longer half-life (about 49 hours) in clients with chronic renal failure, and peak plasma levels occur in about 34 hours.

With darbepoetin alfa and epoetin alfa, dosage is adjusted according to response. With darbepoetin, dosage is adjusted to achieve and maintain a hemoglobin value of approximately 12 g/dL. With epoetin, dosage is adjusted to achieve and maintain a hematocrit value of 30% to

## Age-related Considerations: Use of Hematopoietic and Immunostimulant Drugs

### USE IN CHILDREN

There has been limited experience with hematopoietic and immunostimulant drugs in children (younger than 18 years of age), and the drugs' safety and effectiveness have not been established. *Filgrastim* and *sargramostim* have been used in children with therapeutic and adverse effects similar to those in adults. In clinical trials, filgrastim produced a greater incidence of subclinical spleen enlargement in children than in adults, but whether this affects growth and development or has other long-term consequences is unknown. *Oprelvekin* has been given to a few children with adverse effects similar to those observed in adults. Reports indicate that tachycardia occurs more often in children and that larger doses are needed (eg, a dose of 75 to 100 mcg/kg in children produces similar plasma levels to a dose of 50 mcg/kg in adults). Long-term effects on growth and development are unknown.

Little information is available about the use of interferons in children. *Interferon alfacon-1* (Infergen) is not recommended for use in children.

### USE IN OLDER ADULTS

In general, hematopoietic and immunostimulant agents have the same uses and responses in older adults as in younger adults. As with many other drugs, older adults may be at greater risk for adverse effects, especially if large doses are used. *Oprelvekin* should be used with caution in clients with a history of or risk factors for atrial fibrillation or flutter; these arrhythmias occurred in approximately 10% of clients during clinical trials. In addition, older adults are more likely to have fluid retention, with resultant symptoms of peripheral edema, dyspnea on exertion, and dilutional anemia.

---

36%. Dosage should be reduced when the hematocrit approaches 36% or increases more than 4 points in any 2-week period. Dosage should be increased if hematocrit does not increase by 5 or 6 points after 8 weeks of drug therapy and is below the recommended range. When doses are changed, measurable differences in hematocrit do not occur for 2 to 6 weeks because of the time required for maturation of red blood cells and their release into the circulation. Thus, the hematocrit should be checked twice weekly for at least 2 to 6 weeks after any dosage change. In general, dose adjustments should not be made more often than once monthly.

## Home Care Considerations: Use of Hematopoetic and Immunostimulant Drugs

***ASSESS:*** the client and family's knowledge of condition and ability to comply with the prescribed regimen; quality of life; and need for referral for treatment.

***MONITOR:*** the therapeutic and adverse effects of the drugs; for signs and symptoms of complications; and client's need for additional information and provide that information.

***EDUCATE:*** regarding importance of reading and following dosing instructions and not exceeding recommended dosages without consulting a health care provider. Educate clients or caregivers regarding accurate drug preparation and injection techniques, as well as proper disposal of needles and syringes. Reinforce additional teaching points (see Client Teaching Guidelines: Blood Cell and Immune System Stimulants).

## Colony–stimulating Factors

**Filgrastim** and **sargramostim** are drug formulations of granulocyte colony-stimulating factor (G-CSF) and granulocyte-macrophage colony-stimulating factor (GM-CSF), respectively, produced by recombinant DNA technology. They are used to stimulate blood cell production by the bone marrow in clients with bone marrow transplantation or chemotherapy-induced neutropenia. They can greatly reduce the incidence and severity of infections. GM-CSF is also being used to promote growth of blood vessels (angiogenesis) in clients with ischemic heart disease. The drug apparently promotes growth of arterioles around blocked areas in coronary arteries. It may be more effective than drugs that stimulate capillary growth because arterioles are larger and can carry more blood.

## Interleukins

**Aldesleukin** (Proleukin) is a recombinant DNA version of interleukin-2 (IL-2). It differs from native IL-2 but has the same biologic activity (eg, activates cellular immunity; produces tumor necrosis factor, IL-1, and interferon gamma; and inhibits tumor growth). It is used to treat metastatic renal cell carcinoma and melanoma and is being investigated for use in other types of cancer. The drug is given by IV infusion, after which it is rapidly distributed to extravascular, extracellular spaces and eliminated by metabolism in the kidneys.

Aldesleukin is contraindicated for initial use in clients who have had organ transplantation or those with serious cardiovascular disease (eg, an abnormal thallium stress test, which reflects coronary artery disease) or serious pulmonary disease (eg, abnormal pulmonary function

(*text continues on page 636*)

**DRUG TABLE 35-1**

*Drugs at a Glance*

## Hematopoietic and Immunostimulant Agents

| Generic/Trade Name | Routes and Dosage Ranges | Comments/Uses |
|---|---|---|
| **Hematopoietic Agents** | | |
| **Darbepoetin alfa** (Aranesp) Pregnancy Category C | Sub-Q, IV, 0.45 mcg/kg once weekly, adjusted to achieve and maintain hemoglobin level no greater than 12 g/dL | For anemia associated with chronic renal failure Main advantage over epoetin alfa is that it is given less often |
| **Epoetin alfa** (Epogen, Procrit) Pregnancy Category C | See Prototype Profile 35-1: Epoetin Alfa | |
| **Colony-Stimulating Factors (CSFs)** | | |
| **Filgrastim** (G-CSF) (Neupogen) Pregnancy Category C | Myelosuppressive chemotherapy, Sub-Q injection, IV infusion over 15–30 min, or continuous Sub-Q or IV infusion, 5 mg/kg/d, up to 2 wk until ANC reaches 10,000/mm³ Bone marrow transplantation, IV or Sub-Q infusion, 10 mcg/kg/d initially, then titrated according to neutrophil count (5 mcg/kg/d if ANC >1000/mm³ for 3 consecutive days; stop drug if >1000/mm³ for 6 d. If ANC drops below 1000/mm³, restart filgrastim at 5 mcg/kg/d) Collection of peripheral stem cells, Sub-Q, 10 mcg/kg/d for 6–7 d, with collection on the last 3 days of drug administration Severe, chronic neutropenia, Sub-Q, 5 or 6 mcg/kg, once or twice daily, depending on clinical response and ANC | Used to prevent infection in clients with neutropenia induced by cancer chemotherapy or bone marrow transplantation To mobilize stem cells from bone marrow to peripheral blood, where they can be collected and reinfused after chemotherapy that depresses bone marrow function To treat severe chronic neutropenia Do not give 24 h before or after a dose of cytotoxic chemotherapy Dosage may be increased if indicated by neutrophil count Stop the drug if the ANC exceeds 10,000/mm³ |
| **Pegfilgrastim** (Neulasta) Pregnancy Category C | Sub-Q, 6 mg once per chemotherapy cycle. Do *not* give between 14 d before and 24 h after cytotoxic chemotherapy | To prevent infection in clients with neutropenia induced by cancer chemotherapy |
| **Sargramostim** (GM-CSF) (Leukine) Pregnancy Category C | Bone marrow reconstitution, IV infusion over 2 h, 250 mcg/m²/d, starting 2–4 h after bone marrow infusion and continuing for 21 d Graft failure or delay, IV infusion over 2 h, 250 mcg/m²/d for 14 d Course of treatment may be repeated after 7 d off therapy if engraftment has not occurred Mobilization of stem cells, Sub-Q or IV over 24 h, 250 mcg/m²/d | Used after bone marrow transplantation to promote bone marrow function or to treat graft failure or delayed function Mobilization of stem cells in peripheral blood so they can be collected |
| **Interleukins** | | |
| **Aldesleukin** (interleukin-2) (Proleukin) Pregnancy Category C | IV infusion over 15 min 600,000 IU or 0.037 mg/kg q8h for 14 doses; after 9 d, repeat q8h for 14 doses | Used with metastatic renal cell carcinoma in adults* Adverse reactions are common and may be serious or fatal. Drug administration must be interrupted or stopped for serious toxicity |

*(continued)*

**DRUG TABLE 35-1**

*Drugs at a Glance*

## Hematopoietic and Immunostimulant Agents (Continued)

| Generic/Trade Name | Routes and Dosage Ranges | Comments/Uses |
|---|---|---|
| **Oprelvekin** (Neumega)<br>Pregnancy Category C | Sub-Q, 50 mcg/kg once daily | For prevention of severe thrombocytopenia with antineoplastic chemotherapy that depresses bone marrow function, in clients with nonmyeloid malignancies<br>Start 6–24 h after completion of chemotherapy and continue until postnadir platelet count is 50,000 cells/mm$^3$ or higher, usually 10–21 d<br>Discontinue oprelvekin at least 2 d before the next cycle of chemotherapy |
| *Interferons* | | |
| **Interferon alfa-2a** (Roferon-A)<br>Pregnancy Category C | Chronic hepatitis C: Sub-Q, IM, 3 million IU 3 times weekly for 48–52 wk<br>Hairy cell leukemia: Sub-Q, IM<br>Induction, 3 million IU daily for 16–24 wk<br>Maintenance, 3 million IU three times weekly<br>Kaposi's sarcoma: Sub-Q, IM<br>Induction, 36 million IU daily for 10–12 wk<br>Maintenance, 36 million IU three times weekly<br>Chronic myelogenous leukemia (CML): Sub-Q, IM, 9 million IU daily | Give Sub-Q only when using a prefilled syringe; Sub-Q recommended for clients with platelet counts <50,000/mm$^3$ or who are at risk for bleeding<br>Omit single doses or reduce dosage by 50% if severe adverse reactions occur<br>With CML, drug may be better tolerated if given 3 million IU for 3 d, then 6 million IU for 3 d, then 9 million IU daily |
| **Interferon alfa-2b** (Intron A)<br>Pregnancy Category C | Hairy cell leukemia: Sub-Q, IM<br>Induction and maintenance, 2 million IU/m$^2$ three times weekly up to 6 mo<br>Kaposi's sarcoma: Sub-Q, IM<br>Induction and maintenance: 30 million IU/m$^2$ three times weekly<br>Chronic hepatitis B: Sub-Q, IM, 5 million IU daily or 10 million IU three times weekly (total of 30–35 million IU per wk) for 16 wk<br>Chronic hepatitis C: Sub-Q, IM, 3 million IU three times weekly for 16 wk–24 mo<br>Malignant melanoma induction: IV, 20 million IU/m$^2$ on 5 consecutive days per week for 4 wk; maintenance: Sub-Q, 10 million IU/m$^2$ three times per week for 48 wk<br>Condylomata intralesionally: 1 million IU/lesion (maximum of five lesions) three times weekly for 3 wk | Omit single doses or reduce dosage by 50% if severe adverse reactions occur |
| **Peginterferon alfa-2b** (PEG-Intron)<br>Pregnancy Category C | Sub-Q, 1 mcg/kg once weekly for 1 year | Used with chronic hepatitis C, alone or concurrently with ribavirin<br>Interferon conjugation to polyethylene glycol extends the duration of action |

*(continued)*

| DRUG TABLE 35-1 | *Drugs at a Glance* |
|---|---|

## Hematopoietic and Immunostimulant Agents (Continued)

| Generic/Trade Name | Routes and Dosage Ranges | Comments/Uses |
|---|---|---|
| **Interferon alfa-2b** (Intron A) and **ribavirin** (Rebetron) Pregnancy Category X | Interferon alfa-2b Sub-Q, 3 million IU 3 times weekly Ribavirin PO, 400–600 mg bid | For chronic hepatitis C in clients who have relapsed after interferon therapy The combination is more effective than either drug alone |
| **Interferon alfacon-1** (Infergen) Pregnancy Category C | Sub-Q, 9 mcg three times weekly for 24 wk, with at least 48 h between doses | For use with chronic hepatitis C in adults* |
| **Interferon beta-1a** (Avonex, Rebif) Pregnancy Category C | Avonex IM, 30 mcg once per week Rebif Sub-Q, 8.8 mcg for 2 wk, then 22 mcg for 2 wk, then 44 mcg Give all doses 3 times weekly, with at least 48 h between doses | Managing multiple sclerosis, to reduce frequency of exacerbations |
| **Interferon beta-1b** (Betaseron) Pregnancy Category C | Sub-Q, 0.25 mg every other day | Same as interferon beta-1a, to reduce frequency of exacerbations of multiple sclerosis |
| **Interferon gamma-1b** (Actimmune) Pregnancy Category C | Sub-Q, 50 mcg/m$^2$ if body surface area (BSA) is >0.5 m$^2$; 1.5 mcg/kg if BSA <0.5 m$^2$ three times weekly (eg, Mon, Wed, Fri) | Reducing frequency and severity of serious infections associated with chronic granulomatous disease |
| *Vaccine* | | |
| **Bacillus Calmette-Guérin** (TICE BCG, TheraCys) Pregnancy Category C | Intravesical instillation by urinary catheter, three vials, reconstituted according to manufacturer's instructions, then diluted further in 50 mL of sterile, preservative-free saline solution (total volume per dose, 53 mL). Repeat once weekly for 6 wk, then give one dose monthly for 6–12 mo (TICE BCG) or one dose at 3, 6, 12, 18, and 24 mo (TheraCys) | Bladder cancer Start 7–14 d after bladder biopsy or transurethral resection |

AIDS, acquired immunodeficiency syndrome; ANC, absolute neutrophil count.

*18 years of age and older.

---

## PROTOTYPE PROFILE 35-1

### ℗ Epoetin Alfa (e POE e tin AL fa)

**Drug Class**
*Chemical:* Colony-stimulating factor
*Functional:* Recombinant human erythropoietin

**Trade Names**
Epogen, Procrit

**Therapeutic Indications**
Prevention and treatment of anemia associated with chronic renal failure (CRF), zidovudine therapy, or anticancer chemotherapy. Also used for reduction of blood transfusions in anemic clients undergoing elective noncardiac, nonvascular surgery

Most clients need an iron supplement during epoetin alfa therapy

**Pharmacokinetics**

*Absorption*
Bioavailability Sub-Q: 21% to 31%

*Distribution*
Rapid in plasma; concentrates in the kidney, liver, and bone marrow

*Metabolism*
Some degradation occurs

*(continued)*

**PROTOTYPE PROFILE 35-1**

**P Epoetin Alfa (Continued)**

*Excretion*
Feces, with small amounts in urine

**Pharmacodynamics**
*Onset of Action*
Several days, peak effect in 2 to 3 weeks

*Duration*
Takes 2–6 wk to demonstrate an increase in hemoglobin

**Contraindications/Precautions**
Hypersensitivity to human albumin, mammalian cell-derived products; with caution, with seizures, porphyria, hypertension

**Pregnancy Considerations**
Category C
Unknown excretion in breast milk

**Dosage**
Adjusted to achieve and maintain a hematocrit value of 30%–36%.

CRF: IV, Sub-Q, 50–100 units/kg three times weekly to achieve or maintain a hematocrit of 30%–36%
Zidovudine therapy: IV, Sub-Q, 100 units/kg three times weekly, increased if necessary
Cancer chemotherapy: Sub-Q, 150–300 units/kg three times weekly
Surgery: Sub-Q, 300 units/kg/d for 10 d before surgery, on the day of surgery and for 4 d after surgery

**Adverse Effects**
Hypertension, fever, headache, fatigue, edema, difficulty breathing, rapid weight gain, chest pain, erythrocytosis

**Drug Interactions**
None reported

**Herbal Supplements and Dietary Considerations**
Most clients require iron replacement; should not take other vitamin or iron supplements or make significant changes in the diet without consulting health care provider

---

tests). With aldesleukin, renal and hepatic impairment occurs during therapy. This impairment may be increased if other nephrotoxic or hepatotoxic drugs are taken concomitantly. In addition, drug-induced renal or hepatic impairment may delay metabolism or elimination of other medications and increase risks for adverse effects. It is contraindicated for repeated courses of therapy in clients who had serious toxicity during earlier courses, including the following:

- Cardiac arrhythmias unresponsive to treatment or ventricular tachycardia lasting for five beats or more, recurrent episodes of chest pain with electrocardiographic evidence of angina or myocardial infarction, pericardial tamponade
- Gastrointestinal (GI) bleeding requiring surgery, bowel ischemia or perforation
- Respiratory intubation required longer than 72 hours
- Central nervous system coma or toxic psychosis lasting longer than 72 hours; repetitive or hard-to-control seizures

For clients who experience severe reactions to aldesleukin, dosage reduction is not recommended. Instead, one or more doses should be withheld, or the drug should be discontinued. Withhold the dose for cardiac arrhythmias, hypotension, chest pain, agitation or confusion, sepsis, renal impairment (oliguria, increased serum creatinine), hepatic impairment (encephalopathy, increasing ascites), positive stool guaiac test, or severe dermatitis, until the condition is resolved. The drug should be discontinued for the occurrence of any of the conditions listed as contraindications for repeat courses of aldesleukin

therapy (eg, sustained ventricular tachycardia, angina, myocardial infarction, pulmonary intubation, renal dialysis, coma, and GI bleeding). Dosage reduction is not recommended. Instead, one or more doses should be withheld, or the drug should be discontinued.

**Oprelvekin** (Neumega) is recombinant IL-11, which stimulates platelet production. It is used to prevent severe thrombocytopenia and reduce the need for platelet transfusions in clients with cancer who are receiving chemotherapy that depresses the bone marrow.

## Interferons

**Interferon alfa-2a** and **interferon alfa-2b,** structurally the same except for one amino acid, are used to treat hairy cell leukemia (a type of B-cell leukemia known as hairy cell because the cells are covered with fine, hairlike structures) and Kaposi's sarcoma associated with AIDS. Interferon alfa-2b is also approved for the treatment of viral infections, such as chronic hepatitis and condylomata acuminata (genital warts associated with infection by human papillomavirus). *Interferon alfa-n1* and *interferon alfacon-1* are newer drugs approved for treatment of chronic hepatitis C, a condition that can lead to liver failure. *Interferon gamma* is used to treat chronic granulomatous disease, which involves impaired phagocytosis of ingested microbes and frequent infections. Drug therapy reduces the incidence and severity of infections. *Interferon beta* is used for multiple sclerosis, an autoimmune neurologic disorder in which the drug reduces progression of neurologic dysfunction, prolongs remissions, and reduces the severity of relapses.

Interferons are being investigated for additional uses, especially in cancer and viral infections, including AIDS. In cancer, for example, interferon alfa has demonstrated antitumor effects in non-Hodgkin's lymphoma, chronic myelogenous leukemia, multiple myeloma, malignant melanoma, and renal cell carcinoma. Common solid tumors of the breast, lung, and colon are unresponsive. Interferon alfa-2b is being combined with ribavirin, another antiviral drug, in efforts to increase effectiveness in chronic hepatitis C. In condylomata, interferon alfa-2b is injected directly into the lesions for several weeks, and most of the lesions disappear completely. In chronic myelogenous leukemia (CML), 70% response rates have been reported, and some clients undergo complete remission.

Although the main adverse effects of interferons are flulike symptoms, these drugs may also cause or aggravate serious, life-threatening neuropsychiatric (including depression and some reports of suicide), autoimmune, ischemic, and infectious disorders. These effects usually resolve when the drug is discontinued, but some may persist for months. Clients receiving the drugs should be closely monitored through clinical and laboratory examinations.

Optimal dosages for interferons have not been established. For clients who experience severe adverse reactions with interferon alfa, dosage should be reduced by 50% or administration stopped until the reaction subsides.

## Bacillus Calmette–Guérin

**Bacillus Calmette-Guérin vaccine** is a suspension of attenuated *Mycobacterium bovis*, long used as an immunizing agent against tuberculosis. The drug's immunostimulant properties stem from its ability to stimulate cell-mediated immunity. It is used as a topical agent to treat superficial cancers of the urinary bladder, in which approximately 80% of clients achieve a therapeutic response. BCG is contraindicated in immunosuppressed clients because the live tubercular organisms may cause tuberculosis in this high-risk population.

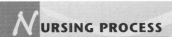

## NURSING PROCESS

### Assessment

- Assess the client's status in relation to conditions for which hematopoietic and immunostimulant drugs are used (eg, infection, neutropenia, cancer).
- Assess nutritional status, including appetite and weight.
- Assess functional abilities in relation to activities of daily living (ADLs).
- Assess adequacy of support systems for outpatients (eg, transportation for clinic visits).
- Assess ability and attitude toward planned drug therapy and associated monitoring and follow-up.
- Assess coping mechanisms of client and significant others in stressful situations.
- Assess client for factors predisposing to infection (eg, skin integrity, invasive devices, cigarette smoking).
- Assess environment for factors predisposing to infection (eg, family or health care providers with infections).
- Assess baseline values of laboratory and other diagnostic test reports to aid monitoring of responses to hematopoietic and immunostimulant drug therapy.

### Nursing Diagnoses

- Risk for Injury: Infection related to drug-induced neutropenia, immunosuppression, malnutrition, chronic disease; bleeding related to anemia or thrombocytopenia
- Risk for Injury: Adverse drug effects
- Activity Intolerance related to weakness, fatigue from debilitating disease, or drug therapy
- Anxiety related to the diagnosis of cancer, hepatitis, multiple sclerosis, or HIV infection
- Deficient Knowledge: Disease process; hematopoietic and immunostimulant drug therapy

### Planning/Goals

*The client will:*

- Participate in interventions to prevent or decrease infection
- Remain afebrile during immunostimulant therapy
- Experience increased immunocompetence as indicated by increased white blood cell (WBC) count (if initially leukopenic) or tumor regression
- Avoid preventable infections
- Experience relief or reduction of disease symptoms
- Maintain independence in ADLs when able; be assisted appropriately when unable
- Maintain adequate levels of nutrition and fluids, rest and sleep, and exercise
- Maintain or increase appetite and weight if initially anorexic and underweight
- Learn to self-administer medications accurately when indicated

### Interventions

- Practice and promote good handwashing techniques by clients and all others in contact with the client.
- Use sterile technique for all injections, IV site care, wound dressing changes, and any other invasive diagnostic or therapeutic measures.
- Screen staff and visitors for signs and symptoms of infection; if infection is noted, do not allow contact with the client.
- Allow clients to participate in self-care and decision making when possible and appropriate.
- Use isolation procedures when indicated, usually when the neutrophil count is below 500/mm$^3$.
- Promote adequate nutrition, with nutritious fluids, supplements, and snacks when indicated.

*(continued)*

## NURSING PROCESS (Continued)

- Promote adequate rest, sleep, and exercise (eg, schedule frequent rest periods, avoid interrupting sleep when possible, individualize exercise or activity according to the client's condition).
- Inform clients about diagnostic test results, planned changes in therapeutic regimens, and evidence of progress.
- Allow family members or significant others to visit clients when feasible.
- Monitor complete blood count (CBC) and other diagnostic test reports for normal or abnormal values.
- Schedule and coordinate drug administration, diagnostic tests, and other elements of care to conserve clients' energy and decrease stress.
- Consult other health care providers (eg, physician, dietitian, social worker) on the client's behalf when indicated.
- Assist clients to learn ways to prevent or reduce the incidence of infections (eg, meticulous personal hygiene, avoiding contact with infected people).
- Assist clients to learn ways to enhance immune mechanisms and other body defenses by healthy lifestyle habits, such as a nutritious diet, adequate rest and sleep, and avoidance of tobacco and alcohol.

- Assist clients or caregivers in learning how to prepare and inject darbepoetin alfa, epoetin alfa, filgrastim, an interferon, or oprelvekin, when indicated.

### Evaluation

- Determine the number and type of infections that have occurred in neutropenic clients.
- Compare current CBC reports with baseline values for changes toward normal levels (eg, WBC count 5000 to 10,000/mm$^3$).
- Compare weight and nutritional status with baseline values for maintenance or improvement.
- Observe and interview for decreased numbers or severity of disease symptoms.
- Observe for increased energy and ability to participate in ADLs.
- Observe and interview outpatients regarding compliance with follow-up care.
- Observe and interview regarding the mental and emotional status of the client and family members.

## CLIENT TEACHING GUIDELINES
## Blood Cell and Immune System Stimulants

### General Considerations

✔ Help your body maintain immune mechanisms and other defenses by healthy lifestyle habits, such as a nutritious diet, adequate rest and sleep, and avoidance of tobacco and alcohol.

✔ Practice meticulous personal hygiene and avoid people and circumstances in which you are exposed to infection.

✔ Keep appointments with health care providers for follow-up care, blood tests, and so forth.

✔ Inform any other physician, dentist, or health care provider about your condition and the medications you are taking.

✔ Several of these medications can be taken at home, even though they are taken by injection. If you are going to self-inject a medication at home, allow sufficient time to learn and practice the techniques under the supervision of a health care provider. Correct preparation and injection are necessary to increase beneficial effects and decrease adverse effects.

✔ With oprelvekin, report the occurrence of ankle edema, shortness of breath, or dizzy spells. Edema and breathing difficulty may be caused by fluid retention, a common adverse effect, and dizziness may result from an irregular heartbeat, which is most likely to occur in older adults.

✔ With interferons, report the occurrence of depression or thoughts of suicide, dizziness, hives, itching, chest tightness, cough, difficulty breathing or wheezing, or

visual problems. These symptoms may require that the drug be stopped or the dosage reduced. In addition, avoid pregnancy (use effective contraceptive methods) and avoid prolonged exposure to sunlight, wear protective clothing, and use sunscreens.

### Self-administration or Caregiver Administration

✔ Take the drugs as prescribed. Although this is important with all medications, it is especially important with these. Obtaining beneficial effects and decreasing adverse effects depend to a great extent on how the drugs are taken.

✔ Use correct techniques to prepare and inject the medications. Instructions for mixing the drugs should be followed exactly.

✔ With interferons:

   ✔ Store in the refrigerator.

   ✔ Do not freeze or shake the drug vial.

   ✔ Do not change brands (changes in dosage may result).

   ✔ Take at bedtime to reduce some common adverse effects (eg, flu-like symptoms such as fever, headache, fatigue, anorexia, nausea, and vomiting).

   ✔ Take acetaminophen (eg, Tylenol, others), if desired, to prevent or decrease fever and headache.

   ✔ Maintain a good fluid intake (eg, 2 to 3 quarts daily).

## DRUG USE IN SPECIFIC SITUATIONS

### Uses in Clients With Cancer

#### Colony-stimulating Factors

Filgrastim and sargramostim are used to restore, promote, or accelerate bone marrow function in clients with cancer who are undergoing chemotherapy or bone marrow transplantation. In cancer chemotherapy, many therapeutic drugs cause bone marrow depression and result in anemia and neutropenia. Neutropenic clients are at high risk for development of infections, often from the normal microbial flora of the client's body or environmental microorganisms, and they may involve bacteria, fungi, and viruses. The client is most vulnerable to infection when the neutrophil count falls below 500/mm³. Filgrastim helps to prevent infection by reducing the incidence, severity, and duration of neutropenia associated with several chemotherapy regimens. Most clients taking filgrastim have fewer days of fever, infection, and antimicrobial drug therapy. In addition, by promoting bone marrow recovery after a course of cytotoxic antineoplastic drugs, filgrastim also may allow higher doses or more timely administration of subsequent antitumor drugs.

When filgrastim is given to prevent infection in neutropenic clients with cancer, the drug should be started at least 24 hours after the last dose of the antineoplastic agent. It should then be continued during the period of maximum bone marrow suppression and the lowest neutrophil count (nadir) and during bone marrow recovery. CBC and platelet counts should be performed twice weekly during therapy, and the drug should be stopped if the neutrophil count exceeds 10,000/mm³. When sargramostim is given to clients with cancer who have had bone marrow transplantation, the drug should be started 2 to 4 hours after the bone marrow infusion and at least 24 hours after the last dose of antineoplastic chemotherapy or 12 hours after the last radiotherapy treatment. CBC should be done twice weekly during therapy, and the neutrophil count should not exceed approximately 20,000/mm³.

Epoetin alfa may be used to prevent or treat anemia in clients with cancer. An adequate intake of iron is required for drug effectiveness. In addition to dietary sources, a supplement is usually necessary.

#### Interleukins

Aldesleukin is a highly toxic drug and contraindicated in clients with preexisting serious cardiovascular or pulmonary impairment. Therefore, when it is used to treat metastatic renal cell carcinoma, clients must be carefully selected, evaluated, and monitored. The drug is most effective in clients with prior nephrectomy and low tumor burden. Still, only about 15% to 25% of clients experience therapeutic responses.

Measures to decrease toxicity are also needed. One strategy is to give the drug by continuous infusion rather than bolus injection. Another is to use cancer-fighting T cells found within tumors. These T cells, called *tumor-infiltrating lymphocytes,* can be removed from the tumors, incubated in vitro with aldesleukin, and reinjected into the client. Tumor-infiltrating lymphocytes return to the tumor and are more active in killing malignant cells than untreated T cells. This technique allows lower and therefore less toxic doses of aldesleukin. Corticosteroids can also decrease toxicity, but their use is not recommended because they also decrease the antineoplastic effects of aldesleukin.

In addition, any preexisting infection should be treated and resolved before initiating aldesleukin therapy because the drug may impair neutrophil function and increase the risk for infections, including septicemia and bacterial endocarditis. Clients with indwelling central IV devices should be given prophylactic antibacterials that are effective against *Staphylococcus aureus* (eg, nafcillin, vancomycin).

Oprelvekin may be used to prevent or treat thrombocytopenia and risks for bleeding in clients with cancer.

#### Interferons

In hairy cell leukemia, interferons normalize WBC counts in 70% to 90% of clients, with or without prior splenectomy. Drug therapy must be continued indefinitely to avoid relapse, which usually develops rapidly after the drug is discontinued. In AIDS-related Kaposi's sarcoma, larger doses are required than in other clinical uses, with resultant increases in toxicity. Interferon alfa is recommended for clients with CD4 cell counts higher than 200/mL (CD4 cells are the helper T cells attacked by the AIDS virus), who have no systemic symptoms, and who have had no opportunistic infections. Approximately 40% of these clients achieve a therapeutic response that lasts 1 to 2 years. In addition to antineoplastic effects, data indicate that viral replication is suppressed in responding clients. Research studies suggest that a combination of interferon alfa and zidovudine, an antiviral drug used in the treatment of AIDS, may have synergistic antineoplastic and antiviral effects. Lower doses of interferon must be used when the drug is combined with zidovudine, to minimize neutropenia.

Interferons may aggravate hepatic impairment. Interferons alfa-2b, alfacon-1, and alfa-n1 are contraindicated in clients with decompensated liver disease (ie, signs and symptoms such as jaundice, ascites, bleeding disorders, or decreased serum albumin), autoimmune hepatitis, a history of autoimmune disease, or posttransplantation immunosuppression. Worsening of liver disease, with jaundice, hepatic encephalopathy, hepatic failure, and death, has occurred in these clients. The drugs should be discontinued in clients with signs and symptoms of liver failure.

## Use of Bacillus Calmette-Guérin With Bladder Cancer

BCG, when instilled into the urinary bladder of clients with superficial bladder cancer, causes remission in up to 82% of clients for an average of 4 years. Early, successful treatment of carcinoma in situ also prevents development of invasive bladder cancer. A specific protocol has been developed for administration of BCG solution, and it should be followed accurately.

## Use in Bone Marrow and Stem Cell Transplantation

*Filgrastim* and *sargramostim* are used to treat clients who undergo bone marrow transplantation for Hodgkin's disease, non-Hodgkin's lymphoma, or acute lymphoblastic leukemia. Before receiving a bone marrow transplant, the client's immune system is suppressed by anticancer drugs or irradiation. After transplantation, it takes 2 to 4 weeks for the engrafted bone marrow cells to mature and begin producing blood cells. During this time, the client has virtually no functioning granulocytes and is at high risk for infection. Sargramostim promotes engraftment and function of the transplanted bone marrow, thereby decreasing risks for infection. If the graft is successful, the granulocyte count starts to rise in approximately 2 weeks. Sargramostim also is used to treat graft failure.

In stem cell transplantation, filgrastim or sargramostim is used to stimulate the movement of hematopoietic stem cells from the bone marrow to circulating blood, where they can be readily collected (in a process called *peripheral blood progenitor cell collection*). Transplantation of large numbers of stem cells can lead to more rapid engraftment and recovery, with less risk for transplant failure and complications.

## Nursing Actions

### Hematopoietic and Immunostimulant Agents

| Nursing Actions | Rationale/Explanation |
|---|---|
| 1. Administer accurately. | For hospitalized clients, the drugs may be prepared for administration in a pharmacy. When nurses prepare the drugs, they should consult the manufacturer's instructions. Outpatients may be taught self-administration techniques. |
| a. Give darbepoetin alfa intravenously (IV) or subcutaneously (Sub-Q) once weekly | Omit the dose if the hemoglobin level is >12g/dL. |
| b. Give epoetin alfa IV or Sub-Q; do not shake the vial; and discard any remainder of multidose vials 21 d after opening. | For clients with chronic renal failure on hemodialysis, epoetin alfa can be given by bolus injection at the end of dialysis. For other patients with an IV line, the drug can be given IV. For patients without an IV line or who are ambulatory, the drug is injected Sub-Q. Shaking can inactivate the medication; the manufacturer does not ensure sterility or stability of multidose vials after 21 days. |
| c. Give filgrastim (Neupogen) according to indication for use:<br>(1) With cancer chemotherapy, give by Sub-Q bolus injection, IV infusion over 15–30 min, or continuous Sub-Q or IV infusion<br>(2) For bone marrow transplantation, give by IV infusion over 4 h or by continuous IV or Sub-Q infusion<br>(3) For collection of stem cells, give as a bolus or a continuous infusion<br>(4) For chronic neutropenia, give Sub-Q | Manufacturer's recommendations |
| d. Give pegfilgrastim (Neulasta) Sub-Q only | |
| e. Give sargramostim by IV infusion over 2 h, after reconstitution with 1 mL sterile water for injection and addition to 0.9% sodium chloride. | Manufacturer's recommendation |
| f. With aldesleukin, review institutional protocols or the manufacturer's instructions for administration. | This drug has limited uses and is rarely given. Thus, most nurses will need to review instructions each time. |
| g. With interferons,<br>(1) Read drug labels carefully to ensure having the correct drug preparation. | Available drugs have similar names but often differ in indications for use, dosages, and routes of administration. |

*(continued)*

## *Nursing Actions*

## Hematopoietic and Immunostimulant Agents (Continued)

| Nursing Actions | Rationale/Explanation |
|---|---|
| (2) Give most interferons Sub-Q, 3 times weekly, on a regular schedule (eg, Mon., Weds., and Fri.), at about the same time of day, at least 48 h apart. | Manufacturer's recommendation |
| (3) Inject interferon for condylomata intralesionally into the base of each wart with a small-gauge needle. For large warts, inject at several points | Manufacturer's recommendation |
| h. With intravesical *Bacillus Calmette-Guérin (BCG):* | |
| (1) Reconstitute solution (see Drugs at a Glance: Hematopoietic and Immunostimulant Agents). | Reconstituted solution should be used immediately or refrigerated. Discard if not used within 2 h. |
| (2) Wear gown and gloves. | |
| (3) Insert a sterile urethral catheter and drain bladder. | |
| (4) Instill medication slowly by gravity. | |
| (5) Remove catheter. | |
| (6) Have the patient lie on abdomen, back, and alternate sides for 15 min in each position. Then, allow to ambulate but ask to retain solution for a total of 2 h before urinating, if able. | |
| (7) Dispose of all equipment in contact with BCG solution appropriately. | BCG contains live mycobacterial organisms and is therefore infectious material. |
| (8) Do not give if catheterization causes trauma (eg, bleeding), and wait 1 wk before a repeat attempt. | |
| **2. Observe for therapeutic effects.** | |
| a. With darbepoetin alfa and epoetin alfa, observe for increased red blood cells, hemoglobin, and hematocrit. | Therapeutic effects depend on the dose and the client's underlying condition. The goal is usually to achieve and maintain a hematocrit between 30% and 36% (with epoetin) or hemoglobin of no more than 12 g/dL (with darbepoetin). With epoetin, it takes 2–6 wk for the hematocrit to change after a dosage change. |
| b. With oprelvekin, observe for maintenance of a normal or near-normal platelet count when used to prevent thrombocytopenia and an increased platelet count or fewer platelet transfusions when used to treat thrombocytopenia. | Platelet counts usually increase in approximately 1 wk and continue to increase for approximately 1 wk after the drug is stopped. Then, counts decrease toward baseline during the next 2 wk. |
| c. With aldesleukin, observe for tumor regression (improvement in signs and symptoms). | Tumor regression may occur as early as 4 wk after the first course of therapy and may continue up to 12 mo. |
| d. With parenteral interferons, observe for improvement in signs and symptoms. | With hairy cell leukemia, hematologic tests may improve within 2 mo, but optimal effects may require 6 mo of drug therapy. With Kaposi's sarcoma, skin lesions may resolve or stabilize over several weeks. With chronic hepatitis, liver function tests may improve within a few weeks. |
| e. With intralesional interferon, observe for disappearance of genital warts. | Lesions usually disappear after several weeks of treatment. |
| **3. Observe for adverse effects.** | |
| a. With darbepoetin alfa and epoetin alfa, observe for nausea, vomiting, diarrhea, arthralgias, and hypertension. | The drugs are usually well tolerated, with adverse effects similar to those of placebo and which may result from the underlying disease processes. |
| b. With oprelvekin, observe for atrial fibrillation or flutter, dyspnea, edema, fever, mucositis, nausea, neutropenia, tachycardia, vomiting | In clinical trials, most adverse events were mild or moderate in severity and reversible after stopping drug administration. Atrial arrhythmias are more likely to occur in older adults. Dyspnea and edema are attributed to fluid retention. |

*(continued)*

## Nursing Actions

## Hematopoietic and Immunostimulant Agents (Continued)

| Nursing Actions | Rationale/Explanation |
|---|---|
| c. With filgrastim, observe for bone pain, erythema at Sub-Q injection sites, and increased serum lactate dehydrogenase, alkaline phosphatase, and uric acid levels. | Bone pain reportedly occurs in 20% to 25% of patients and can be treated with acetaminophen or a nonsteroidal anti-inflammatory drug (NSAID). |
| d. With sargramostim, observe for bone pain, fever, headache, muscle aches, generalized maculopapular skin rash, and fluid retention (peripheral edema, pleural effusion, pericardial effusion). | Pleural and pericardial effusions are more likely at doses greater than 20 mcg/kg/d. Adverse effects occur more often with sargramostim than filgrastim. |
| e. With interferons, observe for acute flu-like symptoms (eg, fever, chills, fatigue, muscle aches, headache), chronic fatigue, depression, leukopenia, and increased liver enzymes. Anemia and depressed platelet and WBC counts may also occur but are infrequent. | Acute effects occur in most patients, increasing with higher doses and decreasing with continued drug administration. Most symptoms can be relieved by acetaminophen. Fatigue and depression occur with long-term administration and are dose-limiting effects. |
| f. With aldesleukin, observe for capillary leak syndrome (hypotension, shock, angina, myocardial infarction, arrhythmias, edema, respiratory distress, gastrointestinal bleeding, renal insufficiency, mental status changes). Other effects may involve most body systems, such as chills and fever, blood (anemia, thrombocytopenia, eosinophilia), central nervous system (CNS) (seizures, psychiatric symptoms), skin (erythema, burning, pruritus), hepatic (cholestasis), endocrine (hypothyroidism), and bacterial infections. In addition, drug-induced tumor breakdown may cause hypocalcemia, hyperkalemia, hyperphosphatemia, hyperuricemia, renal failure, and electrocardiogram changes. | Adverse effects are frequent, often serious, and sometimes fatal. Most subside within 2 to 3 d after stopping the drug. Capillary leak syndrome, which may begin soon after treatment starts, is characterized by a loss of plasma proteins and fluids into extravascular space. Signs and symptoms result from decreased organ perfusion, and most patients can be treated with vasopressor drugs, cautious fluid replacement, diuretics, and supplemental oxygen. |
| g. With intravesical BCG, assess for symptoms of bladder irritation (eg, frequency, urgency, dysuria, hematuria) and systemic symptoms of fever, chills, and malaise. | These effects occur in more than 50% of patients, usually starting a few hours after administration and lasting 2 to 3 d. They can be decreased by phenazopyridine (Pyridium), a urinary tract analgesic, propantheline (Pro-Banthine) or oxybutynin (Ditropan), antispasmodics; and acetaminophen (Tylenol) or ibuprofen (Motrin), analgesic–antipyretic agents. |
| **4. Observe for drug interactions.** | |
| a. Drugs that *increase* effects of sargramostim: | |
| (1) Corticosteroids, lithium | These drugs have myeloproliferative (bone marrow stimulating) effects of their own, which may add to those of sargramostim. |
| b. Drugs that *increase* effects of aldesleukin: | All of the listed drug groups may potentiate adverse effects of aldesleukin. |
| (1) Aminoglycoside antibiotics (eg, gentamicin, others) | Increased nephrotoxicity |
| (2) Antihypertensives | Increased hypotension |
| (3) Antineoplastics (eg, asparaginase, doxorubicin, methotrexate) | Increased toxic effects on bone marrow, heart, and liver. Aldesleukin is usually given as a single antineoplastic agent; its use in combination with other antineoplastic drugs is being evaluated. |
| (4) Opioid analgesics | Increased CNS adverse effects |
| (5) NSAIDs (eg, ibuprofen) | Increased nephrotoxicity |
| (6) Sedative-hypnotics | Increased CNS adverse effects |
| d. Drugs that *decrease* effects of aldesleukin: | |
| (1) Corticosteroids | These drugs should not be given concurrently with aldesleukin, because they decrease the drug's therapeutic anticancer effects. |

## Critical Thinking Exercises

1. The immunizing agent long used against tuberculosis that is also successful in the treatment of bladder cancer through its ability to stimulate cell-mediated immunity is:
   a. Pegfilgrastim (Neulasta)
   b. Sargramostim (Leukine)
   c. Bacillus Calmette-Guérin (BCG) vaccine
   d. Oprelvekin (Neumega)

2. A client has recently received a bone marrow transplant, and the health care provider orders filgrastim (granulocyte-macrophage colony-stimulating factor). Which of the following blood elements will not be stimulated?
   a. Erythrocytes
   b. Eosinophils
   c. Neutrophils
   d. Macrophages

3. Individuals with chronic renal failure can benefit from darbepoetin alfa (Aranesp) because the drug:
   a. Replaces erythropoietin no longer produced by the cells of the kidney
   b. Promotes the kidneys' excretion of elements that impair red blood cell production
   c. Reduces urea, which can destroy circulating red blood cells
   d. Replaces iron stores that improve red blood cell production

4. With darbepoetin and epoetin therapy, clients frequently require:
   a. Hospitalization in an intensive care facility
   b. Bone marrow transplantation
   c. Cardiac monitoring
   d. Supplemental iron

5. Oprelvekin (Neumega) is recombinant IL-11, which stimulates the production of:
   a. Erythrocytes
   b. Platelets
   c. Neutrophils
   d. Macrophages

## SELECTED REFERENCES

Darbepoetin (Aranesp): A long-acting erythropoietin. *The Medical Letter on Drugs and Therapeutics, 43*(1120). New Rochelle, NY: The Medical Letter, Inc.

*Drug facts and comparisons.* (Updated monthly). St. Louis: Facts and Comparisons.

Goldsby, R. A., Kindt, T. J., & Osborne, B. A. (2000). *Kuby Immunology* (4th ed.). New York: WH Freeman and Co.

Guyton, A. C., & Hall, J. E. (2000). *Textbook of medical physiology* (10th ed.). Philadelphia: W. B. Saunders.

Lacy, C. F., Armstrong, L. L., Goldman, M. P., & Lance, L. L. (2003). *Lexi-Comp's drug information handbook* (11th ed.). Hudson, OH: American Pharmaceutical Association.

Moore, M. (2000). Hematopoietic growth factors. In H. D. Humes (Ed.), *Kelley's textbook of internal medicine* (4th ed., pp. 1854–1858). Philadelphia: Lippincott Williams & Wilkins.

Smith, J. W. II, & Urba, W. J. (2000). Principles of biologic therapy. In H. D. Humes (Ed.), *Kelley's textbook of internal medicine* (4th ed., pp. 1849–1854). Philadelphia: Lippincott Williams & Wilkins.

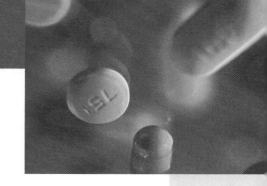

# 36

# Corticosteroids and Immunosuppressants

## OBJECTIVES

*After studying this chapter, the student will be able to:*

1 Review physiologic effects of endogenous corticosteroids.

2 Discuss clinical indications for use of exogenous corticosteroids.

3 Describe characteristics and consequences of immunosuppression.

4 Give characteristics and uses of major immunosuppressant drugs in autoimmune disorders and organ transplantation.

5 Identify adverse effects of immunosuppressant drugs and long-term corticosteroid therapy.

6 Explain the pathophysiologic basis of adverse effects.

7 Apply the nursing process with a client receiving long-term systemic corticosteroid therapy and other immunosuppressant drugs, including teaching needs

## CRITICAL THINKING SCENARIO

*M*argaret Reily, 46 years of age, is scheduled to undergo kidney transplantation this week. After transplantation, she will be on a regimen of immunosuppressive drugs, including corticosteroids and cyclosporine. You are responsible for Ms. Reily's teaching.

✔ Why is lifelong immunosuppression necessary after organ transplantation?

✔ What symptoms might Ms. Reily experience if she rejects her transplanted kidney?

✔ How will you teach Ms. Reily to reduce her risk for infection?

✔ What lifelong measures for medical follow-up and management are necessary for a transplant recipient?

## PROTOTYPE PROFILE

prednisone (Deltasone, Sterapred, Prednisone Inten–sol), p. 648

# OVERVIEW

Corticosteroids and other immunosuppressant drugs interfere with the production or function of immune cells and inhibit the immune response. These drugs are used to decrease an inappropriate or undesirable immune response for conditions that range from treatment of asthma, to management of autoimmune disorders, such as lupus erythematosus or rheumatoid arthritis, to suppression of transplant rejection. The immune response is normally a protective mechanism that helps the body defend itself against potentially harmful external (eg, microorganisms) and internal agents (eg, cancer cells).

# CORTICOSTEROIDS

Corticosteroid drugs are used in nonendocrine disorders to suppress immune responses and to reduce inflammation. Corticosteroids are used with the endocrine disorder, adrenal insufficiency, for replacement of deficient endogenous (within the body) glucocorticoids, along with mineralocorticoids and adrenal sex hormones (see Chap. 20). The term *corticosteroids* actually means all secretions of the adrenal cortex but is used here to designate the glucocorticoids. *Glucocorticoids* are secreted cyclically, with the largest amount being produced in the early morning and the smallest amount during the evening hours (in people with a normal day–night schedule). At the cellular level, glucocorticoids account for most of the characteristics and physiologic effects of the corticosteroids (Box 36-1).

As previously noted, when corticosteroids are administered from sources outside the body (exogenous), they are given mainly for replacement or therapeutic purposes. Replacement involves small doses to correct a deficiency state and restore normal function. Therapeutic purposes involve relatively large doses to exert pharmacologic effects, and such doses are toxic to the body. Drug effects involve extension of the physiologic effects of endogenous corticosteroids and new effects that do not occur with small, physiologic doses. The most frequently desired effects are anti inflammatory, immunosuppressive, antiallergic, and antistress. These are classified as glucocorticoid effects. The most expected adverse effects include increased risk for infection, decreased wound healing, suppression of the hypothalamic-pituitary-adrenal (HPA) axis, osteoporosis, and hyperglycemia.

Corticosteroids are potent anti-inflammatory drugs that act to suppress the immune response at many levels. In many disorders, they relieve signs and symptoms by decreasing the accumulation of lymphocytes and macrophages and the production of cell-damaging cytokines at sites of inflammatory reactions. Because inflammation is a common response to chemical mediators or antigens that cause tissue injury, the anti-inflammatory and

immunosuppressive actions of corticosteroids often overlap and are indistinguishable. Despite this somewhat arbitrary separation, corticosteroid effects on the immune response are emphasized here. In general, the drugs suppress growth of all lymphoid tissue and therefore decrease formation and function of antibodies and T cells. For patients with transplanted tissues, a corticosteroid is usually given with other agents (eg, azathioprine) to prevent acute episodes of graft rejection. Specific effects include the following:

■ Increased numbers of circulating neutrophils (more are released from bone marrow, and fewer leave the circulation to enter inflammatory exudates). In terms of neutrophil functions, corticosteroids increase chemotaxis and release of lysosomal enzymes.

■ Decreased numbers of circulating basophils, eosinophils, and monocytes. The reduced availability of monocytes is considered a major factor in the anti-inflammatory activity of corticosteroids. Functions of monocyte-macrophages are also impaired. Corticosteroids suppress phagocytosis and initial antigen processing (necessary to initiate an immune response), impair migration to areas of tissue injury, and block the differentiation of monocytes to macrophages.

■ Decreased numbers of circulating lymphocytes (immune cells), resulting from impaired production (ie, inhibition of DNA, RNA, and protein synthesis), sequestration in lymphoid tissues, or lysis of the cells. T cells are markedly reduced; B cells are moderately reduced.

■ Impaired function of cellular (T-cell) and humoral (B-cell) immunity. Corticosteroids inhibit the production of immunostimulant cytokines (eg, interleukin-1 [IL-1] and IL-2) required for activation and clonal expansion of lymphocytes and cytotoxic cytokines, such as tumor necrosis factor (TNF) and interferons. When administered for 2 to 3 weeks, the drugs also inhibit immune reactions to antigenic skin tests and reduce serum concentrations of some antibodies (immunoglobulin G [IgG] and IgA, but not IgM).

These drugs are described in Drugs at a Glance 36-1: Corticosteroids; drug use in specific situations is outlined in a subsequent section. However, the use of corticosteroids and other drugs to treat autoimmune disorders or to prevent or treat transplant rejection reactions are the main focus of this chapter. The prototype, **ⓟ prednisone**, is described in Prototype Profile 36-1: Prednisone.

# IMMUNOSUPPRESSANT DRUGS

Other drugs along with corticosteroids are used as immunosuppressants and are diverse agents with often overlapping mechanisms of actions and effects. Numerous disease processes are thought to be initiated or

*(text continues on page 648)*

## BOX 36-1   Effects of Glucocorticoids on Body Processes and Systems

### Carbohydrate Metabolism

- ↑Formation of glucose (gluconeogenesis) by breaking down protein into amino acids. The amino acids are then transported to the liver, where they are acted on by enzymes that convert them to glucose. The glucose is then returned to the circulation for use by body tissues or storage in the liver as glycogen.
- ↓Cell use of glucose, especially in muscle cells. This is attributed to a ↓effect of insulin on the proteins that normally transport glucose into cells and by ↓numbers and functional capacity of insulin receptors.
- Both the ↑production and ↓use of glucose promote higher levels of glucose in the blood (hyperglycemia) and may lead to diabetes mellitus. These actions also increase the amount of glucose stored as glycogen in the liver, skeletal muscles, and other tissues.

### Protein Metabolism

- ↑Breakdown of protein into amino acids (catabolic effect); ↑rate of amino acid transport to the liver and conversion to glucose.
- ↓Rate of new protein formation from dietary and other amino acids (antianabolic effect)
- The combination of ↑breakdown of cell protein and ↓protein synthesis leads to protein depletion in virtually all body cells except those of the liver. Thus, glycogen stores in the body are ↑ and protein stores are ↓.

### Lipid Metabolism

- ↑Breakdown of adipose tissue into fatty acids; the fatty acids are transported in the plasma and used as a source of energy by body cells.
- ↑Oxidation of fatty acids within body cells

### Inflammatory and Immune Responses

- ↓Inflammatory response. Inflammation is the normal bodily response to tissue damage and involves three stages. First, a large amount of plasma-like fluid leaks out of capillaries into the damaged area and becomes clotted. Second, leukocytes migrate into the area. Third, tissue healing occurs, largely by growth of fibrous scar tissue. Normal or physiologic amounts of glucocorticoids probably do not significantly affect inflammation and healing, but large amounts of glucocorticoids inhibit all three stages of the inflammatory process.

  More specifically, corticosteroids stabilize lysosomal membranes (and thereby prevent the release of inflammatory proteolytic enzymes), ↓capillary permeability (and thereby ↓leakage of fluid and proteins into the damaged tissue), ↓the accumulation of neutrophils and macrophages at sites of inflammation (and thereby impair phagocytosis of pathogenic microorganisms and waste products of cellular metabolism), and ↓production of inflammatory chemicals, such as interleukin-1, prostaglandins, and leukotrienes, by injured cells.

- ↓Immune response. The immune system normally protects the body from foreign invaders, and several immune responses overlap inflammatory responses, including phagocytosis. In addition, the immune response stimulates the production of antibodies and activated lymphocytes to destroy the foreign substance. Glucocorticoids impair protein synthesis, including the production of antibodies; ↓the numbers of circulating lymphocytes, eosinophils, and macrophages; and ↓amounts of lymphoid tissue. These effects help to account for the immunosuppressive and antiallergic actions of the glucocorticoids.

### Cardiovascular System

- Help to regulate arterial blood pressure by modifying vascular smooth muscle tone, by modifying myocardial contractility, and by stimulating renal mineralocorticoid and glucocorticoid receptors.
- ↑The response of vascular smooth muscle to the pressor effects of catecholamines and other vasoconstrictive agents.

### Nervous System

- Physiologic amounts help to *maintain normal nerve excitability;* pharmacologic amounts ↓nerve excitability, slow activity in the cerebral cortex, and alter brain wave patterns.
- ↓Secretion of corticotropin-releasing hormone by the hypothalamus and of corticotropin by the anterior pituitary gland. This results in suppression of further glucocorticoid secretion by the adrenal cortex (negative feedback system).

### Musculoskeletal System

- Maintain muscle strength when present in physiologic amounts but cause muscle atrophy (from protein breakdown) when present in excessive amounts.
- ↓Bone formation and growth and ↑bone breakdown. Glucocorticoids also ↓intestinal absorption and ↑renal excretion of calcium. These effects contribute to bone demineralization (osteoporosis) in adults and to ↓linear growth in children.

### Respiratory System

- Maintain open airways. Glucocorticoids do not have direct bronchodilating effects, but help to maintain and restore responsiveness to the bronchodilating effects of endogenous catecholamines, such as epinephrine.
- Stabilize mast cells and other cells to inhibit the release of bronchoconstrictive and inflammatory substances, such as histamine.

### Gastrointestinal System

- ↓Viscosity of gastric mucus. This effect may ↓protective properties of the mucus and contribute to the development of peptic ulcer disease.

↑ increase/increased; ↓, decrease/decreased.

**DRUG TABLE 36-1**

## *Drugs at a Glance*
## Corticosteroids*

| Generic/Trade Name | Routes and Dosage Ranges | Comments |
|---|---|---|
| **Betamethasone** (Celestone, Celestone Soluspan, Luxig, Diprolene, Maxivate) Pregnancy Category C | PO, 0.6–7.2 mg daily initially, gradually reduced to lowest effective dose IM, 0.5–9 mg daily Intraarticular injection, 0.25–2 mL | Often used in women with premature labor to stimulate fetal lung maturation |
| **Cortisone** (Cortone) Pregnancy Category D | PO, 25–300 mg daily, individualized for condition and response | May increase potassium depletion from diuretics; estrogens may increase cortisone effects |
| **Dexamethasone** (Decadron) **Dexamethasone acetate** **Dexamethasone sodium phosphate** Pregnancy Category C | PO, 0.75–9 mg daily in 2–4 doses; higher ranges for serious diseases IM, 8–16 mg (1–2 mL) in single dose, repeated every 1–3 wk if necessary IM, IV, 0.5–9 mg, depending on severity of disease | Interferes with calcium absorption |
| **Hydrocortisone** (Hydrocortone, Cortef) Pregnancy Category C **Hydrocortisone sodium phosphate** **Hydrocortisone sodium succinate** **Hydrocortisone retention enema** (Cortenema) **Hydrocortisone acetate intrarectal foam** (Cortifoam) Pregnancy Category C | PO, 20–240 mg daily, depending on condition and response IV, IM, Sub-Q, 15–240 mg daily in 2 divided doses IV, IM, 100–400 mg initially, repeated at 2-, 4-, or 6-h intervals if necessary Rectally, one enema (100 mg) nightly for 21 d or until optimal response 1 applicatorful 1–2 times daily for 2–3 wk, then once every 2–3 d if needed | Hydrocortisone in conjunction with oral anticoagulants may increase prothrombin time |
| **Methylprednisolone** (Medrol) **Methylprednisolone sodium succinate** (Solu-Medrol) **Methylprednisolone acetate** (Depo-Medrol) Pregnancy Category C | PO, 4–48 mg daily initially, gradually reduced to lowest effective level *Adults:* IV, IM, 10–40 mg initially, adjusted to condition and response Infants and children: IV, IM, not less than 0.5 mg/kg/24 h IM, 40–120 mg once daily | Nervousness and insomnia common adverse effects Acetate salts should not be administered intravenously |
| **Prednisolone** (Delta-Cortef) **Prednisolone acetate** **Prednisolone sodium phosphate** (Hydeltrasol) Pregnancy Category C | PO, 5–60 mg daily initially, adjusted for maintenance IM, 4–60 mg daily initially, adjusted for maintenance IV, IM, PO, 4–60 mg daily initially, adjusted for maintenance | Oral contraceptives may enhance effect of prednisolone |
| **Prednisone** (Deltasone) | See Prototype Profile 36-1: Prednisone | |
| **Triamcinolone** (Aristocort, Kenacort) **Triamcinolone acetonide** (Kenalog-40) **Triamcinolone diacetate** (Aristocort Forte) Pregnancy Category C | PO, 4–48 mg daily initially, reduced for maintenance IM, 2.5–60 mg daily, depending on the disease Reduce dosage and start oral therapy when feasible IM, 20–80 mg initially | Interferes with calcium absorption; may be taken with food to decrease GI distress Give IM injections deep in large muscle mass, avoid the deltoid |

*Respiratory antiasthmatic preparations are outlined in Chapter 37; ophthalmic and dermatologic preparations are discussed in Appendices G and F, respectively.

## PROTOTYPE PROFILE 36-1
### *P* Prednisone (PRED ni sone)

**Drug Class**
*Chemical:* Corticosteroid; glucocorticoid
*Functional:* Anti-inflammatory agent, immunosuppressant agent

**Trade Names**
Deltasone, Sterapred, Prednisone Intensol, others

**Therapeutic Indications**
Treatment of adrenal insufficiency; hypercalcemia; allergic, inflammatory, and autoimmune disorders

**Pharmacokinetics**
*Absorption*
PO: Rapid

*Distribution*
Protein binding 65%–91% (concentration dependent)

*Metabolism*
Hepatic

*Excretion*
Renal

**Pharmacodynamics**
*Onset of Action*
Variable

*Duration*
Variable

**Contraindications/Precautions**
Hypersensitivity, systemic fungal infections; with caution in clients at risk for infections, with infections, diabetes mellitus, hypothyroidism, peptic ulcer disease, inflammatory bowel disorders, hypertension, congestive heart failure, and renal insufficiency

**Pregnancy Considerations**
Category B
Crosses placenta; enters breast milk, compatible

**Dosage**
Not available in parenteral form; taper to wean
*Adults:* Immunosuppression: PO, 5–60 mg daily initially in morning, reduced for maintenance
Physiologic replacement: 4–5 mg/m$^2$/d
*Children:* Immunosuppression or anti-inflammatory effect: 0.05 mg/kg/d
Physiologic replacement: 4–5 mg/m$^2$/d

**Adverse Effects**
Insomnia, nervousness, increased appetite, glucose intolerance, edema, fractures, muscle wasting, seizures

**Drug Interactions**
*Increased Effects*
Risk for GI ulceration with concurrent use with NSAIDs

*Decreased Effects*
Decreased steroid effect with phenytoin, rifampin, barbiturates
Decreased effects of vaccines, toxoids, and salicylates

**Herbal Supplements and Dietary Considerations**
Administer with food or milk to decrease GI irritation; drug interferes with calcium absorption
St. John's wort may decrease prednisone levels
Cat's claw and echinacea have immunostimulant properties and should be avoided

---

aggravated when the immune system perceives the person's own body tissues as harmful invaders and tries to eliminate them. This inappropriate activation of the immune response is a major factor in a growing list of serious diseases believed to involve autoimmune processes, including rheumatoid arthritis, systemic lupus erythematosus, inflammatory bowel disease, and others. To aid understanding of immunosuppressive drug therapy, autoimmunity is described in At the Foundation: Autoimmunity.

An appropriate but undesirable immune response is also elicited when foreign tissue is transplanted into the body. If the immune response is not sufficiently suppressed, the body reacts as with other antigens and attempts to destroy (reject) the foreign organ or tissue. Although numerous advances have been made in transplantation technology, the immune response remains a major factor in determining the success or failure of transplantation.

Older drugs generally depress the immune system (ie, suppress the immune response to all antigens). This greatly increases risks for serious infections with bacteria, viruses, fungi, or protozoa, at any time during the immunosuppressed state. In addition, many immunosuppressant drugs slow the proliferation of activated lymphocytes and damage rapidly dividing nonimmune cells (eg, mucosal, intestinal, and bone marrow hematopoietic stem cells). As a result, serious or life-threatening complications can occur. For example, patients on long-term immunosuppressant drug therapy (eg, with autoimmune disorders and organ transplantation) are at increased risk for infections, cancer (especially lymphoma), hypertension, and metabolic bone disease.

For many reasons, including adverse effects of older drugs and the efforts to develop more effective agents, extensive research has led to the development of drugs that modify the immune response (often called *immunomodulators* or *biologic response modifiers*). As a result, several

## AT THE FOUNDATION: *Autoimmunity*

Autoimmune disorders occur when a person's immune system loses its ability to differentiate between antigens on its own cells (called self-antigens or autoantigens) and antigens on foreign cells. As a result, an undesirable immune response is aroused against host tissues.

The mechanisms by which autoantigens are altered to elicit an immune response are unclear. Genetic susceptibility and possible "triggering" events such as damage by microorganisms or trauma, similarity in appearance between autoantigens and foreign antigens, or a linkage between a foreign antigen and an autoantigen may be involved. Once an autoantigen is changed and perceived as foreign or "nonself," the immune response may involve T lymphocytes in direct destruction of tissue, production of proinflammatory cytokines that recruit and activate phagocytes, and stimulation of B lymphocytes to produce autoantibodies that produce inflammation and tissue damage.

In addition to the factors that activate an immune response, there are also factors that prevent the immune system from "turning off" the abnormal immune or inflammatory process. One of these factors may be a deficient number of suppressor T cells. At present, it is unclear whether suppressor T cells are a separate group or a subpopulation of helper or cytotoxic T cells with suppressive functions.

---

drugs with more specific immunosuppressive actions have been approved in recent years. Most are used in combination with older immunosuppressants for synergistic effects.

Most of the available immunosuppressant drugs inhibit the immune response in a general or nonspecific manner. However, the number of drugs that suppress the immune response to specific antigens is increasing. Newer drugs that target specific components of the immune response rather than causing general suppression of multiple components may lessen the consequences of immunosuppression. In addition to the specific risks or adverse effects of individual immunosuppressant drugs, general risks of immunosuppression include infection and cancer. Infection is a major cause of morbidity and mortality, especially in clients who are neutropenic (neutrophil count <1000/mm$^3$) from cytotoxic immunosuppressant drugs or who have had bone marrow or solid organ transplantation. For the latter group, who must continue lifelong immunosuppression to avoid graft rejection, serious infection is a constant hazard. Extensive efforts are made to prevent infections; if these efforts are unsuccessful and infections occur, they may be fatal unless recognized promptly and treated vigorously. The drugs are described in the following sections and in Drugs at a Glance 36-2: Immunosuppressants.

## INDIVIDUAL IMMUNOSUPPRESSANT DRUGS

Immunosuppressants are discussed here as cytotoxic antiproliferative agents, conventional antirejection agents, antibody preparations, and miscellaneous drugs. This grouping is rather arbitrary because most of the drugs could also fit in one or more other categories (eg, the cytotoxic drugs and most of the antibody preparations are also antirejection drugs; some of the drugs can also be called *anticytokines* because they block the actions of cytokines such as IL-2 and TNF). It is hoped that the chosen groupings will assist the reader in differentiating drug sources, effects, and clinical uses.

## Cytotoxic, Antiproliferative Agents

Cytotoxic, antiproliferative drugs damage or kill cells that are able to reproduce, such as immunologically competent lymphocytes. These drugs are used primarily in cancer chemotherapy. However, in small doses, some also exhibit immunosuppressive activities and are used to treat autoimmune disorders (eg, methotrexate) and to prevent rejection reactions in organ transplantation (azathioprine). These drugs cause generalized suppression of the immune system and can kill lymphocytes and nonlymphoid proliferating cells (eg, bone marrow blood cells, gastrointestinal mucosal cells, and germ cells in gonads).

**Azathioprine** is an antimetabolite that interferes with production of DNA and RNA and thus blocks cellular reproduction, growth, and development. Once ingested, azathioprine is metabolized by the liver to 6-mercaptopurine, a purine analog. The purine analog is then incorporated into the DNA of proliferating cells in place of the natural purine bases, leading to the production of abnormal DNA. Rapidly proliferating cells are most affected, including T and B lymphocytes, which normally reproduce rapidly in response to stimulation by an antigen. The drug acts especially on T cells to block cell division, clonal proliferation, and differentiation.

Azathioprine is well absorbed after oral administration, with peak serum concentrations in 1 to 2 hours and a half-life of less than 5 hours. The mercaptopurine resulting from initial biotransformation is inactivated mainly by the enzyme xanthine oxidase. Impaired liver function may decrease metabolism of azathioprine to its active metabolite and therefore decrease pharmacologic effects.

The drug is used mainly to prevent organ graft rejection and has little effect on acute rejection reactions. It is also used to treat severe rheumatoid arthritis not responsive to conventional treatment. When used to prevent

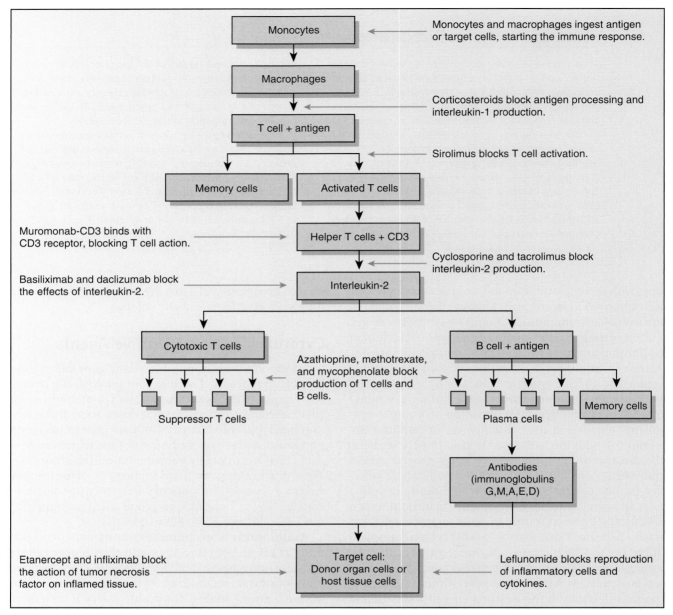

**FIGURE 36–1** Sites of action of immunosuppressants. Available immunosuppressants inhibit the immune response by blocking that response at various sites.

graft rejection, azathioprine is used lifelong. Dosage varies among transplantation centers and types of transplants but depends largely on white blood cell (WBC) and platelet counts.

**Methotrexate** is a folate antagonist. It inhibits dihydrofolate reductase, the enzyme that converts dihydrofolate to the tetrahydrofolate required for biosynthesis of DNA and cell reproduction. The resultant DNA impairment inhibits production and function of immune cells, especially T cells. Methotrexate has long been used in the treatment of cancer. Other uses have evolved from its immunosuppressive effects, including treatment of autoimmune or inflammatory disorders, such as severe arthritis and psoriasis that do not respond to other treat-

ment measures. It is also used (with cyclosporine) to prevent graft-versus-host disease (GVHD) associated with bone marrow transplantation, but it is not approved by the U.S. Food and Drug Administration for this purpose. Lower doses are given for these conditions than for cancers, and adverse drug effects are fewer and less severe.

**Mycophenolate** is similar to azathioprine. It is used for prevention and treatment of rejection reactions with renal, cardiac, and hepatic transplantation. It inhibits proliferation and function of T and B lymphocytes. It has synergistic effects with corticosteroids and cyclosporine and is used in combination with these drugs.

After oral or intravenous (IV) administration, the drug is rapidly broken down to mycophenolic acid, the active

**DRUG TABLE 36-2**

*Drugs at a Glance*

**Immunosuppressants**

| Generic/Trade Name | Routes and Dosage Ranges | Comments |
|---|---|---|
| **Azathioprine** (Imuran)<br>Pregnancy Category D | *Renal transplant:* PO, IV, 3–5 mg/kg/d initially, decreased (1–3 mg/kg/d) for maintenance and in presence of renal impairment<br>*Rheumatoid arthritis:* PO, 1, mg/kg/d (50–100 mg), increased by 0.5 mg/kg/d after 8 wk, then every 5 wk to a maximum dose of 2.5 mg/kg/d. Decrease dosage for maintenance. | To prevent renal transplant rejection<br>For severe rheumatoid arthritis unresponsive to other treatment |
| **Basiliximab** (Simulect)<br>Pregnancy Category B | *Adults:* IV, 20 mg within 2 h before transplantation and 20 mg 4 d after transplantation (total of two doses)<br>*Children (2–15 y):* IV, 12 mg/m$^2$ up to a maximum of 20 mg for two doses as for adults | To prevent renal transplant rejection |
| **Cyclosporine** (Sandimmune, Neoral)<br>Pregnancy Category C | Sandimmune, PO, 15 mg/kg 4–12 h before transplant surgery, then 15 mg/kg once daily for 1–2 wk, then decrease by 5% per week to a maintenance dose of 5–10 mg/kg/d<br>Neoral, PO, the first dose in clients with new transplants is the same as the first oral dose of Sandimmune; later doses are titrated according to the desired cyclosporine blood level<br>IV, 5–6 mg/kg infused over 2–6 h | To prevent rejection of solid organ (eg, heart, kidney, liver) transplant<br>To prevent and treat graft-versus-host disease in bone marrow transplantation |
| **Daclizumab** (Zenapax)<br>Pregnancy Category C | IV, 1 mg/kg over 15 min. First dose within 24 h before transplantation, then a dose every 14 d for four doses (total of five doses) | To prevent renal transplant rejection |
| **Etanercept** (Enbrel)<br>Pregnancy Category B | *Adults:* Sub-Q, 25 mg twice weekly, 72–96 h apart<br>*Children (4–17 y):* Sub-Q, 0.4 mg/kg up to a maximum of 25 mg per dose, twice weekly, 72–96 h apart | For rheumatoid arthritis |
| **Infliximab** (Remicade)<br>Pregnancy Category B | *Crohn's disease, moderate to severe:* IV infusion, 5 mg/kg as a single dose<br>*Crohn's disease, fistulizing:* IV infusion, 5 mg/kg initially and 2 and 6 wk later (total of three doses) | For Crohn's disease, moderate to severe or fistulizing<br>For rheumatoid arthritis |
| **Leflunomide** (Arava)<br>Pregnancy Category X | PO, 100 mg once daily for 3 d, then 20 mg once daily | For rheumatoid arthritis |
| **Lymphocyte immune globulin, antithymocyte globulin, equine** (Atgam)<br>Pregnancy Category C | IV, 15 mg/kg/d for 14 d, then every other day for 14 d (21 doses) | To prevent or treat renal transplant rejection<br>To treat aplastic anemia |
| **Methotrexate (MTX)** (Rheumatrex)<br>Pregnancy Category C | PO, 7.5 mg/wk as single dose, or 2.5 mg q12h for three doses once weekly | For severe rheumatoid arthritis unresponsive to other therapy |
| **Muromonab-CD3** (Orthoclone OKT3)<br>Pregnancy Category C | IV, 5 mg bolus injection once daily for 10–14 d | For treatment of renal, cardiac, and hepatic transplant rejection |

*(continued)*

**DRUG TABLE 36-2**

*Drugs at a Glance*

**Immunosuppressants** (Continued)

| Generic/Trade Name | Routes and Dosage Ranges | Comments |
|---|---|---|
| **Mycophenolate mefetil** (CellCept) Pregnancy Category C | *Renal transplantation:* PO, IV, 1 g twice daily *Cardiac and hepatic transplantation:* PO, IV, 1.5 g twice daily | To prevent renal, cardiac, and hepatic transplant rejection |
| **Sirolimus** (Rapamune) Pregnancy Category C | *Adults:* PO, 6 mg as soon after transplantation as possible, then 2 mg daily *Children >13 y:* PO, 3 mg/m² as loading dose, then 1 mg/m² daily. | To prevent renal transplant rejection |
| **Tacrolimus** (Prograf) Pregnancy Category C | *Adults:* IV infusion, 25–50 mcg/kg/d, starting no sooner than 6 h after transplantation, until the patient can tolerate oral administration, usually 2–3 d PO, 150–200 mcg/kg/d, in two divided doses q12h, with the first dose 8–12 h after stopping the IV infusion *Children:* IV, 50–100 mcg/kg/d PO, 200–300 mcg/kg/d | To prevent liver, kidney, and heart transplant rejection |

component. Mycophenolic acid is further metabolized to inactive metabolites that are eliminated in bile and urine. Neutropenia and thrombocytopenia may occur but are less common and less severe than with azathioprine. Infections with mycophenolate occur at approximately the same rate as with other immunosuppressant drugs. Because of its lesser toxicity, mycophenolate may be preferred over azathioprine, at least in clients who are unable to tolerate azathioprine.

## Conventional Antirejection Agents

Cyclosporine, tacrolimus, and sirolimus are fungal metabolites with strong immunosuppressive effects. Cyclosporine and tacrolimus are chemically unrelated but have a similar action. They inhibit the synthesis of a cytokine, IL-2, which is required for activation of T cells and B cells. Sirolimus is structurally similar to tacrolimus. It inhibits T-cell activation and proliferation in response to several interleukins (eg, IL-2, IL-4, and IL-15). It also inhibits antibody production. Sirolimus and tacrolimus may have stronger immunosuppressant activity than cyclosporine.

By inhibiting helper T-cell proliferation and cytokine expression, these three drugs reduce the activation of various cells involved in graft rejection, including cytotoxic T cells, natural killer cells, macrophages, and B cells. Consequently, they have become a mainstay of heart, liver, kidney, and bone marrow transplantation.

**Cyclosporine** is used to prevent rejection reactions and prolong graft survival after solid organ transplantation (eg, kidney, liver, heart, lung), or to treat chronic rejection in clients previously treated with other immunosuppressive agents. The drug inhibits both cellular and humoral immunity but affects T lymphocytes more than B lymphocytes. With T cells, cyclosporine reduces proliferation of helper and cytotoxic T cells and synthesis of several cytokines (eg, IL-2, interferons). With B cells, cyclosporine reduces production and function to some extent, but considerable activity is retained.

Transplant rejection reactions mainly involve cellular immunity or T cells. With cyclosporine-induced deprivation of IL-2, T cells stimulated by the graft antigen do not undergo clonal expansion and differentiation, and graft destruction is inhibited. In addition to its use in solid organ transplantation, cyclosporine is used to prevent and treat GVHD, a potential complication of bone marrow transplantation. In GVHD, T lymphocytes from the transplanted marrow of the donor mount an immune response against the tissues of the recipient.

Absorption of cyclosporine is slow and incomplete with oral administration. The drug is highly bound to plasma proteins (90%), and approximately 50% is distributed in erythrocytes, so that drug levels in whole blood are significantly higher than those in plasma. Peak plasma levels occur 4 to 5 hours after a dose, and the elimination half-life is 10 to 27 hours. Cyclosporine is metabolized in the liver and excreted in bile; less than 10% is excreted unchanged in urine.

Because the drug is insoluble in water, other solvents are used in commercial formulations. Thus, it is prepared in alcohol and olive oil for oral administration and in alcohol and polyoxyethylated castor oil for IV administration. Anaphylactic reactions, attributed to the castor oil, have occurred with the IV formulation. Neoral is a microemulsion formulation of cyclosporine that is better absorbed than oral Sandimmune. The two formulations are not equivalent and cannot be used interchangeably. Neoral is available in capsules and an oral solution; Sandimmune is available in capsules, oral solution, and an IV solution.

Nephrotoxicity is a major adverse effect. Acute nephrotoxicity commonly occurs and, in some cases, progresses to chronic nephrotoxicity and kidney failure.

**Sirolimus** is used to prevent renal transplant rejection. It acts by inhibiting T-cell activation. It is given concomitantly with a corticosteroid and cyclosporine. It may have synergistic effects with cyclosporine because it has a different mechanism of action. However, the two drugs are metabolized by the same cytochrome P450 3A4 enzymes, and cyclosporine increases blood levels of sirolimus, possibly to toxic levels. Consequently, the drugs should not be given at the same time; sirolimus should be taken 4 hours after a dose of cyclosporine. Sirolimus is contraindicated in patients who are allergic to the drug or who are pregnant or breast-feeding.

Sirolimus is well absorbed with oral administration. Its action has a rapid onset and peaks within 1 hour. It has a long half-life of 62 hours. It is metabolized in the liver and excreted mainly in feces (>90%), with a small amount eliminated in urine (<3%).

Reported adverse effects include abdominal pain, acne, anemia, constipation, diarrhea, edema, headache, hepatotoxicity, hypercholesterolemia, hypertension, insomnia, leukopenia, nausea, nephrotoxicity, skin rash, thrombocytopenia, and tremor. Because of the high risk for infection, with sirolimus as with other immunosuppressant drugs, antimicrobial prophylaxis is recommended for cytomegalovirus (CMV) infection for 3 months and *Pneumocystis carinii* pneumonia for 1 year after transplantation.

**Tacrolimus** (formerly FK506) is similar to cyclosporine in its mechanisms of action, pharmacokinetic characteristics, and adverse effects. It prevents rejection of transplanted organs by inhibiting growth and proliferation of T lymphocytes. Although survival of clients and grafts is approximately the same as with cyclosporine, potential advantages of tacrolimus include less corticosteroid therapy and shorter, less costly hospitalizations.

Tacrolimus is not well absorbed orally; therefore, higher oral doses than IV doses must be given to obtain similar blood levels. With IV administration, action onset is rapid, and peak action occurs in 1 to 2 hours; with oral administration, onset varies, and peak action occurs in 1.5 to 3.5 hours. The drug is well distributed through the body and reaches higher concentrations in erythrocytes than in plasma. It is metabolized in the liver and intestine to several metabolites, which are excreted in bile and urine. It has a half-life of 6 hours. Impaired liver function may slow its metabolism and elimination.

Dosage ranges of tacrolimus vary according to clinical response, adverse effects, and blood concentrations. Serum drug levels are routinely monitored, with therapeutic ranges approximately 10 to 20 ng/mL for 6 months after transplantation, then 5 to 15 ng/mL. Children with transplants metabolize tacrolimus more rapidly than adults with transplants, on a body weight basis. Thus, children require higher doses, based on milligrams per kilogram, to maintain similar plasma drug levels. Dosage does not need to be reduced in renal insufficiency because there is little renal elimination of the drug.

There are numerous potential drug interactions that increase or decrease blood levels and effects of tacrolimus. Because tacrolimus is metabolized mainly by the cytochrome P450 enzymes that metabolize cyclosporine, drug interactions known to alter cyclosporine effects are likely to alter tacrolimus effects. In addition, tacrolimus is a macrolide and may have drug interactions similar to those occurring with erythromycin. Erythromycin is known to increase blood levels and risks for toxicity of several drugs, including oral anticoagulants, digoxin, and theophylline.

The role of tacrolimus in transplantation immunosuppression is not well defined. Because successful liver and intestinal transplantations have been attributed to the drug, some people suggest that tacrolimus may replace cyclosporine as the immunosuppressant of choice for new clients. It may also be useful for clients who do not respond to cyclosporine. In renal transplantation, its role is less clear because high success rates have been achieved with cyclosporine. However, cyclosporine is given with corticosteroids, and tacrolimus may allow corticosteroids to be reduced or stopped, thereby decreasing the adverse effects of long-term corticosteroid therapy. Nephrotoxicity occurs at an approximately equal rate with both drugs.

## Antibody Preparations

Antibody preparations are produced in the laboratory or derived from animals injected with human lymphoid tissue to stimulate an immune response. Such preparations are being extensively used or investigated for use in cancer, transplantation rejection, drug toxicity, Crohn's disease, rheumatoid arthritis, and other diseases. They are also being used in diagnostic imaging technology.

The antibodies may be nonspecific polyclonal or specific monoclonal. *Polyclonal* preparations are a mixture of antibodies (eg, IgA, IgD, IgE, IgG, or IgM) produced by several clones of B lymphocytes. Each clone produces a structurally and functionally different antibody, even though the humoral immune response was induced by a single antigen. *Monoclonal antibodies* are produced in the laboratory by procedures that isolate and clone individual B lymphocytes, resulting in the production of completely identical antibody molecules. The antigen to which the desired antibody will respond is first injected into a mouse. The mouse mounts an immune response in which its B lymphocytes are stimulated to produce a specific antibody against that antigen. The B lymphocytes are then recovered from the spleen of the mouse and mixed with myeloma cells (a cell line that can live forever in culture) in polyethylene glycol. This treatment results in fusion of the cells and produces an antibody-secreting hybridoma, which can be cloned to produce large amounts of the desired antibody. The antibodies can be isolated from the culture and prepared for clinical use. Because the antibodies are proteins and would be destroyed if taken orally, they must be given by injection.

Older animal-derived antibodies (eg, LIG-ATG, muromonab-CD3) are themselves antigenic; they usually elicit human antibodies against the animal cells within 2 weeks. Newer murine (mouse-derived) antibodies (eg, basiliximab) have had human antibodies added by recombinant DNA technology and are less likely to elicit an immune response. However, because the products are proteins, there is some risk for hypersensitivity reactions.

Because they are derived from one cell line or clone, monoclonal antibodies can be designed to suppress the specific components of the immune system that are causing tissue damage in particular disorders. They cause cell destruction by eliciting an antigen–antibody reaction, activating complement, or targeting molecules on the cell surface that are necessary for growth or differentiation of that cell.

Note that the generic names of monoclonal antibodies used as drugs end in *mab* and thus identify their origin.

### Polyclonal Antibody

*Lymphocyte Immune Globulin, Antithymocyte Globulin*
Lymphocyte immune globulin, antithymocyte globulin (LIG-ATG or Atgam) is a nonspecific antibody with activity against all blood cells, although it acts mainly against T lymphocytes. LIG-ATG is obtained from the serum of horses immunized with human thymus tissue or T lymphocytes. It contains antibodies that destroy lymphoid tissues and decrease the number of circulating T cells, thereby suppressing cellular and humoral immune responses. In addition to its high concentration of antibodies against T lymphocytes, the preparation contains low concentrations of antibodies against other blood cells. A skin test is recommended before administration to determine whether the client is allergic to horse serum. Because there is a high risk for anaphylactic reactions in recipients previously sensitized to horse serum, clients with positive skin tests should be desensitized before drug therapy is begun. LIG-ATG may be given for a few weeks to treat rejection reactions after solid organ transplantation, and it may be used to treat aplastic anemia.

### Monoclonal Antibodies

**Basiliximab (Simulect)** and **daclizumab (Zenapax)** are similar drugs. They are humanized IgE (ie, a combination of human and murine antibodies). They are called IL-2 receptor antagonists because they bind to IL-2 receptors on the surface of activated lymphocytes. This action inhibits the ability of IL-2 to stimulate proliferation and cytokine production of lymphocytes, a critical component of the cellular immune response involved in allograft rejection. The drugs are used to prevent organ rejection in clients receiving renal transplants and are given in combination with cyclosporine and a corticosteroid. In clinical trials, adverse effects were consistent with those of transplant status, underlying disease, and concomitant immunosuppressive and other drug therapy. They were also similar to those reported with placebo (ie, basiliximab or daclizumab plus cyclosporine and a corticosteroid, versus placebo plus cyclosporine and a corticosteroid).

**Infliximab** (Remicade) is a humanized IgG monoclonal antibody used to treat rheumatoid arthritis and Crohn's disease. It inhibits a cytokine, TNF-alpha, from binding to its receptors and thus neutralizes its actions. Biologic activities attributed to TNF-alpha include induction of other proinflammatory cytokines (eg, IL-1 and IL-6), increasing leukocyte migration into sites of injury or inflammation, and stimulating neutrophil and eosinophil activity. The ability of infliximab to neutralize TNF-alpha accounts for its anti-inflammatory effects. (It does not neutralize TNF-beta, a related cytokine that uses the same receptors.)

In Crohn's disease, elevated concentrations of TNF-alpha have been found in clients' stools and correlate with episodes of increased disease activity. Infliximab reduces infiltration of inflammatory cells, production of TNF-alpha in inflamed areas of the intestine, and the number of cells that can produce TNF-alpha. It is indicated for clients with moderate to severe disease who do not respond adequately to conventional treatment measures, and for those with draining enterocutaneous fistulas.

Infliximab therapy (ie, anti-TNF therapy) may lead to the formation of autoimmune antibodies and hypersensitivity reactions. Dyspnea, hypotension, and urticaria have occurred. The drug should be administered in settings in which personnel and supplies (eg, epinephrine, antihistamines, corticosteroids) are available for treatment of hypersensitivity reactions, and it should be discontinued if severe reactions occur. In addition, infections developed in approximately 21% of clients in clinical trials, and the drug may aggravate congestive heart failure.

**Muromonab-CD3** (Orthoclone OKT3) is a monoclonal antibody that acts against an antigenic receptor called CD3, which is found on the surface membrane of most T cells in blood and body tissues. *CD* indicates *clusters of differentiation*, or groups of cells with the same surface markers (antigenic receptors). The CD3 molecule is associated with the antigen recognition structure of T cells and is essential for T-cell activation. Muromonab-CD3 binds with its antigen (CD3) and therefore blocks all known functions of T cells containing the CD3 molecule. Because rejection reactions are mainly T-cell–mediated immune responses against antigenic (nonself) tissues, the drug's ability to suppress such reactions accounts for its therapeutic effects in treating renal, cardiac, and hepatic transplant rejection. It is usually given for 10 to 14 days. After treatment, CD3-positive T cells reappear rapidly and reach pretreatment levels within 1 week. The drug's name is derived from its source (murine or mouse cells) and its action (monoclonal antibody against the CD3 antigen). Because the drug is a protein and induces antibodies in most clients, decreased effectiveness and serious allergic reactions may occur if it is readministered later. Second courses of treatment must be undertaken cautiously.

## Miscellaneous Immunosuppressants

**Etanercept** (Enbrel) is a manufactured TNF receptor that binds with TNF and prevents it from binding with its "normal" receptors on cell surfaces. This action inhibits TNF activity in inflammatory and immune responses.

TNF is a naturally occurring cytokine that enhances leukocyte migration into areas of tissue injury and induces the production of other cytokines, such as IL-6. In rheumatoid arthritis, TNF is increased in joint synovial fluid and considered important in joint inflammation and destruction.

The biologic activity of TNF requires its binding to TNF-alpha or TNF-beta receptors on cell surfaces. Etanercept inhibits binding of both TNF-alpha and TNF-beta to cell surface TNF receptors and thereby inactivates TNF.

Etanercept is used to treat moderate to severe rheumatoid arthritis in adults and children who have not received adequate relief of symptoms with other treatments. It can be used in combination with methotrexate in clients who do not respond adequately to methotrexate alone.

**Leflunomide** (Arava) has antiproliferative and anti-inflammatory activities that are attributed to its effects on the immune system. The drug inhibits the synthesis of pyrimidines, which are components of DNA and RNA and therefore important in cell reproduction and growth. Leflunomide is used to treat rheumatoid arthritis in adults. In addition to relieving signs and symptoms, it also slows the progressive destruction of joint tissues.

After oral administration, leflunomide is metabolized to an active metabolite (called M1) that exerts almost all of the drug's effects. M1 has a half-life of about 2 weeks, and a loading dose is usually given for 3 days to achieve therapeutic blood levels more rapidly. It is highly bound to serum albumin and eventually eliminated by further metabolism and renal or biliary excretion. Some of the M1 excreted in bile is reabsorbed, and this contributes to its long half-life. Most adverse effects in clinical trials were similar to those of placebos.

## ■ CORTICOSTEROID USE IN SPECIFIC SITUATIONS

## Adrenal Insufficiency

Adrenal insufficiency is the most clearcut indication for use of a corticosteroid, and even a slight impairment of the adrenal response during severe illness can be lethal if corticosteroid therapy is not provided (see Chap. 20). For example, hypotension is a common symptom in critically ill clients, and hypotension caused by adrenal insufficiency may mimic either hypovolemic or septic shock. If adrenal insufficiency is the cause of the hypotension, administration of corticosteroids can eliminate the need for vasopressor drugs to maintain adequate tissue perfusion.

However, adrenal insufficiency may not be recognized because hypotension and other symptoms also occur with many illnesses. The normal response to illness (eg, pain, hypovolemia) is the increased and prolonged secretion of cortisol. If this does not occur, or if too little cortisol is produced, a state of adrenal insufficiency exists. One way to evaluate a client for adrenal insufficiency is a test in which a baseline serum cortisol level is measured, after which corticotropin is given intravenously to stimulate cortisol production, and the serum cortisol level is measured again in approximately 30 to 60 minutes. Test results are hard to interpret in seriously ill clients, however, because serum cortisol concentrations that would be normal in normal subjects may be low in this population. In addition, a lower-than-expected rise in serum cortisol levels may indicate a normal HPA axis that is already maximally stimulated, or interference with the ability of the adrenal cortex to synthesize cortisol. Thus, a critically ill client may have a limited ability to increase cortisol production in response to stress.

In any client suspected of having adrenal insufficiency, a single IV dose of corticosteroid seems justified. If the client does have adrenal insufficiency, the dose may prevent immediate death and allow time for other diagnostic and therapeutic measures. If the client does not have adrenal insufficiency, the single dose is not harmful.

### Prevention of Acute Adrenocortical Insufficiency

Suppression of the HPA axis may occur with exogenous corticosteroid therapy and may lead to life-threatening inability to increase cortisol secretion when needed to cope with stress. It is most likely to occur with abrupt withdrawal of systemic corticosteroid drugs. The risk for HPA suppression is high with systemic drugs given for more than a few days, although clients vary in degree and duration of suppression with comparable doses, and the minimum dose and duration of therapy that cause suppression are unknown.

When the drugs are given for replacement therapy, adrenal insufficiency is lifelong, and drug administration must be continued. When the drugs are given for purposes other than replacement and then discontinued, the HPA axis usually recovers within several weeks to months, but may take a year. Several strategies have been developed to minimize HPA suppression and risks for acute adrenal insufficiency, including the following:

■ Administer a systemic corticosteroid during high-stress situations (eg, moderate or severe illness, trauma, or surgery) to clients who have received pharmacologic doses for 2 weeks within the previous year or who

(text continues on page 659)

# NURSING PROCESS

## Assessment Related to Initiation of Corticosteroid Therapy

- For a client expected to receive short-term corticosteroid therapy, the major focus of assessment is the extent and severity of symptoms. Such data can then be used to evaluate the effectiveness of drug therapy.
- For a client expected to receive long-term, systemic corticosteroid therapy, a thorough assessment is needed. This may include diagnostic tests for diabetes mellitus, tuberculosis, and peptic ulcer disease because these conditions may develop from or be exacerbated by administration of corticosteroid drugs. If one of these conditions is present, corticosteroid therapy must be altered and other drugs given concomitantly.
- If acute infection is found on initial assessment, it should be treated with appropriate antibiotics either before corticosteroid drugs are started or concomitantly with corticosteroid therapy. This is necessary because corticosteroids may mask symptoms of infection and impair healing. Thus, even minor infections can become serious if left untreated during corticosteroid therapy. If infection occurs during long-term corticosteroid therapy, appropriate antibiotic therapy (as determined by culture of the causative microorganism and antibiotic sensitivity studies) is again indicated. Also, increased doses of corticosteroids are usually indicated to cope with the added stress of the infection.

## Assessment Related to Previous or Current Corticosteroid Therapy

Initial assessment of every client should include information about previous or current treatment with systemic corticosteroids. This can usually be determined by questioning the client or reviewing medical records.

- If the nurse determines that the client has taken corticosteroids in the past, additional information is needed about the specific drug and dosage taken, the purpose and length of therapy, and when therapy was stopped. Such information is necessary for planning nursing care. If the client had an acute illness and received an oral or injected corticosteroid for approximately 1 week or received corticosteroids by local injection or application to skin lesions, no special nursing care is likely to be required. If, however, the client took systemic corticosteroids 2 weeks or longer during the past year, nursing observations must be especially vigilant. Such a client may be at higher risk for development of acute adrenocortical insufficiency during stressful situations. If the client is having surgery, corticosteroid therapy is restarted either before or on the day of surgery and continued, in decreasing dosage, for a few days after surgery. In addition to anesthesia and surgery, potentially significant sources of stress include hospitalization, various diagnostic tests, concurrent infection or other illnesses, and family problems.

  If the client is currently taking a systemic corticosteroid drug, again the nurse must identify the drug, the dosage and schedule of administration, the purpose for which the drug is being taken, and the length of time involved.

Once this basic information is obtained, the nurse can further assess client status and plan nursing care. Some specific factors include the following:

- If the client will undergo anesthesia and surgery, expect that higher doses of corticosteroids will be given for several days. This may be done by changing the drug, the route of administration, and the dosage. Specific regimens vary according to type of anesthesia, surgical procedure, client condition, physician preference, and other variables. A client having major abdominal surgery may be given 300 to 400 mg of hydrocortisone (or the equivalent dosage of other agents) on the day of surgery and then be tapered back to maintenance dosage within a few days.
- Note that additional corticosteroids may be given in other situations as well. One extra dose may be adequate for a short-term stress situation, such as an angiogram or other invasive diagnostic test.
- Using all available data, assess the likelihood of the client's having acute adrenal insufficiency.
- Assess for signs and symptoms of adrenocortical excess and adverse drug effects.
- Assess for signs and symptoms of the disease for which long-term corticosteroid therapy is being given.

## Nursing Diagnoses

- Disturbed Body Image related to cushingoid changes in appearance
- Imbalanced Nutrition: Less Than Body Requirements related to protein and potassium losses
- Imbalanced Nutrition: More Than Body Requirements related to sodium and water retention and hyperglycemia
- Excess Fluid Volume related to sodium and water retention
- Risk for Injury related to adverse drug effects of impaired wound healing; increased susceptibility to infection; weakening of skin and muscles; osteoporosis, gastrointestinal ulceration, diabetes mellitus, hypertension, and acute adrenocortical insufficiency
- Ineffective Coping related to chronic illness, long-term drug therapy and drug-induced mood changes, irritability, and insomnia.
- Deficient Knowledge related to disease process and corticosteroid drug therapy

## Planning/Goals

*The client will:*

- Receive or take the drug correctly
- Receive and practice measures to decrease the need for corticosteroids and minimize adverse effects
- Be monitored regularly for adverse drug effects
- Keep appointments for follow-up care
- Be assisted to cope with body image changes
- Verbalize or demonstrate essential drug information

## Interventions

For clients on long-term, systemic corticosteroid therapy, use supplementary drugs as ordered and nondrug measures to

*(continued)*

## **N**URSING PROCESS (Continued)

decrease dosage and adverse effects of corticosteroid drugs. Some specific measures include the following:

- Help clients to set reasonable goals of drug therapy. For example, partial relief of symptoms may be better than complete relief if the latter requires larger doses or longer periods of treatment with systemic drugs.
- In clients with bronchial asthma and COPD, other treatment measures should be continued during corticosteroid therapy. With asthma, the corticosteroid needs to be given on a regular schedule; inhaled bronchodilators can usually be taken as needed.
- In clients with rheumatoid arthritis, rest, physical therapy, and salicylates or other nonsteroidal anti-inflammatory drugs are continued. Systemic corticosteroid therapy is reserved for severe, acute exacerbations when possible.
- Help clients to identify stressors and to find ways to modify or avoid stressful situations when possible. For example, most clients probably do not think of extreme heat or cold or minor infections as significant stressors. They can be, however, for people taking corticosteroid drugs. This assessment of potential stressors must be individualized because a situation viewed as stressful by one client may not be stressful to another.
- Encourage activity, if not contraindicated, to slow demineralization of bone (osteoporosis). This is especially important in postmenopausal women who are not taking replacement estrogens, because they are very susceptible to osteoporosis. Walking is preferred if the client is able. Range-of-motion exercises are indicated in immobilized or bedfast people. Also, bedfast clients taking corticosteroid drugs should have their positions changed frequently because these drugs thin the skin and increase the risk of pressure ulcers. This risk is further increased if edema also is present.

- Dietary changes may be beneficial in some clients. Salt restriction may help prevent hypernatremia, fluid retention, and edema. Foods high in potassium may help prevent hypokalemia. A diet high in protein, calcium, and vitamin D may help to prevent osteoporosis. Increased intake of vitamin C may help to decrease bleeding in the skin and soft tissues.
- Avoid exposing the client to potential sources of infection by washing hands frequently, using aseptic technique when changing dressings, keeping health care personnel and visitors with colds or other infections away from the client, and following other appropriate measures. Reverse or protective isolation of the client is sometimes indicated, commonly for those who have had organ transplants and are receiving corticosteroids to help prevent rejection of the transplanted organ.
- Handle tissues very gently during any procedures (eg, bathing, assisting out of bed, venipunctures). Because long-term corticosteroid therapy weakens the skin and bones, there are risks of skin damage and fractures with even minor trauma.

### Evaluation

- Interview and observe for relief of symptoms for which corticosteroids were prescribed.
- Interview and observe for accurate drug administration.
- Interview and observe for use of nondrug measures indicated for the condition being treated.
- Interview and observe for adverse drug effects on a regular basis.
- Interview regarding drug knowledge and effects to be reported to health care providers.

---

## CLIENT TEACHING GUIDELINES
## Long-term Corticosteroids

### General Considerations

✔ In most instances, corticosteroids are used to relieve symptoms; they do not cure the underlying disease process. However, they can improve comfort and quality of life.

✔ When taking an oral corticosteroid (eg, prednisone) for longer than 2 weeks, it is extremely important to take the drug as directed. Missing a dose or two, stopping the drug, changing the amount or time of administration, or taking extra drug (except as specifically directed during stress situations) or any other alterations may result in complications. Some complications are relatively minor; several are serious, even life threatening. When these drugs are being discontinued, the dosage is gradually reduced over several weeks. They must not be stopped abruptly.

✔ Wear a special medical alert bracelet or tag or carry an identification card stating the drug being taken; the dosage; the physician's name, address, and telephone number; and instructions for emergency treatment. If an accident or emergency situation occurs, health care providers must know about corticosteroid drug therapy to give additional amounts during the stress of the emergency.

✔ Report to all health care providers consulted that corticosteroid drugs are being taken or have been taken within the past year. Current or previous corticosteroid therapy can influence treatment measures, and such knowledge increases the ability to provide appropriate treatment.

*(continued)*

CLIENT TEACHING GUIDELINES
## Long-term Corticosteroids (Continued)

✔ Maintain regular medical supervision. This is extremely important so that the physician can detect adverse reactions, evaluate disease status, and evaluate drug response and indications for dosage change, as well as other responsibilities that can be carried out only with personal contact between the physician and the client. Periodic blood tests, x-ray studies, and other tests may be performed during long-term corticosteroid therapy.

✔ Take no other drugs, prescription or nonprescription, without notifying the physician who is supervising corticosteroid therapy. Corticosteroid drugs influence reactions to other drugs, and some other drugs interact with corticosteroids either to increase or decrease their effects. Thus, taking other drugs can decrease the expected therapeutic benefits or increase the incidence or severity of adverse effects.

✔ Avoid exposure to infection when possible. Avoid crowds and people known to have an infection. Also, wash hands frequently and thoroughly. These drugs increase the likelihood of infection, so preventive measures are necessary. Also, if infection does occur, healing is likely to be slow.

✔ Practice safety measures to avoid accidents (eg, falls and possible fractures due to osteoporosis, cuts or other injuries because of delayed wound healing, soft tissue trauma because of increased tendency to bruise easily).

✔ Weigh frequently when starting corticosteroid therapy and at least weekly during long-term maintenance. An initial weight gain is likely to occur and is usually attributed to increased appetite. Later weight gains may be caused by fluid retention.

✔ Ask the physician about the amount and kind of activity or exercise needed. As a general rule, being as active as possible helps to prevent or delay osteoporosis, a common adverse effect. However, increased activity may not be desirable for everyone. A client with rheumatoid arthritis, for example, may become too active when drug therapy relieves joint pain and increases mobility.

✔ Follow instructions for other measures used in treatment of the particular condition (eg, other drugs and physical therapy for rheumatoid arthritis). Such measures may allow smaller doses of corticosteroids and decrease adverse effects.

✔ Because the corticosteroid impairs the ability to respond to stress, dosage may need to be temporarily increased with illness, surgery, or other stressful situations. Clarify with the physician predictable sources of stress and the amount of drug to be taken if the stress cannot be avoided.

✔ In addition to stressful situations, report sore throat, fever, or other signs of infection; weight gain of 5 lbs. or more in a week; or swelling in the ankles or elsewhere. These symptoms may indicate adverse drug effects and changes in corticosteroid therapy may be indicated.

✔ Muscle weakness and fatigue or disease symptoms may occur when drug dosage is reduced, withdrawn, or omitted (eg, the nondrug day of alternate-day therapy). Although these symptoms may cause some discomfort, they should be tolerated if possible rather than increasing the corticosteroid dose. If severe, of course, dosage or time of administration may have to be changed.

✔ Dietary changes may be helpful in reducing some adverse effects of corticosteroid therapy. Decreasing salt intake (eg, by not adding table salt to foods and avoiding obviously salty foods, such as many snack foods and prepared sandwich meats) may help decrease swelling. Eating high-potassium foods, such as citrus fruits and juices or bananas, may help prevent potassium loss. An adequate intake of calcium, protein, and vitamin D (meat and dairy products are good sources) may help to prevent or delay osteoporosis. Vitamin C (eg, from citrus fruits) may help to prevent excessive bruising.

✔ Do not object when your physician reduces your dose of oral corticosteroid, with the goal of stopping the drug entirely or continuing with a smaller dose. Long-term therapy should be used only when necessary because of the potential for serious adverse effects, and the lowest effective dose should be given.

✔ With local applications of corticosteroids, there is usually little systemic absorption and few adverse effects, compared with oral or injected drugs. When effective in relieving symptoms, it is better to use a local than a systemic corticosteroid. In some instances, combined systemic and local application allows administration of a lesser dose of the systemic drug.

Commonly used local applications are applied topically to skin disorders, by oral inhalation for asthma, and by nasal inhalation for allergic rhinitis. Although long-term use is usually well tolerated, systemic toxicity can occur if excess corticosteroid is inhaled or if occlusive dressings are used over skin lesions. Thus, a corticosteroid for local application must be applied correctly and not overused.

✔ Corticosteroids are not the same as the steroids often abused by athletes and body builders. Those are anabolic steroids derived from testosterone, the male sex hormone.

### Self-administration or Caregiver Administration

✔ Take an oral corticosteroid with a meal or snack to decrease gastrointestinal upset. However, do not take it with an antacid (eg, Tums, Maalox). Antacids decrease absorption of the corticosteroid and therefore decrease its beneficial effects.

✔ If taking the medication once a day or every other day, take before 9 AM; if taking multiple doses, take at evenly spaced intervals throughout the day.

*(continued)*

## CLIENT TEACHING GUIDELINES
### Long-term Corticosteroids (Continued)

✔ Report to the physician if unable to take a dose orally because of vomiting or some other problem. In some circumstances, the dose may need to be given by injection.

✔ If taking an oral corticosteroid in tapering doses, be sure to follow instructions exactly to avoid adverse effects.

✔ When applying a corticosteroid to skin lesions, do not apply more often than ordered and do not cover with an occlusive dressing unless specifically instructed to do so.

✔ With an intranasal corticosteroid, use on a regular basis (usually once or twice daily) for the best anti-inflammatory effects.

✔ With an oral inhalation corticosteroid, use on a regular schedule for anti-inflammatory effects. The drugs are *not* effective in relieving acute asthma

attacks or shortness of breath and should not be used "as needed" for that purpose. Use metered-dose inhalers as follows (unless instructed otherwise by a health care provider):
1. Shake canister thoroughly.
2. Place canister between lips (both open and pursed lips have been recommended) or outside lips.
3. Exhale completely.
4. Activate canister while taking a slow, deep breath.
5. Hold breath for 10 seconds or as long as possible.
6. Wait at least 1 minute before taking additional inhalations.
7. Rinse mouth after inhalations to decrease the incidence of oral thrush (a fungal infection).
8. Rinse mouthpiece at least once per day.

---

receive long-term systemic therapy (ie, are steroid dependent).

■ Give short courses of systemic therapy for acute disorders, such as asthma attacks, then decrease the dose or stop the drug within a few days.

■ Gradually taper the dose of any systemic corticosteroid. Although specific guidelines for tapering dosage have not been developed, higher doses and longer durations of administration in general require slower tapering, possibly over several weeks. The goal of tapering may be to stop the drug or to decrease the dosage to the lowest effective amount.

■ Use local rather than systemic therapy whenever possible, either alone or in combination with low doses of systemic drugs. Numerous preparations are available for local application, including aerosols, topicals, and intraarticular injections.

■ Use alternate-day therapy, which involves titrating the daily dose to the lowest effective maintenance level, then giving a double dose every other day. This schedule allows rest periods so that adverse effects are decreased while anti-inflammatory effects continue. Symptoms may flare in the long interval between dosing as the drug level falls to a subtherapeutic level.

## Asthma

Corticosteroids are commonly used in the treatment of asthma for anti-inflammatory and other effects, and their use in respiratory conditions is described in detail in Chapter 37. In acute asthma attacks or status asthmaticus unrelieved by an inhaled beta-adrenergic bronchodilator, high doses of systemic corticosteroids are given orally or intravenously along with the bronchodilator for approximately 5 to 10 days. Although these high doses suppress the HPA axis, the suppression lasts for only 1 to 3 days, and other serious adverse effects are avoided.

Thus, systemic corticosteroids are used in short courses as needed and not for long-term treatment. People who regularly use inhaled corticosteroids also need high doses of systemic drugs during acute attacks because aerosols are not effective. As soon as acute symptoms subside, dosage should be tapered to the lowest effective maintenance dose, or the drug should be discontinued.

In chronic asthma, inhaled corticosteroids are drugs of first choice. This recommendation evolved from increased knowledge about the importance of inflammation in the pathophysiology of asthma and the development of aerosol corticosteroids that are effective with minimal adverse effects. Inhaled drugs may be given alone or with systemic drugs. In general, inhaled corticosteroids can replace oral drugs when daily dosage of the oral agent has been tapered to 10 to 15 mg of prednisone or the equivalent dosage of other agents. When a client is being switched from an oral to an inhaled corticosteroid, the inhaled drug should be started during tapering of the oral drug, approximately 1 or 2 weeks before discontinuing or reaching the lowest anticipated dose of the oral drug. When a client requires a systemic corticosteroid, co-administration of an aerosol allows smaller doses of the systemic corticosteroid. Although the inhaled drugs can cause suppression of the HPA axis and adrenocortical function, especially at higher doses, they are much less likely to do so than systemic drugs.

In addition to their anti-inflammatory effects, corticosteroids also increase the effects of adrenergic bronchodilators that are given in asthma and other disorders to prevent or treat bronchoconstriction and bronchospasm. They perform this important function by increasing the number and responsiveness of beta-adrenergic receptors and preventing the tolerance usually associated with chronic administration of adrenergic bronchodilators. Research studies indicate increased responsiveness to beta-adrenergic bronchodilators within 2 hours and increased numbers of beta receptors within 4 hours of cortico-steroid administration.

## Chronic Obstructive Pulmonary Disease

Corticosteroids are more helpful in acute exacerbations than in stable disease. However, oral corticosteroids may improve pulmonary function and symptoms in some clients. For a client with inadequate relief from a bron-chodilator, a trial of a corticosteroid (eg, prednisone, 20 to 40 mg each morning for 5 to 7 days) may be justi-fied. Treatment should be continued only if there is sig-nificant improvement. As in other conditions, the lowest effective dose is needed to minimize adverse drug effects.

Inhaled corticosteroids can also be tried. They pro-duce minimal adverse effects, but their effectiveness in chronic obstructive pulmonary disease (COPD) has not been clearly demonstrated.

## Adult Respiratory Distress Syndrome

Although corticosteroids have been widely used, several well-controlled studies demonstrate that the drugs are not beneficial in early treatment or in prevention of adult respiratory distress syndrome (ARDS). Thus, cortico-steroids should be used in these clients only if there are other specific indications.

## Cancer

Corticosteroids are commonly used in the treatment of lymphomas, lymphocytic leukemias, and multiple myeloma. In these disorders, corticosteroids inhibit cell reproduction and are cytotoxic to lymphocytes. In addition to their anticancer effects in hematologic malignancies, corticosteroids are beneficial in treatment of several signs and symptoms that often accompany cancer. Although the mechanisms of action are unknown and drug and dosage regimens vary widely, corticosteroids are used to treat anorexia, nausea and vomiting, cerebral edema and inflammation associated with brain metastases or radia-tion of the head, spinal cord compression, pain and edema related to pressure on nerves or bone metastases, GVHD after bone marrow transplantation, and other disorders. Clients tend to feel better when taking corticosteroids, although the basic disease process may be unchanged. The following are some guidelines for corticosteroid therapy of cancer and associated symptoms:

*Primary central nervous system (CNS) lymphomas.* Formerly considered rare tumors of older adults, these tumors are being diagnosed more often in younger clients. They are usually associated with chronic immunosuppression from immunosuppressant drugs or from acquired immunodeficiency syndrome (AIDS). Many of these lymphomas are very sensitive to corticosteroids, and therapy is indicated once the diagnosis is established.

*Other central nervous system tumors.* Corticosteroid therapy may be useful in both supportive and definitive treat-ment of brain and spinal cord tumors; neurologic signs and symptoms often improve dramatically within 24 to 48 hours. Corticosteroids help to relieve symp-toms by controlling edema around the tumor, at oper-ative sites, and at sites receiving radiation therapy. Some clients can be tapered off corticosteroids after surgical or radiation therapy; others require continued therapy to manage neurologic symptoms. Adverse effects of long-term corticosteroid therapy may include mental changes ranging from mild agitation to psy-chosis and steroid myopathy (muscle weakness and atrophy), which may be confused with tumor progres-sion. Mental symptoms usually improve if drug dosage is reduced and resolve if the drug is discontinued; steroid myopathy may persist for weeks or months.

*Chemotherapy-induced emesis.* Corticosteroids have strong antiemetic effects; the mechanism is unknown. One effective regimen combines an oral or IV dose of dex-amethasone (10 to 20 mg) with a serotonin antagonist or metoclopramide and is given immediately before the chemotherapeutic drug. This regimen is the treat-ment of choice for chemotherapy with cisplatin, which is a strongly emetic drug.

## Sepsis

Large, well-controlled multicenter studies have shown no beneficial effect from the use of corticosteroids in gram-negative bacteremia, sepsis, or septic shock. In addition, the drugs do not prevent development of ARDS or mul-tiple organ dysfunction syndrome or decrease mortality in clients with sepsis. In addition, clients receiving corti-costeroid therapy for other conditions are at risk for development of sepsis because the drugs impair the abil-ity of WBCs to leave the bloodstream and reach a site of infection.

## Acquired Immunodeficiency Syndrome

Adrenal insufficiency is being increasingly recognized in the AIDS population, and clients should be assessed and treated for it, if indicated. In addition, corticosteroid ther-apy improves survival and decreases risks for respiratory failure with pneumocystosis, a common cause of death in clients with AIDS. The effect of corticosteroids on risks for development of other opportunistic infections or neoplasms is unknown.

## Arthritis

Corticosteroids are the most effective drugs for rapid relief of the pain, edema, and restricted mobility associated with acute episodes of joint inflammation. They are usu-ally given on a short-term basis. When inflammation is limited to three or fewer joints, the preferred route of drug administration is by injection directly into the joint.

Intraarticular injections relieve symptoms in approximately 2 to 8 weeks, and several formulations are available for this route. However, these drugs do not prevent disease progression and joint destruction. As a general rule, a joint should not be injected more often than three times yearly because of risks for infection and damage to intraarticular structures from the injections and from overuse when pain is relieved.

## ■ IMMUNOSUPPRESSANT DRUG USE IN SPECIFIC SITUATIONS

### Tissue and Organ Transplantation

Tissue and organ transplantation usually involves replacing diseased host tissue with healthy donor tissue. The

*(text continues on page 666)*

*Nursing Actions*
## Corticosteroid Drugs

| **Nursing Actions** | **Rationale/Explanation** |
|---|---|
| 1. Administer accurately. | |
| a. Read the drug label carefully to be certain of having the correct preparation for the intended route of administration. | Many corticosteroid drugs are available in several different preparations. For example, hydrocortisone is available in formulations for intravenous (IV) or intramuscular (IM) administration, for intra-articular injection, and for topical application in creams and ointments of several different strengths. These preparations cannot be used interchangeably without causing potentially serious adverse reactions and decreasing therapeutic effects. Some drugs are available for only one use. For example, several preparations are for topical use only; beclomethasone is prepared only for oral and nasal inhalation. |
| b. With oral corticosteroids, | |
| (1) Give single daily doses or alternate day doses between 6 and 9 AM | Early morning administration causes less suppression of hypothalamic–pituitary–adrenal (HPA) function. |
| (2) Give multiple doses at evenly spaced intervals. | |
| (3) If dosage is being tapered, follow the exact schedule. | To avoid adverse effects |
| (4) Give with meals or snacks. | To decrease gastrointestinal (GI) upset |
| (5) With oral budesonide (Entocort EC), ask the client to swallow the drug whole, without biting or chewing. | This drug is formulated to dissolve in the intestine and have local anti-inflammatory effects. Biting or chewing allows it to dissolve in the stomach. |
| (6) Do *not* give these drugs with an antacid containing aluminum or magnesium (eg, Maalox, Mylanta). | The antacids decrease absorption of corticosteroids, with possible reduction of therapeutic effects. |
| c. For IV or IM administration: | |
| (1) Shake the medication vial well before withdrawing medication. | Most of the injectable formulations are suspensions, which need to be mixed well for accurate dosage. |
| (2) Give a direct IV injection over at least 1 min. | To increase safety of administration |
| d. For oral or nasal inhalation of a corticosteroid, check the instruction leaflet that accompanies the inhaler. | These drugs are given by metered dose inhalers or nasal sprays, and correct usage of the devices is essential to drug administration and therapeutic effects. |
| 2. Observe for therapeutic effects. | The primary objective of corticosteroid therapy is to relieve signs and symptoms, because the drugs are not curative. Therefore, therapeutic effects depend largely on the reason for use. |
| a. With adrenocortical insufficiency, observe for absence or decrease of weakness, weight loss, anorexia, nausea, vomiting, hyperpigmentation, hypotension, hypoglycemia, hyponatremia, and hyperkalemia. | These signs and symptoms of impaired metabolism do not occur with adequate replacement of corticosteroids. |
| b. With rheumatoid arthritis, observe for decreased pain and edema in joints, greater capacity for movement, and increased ability to perform usual activities of daily living. | |

*(continued)*

## Nursing Actions

## Corticosteroid Drugs (Continued)

| Nursing Actions | Rationale/Explanation |
|---|---|
| c. With asthma and chronic obstructive pulmonary disease, observe for decrease in respiratory distress and increased tolerance of activity. | |
| d. With skin lesions, observe for decreasing inflammation. | |
| e. When the drug is given to suppress the immune response to organ transplants, therapeutic effect is the absence of signs and symptoms indicating rejection of the transplanted tissue. | |
| 3. Observe for adverse effects. | These are uncommon with replacement therapy but common with long-term administration of the pharmacologic doses used for many disease processes. Adverse reactions may affect every body tissue and organ. |
| a. Adrenocortical insufficiency—fainting, weakness, anorexia, nausea, vomiting, hypotension, shock, and if untreated, death | This reaction is likely to occur in clients receiving daily corticosteroid drugs who encounter stressful situations. It is caused by drug-induced suppression of the HPA axis, which makes the client unable to respond to stress by increasing adrenocortical hormone secretion. |
| b. Adrenocortical excess (hypercorticism or Cushing's disease) | Most adverse effects result from excessive corticosteroids. |
|    (1) "Moon face," "buffalo hump" contour of shoulders, obese trunk, thin extremities | This appearance is caused by abnormal fat deposits in cheeks, shoulders, breasts, abdomen, and buttocks. These changes are more cosmetic than physiologically significant. However, the alterations in self-image can lead to psychological problems. These changes cannot be prevented, but they may be partially reversed if corticosteroid therapy is discontinued or reduced in dosage. |
|    (2) Diabetes mellitus—glycosuria, hyperglycemia, polyuria, polydipsia, polyphagia, impaired healing, and other signs and symptoms | Corticosteroid drugs can cause hyperglycemia and diabetes mellitus or aggravate preexisting diabetes mellitus by their effects on carbohydrate metabolism. |
|    (3) Central nervous system effects—euphoria, psychological dependence, nervousness, insomnia, depression, personality and behavioral changes, aggravation of preexisting psychiatric disorders | Some clients enjoy the drug-induced euphoria so much that they resist attempts to withdraw the drug or decrease its dosage |
|    (4) Musculoskeletal effects—osteoporosis, pathologic fractures, muscle weakness and atrophy, decreased linear growth in children | Demineralization of bone produces thin, weak bones that fracture easily. Fractures of vertebrae, long bones, and ribs are relatively common, especially in postmenopausal women and immobilized clients. Myopathy results from abnormal protein metabolism. Decreased growth in children results from impaired bone formation and protein metabolism. |
|    (5) Cardiovascular, fluid, and electrolyte effects— fluid retention, edema, hypertension, congestive heart failure, hypernatremia, hypokalemia, metabolic alkalosis | These effects result largely from mineralocorticoid activity, which causes retention of sodium and water. They are more likely to occur with older corticosteroids, such as hydrocortisone and prednisone. |
|    (6) Gastrointestinal effects—nausea, vomiting, possible peptic ulcer disease, increased appetite, obesity | |
|    (7) Increased susceptibility to infection and delayed wound healing | Caused by suppression of normal inflammatory and immune processes and impaired protein metabolism |
|    (8) Menstrual irregularities, acne, excessive facial hair | Caused by excessive sex hormones, primarily androgens |
|    (9) Ocular effects—increased intraocular pressure, glaucoma, cataracts | |
|    (10) Integumentary effects—skin becomes reddened, thinner, has stretch marks, and is easily injured | |

## *Nursing Actions*

## Corticosteroid Drugs (Continued)

| Nursing Actions | Rationale/Explanation |
|---|---|
| 4. Observe for drug interactions. | |
|    a. Drugs that *increase* effects of corticosteroids: | |
|      (1) Estrogens, oral contraceptives, ketoconazole, macrolide antibiotics (eg, erythromycin) | These drugs apparently inhibit the enzymes that normally metabolize corticosteroids in the liver. |
|      (2) Diuretics (eg, furosemide, thiazides) | Increase hypokalemia |
|    b. Drugs that *decrease* effects of corticosteroids: | |
|      (1) Antacids, cholestyramine | Decrease absorption |
|      (2) Carbamazepine, phenytoin, rifampin | These drugs induce microsomal enzymes in the liver and increase the rate at which corticosteroids are metabolized or deactivated. |

## Age-related Considerations: Use of Corticosteroids and Immunosuppressants

### USE IN CHILDREN

Corticosteroids are used for the same conditions in children as in adults. Parents and health care providers can monitor drug effects by recording height and weight weekly. Alternate-day therapy (ADT) is less likely to impair normal growth and development than daily administration. In addition, for both systemic and inhaled corticosteroids, each child's dose should be titrated to the lowest effective amount.

Most immunosuppressants are used in children for the same disorders and with similar effects as in adults. Corticosteroids impair growth in children. As a result, some transplantation centers avoid prednisone therapy until a rejection episode occurs. When prednisone is used, administering it every other day may improve growth rates. *Cyclosporine* has been safely and effectively given to children as young as 6 months of age, but extensive studies have not been performed. *Muromonab-CD3* has been used successfully in children as young as 2 years of age; however, safety and efficacy for use in children have not been established. *Mycophenolate* has been used in a few children undergoing renal transplantation. In children with impaired renal function, recommended doses of mycophenolate cause a high incidence of adverse effects. Thus, dosage should be adjusted for the level of renal function. *Tacrolimus* has been used in children younger than 12 years of age who were undergoing liver transplantation. This usage indicates that children require higher doses to maintain therapeutic blood levels than adults because they metabolize the drug more rapidly.

Little information is available about the use of newer immunosuppressants in children. Safety and effectiveness have not been established for *basiliximab, daclizumab, infliximab,* or *leflunomide.* Leflunomide is not recommended for children younger than 18 years of age. *Etanercept* is approved for clients 4 to 17 years of age with juvenile rheumatoid arthritis. In clinical trials, effects in children were similar to those in adults. Most children in a 3-month study had an infection while receiving etanercept. The infections were usually mild and consistent with those commonly seen in outpatient pediatric settings. Children reported abdominal pain, nausea, vomiting, and headache more often than adults. Other medications (eg, a corticosteroid, methotrexate, a nonsteroidal anti-inflammatory drug, or an analgesic) may be continued during treatment.

### USE IN OLDER ADULTS

Corticosteroids are used for the same conditions in older adults as in younger ones. Older adults are especially likely to have conditions that are aggravated by the drugs (eg, congestive heart failure, hypertension, diabetes mellitus, arthritis, osteoporosis, increased susceptibility to infection, and concomitant drug therapy that increases risks for gastrointestinal ulceration and bleeding). Consequently, risk-to-benefit ratios of systemic corticosteroid therapy should be carefully considered, especially for long-term therapy.

When used, lower doses are usually indicated because of decreased muscle mass, plasma volume, hepatic metabolism, and renal excretion in older adults. In addition, therapeutic and adverse responses should be monitored regularly by a health care provider (eg, blood pressure, serum electrolytes, and blood glucose levels at least every 6 months). As in other populations, adverse effects are less likely to occur with oral or nasal inhalations than with oral drugs.

Immunosuppressants are used for the same purposes and produce similar therapeutic and adverse effects in older adults as in younger adults. Because older adults often have multiple disorders and organ impairments, it is especially important that drug choices, dosages, and monitoring tests are individualized. In addition, infections occur more commonly in older adults, and this tendency may be increased with immunosuppressant therapy.

## Home Care Considerations: Use of Corticosteroids and Immunosuppressants

***ASSESS:*** client's understanding of the importance of meticulous environmental cleansing, personal hygiene, and handwashing. Assess medication regimen, serum drug levels, use of Medic Alert device, and quality-of-life considerations.

***MONITOR:*** for compliance with the prescribed regimen, therapeutic and adverse drug effects, especially with changes in drugs or dosages; that client is keeping appointments for observation and follow-up care. Also monitor environment for potential sources of infections, including people with infections, caregivers, water or soil

around live plants, and raw fruits and vegetables. Evaluate client's need for additional information and provide that information

***EDUCATE:*** regarding importance of reading and following medication instructions, not exceeding recommended dosages without consulting a health care provider, and interventions to minimize adverse effects of these drugs and decrease risks for infection. Reinforce additional teaching points regarding specific drug preparations (see Client Teaching Guidelines: Long-Term Corticosteroids; Immunosuppressant Drugs).

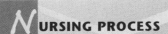

# NURSING PROCESS

## Assessment Related to Use of Immunosuppressants

- Assess clients receiving or anticipating immunosuppressant drug therapy for signs and symptoms of current infection or factors predisposing them to potential infection (eg, impaired skin integrity, invasive devices, cigarette smoking).
- Assess the environment for factors predisposing to infection (eg, family or health care providers with infections, contact with young children, and potential exposure to childhood infectious diseases).
- Assess nutritional status, including appetite and weight.
- Assess baseline values of laboratory and other diagnostic test results to aid monitoring of responses to immunosuppressant drug therapy. With pretransplantation clients, this includes assessing for impaired function of the diseased organ and for abnormalities that need treatment before surgery.
- Assess adequacy of support systems for transplantation recipients.
- Assess post-transplantation clients for surgical wound healing, manifestations of organ rejection, and adverse effects of immunosuppressant drugs.
- Assess clients with autoimmune disorders (eg, rheumatoid arthritis, Crohn's disease) for manifestations of the disease process and responses to drug therapy.

## Nursing Diagnoses

- Risk for Injury: Adverse drug effects
- Risk for Injury: Infection and cancer related to immunosuppression and increased susceptibility
- Deficient Knowledge: Disease process and immunosuppressant drug therapy
- Anxiety related to the diagnosis of serious disease or need for organ transplantation
- Social Isolation related to activities to reduce exposure to infection

## Planning/Goals

The client will:

- Participate in decision making about the treatment plan
- Receive or take immunosuppressant drugs correctly
- Verbalize or demonstrate essential drug information
- Participate in interventions to prevent infection (eg, maintain good hygiene, avoid known sources of infection) while immunosuppressed
- Experience relief or reduction of disease symptoms
- Maintain adequate levels of nutrition and fluids, rest and sleep, and exercise
- Be assisted to cope with anxiety related to the disease process and drug therapy
- Keep appointments for follow-up care
- Have adverse drug effects prevented or recognized and treated promptly
- Maintain diagnostic test values within acceptable limits
- Maintain family and other emotional or social support systems
- Receive optimal instructions and information about the treatment plan, self-care in activities of daily living, reporting adverse drug effects, and other concerns
- Before and after tissue or organ transplantation, receive appropriate care, including prevention or early recognition and treatment of rejection reactions

## Interventions

- Practice and emphasize good personal hygiene and handwashing techniques by clients and all others in contact with clients.
- Use sterile technique for all injections, IV site care, wound dressing changes, and any other invasive diagnostic or therapeutic measures.
- Screen staff and visitors for signs and symptoms of infection; if infection is noted, do not allow contact with the client.
- Report fever and other manifestations of infection *immediately*.

*(continued)*

## NURSING PROCESS (Continued)

- Allow clients to participate in decision making when possible and appropriate.
- Use isolation techniques according to institutional policies, usually after transplantation or when the neutrophil count is below 500/mm³.
- Assist clients to maintain adequate nutrition, rest and sleep, and exercise.
- Inform clients about diagnostic test results, planned changes in therapeutic regimens, and evidence of progress.
- Allow family members or significant others to visit clients when feasible.
- Monitor complete blood count (CBC) and other diagnostic test results related to blood, liver, and kidney function throughout drug therapy. Specific tests vary with the client's health or illness status and the immunosuppressant drugs being taken.
- Schedule and coordinate drug administration to maximize therapeutic effects and minimize adverse effects.
- Consult other health care providers (eg, physician, dietitian, social worker) on the client's behalf when indicated. Multidisciplinary consultation is essential for transplan-

tation clients and desirable for clients with autoimmune disorders.
- Assist clients in learning strategies to manage day-to-day activities during long-term immunosuppression.

### Evaluation

- Interview and observe for accurate drug administration.
- Interview and observe for personal hygiene practices and infection-avoiding maneuvers.
- Interview and observe for therapeutic and adverse drug effects with each client contact.
- Interview regarding knowledge and attitude toward the drug therapy regimen, including follow-up care and symptoms to report to health care providers.
- Determine the number and types of infections that have occurred in the neutropenic client.
- Compare current CBC and other reports with baseline values for acceptable levels, according to the client's condition.
- Observe and interview outpatients regarding compliance with follow-up care.
- Interview and observe for organ function and absence of rejection reactions in post-transplantation clients.

---

## CLIENT TEACHING GUIDELINES
## Immunosuppressant Drugs

### General Considerations

✔ People taking medications that suppress the immune system are at high risk for development of infections. As a result, clients, caregivers, and others in the client's environment need to wash their hands often and thoroughly, practice meticulous personal hygiene, avoid contact with infected people, and practice other methods of preventing infection.

✔ Report adverse drug effects (eg, signs or symptoms of infection such as sore throat or fever, decreased urine output if taking cyclosporine, easy bruising or bleeding if taking azathioprine or methotrexate) to a health care provider.

✔ Try to maintain healthy lifestyle habits, such as a nutritious diet, adequate rest and sleep, and avoiding tobacco and alcohol. These measures enhance immune mechanisms and other body defenses.

✔ Carry identification that lists the drugs being taken; the dosage; the physician's name, address, and telephone number; and instructions for emergency treatment. This information is needed if an accident or emergency situation occurs.

✔ Inform all health care providers that you are taking these drugs.

✔ Maintain regular medical supervision. This is extremely important for detecting adverse drug reactions, evaluating disease status, evaluating drug

responses and indications for dosage change, and having blood tests or other monitoring tests when needed.

✔ Take no other drugs, prescription or nonprescription, without notifying the physician who is managing immunosuppressant therapy. Immunosuppressant drugs may influence reactions to other drugs, and other drugs may influence reactions to the immunosuppressants. Thus, taking other drugs may decrease therapeutic effects or increase adverse effects. In addition, vaccinations may be less effective, and some should be avoided while taking immunosuppressant drugs.

✔ People of reproductive capability who are sexually active should practice effective contraceptive techniques during immunosuppressive drug therapy. With methotrexate, use contraception during and for at least 3 months (men) or one ovulatory cycle (women) after stopping the drug. With mycophenolate, effective contraception should be continued for 6 weeks after the drug is stopped. With sirolimus, effective contraception must be used before, during, and for 12 weeks after drug therapy. The drug was toxic to embryos and fetuses in animal studies.

✔ Wear protective clothing and use sunscreens to decrease exposure of skin to sunlight and risks of skin cancers. Also, methotrexate and sirolimus increase sensitivity to sunlight and may increase sunburn.

*(continued)*

## CLIENT TEACHING GUIDELINES
## Immunosuppressant Drugs (Continued)

### Self-administration

✔ Follow instructions about taking the drugs. This is vital to achieving beneficial effects and decreasing adverse effects. If unable to take a medication, report to the prescribing physician or other health care provider; do not stop unless advised to do so. For transplant recipients, missed doses may lead to transplant rejection; for clients with autoimmune diseases, missed doses may lead to acute flare-ups of symptoms. In addition, take at approximately the same time each day to maintain consistent drug levels in the blood.

✔ Take oral azathioprine in divided doses, after meals, to decrease stomach upset.

✔ With cyclosporine, use the same oral solution consistently. The two available solutions (Neoral and Sandimmune) are not equivalent and cannot be used interchangeably. If a change in formulation is necessary, it should be made cautiously and only under supervision of the prescribing physician.

Measure oral cyclosporine solution with the dosing syringe provided; add to orange or apple juice that is at room temperature (avoid grapefruit juice); stir well and drink at once (do not allow diluted solution to stand before drinking). Use a glass container, not plastic. Rinse the glass with more diluent to ensure the total dose is taken. Do not rinse the dosing syringe with water or other cleaning agents. Take on a consistent schedule with regard to time of day and meals.

These are the manufacturer's recommendations. Mixing with orange or apple juice improves taste; grapefruit juice should not be used because it affects metabolism of cyclosporine. The amount of fluid should be large enough to increase palatability, especially for children, but small enough to be consumed quickly. Rinsing ensures the entire dose is taken.

✔ Take mycophenolate on an empty stomach; food decreases the amount of active drug by 40%. Do not crush mycophenolate tablets and do not open or crush the capsules.

✔ Take sirolimus consistently with or without food; do *not* mix or take the drug with grapefruit juice. Grapefruit juice inhibits metabolism and increases adverse effects. If also taking cyclosporine, take the sirolimus 4 hours after a dose of cyclosporine.

If taking the oral solution, use the syringe that comes with the medication to measure and withdraw the dose from the bottle. Empty the dose into a glass or plastic container with at least 2 oz ($1/4$ cup or 60 mL) of water or orange juice. *Do not use any other liquid to dilute the drug.* Stir the mixture vigorously, and drink it immediately. Refill the container with at least 4 oz (1/2 cup or 120 mL) of water or orange juice, stir vigorously, and drink at once.

✔ Take tacrolimus with food to decrease stomach upset.

✔ If giving or taking an injected drug (eg, etanercept), be sure you understand how to mix and inject the medication correctly. For example, with etanercept, rotate injection sites, give a new injection at least 1 inch from a previous injection site, and do not inject the medication into areas where the skin is tender, bruised, red, or hard. When possible, practice the required techniques and perform at least the first injection under supervision of a qualified health care professional.

---

goal of such treatment is to save or enhance the quality of the host's life. Skin and renal grafts are commonly and successfully performed; heart, liver, lung, pancreas, and bone marrow transplantations are increasing. Although numerous factors affect graft survival, including the degree of matching between donor tissues and recipient tissues, drug-induced immunosuppression is a major part of transplantation technology. The goal is to provide adequate, but not excessive, immunosuppression. If immunosuppression is inadequate, graft rejection reactions occur with solid organ transplantation, and GVHD occurs with bone marrow transplantation. If immunosuppression is excessive, the client develops serious infections and other adverse effects because the drug actions that slow the proliferation of activated lymphocytes also affect any rapidly dividing nonimmune cells (eg epithelial cells of the gastrointestinal tract and hematopoietic stem cells of the bone marrow). Serious complications can occur.

## Rejection Reactions With Solid Organ Transplantation and Graft-Versus-Host Disease

A rejection reaction occurs when the host's immune system is stimulated to destroy the transplanted organ. The immune cells of the transplant recipient attach to the donor cells of the transplanted organ and react against the antigens of the donor organ. The rejection process involves T and B lymphocytes, antibodies, multiple cytokines, and inflammatory mediators. In general, T-cell activation and proliferation are more important in the rejection reaction than B-cell activation and formation of antibodies. Cytotoxic and helper T cells are activated; activated helper T cells stimulate B cells to produce antibodies and lead to a delayed hypersensitivity reaction. The initial target of the recipient antibodies is the blood vessels of the transplanted organ. The antibodies can injure the transplanted organ by activating complement, producing antigen–antibody complexes, or causing antibody-mediated tissue breakdown. This reaction can destroy the solid organ graft within 2 weeks unless the recipient's immune system is adequately suppressed by immunosuppressant drugs.

Rejection reactions are designated as hyperacute, acute, or chronic, depending on the time elapsed between transplantation and rejection. *Hyperacute* reactions occur within 24 hours. This rare type of reaction occurs in recipients who have previously formed antibodies against antigens in the graft. The antibodies bind to the graft and induce intense inflammation with extensive infiltration of neutrophils into the grafted tissue. The inflammatory reaction causes massive blood clots within the capillaries and prevents vascularization and function of the graft. *Acute* reactions, which may occur from 10 days to a few months after transplantation, mainly involve a cellular response with the proliferation of T lymphocytes. Characteristics include signs of organ failure and vasculitis lesions that often lead to arterial narrowing or obliteration. Treatment with immunosuppressant drugs is usually effective in ensuring short-term survival of the transplant, but does not prevent chronic rejection. *Chronic* reactions, which may occur after months or years of normal function, are caused by both cellular and humoral immunity and do not respond to increased immunosuppressive drug therapy. Characteristics include fibrosis of blood vessels and progressive failure of the transplanted organ.

Rejection reactions produce general manifestations of inflammation and specific manifestations depending on the organ involved. With renal transplantation, for example, acute rejection reactions produce fever, flank tenderness over the graft organ site, and symptoms of renal failure (eg, increased serum creatinine, decreased urine output, edema, weight gain, hypertension). Chronic rejection reactions are characterized by a gradual increase in serum creatinine levels over approximately 4 to 6 months.

## Bone Marrow Transplantation and Graft–Versus–Host Disease

With bone marrow transplantation, the donor bone marrow mounts an immune response (mainly by stimulating T lymphocytes) against antigens on the host's tissues, producing GVHD. Tissue damage is produced directly by the action of cytotoxic T cells or indirectly through the release of inflammatory mediators such as complement and cytokines such as TNF-alpha and interleukins.

Acute GVHD occurs in 30% to 50% of clients, usually within 6 weeks. Signs and symptoms include delayed recovery of blood cell production in the bone marrow, skin rash, liver dysfunction (indicated by increased alkaline phosphatase, aminotransferases, and bilirubin), and diarrhea. The skin reaction is usually a pruritic maculopapular rash that begins on the palms and soles and may extend over the entire body. Liver involvement can lead to bleeding disorders and coma.

Chronic GVHD occurs when symptoms persist or occur 100 days or more after transplantation. It is characterized by abnormal humoral and cellular immunity, severe skin disorders, and liver disease. Chronic GVHD appears to be an autoimmune disorder in which activated T cells perceive autoantigens as foreign antigens.

## Combination Immunosuppressant Drug Therapy With Transplantation

Most immunosuppressants are used to prevent rejection of transplanted tissues. The rejection reaction involves T and B lymphocytes, multiple cytokines, and inflammatory mediators. Thus, drug combinations are rational because they act on different components of the immune response and often have overlapping and synergistic effects. They may also allow lower doses of individual drugs, which usually cause fewer or less severe adverse effects. For example, most organ transplantation centers use a combination regimen (eg, azathioprine, a corticosteroid, and either cyclosporine, sirolimus, or tacrolimus) for prevention and treatment of rejection reactions. Once the transplanted tissue is functioning and rejection has been successfully prevented or treated, it often is possible to maintain the graft with fewer drugs or lower drug dosages. Some recommendations to increase safety or effectiveness of drug combinations include the following:

- *Lymphocyte immune globulin, antithymocyte globulin* is usually given with azathioprine and a corticosteroid.
- *Azathioprine* is usually given with cyclosporine and prednisone.
- *Basiliximab* and *daclizumab* are given with cyclosporine and a corticosteroid.
- *Corticosteroids* may be given alone or included in multidrug regimens with cyclosporine and muromonab-CD3. A corticosteroid should always accompany cyclosporine administration, to enhance immunosuppression. In prophylaxis of organ transplant rejection, the combination seems more effective than azathioprine alone or azathioprine and a corticosteroid. A corticosteroid may not be required, at least long-term, with tacrolimus.
- *Cyclosporine* should be used cautiously with immunosuppressants other than corticosteroids to decrease risks for excessive immunosuppression and its complications.
- *Methotrexate* may be used alone or with cyclosporine for prophylaxis of GVHD after bone marrow transplantation.
- *Muromonab-CD3* may be given cautiously with reduced numbers or dosages of other immunosuppressants. When co-administered with prednisone and azathioprine, the maximum daily dose of prednisone is 0.5 mg/kg, and the maximum for azathioprine is 25 mg. When muromonab-CD3 is co-administered with cyclosporine, cyclosporine dosage should be reduced or the drug temporarily discontinued. If discontinued, cyclosporine is restarted 3 days before completing the course of muromonab-CD3 therapy, to resume a maintenance level of immunosuppression.

- *Mycophenolate* is used with cyclosporine and a corticosteroid. It may be used instead of azathioprine.
- *Sirolimus* is used with cyclosporine and a corticosteroid.
- *Tacrolimus* is substituted for cyclosporine in some long-term immunosuppressant regimens. An advantage of tacrolimus is that corticosteroid therapy can often be discontinued, with the concomitant elimination of the adverse effects associated with the long-term use of corticosteroids.

### Laboratory Monitoring

With *azathioprine*, bone marrow depression (eg, severe leukopenia or thrombocytopenia) may occur. To monitor bone marrow function, complete blood cell (CBC) and platelet counts should be checked weekly during the first month, every 2 weeks during the second and third months, then monthly. If dosage is changed or a client's health status worsens at any time during therapy, more frequent blood tests are needed.

With oral *cyclosporine*, blood levels are monitored periodically for low or high values. Subtherapeutic levels may lead to organ transplant rejection. They are more likely to occur with the Sandimmune formulation than with Neoral because Sandimmune is poorly absorbed. High levels increase adverse effects. The blood levels are used to regulate dosage. In addition, renal (serum creatinine, blood urea nitrogen) and liver (bilirubin, aminotransferase enzymes) function tests should be performed regularly to monitor for nephrotoxicity and hepatotoxicity.

With *leflunomide*, renal and liver functions tests should be done periodically.

With *methotrexate*, CBC and platelet counts and renal and liver function tests should be done periodically.

With *muromonab-CD3*, WBC and differential counts should be performed periodically.

With *mycophenolate*, a CBC is recommended weekly during the first month, twice monthly during the second and third months, and monthly during the first year.

With *sirolimus*, serum drug levels should be monitored in patients who are likely to have altered drug metabolism (eg, those 13 years of age and older who weigh less than 40 kg; those with impaired hepatic function; and those who also are receiving enzyme-inducing or enzyme-inhibiting drugs). Trough concentrations of 15 ng/mL or more are associated with increased frequency of adverse effects. In addition, tests related to hyperlipidemia and renal function should also be performed periodically.

With *tacrolimus*, periodic measurements of serum creatinine, potassium, and glucose are recommended to monitor for the adverse effects of nephrotoxicity, hyperkalemia, and hyperglycemia.

(text continues on page 674)

## Nursing Actions
## Immunosuppressants

| Nursing Actions | Rationale/Explanation |
|---|---|
| 1. Administer accurately. | |
| a. For prepared intravenous (IV) solutions, check for appropriate dilution, discoloration, particulate matter, and expiration time. If okay, give by infusion pump, for the recommended time. | IV drugs should be reconstituted and diluted in a pharmacy, and the manufacturers' instructions should be followed exactly. Once mixed, most of these drugs are stable only for a few hours and some do not contain preservatives. |
| b. Give oral **azathioprine** in divided doses, after meals; give IV drug by infusion, usually over 30 to 60 min. | To decrease nausea and vomiting with oral drug |
| c. With **basiliximab**, infuse through a peripheral or central vein over 20–30 min. Use the reconstituted solution within 4 h at room temperature or 24 h if refrigerated. | The first dose is given within 2 h before transplantation surgery and the second dose 4 d after transplantation. |
| d. With **IV cyclosporine**, infuse over 2–6 h. | IV drug is given to patients who are unable to take it orally; resume oral administration when feasible. |
| e. With **oral cyclosporine** solutions, measure doses with the provided syringe; add to room temperature orange or apple juice (avoid grapefruit juice); stir well and have the patient drink at once (do not allow diluted solution to stand before drinking). Use a glass container, not plastic. Rinse the glass with more juice to ensure the total dose is taken. Do not rinse the dosing syringe with water or other cleaning agents. Give on a consistent schedule in relation to time of day and meals. | These are the manufacturers' recommendations. Mixing with orange or apple juice improves taste; grapefruit juice should not be used because it affects metabolism of cyclosporine. The amount of fluid should be large enough to increase palatability, especially for children, but small enough to be consumed quickly. Rinsing ensures the entire dose is taken. Oral cyclosporine may be given to clients who have had an anaphylactic reaction to the IV preparation, because the reaction is attributed to the oil diluent rather than the drug. |

*(continued)*

## Nursing Actions

## Immunosuppressants (Continued)

| Nursing Actions | Rationale/Explanation |
|---|---|
| f. Infuse reconstituted and diluted **daclizumab** through a peripheral or central vein over 15 min. Once mixed, use within 4 h or refrigerate up to 24 h. | The first dose is given approximately 24 h before transplantation, followed by a dose every 2 wk for four doses (total of five doses). |
| g. With **etanercept**, slowly inject 1 mL of the supplied Sterile Bacteriostatic Water for Injection into the vial, without shaking (to avoid excessive foaming). Give subcutaneously, rotating sites so that a new dose is injected at least 1 inch from an old site and never into areas where the skin is tender, bruised, red, or hard. | This drug may be administered at home, by a client or a caregiver, with appropriate instructions and supervised practice in mixing and injecting the drug. |
| h. Infuse reconstituted and diluted **infliximab** over approximately 2 h, starting within 3 h of preparation (contains no antibacterial preservatives). | Infliximab should be prepared in a pharmacy because special equipment is required for administration. |
| i. Give **lymphocyte immune globulin, antithymocyte globulin** (diluted to a concentration of 1 mg/mL) into a large or central vein, using an in-line filter and infusion pump, over at least 4 h. Once diluted, use within 24 h. | Manufacturer's recommendations. Using a high-flow vein decreases phlebitis and thrombosis at the IV site. The filter is used to remove any insoluble particles. |
| j. Give **muromonab-CD3** in an IV bolus injection once daily. Do not give by IV infusion or mix with other drug solutions. | Manufacturer's recommendations |
| k. Infuse **IV mycophenolate** over approximately 2 h, within 4 h of solution preparation (contains no antibacterial preservatives). | The IV drug must be reconstituted and diluted with 5% dextrose to a concentration of 6 mg/mL (1 g in 140 mL or 1.5 g in 210 mL). Handle the drug cautiously to avoid contact with skin and mucous membranes. If such contact occurs, wash thoroughly with soap and water; rinse eyes with plain water. |
| l. Give **oral mycophenolate** on an empty stomach. Do not crush the tablets, do not open or crush the capsules, and ask clients to swallow the capsules whole, without biting or chewing. | Food decreases absorption. Avoid inhaling the powder from the capsules or getting on skin or mucous membranes. Such contacts produced teratogenic effects in animals. |
| m. With **sirolimus**, give 4 h after a dose of cyclosporine; give consistently with or without food; and do not give with grapefruit juice. With oral sirolimus solution, use the amber oral dose syringe to withdraw a dose from the bottle; empty the dose into a glass or plastic container with at least 60 mL of water or orange juice (do not use any other diluent); stir the mixture vigorously and ask the patient to drink it immediately; refill the container with at least 120 mL of water or orange juice; stir vigorously and ask the patient to drink all of the fluid. | Serum drug levels of sirolimus are increased if the two drugs are taken at the same time; consistent timing in relation to food provides more consistent absorption and blood levels; grapefruit juice inhibits the enzymes that metabolize sirolimus, thereby increasing blood levels of drug and increasing risks of toxicity. Manufacturer's recommendations |
| n. Give **IV tacrolimus** as a continuous infusion by infusion pump. | |
| o. Give the first dose of **oral tacrolimus** 8–12 h after stopping the IV infusion. | Oral tacrolimus can usually be substituted for IV drug 2–3 d after transplantation. |
| 2. **Observe for therapeutic effects.** | |
| a. When a drug is given to suppress the immune response to organ transplants, therapeutic effect is the absence of signs and symptoms indicating rejection of the transplanted tissue. | |
| b. When azathioprine or methotrexate is given for rheumatoid arthritis, observe for decreased pain. | With azathioprine, therapeutic effects usually occur after 6–8 wk. If no response occurs within 12 wk, other treatment measures are indicated. With methotrexate, therapeutic effects usually occur within 3–6 wk. |

*(continued)*

## Nursing Actions

## Immunosuppressants (Continued)

| Nursing Actions | Rationale/Explanation |
|---|---|
| c. When etanercept is given for rheumatoid arthritis, observe for decreased symptoms and less joint destruction on x-ray reports.<br><br>d. When infliximab is given for rheumatoid arthritis or Crohn's disease, observe for decreased symptoms. | |
| 3. **Observe for adverse effects.**<br>a. Observe for infection (fever, sore throat, wound drainage, productive cough, dysuria, and so forth). | Frequency and severity increase with higher drug dosages. Risks are high in immunosuppressed clients. Infections may be caused by almost any microorganism and may affect any part of the body, although respiratory and urinary tract infections may occur more often. |
| b. With azathioprine, observe for:<br>(1) Bone marrow depression (anemia, leukopenia, thrombocytopenia, abnormal bleeding). | The incidence of adverse effects is high in renal transplant recipients. Dosage reduction or stopping azathioprine may be indicated. |
| (2) Nausea and vomiting | Can be reduced by dividing the daily dosage and giving after meals |
| c. With basiliximab and daclizumab, observe for gastrointestinal (GI) disorders (nausea, vomiting, diarrhea, heartburn, abdominal distention) | GI symptoms were often reported in clinical trials. Although adverse effects involving all body systems were reported, the number and type were similar for basiliximab, daclizumab, and placebo groups. All patients were also receiving cyclosporine and a corticosteroid. |
| d. With cyclosporine, observe for:<br>(1) Nephrotoxicity (increased serum creatinine and blood urea nitrogen [BUN], decreased urine output, edema, hyperkalemia) | This is a major adverse effect, and it may produce signs and symptoms that are difficult to distinguish from those caused by renal graft rejection. Rejection usually occurs within the first month after surgery. If it occurs, dosage must be reduced and the patient observed for improved renal function.<br>Also, note that graft rejection and drug-induced nephrotoxicity may be present simultaneously. The latter may be decreased by reducing dosage. Nephrotoxicity often occurs 2–3 mo after transplantation and results in a stable but decreased level of renal function (BUN of 35–45 mg/dL and serum creatinine of 2.0–2.5 mg/dL). |
| (2) Hepatotoxicity (increased serum enzymes and bilirubin) | The reported incidence is less than 8% after kidney, heart, or liver transplantation. It usually occurs during the first month, when high doses are used, and decreases with dosage reduction. |
| (3) Hypertension | This is especially likely to occur in clients with heart transplants and may require antihypertensive drug therapy.<br>Do not give a potassium-sparing diuretic as part of the antihypertensive regimen because of increased risk of hyperkalemia. |
| (4) Anaphylaxis (with IV cyclosporine) (urticaria, hypotension or shock, respiratory distress) | This is rare but may occur. The allergen is thought to be the polyoxyethylated castor oil because people who had allergic reactions with the IV drug have later taken oral doses without allergic reactions. During IV administration, observe the client continuously for the first 30 min and often thereafter. Stop the infusion if a reaction occurs, and give emergency care (eg, epinephrine 1:1000). |
| (5) Central nervous system (CNS) toxicity (confusion, depression, hallucinations, seizures, tremor) | These effects are relatively uncommon and may be caused by factors other than cyclosporine (eg, nephrotoxicity). |

*(continued)*

## *Nursing Actions*

## Immunosuppressants (Continued)

| *Nursing Actions* | *Rationale/Explanation* |
|---|---|
| (6) Other (gingival hyperplasia, hirsutism) | Gingival hyperplasia can be minimized by thorough oral hygiene. |
| e. With infliximab, observe for:<br>(1) Infusion reactions (fever, chills, pruritus, urticaria, chest pain)<br>(2) GI upset (nausea, vomiting, abdominal pain)<br>(3) Respiratory symptoms (bronchitis, chest pain, coughing, dyspnea) | |
| f. With leflunomide, observe for:<br>(1) GI upset (nausea, diarrhea)<br>(2) Hepatotoxicity (elevation of transaminases)<br>(3) Skin disorders (alopecia, rash) | The drug was, in general, well tolerated in clinical trials, with the number and type of most adverse effects similar to those occurring with placebo. |
| g. With lymphocyte immune globulin, antithymocyte globulin, observe for:<br>(1) Anaphylaxis (chest pain, respiratory distress, hypotension, or shock) | An uncommon but serious allergic reaction to the animal protein in the drug that may occur anytime during therapy. If it occurs, stop the drug infusion, inject 0.3 mL epinephrine 1:1000, and provide other supportive emergency care as indicated. |
| (2) Chills and fever | Fever occurs in approximately 50% of clients; it may be decreased by premedicating with acetaminophen, an antihistamine, or a corticosteroid. |
| h. With methotrexate, observe for:<br>(1) GI disorders (nausea, vomiting, diarrhea, ulcerations, bleeding)<br>(2) Bone marrow depression (anemia, neutropenia, thrombocytopenia) | Monitor complete blood count (CBC) regularly. Bone marrow depression is less likely to occur with the small doses used for inflammatory disorders than with doses used in cancer chemotherapy. |
| (3) Hepatotoxicity (yellow discoloration of skin or eyes, dark urine, elevated liver aminotransferases) | Long-term, low-dose methotrexate may produce fatty changes, fibrosis, necrosis, and cirrhosis in the liver. |
| i. With muromonab-CD3, observe for:<br>(1) An acute reaction called the cytokine release syndrome (high fever, chills, chest pain, dyspnea, hypertension, nausea, vomiting, diarrhea) | This reaction is attributed to the release of cytokines by activated lymphocytes or monocytes. Symptoms may range from "flu-like" to a less frequent but severe, shock-like reaction that may include serious cardiovascular and CNS disorders. |
| (2) Hypersensitivity (edema, difficulty in swallowing or breathing, skin rash, urticaria, rapid heartbeat) | Symptoms usually occur within 30–60 min after administration of a dose, especially the first dose, and may last several hours. The reaction usually subsides with later doses, but may recur with dosage increases or restarting after a period without the drug. |
| (3) Nausea, vomiting, diarrhea | Patients experiencing a hypersensitivity reaction should receive immediate treatment. |
| j. With mycophenolate, observe for:<br>(1) GI effects (nausea, vomiting, diarrhea) | GI effects are more likely when mycophenolate is started and may subside if dosage is reduced. |
| (2) Hematologic effects (anemia, neutropenia) | Monitor CBC reports regularly. Up to 2% of renal and 2.8% of cardiac transplant recipients taking mycophenolate have severe neutropenia (absolute neutrophil count <500/mm³). The neutropenia may be related to mycophenolate, concomitant medications, viral infections, or a combination of these causes. If a client has neutropenia, interrupt drug administration or reduce the dose and initiate appropriate treatment as soon as possible. |

*(continued)*

## *Nursing Actions*
## Immunosuppressants (Continued)

| Nursing Actions | Rationale/Explanation |
|---|---|
| (3) CNS effects (dizziness, headache, insomnia) | |
| k. With sirolimus, observe for: | Most reactions were common (ie, occurred in >10% of recipients). However, patients were also receiving cyclosporine and a corticosteroid. |
|   (1) GI effects—abdominal pain, nausea, vomiting, constipation, diarrhea, hepatotoxicity | |
|   (2) Hematologic effects—anemia, leukopenia, thrombocytopenia, hypercholesterolemia | |
|   (3) Cardiovascular effects—edema, hypertension | |
|   (4) CNS effects—insomnia, headache, tremor | |
| l. With tacrolimus, observe for: | |
|   (1) Nephrotoxicity—increased serum creatinine, decreased urine output | Nephrotoxicity has occurred in one third or more of liver transplant recipients who received tacrolimus. The risk is greater with higher doses. |
|   (2) Neurotoxicity—minor effects include insomnia, mild tremors, headaches, photophobia, nightmares; major effects include confusion, seizures, coma, expressive aphasia, psychosis, and encephalopathy. | Neurologic symptoms are common and occur in approximately 10%–20% of clients receiving tacrolimus. |
|   (3) Infection—cytomegalovirus (CMV) infection and others | CMV infection commonly occurs. |
|   (4) Hyperglycemia | Glucose intolerance may require insulin therapy. |
| **4. Observe for drug interactions.** | Drug interactions have not been reported with the newer biologic immunosuppressants (basiliximab, daclizumab, etanercept, infliximab). |
| a. Drugs that *increase* effects of azathioprine: | |
|   (1) Allopurinol | Inhibits hepatic metabolism, thereby increasing pharmacologic effects. If the two drugs are given concomitantly, the dose of azathioprine should be reduced drastically to 25%–35% of the usual dose. |
|   (2) Corticosteroids | Increased immunosuppression and risk of infection |
| b. Drugs that *increase* effects of cyclosporine: | |
|   (1) Aminoglycoside antibiotics (eg, gentamicin), antifungals (eg, amphotericin B) | Increased risk of nephrotoxicity. Avoid other nephrotoxic drugs when possible. |
|   (2) Antifungals (fluconazole, itraconazole), calcium channel blockers (diltiazem, nicardipine, verapamil), macrolide antibiotics (erythromycin, clarithromycin), cimetidine | Decreased hepatic metabolism, increased serum drug levels, and increased risk of toxicity |
| c. Drugs that *decrease* effects of cyclosporine: | |
|   (1) Enzyme inducers, including anticonvulsants (carbamazepine, phenytoin), rifampin, trimethoprim-sulfamethoxazole | Enzyme-inducing drugs stimulate hepatic metabolism of cyclosporine, thereby reducing blood levels. If concurrent administration is necessary, monitor cyclosporine blood levels to avoid subtherapeutic levels and decreased effectiveness. |
| d. Drugs that *increase* effects of leflunomide: | |
|   (1) Rifampin | Rifampin induces liver enzymes and accelerates metabolism of leflunomide to its active metabolite. |
|   (2) Hepatotoxic drugs (eg, methotrexate) | Additive hepatotoxicity |
| e. Drugs that *decrease* effects of leflunomide: | |
|   (1) Charcoal | These drugs may be used to lower blood levels of leflunomide. |
|   (2) Cholestyramine | |

*(continued)*

## Nursing Actions

## Immunosuppressants (Continued)

| Nursing Actions | Rationale/Explanation |
|---|---|
| f. Drugs that *increase* effects of methotrexate:<br>  (1) Probenecid<br>  (2) Salicylates<br>  (3) Sulfonamides<br><br><br><br>  (4) Nonsteroidal anti-inflammatory drugs (NSAIDs)<br><br><br><br>  (5) Procarbazine<br>  (6) Alcohol and other hepatotoxic drugs<br>g. Drug that *decreases* effects of methotrexate:<br>  (1) Folic acid | Probenecid, salicylates, and sulfonamides may increase both therapeutic and toxic effects. The mechanism is unknown, but may involve slowing of methotrexate elimination through the kidneys or displacement of methotrexate from plasma protein-binding sites.<br>NSAIDs are often used concomitantly with methotrexate by clients with rheumatoid arthritis. There may be an increased risk of GI ulceration and bleeding.<br>Procarbazine may increase nephrotoxicity; hepatotoxic drugs increase hepatotoxicity.<br><br>Methotrexate acts by blocking folic acid. Its effectiveness is decreased by folic acid supplementation, alone or in multivitamin preparations. |
| h. Drugs that *increase* effects of mycophenolate:<br>  (1) Acyclovir, ganciclovir<br><br>  (2) Probenecid, salicylates<br>i. Drug that *decreases* effects of mycophenolate:<br>  (1) Cholestyramine | Increase blood levels of mycophenolate, probably by decreasing renal excretion<br>Increase blood levels<br><br>Decreases absorption |
| j. Drugs that *increase* effects of sirolimus:<br>  (1) Cyclosporine<br><br>  (2) CYP3A4 enzyme inhibitors—Azole antifungal drugs (eg, fluconazole, itraconazole), calcium channel blockers (eg, diltiazem, nicardipine, verapamil), macrolide antibiotics (eg, erythromycin, clarithromycin), protease inhibitors (eg, ritonavir, indinavir), cimetidine | Increases blood levels of sirolimus and should not be given at same time (give sirolimus 4 h after a dose of cyclosporine)<br>These drugs inhibit metabolism of sirolimus, which increases blood levels and risks of toxicity. |
| k. Drugs that *decrease* effects of sirolimus:<br>  (1) Enzyme inducers—anticonvulsants (eg, carbamazepine, phenytoin), rifamycins (eg, rifampin, rifabutin, rifapentine), St. John's wort | These drugs speed up the metabolism and elimination of sirolimus. |
| l. Drugs that *increase* effects of tacrolimus:<br>  (1) Nephrotoxic drugs (eg, aminoglycoside antibiotics, amphotericin B, cisplatin, NSAIDs)<br>  (2) Antifungals (clotrimazole, fluconazole, itraconazole); erythromycin and other macrolides; calcium channel blockers (diltiazem, verapamil), cimetidine, danazol, methylprednisolone, metoclopramide<br>  (3) Angiotensin-converting enzyme inhibitors, potassium supplements | Increased risk of nephrotoxicity<br><br>These drugs may increase blood levels of tacrolimus, probably by inhibiting or competing for hepatic drug-metabolizing enzymes<br><br>Increased risk of hyperkalemia. Serum potassium levels should be monitored closely. |
| m. Drugs that *decrease* effects of tacrolimus:<br>  (1) Antacids<br><br><br><br><br>  (2) Enzyme inducers—carbamazepine, phenytoin, rifampin, rifabutin | With oral tacrolimus, antacids adsorb the drug or raise the pH of gastric fluids and increase its degradation. If ordered concomitantly, an antacid should be given at least 2 h before or after tacrolimus.<br>Induction of drug-metabolizing enzymes in the liver may accelerate metabolism of tacrolimus and decrease its blood levels. |

## Critical Thinking Exercises

**1.** To decrease gastrointestinal upset, a client should be instructed to take an oral corticosteroid with any of the following except:

   **a.** An antacid
   **b.** Crackers
   **c.** A piece of fruit
   **d.** A meal

**2.** The client has been prescribed prednisone, 10 mg orally once a day. At what time of day should the drug be scheduled to be administered?

   **a.** 8 AM
   **b.** 12 PM
   **c.** 4 PM
   **d.** 8 PM

**3.** The dosage of sirolimus would need to be increased if a client were also receiving any of the following drugs, except:

   **a.** Phenytoin
   **b.** Carbamazepine
   **c.** Rifampin
   **d.** Cyclosporine

**4.** Cytotoxic, antiproliferative drugs are not the drugs of first choice for immunosuppressive therapy because they:

   **a.** Are too specific to be effective
   **b.** Cause sterility
   **c.** Cause gastrointestinal upset
   **d.** Are toxic to lymphocytes and nonlymphoid proliferating cells

**5.** The nurse is outlining discharge instructions for a client taking oral cyclosporine. To avoid increased plasma levels, the nurse should instruct the client to avoid taking the drug with:

   **a.** Skim milk
   **b.** Apple juice
   **c.** Grapefruit juice
   **d.** Orange juice

## SELECTED OREFERENCES

Chong, A. S., Huang, W., Liu, W., Luo, J., Shen, J., Xu, W., et al. (1999). In vivo activity of leflunomide: Pharmacokinetic analyses and mechanism of immunosuppression. *Transplantation, 68,* 100–109.

*Drug facts and comparisons.* (Updated monthly). St. Louis: Facts and Comparisons.

Goldsby, R. A., Kindt, T. J., & Osborne, B. A. (2000). *Kuby Immunology* (4th ed.). New York: WH Freeman and Co.

Guyton, A. C., & Hall, J. E. (Eds.). (2000). *Textbook of medical physiology* (10th ed.). Philadelphia: W. B. Saunders.

Hoffmeister, A. M., & Tietze, K. J. (2000). Adrenocortical dysfunction and clinical use of steroids. In E. T. Herfindal & D. R. Gourley (Eds.), *Textbook of therapeutics: Drug and disease management* (7th ed., pp. 305–324). Philadelphia: Lippincott Williams & Wilkins.

Humes, H. D. (Ed.). (2000). *Kelley's textbook of internal medicine* (4th ed.). Philadelphia: Lippincott Williams & Wilkins.

Johnson, H. J. (2000). Transplantation. In E. T. Herfindal & D. R. Gourley (Eds.), *Textbook of therapeutics: Drug and disease management* (7th ed., pp. 2095–2116). Philadelphia: Lippincott Williams & Wilkins.

Lacy, C. F., Armstrong, L. L., Goldman, M. P., & Lance, L. L. (2003). *Lexi-Comp's drug information handbook* (11th ed.). Hudson, OH: American Pharmaceutical Association.

Porth, C. M. (2002). *Pathophysiology: Concepts of altered health states* (6th ed.). Philadelphia: Lippincott Williams & Wilkins.

# Drugs Affecting the Respiratory System

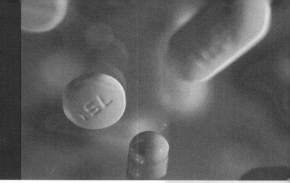

## 37

# Bronchodilating and Other Antiasthmatic Drugs

## OBJECTIVES

*After studying this chapter, the student will be able to:*

1 Describe the main pathophysiologic characteristics of asthma and other bronchoconstrictive disorders.

2 Give the uses and effects of bronchodilating drugs, including adrenergics, ipratropium, and theophylline.

3 Differentiate between short-acting and long-acting inhaled beta$_2$-adrenergic agonists in terms of uses and nursing process implications.

4 Discuss the uses of anti-inflammatory drugs, including corticosteroids, leukotriene modifiers, and mast cell stabilizers.

5 Identify reasons for using inhaled drugs when possible.

6 Differentiate between "quick relief" and long-term control of asthma symptoms.

7 Discuss the use of antiasthmatic drugs in special populations.

8 Teach clients self-care and long-term control measures.

## CRITICAL THINKING SCENARIO

Gwen, a 12-year-old middle school student, was recently diagnosed with asthma. She uses two inhalers four times a day, in addition to using a rescue inhaler during periods of dyspnea. She also is taking peak flow measurements. As the school nurse, you are responsible for overseeing Gwen's care while she is in school.

✔ How might the developmental level of a 12-year-old affect Gwen's feelings about having asthma and complying with treatment?

✔ What asthma triggers might be present in the school environment?

✔ School regulations usually require that all medication be kept in the nurse's office. What effect might this have if Gwen experiences an asthma attack?

✔ Develop an educational program on asthma for middle school–aged students. How might Gwen and other students with asthma participate?

### PROTOTYPE PROFILES

**albuterol** (Proventil, Ventolin, AccuNeb, Volmax, Proventil Repetab), p. 684

**theophylline** (Aminophylline, Theo–Dur), p. 686

# OVERVIEW

The drugs described in this chapter are used to treat respiratory disorders characterized by bronchoconstriction, inflammation, mucosal edema, and excessive mucus production (asthma, bronchitis, and emphysema). Asthma is emphasized because of its widespread prevalence, especially in urban populations. Compared with whites, African Americans and Hispanics have a higher prevalence, and African Americans have a higher death rate from asthma. However, the differences are usually attributed to urban living and lesser access to health care rather than race or ethnic group. Occupational asthma (ie, asthma resulting from repeated and prolonged exposure to industrial inhalants) is also a major health problem. Persons with occupational asthma often have symptoms while in the work environment, with improvement on days off and during vacations. Symptoms sometime persist after termination of exposure. Asthma may occur at any age but is especially common in children and older adults. Discussion of asthma as it relates to age is summarized in Age-related Considerations. Children who are exposed to allergens and airway irritants such as tobacco smoke during infancy are at high risk for development of asthma.

## Asthma

Asthma is an airway disorder characterized by bronchoconstriction (also called *bronchospasm*), inflammation, and hyperreactivity to various stimuli. Resultant symptoms include dyspnea, wheezing, chest tightness, cough, and sputum production. Wheezing is a high-pitched, whistling sound caused by turbulent airflow through an obstructed airway. Thus, any condition that produces significant airway occlusion can cause wheezing. However, a chronic cough may be the only symptom in some people. Symptoms vary in incidence and severity from occasional episodes of mild respiratory distress, with normal functioning between "attacks," to persistent, daily, or continual respiratory distress if not adequately controlled. Inflammation and damaged airway mucosa are chronically present, even when clients appear symptom free.

Acute symptoms of asthma may be precipitated by numerous stimuli, and hyperreactivity to such stimuli may initiate both inflammation and bronchoconstriction. A discussion of the pathophysiology involved in bronchospasm is described in At the Foundation: The Mechanisms of Bronchoconstriction. Viral infections of the respiratory tract are often the causative agents, especially in infants and young children, whose airways are

## Age-related Considerations: Bronchodilating and Other Antiasthmatic Drugs

### USE IN CHILDREN

The American Academy of Pediatrics endorses the clinical practice guidelines established by the National Asthma Education and Prevention Program (see Box 37-1). In general, antiasthmatic medications are used in children and adolescents for the same indications as for adults. With adrenergic bronchodilators, recommendations for use vary according to route of administration, age of the child, and specific drug formulations. However, even infants and young children can be treated effectively with aerosolized or nebulized drugs. In addition, some oral drugs can be given to children as young as 2 years and most can be given to children 6 to 12 years of age.

With theophylline, use in children should be closely monitored because dosage needs and rates of metabolism vary widely. In children younger than 6 months, especially premature infants and neonates, drug elimination may be prolonged because of immature liver function. Except for preterm infants with apnea, theophylline preparations are not recommended for use in this age group. Children 6 months to 16 years of age, approximately, metabolize theophylline more rapidly than younger or older clients. Thus, they may need higher doses than adults in proportion to size and weight. If the child is obese, the dosage should be calculated on the basis of lean or ideal body weight because the drug is not highly distributed in fatty tissue. Long-acting dosage forms are not recommended for children younger than 6 years of age. Children may

become hyperactive and disruptive from the CNS-stimulating effects of theophylline. Tolerance to these effects usually develops with continued use of the drug.

Corticosteroids are being used earlier in children as in adults, and inhaled corticosteroids are first-line drugs for treatment of persistent bronchoconstrictive disorders. The effectiveness and safety of inhaled corticosteroids in children older than 3 years of age is well established; few data are available on the use of inhaled drugs in those younger than 3 years. Major concerns about long-term use in children include decreased adrenal function, growth, and bone mass. Most are given by inhalation. Dosage, type of inhaler device, and characteristics of individual drugs influence the extent and severity of these systemic effects.

Adrenal insufficiency is most likely to occur with systemic or high doses of inhaled corticosteroids. Dose-related inhibition of growth has been reported in short and intermediate studies but long-term studies have found few, if any, decreases in expected adult height. Inhaled corticosteroids have not been associated with significant decreases in bone mass, but more studies of high doses and of drug therapy in adolescents are needed. Bone growth should be monitored closely in children taking corticosteroids. Although inhaled corticosteroids are the most effective anti-inflammatory medications available for asthma, high doses in children are still of concern. The risk of high doses

*(continued)*

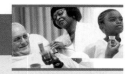

## Age-related Considerations: Bronchodilating and Other Antiasthmatic Drugs (Continued)

is especially great in children with other allergic conditions that require topical corticosteroid drugs. Using the lowest effective dose, administration techniques that minimize swallowed drug, and other antiasthmatic drugs to reduce corticosteroid dose can decrease the risk.

Leukotriene modifiers have not been extensively studied in children and adolescents. With montelukast, the 10-mg film-coated tablet is recommended for adolescents 15 years of age and older, and the 4-mg chewable tablet is recommended for children 2 to 5 years of age. Safety and effectiveness of zafirlukast in children younger than 12 years have not been established.

Cromolyn aerosol solution may be used in children 5 years of age and older, and nebulizer solution is used with children 2 years and older. Nedocromil is not established as safe and effective in children younger than 12 years of age.

### USE IN OLDER ADULTS

Older adults often have chronic pulmonary disorders for which bronchodilators and antiasthmatic medications are used. As with other populations, administering the medications by inhalation and giving the lowest effective dose decrease adverse effects. The main risks with adrenergic

bronchodilators are excessive cardiac and CNS stimulation.

Theophylline use must be carefully monitored because drug effects are unpredictable. On the one hand, cigarette and marijuana smoking and drugs that stimulate drug-metabolizing enzymes in the liver (eg, phenobarbital, phenytoin) increase the rate of metabolism and therefore dosage requirements. On the other hand, impaired liver function, decreased blood flow to the liver, and some drugs (eg, cimetidine, erythromycin) impair metabolism and therefore decrease dosage requirements. Adverse effects include cardiac and CNS stimulation. Measuring serum drug levels and adjusting dosage to maintain therapeutic levels of 5 to 15 mcg/mL can increase safety. If the client is obese, dosage should be based on lean or ideal body weight because theophylline is not highly distributed in fatty tissue.

Corticosteroids increase the risks for osteoporosis and cataracts in older adults. Leukotriene modifiers usually are well tolerated by older adults, with pharmacokinetics and effects similar to those in younger adults. With zafirlukast, however, blood levels are higher and elimination is slower than in younger adults. Zileuton is contraindicated in older adults with underlying hepatic dysfunction.

---

small and easily obstructed. Asthma symptoms may persist for days or weeks after the viral infection resolves. In about 25% of clients with asthma, aspirin and other nonsteroidal anti-inflammatory drugs (NSAIDs) can precipitate an attack. Some clients are allergic to sulfites and may experience life-threatening asthma attacks if they ingest foods processed with these preservatives (eg, beer, wine, dried fruit). The U.S. Food and Drug Administration (FDA) has banned the use of sulfites on foods meant to be served raw, such as open salad bars. Clients with severe asthma should be cautioned against ingesting food and drug products containing sulfites or metabisulfites.

---

### AT THE FOUNDATION: *The Mechanisms of Bronchoconstriction*

Bronchoconstriction involves strong muscle contractions that narrow the airways. Airway smooth muscle extends from the trachea through the bronchioles. It is wrapped around the airways in a spiral pattern, and contraction causes a sphincter-type action that can completely occlude the airway lumen. Bronchoconstriction is aggravated by inflammation, mucosal edema, and excessive mucus and may be precipitated by the numerous stimuli described above.

When lung tissues are exposed to causative stimuli, mast cells release substances that cause bronchoconstriction and inflammation. Mast cells are found throughout the body in connective tissues and are abundant in tissues surrounding capillaries in the lungs. When sensitized mast cells in the lungs or eosinophils in the blood are exposed to allergens or irritants, multiple cytokines and other chemical mediators (eg, acetylcholine, cyclic guanosine monophosphate [GMP], histamine, interleukins, leukotrienes, prostaglandins,

and serotonin) are synthesized and released. These chemicals act directly on target tissues of the airways, causing smooth muscle constriction, increased capillary permeability and fluid leakage, and changes in the mucus-secreting properties of the airway epithelium.

Bronchoconstrictive substances are antagonized by cyclic adenosine monophosphate (cAMP). cAMP is an intracellular substance that initiates various intracellular activities, depending on the type of cell. In lung cells, cAMP inhibits release of bronchoconstrictive substances and thus indirectly promotes bronchodilation. In mild to moderate asthma, bronchoconstriction is usually recurrent and reversible, either spontaneously or with drug therapy. In advanced or severe asthma, airway obstruction becomes less reversible and worsens because chronically inflamed airways undergo structural changes (eg, fibrosis, enlarged smooth muscle cells, and enlarged mucus glands), called "airway remodeling," that inhibit their function.

Gastroesophageal reflux disease (GERD), a common disorder characterized by heartburn and esophagitis, is also associated with asthma. Asthma that worsens at night may be associated with nighttime acid reflux. The reflux of acidic gastric contents into the esophagus is thought to initiate a vagally mediated, reflex type of bronchoconstriction. (Asthma may also aggravate GERD because antiasthma medications that dilate the airways also relax muscle tone in the gastroesophageal sphincter and may increase acid reflux.) Additional precipitants may include allergens (eg, pollens, molds, others), airway irritants and pollutants (eg, chemical fumes, cigarette smoke, automobile exhaust), cold air, and exercise. Acute episodes of asthma may last minutes to hours.

### National Asthma Education and Prevention Program

Because of asthma's significance as a public health problem, the National Heart, Lung, and Blood Institute (NHLBI) of the National Institutes of Health (NIH) established the National Asthma Education and Prevention Program (NAEPP), along with "Guidelines for the Diagnosis and Management of Asthma." These guidelines (Box 37-1) were updated in 1997, and selected aspects, mainly related to children, were updated in 2002. The guidelines are the current standard of care for adults and children with asthma. Additional information can be obtained on the Internet at http://www.nhlbi.nih.gov.

## Chronic Bronchitis and Emphysema

*Chronic bronchitis* and *emphysema*, commonly called *chronic obstructive pulmonary disease* (COPD), usually develop after long-standing exposure to airway irritants such as cigarette smoke. In these conditions, bronchoconstriction and inflammation are more constant and less reversible than with asthma. Anatomic and physiologic changes occur over several years and lead to increasing dyspnea and activity intolerance. These conditions usually affect middle-aged or older adults.

## ▨ DRUG THERAPY

Two major groups of drugs used to treat asthma, acute and chronic bronchitis, and emphysema are bronchodilators and anti-inflammatory drugs. All of the drugs discussed in this chapter are used in the home setting. Points to consider when assisting clients in using the drugs safely and effectively in the home are discussed in Home Care Considerations. Bronchodilators are used to prevent and treat bronchoconstriction; anti-inflammatory drugs are used to prevent and treat inflammation of the airways. Reducing inflammation also reduces bronchoconstriction by decreasing mucosal edema and mucus secretions that narrow airways and by decreasing airway hyperreactivity to various stimuli. The drugs are described in the following sections; pharmacokinetic characteristics of inhaled drugs are listed in Table 37-1, and dosage ranges are listed in Drugs at a Glance 37-1: Bronchodilating Agents, and Drugs at a Glance 37-2: Anti-inflammatory Antiasthmatic Drugs.

## Bronchodilators

### Adrenergics

Adrenergic drugs (see Chap. 16) stimulate beta$_2$-adrenergic receptors in the smooth muscle of bronchi and bronchioles. The receptors, in turn, stimulate the enzyme adenyl cyclase to increase production of cyclic adenosine monophosphate (cAMP). The increased cAMP produces bronchodilation. Some beta-adrenergic drugs (eg, epinephrine) also stimulate beta$_1$-adrenergic receptors in the heart to increase the rate and force of contraction. Cardiac stimulation is an adverse effect when the drugs are given for bronchodilation. These drugs are contraindicated in clients with cardiac tachydysrhythmias and severe coronary artery disease; they should be used cautiously in clients with hypertension, hyperthyroidism, diabetes mellitus, and seizure disorders.

**Epinephrine** may be injected subcutaneously in an acute attack of bronchoconstriction, with therapeutic effects occurring in approximately 5 minutes and lasting for approximately 4 hours. However, an inhaled selective beta$_2$ agonist is the drug of choice in this situation. Epinephrine is also available without prescription in a pressurized aerosol form (eg, Primatene). Almost all over-the-counter aerosol products promoted for use in asthma contain epinephrine. These products are often abused and may delay the client from seeking medical attention. Clients should be cautioned that excessive use may produce hazardous cardiac stimulation and other adverse effects.

Ⓟ **Albuterol, bitolterol, levalbuterol,** and **pirbuterol** are short-acting beta$_2$-adrenergic agonists used for prevention and treatment of bronchoconstriction. Of this group, albuterol serves as the prototype (see Prototype Profile 37-1: Albuterol). These drugs act more selectively on beta$_2$ receptors and cause less cardiac stimulation than epinephrine. Most often taken by inhalation, they are also the most effective bronchodilators and are the treatment of first choice to relieve acute asthma. Because the drugs can be effectively delivered by aerosol or nebulization, even to young children and clients on mechanical ventilation, there is seldom a need to give epinephrine or other nonselective adrenergic drugs by injection.

The beta$_2$ agonists are usually self-administered by metered-dose inhalers (MDIs). Although most drug references still list a regular dosing schedule (eg, every 4 to 6 hours), asthma experts recommend that the drugs be used when needed (eg, to treat acute dyspnea or prevent dyspnea during exercise). If these drugs are overused, they lose their bronchodilating effects because the beta$_2$-adrenergic receptors become unresponsive to stimula-

BOX
37-1
## National Asthma Education and Prevention Program (NAEPP) Expert Panel Guidelines*

### Definition
Asthma is "a chronic inflammatory disorder of the airways in which many cells and cellular elements play a role, in particular, mast cells, eosinophils, T lymphocytes, macrophages, neutrophils, and epithelial cells."

### Goals of Therapy
1. Minimal or no chronic symptoms day or night
2. Minimal or no exacerbations
3. No limitations on activities; for children, no school/parent's work missed
4. Minimal use of short-acting inhaled beta$_2$ agonist (<1 time per day, <1 canister/month)
5. Minimal or no adverse effects from medications

### General Recommendations
- Establish and teach patients/parents/caregivers about quick relief measures and long-term control measures. Assist to identify and control environmental factors that aggravate asthma.
- For acute attacks, gain control as quickly as possible (a short course of systemic corticosteroids may be needed); then step down to the least medication necessary to maintain control.
- Review the treatment regimen every 1 to 6 months. If control is adequate and goals are being met, a gradual stepwise reduction in medication may be possible. If control is inadequate, the treatment regimen may need to be changed. For example, frequent or increasing use of a short-acting beta$_2$ agonist (>2 times a week with intermittent asthma; daily or increasing use with persistent asthma) may indicate the need to initiate or increase long-term control therapy. However, first reassess patients' medication techniques (eg, correct use of inhalers), adherence, and environmental control measures.

### Quick Relief for Acute Exacerbations
- **Adults and children > 5 years:** Short-acting, inhaled, beta$_2$ agonist, 2–4 puffs as needed. If symptoms are severe, patients may need up to 3 treatments at 20-minute intervals or a nebulizer treatment. A short course of a systemic corticosteroid may also be needed.
- **Children 5 years and younger:** Short-acting beta$_2$ agonist by nebulizer or face mask and spacer or holding chamber. Alternative: oral beta$_2$ agonist. With viral respiratory infections, the beta$_2$ agonist may be needed q4–6h up to 24 hours or longer and a systemic corticosteroid may be needed.

### Long-term Control
- **Step 1 Mild Intermittent** (symptoms 2 days/week or less or 2 nights/month or less): No daily medication needed; treat acute exacerbations with an inhaled beta$_2$ agonist and possibly a short course of a systemic corticosteroid.
- **Step 2 Mild Persistent** (symptoms >2/week but <1×/day or >2 nights/month):
  - **Adults and children > 5 years:** Low-dose inhaled corticosteroid. Alternatives: cromolyn or nedocromil,

a leukotriene modifier, or sustained-release theophylline to maintain a serum drug level of 5–15 mcg/mL.
- **Children 5 years and younger:** Administer the inhaled corticosteroid by a nebulizer or metered-dose inhaler (MDI) with a holding chamber. Alternatives: cromolyn (via nebulizer or MDI with holding chamber) or a leukotriene modifier.
- **Step 3 Moderate Persistent** (symptoms daily and >1 night/week):
  - **Adults and children > 5 years:** Low- to medium-dose inhaled corticosteroid and a long-acting beta$_2$ agonist. Alternatives: increase corticosteroid dose or continue low to medium dose of corticosteroid and add a leukotriene modifier or theophylline.
  - **Children < 5 years:** Low-dose inhaled corticosteroid and a long-acting beta$_2$ agonist or medium dose inhaled corticosteroid.
- **Step 4 Severe Persistent** (symptoms continual during daytime hours and frequent at night):
  - **Adults and children > 5 years:** High-dose inhaled corticosteroid and long-acting beta$_2$ agonist and, if necessary, a systemic corticosteroid (2 mg/kg/d, not to exceed 60 mg/d). Reduce systemic corticosteroid when possible.
  - **Children < 5 years:** Same as for adults and older children.

### Low (L), Medium (M), and High (H) Doses of Inhaled Corticosteroids:

|  | Adults (mcg) | Children (12 y and younger) (mcg) |
|---|---|---|
| Beclomethasone (42 or 84 mcg/puff) | L: 168–504 M: 504–840 H: >840 | L: 84–336 M: 336–672 H: >672 |
| Beclomethasone (40–80 mcg/puff) | L: 80–240 M: 240–480 H: >480 | L: 80–160 M: 160–320 H: >320 |
| Budesonide (200 mcg/ inhalation) | L: 200–600 M: 600–1200 H: >1200 | L: 200–400 M: 400–800 H: >800 |
| Budesonide inhalation suspension for nebulization (child dose only) |  | L: 0.5 mg M: 1.0 mg H: 2.0 mg |
| Flunisolide (250 mcg/puff) | L: 500–1000 M: 1000–2000 H: >2000 | L: 500–750 M: 1000–1250 H: >1250 |
| Fluticasone aerosol (44, 110, or 220 mcg/puff) | L: 88–264 M: 264–660 H: >660 | L: 88–176 M: 176–440 H: >440 |
| Fluticasone powder (50, 100, or 250 mcg/puff) | L: 100–300 M: 300–600 H: >600 | L: 100–200 M: 200–400 H: >400 |
| Triamcinolone acetonide (100 mcg/puff) | L: 400–1000 M: 1000–2000 H: >2000 | L: 400–800 M: 800–1200 H: >1200 |

*Adapted from NAEPP Expert Panel Report 2 (NIH Publication No. 97-4051, 1997) and the Update on Selected Topics 2002 (NIH Publication No. 02-5075).

## Home Care Considerations: Use of Bronchodilating and Other Antiasthmatic Drugs

***ASSESS:*** knowledge level of client and caregiver; client's medication techniques (eg, correct use of inhalers), adherence, environmental control measures, use of MedicAlert device, and quality-of-life considerations.

***MONITOR:*** vital signs, serum plasma levels, effectiveness of therapy, and adverse effects.

***EDUCATE:*** regarding appropriate use, especially correct use of nebulizers, importance of consulting health care provider before taking OTC medications, interventions to reduce side effects; how to store medications out of reach of children, and to replace medications to ensure a constant supply. Also, assist clients to recognize and treat (or get help for) exacerbations before respiratory distress becomes severe. Instruct on the importance of smoking cessation. Stress the importance of women to consult with health care provider if contemplating pregnancy if taking aminophylline. Emphasize the importance of not exceeding the prescribed dose, not crushing long-acting formulations, reporting adverse effects, and keeping appointments for follow-up care; reinforce NAEPP Panel Guidelines (see Box 37-1) and additional teaching points (see Client Teaching Guidelines: Antiasthmatic Drugs).

tion. This tolerance does not occur with the long-acting beta$_2$ agonists.

**Formoterol and salmeterol** are long-acting beta$_2$-adrenergic agonists used only for *prophylaxis* of acute bronchoconstriction. They are not effective in acute attacks because they have a slower onset of action than the short-

acting drugs (up to 20 minutes for salmeterol). Effects last 12 hours, and the drug should *not* be taken more frequently. If additional bronchodilating medication is needed, a short-acting agent (eg, albuterol) should be used.

**Isoproterenol** is a short-acting bronchodilator and cardiac stimulant. When used for treatment of bronchospasm, isoproterenol is given by inhalation, alone or in combination with other agents.

**Metaproterenol** is a relatively selective, intermediate-acting beta$_2$-adrenergic agonist that may be given orally or by MDI. It is used to treat acute bronchospasm and to prevent exercise-induced asthma. In high doses, metaproterenol loses some of its selectivity and may cause cardiac and central nervous system (CNS) stimulation.

**Terbutaline** is a relatively selective beta$_2$-adrenergic agonist that is a long-acting bronchodilator. When given subcutaneously, terbutaline loses its selectivity and has little advantage over epinephrine. Muscle tremor is the most frequent side effect with this agent.

### Anticholinergics

Anticholinergics (see Chap. 19) block the action of acetylcholine in bronchial smooth muscle when given by inhalation. This action reduces intracellular guanosine monophosphate (GMP), a bronchoconstrictive substance.

**Ipratropium** was formulated to be taken by inhalation for maintenance therapy of bronchoconstriction associated with chronic bronchitis and emphysema. Improved pulmonary function usually occurs in a few minutes. Ipratropium acts synergistically with adrenergic bronchodilators and may be used concomitantly. It improves lung function about 10% to 15% over an inhaled beta$_2$ agonist alone. Ipratropium may also be used

*(text continues on page 685)*

### TABLE 37-1   Pharmacokinetics of Selected Inhaled Antiasthma Medications

| Generic Name | Onset (min) | Peak (hours) | Duration (hours) | Metabolism/Excretion | Half-life (h) |
|---|---|---|---|---|---|
| *Adrenergics* | | | | | |
| **Albuterol** | 5 | 1.5–2 | 3–6 | Liver/urine | 2–4 |
| **Bitolterol** | 2–4 | 0.5–2 | 5–8 | Liver/lungs | 3 |
| **Levalbuterol** | 5 | 1 | 6–8 | Liver/urine | 4–6 |
| **Pirbuterol** | 5 | | 5 | Liver, tissue/urine | ND |
| **Salmeterol** | 13–20 | 3–4 | 7.5–17 | Liver/feces | ND |
| *Anticholinergic* | | | | | |
| **Ipratropium** | 15 | 1–2 | 3–4 | | 1.6 |
| *Corticosteroids* | | | | | |
| **Beclomethasone** | Rapid | 1–2 wk | | Liver/feces | 3–15 |
| **Budesonide** | Immediate | Rapid | 8–12 | Liver/urine (60%) & feces | 2.8 |
| **Flunisolide** | Slow | 10–30 | 4–6 | Liver/renal (50%), feces (40%) | 1–2 |
| **Fluticasone** | Slow | | 24 | Liver/feces & urine | 3.1 |

ND, not determined.

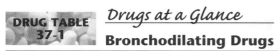

## Drugs at a Glance

**DRUG TABLE 37-1**

## Bronchodilating Drugs

| Generic/Trade Name | Routes and Dosage Ranges | Comments |
|---|---|---|
| **Bronchodilators** | | |
| *Adrenergics* | | |
| **Epinephrine** (Adrenalin, Bronkaid) <br> Pregnancy Category C | *Adults:* Aqueous solution (epinephrine 1:1000), Sub-Q, 0.2–0.5 mL; dose may be repeated after 20 min if necessary <br> Inhalation by inhaler, 1–2 inhalations 4–6 times per day <br> Inhalation by nebulizer, 0.25–0.5 mL of 2.25% racemic epinephrine in 2.5 mL normal saline <br> *Children:* Aqueous solution (epinephrine 1:1000), Sub-Q, 0.01 mL/kg q4h as needed. A single dose should not exceed 0.5 mL. <br> Inhalation, same as adults for both inhaler and nebulizer | Use phentolamine as antidote for extravasation |
| **Albuterol** (Proventil, Ventolin, AccuNeb, Volmax, Proventil Repetab) | See Prototype Profile 37-1: Albuterol | |
| **Bitolterol** (Tornalate) <br> Pregnancy Category C | *Adults:* Aerosol, two inhalations (0.37 mg/puff) at least 1–3 min apart, followed by a third if necessary; nebulizing solution, 1 mg via intermittent flow, 2.5 mg via continuous flow <br> Aerosol, prophylaxis, two inhalations q8h; maximum recommended dose, three inhalations q6h or two inhalations q4h <br> *Children:* >12 y: Same as adults <br> <12 y: Dosage not established | Shake inhaler well before administration |
| **Formoterol** (Foradil) <br> Pregnancy Category C | *Adults:* Oral inhalation by special inhaler (Aerolizer), 12 mcg (contents of 1 capsule) twice daily, q12h <br> *Children:* 5 y and older, same as adults | Do not swallow drug capsule; use only with special inhaler dedicated to this medication |
| **Isoproterenol** (Isuprel) <br> Pregnancy Category C | *Adults:* Inhalation by nebulizer, 0.25–0.5 mL of 1:200 Isuprel solution in 2.5 mL saline <br> Inhalation by inhaler,* one or two inhalations (0.075–0.125 mg/puff) four times per day; maximum dose, three inhalations per attack of bronchospasm <br> *Children:* Same as adults | Assess heart rate, respiratory rate, blood pressure <br> Shake inhaler well before administration <br> If two inhalations are ordered per dose, wait at least 1 min between inhalation (best delivered 10 min after first inhalation) |
| **Levalbuterol** (Xopenex) <br> Pregnancy Category C | *Adults:* Nebulizer, 0.63–1.25 mg 3 times daily, q6–8h <br> *Children:* 12 y and older, same as adults <br> 6–11 y: Nebulizer, 0.31 mg 3 times daily, q6–8h | Tolerance may develop with overuse |

*(continued)*

**DRUG TABLE 37-1**

_Drugs at a Glance_

**Bronchodilating Drugs** (Continued)

| Generic/Trade Name | Routes and Dosage Ranges | Comments |
|---|---|---|
| **Metaproterenol** (Alupent)<br>Pregnancy Category C | _Adults:_ Inhalation,* 1–3 puffs (0.65 mg/dose), four times per day; maximum dose, 12 inhalations/d<br>PO, 10–20 mg q6–8h<br>_Children:_ Inhalation, not recommended for use in children <12 y<br>9 y or less or weight under 27 kg, PO, 10 mg q6–8h<br>>9 y or weight over 27 kg, PO, 20 mg q6–8h | Do not use solutions for nebulization if brown in color or precipitated<br>Shake inhaler well before administration |
| **Pirbuterol** (Maxair)<br>Pregnancy Category C | _Adults:_ Inhalation,* two puffs (0.4 mg/dose), four to six times per day; maximum dose, 12 inhalations/d<br>_Children:_ >12 y: Same as adults; not recommended for use in children <12 y | Assess heart rate, respiratory rate, blood pressure<br>Shake inhaler well before administration |
| **Salmeterol** (Serevent)<br>Pregnancy Category C | _Adults:_ Aerosol: 2 inhalations (42 mcg), q12h<br>Inhalation powder: 1 inhalation (50 mcg) q12h<br>_Children:_ Aerosol: 12 y and older, same as adults; <12 y, dosage not established<br>Inhalation powder: 4 y and older, same as adults | _Not_ to be used for relief of acute attacks<br>Shake inhaler well before administration |
| **Terbutaline** (Brethine)<br>Pregnancy Category B | _Adults:_ PO, 2.5–5 mg q6–8h; maximum dose, 15 mg/d<br>Sub-Q, 0.25 mg, repeated in 15–30 min if necessary, q4–6h<br>Inhalation,* two inhalations (400 mcg/dose) q4–6h<br>_Children:_ PO, 2.5 mg three times per day for children 12 y and older; maximum dose, 7.5 mg/d<br>Sub-Q dosage not established<br>Inhalation, same as adults for children 12 y and older | Observe client for wheezing after administration and call health care provider if this occurs |
| _Anticholinergic_ | | |
| **Ipratropium bromide** (Atrovent)<br>Pregnancy Category B | _Adults:_ Two inhalations (36 mcg) from the metered-dose inhaler four times per day<br>_Children:_ Dosage not established | Shake inhaler well before administration, wait 1 min between inhalations, close eyes while administering because contact with eyes may cause temporary blurred vision |
| _Xanthines_<br>Aminophylline | See Prototype Profile 37-2: Aminophylline | |
| _Combination Drugs_ | | |
| **Fluticasone, salmeterol** (Advair)<br>Pregnancy Category C | _Adults:_ Oral inhalation, one inhalation, twice daily<br>_Children:_ 12 y and older: same as adults | Shake inhaler well before administration |
| **Ipratropium, albuterol** (Combivent, DuoNeb)<br>Pregnancy Category C | _Adults:_ Aerosol: 2 inhalations 4 times daily<br>Nebulizing solution: 1 vial 4 times daily, increased to 6 times daily if necessary<br>_Children:_ Dosage not established | |

*Short-acting adrenergic bronchodilators are used mainly by inhalation, as needed, rather than on a regular schedule.

## DRUG TABLE 37-2

### *Drugs at a Glance*
### Anti-inflammatory Antiasthmatic Drugs

| Generic/Trade Name | Routes and Dosage Ranges | Comments |
|---|---|---|
| **Corticosteroids** | | |
| **Beclomethasone** (Beclovent, Vanceril)<br>Pregnancy Category C | *Adults:* Oral inhalation, two inhalations (0.84 mg/dose) three or four times daily; maximum, 20 inhalations/24 h<br>*Children:* 6–12 y: Oral inhalation, one or two inhalations three or four times per day; maximum dose, 10 inhalations/24 h | Shake inhaler well before administration<br>Rinse mouth after inhalation to prevent oral *Candida* infection |
| **Budesonide** (Entocort, Rhinocort, Pulmicort Respules, Pulmocort Turbuhaler)<br>Pregnancy Category C; B (Pulmocort Turbuhaler) | *Adults:* Oral inhalation, 200–400 µg twice daily<br>*Children:* <6 y: Oral inhalation, 200 mcg twice daily | Rinse mouth after inhalation to prevent oral *Candida* infection (wash face if using face mask) |
| **Flunisolide** (AeroBid, Nasarel)<br>Pregnancy Category C | *Adults:* Oral inhalation, two inhalations (0.50 mg/dose) twice daily, morning and evening; maximum dose, four inhalations twice daily (2 mg)<br>*Children:* 6–15 y: Oral inhalation, two inhalations twice daily | |
| **Fluticasone** aerosol (Flovent)<br>Fluticasone powder (Flovent Rotadisk)<br>Pregnancy Category C | *Adults:* Aerosol, 220–440 mcg twice daily<br>Powder, 100–500 mcg twice daily<br>*Children:* Aerosol dosage not established<br>4–11 y: Powder, 50–100 mcg twice daily | Rinse mouth after inhalation to prevent oral *Candida* infection; avoid contact with eyes<br>Do not use a spacer with powder form |
| **Hydrocortisone** sodium phosphate and sodium succinate<br>Pregnancy Category C | *Adults:* IV, 100–200 mg q4–6h initially, then decreased or switched to an oral dosage form<br>*Children:* IV, 1–5 mg/kg q4–6h | Drug interferes with calcium absorption<br>St. John's wort may decrease cortisone levels with concomitant use |
| **Methylprednisolone** sodium succinate<br>Pregnancy Category C | *Adults:* IV, 10–40 mg q4–6h for 48–72 h<br>*Children:* IV, 0.5 mg/kg q4–6h | Assess blood pressure, and serum electrolytes and glucose |
| **Prednisone**<br>Pregnancy Category B | *Adults:* PO, 20–60 mg/d<br>*Children:* PO, 2 mg/kg/d initially | See Prototype Profile 36-1: Prednisone, Chap. 36 |
| **Triamcinolone** (Azmacort)<br>Pregnancy Category C | *Adults:* Oral inhalation, two inhalations three or four times per day; maximum dose, 16 inhalations/24 h<br>*Children:* 6–12 y: one or two inhalations three or four times per day; maximum dose, 12 inhalations/24 h | Clear nasal passages before inhalation; not for use during acute asthmatic attacks |
| **Leukotriene Modifiers** | | |
| **Montelukast** (Singulair)<br>Pregnancy Category B | *Adults:* PO, 10 mg once daily in the evening or at bedtime<br>*Children:* 15 y and older: Same as adults<br>6–14 y: PO, 5 mg once daily in the evening<br>2–5 y: 4 mg once daily | Administer within 15 min of opening packet; not for use during acute asthmatic attacks |

*(continued)*

**DRUG TABLE 37-2**

*Drugs at a Glance*

## Anti-inflammatory Antiasthmatic Drugs (Continued)

| Generic/Trade Name | Routes and Dosage Ranges | Comments |
|---|---|---|
| **Zafirlukast** (Accolate)<br>Pregnancy Category B | *Adults:* PO, 20 mg twice daily, 1 h before or 2 h after a meal<br>*Children:* 12 y and older: Same as adults<br>5–11 y: PO, 10 mg twice daily | Should be taken on an empty stomach; not for use during acute asthmatic attacks |
| **Zileuton** (Zyflo)<br>Pregnancy Category C | *Adults:* PO, 600 mg four times daily<br>*Children:* 12 y and older: Same as adults<br><12 y: Dosage not established | Altered liver function test may occur with administration; not for use during acute asthmatic attacks |
| ***Mast Cell Stabilizers*** | | |
| **Cromolyn** (Intal)<br>Pregnancy Category B | *Adults:* Nebulizer solution, oral inhalation, 20 mg four times daily<br>Aerosol spray, oral inhalation, two sprays four times daily<br>*Children:* 2 y and older: Same as adults<br>5 y and older: Same as adults | Should take 30 min before meals; not for use during acute asthmatic attacks |
| **Nedocromil** (Tilade)<br>Pregnancy Category B | *Adults:* Inhalation, 4 mg q6–12h<br>*Children:* >12 y: Same as adults | Not for use during acute asthmatic attacks |

---

## PROTOTYPE PROFILE 37-1

### P Albuterol (al BYOO ter ole)

**Drug Class**
*Chemical:* Beta$_2$ Agonist
*Functional:* Bronchodilator

**Trade Names**
Proventil, Ventolin, AccuNeb, Volmax, Proventil Repetab

**Therapeutic Indications**
Relaxes bronchial smooth muscle through action on beta$_2$ receptors

**Pharmacokinetics**
*Absorption*
Well absorbed

*Distribution*
Protein binding unknown

*Metabolism*
Hepatic

*Excretion*
Urine

**Pharmacodynamics**
*Onset of Action*
PO, 30 min; inhalation, 5 min

*Duration*
PO, 4–6 h; inhalation, 3–6 h

**Contraindications/Precautions**
Hypersensitivity; with caution with cardiovascular disease, diabetes, hyperthyroidism, hypokalemia, pregnancy, or convulsive disorders

**Pregnancy Considerations**
Category C
Crosses placenta. Tocolytic effects, fetal tachycardia, fetal hypoglycemia (secondary to maternal hyperglycemia) reported with oral and IV routes; evidence suggests that administration is safe during pregnancy, but benefits of use should outweigh possible risks

**Dosage**
*Adults:* Inhalation* aerosol (90 mcg/actuation): 1–2 oral inhalations q4–6h; prevention of exercise-induced bronchospasm, 2 inhalations 1 min before exercise
Inhalation solution via nebulizer, 2.5 mg 3–4 times daily (in 2.5-mL sterile saline, over 5–15 min)
Regular tablets: PO, 2–4 mg 3–4 times daily
Extended release tablets: Volmax, PO, 8 mg q12h; Proventil Repetabs, PO, 4–8 mg q12h, initially. Increase if necessary to a maximum of 32 mg/d, in divided doses, q12h (both Volmax and Proventil Repetab)

*(continued)*

## PROTOTYPE PROFILE 37-1
### *P* Albuterol (Continued)

*Children:* Inhalation aerosol: 4 y and older (12 y and older for Proventil), same as adults

Nebulizer solution, 12 y and older, same as adults; 2–12 y (AccuNeb), 1.25 mg 3–4 times daily, as needed, over 5–15 min

Regular tablets: 12 y and older, same as adults; 6–12 y, 2 mg 3–4 times daily

Extended release tablets: 12 y and older, same as adults: 6–12 y: PO, 4 mg q12h initially; increase if necessary to a maximum of 24 mg/d, in divided doses, q12h (both Volmax and Proventil Repetab)

### Adverse Effects

CNS stimulation, dizziness, nervousness, tremor, angina, tachycardia, hypertension

### Drug Interactions
*Increased Effects*

Duration of bronchodilation with inhaled ipratropium

Cardiovascular effects with sympathomimetics, monoamine oxidase inhibitors, and tricyclic anti-depressants

Risk for malignant dysrhythmias with inhaled anesthetics

*Decreased Effects*

Albuterol effects with concurrent use of nonselective beta-adrenergic blockers

### Herbal Supplements and Dietary Considerations

Avoid ephedra and yohimbe because they may cause CNS stimulation

Limit caffeine because it may cause CNS stimulation

---

*Short-acting adrenergic bronchodilators are used mainly by inhalation, as needed, rather than on a regular schedule.

---

to treat rhinorrhea associated with allergic rhinitis and the common cold. It is available as a nasal spray for such use. Ipratropium is poorly absorbed and produces few systemic effects. However, cautious use is recommended in clients with narrow-angle glaucoma and prostatic hypertrophy. The most common adverse effects are cough, nervousness, nausea, gastrointestinal upset, headache, and dizziness.

## Xanthines

The main xanthine used clinically is **theophylline.** Despite many years of use, the drug's mechanism of action is unknown. Various mechanisms have been proposed, such as inhibiting phosphodiesterase enzymes that metabolize cAMP, increasing endogenous catecholamines, inhibiting calcium ion movement into smooth muscle, inhibiting prostaglandin synthesis and release, and inhibiting the release of bronchoconstrictive substances from mast cells and leukocytes. In addition to bronchodilation, other effects that may be beneficial in asthma and COPD include inhibiting pulmonary edema by decreasing vascular permeability, increasing the ability of cilia to clear mucus from the airways, strengthening contractions of the diaphragm, and decreasing inflammation. Theophylline also increases cardiac output, causes peripheral vasodilation, exerts a mild diuretic effect, and stimulates the CNS. The cardiovascular and CNS effects are adverse effects. Serum drug levels should be monitored to help regulate dosage and avoid adverse effects. Theophylline preparations are contraindicated in clients with acute gastritis and peptic ulcer disease; they should be used cautiously in those with cardiovascular disorders that could be aggravated by drug-induced cardiac stimulation.

Theophylline was formerly used extensively in the prevention and treatment of bronchoconstriction associated with asthma, bronchitis, and emphysema. It is considered a prototype, although it is now considered a second-line agent that may be added in severe disease inadequately controlled by first-line drugs (see Prototype Profile 37-2: Theophylline). Numerous dosage forms of theophylline are available. Theophylline ethylenediamine (aminophylline) contains approximately 85% theophylline and is the only formulation that can be given intravenously. However, intravenous aminophylline is not recommended for emergency treatment of acute asthma because studies indicate little, if any, added benefit in adults or children. Oral theophylline preparations may be used for long-term treatment. Most formulations contain anhydrous theophylline (100% theophylline) as the active ingredient, and sustained-action tablets (eg, Theo-Dur, Theobid) are more commonly used than other formulations.

## Anti-inflammatory Agents
### Corticosteroids

Corticosteroids (see Chap. 36) are used in the treatment of acute and chronic asthma and other bronchoconstrictive disorders, in which they have two major actions. First, they suppress inflammation in the airways by inhibiting the following processes: movement of fluid and protein into tissues; migration and function of neutrophils and eosinophils; synthesis of histamine in mast cells; and production of proinflammatory substances (eg, prostaglandins, leukotrienes, several interleukins, and others). Beneficial effects of suppressing airway inflammation include decreased mucus secretion, decreased edema

## PROTOTYPE PROFILE 37-2

### *P* Theophylline (thee OFF i lin)

### Drug Class
**Chemical:** Xanthine; methylxanthine
**Functional:** Bronchodilator

### Trade Names
Aminophylline, Theo-Dur, others

### Therapeutic Indications
Bronchodilator in airway obstruction due to asthma, chronic bronchitis, and emphysema

### Pharmacokinetics
*Absorption*
Well absorbed

*Distribution*
Plasma protein binding: 60%
Crosses placenta, enters breast milk

*Metabolism*
Liver; metabolism increased in smokers

*Excretion*
Kidneys

### Pharmacodynamics
*Onset of Action*
PO, 30 min; PO-SR, 1–3 h; IV: rapid

*Duration*
PO, 6 h; PO-SR, 8–24 h; IV: 6–8 h

### Contraindications/Precautions
Hypersensitivity, uncontrolled dysrhythmias, seizure disorders; with caution, peptic ulcer disease, hypertension, hyperthyroidism, tachydysrhythmias, liver dysfunction, and pulmonary edema

### Pregnancy Considerations
Category C
Crosses the placenta; enters breast milk; compatible

### Dosage
*To maintain serum drug level at 5–15 mcg/mL*

*Short-acting theophylline (Aminophylline)*
*Adults:* PO, 500 mg initially, then 200–300 mg q6–8h; IV infusion, 6 mg/kg over 30 min, then 0.1–1.2 mg/kg/h

*Long-acting Theophylline (Theo-Dur, others)*
PO, 150–300 mg q8–12h; maximal dose 13 mg/kg or 900 mg daily, whichever is less
*Children:* PO, 7.5 mg/kg initially, then 5–6 mg/kg q6–8h; IV infusion, 6 mg/kg over 30 min, then 0.6–0.9 mg/kg/h
PO, 100–200 mg q8–12h; maximal dose, 24 mg/kg/d

### Adverse Effects
Irritability, tachycardia, palpitations, insomnia, nausea, vomiting, anorexia, seizures, dysrhythmias

### Drug Interactions
*Increased Effects*
Increased serum levels with propranolol and other beta blockers, erythromycin, cimetidine, allopurinol, ciprofloxacin, oral contraceptives, isoniazid, loop diuretics, ephedrine, influenza virus vaccine, calcium channel blockers, disulfiram, and thyroid hormones

*Decreased Effects*
Drug effects with corticosteroids

### Herbal Supplements and Dietary Considerations
Changes in diet may alter the elimination of theophylline; increased drug elimination with charbroiled foods, smoking, high-protein, low-carbohydrate diets
Avoid excessive amounts of caffeine

SR, sustained release.

---

of airway mucosa, and repair of damaged epithelium, with subsequent reduction of airway reactivity. A second action is to increase the number and sensitivity of beta₂-adrenergic receptors, which restores or increases the effectiveness of beta₂-adrenergic bronchodilators. The number of beta₂ receptors increases within approximately 4 hours, and improved responsiveness to beta₂ agonists occurs within approximately 2 hours.

In acute, severe asthma, a systemic corticosteroid in relatively high doses is indicated in clients whose respiratory distress is not relieved by multiple doses of an inhaled beta₂ agonist (eg, every 20 minutes for 3 to 4 doses). The corticosteroid may be given intravenously or orally, and intravenous administration offers no therapeutic advantage over oral administration. Once the drug is started, pulmonary function usually improves in 6 to 8 hours. Most clients achieve substantial benefit

within 48 to 72 hours, and the drug is usually continued for 7 to 10 days. Multiple doses are usually given because studies indicate that maintaining the drug concentration at steroid receptor sites in the lung is more effective than high single doses. High single or pulse doses do not increase therapeutic effects; they may increase the risk for myopathy and other adverse effects, however. In some infants and young children with acute, severe asthma, oral prednisone for 3 to 10 days has relieved symptoms and prevented hospitalization.

In chronic asthma, a corticosteroid is usually taken by inhalation, on a daily schedule. It is often given concomitantly with one or more bronchodilators and may be given with another anti-inflammatory drug such as a leukotriene modifier or a mast cell stabilizer. In some instances, the other drugs allow smaller doses of the corticosteroid. For acute flare-ups of symptoms during treatment of chronic asthma, a systemic corticosteroid may be needed temporarily to regain control.

In early stages of the progressive disease, clients with COPD are unlikely to need corticosteroid therapy. In later stages, however, they usually need periodic short-course therapy for episodes of respiratory distress. When needed, the corticosteroid is given orally or parenterally because effectiveness of inhaled corticosteroids has not been established in COPD. In end-stage COPD, clients often become steroid dependent and require daily doses because any attempt to reduce dosage or stop the drug results in respiratory distress. Such clients experience numerous serious adverse effects of prolonged systemic corticosteroid therapy.

Corticosteroids should be used with caution in clients with peptic ulcer disease, inflammatory bowel disease, hypertension, congestive heart failure, and thromboembolic disorders. However, they cause fewer and less severe adverse effects when taken in short courses or by inhalation than when taken systemically for long periods of time.

**Beclomethasone, budesonide, flunisolide, fluticasone,** and **triamcinolone** are topical corticosteroids for inhalation. Topical administration minimizes systemic absorption and adverse effects. These preparations may substitute for or allow reduced dosage of systemic corticosteroids. In people with asthma who are taking an oral corticosteroid, the oral dosage is reduced slowly (over

weeks to months) when an inhaled corticosteroid is added. The goal is to give the lowest oral dose necessary to control symptoms. Beclomethasone, flunisolide, and fluticasone also are available in nasal solutions for treatment of allergic rhinitis, which may play a role in bronchoconstriction. Because systemic absorption occurs in clients using inhaled corticosteroids (about 20% of a dose), high doses should be reserved for those otherwise requiring oral corticosteroids.

**Hydrocortisone, prednisone,** and **methylprednisolone** are given to clients who require systemic corticosteroids. Prednisone is given orally; hydrocortisone and methylprednisolone may be given intravenously to clients who are unable to take an oral medication.

### Leukotriene Modifiers

Leukotrienes are strong chemical mediators of bronchoconstriction and inflammation, the major pathologic features of asthma. They can cause sustained constriction of bronchioles and immediate hypersensitivity reactions. They also increase mucus secretion and mucosal edema in the respiratory tract. Leukotrienes are formed by the lipoxygenase pathway of arachidonic acid metabolism (see Fig. 37-1) in response to cellular injury. They are designated by LT, the letter B, C, D, or E, and the number of chemical bonds in their structure (eg, LTB4, LTC4, and LTE4, also called *slow-releasing substances of anaphylaxis*

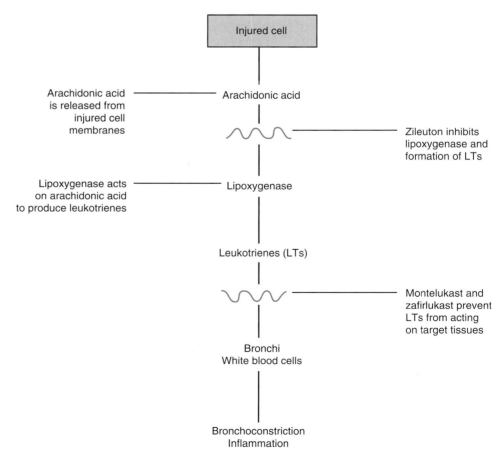

**FIGURE 37-1** Formation of leukotrienes and actions of leukotriene modifying drugs.

or SRS-A, because they are released more slowly than histamine).

Leukotriene modifier drugs were developed to counteract the effects of leukotrienes and are indicated for long-term treatment of asthma in adults and children. The drugs help to prevent acute asthma attacks induced by allergens, exercise, cold air, hyperventilation, irritants, and aspirin or NSAIDs. They are not effective in relieving acute attacks. However, they may be continued concurrently with other drugs during acute episodes.

The leukotriene modifiers include three agents with two different mechanisms of action. **Zileuton** inhibits lipoxygenase and thereby reduces formation of leukotrienes; **montelukast** and **zafirlukast** are leukotriene receptor antagonists. Zileuton is used infrequently because it requires multiple daily dosing, may cause hepatotoxicity, and may inhibit the metabolism of drugs metabolized by the cytochrome P450 3A4 enzymes. Zafirlukast and montelukast improve symptoms and pulmonary function tests (PFTs), decrease nighttime symptoms, and decrease the use of beta$_2$ agonists. They are effective with oral administration, can be taken once or twice a day, can be used with bronchodilators and corticosteroids, and elicit a high degree of client adherence and satisfaction. However, they are less effective than low doses of inhaled corticosteroids.

Montelukast and zafirlukast are well absorbed with oral administration. They are metabolized in the liver by the cytochrome P450 enzyme system and may interact with other drugs metabolized by this system. Most metabolites are excreted in the feces. Zafirlukast is excreted in breast milk and should not be taken during lactation. The most common adverse effects reported in clinical trials were headache, nausea, diarrhea, and infection.

Zileuton is well absorbed, highly bound to serum albumin (93%), and metabolized by the cytochrome P450 liver enzymes; metabolites are excreted mainly in urine. It is contraindicated in clients with active liver disease or substantially elevated liver enzymes (three times the upper limit of normal values). When used, hepatic aminotransferase enzymes should be monitored during therapy, and the drug should be discontinued if enzyme levels reach five times the normal values or if symptoms of liver dysfunction develop. Elevation of liver enzymes was the most serious adverse effect during clinical trials; other adverse effects include headache, pain, and nausea. In addition, zileuton increases serum concentrations of propranolol, theophylline, and warfarin.

### Mast Cell Stabilizers

**Cromolyn** and **nedocromil** stabilize mast cells and prevent the release of bronchoconstrictive and inflammatory substances when mast cells are confronted with allergens and other stimuli. The drugs are indicated only for prophylaxis of acute asthma attacks in clients with chronic asthma; they are not effective in acute bronchospasm or status asthmaticus and should not be used in these conditions. Use of one of these drugs may allow reduced dosage of bronchodilators and corticosteroids.

The drugs are taken by inhalation. Cromolyn is available in a metered-dose aerosol and a solution for use with a power-operated nebulizer. A nasal solution is also available for prevention and treatment of allergic rhinitis. Nedocromil is available in a metered-dose aerosol.

Mast cell stabilizers are contraindicated in clients who are hypersensitive to the drugs. They should be used with caution in clients with impaired renal or hepatic function. Also, the propellants in the aerosols may aggravate coronary artery disease or dysrhythmias.

## Herbal and Dietary Supplements

Numerous preparations are promoted to relieve symptoms of asthma, and clients with asthma are increasingly using alternative and complementary therapies. Some herbs have a pharmacologic basis for effect. However, most are less potent or more toxic than traditional asthma medications. For example, caffeine is a xanthine and therefore has bronchodilating effects similar to, but weaker than, those of theophylline. Caffeine-containing products, including coffee and tea, may slightly enhance bronchodilation. However, they also increase the adverse effects associated with adrenergic bronchodilators or theophylline (eg, symptoms of excessive cardiac and CNS stimulation such as tachycardia, dysrhythmias, insomnia, nervousness). Ephedra (ma huang), an adrenergic-type product, may also have bronchodilating effects. However, it also causes excessive cardiac and CNS stimulation, and deaths have been reported. It is not recommended for any use, by anyone.

In general, herbal and dietary therapies in asthma, as in other disorders, have not been studied in controlled clinical trials and should be avoided. Because asthma can result in death in a matter of minutes, clients should be counseled *not* to use dietary or herbal supplements in place of prescribed bronchodilating and anti-inflammatory medications. Delays in appropriate treatment can have serious, even fatal, consequences.

## ■ MANAGEMENT CONSIDERATIONS

### Drug Selection and Administration

Choice of drug and route of administration are determined largely by the severity of the disease process and the client's response to therapy. Some guidelines include the following:

1. A selective, short-acting, inhaled beta$_2$-adrenergic agonist (eg, albuterol) is the initial drug of choice for acute bronchospasm.
2. Because aerosol products act directly on the airways, drugs given by inhalation can usually be given in

*(text continues on page 691)*

# NURSING PROCESS

## Assessment

Assess the client's pulmonary function:

- General assessment factors include rate and character of respiration, skin color, arterial blood gas analysis, and pulmonary function tests. Abnormal breathing patterns (eg, rate below 12 or above 24 per minute, dyspnea, cough, orthopnea, wheezing, "noisy" respirations) may indicate respiratory distress. Severe respiratory distress is characterized by tachypnea, dyspnea, use of accessory muscles of respiration, and hypoxia. Early signs of hypoxia include mental confusion, restlessness, anxiety, and increased blood pressure and pulse rate. Late signs include cyanosis and decreased blood pressure and pulse. Hypoxemia is confirmed if arterial blood gas analysis shows decreased partial pressure of oxygen ($Po_2$).
- In acute bronchospasm, a medical emergency, the client is in obvious and severe respiratory distress. A characteristic feature of bronchospasm is forceful expiration or wheezing.
- If the client has chronic asthma, try to determine the frequency and severity of acute attacks, factors that precipitate or relieve acute attacks, antiasthmatic medications taken occasionally or regularly, allergies, and condition between acute attacks, such as restrictions in activities of daily living due to asthma.
- If the client has chronic bronchitis or emphysema, assess for signs of respiratory distress, hypoxia, cough, amount and character of sputum, exercise tolerance (eg, dyspnea on exertion, dyspnea at rest), medications, and nondrug treatment measures (eg, breathing exercises, chest physiotherapy).

## Nursing Diagnoses

- Impaired Gas Exchange related to bronchoconstriction and excessive mucus production
- Activity Intolerance related to impaired gas exchange and fatigue
- Risk for Injury: Severe bronchospasm with asthma and adverse effects with antiasthmatic drugs
- Noncompliance: Overuse of adrenergic bronchodilators
- Deficient Knowledge: Factors precipitating bronchoconstriction and strategies to avoid precipitating factors.
- Deficient Knowledge: Accurate self-administration of drugs, including use of inhalers

## Planning/Goals

*The client will:*
- Self-administer bronchodilating and other drugs accurately
- Experience relief of symptoms
- Avoid preventable adverse drug effects
- Avoid overusing bronchodilating drugs
- Avoid exposure to stimuli that cause bronchospasm when possible
- Avoid respiratory infections when possible

## Interventions

Use measures to prevent or relieve bronchoconstriction when possible. General measures include those to prevent respiratory disease or promote an adequate airway. Some specific measures include the following:

- Use mechanical measures for removing excessive respiratory tract secretions and preventing their retention. Effective measures include coughing, deep breathing, percussion, and postural drainage.
- Help the client identify and avoid exposure to conditions that precipitate bronchoconstriction. For example, allergens may be removed from the home, school, or work environment; cigarette smoke should be avoided when possible. When bronchospasm is precipitated by exercise, prophylaxis by prior inhalation of bronchodilating agents is better than avoiding exercise, especially in children.
- Assist clients with asthma to identify early signs of difficulty, including increased need for beta-adrenergic agonists, activity limitations, and waking at night with asthma symptoms.
- Monitor peak expiratory flow rate (PEFR) when indicated. Portable meters are available for use in clinics, physicians' offices, and clients' homes. This is an objective measure of airflow/airway obstruction and helps to evaluate the client's treatment regimen.
- Assist clients with moderate to severe asthma in obtaining meters and learning to measure PEFR. Clients with a decreased PEFR may need treatment to prevent acute, severe respiratory distress.
- Assist clients and at least one family member in managing acute attacks of bronchoconstriction, including when to seek emergency care.
- Try to prevent or reduce anxiety, which may aggravate bronchospasm. Stay with the client during an acute asthma attack if feasible. Clients experiencing severe and prolonged bronchospasm (status asthmaticus) should be admitted or transferred to a hospital intensive care unit.
- With any clients who smoke cigarettes, encourage cessation of smoking and provide information, resources, and assistance in doing so. Emphasize the health benefits of improved respiratory function.

## Evaluation

- Observe for relief of symptoms and improved arterial blood gas values.
- Interview and observe for correct drug administration, including use of inhalers.
- Interview and observe for tachydysrhythmias, nervousness, insomnia, and other adverse drug effects.
- Interview about and observe behaviors to avoid stimuli that cause bronchoconstriction and respiratory infections.

## CLIENT TEACHING GUIDELINES
## Antiasthmatic Drugs

### General Considerations

✔ Asthma and other chronic lung diseases are characterized by constant inflammation of the airways and periodic or persistent labored breathing from constriction or narrowing of the airways. Antiasthmatic drugs are often given in combination to combat these problems. Thus, it is extremely important to know the type and purpose of each drug.

✔ Except for the short-acting, inhaled bronchodilators (eg, albuterol), antiasthmatic medications are used long term to control symptoms and prevent acute asthma attacks. This means they must be taken on a regular schedule and continued when symptom free.

✔ When an asthma attack (ie, acute bronchospasm with shortness of breath, wheezing respirations, cough) occurs, the only fast-acting, commonly used medication to relieve these symptoms is an inhaled, short-acting bronchodilator (eg, albuterol). Other inhaled and oral drugs are not effective and should not be used.

✔ Try to prevent symptoms. For example, respiratory infections can precipitate difficulty in breathing. Avoiding infections (eg, by good handwashing, avoiding people with infections, annual influenza vaccinations, and other measures) can prevent acute asthma attacks. If you are allergic to tobacco smoke, perfume, or flowers, try to avoid or minimize exposure.

✔ A common cause of acute asthma attacks is not taking medications correctly. Some studies indicate that one third to two thirds of clients with asthma do not comply with instructions for using their medications. Factors that contribute to noncompliance with drug therapy include long-term use, expense, and adverse effects. If you have difficulty taking medications as prescribed, discuss the situation with a health care provider. Cheaper medications or lower doses may be effective alternatives. Just stopping the medications may precipitate acute breathing problems.

✔ If unable to prevent symptoms, early recognition and treatment may help prevent severe distress and hospitalizations. Signs of impending difficulty include increased needs for bronchodilator inhalers, activity limitations, waking at night because of asthma symptoms, and variability in the peak expiratory flow rate (PEFR), if you use a PEFR meter at home. The first treatment is to use a short-acting, inhaled bronchodilator. If this does not improve breathing, seek emergency care.

✔ Keep adequate supplies of medications on hand. Missing a few doses of long-term control or "preventive" medications may precipitate an acute asthma attack; not using an inhaled bronchodilator for early breathing difficulty may lead to more severe problems and the need for emergency treatment or hospitalization.

✔ Be sure you can use your metered-dose inhalers correctly. According to several research studies, many patients do not.

✔ Drinking 2 to 3 quarts of fluids daily helps thin secretions in the throat and lungs and makes them easier to remove.

✔ Avoid tobacco smoke and other substances that irritate breathing passages (eg, aerosol hair spray, antiperspirants, cleaning products, and automobile exhaust) when possible.

✔ Avoid excessive intake of caffeine-containing fluids such as coffee, tea, and cola drinks. These beverages may increase bronchodilation but also may increase heart rate and cause palpitations, nervousness, and insomnia with bronchodilating drugs.

✔ Take influenza vaccine annually and pneumococcal vaccine at least once if you have chronic lung disease.

✔ Inform all health care providers about the medications you are taking and do not take over-the-counter drugs or herbal supplements without consulting a health care provider. Some drugs can decrease beneficial effects or increase adverse effects of antiasthmatic medications. For example, over-the-counter nasal decongestants, asthma remedies, cold remedies, and antisleep medications can increase the rapid heartbeat, palpitations, and nervousness often associated with bronchodilators. With herbal remedies, none are as effective as standard antiasthmatic medication, and they may cause serious or life-threatening adverse effects. Preparations containing ephedra (also called ma huang or herbal ecstasy) are especially dangerous and not recommended for use by anyone, for any purpose.

### Self-administration

✔ Follow instructions carefully. Better breathing with minimal adverse effects depends on accurate use of prescribed medications. If help is needed with metered-dose inhalers, consult a health care provider.

✔ Use short-acting bronchodilator inhalers as needed, not on a regular schedule. If desired effects are not achieved or if symptoms worsen, inform the prescribing physician. Do not increase dosage or frequency of taking medication. Overuse increases adverse drug effects and decreases drug effectiveness.

✔ If taking formoterol or salmeterol, which are long-acting, inhaled bronchodilators, do not use more often than every 12 hours. If constricted breathing occurs, use a short-acting bronchodilator inhaler between doses of a long-acting drug. Salmeterol does not relieve acute shortness of breath because it takes approximately 20 minutes to start acting and 1 to 4 hours to achieve maximal bronchodilating effects.

✔ If taking an oral or inhaled corticosteroid, take on a regular schedule, approximately the same time each day. The purpose of these drugs is to relieve inflammation in the airways and prevent acute respiratory distress. They are not effective unless taken regularly.

*(continued)*

**CLIENT TEACHING GUIDELINES**
## Antiasthmatic Drugs (Continued)

✔ If taking oral theophylline, take fast-acting preparations before meals with a full glass of water, at regular intervals around the clock. If gastrointestinal upset occurs, take with food. Take long-acting preparations every 8 to 12 hours; do not chew or crush.

✔ Take zafirlukast 1 hour before or 2 hours after a meal; montelukast and zileuton may be taken with or without food. Take montelukast in the evening or at bedtime. This schedule provides maximum beneficial effects during the night and early morning, when asthma symptoms often occur or worsen.

✔ Use inhalers correctly:

1. Shake well immediately before each use.
2. Remove the cap from the mouthpiece.
3. Exhale to the end of a normal breath.
4. With the inhaler in the upright position, place the mouthpiece just inside the mouth, and use the lips to form a tight seal or hold the mouthpiece approximately two finger-widths from the open mouth.
5. While pressing down on the inhaler, take a slow, deep breath for 3 to 5 seconds, hold the breath for approximately 10 seconds, and exhale slowly.
6. Wait 3 to 5 min before taking a second inhalation of the drug.
7. Rinse the mouth with water after each use.
8. Rinse the mouthpiece and store the inhaler away from heat.
9. If you have difficulty using an inhaler, ask your physician about a spacer device (a tube attached to the inhaler that makes it easier to use).

---

smaller doses and produce fewer adverse effects than oral or parenteral drugs.

3. Ipratropium, the anticholinergic bronchodilator, is most useful in the long-term management of COPD. It is ineffective in relieving acute bronchospasm by itself, but it adds to the bronchodilating effects of adrenergic drugs.

4. Theophylline is used less often than formerly and is now considered a second-line drug. When used, it is usually given orally in an extended-release formulation for chronic disorders, such as COPD. Intravenous aminophylline is no longer used to treat acute asthma attacks.

5. Cromolyn and nedocromil are used prophylactically; they are ineffective in acute bronchospasm.

6. Because inflammation has been established as a major component of asthma, an inhaled corticosteroid is being used early in the disease process, often with a bronchodilator or mast cell stabilizer. In acute episodes of bronchoconstriction, a corticosteroid is often given orally or intravenously for several days.

In chronic disorders, inhaled corticosteroids should be taken on a regular schedule. These drugs may be effective when used alone or with relatively small doses of an oral corticosteroid. Optimal schedules of administration are not clearly established, but more frequent dosing (eg, every 6 hours) may be more effective than less frequent dosing (eg, every 12 hours), even if the total amount is the same. As with systemic glucocorticoid therapy, the recommended dose is the lowest amount required to control symptoms. High doses suppress adrenocortical function, but much less than systemic drugs. Small doses may impair bone metabolism and predispose adults to osteoporosis by decreasing calcium deposition and increasing calcium resorption from bone. In children, chronic administration of corticosteroids may retard growth. Local adverse effects (oropharyngeal candidiasis, hoarseness) can be decreased by reducing the dose, administering less often, rinsing the mouth after use, or using a spacer device. These measures decrease the amount of drug deposited in the oral cavity. The inhaled drugs are well tolerated with chronic use.

7. A common regimen for treatment of moderate asthma is an inhaled corticosteroid on a regular schedule, two to four times daily, and a short-acting, inhaled beta$_2$-adrenergic agonist as needed for prevention or treatment of bronchoconstriction. For more severe asthma, an inhaled corticosteroid is continued, and both a short-acting and a long-acting beta$_2$ agonist may be given. A leukotriene modifier may also be added to the regimen, to control symptoms further and to reduce the need for corticosteroids and inhaled bronchodilators.

8. Multidrug regimens are commonly used, and one advantage is that smaller doses of each agent can usually be given. This may decrease adverse effects and allow dosages to be increased when exacerbation of symptoms occurs. Available combination inhalation products include Combivent (albuterol

---

**? How Can You Avoid
This Medication Error?**

Keith Wilson, 66 years of age, has worsening chronic obstructive pulmonary disease. At his last office visit, his physician added ipratropium bromide (Atrovent) and beclomethasone (Vanceril) to his beta-adrenergic (Alupent) inhaler. He visits the office complaining of severe dyspnea. You quickly grab his Atrovent inhaler to administer a PRN dose and try to get him to relax. What drug error has occurred, and how could this error be avoided?

and ipratropium) and Advair (salmeterol and fluticasone). Advair, which was developed to treat both inflammation and bronchoconstriction, was more effective than the individual components at the same doses and as effective as concurrent use of the same drugs at the same doses. In addition, the combination reduced the corticosteroid dose by 50% and was more effective than higher doses of fluticasone alone in reducing asthma exacerbations. The combination improved symptoms within 1 week. Additional combination products are likely to be marketed and may improve client compliance with prescribed drug therapy.

## Dosage Factors

Dosage of antiasthmatic drugs must be individualized to attain the most therapeutic effects and the fewest adverse effects. Larger doses of bronchodilators and corticosteroids (inhaled, systemic, or both) are usually required to relieve the symptoms of acute, severe bronchoconstriction or status asthmaticus. Then, doses should be reduced to the smallest effective amounts for long-term control.

Dosage of theophylline preparations should be based mainly on serum theophylline levels (therapeutic range is 5 to 15 mcg/mL; toxic levels are 20 mcg/mL or above). Blood for serum levels should be drawn 1 to 2 hours after immediate-release dosage forms and about 4 hours after sustained-release forms. In addition, children and cigarette smokers usually need higher doses to maintain therapeutic blood levels because they metabolize theophylline rapidly, and clients with liver disease, congestive heart failure, chronic pulmonary disease, or acute viral infections usually need smaller doses because these conditions impair theophylline metabolism. For obese clients, theophylline dosage should be calculated on the basis of lean or ideal body weight because theophylline is not highly distributed in fatty tissue.

## ■ DRUG USE IN SPECIFIC SITUATIONS

### Drug Toxicity and Overdose

Signs and symptoms of overdose and toxicity are probably most likely to occur when clients with acute or chronic bronchoconstrictive disorders overuse bronchodilators in their efforts to relieve dyspnea. General management of acute poisoning includes early recognition of signs and symptoms, stopping the causative drug, and instituting other treatment measures as indicated. Specific measures include the following:

- **Bronchodilator overdose.** With inhaled or systemic adrenergic bronchodilators, major adverse effects are excessive cardiac and CNS stimulation. Symptoms of cardiac stimulation include angina, tachycardia, and palpitations; serious dysrhythmias and cardiac arrest have also been reported. Symptoms of CNS stimulation include agitation, anxiety, insomnia, seizures, and tremors. Severe overdoses may cause delirium, collapse, and coma. In addition, hypokalemia, hyperglycemia, and hypotension or hypertension may occur. Management includes discontinuing the causative medications and using general supportive measures (emesis, gastric lavage, or activated charcoal may be useful with oral drugs). For cardiac symptoms, monitor blood pressure, pulse, and electrocardiogram (ECG). Cautious use of a beta-adrenergic blocking drug (eg, propranolol) may be indicated. However, a nonselective beta-blocker may induce bronchoconstriction.

- **Theophylline overdose.** Signs and symptoms include anorexia, nausea, vomiting, agitation, nervousness, insomnia, tachycardia and other dysrhythmias, and tonic-clonic convulsions. Ventricular dysrhythmias or convulsions may be the first sign of toxicity. Serious adverse effects rarely occur at serum drug levels of less than 20 mcg/mL. Overdoses with sustained-release preparations may cause a dramatic increase in serum drug concentrations much later (12 hours or longer) than the immediate-release preparations. Early treatment helps but does not prevent these delayed increases in serum drug levels.

  In clients without seizures, induce vomiting unless the level of consciousness is impaired. In these clients, precautions to prevent aspiration are needed, especially in children. If overdose is identified within an hour of drug ingestion, gastric lavage may be helpful if unable to induce vomiting or if vomiting is contraindicated. Administration of activated charcoal and a cathartic is also recommended, especially for overdoses of sustained-release formulations.

  In clients with seizures, treatment includes securing the airway, giving oxygen, injecting intravenous diazepam (0.1 to 0.3 mg/kg, up to 10 mg), monitoring vital signs, maintaining blood pressure, providing adequate hydration, and monitoring serum theophylline levels until below 20 mcg/mL. Also, symptomatic treatment of dysrhythmias may be needed.

- **Leukotriene modifiers and mast cell stabilizers.** These drugs seem relatively devoid of serious toxicity. There have been few reports of toxicity in humans and little clinical experience in managing it. If toxicity occurs, general supportive and symptomatic treatment is indicated.

## Status Asthmaticus

Acute, severe asthma (status asthmaticus) is characterized by severe respiratory distress and requires emergency treatment. Beta$_2$ agonists should be given in high doses and as often as every 20 minutes for 1 to 2 hours (by MDIs with spacer devices or by compressed-air nebulization). However, high doses of nebulized albuterol have been associated with tachycardia, hypokalemia, and hyperglycemia. Once symptoms are controlled, dosage can usually be reduced and dosing intervals extended. High doses of systemic corticosteroids are also given for several days, intravenously or orally. If the client is able to take an oral drug, there is no therapeutic advantage to intravenous administration.

When respiratory function improves, efforts to prevent future episodes are needed. These efforts may include identifying and avoiding suspected triggers, evaluation and possible adjustment of the client's treatment regimen, and assessment of the client's adherence to the prescribed regimen.

## Nursing Actions
## Drugs for Asthma and Other Bronchoconstrictive Disorders

| Nursing Actions | Rationale/Explanation |
|---|---|
| **1. Administer accurately.** | |
| a. Be sure clients have adequate supplies of inhaled bronchodilators and corticosteroids available for self-administration. Observe technique of self-administration for accuracy and assist if needed. | |
| b. Give immediate-release oral theophylline before meals with a full glass of water, at regular intervals around the clock. If gastrointestinal upset occurs, give with food. | To promote dissolution and absorption. Taking with food may decrease nausea and vomiting. |
| c. Give sustained-release theophylline q8–12h, with instructions not to chew or crush. | Sustained-release drug formulations should never be chewed or crushed because doing so causes immediate release of potentially toxic doses. |
| d. Give zafirlukast 1 h before or 2 h after a meal; montelukast and zileuton may be given with or without food. | The bioavailability of zafirlukast is reduced approximately 40% if taken with food. Food does not significantly affect the bioavailability of montelukast and zileuton. |
| e. Give montelukast in the evening or at bedtime | This schedule provides high drug concentrations during the night and early morning, when asthma symptoms tend to occur or worsen. |
| **2. Observe for therapeutic effects.** | |
| a. Decreased dyspnea, wheezing, and respiratory secretions | Relief of bronchospasm and wheezing should be evident within a few minutes after giving subcutaneous epinephrine, IV aminophylline, or aerosolized adrenergic bronchodilators. |
| b. Reduced rate and improved quality of respirations | |
| c. Reduced anxiety and restlessness | |
| d. Therapeutic serum levels of theophylline (5–15 mcg/mL) | |
| e. Improved arterial blood gas levels (normal values: $Po_2$ 80 to 100 mm Hg; $Pco_2$ 35 to 45 mm Hg; pH, 7.35 to 7.45) | |
| f. Improved exercise tolerance | |
| g. Decreased incidence and severity of acute attacks of bronchospasm with chronic administration of drugs | |
| **3. Observe for adverse effects.** | |
| a. With adrenergic bronchodilators, observe for tachycardia, arrhythmias, palpitations, restlessness, agitation, insomnia. | These signs and symptoms result from cardiac and central nervous system (CNS) stimulation. |
| b. With ipratropium, observe for cough or exacerbation of symptoms. | Ipratropium produces few adverse effects because it is not absorbed systemically. |
| c. With xanthine bronchodilators, observe for tachycardia, arrhythmias, palpitations, restlessness, agitation, insomnia, nausea, vomiting, convulsions. | Theophylline causes cardiac and CNS stimulation. Convulsions occur at toxic serum concentrations (>20 mcg/mL). They may occur without preceding symptoms of toxicity and may result in death. IV diazepam (Valium) may be used to control seizures. Theophylline also stimulates the chemoreceptor trigger zone in the medulla oblongata to cause nausea and vomiting. |

(continued)

## Nursing Actions

### Drugs for Asthma and Other Bronchoconstrictive Disorders (Continued)

| Nursing Actions | Rationale/Explanation |
|---|---|
| d. With inhaled corticosteroids, observe for hoarseness, cough, throat irritation, and fungal infection of mouth and throat. | Inhaled corticosteroids are unlikely to produce the serious adverse effects of long-term systemic therapy (see Chap. 24). |
| e. With leukotriene inhibitors, observe for headache, infection, nausea, pain, elevated liver enzymes (eg, alanine aminotransferase [ALT]), and liver dysfunction. | These drugs are usually well tolerated. A highly elevated ALT and liver dysfunction are more likely to occur with zileuton. |
| f. With cromolyn, observe for dysrhythmias, hypotension, chest pain, restlessness, dizziness, convulsions, CNS depression, anorexia, nausea and vomiting. Sedation and coma may occur with overdosage. | Some of the cardiovascular effects are thought to be caused by the propellants used in the aerosol preparation. |
| **4. Observe for drug interactions.** | |
| a. Drugs that *increase* effects of bronchodilators: | |
| (1) Monoamine oxidase inhibitors | These drugs inhibit the metabolism of catecholamines. The subsequent administration of bronchodilators may increase blood pressure. |
| (2) Erythromycin, clindamycin, cimetidine | These drugs may decrease theophylline clearance and thereby increase plasma levels. |
| b. Drugs that *decrease* effects of bronchodilators: | |
| (1) Lithium | Lithium may increase excretion of theophylline and therefore decrease therapeutic effectiveness. |
| (2) Phenobarbital | This drug may increase the metabolism of theophylline by way of enzyme induction. |
| (3) Propranolol, other nonselective beta blockers | These drugs may cause bronchoconstriction and oppose effects of bronchodilators. |
| c. Drugs that alter effects of zafirlukast: | |
| (1) Aspirin | Increases blood levels |
| (2) Erythromycin, theophylline | Decrease blood levels |

### ? How Can You Avoid This Medication Error?

**Answer:** Only short-acting beta-adrenergic bronchodilators should be used for acute dyspnea. Alupent, not Atrovent, is indicated. When patients have more than one inhaler, they should be taught which inhaler to use in emergency situations. The canister should be a different color (many manufacturers consider this) or clearly marked with tape, so that quick identification can occur in an emergency. Additional teaching may be indicated for the nurse and the patient regarding the action of each inhaler.

### Critical Thinking Exercises

1. The nurse checks the results of a serum theophylline level before administration of a scheduled dose. The level is 16 mg/mL. The nurse should:
   a. Hold the drug and contact the health care provider
   b. Administer the dose as scheduled
   c. Recognize that the level is subtherapeutic and inform the health care provider
   d. Hold the drug and monitor for signs of cardiac dysrhythmias, anorexia, and seizure activity

2. A client who is taking theophylline reports that she is continuing to smoke. What effect will smoking have on serum theophylline levels?
   a. Decreased theophylline levels
   b. Increased theophylline levels
   c. No effect
   d. Decreased reliability of calculated levels

3. A client with asthma begins experiencing wheezing and demonstrates signs of an acute asthmatic attack. Which inhaler can the nurse anticipate would be most effective in relieving her acute symptoms?

   a. Montelukast (Singulair)
   b. Triamcinolone (Azmacort)
   c. Nedocromil (Tilade)
   d. Albuterol (Proventil)

4. The most frequent adverse effect with the use of a glucocorticoid inhaler is:

   a. Oral *Candida* species infection
   b. Glucose intolerance
   c. Osteoporosis
   d. Fluid retention

5. The nurse is teaching a client about administering beta$_2$-adrenergic agonists and glucocorticoid inhalers. How should the nurse instruct the client to administer the inhalers?

   a. Administer the glucocorticoid inhaler first, followed by the beta$_2$-adrenergic agonist inhaler
   b. Administer the beta$_2$-adrenergic agonist inhaler first, followed by the glucocorticoid inhaler
   c. Inhalers can be used in any sequence
   d. Administration of the inhalers should be spaced 4 hours apart

## SELECTED REFERENCES

Allen, D. B. (2002). Inhaled corticosteroid therapy for asthma in preschool children: Growth issues. *Pediatrics, 109*(2), 373–380.

Allen, D. B. (2002). Safety of inhaled corticosteroids in children. *Pediatric Pulmonology, 33,* 208–220.

American Academy of Pediatrics. Practice guideline endorsement. *Guidelines for the diagnosis and management of asthma.* (2002). [On-line.] Available: http://www.aap.org/policy/astmaref.html. Accessed December 27, 2003.

Blake, K. (2000). Asthma. In E. T. Herfindal & D. R. Gourley (Eds.), *Textbook of therapeutics: Drug and disease management* (7th ed., pp. 727–764). Philadelphia: Lippincott Williams & Wilkins.

Cockcroft, D. W. (1999). Pharmacologic therapy for asthma: Overview and historical perspective. *Journal of Clinical Pharmacology, 39,* 216–222.

Dhand, R. (2000). MDIs and dry powder inhalers: Maximizing benefits, avoiding pitfalls—metered dose inhalers. *Consultant, 40*(3), 501–509.

*Drug facts and comparisons.* (Updated monthly). St. Louis: Facts and Comparisons.

Fulco, P. P., Lone, A. A., & Pugh, C. B. (2002). Intravenous versus oral corticosteroids for treatment of acute asthma exacerbations. *Annals of Pharmacotherapy, 36,* 565–570.

Gallagher, C. (2002). Childhood asthma: Tools that help parents manage it. *American Journal of Nursing, 102*(8), 71–83.

Kelly, H. W., & Sorkness, C. A. (2002). Asthma. In J. T. DiPiro, R. L. Talbert, G. C. Yee, G. R. Matzke, B. G. Wells, & L. M. Posey (Eds.), *Pharmacotherapy: A pathophysiologic approach* (4th ed., pp. 475–510). New York: McGraw-Hill.

Lazarus, S. C., Boushey, H. A., Fahy, J. V., Chinchilli, V. M., Lemanski, R. F., Sorkness, C. A., et al. (2001). Long-acting beta$_2$-agonist monotherapy vs. continued therapy with inhaled corticosteroids in patients with persistent asthma: A randomized controlled trial. *Journal of the American Medical Association, 285*(20), 2583–2593.

Lemanske, R. F., Jr. (2002). Inflammation in childhood asthma and other wheezing disorders. *Pediatrics, 109*(2), 368–372.

Lacy, C. F., Armstrong, L. L., Goldman, M. P., & Lance, L. L. (2003). *Lexi-Comp's drug information handbook* (11th ed.). Hudson, OH: American Pharmaceutical Association.

National Asthma Education and Prevention Program. Expert Panel Report 2: *Guidelines for the diagnosis and management of asthma.* Bethesda, MD: National Institutes of Health, National Heart, Lung, and Blood Institute, 1997. (Clinical Practice Guidelines. NIH Pub. No. 97-4051, Feb. 1997). *Update on selected topics 2002* (NIH Pub. No. 02-5075, June, 2002).

Pope, B. B. (2002). Patient Education Series: Asthma. *Nursing 2002, 32*(5), 44–45.

Porth, C. M. (Ed.). (2002). *Pathophysiology: Concepts of altered health states* (6th ed.). Philadelphia: Lippincott Williams & Wilkins.

Sorkness, C. A. (2001). Leukotriene receptor antagonists in the treatment of asthma. *Pharmacotherapy, 21*(2 Pt 3), 34S–37S.

Togger, D. A., & Brenner, P. S. (2001). Metered dose inhalers. *American Journal of Nursing, 101*(10), 26–32.

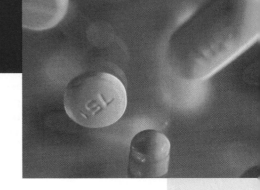

# 38

# Antihistamines

## OBJECTIVES

*After studying this chapter, the student will be able to:*

1 Delineate effects of histamine on selected body tissues.

2 Differentiate histamine receptors.

3 Describe the types of hypersensitivity or allergic reactions.

4 Discuss allergic rhinitis, allergic contact dermatitis, and drug allergies as conditions for which antihistamines are commonly used.

5 Identify the effects of histamine that are blocked by histamine-1 receptor antagonist drugs.

6 Differentiate first- and second-generation antihistamines.

7 Describe antihistamines in terms of indications for use, adverse effects, and nursing process implications.

8 Discuss the use of antihistamines in special populations.

## CRITICAL THINKING SCENARIO

*Y*ou are working at the college health center. Brad, a freshman, comes to the clinic complaining of seasonal pollen allergies that have worsened significantly since his relocation at college. He has been self-treating with over-the-counter (OTC) medications that a friend in his dormitory gave him.

✔ How would you assess Brad's allergy history and factors that may have increased Brad's allergic response?

✔ What would you teach Brad about his allergic response and how antihistamines work?

✔ How would you inform Brad on the correct use of OTC allergy medications to manage symptoms, including side effects and interactions?

✔ What are some nonpharmacologic methods Brad might use to prevent or limit allergic reactions?

## PROTOTYPE PROFILES

**diphenhydramine** (Benadryl), p. 704

**loratadine** (Claritin), p. 705

# OVERVIEW

Antihistamines are drugs that antagonize the action of histamine. Thus, to understand the use of these drugs, it is necessary to understand histamine and its effects on body tissues, characteristics of allergic reactions, and selected conditions for which antihistamines are used. Histamine effects on body tissues are described in At the Foundation: Histamine and Its Receptors; allergic reactions and select conditions are described below.

# HYPERSENSITIVITY (ALLERGIC) REACTIONS

Hypersensitivity or allergic reactions are immune responses in which a person's body overreacts to an environmental or ingested substance that does not cause a reaction in most people. That is, the person is hypersensitive or allergic to the substance (called an *antigen* or *allergen*). Allergic reactions may result from specific antibodies, sensitized T lymphocytes, or both, formed during exposure to an antigen.

## Types of Allergic Reactions

■ *Type I* (also called immediate hypersensitivity because it occurs within minutes of exposure to the antigen) is an immunoglobulin E (IgE)-induced response that causes release of histamine and other mediators. For example, *anaphylaxis* is a type I response that may be mild (characterized mainly by urticaria, other dermatologic manifestations, or rhinitis) or severe and life threatening (characterized by respiratory distress and cardiovascular collapse). It is uncommon and does not occur on first exposure to an antigen; it occurs with a second or later exposure, after antibody formation was induced by an earlier exposure. Severe anaphylaxis (sometimes called *anaphylactic shock*) is characterized by cardiovascular collapse from profound vasodilation and pooling of blood in the splanchnic system so that the patient has severe hypotension and functional hypovolemia. Respiratory distress often occurs from laryngeal edema and bronchoconstriction. Urticaria often occurs because the skin has many mast cells to release histamine. Anaphylaxis is a systemic reaction that usually involves the respiratory, cardiovascular, and dermatologic systems. Severe anaphylaxis may be fatal if not treated promptly and effectively.

■ *Type II* responses are mediated by IgG or IgM. They produce direct damage to the cell surface. These cytotoxic reactions include blood transfusion reactions, hemolytic disease of newborns, autoimmune hemolytic anemia, and some drug reactions.

■ *Type III* is an IgG- or IgM-mediated reaction characterized by formation of antigen–antibody complexes that induce an acute inflammatory reaction in the tissues. *Serum sickness*, the prototype of these reactions, occurs when excess antigen combines with antibodies

---

**AT THE FOUNDATION:** *Histamine and Its Receptors*

Histamine is the first chemical mediator to be released in immune and inflammatory responses. It is synthesized and stored in most body tissues, with high concentrations in tissues exposed to environmental substances (eg, the skin and mucosal surfaces of the eye, nose, lungs, and GI tract). It is also found in the CNS. In these tissues, histamine is located mainly in secretory granules of mast cells (tissue cells surrounding capillaries) and basophils (circulating blood cells).

Histamine is discharged from mast cells and basophils in response to certain stimuli (eg, allergic reactions, cellular injury, extreme cold). Once released, it diffuses rapidly into other tissues, where it interacts with histamine receptors on target organs, called $H_1$ and $H_2$. $H_1$ receptors are located mainly on smooth muscle cells in blood vessels and the respiratory and GI tracts. When histamine binds with these receptors and stimulates them, effects include the following:

• Contraction of smooth muscle in the bronchi and bronchioles (producing bronchoconstriction and respiratory distress)
• Stimulation of vagus nerve endings to produce reflex bronchoconstriction and cough

• Increased permeability of veins and capillaries, which allows fluid to flow into subcutaneous tissues and form edema.
• Increased secretion of mucous glands. Mucosal edema and increased nasal mucus produce the nasal congestion characteristic of allergic rhinitis and the common cold.
• Stimulation of sensory peripheral nerve endings to cause pain and pruritus. Pruritus is especially prominent with allergic skin disorders.
• Dilation of capillaries in the skin, to cause flushing

When $H_2$ receptors are stimulated, the main effects are increased secretion of gastric acid and pepsin, increased rate and force of myocardial contraction, and decreased immunologic and proinflammatory reactions (eg, decreased release of histamine from basophils, decreased movement of neutrophils and basophils into areas of injury, inhibited T- and B-lymphocyte function). Stimulation of both $H_1$ and $H_2$ receptors causes peripheral vasodilation (with hypotension, headache, and skin flushing) and increases bronchial, intestinal, and salivary secretion of mucus.

to form immune complexes. The complexes then diffuse into affected tissues, where they cause tissue damage by activating the complement system and initiating the inflammatory response. If small amounts of immune complexes are deposited locally, the antigenic material can be phagocytized and digested by white blood cells and macrophages without tissue destruction. If large amounts are deposited locally or reach the bloodstream and become deposited in blood vessel walls, the lysosomal enzymes released during phagocytosis may cause permanent tissue destruction.

■ *Type IV* hypersensitivity (also called delayed hypersensitivity because it usually occurs several hours or days after exposure to the antigen) is a cell-mediated response in which sensitized T lymphocytes react with an antigen to cause inflammation mediated by release of lymphokines, direct cytotoxicity, or both.

## Allergic Rhinitis

Allergic rhinitis is inflammation of nasal mucosa caused by a type I hypersensitivity reaction to inhaled allergens. It is a very common disorder characterized by nasal congestion, itching, sneezing, and watery drainage. Itching of the throat, eyes, and ears often occurs as well.

There are two types of allergic rhinitis. Seasonal disease (often called hay fever) produces acute symptoms in response to the protein components of airborne pollens from trees, grasses, and weeds, mainly in spring or fall. Perennial disease produces chronic symptoms in response to nonseasonal allergens such as dust mites, animal dander, and molds. Actually, mold spores can cause both seasonal and perennial allergies because they are present year round, with seasonal increases. Some people have both types, with chronic symptoms plus acute seasonal symptoms.

People with a personal or family history of other allergic disorders are likely to have allergic rhinitis. Once the nasal mucosa is inflamed, nonallergenic irritants such as tobacco smoke, strong odors, air pollution, and climatic changes can worsen symptoms.

Allergic rhinitis is an immune response in which normal nasal breathing and filtering of air brings inhaled antigens into contact with mast cells and basophils in nasal mucosa, blood vessels, and submucosal tissues. With initial exposure, the inhaled antigens are processed by lymphocytes that produce IgE, an antigen-specific antibody that binds to mast cells. With later exposures, the IgE interacts with inhaled antigens and triggers the breakdown of the mast cell. This breakdown causes the release of histamine and other inflammatory mediators such as prostaglandins and leukotrienes (Fig. 38-1). These mediators, of which histamine may be the most important, dilate and engorge blood vessels to produce

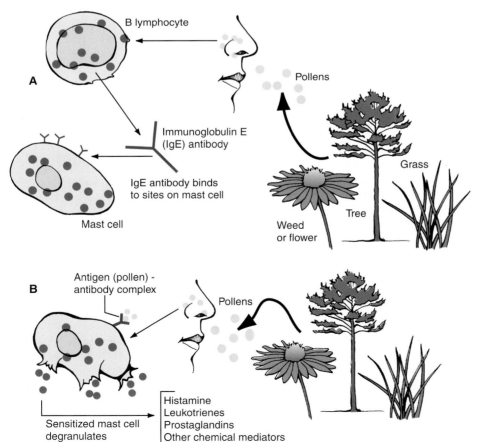

FIGURE 38-1 Type I hypersensitivity reaction: allergic rhinitis. (A) The first exposure of mast cells in nasal mucosa to inhaled antigens (eg, pollens from weeds, grasses, trees) leads to the formation of immunoglobulin E (IgE) antibody molecules. These molecules then bind to the surface membranes of mast cells. This process sensitizes mast cells to the effects of inhaled antigens (allergens). (B) When sensitized mast cells are re-exposed to inhaled pollens or other antigens, they release histamine and other chemical mediators which then act on nasal mucosa to produce characteristic symptoms of allergic rhinitis.

nasal congestion, stimulate secretion of mucus, and attract inflammatory cells (eg, eosinophils, lymphocytes, monocytes, macrophages). In people with allergies, mast cells and basophils are increased in both number and reactivity. Thus, they may be capable of releasing large amounts of histamine and other mediators.

Allergic rhinitis that is not effectively treated may lead to chronic fatigue, impaired ability to perform usual activities of daily living, difficulty sleeping, sinus infections, postnasal drip, cough, and headache. In addition, this condition is a strong risk factor for asthma.

## Allergic Contact Dermatitis

Allergic contact dermatitis is a type IV hypersensitivity reaction resulting from direct contact with antigens to which a person has previously become sensitized (eg, poison ivy or poison oak, cosmetics, hair dyes, metals, drugs applied topically to the skin). This reaction, which may be acute or chronic, usually occurs more than 24 hours after reexposure to an antigen and may last from days to weeks.

Affected areas of the skin are usually inflamed, warm, edematous, intensely pruritic, and tender to touch. Skin lesions are usually erythematous macules, papules, and vesicles (blisters) that may drain, develop crusts, and become infected. Lesion location may indicate the causative antigen.

## Allergic Drug Reactions

Virtually any drug may induce an immunologic response in susceptible people, and any body tissues may be affected. Allergic drug reactions are complex and diverse and may include any of the types of hypersensitivity described previously. A single drug may induce one or more of these states and multiple symptoms. There are no specific characteristics that identify drug-related reactions, although some reactions commonly attributed to drugs (eg, skin rashes, drug fever, hematologic reactions, hepatic reactions) rarely occur with plant pollens and other naturally occurring antigens. Usually, however, the body responds to a drug as it does to other foreign materials (antigens). In addition, coloring agents, preservatives, and other additives, rather than the drug itself, may cause some reactions.

Allergic drug reactions should be considered when new signs and symptoms develop or when they differ from the usual manifestations of the illness being treated, especially if a reaction:

- Follows ingestion of a drug, especially one known to produce allergic reactions
- Is unpredictable and occurs in only a few clients when many clients receive the suspected drug
- Occurs approximately 7 to 10 days after initial exposure to the suspected drug (to allow antibody production)

- Follows a previous exposure to the same or similar drug (sensitizing exposure)
- Occurs minutes or hours after a second or subsequent exposure
- Occurs after small doses (reduces the likelihood that the reaction is due to dose-related drug toxicity)
- Occurs with other drugs that are chemically or immunologically similar to the suspected drug
- Produces signs and symptoms that differ from the usual pharmacologic actions of the suspected drug
- Produces signs and symptoms usually considered allergic in nature (eg, anaphylaxis, urticaria, serum sickness)
- Produces similar signs and symptoms to previous allergic reactions to the same or a similar drug
- Increases eosinophils in blood or tissue
- Resolves within a few days of discontinuing the suspected drug

Virtually all drugs have been implicated in **anaphylactic reactions.** Penicillins and other antimicrobials, radiocontrast media, aspirin and other nonsteroidal antiinflammatory drugs, and antineoplastics such as asparaginase and cisplatin are more common offenders. Less common causes include anesthetics (local and general), opioid analgesics, skeletal muscle relaxants used with general anesthetics, and vaccines. Approximately 10% of severe anaphylactic reactions are fatal. In many cases, it is unknown whether clinical manifestations are immunologic or nonimmunologic in origin.

**Serum sickness** is a delayed hypersensitivity reaction most often caused by drugs, such as antimicrobials. In addition, many drugs that produce anaphylaxis also produce serum sickness. With initial exposure to the antigen, symptoms usually develop within 7 to 10 days and include urticaria, lymphadenopathy, myalgia, arthralgia, and fever. The reaction usually resolves within a few days but may be severe or even fatal. With repeated exposure to the antigen, after prior sensitization of the host, accelerated serum sickness may develop within 2 to 4 days, with similar but often more severe signs and symptoms.

**Systemic lupus erythematosus** (SLE) is an autoimmune disorder that may be induced by hydralazine, procainamide, isoniazid, and other drugs. Clinical manifestations vary greatly, depending on the location and severity of the inflammatory and immune processes, and may include skin lesions, fever, pneumonia, anemia, arthralgia, arthritis, nephritis, and others. Drug-induced lupus produces less renal and CNS involvement than idiopathic SLE.

**Fever** often occurs with allergic drug reactions. It may occur alone, with a skin rash and eosinophilia, or with other drug-induced allergic reactions such as serum sickness, SLE, vasculitis, and hepatitis.

**Dermatologic conditions** (eg, skin rash, urticaria, inflammation) commonly occur with allergic drug reactions and may be the first and most visible manifestations.

## Pseudoallergic Drug Reactions

Pseudoallergic drug reactions resemble immune responses (because histamine and other chemical mediators are released), but they do not produce antibodies or sensitized T lymphocytes. **Anaphylactoid reactions** are like anaphylaxis in terms of immediate occurrence, symptoms, and life-threatening severity. The main difference is that they are not antigen–antibody reactions and therefore may occur on first exposure to the causative agent. The drugs bind directly to mast cells, activate the cells, and cause the release of histamine and other vasoactive chemical mediators. Contrast media for radiologic diagnostic tests are often implicated.

## ■ ANTIHISTAMINES

The term *antihistamine* generally indicates classic or traditional drugs. With increased knowledge about histamine receptors, these drugs are often called histamine-1 (H₁) receptor antagonists. These drugs prevent or reduce most of the physiologic effects that histamine normally induces at H₁ receptor sites. Thus, they accomplish the following:

- Inhibit smooth muscle constriction in blood vessels and the respiratory and gastrointestinal (GI) tracts
- Decrease capillary permeability
- Decrease salivation and tear formation

The drugs are similar in effectiveness as histamine antagonists but differ in adverse effects. These are the antihistamines discussed in this chapter. Cimetidine (Tagamet), ranitidine (Zantac), famotidine (Pepcid), and nizatidine (Axid) are H₂ receptor antagonists or blocking agents used to prevent or treat peptic ulcer disease. These are discussed in Chapter 47. Appropriate dosages are required for safe drug use of H₁ antagonists in children and older adults. The Age-related Considerations outline current thoughts about the use of these drugs. Antihistamines are often taken in the home setting, especially for allergic rhinitis and other allergic disorders. Home Care Considerations focus on overall assessment, monitoring, and education concerns in these clients. Selected H₁ antagonists are described in the following sections and in Drugs at a Glance 38-1: Commonly Used Antihistamines.

## First-Generation Histamine-1 Receptor Antagonists

These chemically diverse antihistamines (also called *nonselective* or *sedating agents*) bind to both central and peripheral H₁ receptors and can cause central nervous system (CNS) depression or stimulation. They usually cause CNS depression (drowsiness, sedation) with therapeutic doses and may cause CNS stimulation (anxiety, agitation) with excessive doses, especially in children. They also have substantial anticholinergic effects (eg,

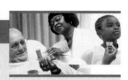

### Age-related Considerations: Use of Antihistamines

#### USE IN CHILDREN

First-generation antihistamines (eg, diphenhydramine) may cause drowsiness and decreased mental alertness in children as in adults. Young children may experience paradoxical excitement. These reactions may occur with therapeutic dosages. In overdosage, hallucinations, convulsions, and death may occur. Close supervision and appropriate dosages are required for safe drug usage in children.

**Diphenhydramine** is not recommended for use in newborn infants (premature or full-term) or children with chickenpox or a flulike infection. When used in young children, doses should be small because of drug effects on the brain and nervous system. **Promethazine** should not be used in children with hepatic disease, Reye's syndrome, a history of sleep apnea, or a family history of sudden infant death syndrome.

The second-generation drugs vary in recommendations for use according to age groups. **Cetirizine** and **loratadine** may be used in children 2 years and older. Syrup formulations are available for use in younger children. **Azelastine** may be used in children 5 years and older; **fexofenadine** may be used in children 6 years of age and older; and **desloratadine** may be used in children 12 years and older.

#### USE IN OLDER ADULTS

First-generation antihistamines (eg, **diphenhydramine**) may cause confusion (with impaired thinking, judgment, and memory), dizziness, hypotension, sedation, syncope, unsteady gait, and paradoxical CNS stimulation in older adults. These effects, especially sedation, may be misinterpreted as senility or mental depression. Older men with prostatic hypertrophy may have difficulty voiding while taking these drugs. Some of these adverse reactions derive from anticholinergic effects of the drugs and are likely to be more severe if the client is also taking other drugs with anticholinergic effects (eg, tricyclic antidepressants, older antipsychotic drugs, some antiparkinson drugs). Despite the increased risk for adverse effects, however, diphenhydramine is sometimes prescribed as a sleep aid for occasional use in older adults. As with many other drugs, smaller-than-usual dosages are indicated.

In general, second-generation antihistamines should be used for older adults. They are much safer because they do not impair consciousness, thinking, or ability to perform activities of daily living (eg, driving a car or operating various machines).

## Home Care Considerations: Use of Antihistamines

**ASSESS:** knowledge level of client and caregiver, client's medication techniques (eg, correct use of inhalers), adherence, environmental control measures, and quality-of-life considerations.

**MONITOR:** vital signs, serum plasma levels, effectiveness of therapy, and adverse effects.

**EDUCATE:** to take as directed, not exceed recommended dose; to avoid use of other depressants, alcohol, or sleep-inducing medications without being prescribed by health care provider; to use caution when driving or engaging in tasks requiring mental alertness; to perform frequent mouth care—chewing gum or sucking hard candy may minimize dry mouth; to report nausea and vomiting, change in urinary pattern, or blurred vision; to take adequate fluids to thin thickened secretions. Educate on interventions to reduce side effects; how to store medications out of reach of children, and to replace medications to ensure a constant supply. Also, assist clients to recognize and treat (or get help for) exacerbations before respiratory distress becomes severe. Instruct on the importance of smoking cessation. In a client with an allergic disorder, identify and alleviate environmental allergens (eg, cigarette smoke, animal dander, dust mites).

cause dry mouth, urinary retention, constipation, blurred vision).

**Brompheniramine, chlorpheniramine** (Chlor-Trimeton), and **dexchlorpheniramine** (Polaramine) cause minimal drowsiness. ℗ **Diphenhydramine** (Benadryl), the prototype of first-generation antihistamines, causes a high incidence of drowsiness and anticholinergic effects (see Prototype Profile 38-1: Diphenhydramine). **Hydroxyzine** (Vistaril) and **promethazine** (Phenergan) are strong CNS depressants and cause extensive drowsiness.

First-generation antihistamines are usually well absorbed after oral administration. Immediate-release oral forms act within 15 to 60 minutes and last 4 to 6 hours. Enteric-coated or sustained-release preparations last 8 to 12 hours. Most drugs are given orally; a few may be given parenterally. These drugs are primarily metabolized by the liver, with metabolites and small amounts of unchanged drug excreted in urine within 24 hours. Several of these drugs are available without prescription. **Brompheniramine** is available only in multi-ingredient preparations (eg, several Dimetapp formulations); **chlorpheniramine** and **diphenhydramine** are available alone and in combination with adrenergic nasal decongestants, analgesics, and allergy, cold, and sinus remedies.

## Second-Generation Histamine-1 Receptor Antagonists

Second-generation $H_1$ antagonists (also called selective or nonsedating agents) were developed mainly to produce less sedation than the first-generation drugs. They cause less CNS depression because they are selective for peripheral $H_1$ receptors and do not cross the blood–brain barrier. Previously, these drugs have been available only by prescription. However, in 2002, the U.S. Food and Drug Administration (FDA) approved the OTC sales of loratadine (Claritin, Alavert).

**Azelastine** (Astelin) is the only antihistamine formulated as a nasal spray for topical use. When applied to nasal mucosa, it produces peak levels in 2 to 3 hours and lasts 12 to 24 hours. It is metabolized in the liver to an active metabolite and is excreted mainly in feces. The other drugs are well absorbed with oral administration and have a rapid onset of action. **Cetirizine** (Zyrtec) is an active metabolite of hydroxyzine that causes less drowsiness than hydroxyzine. It reaches maximal serum concentration in 1 hour and is about 93% protein bound. About half of a dose is metabolized in the liver; the other half is excreted unchanged in the urine. **Fexofenadine** (Allegra) reaches peak serum concentrations in about 2.5 hours, it is 60% to 70% protein bound, and 95% is excreted unchanged in bile and urine. With ℗ **loratadine** (Claritin, Alavert), the prototype, effects occur within 1 to 3 hours, reach a maximum in 8 to 12 hours, and last 24 hours or longer (see Prototype Profile 38-2: Loratadine). It is metabolized in the liver, and its long duration of action is due, in part, to an active metabolite. Loratadine's patent expired in December 2002, clearing the way for generic formulations. **Desloratadine** (Clarinex), an active metabolite of loratadine and marketed by the manufacturer of Claritin, seems to offer no advantage over loratadine or other second-generation drugs. For most people, a second-generation drug is the first drug of choice. However, they are quite expensive. If costs are prohibitive for a client, a first-generation drug may be used with minimal daytime sedation if taken at bedtime or in low initial doses, with gradual increases over 1 or 2 weeks. Azelastine nasal spray also causes little sedation, but it leaves an unpleasant taste. Overall, safety should be the determining factor. Some studies have shown cognitive and performance impairment with the first-generation drugs even when the person does not feel drowsy or impaired.

## Mechanism of Action

Antihistamines are structurally related to histamine and occupy the same receptor sites as histamine, which prevents histamine from acting on target tissues (Fig. 38-2).

*(text continues on page 704)*

**DRUG TABLE 38-1**

*Drugs at a Glance*

## Commonly Used Antihistamines

| Generic/Trade Name | Routes and Dosage Ranges | Comments |
|---|---|---|
| **First Generation** | | |
| **Azelastine** (Astelin, Optiver) Pregnancy Category C | Allergic rhinitis *Adults:* Nasal inhalation, two sprays per nostril q12h *Children:* ≥12 y: Same as adults | Avoid spraying in eyes; drowsiness is possible in some clients |
| **Chlorpheniramine** (Chlor-Trimeton) Pregnancy Category C | Allergic rhinitis *Adults:* PO, 4 mg q4–6h; maximal dose, 24 mg in 24h Timed-release forms, PO, 8 mg q8–12h or 12 mg q12h; maximal dose, 24 mg in 24h *Children:* ≥12 y: Same as adults 6–12 y: PO, 2 mg q4–6h; maximal dose, 12 mg in 24h 2–6 y: PO, 1 mg q4–6h Timed-release forms, ≥12 y: PO, 8 mg q8–12h or 12 mg q12h; maximal dose, 24 mg in 24h | Often compounded in combination with other drugs |
| **Clemastine** (Tavist) Pregnancy Category B | Allergic rhinitis *Adults:* PO, 1.34 mg twice daily, increased up to a maximum of 8.04 mg daily, if necessary Urticaria/angioedema, PO, 2.68 mg one to three times daily *Children:* 6–12 y (syrup only): PO, 0.67 mg twice daily, increased up to a maximum of 4.02 mg daily, if necessary Urticaria/angioedema, 6–12 y (syrup only): PO, 1.34 mg twice daily | May cause drowsiness and impair judgment. Keep side rails up in hospitalized client after administration and institute other safety measures |
| **Cyproheptadine** (Periactin) Pregnancy Category B | Hypersensitivity reactions *Adults:* PO, 4 mg q8h initially, increase if necessary. Maximal dose 0.5 mg/kg/d *Children:* (Calculate total daily dosage as 0.25 mg/kg or 8 mg/m$^2$) 7–14 y: PO, 4 mg q8–12h; maximal dose, 16 mg/d 2–6 y: 2 mg q8–12h; maximal dose, 12 mg/d < 2 y: Safety and efficacy not established | May stimulate weight gain. May cause drowsiness; institute safety measures |
| **Dexchlorpheniramine** (Polaramine) Pregnancy Category B | Hypersensitivity reactions *Adults:* Regular tablets and syrup, PO, 2 mg q4–6h Timed-release tablets, PO, 4–6 mg at bedtime or q8–12h *Children:* ≥12 y: Same as adults 6–11 y: PO, 1 mg q4–6h 2–5 y: PO, 0.5 mg q4–6h Timed-release tablets, ≥12 y: Same as adults 6–12 y: 4 mg once daily, at bedtime | Do not use timed-release form in children <6 y |

*(continued)*

**DRUG TABLE 38-1**

*Drugs at a Glance*

## Commonly Used Antihistamines (Continued)

| Generic/Trade Name | Routes and Dosage Ranges | Comments |
|---|---|---|
| **Diphenhydramine** (Benadryl) | See Prototype Profile 38-1: Diphenhydramine | |
| **Hydroxyzine** (Vistaril, Atarax)<br>Pregnancy Category C | Pruritus, Antiemetic, Sedation<br>*Adults:* PO, 25 mg q6–8h; IM, 25–100 mg as needed<br>*Children:* >6 y: PO, 50–100 mg daily in divided doses<br><6 y: PO, 50 mg daily in divided doses | Although not recommended in product labeling, may be ordered as a short (15–30 min) IV infusion |
| **Phenindamine** (Nolahist)<br>Pregnancy Category B | Allergic rhinitis<br>*Adults:* PO, 25 mg q4–6h; maximal dose 150 mg in 24 h<br>*Children:* ≥12 y: Same as adults<br>6–11 y: PO, 12.5 mg q4–6h; maximal dose 75 mg in 24 h | |
| **Promethazine** (Phenergan)<br>Pregnancy Category C | Hypersensitivity reactions, sedation, antiemetic, motion sickness<br>*Adults:* PO, IM, rectally, 25 mg q4–6h as needed<br>*Children:* ≥2 y: 12.5 mg q4–6h as needed | Alters the flare response in intradermal allergen tests<br>Avoid IV administration, but if necessary, dilute to a maximum concentration of 25 mg/mL and infuse at maximum rate of 25 mg/min. IV administration may cause transient fall in blood pressure |
| **Tripelennamine** (PBZ)<br>Pregnancy Category B | Hypersensitivity reactions<br>*Adults:* PO, 25–50 mg q4–6h<br>Extended-release tablets, PO, 100 mg q12h<br>*Children:* PO, 5 mg/kg/d or 150 mg/m$^2$/d in four to six divided doses<br>Do not use extended-release tablets | Do not crush extended-release tablets |
| ***Second Generation***<br>**Cetirizine** (Zyrtec)<br>Pregnancy Category B | Allergic rhinitis, chronic idiopathic urticaria<br>*Adults:* PO, 5–10 mg once daily<br>Renal or hepatic impairment: PO, 5 mg once daily<br>*Children:* ≥6 y: Same as adults | Use with caution in renal or liver disease, in breast-feeding mothers, and in the elderly<br>Alcohol may increase CNS effects |
| **Desloratadine** (Clarinex)<br>Pregnancy Category C | Allergic rhinitis, chronic idiopathic urticaria<br>*Adults:* PO, 5 mg once daily<br>Renal and hepatic impairment: PO, 5 mg every other day<br>*Children:* 12 y and older: Same as adults<br><12 y: Dosage not established | Use with caution in pregnant women; not recommended for mothers who are breast-feeding |
| **Fexofenadine** (Allegra)<br>Pregnancy Category C | Allergic rhinitis<br>*Adults:* PO, 60 mg twice daily<br>Renal impairment: PO, 60 mg once daily<br>*Children:* ≥12 y: Same as adults<br>6–11 y: PO, 30 mg twice daily | Report nausea, drowsiness, increased pain or cramping with menstruation while taking drug |
| **Loratadine** (Claritin, Alavert) | See Prototype Profile 38-2: Loratadine | |

## PROTOTYPE PROFILE 38-1

### ℗ Diphenhydramine (dye fen HYE dra meen)

**Drug Class**
*Chemical:* Antihistamine
*Functional:* Antihistamine

**Trade Names**
Benadryl, others

**Therapeutic Indications**
Hypersensitivity reactions (allergic rhinitis, conjunctivitis, dermatitis), motion sickness, parkinsonism, insomnia, antitussive (syrup only)

**Pharmacokinetics**
*Absorption*
Bioavailability PO: 40%–60%

*Distribution*
Plasma protein binding: 78%
Enters breast milk; incompatible

*Metabolism*
Primarily hepatic, with significant first-pass effect; minimal metabolism through renal and pulmonary systems

*Excretion*
Urine

**Pharmacodynamics**
*Onset of Action*
Maximum sedative effect in 1–3 h

*Duration*
4–7 h; in elderly, half-life may extend to 13.5 h

**Contraindications/Precautions**
Hypersensitivity, acute asthma, neonates; with caution, in tasks requiring mental alertness, angle-closure glaucoma, urinary tract obstruction, hyperthyroidism, cardiovascular disease (including tachycardia and hypertension), and pyloroduodenal obstruction

**Pregnancy Considerations**
Category B
Enters breast milk; do not breast feed

**Dosage**
*Adults:* hypersensitivity reaction, motion sickness, parkinsonism: PO, 25–60 mg q4–8h; IV or deep IM, 10–50 mg, increase as necessary to a maximum daily dose of 400 mg
Insomnia: PO, 50 mg at bedtime
Syrup for cough: PO, 25 mg (10 mL) q4h, not to exceed 100 mg (40 mL) in 24h
*Children:* hypersensitivity reaction, motion sickness with weight >10 kg (22 lb): PO, 12.5–25 mg q6–8h, 5 mg/kg/d, or 150 mg/m²/d. Maximum daily oral or parenteral dosage 300 mg
Insomnia, ≥12 y: Same as adults
Syrup for cough 6–12 y: PO, 12.5 mg (5 mL) q4h, not to exceed 50 mg (20 mL) in 24 h
2–6 y: PO, 6.25 mg (2.5 mL) q4h, not to exceed 25 mg (10 mL) in 24 h

**Adverse Effects**
Sedation, gait disturbances, hypotension, tachycardia, dry mouth, urinary retention, blurred vision, constipation, and thickening of bronchial secretions

**Drug Interactions**
*Increased Effects*
Increased respiratory depression and sedation with CNS depressants, including alcohol
Central and/or peripheral anticholinergic syndrome with concurrent use with quinidine, procainamide, tricyclic antidepressants, disopyramide
Risk for disulfiram reactions with concurrent use of metronidazole and chlorpropamide with syrup form, which contains alcohol
Increased absorption of digoxin with concurrent use

*Decreased Effects*
Concurrent use with levodopa decreases the amount of absorption of levodopa through increased degradation of levodopa
Decreased therapeutic effects of neuroleptic and cholinergic agents with concurrent use

**Herbal Supplements and Dietary Considerations**
Avoid alcohol, St. John's wort, valerian, kava kava, gotu kola because they may increase CNS depression

---

Thus, the drugs are effective in inhibiting vascular permeability, edema formation, bronchoconstriction, and pruritus associated with histamine release. They do not prevent histamine release or reduce the amount released.

## Indications for Use

Antihistamines are used for a variety of allergic and non-allergic disorders to prevent or reverse target organ inflammation and its effects on organ function. The drugs can relieve symptoms but do not relieve the hypersensitivity. Choosing an antihistamine is based on the desired effect, duration of action, adverse effects, and other characteristics of available drugs. For treatment of acute allergic reactions, a rapid-acting agent of short duration is preferred. For chronic allergic symptoms (eg, allergic rhinitis), long-acting preparations provide more consistent relief. A client may respond better to one antihistamine than to another. Thus, if one does not relieve symptoms or produces excessive sedation, another may be effective. For treatment of the common cold, studies have demon-

## PROTOTYPE PROFILE 38-2

### Ⓟ Loratadine (lor AT a deen)

**Drug Class**
*Chemical:* Antihistamine
*Functional:* Antihistamine

**Trade Names**
Claritin, Alavert

**Therapeutic Indications**
Relief of nasal and other symptoms of seasonal allergic rhinitis

**Pharmacokinetics**
*Absorption*
Rapid

*Distribution*
Enters breast milk in significant amounts

*Metabolism*
Hepatic

*Excretion*
Urine and feces

**Pharmacodynamics**
*Onset of Action*
1–3 h

*Duration*
>24 h

**Contraindications/Precautions**
Hypersensitivity; with caution, in renal and liver impairment, children < 2 y because safety and efficacy have not been established

**Pregnancy Considerations**
Category B
Enters breast milk; compatible

**Dosage**
*Adults:* PO, 10 mg once daily
*Children:* ≥ 6 y: PO, 10 mg once daily
2–5 y: PO, 5 mg once daily

**Adverse Effects**
Headache, fatigue, nervousness, somnolence, wheezing, and tachycardia

**Drug Interactions**

*Increased Effects*
Increased toxicity with other antihistamines, alcohol, and procarbazine
Increased plasma concentration of drug with concurrent use with erythromycin, ketoconazole, and protease inhibitors

*Decreased Effects*
None reported

**Herbal Supplements and Dietary Considerations**
St. John's wort may decrease loratadine levels
Take on an empty stomach; food increases bioavailability and delays peak action
Avoid alcohol as may increase central nervous system depression
Alavert contains phenylalanine

---

strated that antihistamines do not relieve symptoms and are not recommended. However, an antihistamine is often included in prescription and OTC combination products for the common cold. General indications for specific conditions and situations include:

- **Allergic rhinitis.** Of people with seasonal allergic rhinitis, 75% to 95% experience some relief of sneezing, rhinorrhea, nasal congestion, and conjunctivitis with the use of antihistamines. People with perennial allergic rhinitis usually experience decreased nasal congestion and drying of nasal mucosa. However, many people require an additional drug to relieve symptoms. Cromolyn, ipratropium, and several corticosteroids are available in intranasal preparations for this purpose. These drugs, with dosage ranges for adults and children, are listed in Drugs at a Glance 38-2: Intranasal Drugs for Allergic Rhinitis.

- **Anaphylaxis.** Antihistamines are helpful in treating urticaria and pruritus but are not effective in treating bronchoconstriction and hypotension. Epinephrine, rather than an antihistamine, is the drug of choice for treating severe anaphylaxis.

- **Allergic conjunctivitis.** This condition, which is characterized by redness, itching, and tearing of the eyes, is often associated with allergic rhinitis. Antihistamine eye medications may be given (see Appendix G).

- **Drug allergies and pseudoallergies.** Antihistamines may be given to prevent or treat reactions to drugs. When used for prevention, they should be given before exposure (eg, before a diagnostic test that uses an iodine preparation as a contrast medium; before an intravenous infusion of amphotericin B). When used for treatment, giving an antihistamine and stopping the causative drug usually relieve signs and symptoms within a few days.

- **Transfusions of blood and blood products.** Premedication with an antihistamine is often used to prevent allergic reactions.

- **Dermatologic conditions.** Antihistamines are the drugs of choice for treatment of allergic contact dermatitis and acute urticaria (a vascular reaction of the skin characterized by papules or wheals and severe itching, often called *hives*). Urticaria often occurs because the skin has many mast cells to release histamine. Other indications

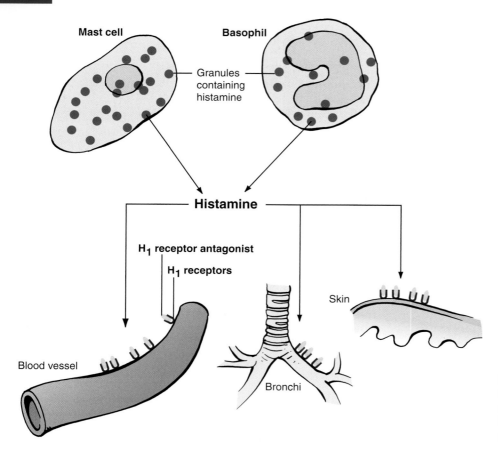

**FIGURE 38–2** Action of antihistamine drugs. Histamine₁ ($H_1$) receptor antagonists bind to $H_1$ receptors. This prevents histamine from binding to its receptors and acting on target tissues.

**DRUG TABLE 38-2**

*Drugs at a Glance*

## Intranasal Drugs for Allergic Rhinitis

| Generic/Trade Name | Routes and Dosage Ranges | Comments |
|---|---|---|
| **Anticholinergic** | | |
| **Ipratropium** (Atrovent nasal spray) Pregnancy Category B | *Adults:* 2 sprays (42 mcg or 84 mcg) per nostril 2–4 times daily *Children:* 12 y and older: Same as adults | Shake inhaler well before administration, wait 1 min between inhalations, close eyes while administering because contact with eyes may cause temporary blurred vision |
| **Corticosteroids** | | |
| **Beclomethasone** (Beconase, Vancenase) Pregnancy Category C | *Adults:* 1 inhalation (42 mcg) in each nostril 2–4 times daily *Children:* 12 y and older: Same as adults 6–12 y: 1 inhalation in each nostril 3 times daily | Shake inhaler well before administration Rinse mouth after inhalation to prevent oral *Candida* infection |
| **Budesonide** (Rhinocort) Pregnancy Category C | *Adults:* 256 mcg daily as 2 sprays per nostril twice daily or 4 sprays per nostril once daily *Children:* 6 y and older: Same as adults | Rinse mouth after inhalation to prevent oral *Candida* infection (wash face if using face mask) |
| **Flunisolide** (Nasalide, Nasarel) Pregnancy Category C | *Adults:* 2 sprays (50 mcg) in each nostril 2 times daily; increase to 3 times daily if necessary *Children:* 6–14 y: 1 spray (25 mcg) in each nostril 3 times daily or 2 sprays per nostril (50 mcg) 2 times daily | |

*(continued)*

**DRUG TABLE 38-2**

*Drugs at a Glance*

**Intranasal Drugs for Allergic Rhinitis** (Continued)

| Generic/Trade Name | Routes and Dosage Ranges | Comments |
|---|---|---|
| **Fluticasone** (Flonase) Pregnancy Category C | *Adults:* 2 sprays (50 mcg each) per nostril once daily (200 mcg daily) *Children:* 4 y and older: 1 spray per nostril per day (100 mcg daily) | Rinse mouth after inhalation to prevent oral *Candida* infection; avoid contact with eyes Do not use a spacer with powder form |
| **Mometasone furoate** (Nasonex) Pregnancy Category C | *Adults:* 2 sprays (50 mcg each) per nostril once daily (200 mcg daily) *Children:* 12 y and older: Same as adults 3–11 y: 1 spray per nostril once daily (100 mcg daily) | Prime pump before using for first time; reprime after a maximum of 1 week; shake well before administration; protect from light |
| **Triamcinolone** (Nasacort, Nasacort AQ) Pregnancy Category C | *Adults:* 2 sprays (55 mcg/spray) in each nostril once daily *Children:* 6 y and older: Same as adults initially, then reduce to 1 spray per nostril per day | Clear nasal passages before inhalation |
| *Mast Cell Stabilizer* | | |
| **Cromolyn** (Nasalcrom) Pregnancy Category B | *Adults:* 1 spray in each nostril 3–6 times daily, q4–6h *Children:* 6 y and older: Same as adults | Should take 30 min before meals |

for use include drug-induced skin reactions, pruritus ani, and pruritus vulvae. Systemic drugs are used; topical preparations are not recommended because they often induce skin rashes themselves. With pruritus, oral cyproheptadine (Periactin) and hydroxyzine (Atarax) are especially effective.

■ **Miscellaneous.** Some antihistamines are commonly used for nonallergic disorders, such as motion sickness, nausea and vomiting (eg, promethazine, hydroxyzine; see Chap. 48), and sleep (eg, diphenhydramine). The active ingredient in OTC sleep aids (eg, Compoz, Sominex) is a sedating antihistamine. Antihistamines are also common ingredients in OTC cold remedies (see Chap. 39).

## Contraindications to Use

Antihistamines are contraindicated or must be used with caution in clients with hypersensitivity to the drugs, narrow-angle glaucoma, prostatic hypertrophy, stenosing peptic ulcer, and bladder neck obstruction, and during pregnancy.

## NURSING PROCESS

### Assessment

● Assess the client's condition in relation to disorders for which antihistamines are used. For the client with known allergies, try to determine the factors that precipitate or relieve allergic reactions and specific signs and symptoms experienced during a reaction.

● Assess every client for a potential hypersensitivity reaction. For example, it is standard practice on first contact to ask a client if he or she has any food, drug, or other allergies. The health care provider is likely to get more complete information by asking clients about allergic reactions to specific drugs (eg, antibiotics such as penicillin, local anesthetics) rather than asking if they are allergic to or cannot take any drugs.

  If a drug allergy is identified, ask about specific signs and symptoms as well as any drugs currently taken. With previ-

ous exposure and sensitization to the same or a similar drug, immediate allergic reactions may occur. With a new drug, antibody formation and allergic reactions usually require a week or longer. Most reactions appear within a month of starting a drug.

  When a suspected allergic reaction occurs (eg, skin rash, fever, edema, dyspnea), interview the client or consult medical records about the drug, dose, route, and time of administration. In addition, evaluate all the drugs a client is taking as a potential cause of the reaction. This assessment may involve searching drug literature to see if the suspected drug is associated with allergic reactions and discussion with physicians and pharmacists.

### Nursing Diagnoses

● Risk for Injury related to drowsiness with first-generation antihistamines

- Deficient Knowledge: Safe and accurate drug use
- Deficient Knowledge: Strategies for minimizing exposure to allergens and irritants

### Planning/Goals

*The client will:*

- Experience relief of symptoms
- Take antihistamines accurately
- Avoid hazardous activities if sedated from antihistamines
- Avoid preventable adverse drug effects
- Avoid taking sedative-type antihistamines with alcohol or other sedative drugs

### Interventions

- For clients with known allergies, assist in identifying and avoiding precipitating factors when possible. If it is a drug allergy, encourage the client to carry a medical alert device that identifies the drug.
- Monitor the client closely for excessive drowsiness during the first few days of therapy with antihistamines known to cause sedation.

- Encourage a fluid intake of 2000 to 3000 mL daily, if not contraindicated.
- Because antihistamines are most effective before exposure to the stimulus that causes histamine release, assist clients in learning when to take the drugs (eg, during seasons of high pollen and mold counts).
- When indicated, obtain an order and administer an antihistamine before situations known to elicit allergic reactions (eg, blood transfusions, diagnostic tests that involve contrast media).
- For clients who have experienced an allergic or pseudo-allergic drug reaction, assist them in learning about the drug thought responsible (including the generic and commonly used trade names), suitable alternatives for future drug therapy, and potential sources of the drug.

### Evaluation

- Observe for relief of symptoms.
- Interview and observe for correct drug usage.
- Interview and observe for excessive drowsiness.

---

## CLIENT TEACHING GUIDELINES
## Antihistamines

### General Considerations

✔ Some antihistamines should not be taken by people with glaucoma, peptic ulcer, urinary retention, or pregnancy. Inform your physician if you have any of these conditions or, for over-the-counter (OTC) antihistamines, read the label to see if you should avoid a particular drug.

✔ Antihistamines may dry and thicken respiratory tract secretions and make them more difficult to remove. Thus, do not take diphenhydramine (Benadryl), which is available OTC, if you have active asthma, bronchitis, or pneumonia.

✔ Some antihistamines cause drowsiness or dizziness and impair mental alertness, judgment, and physical coordination, especially during the first few days. Do not smoke, drive a car, operate machinery, or perform other tasks requiring alertness and physical dexterity until drowsiness has worn off, to avoid injury.

✔ Avoid using sedating antihistamines with other sedative-type drugs (eg, alcohol, medications to relieve nervousness or produce sleep), to avoid adverse effects and dangerous drug interactions. Alcohol and other drugs that depress brain function may cause excessive sedation, respiratory depression, and death.

✔ Do not take more than one antihistamine at a time (eg, two prescription drugs, two OTC drugs, or a combination of prescription and OTC drugs) because adverse effects are likely. If you do not know whether a particular medication is an antihistamine, consult a health care provider. For example, many OTC cold remedies and "nighttime" or "PM" allergy or sinus preparations contain an antihistamine. In addition, the active ingredient in OTC sleep aids is a sedating antihistamine, usually diphenhydramine (Benadryl).

✔ Avoid prolonged exposure to sunlight and use sunscreens and protective clothing; some antihistamines may increase sensitivity to sunlight and risks of skin damage from sunburn.

✔ Report adverse effects, such as excessive drowsiness. The physician may be able to change drugs or dosages to decrease adverse effects.

✔ Store antihistamines out of reach of children to avoid accidental ingestion.

✔ If you experience an allergic reaction to a medication, obtain information about the drug thought responsible (including its various names), acceptable alternatives for future drug therapy, and potential sources of the drug. In addition, read the list of ingredients on labels of OTC drug preparations, inform all health care providers about the drug reaction before taking any newly prescribed drug, and wear a medical alert device that lists drugs to be avoided. Note that people may be allergic to additives (eg, dyes, binders, others) rather than the active drug.

### Self-administration

✔ Take antihistamines only as prescribed or as instructed on packages of OTC preparations to increase beneficial effects and decrease adverse effects. If you miss a dose, do not take a double dose.

✔ Take most antihistamines with meals to decrease stomach upset. Take loratadine (Claritin) on an empty stomach for better absorption; cetirizine (Zyrtec) and desloratadine (Clarinex) may be taken with or without food.

✔ Do not chew or crush sustained-release tablets and do not open sustained-release capsules. Such actions can cause rapid drug absorption, high blood levels, and serious adverse effects, rather than the slow absorption and prolonged action intended with these products.

## ? How Can You Avoid This Medication Error?

You are the phone resource nurse for an urgent care center. Mrs. Doe calls you, very upset, explaining that her 2-year-old son has just swallowed what was remaining in a bottle of an over-the-counter (OTC) cold remedy. What advice should you give Mrs. Doe? How can this error be prevented in the future?

## *Nursing Actions*
## Antihistamines

| Nursing Actions | Rationale/Explanation |
|---|---|
| 1. Administer accurately. | |
| a. Give most oral antihistamines with food; give loratadine on an empty stomach; give cetirizine with or without food. | To decrease gastrointestinal (GI) effects of the drugs |
| b. Give intramuscular antihistamines deeply into a large muscle mass. | To decrease tissue irritation |
| c. Inject intravenous (IV) antihistamines slowly, over a few minutes. | Severe hypotension may result from rapid IV injection. |
| d. When a drug is used to prevent motion sickness, give it 30–60 min before travel. | |
| 2. Observe for therapeutic effects. | Therapeutic effects depend on the reason for use. |
| a. A verbal statement of therapeutic effect (relief of symptoms) | |
| b. Decreased nausea and vomiting when given for antiemetic effects | |
| c. Decreased dizziness and nausea when taken for motion sickness | |
| d. Drowsiness or sleep when given for sedation | |
| 3. Observe for adverse effects. | |
| a. First-generation drugs | |
| (1) Sedation | Drowsiness due to central nervous system (CNS) depression is the most common adverse effect. |
| (2) Paradoxical excitation—restlessness, insomnia, tremors, nervousness, palpitations | This reaction is more likely to occur in children. It may result from the anticholinergic effects of antihistamines. |
| (3) Convulsive seizures | Antihistamines, particularly the phenothiazines, may lower the seizure threshold. |
| (4) Dryness of mouth, nose, and throat, blurred vision, urinary retention, constipation | Due to anticholinergic effects |
| (5) GI distress—anorexia, nausea, vomiting | |
| b. Second-generation drugs | Adverse effects are few and mild. |
| (1) Drowsiness | Drowsiness and dry mouth are more likely to occur with cetirizine; headache is more likely to occur with loratadine; desloratadine and fexofenadine reportedly produce minimal adverse effects. |
| (2) Dry mouth | |
| (3) Fatigue | |
| (4) Headache | |
| (5) GI upset | |
| 4. Observe for drug interactions. | Note: No documented drug interactions have been reported with intranasal azelastine or oral cetirizine or desloratadine. |
| a. Drugs that *increase* effects of first-generation antihistamines: | |

*(continued)*

## Nursing Actions

### Antihistamines (Continued)

| Nursing Actions | Rationale/Explanation |
|---|---|
| (1) Alcohol and other CNS depressants (eg, anti-anxiety and antipsychotic agents, opioid analgesics, sedative-hypnotics) | Additive CNS depression. Concomitant use may lead to drowsiness, lethargy, stupor, respiratory depression, coma, and death. |
| (2) Monoamine oxidase inhibitors | Inhibit metabolism of antihistamines, leading to an increased duration of action; increased incidence and severity of sedative and anticholinergic adverse effects. |
| (3) Tricyclic antidepressants | Additive anticholinergic side effects |
| b. Drugs that *increase* effects of loratadine: | All of these drugs increase plasma levels of loratadine by decreasing its metabolism. |
| (1) Macrolide antibacterials (azithromycin, clarithromycin, erythromycin) | |
| (2) Azole antifungals (fluconazole, itraconazole, ketoconazole, miconazole) | |
| (3) Cimetidine | |
| c. Drugs that may *decrease* effects of fexofenadine: | |
| (1) Rifampin | Rifampin may induce enzymes that accelerate metabolism of fexofenadine. |

### ? How Can You Avoid This Medication Error?

**Answer:** Mrs. Doe needs to induce her son to vomit to prevent additional absorption of the cold remedy. Syrup of ipecac can be used to promote vomiting, which usually occurs 20 to 30 minutes after ingestion. If vomiting cannot be induced, instruct Mrs. Doe to bring her son to the urgent care center where gastric lavage can be used to empty the stomach.

Question Mrs. Doe regarding the time that has elapsed since ingestion, the amount of the medication ingested, medications contained in the cold remedy, and any symptoms her son is exhibiting.

Teaching is essential to prevent future accidental poisonings. All medication, even OTC and herbal remedies, must be kept out of reach of all children and have childproof tops. Toddlers are especially prone to accidental poisoning because they are inquisitive, like to put things in their mouths, and cannot understand the danger such a situation poses. Children need constant supervision and should not be left alone. Make sure that Mrs. Doe has syrup of ipecac on hand and the phone number of the poison control center posted.

### Critical Thinking Exercises

1. The only antihistamine formulated as a nasal spray for topical use is:
   a. Azelastine (Astelin)
   b. Desloratadine (Clarinex)
   c. Loratadine (Claritin, Alavert)
   d. Cetirizine (Zyrtec)

2. Allergic contact dermatitis results from direct contact with antigens to which a person has previously become sensitized. This is what type hypersensitivity reaction?
   a. Type I allergic reaction
   b. Type II allergic reaction
   c. Type III allergic reaction
   d. Type IV allergic reaction

3. Second-generation $H_1$ antagonists differ from first-generation $H_1$ antagonists in that they:
   a. Cause more CNS depression
   b. Have always been available without a prescription
   c. Bind to central $H_1$ receptors
   d. Do not cross the blood–brain barrier

4. The drug of choice for treating severe anaphylaxis is:
   a. Loratadine (Claritin, Alavert)
   b. Chlorpheniramine (Chlor-Trimeton)
   c. Fexofenadine (Allegra)
   d. Epinephrine (Adrenalin, Bronkaid)

**5.** Studies have demonstrated that antihistamines do not relieve symptoms of:
   a. Allergic rhinitis
   b. Allergic conjunctivitis
   c. The common cold
   d. Allergic contact dermatitis

## SELECTED REFERENCES

Desloratadine (Clarinex). *The Medical Letter on Drugs and Therapeutics, 44*(Issue 1126, March 18, 2002). New Rochelle, NY: The Medical Letter, Inc.

*Drug facts and comparisons.* (Updated monthly). St. Louis: Facts and Comparisons.

Guyton, A. C., & Hall, J. E. (2000). *Textbook of medical physiology* (10th ed.). Philadelphia: W. B. Saunders.

Hussex, T. C. (2002). Allergic rhinitis: a focus on nonprescription therapy. *Pharmacy Times, 68*(5), 63–67.

Kim, R. B. (Ed.). (2001). *Handbook of adverse drug interactions.* New Rochelle, NY: The Medical Letter, Inc.

Lacy, C. F., Armstrong, L. L., Goldman, M. P., & Lance, L. L. (2003). *Lexi-Comp's drug information handbook* (11th ed.). Hudson, OH: American Pharmaceutical Association.

Porth, C. M. (Ed.). (2002). *Pathophysiology: Concepts of altered health states* (6th ed.). Philadelphia: Lippincott Williams & Wilkins.

Sampey, C. S., & Follin, S. L. (2001). Second generation antihistamines: The OTC debate. *Journal of the American Pharmaceutical Association, 43*(3), 454–457.

Terr, A. I. (2000). Approach to the patient with allergies. In H. D. Humes (Ed.), *Kelley's textbook of internal medicine* (4th ed., pp. 1340–1346). Philadelphia: Lippincott Williams & Wilkins.

# Drugs Affecting the Cardiovascular System

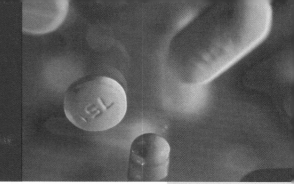

## 39

# Drug Therapy of Heart Failure

## OBJECTIVES

*After studying this chapter, the student will be able to:*

1　Describe major manifestations of heart failure (HF).

2　Differentiate the types of drugs used to treat HF.

3　List characteristics of digoxin in terms of effects on myocardial contractility and cardiac conduction, indications for use, and nursing process implications.

4　Differentiate digitalizing and maintenance doses of digoxin.

5　Identify therapeutic and excessive serum digoxin levels.

6　Identify clients at risk for development of digoxin toxicity.

7　Discuss interventions to prevent or minimize digoxin toxicity.

8　Explain the roles of potassium chloride, lidocaine, atropine, and digoxin immune fab in the management of digoxin toxicity.

9　Teach clients ways to increase safety and effectiveness of digoxin.

## CRITICAL THINKING SCENARIO

*E*lmer Sweeney, a 68-year-old retired plumber, was recently hospitalized with heart failure and started on captopril, an angiotensin-converting enzyme (ACE) inhibitor. You are a staff nurse assigned to his care. He has many questions about his new diagnosis and the captopril.

✔ Physiologically, what happens when the heart fails to pump adequately, and what symptoms are seen in the client?

✔ How do ACE inhibitors decrease the workload of the heart?

✔ What criteria (objective and subjective) will you use to evaluate whether the ACE inhibitor is effectively managing Mr. Sweeney's heart failure?

## PROTOTYPE PROFILE

digoxin (Lanoxin), p. 720

# HEART FAILURE

Heart failure (HF), also called congestive heart failure (CHF), is a common condition that occurs when the heart cannot pump enough blood to meet tissue needs for oxygen and nutrients (see At the Foundation: Heart Failure). It may result from impaired myocardial contraction during systole (systolic dysfunction), impaired relaxation and filling of ventricles during diastole (diastolic dysfunction), or a combination of systolic and diastolic dysfunction. Heart failure is also classed as left sided or right sided, and symptoms vary as a result of the ventricle affected.

## Signs and Symptoms

When compensatory mechanisms are successful, clients usually have no symptoms at rest and no edema; dyspnea and fatigue occur only with activities involving moderate or higher levels of exertion. When compensatory mechanisms fail, the symptoms associated with HF are the result of an increase in blood in the ventricle at the end of diastole (preload) and increased peripheral vascular resistance (afterload). Symptoms that occur with minimal exertion or at rest and are accompanied by distention of the jugular vein and ankle edema (from congestion of veins and leakage of fluid into tissues) reflect decompensation. Acute, severe cardiac decompensation is manifested by pulmonary edema, a medical emergency that requires immediate treatment. Clients with chronic HF are often described according to the New York Heart Association classification categories that separate clients into four groups according to symptoms and activity tolerance (Box 39-1). These categories are often used to help evaluate results of therapy and to indicate a client's functional status.

## Management Goals and Measures

The goals for clients with asymptomatic (compensated) HF are to maintain function as nearly normal as possible and to prevent symptomatic (acute, congestive, or decompensated) HF, hospitalizations, and death. When symptoms or decompensation occurs, the goals are to relieve symptoms, restore function, and prevent progressive cardiac deterioration.

# NONPHARMACOLOGIC MANAGEMENT MEASURES

Nonpharmacologic measures to manage HF are an integral part of the course of therapy. Strategies to control diet, manage weight, and improve activity are frequently employed and include the following:

1. Prevent or treat conditions that precipitate cardiac decompensation and failure (eg, fluid and sodium retention, factors that impair myocardial contractility or increase cardiac workload).
2. Restrict dietary sodium intake to reduce edema and other symptoms and allow a decrease in diuretic dosage. A common order, "no added salt," may be accomplished by avoiding obviously salty foods (eg, ham, potato chips, snack foods) and by not

---

**AT THE FOUNDATION:** *Heart Failure*

At the cellular level, HF stems from dysfunction of contractile myocardial cells and the endothelial cells that line the heart and blood vessels. This dysfunction impairs pumping ability or increases the workload of the heart so that an adequate cardiac output cannot be maintained. As the heart fails, the low cardiac output and inadequately filled arteries activate the neurohormonal system by several feedback mechanisms: (1) increased sympathetic activity and circulating catecholamines (neurohormones), which increases the force of myocardial contraction, increases heart rate, and causes vasoconstriction; and (2) activation of the renin-angiotensin-aldosterone (RAA) system that raises filling pressures inside the heart, increases stretch and stress on the myocardial wall, and predisposes the heart to subendocardial ischemia. In addition, clients with severe HF have constricted arterioles in cerebral, myocardial, renal, hepatic, and mesenteric vascular beds. This results in increased organ hypoperfusion and dysfunction.

Venous vasoconstriction limits venous capacitance, resulting in venous congestion and increased diastolic ventricular filling pressures (preload). Angiotensin II (a component of the RAA system) also promotes sodium and water retention by stimulating aldosterone release from the adrenal cortex and the release of vasopressin (antidiuretic hormone) from the posterior pituitary gland.

All of these mechanisms combine to increase blood volume and pressure in the heart chambers, stretch muscle fibers, and produce dilation, hypertrophy, and changes in the shape of the heart (a process called *cardiac* or *ventricular remodeling*) that make it contract less efficiently. Overall, the compensatory mechanisms increase preload (amount of venous blood returning to the heart), workload of the heart, afterload (amount of resistance in the aorta and peripheral blood vessels that the heart must overcome to pump effectively), and blood pressure. These compensatory mechanisms that initially preserve cardiac function result in progressive deterioration of myocardial function over time.

**BOX 39-1    New York Heart Association Classification of Patients with Heart Disease**

**Class I.** No limitations of physical activity; ordinary physical activity does not cause dyspnea, fatigue, or palpitations.

**Class II.** Slight limitations of physical activity. Patients are comfortable at rest but have dyspnea, fatigue, palpitations, or chest pain (angina) with ordinary physical activity.

**Class III.** Marked limitations of physical activity. Patients are comfortable at rest but develop symptoms with less than ordinary physical activity.

**Class IV.** Patients are unable to perform any physical activity without discomfort. Symptoms of heart failure or angina are present even at rest. If any physical activity is undertaken, discomfort increases.

adding salt during cooking or eating. For clients with more severe HF, dietary intake may be more restricted (eg, no more than 2 g daily). A major source of sodium intake is table salt: a level teaspoonful contains 2300 mg of sodium.

3. If hyponatremia (serum sodium <130 mEq/L) develops from sodium restrictions and diuretic therapy, fluids may need to be restricted (eg, 1.5 L/day or less) until the serum sodium level increases. Severe hyponatremia (<125 mEq/L) may lead to dysrhythmias.

4. For clients who are obese, weight loss is desirable to decrease systemic vascular resistance and myocardial oxygen demand.

5. Reduce physical activity in clients with symptomatic HF. This decreases the workload and oxygen consumption of the myocardium. If bed rest is instituted, antithrombotic measures, such as compression stockings or devices or heparin therapy, should be prescribed to prevent deep vein thrombosis.

## DRUG THERAPY OF HEART FAILURE

Pharmacologic management of HF continues to evolve as the pathophysiologic mechanisms are better understood and research studies indicate more effective regimens. Oxygen as a drug may be used, as needed, to relieve dyspnea, improve oxygen delivery, reduce the work of breathing, and decrease constriction of pulmonary blood vessels (which is a compensatory measure in clients with hypoxemia). Combinations of drugs are commonly used in efforts to improve circulation, alter the compensatory mechanisms, and reverse heart damage. Most of the drugs used to treat HF are also used in other disorders and are discussed in other chapters; their effects in HF are described in Box 39-2. The primary focus of this chapter is inotropic agents, which include digoxin, a cardiac glycoside, and the phosphodiesterase inhibitors, inamrinone and milrinone. These drugs are discussed in the following sections and in Drugs at a Glance 39-1: Drugs for Heart Failure. Two new classifications of drugs, human natriuretic peptides and endothelin receptor antagonists, are also presented. Discussion of specific management considerations in children and older adults is found in Age-related Considerations: Digoxin.

A combination of drugs is the standard of care for both acute and chronic HF. Specific drug components depend on the client's symptoms and hemodynamic status.

1. For **acute HF**, the first drugs of choice may include an intravenous (IV) loop diuretic, a cardiotonic-inotropic agent (eg, digoxin, dobutamine, or milrinone), and vasodilators (eg, nitroglycerin and hydralazine or nitroprusside). This combination reduces preload and afterload and increases myocardial contractility.

2. For **chronic HF**, an ACE inhibitor or angiotensin receptor blocker (ARB) and a diuretic are the basic standard of care. Digoxin, a beta-adrenergic blocking agent, and spironolactone may also be added. Although the use of digoxin in clients with normal sinus rhythm has been questioned, studies indicate improved ejection fraction and exercise tolerance in clients who receive digoxin. In addition, in clients stabilized on digoxin, a diuretic, and an ACE inhibitor or ARB, symptoms worsen if digoxin is discontinued.

   Overall, these drugs improve clients' quality of life by decreasing their symptoms and increasing their ability to function in activities of daily living. They also decrease hospitalizations and deaths from HF.

3. **Electrolyte balance** must be monitored and maintained during digoxin therapy, particularly normal serum levels of potassium (3.5 to 5 mEq/L), magnesium (1.5 to 2.5 mg/100 mL), and calcium (8.5 to 10 mg/100 mL). Hypokalemia and hypomagnesemia increase cardiac excitability and ectopic pacemaker activity, leading to dysrhythmias; hypercalcemia enhances the effects of digoxin. These electrolyte abnormalities increase the risk for digoxin toxicity. Hypocalcemia increases excitability of nerve and muscle cell membranes and causes myocardial contraction to be weak (leading to a decrease in digoxin effect).

   In acute HF, there is a substantial risk for hypokalemia because large doses of potassium-losing diuretics are often given. Serum potassium levels should be monitored regularly, and supplemental potassium may be needed. In chronic HF, hypokalemia may be less likely to occur than formerly because lower doses of potassium-losing diuretics are usually being given. In addition, there may be more extensive use *(text continues on page 718)*

## BOX 39-2    Drugs Used to Treat Heart Failure

### Adrenergics

Dopamine or dobutamine (see Chaps. 16 and 42) may be used in acute, severe heart failure (HF) when circulatory support is required, usually in a critical care unit. Given by IV infusion, these drugs strengthen myocardial contraction (inotropic or cardiotonic effects) and increase cardiac output. Dosage or flow rate is titrated to hemodynamic effects; minimal effective doses are recommended because of vasoconstrictive effects. The drugs also cause tachycardia and hypertension and increase cardiac workload and oxygen consumption.

### Angiotensin-Converting Enzyme (ACE) Inhibitors

Captopril and other ACE inhibitors (see Chap. 43) are drugs of first choice in treating patients with all four New York Heart Association (NYHA) classifications of chronic HF. For patients with moderate or severe symptomatic HF (NYHA class III or IV), the standard of care includes an ACE inhibitor (or an ARB) and a loop diuretic, with or without digoxin.

These drugs improve cardiac function and decrease mortality. They also relieve symptoms, increase exercise tolerance, and delay further impairment of myocardial function and progression of HF (ie, ventricular remodeling). They act mainly to decrease activation of the renin–angiotensin–aldosterone system, a major pathophysiologic mechanism in HF. More specifically, the drugs prevent inactive angiotensin I from being converted to angiotensin II. Angiotensin II produces vasoconstriction and retention of sodium and water; inhibition of angiotensin II decreases vasoconstriction and retention of sodium and water. Thus, major effects of the drugs are dilation of both veins and arteries, decreased preload and afterload, decreased workload of the heart, and increased perfusion of body organs and tissues.

An ACE inhibitor is usually given in combination with a diuretic. All of the drugs have similar effects, but captopril, enalapril, lisinopril, quinapril, and ramipril are FDA-approved for treatment of HF. Some clinicians use captopril initially because it has a short half-life and is rapidly eliminated when stopped, then switch to a long-acting drug if captopril is tolerated by the client. Digoxin, a beta-adrenergic blocking agent, or spironolactone may be added to the ACE inhibitor/diuretic regimen.

During ACE inhibitor therapy, clients usually need to see a health care provider frequently for dosage titration and monitoring of serum creatinine and potassium levels for increases. Elevated creatinine levels may indicate impaired renal function, in which case dosage needs to be reduced; elevated potassium levels indicate hyperkalemia, an adverse effect of the drugs.

### Angiotensin Receptor Blockers (ARBs)

Losartan and other angiotensin receptor blockers (see Chap. 43) are similar to the ACE inhibitors in their effects on cardiac function, although they are not FDA approved for treatment of HF. Valsartan recently received FDA approval for management of clients with HF who are unable to tolerate an ACE inhibitor (eg, development of a cough, a common adverse effect of ACE inhibitors).

### Beta-Adrenergic Blocking Agents

Although beta blockers (see Chaps. 17, 40, and 43) were formerly considered contraindicated, numerous research studies indicate they decrease morbidity (ie, symptoms and hospitalizations) and mortality in clients with chronic HF. The change evolved from a better understanding of chronic HF (ie, that it involves more than a weak pumping mechanism).

Beta blockers suppress activation of the sympathetic nervous system and the resulting catecholamine excess that eventually damages myocardial cells, reduces myocardial beta receptors, and reduces cardiac output. As a result, over time, ventricular dilatation and enlargement (ventricular remodeling) regress, the heart returns toward a more normal shape and function, and cardiac output increases. Most studies were done with clients in NYHA class II or III; effects in class IV clients are being studied.

Beta blockers are not recommended for clients in acute HF because of the potential for an initial decrease in myocardial contractility. A beta blocker is started once normal blood volume is restored and edema and other symptoms are relieved. The goal of beta blocker therapy is to shrink the ventricle back to its normal size (reverse remodeling). The beta blocker is added to the ACE inhibitor/diuretic regimen, usually near the end of a hospital stay or as outpatient therapy. Most studies have been done with bisoprolol, carvedilol, or metoprolol; it is not yet known whether some beta blockers are more effective than others. When one of the drugs is used in clients with chronic HF, recommendations include starting with a low dose (because symptoms may initially worsen in some clients), titrating the dose upward at approximately 2-week intervals, and monitoring closely. Significant hemodynamic improvement usually requires 2 to 3 months of therapy, but effects are long lasting. Beneficial effects can be measured by increases in the left ventricular ejection fraction (ie, cardiac output).

### Diuretics

Diuretics (see Chap. 44) are used in treating both acute and chronic HF. Thiazides (eg, hydrochlorothiazide) can be used for mild diuresis in clients with normal renal function; loop diuretics (eg, furosemide) should be used in clients who need strong diuresis or who have impaired renal function.

In acute HF, which is characterized by fluid accumulation, a diuretic is the initial treatment. It acts to decrease plasma volume (extracellular fluid volume) and increase excretion of sodium and water, thereby decreasing preload. With early or mild HF, starting or increasing the dose of an oral thiazide may be effective. With moderate to severe HF (pulmonary edema), an IV loop diuretic is indicated. IV furosemide also has a vasodilatory effect that helps relieve vasoconstriction (afterload). Although diuretic therapy relieves symptoms, it does not improve left ventricular function and decrease mortality rates. Some clients may also need drugs to increase myocardial contractility and vasodilators to decrease preload, afterload, or both.

In chronic HF, an oral diuretic is a common component of treatment regimens. Depending on the severity of symptoms

*(continued)*

## BOX 39-2 Drugs Used to Treat Heart Failure (Continued)

or degree of HF, the regimen may also include an ACE inhibitor or ARB, a beta blocker, and digoxin.

Potassium-sparing diuretics (eg, amiloride, triamterene) are often given concurrently with potassium-losing diuretics (eg, thiazides or loop diuretics) to help maintain normal serum potassium levels. Concomitant use of ACE inhibitors and nonsteroidal anti-inflammatory drugs and the presence of diabetes mellitus increase risks of hyperkalemia.

With all diuretic therapy, serum potassium levels must be measured periodically to monitor for hypokalemia and hyperkalemia. Both hypokalemia and hyperkalemia are cardiotoxic or impair heart function.

### Aldosterone Antagonist

Increasingly, spironolactone is also being added for clients with moderate to severe HF. Increased aldosterone, a major factor in the pathophysiology of HF, results in increased interstitial fibrosis that may decrease systolic function and increase the risk of ventricular dysrhythmias. Spironolactone is an aldosterone antagonist that reduces the aldosterone-induced retention of sodium and water and impaired vascular function. Although ACE inhibitors also decrease aldosterone initially, this effect is transient. Spironolactone is given in a daily dose of 12.5 to 25 mg, along with standard doses of an ACE inhibitor, a loop diuretic, and usually digoxin. In clients with adequate renal function (ie, serum creatinine 2.5 mg/dL or less), the addition of spironolactone usually allows smaller doses of loop diuretics and potassium supplements. Overall, studies indicate that the addition of spironolactone improves cardiac function and reduces symptoms, hospitalizations, and mortality.

### Vasodilators

Vasodilators are essential components of treatment regimens for HF, and the beneficial effects of ACE inhibitors and angiotensin receptor antagonists stem significantly from their vasodilating effects (ie, preventing or decreasing angiotensin-induced vasoconstriction). Other vasodilators may also be used. Venous dilators (eg, nitrates) decrease preload; arterial dilators (eg, hydralazine) decrease afterload. Isosorbide dinitrate and hydralazine may be combined to decrease both preload and afterload. The combination has similar effects to those of an ACE inhibitor or an ARB, but may not be as well tolerated by clients. Nitrates are discussed in Chapter 41; hydralazine and other vasodilators are discussed in Chapter 43.

Oral vasodilators usually are used in clients with chronic HF and parenteral agents are reserved for those who have severe HF or are unable to take oral medications. They should be started at low doses, titrated to desired hemodynamic effects, and discontinued slowly to avoid rebound vasoconstriction.

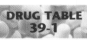

### DRUG TABLE 39-1 · Drugs at a Glance

## Drugs for Heart Failure

| Generic/Trade Name | Routes and Dosage Ranges | Comments |
|---|---|---|
| **Inotropic Agents** | | |
| *Cardiac Glycoside* | | |
| **Digoxin** (Lanoxin) | See Prototype Profile 39-1: Digoxin | |
| *Phosphodiesterase Inhibitor* | | |
| **Inamrinone** (Inocor)<br>Pregnancy Category C | *Adults:* IV injection (loading dose), 0.75 mg/kg slowly, over 2–3 min<br>IV infusion (maintenance dose), 5–10 mcg/kg/min, diluted in 0.9% or 0.45% NaCl solution to a concentration of 1–3 mg/mL. May give another bolus dose 30 min after start of therapy. Maximum dose, 10 mg/kg/d<br>*Children:* ≥1 y: Same as adult<br>Infants: IV injection (loading dose), 3–4.5 mcg/kg, in divided doses. IV infusion (maintenance dose), 10 mcg/kg/min<br>Neonates: IV injection (loading dose), 3–4.5 mcg/kg, in divided doses. IV infusion (maintenance dose), 3–5 mcg/kg/min | Infrequently used as short-term therapy as a last resort in clients with intractable heart failure<br>Long-term therapy has been associated with increased risk for hospitalization and death<br>Monitor liver function. If significant increases in liver enzymes and clinical symptoms occur, inamrinone should be discontinued. A reduction of dosage may be indicated with smaller increases in liver enzymes without clinical symptoms<br>Observe for dysrhythmias and dose-dependent thrombocytopenia |

*(continued)*

**DRUG TABLE 39-1**

*Drugs at a Glance*

**Drugs for Heart Failure** (Continued)

| Generic/Trade Name | Routes and Dosage Ranges | Comments |
|---|---|---|
| **Milrinone** (Primacor)<br>Pregnancy Category C | *Adults:* IV bolus infusion (loading dose), 50 mcg/kg over 10 min<br>IV continuous infusion (maintenance dose), 0.375–0.75 mcg/kg/min, diluted in 0.9% or 9.45% NaCl or 5% dextrose solution<br>*Children:* Safety and dosing not established | With milrinone, which is also excreted primarily by the kidneys, renal impairment significantly increases elimination half-life, drug accumulation, and adverse effects. Dosage should be reduced according to creatinine clearance (see manufacturer's instructions). Cardiac and blood pressure monitor indicated because dysrhythmias and hypotension are adverse reactions |
| *Human B-type Natriuretic Peptide* | | |
| **Nesiritide** (Natrecor)<br>Pregnancy Category C | *Adults:* IV bolus infusion (loading dose), 2 mcg/kg followed by continuous infusion of 0.01 mcg/kg/min. Use for >48 hours not studied<br>*Children:* Safety and dosing not established | Use cautiously in clients with hypotension, particularly at higher dosages; effects may be additive with other agents known to cause hypotension. No dosage adjustment required with renal impairment |

of potassium-sparing diuretics (eg, amiloride or triamterene) and spironolactone. Note, however, that it is important to prevent hyperkalemia because it is cardiotoxic.

Several drugs are used to treat acute HF, and a combination of an ACE inhibitor or ARB and a diuretic is first-line therapy for chronic failure. Increasingly, digoxin, a beta-adrenergic blocking agent, or spironolactone is being added to the ACE inhibitor or ARB and diuretic regimen.

Home care is an essential component in the management of chronic heart failure. Guidelines for ongoing evaluation and intervention are addressed in Home Care Considerations.

## Digoxin

**Ⓟ Digoxin (Lanoxin)** is the only commonly used digitalis glycoside and is considered the prototype. Key infor-

## Age-related Considerations: Use of Digoxin

### USE IN CHILDREN

The response to a given dose of digoxin varies with age, size, and renal and hepatic function. There may be little difference between a therapeutic dose and a toxic dose. Very small amounts are often given to children. These factors increase the risk for dosage errors in children. In a hospital setting, institutional policies may require that each dose be verified with another nurse before it is administered. ECG monitoring is desirable when digoxin therapy is started. In general, divided daily doses should be given to infants and children younger than 10 years, and adult dosages adjusted to their weight should be given to children older than 10 years of age. Larger doses are usually needed to slow a too-rapid ventricular rate in children with atrial fibrillation or atrial flutter (see Chap. 40). Differences in bioavailability of different preparations (parenterals, capsules, elixirs, and tablets) must be considered when switching from one preparation to another.

Neonates vary in tolerance of digoxin, depending on their degree of maturity. Premature infants are especially sensitive to drug effects. Dosage must be reduced, and digi-

talization should be even more individualized and cautiously approached than in more mature infants and children. Early signs of toxicity in newborns are undue slowing of sinus rate, sinoatrial arrest, and prolongation of the PR interval.

### USE IN OLDER ADULTS

Reduced dosages are usually required because of decreased liver or kidney function, decreased lean body weight, and advanced cardiovascular disease. All of these characteristics are common and are a frequent cause of adverse effects in older adults. Impaired renal function leads to slower drug excretion and increased risk for accumulation. Dosage must be reduced by approximately 50% with renal failure or concurrent administration of amiodarone, quinidine, nifedipine, or verapamil. These drugs increase serum digoxin levels and increase risks for toxicity if dosage is not reduced. The most commonly recommended dose is 0.125 mg daily. Antacids decrease absorption of oral digoxin and should not be given at the same time.

## Home Care Considerations: Management of Heart Failure

**ASSESS:** for the presence of HF symptoms, client's understanding regarding the different types of drugs and their different actions and responses.

**MONITOR:** clients' responses to the drug and changes in conditions or drug therapy that increase risks for toxicity.

**EDUCATE:** how to use the drug effectively and about circumstances for which the client should seek emergency care (see Client Teaching Guidelines: Digoxin). Accurate dosing is vitally important because underuse may cause recurrence of symptoms and overuse may cause toxicity. Either condition may be life threatening and require emergency care; changing drugs or dosages can upset the balance of cardiovascular function and lead to acute and severe symptoms that require hospitalization and may even cause death from HF. If unable to take the medications for any reason, clients or caregivers should notify the prescribing health care provider and be instructed not to wait until symptoms become severe before seeking care.

mation about this prototype can be found in Prototype Profile 39-1: Digoxin. In the following discussion, the terms *digitalization* and *digitalis toxicity* refer to digoxin.

### General Characteristics

When digoxin is given orally, absorption varies among available preparations. Lanoxicaps, which are liquid-filled capsules, and the elixir used for children are better absorbed than tablets. With tablets, the most frequently used formulation, differences in bioavailability are important because a person who is stabilized on one formulation may be underdosed or overdosed if another formulation is taken. Differences are attributed to the rate and extent of tablet dissolution rather than amounts of digoxin. In addition to drug dosage forms, other factors that may decrease digoxin absorption include the presence of food in the gastrointestinal (GI) tract, delayed gastric emptying, malabsorption syndromes, and concurrent administration of some drugs (eg, antacids).

### Mechanisms of Action

In HF, digoxin exerts a cardiotonic or positive inotropic effect that improves the pumping ability of the heart. Increased myocardial contractility allows the ventricles to empty more completely with each heartbeat. With improved cardiac output, decreases in heart size, heart rate, end-systolic and end-diastolic pressures, vasoconstriction, sympathetic nerve stimulation, and venous congestion result. The mechanism by which digoxin increases the force of myocardial contraction is thought to be inhibition of $Na^+$-$K^+$-adenosine triphosphatase ($Na^+$-$K^+$-ATPase), an enzyme in cardiac cell membranes that decreases the movement of sodium out of myocardial

cells after contraction. As a result, calcium enters the cell in exchange for sodium, causing additional calcium to be released from intracellular binding sites. With the increased intracellular concentration of free calcium ions, more calcium is available to activate the contractile proteins actin and myosin, and to increase myocardial contractility. This promotes increased force of cardiac contraction (positive inotropic effect), cardiac output, and tissue perfusion. Overall, digoxin helps to relieve symptoms and decrease hospitalizations, but does not prolong survival. In HF, it is given concomitantly with a diuretic and an ACE inhibitor or ARB.

In atrial dysrhythmias, digoxin slows the rate of ventricular contraction (negative chronotropic effect). Negative chronotropic effects are probably caused by several factors. First, digoxin has a direct depressant effect on cardiac conduction tissues, especially the atrioventricular node. This action decreases the number of electrical impulses allowed to reach the ventricles from supraventricular sources. Second, digoxin indirectly stimulates the vagus nerve. Third, increased efficiency of myocardial contraction and vagal stimulation decrease compensatory tachycardia that results from the sympathetic nervous system response to inadequate circulation.

### Digitalization

In the heart, maximum drug effect of digoxin occurs when a steady-state tissue concentration has been achieved. This occurs in approximately 1 week (five half-lives) unless loading doses are given for more rapid effects. Traditionally, a loading dose is called a *digitalizing dose*. Digitalization (administration of an amount sufficient to produce therapeutic effects) may be accomplished rapidly by giving divided doses over a 24-hour period in a total dose larger than the usual maintenance dose. Maintenance doses, which are much smaller than digitalizing doses, may be safely used to initiate digoxin therapy and are always used for long-term therapy.

Smaller doses (loading and maintenance) should be given to clients who are elderly or have hypothyroidism. Because metabolism and excretion of digoxin are delayed in such people, the drug may accumulate and cause toxicity if dosage is not reduced. Dosage also should be reduced in clients with hypokalemia, extensive myocardial damage, or cardiac conduction disorders. These conditions increase risks for digoxin-induced dysrhythmias.

Digoxin dosage must be reduced by approximately half in clients with renal failure, to avoid drug accumulation and toxicity. Dosage should be based on signs and symptoms of toxicity, creatinine clearance, and serum drug levels.

### Digoxin Toxicity

Digoxin has a low therapeutic index (ie, a dose adequate for therapeutic effects may be accompanied by signs of toxicity). Digoxin toxicity may result from many contributing factors:

## PROTOTYPE PROFILE 39-1
### *P* Digoxin (di JOKS in)

**Drug Class**
*Chemical:* Cardiac glycoside
*Functional:* Antidysrhythmic agent, class IV

**Trade Names**
Lanoxin, Digitek, Lanoxicaps

**Therapeutic Indications**
Management of HF, atrial fibrillation, and atrial flutter. Digoxin may be used in acute or chronic conditions, for digitalization, or for maintenance therapy

**Pharmacokinetics**
*Absorption*
PO: Tablet, 60%–70%; capsule, 90%–100%; liquid, 90%

*Distribution*
Plasma protein binding: 25%

*Metabolism*
Half-life 36 hours

*Excretion*
70% by urine; 30% by liver metabolism

**Pharmacodynamics**
Therapeutic plasma levels: 0.5–2 ng/mL

*Onset of Action*
Onset of action is ½ to 2 h after oral administration and 10 to 30 min after IV injection

*Duration*
2 to 4 days

**Contraindications**
Severe myocarditis, ventricular tachycardia, or ventricular fibrillation.
Must be used with caution in clients with acute myocardial infarction, heart block, Adams-Stokes syndrome, Wolff-Parkinson-White syndrome (risk for fatal dysrhythmias), electrolyte imbalances (hypokalemia, hypomagnesemia, hypercalcemia), and renal impairment

**Side Effects/Adverse Reactions**
Anorexia, nausea and vomiting, yellow-green vision, photophobia, drowsiness, and confusion

**Pregnancy Considerations**
Category C
Crosses placenta; small amounts found in breast milk

**Dosage**
Digitalizing dose, PO
*Adults and children > 10 y:* 0.75–1 mg in 3 or 4 divided doses over 24 h; IV, 0.5–0.75 mg in divided doses over 24 h
Maintenance dose, PO, IV, 0.125–0.5 mg/d (average, 0.25 mg)
*Children 2–10 y:* Digitalizing dose, PO, 0.02–0.04 mg/kg in 4 divided doses over 24 h. Maintenance dose, PO, IV, approximately 20%–35% of the digitalizing dose or a maximum dose of 100–150 mcg/d
*Children 1 mo–2 y:* Digitalizing dose, PO, 0.035–0.06 mg/kg in 4 divided doses over 24 h; IV, 0.035–0.05 mg/kg in 4 divided doses over 24 h
Maintenance dose, PO, IV, approximately 20%–35% of the digitalizing dose
*Newborns:* Digitalizing dose, PO, 0.025–0.035 mg/kg in 4 divided doses over 24 h
Maintenance dose, PO, IV, approximately 20%–35% of the digitalizing dose
Because of variations in the degree of renal metabolism, clients vary widely in the dosages required to maintain a therapeutic response

**Drug Interactions**
*Increased*
Serum digoxin level with verapamil, quinidine, and flecainide

*Decreased*
Absorption with antacids and cholestyramine
Increased risk for digoxin toxicity with loop and thiazide diuretics (secondary to hypokalemia)

**Herbal Supplements and Dietary Considerations**
Ephedra may increase cardiac stimulation and worsen dysrhythmias. Natural licorice blocks the effects of spironolactone and causes sodium retention and potassium loss, effects that may worsen HF and potentiate the effects of digoxin. Hawthorn should be used cautiously because it may increase the effects of ACE inhibitors and digoxin. Use of ginseng can result in digoxin toxicity. Clients may use herbs such as dandelion root and juniper berries for their diuretic effect. Herbal and dietary supplements should not be taken instead of prescribed drug therapies.
Administer with food; food may delay but does not affect the extent of absorption.

- Accumulation of larger-than-necessary maintenance doses
- Rapid loading or digitalization, whether by one or more large doses or frequent administration of small doses
- Impaired renal function, which delays excretion of digoxin
- Age extremes (young or old)

- Electrolyte imbalance (eg, hypokalemia, hypomagnesemia, hypercalcemia)
- Hypoxia due to heart or lung disease, which increases myocardial sensitivity to digoxin
- Hypothyroidism, which slows digoxin metabolism and may cause accumulation
- Concurrent management with other drugs affecting the heart, such as quinidine, verapamil, or nifedipine

**? How Can You Avoid This Medication Error?**

Mr. Bello, a 75-year-old nursing home resident, currently takes digoxin 0.25 mg qd and Lasix 20 mg bid to treat his congestive heart failure. During your morning assessment he tells you his stomach is upset and he would like some Maalox. You explain that you cannot give him the Maalox with the digoxin because it will impact drug absorption. Because the digoxin is more important, he should take that first. Did this nurse make a good decision?

Recognition of digoxin toxicity may be difficult because of nonspecific early manifestations (eg, anorexia, nausea, confusion) and the similarity between the signs and symptoms of heart disease for which digoxin is given and the signs and symptoms of digoxin intoxication. Continued atrial fibrillation with a rapid ventricular response may indicate inadequate dosage. However, other dysrhythmias may indicate toxicity. Premature ventricular contractions commonly occur. Serum drug levels and electrocardiograms (ECGs) may be helpful in verifying suspected toxicity. Serum digoxin levels should be drawn just before a dose. Drug distribution to tissues requires about 6 hours after a dose is given; if the blood is drawn before 6 hours, the level may be high.

When signs and symptoms of digoxin toxicity occur, management may include any or all of the following interventions, depending on the client's condition:

1. Digoxin should be discontinued, not just reduced in dosage. Most clients with mild or early toxicity recover completely within a few days after the drug is stopped.
2. If serious cardiac dysrhythmias are present, several drugs may be used, including the following:
   a. **Potassium chloride** may be given if serum potassium level is low. It is a myocardial depressant that acts to decrease myocardial excitability. The dose depends on the severity of toxicity, serum potassium level, and client response. Potassium is contraindicated in renal failure and should be used with caution in the presence of cardiac conduction defects.
   b. **Lidocaine,** an antiarrhythmic local anesthetic agent used to decrease myocardial irritability, may be used.
   c. **Atropine** or **isoproterenol** is used in the management of bradycardia or conduction defects.
   d. **Other antiarrhythmic drugs** may be used, but are in general less effective in digoxin-induced dysrhythmias than in dysrhythmias due to other causes.
   e. **Digoxin immune fab** (Digibind) is a digoxin-binding antidote derived from antidigoxin antibodies produced in sheep. It is recommended only for serious toxicity. It combines with digoxin and pulls digoxin out of tissues and into the bloodstream. This causes serum digoxin levels to remain high, but the drug is bound to the antibody and therefore inactive. Digoxin immune fab is given intravenously, as a bolus injection if the client is in danger of immediate cardiac arrest, but preferably over 15 to 30 minutes. Dosage varies and is calculated according to the amount of digoxin ingested or serum digoxin levels (see manufacturer's instructions).

## Phosphodiesterase Inhibitors

**Inamrinone** (Inocor), formerly amrinone, and **milrinone IV** (Primacor) are cardiotonic-inotropic agents used in short-term management of acute, severe HF that is not controlled by digoxin, diuretics, and vasodilators. The drugs increase levels of cyclic adenosine monophosphate (cAMP) in myocardial cells by inhibiting phosphodiesterase, the enzyme that normally metabolizes cAMP. They also relax vascular smooth muscle to produce vasodilation and decrease preload and afterload. In HF, inotropic and vasodilator effects increase cardiac output. The effects of these drugs are additive to those of digoxin and may be synergistic with those of adrenergic drugs (eg, dobutamine). There is a time delay before the drugs reach therapeutic serum levels and interindividual variability in therapeutic doses.

Compared with inamrinone, milrinone is more potent as an inotropic agent and causes fewer adverse effects. Both drugs are given intravenously by bolus injection followed by continuous infusion. Flow rate is titrated to maintain adequate circulation. Milrinone can be used alone or with other drugs such as dobutamine and nitroprusside. Its dosage should be reduced in the presence of renal impairment. Dose-limiting adverse effects of the drugs include tachycardia, atrial or ventricular dysrhythmias, and hypotension. Hypotension is more likely to occur in clients who are hypovolemic. Milrinone has a long half-life of approximately 80 hours and may accumulate with prolonged infusions.

## Human B–type Natriuretic Peptide

**Nesiritide** (Natrecor) is the first in this new class of drugs, to be used in the management of acute HF. Produced by recombinant DNA technology, nesiritide is identical to endogenous human B-type natriuretic peptide, which is secreted primarily by the ventricles in response to fluid and pressure overload. This drug acts to compensate for deteriorating cardiac function by reducing preload and afterload, increasing diuresis and secretion of sodium, suppressing the renin-angiotensin-aldosterone system, and decreasing secretion of neurohormones, endothelin, and norepinephrine. Onset of action is immediate, with peak effects attained in 15 minutes with a bolus dose followed by continuous IV infusion. Administration should be by a separate IV line because nesiritide is incompatible with many other drugs. Hemodynamic monitoring of pulmonary artery pressure is indicated to determine drug effectiveness. Clearance of the drug is proportional to body weight and partially by the kidneys; however, no adjustment in dosing is required for age, gender, race-ethnicity, or renal function impairment. Clinical studies have not been conducted on the use of nesiritide for more than 48 hours.

## Endothelin Receptor Antagonists

This new class of drugs relaxes blood vessels and improves blood flow by targeting endothelin-1 (a neurohormone) that is produced in excess in HF. Endothelin-1 causes blood vessels to constrict, forcing the ailing heart to work harder to pump blood through the narrowed vessels. Studies indicate that endothelin antagonist drugs improve heart function, as measured by cardiac index; animal studies indicate that structural changes of HF (eg, hypertrophy) may be reversed by the drugs. Currently, one endothelin receptor antagonist, bosentan (Tracleer), is FDA approved, but only for treatment of pulmonary hypertension. Additional data are being collected to support specific indications for these drugs in the management of HF.

*(text continues on page 725)*

---

## NURSING PROCESS

### Assessment

Assess clients for current or potential HF:

- Identify risk factors for HF:
  - **Cardiovascular disorders:** atherosclerosis, hypertension, coronary artery disease, myocardial infarction, cardiac dysrhythmias, and cardiac valvular disease.
  - **Noncardiovascular disorders:** severe infections, hyperthyroidism, pulmonary disease (eg, cor pulmonale–right-sided HF resulting from lung disease)
  - **Other factors:** excessive amounts of IV fluids, rapid infusion of IV fluids or blood transfusions, advanced age
  - A **combination** of any of the preceding factors
- Interview and observe for signs and symptoms of chronic HF. Within the clinical syndrome of HF, clinical manifestations vary from few and mild to many and severe, including the following:
  - **Mild HF.** Common signs and symptoms of mild HF are ankle edema, dyspnea on exertion, and fatigue with ordinary physical activity. Edema results from increased venous pressure, which allows fluids to leak into tissues; dyspnea and fatigue result from tissue hypoxia.
  - **Moderate or severe HF.** More extensive edema, dyspnea, and fatigue at rest are likely to occur. Additional signs and symptoms include orthopnea, postnocturnal dyspnea, and cough (from congestion of the respiratory tract with venous blood); mental confusion (from cerebral hypoxia); oliguria and decreased renal function (from decreased blood flow to the kidneys); and anxiety.
- Observe for signs and symptoms of acute HF. Acute pulmonary edema indicates acute HF and is a medical emergency. Causes include acute myocardial infarction, cardiac dysrhythmias, severe hypertension, acute fluid or salt overload, and certain drugs (eg, quinidine and other cardiac depressants, propranolol and other anti-adrenergics, and phenylephrine, norepinephrine, and other alpha-adrenergic stimulants). Pulmonary edema occurs when left ventricular failure causes blood to accumulate in pulmonary veins and tissues. As a result, the person experiences severe dyspnea, hypoxia, hypertension, tachycardia, hemoptysis, frothy respiratory tract secretions, and anxiety.

Assess clients for signs and symptoms of atrial tachydysrhythmias:

- Record the rate and rhythm of apical and radial pulses. Atrial fibrillation, the most common atrial dysrhythmia, is characterized by tachycardia, pulse deficit (faster apical rate than radial rate), and a very irregular rhythm. Fatigue, dizziness, and fainting may occur.
- Check the electrocardiogram (ECG) for abnormal P waves, rapid rate of ventricular contraction, and QRS complexes of normal configuration but irregular intervals.

Assess baseline vital signs; weight; edema; laboratory results for potassium, magnesium, and calcium levels; and other tests of cardiovascular function when available.

Assess a baseline ECG before digoxin therapy when possible. If a client is in normal sinus rhythm, later ECGs may aid recognition of digitalis toxicity (ie, drug-induced dysrhythmias). If a client has an atrial tachydysrhythmia and is receiving digoxin to slow the ventricular rate, later ECGs may aid recognition of therapeutic and adverse effects. For clients who are already receiving digoxin at the initial contact, a baseline ECG can still be valuable because changes in later ECGs may promote earlier recognition and management of drug-induced dysrhythmias.

### Nursing Diagnoses

- Ineffective Tissue Perfusion related to decreased cardiac output
- Anxiety related to chronic illness and lifestyle changes
- Impaired Gas Exchange related to venous congestion and fluid accumulation in lungs
- Imbalanced Nutrition: Less Than Body Requirements related to digoxin-induced anorexia, nausea, and vomiting
- Noncompliance related to the need for long-term drug therapy and regular medical supervision
- Deficient Knowledge: Managing drug therapy regimen safely and effectively

### Planning/Goals

*The client will:*

- Take digoxin and other medications safely and accurately
- Experience improved breathing and less fatigue and edema

*(continued)*

## NURSING PROCESS (Continued)

- Maintain serum digoxin levels within therapeutic ranges
- Be closely monitored for therapeutic and adverse effects, especially during digitalization, when dosage is being changed, and when other drugs are added to or removed from the management regimen
- Keep appointments for follow-up monitoring of vital signs, serum potassium levels, serum digoxin levels, and renal function

### Interventions

Use measures to prevent or minimize HF and atrial dysrhythmias. In the broadest sense, preventive measures include sensible eating habits (a balanced diet, avoiding excess saturated fat and salt, weight control), avoiding cigarette smoking, and regular exercise. In the client at risk for development of HF and dysrhythmias, preventive measures include the following:

- Treatment of hypertension
- Avoidance of hypoxia
- Weight control
- Avoidance of excess sodium in the diet

- Avoidance of fluid overload, especially in elderly clients
- Maintenance of management programs for HF, atrial dysrhythmias, and other cardiovascular or noncardiovascular disorders

Monitor vital signs, weight, urine output, and serum potassium regularly, and compare with baseline values.

Monitor ECG when available, and compare with baseline or previous tracings.

### Evaluation

- Interview and observe for relief of symptoms (weight loss, increased urine output, less extremity edema, easier breathing, improved activity tolerance and self-care ability, slower heart rate).
- Observe serum drug levels for normal or abnormal values, when available.
- Interview regarding compliance with instructions for taking the drug.
- Interview and observe for adverse drug effects, especially cardiac dysrhythmias.

## CLIENT TEACHING GUIDELINES
## Digoxin

### General Considerations

✔ This drug is prescribed for two types of heart disease. One type is heart failure, in which digoxin strengthens your heartbeat and helps to relieve such symptoms as ankle swelling, shortness of breath, and fatigue. The other type is a fast heartbeat called atrial fibrillation, in which digoxin slows the heartbeat and decreases symptoms such as fatigue. Because these are chronic conditions, digoxin therapy is usually long term. Ask your health care provider why you are being given digoxin and what effects you can expect, both beneficial and adverse.

✔ It is extremely important to take digoxin (and other cardiovascular medications) as prescribed, usually once daily. The drug must be taken regularly to maintain therapeutic blood levels, but overuse can cause serious adverse effects.

✔ Precautions to increase the drug's safety and effectiveness include the following:

✔ As a general rule, do not miss a dose. It is helpful to develop a routine of taking the medication at approximately the same time each day and maintaining a written record, such as a dated checklist. If you forget a dose at the usual time and remember it within a few hours (approximately 6), go ahead and take the daily dose.

✔ Do not take an extra dose. For example, do not take a double dose to make up for a missed dose.

✔ Do not take other prescription or nonprescription (eg, antacids, cold remedies, diet pills) drugs without consulting the health care provider who prescribed digoxin. Many drugs interact with digoxin to increase or decrease its effects.

✔ You will need periodic physical examinations, electrocardiograms, and blood tests to check digoxin and electrolyte (sodium, potassium, magnesium) levels to monitor your response to digoxin and see whether changes in dosage are needed.

✔ Digoxin is often one drug in a management regimen of several drugs for heart disease. The drugs are all needed to help the heart and blood vessels work better. Together, the drugs help maintain a balance in the cardiovascular system. As a result, changing any aspect of one of the drugs can upset the balance and lead to symptoms. For example, stopping one drug because of adverse effects can lead to problems. If you think a drug needs to be stopped or its dosage reduced, talk with a health care provider. Do not make changes on your own; serious illness or even death could result.

✔ Small doses (eg, 0.125 milligrams [125 micrograms] daily or every other day) are usually given to older adults, and other people with impaired kidney function. Digoxin is eliminated through the kidneys; it can accumulate and cause adverse effects if dosage is not reduced with kidney impairment.

*(continued)*

## CLIENT TEACHING GUIDELINES
**Digoxin** (Continued)

✔ You may need to limit your salt (sodium chloride) intake and get an adequate supply of potassium. Follow your health care provider's recommendations about any diet changes. People taking digoxin are often taking a diuretic, a drug that increases urine production and loss of sodium and potassium from the body. If potassium levels get too low, adverse effects of digoxin are more likely to occur. However, too much potassium can also be harmful. Do not use salt substitutes (potassium chloride) without consulting a health care provider.

✔ Report adverse drug effects (eg, undesirable changes in heart rate or rhythm, nausea and vomiting, or visual problems) to a health care provider. These symptoms may indicate that digoxin dosage needs to be reduced.

✔ Use the same brand and type of digoxin all the time. For example, whether using generic digoxin or trade-name Lanoxin tablets, get the same one each time a prescription is refilled. In addition, there is a capsule form and a liquid form. These forms and concentrations are different and cannot be used interchangeably. Under-

doses and overdoses may occur. Lanoxin tablets are the most commonly used formulation.

### Self-administration or Caregiver Administration

✔ If instructed to do so by your health care provider, count your pulse before each dose. In some circumstances, you may be advised to skip that scheduled dose. *Do not* skip doses unless specifically instructed to do so.

✔ Take or give digoxin tablets approximately the same time each day to maintain more even blood levels and help in remembering to take the drug. The tablets may be crushed and can be taken with or after food, if desired, although milk and dairy products may delay absorption.

✔ Digoxin capsules should be swallowed whole.

✔ If taking or giving a liquid form of digoxin, it is extremely important to measure it accurately. A few drops more could produce overdosage, with serious adverse effects; a few drops less could produce underdosage, with a loss or decrease of therapeutic effects.

## *Nursing Actions*

## Cardiotonic-Inotropic Drugs

| Nursing Actions | Rationale/Explanation |
|---|---|
| 1. Administer accurately. | |
| a. With digoxin: | |
| (1) Read the drug label and the health care provider's order carefully when preparing a dose. | For accurate administration |
| (2) Give only the ordered dosage form (eg, tablet, Lanoxicap, or elixir). | Digoxin formulations vary in concentration and bioavailability and *cannot* be used interchangeably. |
| (3) Check the apical pulse before each dose. If the rate is below 60 in adults or 100 in children, omit the dose, and notify the health care provider. | Bradycardia is an adverse effect. |
| (4) Have the same nurse give digoxin to the same clients when possible because it is important to detect changes in rate and rhythm (see *Observe for therapeutic effects* and *Observe for adverse effects,* later). | |
| (5) Give oral digoxin with food or after meals. | This may minimize gastric irritation and symptoms of anorexia, nausea, and vomiting. However, these symptoms probably arise from drug stimulation of chemoreceptors in the medulla rather than a direct irritant effect of the drug on the gastrointestinal (GI) tract. |
| (6) Inject intravenous (IV) digoxin slowly (over at least 5 min). | Digoxin should be given slowly because the diluent, propylene glycol, has toxic effects on the cardiac conduction system if given too rapidly. Digoxin may be given undiluted or diluted with a fourfold or greater volume of sterile water for injection, 0.9% sodium chloride injection, or 5% dextrose injection. If diluted, use the solution immediately. |

*(continued)*

*Nursing Actions*

## Cardiotonic-Inotropic Drugs (Continued)

| Nursing Actions | Rationale/Explanation |
|---|---|
| b. With inamrinone: | |
| (1) Give undiluted or diluted to a concentration of 1 to 3 mg/mL. | Manufacturer's recommendations |
| (2) Dilute with 0.9% or 0.45% sodium chloride solution; use the diluted solution within 24 h. Do not dilute with solutions containing dextrose. | Inamrinone may be injected into IV tubing containing a dextrose solution because contact is brief. However, a chemical interaction occurs with prolonged contact. |
| (3) Give bolus injections into the tubing of an IV infusion, over 2 to 3 min. | |
| (4) Administer maintenance infusions at a rate of 5 to 10 mcg/kg/min. | |
| c. With milrinone: | |
| (1) Dilute with 0.9% or 0.45% sodium chloride or 5% dextrose solution; use the diluted solution within 24 h. | Manufacturer's recommendations |
| (2) Give the loading dose by bolus infusion over 10 min. | |
| (3) Give maintenance infusions at a standard rate of 0.5 mcg/kg/min; this rate may be increased or decreased according to response. | Manufacturer's recommendations |
| d. With nesiritide: | |
| (1) Dilute with 5 mL of 0.9% or 0.45% sodium chloride or 5% dextrose solution from a 250 mL IV container; add mixed drug to the container and use diluted solution within 24 h. | Manufacturer's recommendations |
| (2) Prime infusion tubing with 25 mL prior to connecting to the patient; withdraw a bolus loading dose from infusion solution. | Manufacturer's recommendations |
| (3) Give a bolus injection of 2 mcg/kg over 1 minute. | |
| (4) Give the maintenance infusion at a rate of 0.01 mcg/kg/min. | |
| (5) Do not mix with any other drug solution; administer through a separate line. | Incompatible with most drugs |
| 2. **Observe for therapeutic effects.** | |
| a. When the drugs are given in heart failure (HF), observe for: | |
| (1) Fewer signs and symptoms of pulmonary congestion (dyspnea, orthopnea, cyanosis, cough, hemoptysis, crackles, anxiety, restlessness) | The pulmonary symptoms that develop with HF are a direct result of events initiated by inadequate cardiac output. The left side of the heart is unable to accommodate incoming blood flow from the lungs. The resulting back pressure in pulmonary veins and capillaries causes leakage of fluid from blood vessels into tissue spaces and alveoli. Fluid accumulation may result in severe respiratory difficulty and pulmonary edema, a life-threatening development. The improved strength of myocardial contraction resulting from cardiotonic-inotropic drugs reverses this potentially fatal chain of events. |
| (2) Decreased edema—absence of pitting, decreased size of ankles or abdominal girth, decreased weight | Diuresis and decreased edema result from improved circulation and increased renal blood flow. |
| (3) Increased tolerance of activity | Indicates a more adequate supply of blood to tissues |

*(continued)*

## Nursing Actions

## Cardiotonic-Inotropic Drugs (Continued)

| Nursing Actions | Rationale/Explanation |
|---|---|
| b. When digoxin is given in atrial dysrhythmias, observe for:<br>  (1) Gradual slowing of the heart rate to 70 to 80 beats/min<br>  (2) Elimination of the pulse deficit<br>  (3) Change in rhythm from irregular to regular | In clients with atrial fibrillation, slowing of the heart rate and elimination of the pulse deficit are clinical indicators that digitalization has been achieved. |
| 3. Observe for adverse effects.<br>  a. With digoxin observe for: | There is a high incidence of adverse effects with digoxin therapy. Therefore, every client receiving digoxin requires close observation. Severity of adverse effects can be minimized with early detection and treatment. |
|   (1) Cardiac dysrhythmias: | Digoxin toxicity may cause any type of cardiac dysrhythmia. These are the most serious adverse effects associated with digoxin therapy. They are detected as abnormalities in electrocardiograms and in pulse rate or rhythm. |
|     (a) Premature ventricular contractions (PVCs) | PVCs are among the most common digoxin-induced dysrhythmias. They are not specific for digoxin toxicity because there are many possible causes. They are usually perceived as "skipped" heartbeats. |
|     (b) Bradycardia | Excessive slowing of the heart rate is an extension of the drug's therapeutic action of slowing conduction through the atrioventricular (AV) node and probably depressing the sinoatrial node as well. |
|     (c) Paroxysmal atrial tachycardia with heart block<br>     (d) AV nodal tachycardia<br>     (e) AV block (second- or third-degree heart block) | ECG is necessary for identification of nodal rhythms and heart block. |
|   (2) Anorexia, nausea, vomiting | These GI effects commonly occur with digoxin therapy. Because they are caused at least in part by stimulation of the vomiting center in the brain, they occur with parenteral and oral administration. The presence of these symptoms raises suspicion of digitalis toxicity, but they are not specific because many other conditions may cause anorexia, nausea, and vomiting. Also, clients receiving digoxin are often taking other medications that cause these side effects, such as diuretics and potassium supplements. |
|   (3) Headache, drowsiness, confusion | These central nervous system effects are most common in older adults. |
|   (4) Visual disturbances (eg, blurred vision, photophobia, altered perception of colors, flickering dots) | These are due mainly to drug effects on the retina and may indicate acute toxicity. |
| b. With inamrinone, observe for:<br>  (1) Thrombocytopenia | Thrombocytopenia is more likely to occur with prolonged therapy and is usually reversible if dosage is reduced or the drug is discontinued. |
|   (2) Anorexia, nausea, vomiting, abdominal pain | GI symptoms can be decreased by reducing drug dosage. |
|   (3) Hypotension | Hypotension probably results from vasodilatory effects of inamrinone. |
|   (4) Hepatotoxicity | If marked changes in liver enzymes occur in conjunction with clinical symptoms, the drug should be discontinued. |
| c. With milrinone, observe for ventricular dysrhythmias, hypotension, and headache | Ventricular dysrhythmias reportedly occur in 12% of clients; hypotension and headache in approximately 3% of clients. |
| d. With nesiritide, observe for hypotension, headache, nausea, back pain, ventricular tachycardia, dizziness, anxiety, insomnia, bradycardia, and vomiting. | Hypotension occurs in approximately 11% of clients; headache in 8%; nausea and back pain in 4%; and other adverse effects in 1 to 3%. |

*(continued)*

## Nursing Actions

### Cardiotonic-Inotropic Drugs (Continued)

| Nursing Actions | Rationale/Explanation |
|---|---|
| 4. Observe for drug interactions. | Most significant drug interactions increase risks of toxicity. Some alter absorption or metabolism to produce under-digitalization and decreased therapeutic effect. |
| a. Drugs that *increase* effects of digoxin: | |
| (1) Adrenergic drugs (eg, ephedrine, epinephrine, isoproterenol) | Increase risks of cardiac dysrhythmias |
| (2) Antidysrhythmics (eg, amiodarone, propafenone, quinidine) | Decrease clearance of digoxin, thereby increasing serum digoxin levels and risks of toxicity. Dosage of digoxin should be reduced if one of these drugs is given concurrently (25% with propafenone and 50% with amiodarone and quinidine). |
| (3) Anticholinergics | Increase absorption of oral digoxin by slowing transit time through the GI tract |
| (4) Calcium preparations | Increase risks of cardiac dysrhythmias. IV calcium salts are contraindicated in digitalized clients. |
| (5) Calcium channel blockers (eg, diltiazem, felodipine, nifedipine, verapamil) | Decrease clearance of digoxin, thereby increasing serum digoxin levels and risks of toxicity. Dosage of digoxin should be reduced 25% if verapamil is given concurrently. |
| b. Drugs that *decrease* effects of digoxin: | |
| (1) Antacids, cholestyramine, colestipol, laxatives, oral aminoglycosides (eg, neomycin) | Decrease absorption of oral digoxin |

---

### ? How Can You Avoid This Medication Error?

**Answer:** There is no indication in this situation that the nurse collected important information to make a sound decision regarding the safe administration of the digoxin. Nausea and vomiting often are the first and sometimes only symptoms of digoxin toxicity. Digoxin has a very narrow therapeutic window, so cumulative effects can cause toxicity, especially when an elderly patient has poor kidney function.

It is important that the nurse take an apical pulse for a full minute to detect new dysrhythmias, especially brady-cardia, prior to administering digoxin. Because this patient is receiving Lasix, the nurse should also check the potassium level inasmuch as digoxin toxicity is more likely if the patient is hypokalemic. The nurse is right that digoxin should not be administered with antacids because concurrent administration will impact drug absorption. If assessment data support the likelihood of digoxin toxicity, a digoxin level can be drawn to confirm or rule out toxicity.

### Critical Thinking Exercises

1. A 56-year-old client develops digoxin toxicity 1 month after beginning 0.125 mg of digoxin, PO daily. Which factors affect the duration of such an adverse reaction?

   a. Daily drug dosage
   b. Half-life of the drug
   c. Form of the drug prescribed
   d. Duration of therapy

2. A 44-year-old client develops blurring of vision with flickering dots in his visual fields while taking digoxin. The nurse recognizes that the visual changes may indicate:

   a. A need for a visual exam
   b. Adjustment of the retina to the drug
   c. Acute toxicity
   d. Therapeutic effects

3. What is the onset of action of an IV dose of digoxin?

   a. 10 to 30 minutes
   b. 30 to 60 minutes
   c. 60 to 90 minutes
   d. 90 to 120 minutes

4. Mr. Smith, age 74 years, comes to the emergency department complaining of shortness of breath, anxiety, and a rapid heartbeat. The ECG reveals atrial fibrillation with a ventricular response of 140 beats/minute. The physician prescribes digoxin (Lanoxin), 0.5 mg IV as a loading dose followed by 0.25 mg PO daily. The client's wife asks why he is getting a loading dose. The nurse's response is based on the understanding that the loading dose:

   a. Provides for more rapid effects of the drug
   b. Is used because digoxin is poorly absorbed from the GI tract
   c. Determines the client's tolerance to the drug
   d. Is based on the drug's excretion by the liver

5. A 1-week-old infant is prescribed digoxin. Which electrolyte imbalance will place her at greater risk for digoxin toxicity?

   a. Hyponatremia
   b. Hyperkalemia
   c. Hypocalcemia
   d. Hypokalemia

## SELECTED REFERENCES

Carelock, J., & Clark, A. P. (2001). Heart failure: Pathophysiologic mechanisms. *American Journal of Nursing, 101*(12), 26–33.

Cody, R. J. (2000). Approach to the patient with heart failure. In H. D. Humes (Ed.), *Kelley's textbook of internal medicine* (4th ed., pp. 374–381). Philadelphia: Lippincott Williams & Wilkins.

*Drug facts and comparisons.* (Updated monthly). St. Louis: Facts and Comparisons.

Ewald, G. A., & Rogers, J. G. (2001). Heart failure, cardiomyopathy, and valvular heart disease. In S. N. Ahya, K. Flood, & S. Paranjothi (Eds.), *The Washington manual of medical therapeutics* (30th ed., pp. 131–152). Philadelphia: Lippincott Williams & Wilkins.

Johnson, J. A., Parker, R. B., & Patterson, J. H. (2002). Heart failure. In J. T. DiPiro, R. L. Talbert, G. C. Yee, G. R. Matzke, B. G. Wells, & L. M. Posey (Eds.), *Pharmacotherapy: A pathophysiologic approach* (4th ed., pp. 185–218). New York: McGraw-Hill.

Lacy, C. F., Armstrong, L. L., Goldman, M. P., & Lance, L. L. (2003). *Lexi-Comp's drug information handbook* (11th ed.). Hudson, OH: American Pharmaceutical Association.

Karch, A. M. (2003). *Lippincott's nursing drug guide.* Philadelphia: Lippincott Williams & Wilkins.

North American Nursing Diagnosis Association. (2001). *Nursing diagnoses: Definitions & classification 2001–2002.* Philadelphia: Author.

Porth, C. M. (2002). *Pathophysiology: Concepts of altered health states* (6th ed., pp. 547–556). Philadelphia: Lippincott Williams & Wilkins.

Skidmore-Roth, L. (2001). *Mosby's handbook of herbs & natural supplements.* St. Louis: Mosby.

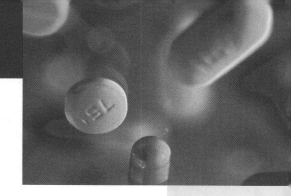

# 40

# Antidysrhythmic Drugs

## OBJECTIVES

*After studying this chapter, the student will be able to:*

1 Differentiate between supraventricular and ventricular dysrhythmias in terms of etiology and hemodynamic effects.

2 Discuss the roles of beta-adrenergic blocking agents, calcium channel blockers, digoxin, and quinidine in the management of supraventricular tachydysrhythmias.

3 Give the effects of lidocaine in the management of ventricular tachycardia.

4 Describe adverse effects and nursing process implications related to the use of selected antidysrhythmic drugs.

## CRITICAL THINKING SCENARIO

Leon Fitzgerald, 79 years old, was recently diagnosed with atrial fibrillation. His heart rate is irregularly irregular, ranging between 120 and 160 beats/minute. At times, Mr. Fitzgerald is very symptomatic, experiencing weakness, dizziness, and syncope. His health care provider prescribes verapamil, a calcium channel blocker.

✔ What is the emotional impact of a diagnosis of a serious cardiac problem, such as a dysrhythmia?

✔ How does atrial fibrillation affect cardiac function and the ability to oxygenate effectively?

✔ How might the resulting symptoms of weakness, dizziness, and syncope affect Mr. Fitzgerald's daily functioning?

✔ How does verapamil acts to improve cardiac function?

## PROTOTYPE PROFILES

quinidine (Quinaglute, others), p. 743

lidocaine (Xylocaine, others), p. 744

# OVERVIEW

Antidysrhythmic agents are diverse drugs used for prevention and management of cardiac dysrhythmias. Dysrhythmias, also called arrhythmias, are abnormalities in heart rate or rhythm. They become significant when they interfere with cardiac function and ability to perfuse body tissues. To aid in understanding of dysrhythmias and antidysrhythmic drug therapy, the physiology of cardiac conduction and contractility is reviewed in At the Foundation: Cardiac Electrophysiology.

# CARDIAC DYSRHYTHMIAS

Cardiac dysrhythmias can originate in any part of the conduction system or from atrial or ventricular muscle. They result from disturbances in electrical impulse formation (automaticity), conduction (conductivity), or both. The characteristic of automaticity allows myocardial cells other than the sinoatrial (SA) node to depo-

larize and initiate the electrical impulse that culminates in atrial and ventricular contraction. This may occur when the SA node fails to initiate an impulse or does so too slowly. When the electrical impulse arises anywhere other than the SA node, it is an abnormal or ectopic focus. If the ectopic focus depolarizes at a rate faster than the SA node, the ectopic focus becomes the dominant pacemaker. Ectopic pacemakers may arise in the atria, atrioventricular (AV) node, Purkinje fibers, or ventricular muscle. They may be activated by hypoxia, ischemia, or hypokalemia. Ectopic foci indicate myocardial irritability (increased responsiveness to stimuli) and potentially serious impairment of cardiac function.

Dysrhythmias may be mild or severe, acute or chronic, episodic or relatively continuous. They are clinically significant if they interfere with cardiac function (ie, the heart's ability to pump sufficient blood to body tissues). Nonpharmacologic management is preferred, at least initially, for several dysrhythmias. For example, sinus tachycardia usually results from such disorders as infection, anxiety, or hypotension, and management should

---

**AT THE FOUNDATION:** *Cardiac Electrophysiology*

Specialized conductive tissue in the heart can generate and conduct an electrical impulse through specialized pacemaker cells that comprise a conduction system. Normally, electrical impulses originate in the SA node and are transmitted to atrial muscle, where they cause atrial contraction, and then to the AV node, bundle of His, bundle branches, Purkinje fibers, and ventricular muscle, where they cause ventricular contraction. These activities commonly result in effective cardiac contraction and distribution of blood throughout the body.

Four properties exist in cardiac muscle: automaticity, excitability, rhythmicity, and conductivity. *Automaticity* is the heart's ability to generate an electrical impulse. Any part of the conduction system can spontaneously start an impulse, but the SA node normally has the highest degree of automaticity and spontaneous impulse formation. With its faster rate of electrical discharge or depolarization than other parts of the conduction system, the SA node serves as pacemaker and controls heart rate and rhythm.

Initiation of an electrical impulse depends on the movement of sodium and calcium ions into a myocardial cell and movement of potassium ions out of the cell. Normally, the cell membrane becomes more permeable to sodium and opens pores or channels to allow its rapid movement into the cell. Calcium ions follow sodium ions into the cell at a slower rate. As sodium and calcium ions move into cells, potassium ions move out of cells. The movement of the ions changes the membrane from its resting state of electrical neutrality to an activated state of electrical energy buildup. When the electrical energy is discharged (depolarization), muscle contraction occurs.

The ability of a cardiac muscle cell to respond to an electrical stimulus is called *excitability* or *irritability*. The stimulus must reach a certain intensity or threshold to cause contraction. After contraction, sodium and calcium ions return to the extracellular space, potassium ions return to the intracellular space, muscle relaxation occurs, and the cell prepares for the next electrical stimulus and contraction.

Following contraction, there is also a period of decreased excitability (called the *absolute refractory period*) during which the cell cannot respond to a new stimulus. Before the resting membrane potential is reached, a stimulus greater than normal can evoke a response in the cell. This period is called the *relative refractory period*.

### Conductivity

*Conductivity* is the ability of cardiac tissue to transmit electrical impulses. Although the electrophysiology of a single myocardial cell can assist understanding of the process, the orderly, rhythmic transmission of impulses to all cells is needed for effective myocardial contraction.

The cardiac conduction system is shown in Figure 40-1.

The ability of the heart to beat regularly is the result of the inherent *rhythmicity* of cardiac muscle. Within the heart, specialized cells generate repetitive self-induced action potentials that spread through the conducting system of the heart and into the muscle to cause a contraction. No nerves are located inside the heart itself, and no outside regulatory mechanisms are necessary to stimulate the muscle to rhythmically contract.

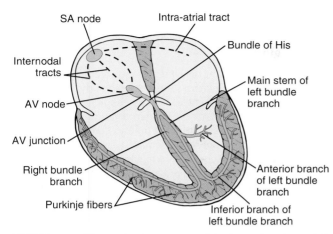

**FIGURE 40-1** The conducting system of the heart. Impulses originating in the SA node are transmitted through the atria, into the AV node to the bundle of His, and by way of Purkinje fibers through the ventricles.

attempt to relieve the underlying cause. For paroxysmal supraventricular tachycardia (PSVT) with mild or moderate symptoms, Valsalva's maneuver, carotid sinus massage, or other measures to increase vagal tone are preferred. For ventricular fibrillation, immediate defibrillation by electrical countershock is the initial management of choice. In addition, other current technology allows clinicians to insert pacemakers and defibrillators

(eg, ICD) to control bradydysrhythmias or tachydysrhythmias and to use radio waves (radiofrequency catheter ablation) or surgery to destroy arrhythmogenic foci. Dysrhythmias are usually categorized by rate, location, or patterns of conduction. Common types of dysrhythmias are described in Table 40-1.

## ■ ANTIDYSRHYTHMIC DRUGS

Antidysrhythmic drugs alter the heart's electrical conduction system. Atropine for bradydysrhythmias is discussed in Chapter 19; digoxin and its use in treating atrial fibrillation (AF) are discussed in Chapter 39. The focus of this chapter is on the drugs used for tachydysrhythmias. These drugs are described in the following sections and listed in Drugs at a Glance 40-1: Antidysrhythmic Drugs. Discussion of management considerations in children and older adults is found in Age-related Considerations.

### Mechanisms of Action

Drugs used for rapid dysrhythmias mainly *reduce automaticity* (spontaneous depolarization of myocardial cells, including ectopic pacemakers), *slow conduction* of electrical impulses through the heart, and *prolong the refractory period* of myocardial cells (thus they are less

*(text continues on page 737)*

| **TABLE 40-1   Common Dysrhythmias** | | |
|---|---|---|
| **Dysrhythmia** | **Characteristics of Rhythm** | **Clinical Significance** |
| ***Sinus Dysrhythmias*** | | |
| Sinus bradycardia (SB) | Rhythm: regular<br>P waves: normal<br>**AV rates: <60 beats/min**<br>PR interval: within normal limits<br>(0.12–0.20 sec)<br>QRS complex: within normal limits<br>(0.06–0.10 sec) | Significance is based on severity of underlying cause and duration. May occur in healthy young adults, especially in athletes and during sleep. Bradycardia can decrease cardiac output unless stroke volume increases as a compensatory mechanism. |

*(continued)*

**TABLE 40-1   Common Dysrhythmias** (Continued)

| Dysrhythmia | Characteristics of Rhythm | Clinical Significance |
|---|---|---|
| Sinus tachycardia (ST) | Rhythm: regular<br>P waves: normal<br>**AV rates: >100 beats/min**<br>PR interval: within normal limits<br>QRS complex: within normal limits | Usually significant only if severe or prolonged. Sinus tachycardia increases the workload of the heart and may lead to heart failure or angina pectoris by increasing myocardial oxygen consumption and shortening diastolic filling time so that coronary arteries may not have adequate filling time between heartbeats. Thus, additional blood flow to the myocardium is required at the same time that a decreased blood supply is delivered. |

*Atrial Dysrhythmias*

| | | |
|---|---|---|
| Premature atrial contractions (PACs) | Rhythm: Irregular due to prematurity of PACs<br>**P waves: P wave associated with PAC is premature,** and often abnormal in size, shape, or direction<br>AV rates: > determined by underlying rhythm<br>PR interval: typically different from that of underlying rhythm<br>QRS complex: within normal limits | Common in individuals with a normal or diseased heart. The underlying cause of the beats determines the clinical significance. PACs may warn of or initiate a more significant atrial dysrhythmia (ie, atrial flutter or atrial fibrillation) or the development of heart failure (due to stretch of the myocardium) |

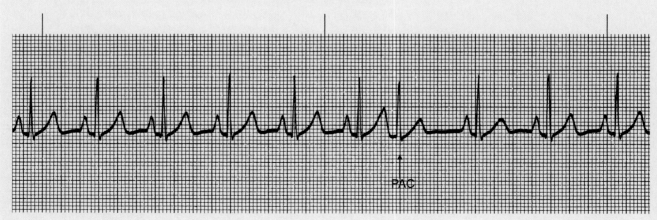

PAC

*(continued)*

**TABLE 40-1    Common Dysrhythmias** (Continued)

| Dysrhythmia | Characteristics of Rhythm | Clinical Significance |
|---|---|---|
| Atrial fibrillation (AF) | Rhythm: irregular (appears more regular with very rapid ventricular rates)<br>**P waves: not identifiable; appear as fibrillation waves**<br>AV rates: atrial rate not measurable; ventricular rate varies with the number of impulses that are conducted through AV node<br>PR interval: not measurable<br>QRS complex: within normal limits<br>Comment: ST-segment depression and T-wave inversion present on representative strip | The lack of atrial contraction in AF impairs ventricular filling, decreases cardiac output (by as much as 30% through loss of "atrial kick"), and may lead to the formation of atrial thrombi, with a high potential for embolization. |

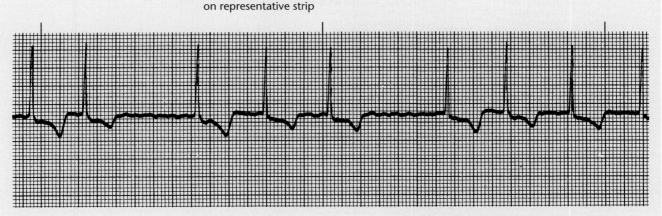

| Atrial flutter | Rhythm: regular or irregular depending on conduction ratios<br>**P waves: normal with sawtooth appearance (flutter or f waves)**<br>AV rates: atrial rate 250–400 beats/min; ventricular rate varies with the number of impulses that are conducted through AV node (will be less than atrial rate)<br>PR interval: not measurable<br>QRS complex: within normal limits<br>Comment: flutter waves marked with Fs in representative strip | Possible rapid ventricular response increases myocardial oxygen consumption and cardiac workload and decreases cardiac output. The rapidly contracting atria are inefficient in emptying their contents, resulting in a loss of "atrial kick," and may lead to the formation of atrial thrombi, with a high potential for embolization. |

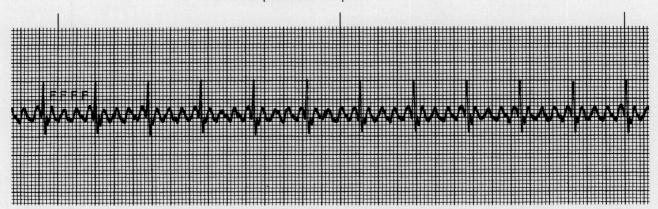

*(continued)*

## TABLE 40-1 Common Dysrhythmias (Continued)

| Dysrhythmia | Characteristics of Rhythm | Clinical Significance |
|---|---|---|
| *Atrioventricular (AV) Blocks* | | |
| First-degree AV block | Regular rhythm<br>P waves normal (one P wave to each QRS)<br>AV rates < 60 beats/min<br>PR interval: **prolonged (>0.20 sec)**<br>QRS complex: within normal limits | Heart block involves impaired conduction of the electrical impulse through the AV node. With first-degree heart block, conduction is slowed, but not significantly. Clinical concern relates to the effect of the block on heart rate. |

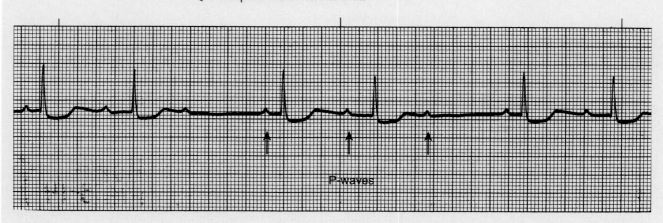

P-wave

| | | |
|---|---|---|
| Second-degree AV block<br>  *Mobitz type 1*<br>  *(Wenckebach's phenomenon)* | Rhythm: regular atrial; irregular ventricular<br>P waves normal<br>AV rates: Atrial: rate determined by underlying rhythm; ventricular: dependent on the number of impulses successfully conducted through AV node **(ventricular rate always less than atrial rate)**<br>PR interval: **varies and progressively lengthens until a P wave occurs without a corresponding QRS complex**<br>QRS complex: within normal limits | With second-degree heart block, every second, third, or fourth atrial impulse is blocked and does not reach the ventricles (2:1, 3:1, or 4:1 block). Thus, atrial and ventricular rates differ. Second-degree heart block may interfere with cardiac output and has been divided into two types (Mobitz type I, or Wenckebach's phenomenon, and Mobitz type II). Mobitz type I is transient in nature and has been associated with individuals with acute inferior wall MI or digoxin toxicity and usually does not require temporary pacing. May also occur in athletes at rest due to increased vagal tone. |

P-waves

*(continued)*

## TABLE 40-1    Common Dysrhythmias (Continued)

| Dysrhythmia | Characteristics of Rhythm | Clinical Significance |
| --- | --- | --- |
| *Mobitz type II* | Rhythm: regular atrial and ventricular rhythm<br>P waves normal<br>AV rates: Atrial: rate determined by underlying rhythm; ventricular: dependent on the number of impulses successfully conducted through AV node (**ventricular rate always less than atrial rate**)<br>**PR interval: remains constant,** but may be normal or prolonged<br>QRS complex: normal if block located in bundle of His; wide if block is in bundle branches | Mobitz type II occurs in clients with anterior wall MI, may progress to third-degree block, and often requires cardiac pacing because it is unpredictable in nature and is associated with a high mortality rate. |

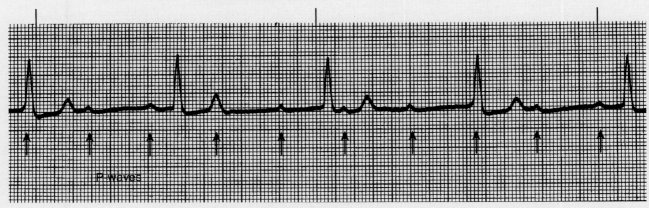

P-waves

| | | |
| --- | --- | --- |
| Third-degree AV block | Rhythm: atrial regular; ventricular regular<br>P waves: normal; **no constant relationship between P waves and QRS complexes (P waves "marching through" QRS complexes)**<br>AV rates:<br>PR interval: varies significantly, no correlation of P waves to QRS complex<br>QRS complex: normal if block located in bundle of His; wide if block in bundle branches | Third-degree is the most serious type of heart block because no impulses reach the ventricles. As a result, AV dissociation occurs, and the ventricles beat independently at a rate less than 40 beats/min. This slow ventricular rate severely reduces cardiac output and hemodynamic stability. |

P-waves

*(continued)*

**TABLE 40-1    Common Dysrhythmias** (Continued)

| Dysrhythmia | Characteristics of Rhythm | Clinical Significance |
| --- | --- | --- |

*Ventricular Dysrhythmias*

| Premature ventricular complexes (PVCs) | Rhythm: Irregular owing to prematurity of PVCs<br>P waves: none associated with PVC because complex originates in ventricle<br>AV rates: rate of underlying rhythm<br>PR interval: not measurable<br>**QRS complex: premature and wide (0.12 sec or greater)**<br>Comment: PVCs are multifocal on representative strip | PVCs occur in healthy individuals as well as those with heart disease and may cause no symptoms. PVCs are considered serious if they produce significant symptoms (eg, anginal pain, dyspnea, or syncope), occur more than 5 times per minute, are coupled or grouped, are multifocal, or occur during the resting phase of the cardiac cycle (R-on-T phenomenon). Serious PVCs indicate a high degree of myocardial irritability and may lead to life-threatening ventricular tachycardia, ventricular fibrillation, or asystole. |

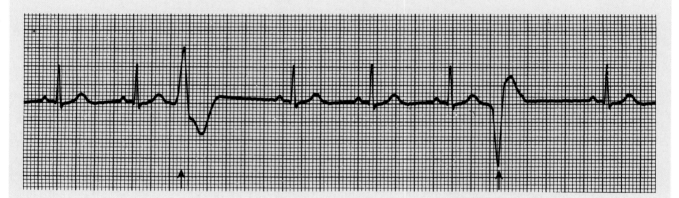

| Ventricular tachycardia (VT) | **Rhythm: regular but originates in ventricle**<br>P waves: absent<br>**AV rates: atrial rate not present; ventricular rate: 140–250 beats/min**<br>PR interval: not measurable<br>QRS complex: wide (0.12 sec or greater) | VT may be sustained (lasts longer than 30 sec or requires termination because of hemodynamic collapse) or nonsustained (stops spontaneously in less than 30 sec). Occasional brief episodes of VT may be asymptomatic; frequent or relatively long episodes may result in hemodynamic collapse, a life-threatening situation. An acute episode most often occurs during an acute MI. Other precipitating factors include severe electrolyte imbalances (eg, hypokalemia), hypoxemia, or digoxin toxicity. |

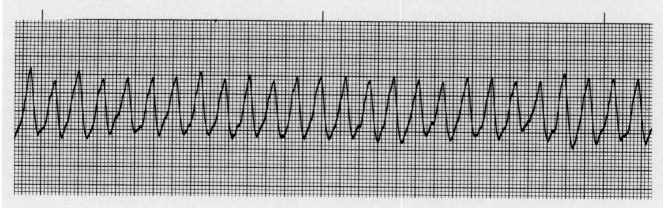

*(continued)*

## TABLE 40-1 Common Dysrhythmias (Continued)

| Dysrhythmia | Characteristics of Rhythm | Clinical Significance |
|---|---|---|
| Ventricular fibrillation (VF) | **Rhythm: irregular and chaotic**<br>P waves: absent<br>AV rates: no P wave or QRS complexes present<br>PR interval: not measurable<br>QRS complex: absent | VF produces no myocardial contraction, so that there is no cardiac output and sudden cardiac death occurs. Death results unless effective cardio-pulmonary resuscitation or defibrillation is instituted within approximately 4 to 6 min. VF most often occurs in clients with ischemic heart disease, especially acute MI. |
| Asystole | **Rhythm: absent**<br>P waves: absent<br>AV rates: no P wave or QRS complexes present<br>PR interval: not measurable<br>QRS complex: absent<br>Comment: one ventricular complex leading to ventricular asystole on representative strip | Asystole produces no myocardial contraction, so that there is no cardiac output and sudden cardiac death occurs. Death results unless effective cardio-pulmonary resuscitation or defibrillation is instituted within approximately 4 to 6 min. |

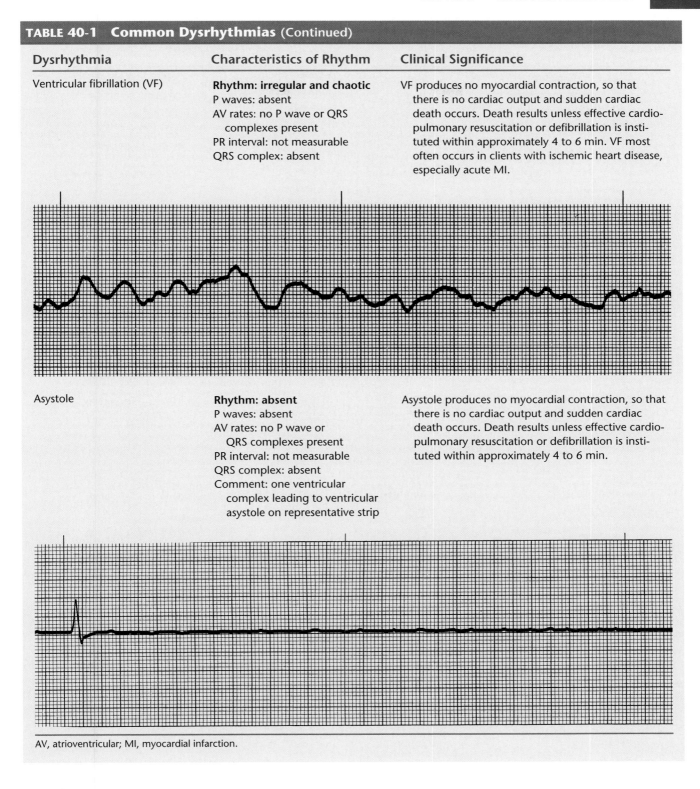

AV, atrioventricular; MI, myocardial infarction.

likely to be prematurely activated by adjacent cells). Several different groups of drugs perform one or more of these actions. They are classified according to their mechanisms of action and effects on the conduction system, even though they differ in other respects. Additionally, some drugs have characteristics of more than one classification. General trends and considerations for drug therapy of supraventricular and ventricular dysrhythmias are described in the following sections.

## General Trends and Considerations

Clinical use of antidysrhythmic drugs for tachydysrhythmias has undergone significant changes. One change is

**DRUG TABLE 40-1**

*Drugs at a Glance*

## Antidysrhythmic Drugs

| Drugs for Tachydysrhythmias | Routes and Dosage Ranges | Comments |
|---|---|---|
| **Class I Sodium Channel Blockers** | | |
| *Class 1a: Treatment of Symptomatic Premature Ventricular Contractions, Supraventricular Tachycardia, and Ventricular Tachycardia; Prevention of Ventricular Fibrillation* | | |
| **Quinidine** (Cardioquin, Quinaglute) | See Prototype Profile 40-1: Quinidine | |
| **Procainamide** (Pronestyl, Procanbid) Pregnancy Category C | *Adults:* PO, 1 g loading dose initially, then 250–500 mg q3–4h (q6h for sustained-release tablets) IM loading dose, 500–1000 mg followed by oral maintenance doses IV, 25–50 mg/min; maximum dose, 1000 mg *Children:* PO, 50 mg/kg/d in 4–6 divided doses | |
| **Disopyramide** (Norpace) Pregnancy Category C | *Adults:* PO, loading dose, 300 mg, followed by 150 mg q6h; usual dose, PO, 400–800 mg/d in 4 divided doses | Low toxic: therapeutic ratio so risk of adverse effects high Erythromycin and rifampin decrease levels; phenytoin increases metabolism |
| *Class 1b: Treatment of Symptomatic Premature Ventricular Contractions and Ventricular Tachycardia; Prevention of Ventricular Fibrillation* | | |
| **Lidocaine** (Xylocaine) | See Prototype Profile 40-2: Lidocaine | |
| **Mexiletine** (Mexitil) Pregnancy Category C | *Adults:* PO, 200 mg q8h initially, increased by 50–100 mg every 2–3 d if necessary to a maximum of 1200 mg/d | |
| **Tocainide** (Tonocard) Pregnancy Category C | *Adults:* PO, 400 mg q8h initially, increased up to 1800 mg/d in three divided doses if necessary | Dizziness and falls more likely to occur with elderly |
| **Phenytoin** (Dilantin) Pregnancy Category D | *Adults:* PO, loading dose 13 mg/kg (approximately 1000 mg) first day, 7.5 mg/kg second and third days; maintenance dose 4–6 mg/kg/d (average 400 mg) in 1 or 2 doses starting on the fourth day IV, 100 mg every 5 min until the dysrhythmia is reversed or toxic effects occur; maximum dose, 1 g/24 h | See Prototype Profile 11-1: Phenytoin in Chapter 11 |
| *Class 1c: Treatment of Life-threatening Ventricular Tachycardia or Fibrillation and Supraventricular Tachycardia Unresponsive to Other Drugs* | | |
| **Flecainide** (Tambocor) Pregnancy Category C | *Adults:* PO, 100 mg q12h initially, increased by 50 mg q12h every 4 d until effective; maximum dose, 400 mg/d | Take around-the-clock exactly as directed |
| **Propafenone** (Rythmol) Pregnancy Category C | *Adults:* PO, 150 mg q8h initially, increased to a maximum dose of 1200 mg/d if necessary; usual maintenance dose 150–300 mg q8h | Clients with bronchospastic disease should generally not take this drug |

*(continued)*

**DRUG TABLE 40-1**

*Drugs at a Glance*

## Antidysrhythmic Drugs (Continued)

| Drugs for Tachydysrhythmias | Routes and Dosage Ranges | Comments |
|---|---|---|
| **Class 1 Miscellaneous: *Treatment of Life-Threatening Ventricular Dysrhythmias*** | | |
| **Moricizine** (Ethmozine) Pregnancy Category B | *Adults:* PO, 200–300 mg q8h | Concurrent use may decrease level of diltiazem or aminophylline; food decreases peak serum concentration of drug |
| **Class II Beta Blockers: *Treatment of Supraventricular Tachycardia*** | | |
| **Acebutolol** (Sectral) Pregnancy Category B | *Adults:* PO, 200 mg twice daily, increased gradually until optimal response is obtained (usually 600–1200 mcg/d) | Stopping drug abruptly may worsen angina and myocardial infarction |
| **Esmolol** (Brevibloc) Pregnancy Category C | *Adults:* IV infusion, 500 mcg/kg/min initially as a loading dose, followed by a maintenance dose of 50 mcg/kg/min over 4 min. Repeat the same loading dose, and increase maintenance doses in 50 mcg/kg increments every 5–10 min until therapeutic effects are obtained. Average maintenance dose, 100 mcg/kg/min. | Administered IV in emergency situations |
| **Propranolol** (Inderal) Pregnancy Category C | *Adults:* IV injection, 1–3 mg at a rate of 1 mg/min PO, 10–20 mg three or four times per day | See Prototype Profile 41-1: Propranolol in Chapter 41 |
| **Sotalol** (Betapace) Pregnancy Category B | *Adults:* PO, 80 mg q12h initially, titrated to response; average dose; 160–320 mg daily. See manufacturer's recommendations for dosing in renal failure. | Should not be stopped abruptly |
| **Class III Potassium Channel Blockers: *Treatment of Ventricular Tachycardia and Fibrillation; Conversion of Atrial Fibrillation or Flutter to Sinus Rhythm; Maintenance of Sinus Rhythm (Amiodarone)*** | | |
| **Amiodarone** (Cordarone) Pregnancy Category D | *Adults:* Loading dose, IV, 150 mg over 10 min (15 mg/min), then 360 mg over the next 6 h (1 mg/min), then 540 mg over the next 18 h (0.5 mg/min) Maintenance dose, IV, 720 mg/24 h (0.5 mg/min) Loading dose, PO, 800–1600 mg/d for 1–3 wk, with a gradual decrease to 600–800 mg/d for 1 mo Maintenance dose, PO, 400 mg/d | Administer oral preparations consistently with regard to time and meals |
| **Dofetilide** (Tikosyn) Pregnancy Category C | *Adults:* PO, 500 mcg twice daily with creatinine clearance > 60 mL/min, adjusted to manage adverse effects | Capsules should not be opened |
| **Bretylium** (Bretylol) Pregnancy Category C | *Adults:* IM, 5 mg/kg, repeated in 1–2 h then q6–8h IV, 5–10 mg/kg (diluted in at least 50 mL of IV fluid and infused over 10–20 min). During cardiopulmonary resuscitation, IV 5 mg/kg given by direct injection (undiluted); may be repeated every 15–30 min to a maximum total dose of 30 mg/kg. | May cause nausea or vomiting; elderly at high risk for hypotension |

*(continued)*

## *Drugs at a Glance*

### Antidysrhythmic Drugs (Continued)

| Drugs for Tachydysrhythmias | Routes and Dosage Ranges | Comments |
|---|---|---|
| **Ibutilide** (Corvert) Pregnancy Category C | *Adults:* Weight ≥60 kg: IV infusion over 10 min, 1 mg Weight <60 kg: IV infusion over 10 min, 0.01 mg/kg The dose can be repeated once, after 10 min, if necessary. | Only administered IV: requires cardiac monitoring with infusion and for 4h after |
| *Class IV Calcium Channel Blockers:* **Treatment of Supraventricular Tachycardia** | | |
| **Diltiazem** (Cardizem) Pregnancy Category C | *Adults:* IV injection, 0.25 mg/kg (average dose 20 mg) over 2 min. A second dose of 0.35 mg/kg (average, 25 mg) may be given in 15 min, and an IV infusion of 5–15 mg/h may be given up to 24 h, if necessary. | Serum drug levels may be elevated if taken with food |
| **Verapamil** (Calan, Isoptin) Pregnancy Category C | *Adults:* PO, 40–120 mg q6–8h IV, 5–10 mg initially, then 10 mg 30 min later, if necessary *Children <1 y:* IV injection, 0.1–0.2 mg/kg (usual range, 0.75–2.0 mg for a single dose) over 2 min with continuous ECG monitoring *1–15 y:* IV injection, 0.1–0.3 mg/kg (usual range 2–5 mg for a single dose) over 2 min with continuous ECG monitoring; repeat in 30 min if necessary | Grapefruit juice may increase the serum concentration of verapamil |
| *Unclassified:* **Adenosine Is Used to Treat Supraventricular Tachycardia; Magnesium Sulfate Is Used to Treat Torsades de Pointes** | | |
| **Adenosine** (Adenocard) Pregnancy Category C | *Adults:* IV, 6 mg given rapidly over 1–2 sec. If first dose does not slow the supraventricular tachycardia within 1–2 min, give 12 mg rapidly, and repeat one time, if necessary. | Geriatric clients more sensitive to effects |
| **Magnesium sulfate** Pregnancy Category B | *Adults:* IV, 1–2 g (2–4 mL of 50% solution), diluted in 10 mL of 5% dextrose solution | Continuous cardiac monitoring essential |

that the goal of drug therapy is to prevent or relieve symptoms or prolong survival, not just suppress dysrhythmias. This change resulted from studies in which clients treated for some dysrhythmias had a higher mortality rate than clients who did not receive antidysrhythmic drug therapy due to prodysrhythmic effects (ie, worsening existing dysrhythmias or causing new dysrhythmias). Overall, there is decreasing use of class I drugs (eg, quinidine) and increasing use of class II (beta blockers) and class III drugs (eg, amiodarone).

Rational drug therapy for cardiac dysrhythmias requires accurate identification of the dysrhythmia, understanding of the basic mechanisms causing the dysrhythmia, observation of the hemodynamic and electrocardiogram (ECG) effects of the dysrhythmia, knowledge of the pharmacologic actions of specific antidysrhythmic drugs, and the expectation that therapeutic effects will outweigh potential adverse effects. Even when these criteria are met, antidysrhythmic drug therapy is somewhat empiric. Although some dysrhythmias usually respond to particular drugs, different drugs or combinations of drugs are often required. Antidysrhythmic drug therapy in clients with renal or hepatic impairment should be very cautious, with close monitoring of drug effects (eg, plasma drug levels,

## Age-related Considerations: Use of Antidysrhythmic Drugs

### USE IN CHILDREN

Antidysrhythmic drugs are less often needed, and this drug therapy is also less clearcut, in children than in adults; use of these drugs has decreased with increased use of catheter ablative techniques. The only antidysrhythmic drug that is approved by the FDA for use in children is digoxin. However, pediatric cardiologists have used various drugs and developed guidelines for their use, especially dosages.

Supraventricular tachydysrhythmias are the most common sustained dysrhythmias in children. IV **adenosine, digoxin, procainamide,** or **propranolol** can be used acutely to terminate supraventricular tachydysrhythmias. IV verapamil is contraindicated in infants and small children, although it can be used cautiously in older children. **Digoxin** or a **beta blocker** may be used for long-term management of supraventricular tachydysrhythmias.

**Propranolol** is the beta blocker most commonly used in children. It is one of the few antidysrhythmic drugs available in a liquid solution. Propranolol has a shorter half-life (3 to 4 hours) in infants than in children older than 1 to 2 years of age and adults (6 hours). When given intravenously, antidysrhythmic effects are rapid, and clients require careful monitoring for bradycardia and hypotension. **Esmolol** is

being used more frequently to treat tachydysrhythmias in children, especially those occurring after surgery.

**Lidocaine** may be used to treat ventricular dysrhythmias precipitated by cardiac surgery or digitalis toxicity. Because of their prodysrhythmic effects, class I or III drugs are usually started in a hospital setting, at lower dosage ranges. Prodysrhythmia is more common in children with structural heart disease or significant dysrhythmias. In general, serum levels should be monitored with class IA and IC drugs and with IV lidocaine. Flecainide is the class IC drug most commonly used in children. Class III drugs are used in pediatrics mainly to treat life-threatening refractory tachydysrhythmias.

### USE IN OLDER ADULTS

Cardiac dysrhythmias are common in older adults, but in general only those causing symptoms of circulatory impairment should be treated with antidysrhythmic drugs. Compared with younger adults, older adults are more likely to experience serious adverse drug effects, including aggravation of existing dysrhythmias, production of new dysrhythmias, hypotension, and heart failure.

---

ECG changes, symptoms that may indicate drug toxicity). The kidneys excrete most antidysrhythmic drugs and their metabolites. As a general rule, dosage of most antidysrhythmics, except adenosine, amiodarone, ibutilide, and mexiletine, will require dosage reduction with renal impairment. Home care is an essential component in the management of dysrhythmias. Guidelines for strategies for ongoing evaluation and intervention are addressed in Home Care Considerations.

## Home Care Considerations: Use of Antidysrhythmic Drugs

***ASSESS:*** the client's physical, mental, and functional status, compliance with drug therapy, and presence of side effects.

***MONITOR:*** pulse and blood pressure and evaluation of drug effects (eg, plasma drug levels, ECG changes, symptoms that may indicate drug toxicity).

***EDUCATE:*** how to use, store, and replace medications to ensure a constant supply; about circumstances for which the client should report symptoms (eg, dizziness or fainting, chest pain). Also include the importance of avoiding over-the-counter drugs unless discussed with a health care provider. Reinforce additional teaching points (see Client Teaching Guidelines: Antidysrhythmic Drugs).

## Management of Supraventricular Tachydysrhythmias

1. **Propranolol** and other beta blockers are being increasingly used for tachydysrhythmias, especially in clients with myocardial infarction, heart failure, or exercise-induced dysrhythmias. In addition to controlling dysrhythmias, the drugs decrease the mortality rate in these clients. Also, a beta blocker is the drug of choice for management of a rapid heart rate that is causing angina or other symptoms in a client with known coronary artery disease.

2. **AF** is the most common dysrhythmia. Management may involve conversion to normal sinus rhythm (NSR) by electrical or pharmacologic means or long-term drug therapy to slow the rate of ventricular response. Advantages of conversion to NSR include improvement of symptoms and decreased risk for heart failure or thromboembolic problems. If pharmacologic conversion is chosen, intravenous (IV) **adenosine, dofetilide, ibutilide, verapamil,** or **diltiazem** may be used. Once converted to NSR, clients usually require long-term drug therapy to maintain NSR. Low-dose **amiodarone** seems to be emerging as the drug of choice for preventing recurrent AF after electrical or pharmacologic conversion. The low doses cause fewer adverse effects than the higher ones used for life-threatening ventricular dysrhythmias.

When clients are not converted to NSR, drugs are given to slow the heart rate. This strategy is used for clients who:

a. Have chronic AF but are asymptomatic
b. Have had AF for longer than 1 year
c. Are elderly
d. Have not responded to multiple drugs

In addition to amiodarone, other drugs used to slow the heart rate include a **beta blocker, digoxin, verapamil,** or **diltiazem.** In most clients, a beta blocker, verapamil, or diltiazem may be preferred. In clients with heart failure, digoxin may be preferred. In addition, one of the class IC agents, **flecainide** or **propafenone,** may be used to suppress paroxysmal atrial flutter and fibrillation in clients with minimal or no heart disease.

3. IV **adenosine, ibutilide, verapamil,** or **diltiazem** may be used to convert PSVT to NSR. These drugs block conduction across the AV node.

## Management of Ventricular Dysrhythmias

1. Treatment of asymptomatic premature ventricular contractions (PVCs) and nonsustained ventricular tachycardia (formerly standard practice with lidocaine in post–myocardial infarction clients) is no longer recommended.
2. Antidysrhythmics may be used to control a ventricular rate that is so fast or irregular that cardiac output is impaired. Decreased cardiac output leads to symptoms of decreased systemic, cerebral, and coronary circulation. A **beta blocker** may be preferred as a first-line drug for symptomatic ventricular dysrhythmias. **Amiodarone, bretylium, flecainide, propafenone,** and **sotalol** are also used in the management of life-threatening ventricular dysrhythmias, such as sustained ventricular tachycardia, which may cause cardiac arrest. Class I agents (eg, **lidocaine, mexiletine, tocainide**) may be used in clients with structurally normal hearts. Lidocaine may also be used for treating digoxin-induced ventricular dysrhythmias.
3. **Amiodarone, sotalol,** or a **beta blocker** may be used to prevent recurrence of ventricular tachycardia or fibrillation in clients resuscitated from cardiac arrest.

## CLASSIFICATIONS AND INDIVIDUAL DRUGS

### Class I Sodium Channel Blockers

Class I drugs block the movement of sodium into cells of the cardiac conducting system. This results in a membrane-stabilizing effect and decreased formation and conduction of electrical impulses. Class I agents do not prolong survival in any group of clients, and their clinical use is declining, mainly because of prodysrhythmic effects with resultant increased mortality rates. The higher mortality rates occur most often in clients with significant structural heart disease; therefore, clinicians recommend restricting this class to clients without structural heart disease, who are less likely to experience increased mortality than others.

### Class IA

Class IA drugs have a broad spectrum of antidysrhythmic effects and are used for both supraventricular and ventricular dysrhythmias. **Quinidine** is the prototype and is highlighted in the Prototype Profile 40-1: Quinidine.

Each quinidine salt differs in the amount of active drug (quinidine base) it contains and in the rate of absorption with oral administration. Three salts are available—sulfate, gluconate, and polygalacturonate—and the molecular weights differ. A 200-mg dose of sulfate provides an equivalent amount of quinidine as 267 mg of gluconate or polygalacturonate. The sulfate salt's (83% quinidine base) peak effect occurs in 0.5 to 1.5 hours (4 hours for sustained-release forms). The gluconate salt's (62% quinidine base) peak effect occurs in 3 to 4 hours. The polygalacturonate salt's (60% quinidine base) peak effect occurs in about 6 hours. Quinidine preparations are usually given orally. The gluconate and polygalacturonate salts reportedly cause less gastrointestinal (GI) irritation than quinidine sulfate; this is probably related to their lower quinidine content. Oral extended-action preparations of quinidine (Quinidex Extentabs, Quinaglute Dura-Tabs) also are available.

**Disopyramide** is similar to quinidine in pharmacologic actions and may be given orally to adults with ventricular tachydysrhythmias. It is well absorbed after oral administration and reaches peak serum levels (2 to 8 mcg/mL) within 30 to 60 minutes. Drug half-life is 5 to 8 hours. The kidneys and the liver, in almost equal proportions, excrete disopyramide; thus, the dosage must be reduced in clients with renal insufficiency or hepatic failure.

**Procainamide** is related to the local anesthetic procaine and is similar to quinidine in actions and uses. Quinidine may be preferred for long-term use because procainamide produces a high incidence of adverse effects, including a syndrome resembling lupus erythematosus. Procainamide has a short duration of action (3 to 4 hours); sustained-release tablets (Procanbid) prolong action to about 6 hours. Therapeutic serum levels are 4 to 8 mcg/mL.

### Class IB

**Lidocaine,** a local anesthetic, is the prototype of class IB. Key information about this prototype can be found in

## PROTOTYPE PROFILE 40-1
### P Quinidine (KWIN I deen)

**Drug Class**
*Chemical:* Class I antidysrhythmic agent
*Functional:* Antidysrhythmic agent

**Trade Names**
Quinaglute, Dura-Tabs, Quinidex Extentabs, Cardioquin

**Therapeutic Indications**
Reduces automaticity, slows conduction, and pro-longs the refractory period; maintain NSR in clients with AF or flutter who have been converted to NSR with digoxin or electrical cardioversion. However, such use is declining because clients may have recurrent AF and have higher mortality rates with long-term quinidine therapy.

**Pharmacokinetics**
Therapeutic plasma levels: 2–5 mcg/mL

*Absorption*
Rapidly absorbed from GI tract

*Distribution*
Plasma protein binding: Adults—80%–90%; Newborns—60%–70%

*Metabolism*
Extensively in the liver (50%–90%)

*Excretion*
Urine

**Pharmacodynamics**
*Onset of Action*
Rapid; peak response to quinidine sulfate occurs in 30–90 min; with quinidine gluconate 3–4 h

*Duration*
>6–8 h

**Contraindications/Precautions**
Hypersensitivity to quinidine; severe, uncompensated heart failure or heart block; myasthenia gravis; concurrent use of quinolone antibiotic

**Pregnancy Considerations**
Category C; crosses placenta
Enters breast milk/compatible

**Dosage**
Expressed in terms of the salt. Three salts available: sulfate, gluconate, and polygalacturonate; molecular weights differ—200-mg dose of sulfate provides an equivalent amount of quinidine as 267 mg of gluconate or polygalacturonate.
PO quinidine sulfate, *Adults:* 200–400 mg every 4–6 h
PO quinidine gluconate, *Adults:* 324–648 mg every 8–12 h
IM injections painful and produce erratic absorption
IV, 200–400 mg dose, diluted and given to a rate ≤10 mg/min with cardiac monitoring

**Side Effects/Adverse Reactions**
QT prolongation, diarrhea, cinchonism, stomach cramping, nausea, vomiting, lightheadedness, palpitation, headache

**Drug Interactions**
*Increased Effects*
Digoxin levels (can double)
Effects of warfarin; other atropine-like drugs

*Decreased Effects*
Analgesic efficacy of codeine may be decreased

**Herbal Supplements and Dietary Considerations**
St. John's wort may decrease serum concentrations; ephedra may worsen dysrhythmias
Administer with food or milk to decrease GI upset; rate and extent of absorption may be altered by dietary salt intake (decreased salt intake increases drug's serum concentration); ingestion of grapefruit juice may decrease absorption

---

Prototype Profile 40-2: Lidocaine. It is the drug of choice for treating serious ventricular dysrhythmias associated with acute myocardial infarction, cardiac surgery, cardiac catheterization, and electrical cardioversion. Lidocaine decreases myocardial irritability (automaticity) in the ventricles. It has little effect on atrial tissue and is not useful in treating atrial dysrhythmias. It differs from quinidine in that:

1. It must be given by injection due to extensive first-pass effect orally.
2. It does not decrease AV conduction or myocardial contractility with usual therapeutic doses.

3. It has a rapid onset and short duration of action. After IV administration of a bolus dose, therapeutic effects occur within 1 to 2 minutes and last approximately 20 minutes. This characteristic is advantageous in emergency management but limits lidocaine use to acute care settings.
4. It has no significant anticholinergic properties.
5. It is metabolized in the liver. Dosage must be reduced in clients with hepatic insufficiency or heart failure to avoid drug accumulation and toxicity.
6. It is less likely to cause heart block, cardiac asystole, ventricular dysrhythmias, and heart failure.

## PROTOTYPE PROFILE 40-2
### P Lidocaine (LYE doe kane)

**Drug Class**
*Chemical:* Class I antidysrhythmic agent
*Functional:* Antidysrhythmic agent

**Trade Name**
Xylocaine, and others

**Therapeutic Indications**
Acute treatment of ventricular dysrhythmias from myocardial infarction

**Pharmacokinetics**
Therapeutic plasma levels: 1.5–6 mcg/mL

*Absorption*
Ineffective orally (extensive first-pass effect)
Intravenous

*Distribution*
Plasma protein binding: Adults 60%–80%

*Metabolism*
Rapid metabolism in liver

*Excretion*
Urine

**Pharmacodynamics**
*Onset of Action*
IV bolus, 45–90 sec

*Duration*
IV, 10–20 min

**Contraindications/Precautions**
Hypersensitivity to lidocaine; Stokes-Adams syndrome; Wolff-Parkinson-White syndrome; severe degrees of heart block in the absence of a cardiac pacemaker

**Pregnancy Considerations**
Category B (by manufacturer); C (by expert analysis)
Crosses placental barrier
Enters breast milk (compatible)

**Dosage**
IV, Use only lidocaine injection without preservative
*Adults:* IV bolus, 50–100 mg with second bolus in 5 min followed by continuous infusion at rate of 1–4 mg/min
*Children:* IV bolus, 1 mg/kg/dose followed by infusion 30 mcg/kg/min

**Side Effects/Adverse Reactions**
Drowsiness, confusion, paresthesias, hypotension, bradycardia, apprehension, convulsions, coma

**Drug Interactions**
*Increased*
Serum levels of lidocaine with cimetidine or propranolol as well as digoxin, diltiazem, erythromycin, ethanol, verapamil

*Decreased*
None reported

**Herbal Supplements and Dietary Considerations**
St. John's wort may decrease lidocaine levels

---

Therapeutic serum levels of lidocaine are 1.5 to 6 mcg/mL. Lidocaine may be given intramuscularly in emergencies when IV administration is impossible. When given intramuscularly, therapeutic effects occur in about 15 minutes and last about 90 minutes. Lidocaine is contraindicated in clients allergic to related local anesthetics (eg, procaine). Anaphylactic reactions may occur in sensitized individuals.

**Mexiletine** and **tocainide** are oral analogs of lidocaine with similar pharmacologic actions. They are used to suppress ventricular fibrillation or ventricular tachycardia. They are well absorbed from the GI tract, and peak serum levels are obtained within 3 hours. Taking the drug with food delays but does not decrease absorption.

**Phenytoin,** an anticonvulsant (see Chap. 11), may be used to treat dysrhythmias produced by digoxin intoxication. Phenytoin decreases automaticity and improves conduction through the AV node. Decreased automaticity helps control dysrhythmias, whereas enhanced conduction may improve cardiac function. Further, because heart block may result from digoxin, quinidine, or procainamide, phenytoin may relieve dysrhythmias without intensifying heart block. Phenytoin is not a cardiac depressant. Its only quinidine-like action is to suppress automaticity; otherwise, it counteracts the effects of quinidine and procainamide largely by increasing the rate of conduction. Phenytoin also has a longer half-life (22 to 36 hours) than other antidysrhythmic drugs. Given intravenously, a therapeutic plasma level (10 to 20 mcg/mL) can be obtained rapidly. Given orally, however, the drug may not reach a steady-state concentration for approximately 1 week unless loading doses are given initially.

## Class IC

**Flecainide** and **propafenone** are oral agents that greatly decrease conduction in the ventricles. They may initiate new dysrhythmias or aggravate preexisting dysrhythmias, sometimes causing sustained ventricular tachycardia or ventricular fibrillation. These effects are more likely to occur with high doses and rapid dose increases. The drugs are recommended for use only in life-threatening ventricular dysrhythmias.

## Class II Beta–Adrenergic Blockers

These agents (see Chap. 17) exert antidysrhythmic effects by blocking sympathetic nervous system stimulation of beta receptors in the heart and decreasing risks for ventricular fibrillation. Blockage of receptors in the SA node and ectopic pacemakers decreases automaticity, and blockage of receptors in the AV node increases the refractory period. The drugs are effective for management of supraventricular dysrhythmias and those resulting from excessive sympathetic activity. Thus, they are most often used to slow the ventricular rate of contraction in supraventricular tachydysrhythmias (eg, AF, atrial flutter, PSVT).

As a class, beta blockers are being used more extensively because of their effectiveness and their ability to reduce mortality in a variety of clinical settings, including post–myocardial infarction and heart failure. Reduced mortality may result from the drugs' ability to prevent ventricular fibrillation. Only four of the beta blockers (acebutolol, esmolol, propranolol, and sotalol) marketed in the United States are approved by the U.S. Food and Drug Administration (FDA) for management of dysrhythmias.

**Acebutolol** may be given orally for chronic therapy to prevent ventricular dysrhythmias, especially those precipitated by exercise. **Esmolol** has a rapid onset and short duration of action. It is given intravenously for supraventricular tachydysrhythmias, especially during anesthesia, surgery, or other emergency situations when the ventricular rate must be reduced rapidly. It is not used for chronic therapy. **Propranolol** may be given orally for chronic therapy to prevent ventricular dysrhythmias, especially those precipitated by exercise. It may be given intravenously for life-threatening dysrhythmias or those occurring during anesthesia. **Sotalol** is a noncardioselective beta blocker (class II) that also has properties of class III antidysrhythmic drugs.

## Class III Potassium Channel Blockers

These drugs act to prolong duration of the action potential, slow repolarization, and prolong the refractory period in both atria and ventricles. Although the drugs share a common mechanism of action, they are very different drugs. As with beta blockers, clinical use of class III agents is increasing because they are associated with less ventricular fibrillation and decreased mortality compared with class I drugs.

Although classified as a potassium channel blocker, **amiodarone** also has electrophysiologic characteristics of sodium channel blockers, beta blockers, and calcium channel blockers. Thus, it has vasodilating effects and decreases systemic vascular resistance; it prolongs conduction in all cardiac tissues and decreases heart rate; and it decreases contractility of the left ventricle.

Intravenous and oral amiodarone differ in their electrophysiologic effects. When given intravenously, the major effect is slowing conduction through the AV node and prolonging the effective refractory period. Thus, it is given intravenously mainly for acute suppression of refractory, hemodynamically destabilizing ventricular tachycardia and ventricular fibrillation. It is given orally to treat recurrent ventricular tachycardia or ventricular fibrillation and to maintain an NSR after conversion of AF and flutter. Low doses (100 to 200 mg/day) may prevent recurrence of AF with less toxicity than higher doses of amiodarone or usual doses of other agents, including quinidine.

Amiodarone is extensively metabolized in the liver and produces active metabolites. The drug and its metabolites accumulate in the liver, lung, fat, skin, and other tissues. With IV administration, the onset of action usually occurs within several hours. With oral administration, the action may be delayed from a few days up to a week or longer. Because of its long serum half-life, loading doses are usually given, and higher loading doses reduce the time required for therapeutic effects. Also, effects may persist for several weeks after the drug is discontinued.

Adverse effects include hypothyroidism, hyperthyroidism, pulmonary fibrosis, myocardial depression, hypotension, bradycardia, hepatic dysfunction, central nervous system (CNS) disturbances (depression, insomnia, nightmares, hallucinations), peripheral neuropathy and muscle weakness, bluish discoloration of skin and corneal deposits that may cause photosensitivity, appearance of colored halos around lights, and reduced visual acuity. Most adverse effects are considered dose dependent and reversible.

When oral amiodarone is used long term, it also increases the effects of numerous drugs, including anticoagulants, beta blockers, calcium channel blockers, class I antidysrhythmics (quinidine, flecainide, lidocaine, procainamide), cyclosporine, digoxin, methotrexate, phenytoin, and theophylline.

**Bretylium** initially increases release of catecholamines and therefore increases heart rate, blood pressure, and myocardial contractility. This is followed in a few minutes by a decrease in vascular resistance, blood pressure, and heart rate. It is used primarily in critical care settings for acute control of recurrent ventricular fibrillation, especially in clients with recent myocardial infarction. It is given by IV infusion, with a loading dose followed by a maintenance dose, or in repeated IV injections. Because it is excreted almost entirely by the kidney, drug half-life is prolonged with renal impairment, and the dosage must be reduced. Adverse effects include hypotension and dysrhythmias.

**Ibutilide** is indicated for management of recent onset of AF or atrial flutter, in which the goal is conversion to NSR. The drug enhances the efficacy of cardioversion. Ibutilide is structurally similar to sotalol but lacks clinically significant beta-blocking activity. Ibutilide is widely distributed and has an elimination half-life of about 6 hours. Most of a dose is metabolized, and the metabolites are excreted in urine and feces. Adverse effects include supraventricular and ventricular dysrhythmias (particularly torsades de pointes) and hypotension. Ibutilide should be administered in a setting with personnel and equipment available for emergency use.

**Dofetilide** is indicated for the maintenance of normal sinus rhythm in symptomatic clients who are in AF for longer than 1 week. Adverse effects increase with decreasing creatinine clearance levels; hence, renal function must be assessed, and initial dosage is dependent on creatinine clearance levels. High doses in clients with renal dysfunction result in drug accumulation and prodysrhythmias (torsades de pointes). The drug has an elimination half-life of approximately 8 hours, with the kidneys being the major route of elimination. The drug should initially be administered in a setting with personnel and equipment available for emergency use.

**Sotalol** has both beta-adrenergic blocking and potassium channel blocking activity. Beta-blocking effects predominate at lower doses, and class III effects predominate at higher doses. The drug is well absorbed after oral administration, and peak serum level is reached in 2 to 4 hours. It has an elimination half-life of approximately 12 hours, and 80% to 90% is excreted unchanged by the kidneys. Sotalol is approved for prevention or management of ventricular tachycardia and fibrillation. It has also been used, usually in smaller doses, to prevent or treat AF. However, it is less effective than amiodarone in the prophylaxis of AF. It is contraindicated in clients with asthma, sinus bradycardia, heart block, cardiogenic shock, heart failure, and previous hypersensitivity to sotalol. Dosage should be individualized, reduced with renal impairment, and increased slowly (eg, every 2 to 3 days with normal renal function, at longer intervals with impaired renal function). Arrhythmogenic effects are most likely to occur when therapy is started or when dosage is increased. Heart failure may occur in clients with markedly depressed left ventricular systolic function. Most adverse effects are attributed to beta-blocking activity.

Like amiodarone, sotalol may be preferred over a class I agent because it is more effective in reducing recurrent ventricular tachycardia, ventricular fibrillation, and death.

## Class IV Calcium Channel Blockers

Calcium channel blockers (see Chap. 40) block the movement of calcium into conductile and contractile myocardial cells. As antidysrhythmic agents, they act primarily against tachycardias at SA and AV nodes because the cardiac cells and slow channels that depend on calcium influx are found mainly at these sites. Thus, they reduce automaticity of the SA and AV nodes, slow conduction, and prolong the refractory period in the AV node. They are effective only in supraventricular tachycardias.

**Diltiazem** and **verapamil** are the only calcium channel blockers approved for management of dysrhythmias. Both drugs may be given intravenously to terminate acute PSVT, usually within 2 minutes, and in AF and atrial flutter. They are also effective in exercise-related tachycardias. When given intravenously, the drugs act within 15 minutes and last up to 6 hours. Oral verapamil may be used in the chronic management of the aforementioned dysrhythmias. Diltiazem and verapamil are metabolized by the liver, and metabolites are primarily excreted by the kidneys. The drugs are contraindicated in digoxin toxicity because they may worsen heart block. If used with propranolol or digoxin, caution must be exercised to avoid further impairment of myocardial contractility. *Do not use* IV verapamil with IV propranolol; potentially fatal bradycardia and hypotension may occur.

## Unclassified

**Adenosine,** a naturally occurring component of all body cells, differs chemically from other antidysrhythmic drugs but acts like the calcium channel blockers. It depresses conduction at the AV node and is used to restore NSR in clients with PSVT; it is ineffective in other dysrhythmias. The drug has a very short duration of action (serum half-life is less than 10 seconds) and a high degree of effectiveness. It must be given by a rapid bolus injection, preferably through a central venous line. If given slowly, it is eliminated before it can reach cardiac tissues and exert its action.

**Magnesium sulfate** is given intravenously in the management of several dysrhythmias, including prevention of recurrent episodes of torsades de pointes and management of digitalis-induced dysrhythmias. Its antidysrhythmic effects may derive from imbalances of magnesium, potassium, and calcium.

Hypomagnesemia increases myocardial irritability and is a risk factor for both atrial and ventricular dysrhythmias. Thus, serum magnesium levels should be monitored in clients at risk and replacement therapy instituted when indicated. However, in some instances, the drug seems to have antidysrhythmic effects even when serum magnesium levels are normal.

*(text continues on page 750)*

## NURSING PROCESS

### Assessment

Assess the client's condition in relation to cardiac dysrhythmias:

- Identify conditions or risk factors that may precipitate dysrhythmias. These include the following:
  - Hypoxia
  - Electrolyte imbalances (eg, hypokalemia, hypomagnesemia)
  - Acid–base imbalances
  - Ischemic heart disease (angina pectoris, myocardial infarction)
  - Cardiac valvular disease
  - Febrile illness
  - Respiratory disorders (eg, chronic lung disease)
  - Exercise
  - Emotional upset
  - Excessive ingestion of caffeine-containing beverages (eg, coffee, tea, colas)
  - Cigarette smoking
  - Drug therapy with digoxin, antidysrhythmic drugs, CNS stimulants, anorexiants, and tricyclic antidepressants
  - Hyperthyroidism
- Observe for clinical signs and symptoms of dysrhythmias. Mild or infrequent dysrhythmias may be perceived by the client as palpitations or skipped heartbeats. More severe dysrhythmias may produce manifestations that reflect decreased cardiac output and other hemodynamic changes, as follows:
  - Hypotension, bradycardia or tachycardia, and irregular pulse
  - Shortness of breath, dyspnea, and cough from impaired respiration
  - Syncope or mental confusion from reduced cerebral blood flow
  - Chest pain from decreased coronary artery blood flow. Angina pectoris or myocardial infarction may occur.
  - Oliguria from decreased renal blood flow
- When electrocardiograms (ECGs) are available (eg, 12-lead ECG or continuous ECG monitoring), assess for indications of dysrhythmias.

### Nursing Diagnoses

- Decreased Cardiac Output related to ineffective pumping action of the heart
- Ineffective Tissue Perfusion, cerebral and peripheral, related to compromised cardiac output or drug-induced hypotension
- Activity Intolerance related to weakness and fatigue
- Impaired Gas Exchange related to decreased tissue perfusion
- Anxiety related to potentially serious illness

- Deficient Knowledge: Pharmacologic and nonpharmacologic management of dysrhythmias
- Excess Fluid Volume: Peripheral edema and pulmonary congestion related to decreased cardiac output

### Planning/Goals

*The client will:*

- Receive or take antidysrhythmic drugs accurately
- Avoid conditions that precipitate dysrhythmias, when feasible
- Experience improved heart rate, circulation, and activity tolerance
- Be closely monitored for therapeutic and adverse drug effects
- Avoid preventable adverse drug effects
- Have adverse drug effects promptly recognized and treated if they occur
- Keep follow-up appointments for monitoring responses to treatment measures

### Interventions

Use measures to prevent or minimize dysrhythmias:

- Treat underlying disease processes that contribute to dysrhythmia development. These include cardiovascular (eg, acute myocardial infarction) and noncardiovascular (eg, chronic lung disease) disorders.
- Prevent or treat other conditions that predispose to dysrhythmias (eg, hypoxia, electrolyte imbalance).
- Help the client avoid cigarette smoking, overeating, excessive coffee drinking, and other habits that may cause or aggravate dysrhythmias. Long-term supervision and counseling may be needed.
- For the client receiving antidysrhythmic drugs, implement the preceding measures to minimize the incidence and severity of acute dysrhythmias, and help the client comply with drug therapy.
- Monitor heart rate and rhythm and blood pressure every 4 to 6 hours.
- Check laboratory reports of serum electrolytes and serum drug levels when available. Report abnormal values.

### Evaluation

- Check vital signs for improved heart rate and rhythm.
- Interview and observe for relief of symptoms and improved functioning in activities of daily living.
- Interview and observe for hypotension and other adverse drug effects.
- Interview and observe for compliance with instructions for taking antidysrhythmic drugs and other aspects of care.

**CLIENT TEACHING GUIDELINES**
## Antidysrhythmic Drugs

### General Considerations

✔ A fast heartbeat normally occurs in response to exercise, fever, and other conditions so that more blood can be pumped and carried to body tissues. An irregular heartbeat occurs occasionally in most individuals. However, when you are prescribed a long-term medication to slow or regularize your heartbeat, this means that you have a potentially serious condition. In addition, the medications can cause potentially serious adverse effects. Thus, it is extremely important that you take the medications exactly as prescribed. Taking extra doses is dangerous; skipping doses or waiting longer between doses may lead to loss of control of the heart problem.

✔ You may be given a drug classified as an antidysrhythmic or a drug from another group that has antidysrhythmic effects (eg, a beta blocker such as propranolol, a calcium channel blocker such as verapamil or diltiazem, or digoxin). Instructions should be provided for the specific drug ordered.

✔ Be sure you know the names (generic and brand) of the medication, why you are receiving it, and what effects you can expect (therapeutic and adverse).

✔ You will need continued medical supervision, along with periodic measurements of heart rate and blood pressure, blood tests, and electrocardiograms.

✔ Try to learn the triggers for your irregular heartbeats and avoid them when possible (eg, excessive caffeinated beverages, strenuous or excessive exercise).

✔ Avoid over-the-counter cold and asthma remedies, appetite suppressants, and antisleep preparations. These drugs are stimulants that can cause or aggravate irregular heartbeats.

### Self-administration or Caregiver Administration

✔ Take or give medications at evenly spaced intervals to maintain adequate blood levels.

✔ Take or give amiodarone, mexiletine, quinidine, and tocainide with food to decrease gastrointestinal symptoms.

✔ Do not crush or chew sustained-release tablets or capsules.

✔ Report dizziness or fainting spells. This may mean the medication is decreasing your blood pressure, which is more likely to occur when starting or increasing the dose of an antidysrhythmic drug. Drug dosage may need to be adjusted.

---

## *Nursing Actions*
## Antidysrhythmic Drugs

| Nursing Actions | Rationale/Explanation |
|---|---|
| 1. Administer accurately. | |
| a. Check apical and radial pulses before each dose. Withhold the dose and report to the physician if marked changes are noted in rate, rhythm, or quality of pulses. | Bradycardia may indicate impending heart block or cardiovascular collapse. |
| b. Check blood pressure at least once daily in hospitalized clients. | To detect hypotension, which is most likely to occur when antidysrhythmic drug therapy is being initiated or altered. |
| c. During intravenous (IV) administration of antidysrhythmic drugs, maintain continuous cardiac monitoring and check blood pressure about every 5 min. | For early detection of hypotension and impending cardiac collapse. These drug side effects are more likely to occur with IV use. |
| d. Give oral drugs at evenly spaced intervals. | To maintain adequate blood levels |
| e. With oral amiodarone, give once daily or in two divided doses if stomach upset occurs. | |
| f. With IV amiodarone, mix and give loading and maintenance infusions according to the manufacturer's instructions. | Specific instructions are required for accurate mixing and administration, partly because concentrations and infusion rates vary. The drug should be given in a critical care setting, by experienced personnel, preferably through a central venous catheter. |
| g. Give mexiletine, quinidine, and tocainide with food. | To decrease gastrointestinal (GI) symptoms |

*(continued)*

## Nursing Actions

## Antidysrhythmic Drugs (Continued)

| Nursing Actions | Rationale/Explanation |
|---|---|
| h. Give lidocaine parenterally only, as a bolus injection or a continuous drip. Use only solutions labeled "For cardiac dysrhythmias," and do not use solutions containing epinephrine. Give an IV bolus over 2 min. | Lidocaine solutions that contain epinephrine are used for local anesthesia only. They should never be given intravenously in cardiac dysrhythmias because the epinephrine can cause or aggravate dysrhythmias. Rapid injection (within approximately 30 sec) produces transient blood levels several times greater than therapeutic range limits. Therefore, there is increased risk of toxicity without a concomitant increase in therapeutic effectiveness. |

2. **Observe for therapeutic effects.**
   a. Conversion to normal sinus rhythm
   b. Improvement in rate, rhythm, and quality of apical and radial pulses and the electrocardiogram (ECG)
   c. Signs of increased cardiac output—blood pressure near normal range, urine output more adequate, no complaints of dizziness.

   d. Serum drug levels (mcg/mL) within therapeutic ranges.

   Class IA
   | Quinidine | 2–6 |
   |---|---|
   | Disopyramide | 2–8 |
   | Procainamide | 4–8 |

   Class IB
   | Lidocaine | 1.5–6 |
   |---|---|
   | Mexiletine | 0.5–2 |
   | Phenytoin | 10–20 |
   | Tocainide | 4–10 |

   Class IC
   | Flecainide | 0.2–1 |
   |---|---|
   | Propafenone | 0.06–1 |

   Class II
   | Propranolol | 0.05–0.1 |
   |---|---|

   Class III
   | Amiodarone | 0.5–2.5 |
   |---|---|
   | Bretylium | 0.5–1.5 |

   Class IV
   | Verapamil | 0.08–0.3 |
   |---|---|

After a single oral dose, peak plasma levels are reached in approximately 1–4 h with quinidine, procainamide, and propranolol and in 6–12 h with phenytoin. Equilibrium between plasma and tissue levels is reached in 1 or 2 d with quinidine, procainamide, and propranolol; in approximately 1 wk with phenytoin; in 1–3 wk with amiodarone; and in just a few minutes with IV lidocaine.

Serum drug levels must be interpreted in light of the client's clinical status.

3. **Observe for adverse effects.**
   a. Heart block—may be indicated on the ECG by a prolonged PR interval, prolonged QRS complex, or absence of P waves

   *Owing to depressant effects on the cardiac conduction system*

   b. Dysrhythmias—aggravation of existing dysrhythmia, tachycardia, bradycardia, premature ventricular contractions, ventricular tachycardia or fibrillation

   *Because they affect the cardiac conduction system, antidysrhythmic drugs may worsen existing dysrhythmias or cause new dysrhythmias.*

   c. Hypotension

   *Owing to decreased cardiac output*

   d. Additional adverse effects with specific drugs:
      (1) Disopyramide—mouth dryness, blurred vision, urinary retention, other anticholinergic effects

   *These effects commonly occur.*

*(continued)*

## Nursing Actions

### Antidysrhythmic Drugs (Continued)

| Nursing Actions | Rationale/Explanation |
|---|---|
| (2) Lidocaine—drowsiness, paresthesias, muscle twitching, convulsions, changes in mental status (eg, confusion), hypersensitivity reactions (eg, urticaria, edema, anaphylaxis) | Most adverse reactions result from drug effects on the central nervous system (CNS). Convulsions are most likely to occur with high doses. Hypersensitivity reactions may occur in individuals who are allergic to related local anesthetic agents. CNS changes are caused by depressant effects. |
| (3) Phenytoin—nystagmus, ataxia, slurring of speech, tremors, drowsiness, confusion, gingival hyperplasia | |
| (4) Propranolol—weakness or dizziness, especially with activity or exercise | The beta-adrenergic blocking action of propranolol blocks the normal sympathetic nervous system response to activity and exercise. Clients may have symptoms caused by deficient blood supply to body tissues. |
| (5) Quinidine—hypersensitivity and cinchonism (tinnitus, vomiting, severe diarrhea, vertigo, headache) | |
| (6) Tocainide—lightheadedness, dizziness, nausea, paresthesia, tremor | These are the most frequent adverse effects. They may be reversed by decreasing dosage, administering with food, or discontinuing the drug. |
| **4. Observe for drug interactions.** | |
| a. Drugs that *increase* effects of antidysrhythmics: | These drugs may potentiate therapeutic effects or increase risk of toxicity. |
| (1) Antidysrhythmic agents | When antidysrhythmic drugs are combined, there are additive cardiac depressant effects. |
| (2) Antihypertensives, diuretics, phenothiazine antipsychotic agents | Additive hypotension |
| (3) Cimetidine | Increases effects by inhibiting hepatic metabolism of quinidine, procainamide, lidocaine, tocainide, flecainide, and phenytoin |
| b. Drugs that *decrease* effects of antidysrhythmic agents: | |
| (1) Atropine sulfate | Atropine is used to reverse propranolol-induced bradycardia. |
| (2) Phenytoin, rifampin | Decrease effects by inducing drug-metabolizing enzymes in the liver and accelerating the metabolism of quinidine, disopyramide, and mexiletine |

## Critical Thinking Exercises

1. While Mr. Smith is receiving quinidine, the nurse should monitor his ECG for:
   a. Peaked P wave
   b. Elevated ST segment
   c. Inverted T wave
   d. Prolonged QT interval

2. Ms. Ferguson, age 58 years, is admitted to the coronary care unit for treatment of an acute anterior myocardial infarction. That evening, she experiences frequent premature ventricular contractions. The physician tells the nurse to prepare an IV bolus dose of lidocaine. Why is lidocaine administered intravenously instead of orally?

   a. Lidocaine absorption is too erratic when administered orally.
   b. Lidocaine is inactivated by gastric secretions.
   c. Most of an absorbed oral dose undergoes first-pass metabolism in the liver.
   d. Onset of action for oral lidocaine is more than 1 one hour.

3. Which common adverse reaction does propranolol and other class II antiarrhythmics cause?
   a. Bradycardia
   b. Seizures
   c. Hypertension
   d. Frequent premature atrial contractions

4. Mr. Rubin, age 63 years, is about to be discharged from the hospital after treatment for recurrent ventricular fibrillation unresponsive to other agents. To prevent further ventricular ectopy, the health care provider prescribes amiodarone (Cordarone), 1000 mg PO daily as a loading dose for 2 weeks. Why is such a large loading dose required?

a. Most of the drug is destroyed in the GI tract.
b. Males require larger dosages because of their higher metabolism.
c. A history of ventricular arrhythmia necessitates a higher dose.
d. The drug has a long serum half-life.

## SELECTED REFERENCES

Bauman, J. L., & Schoen, M. D. (2002). The arrhythmias. In J. T. DiPiro, R. L. Talbert, G. C. Yee, G. R. Matzke, B. G. Wells, & L. M. Posey (Eds.), *Pharmacotherapy: A pathophysiologic approach* (5th ed., pp. 273–304). New York: McGraw-Hill.

Brater, D. C. (2000). Clinical pharmacology of cardiovascular drugs. In H. D. Humes (Ed.), *Kelley's textbook of internal medicine* (4th ed., pp. 651–672). Philadelphia: Lippincott Williams & Wilkins.

*Drug facts and comparisons.* (Updated monthly). St. Louis: Facts and Comparisons.

Faddis, M. N. (2001). Cardiac arrhythmias. In S. N. Ahya, K. Flood, & S. Paranjothi (Eds.), *The Washington manual of medical therapeutics* (30th ed., pp. 96–130). Philadelphia: Lippincott Williams & Wilkins.

Feller, D. B., & Grauer, K. (2002). Atrial fibrillation: How best to use rate control and anticoagulation. *Consultant, 42*(4), 526–531.

Guyton, A. C., & Hall, J. E. (2000). *Textbook of medical physiology* (10th ed.). Philadelphia: W. B. Saunders.

Haugh, K. H. (2002). Antidysrhythmic agents at the turn of the twenty-first century: A current review. *Critical Care Nursing Clinics of North America, 14*(1), 53–69.

Lacy, C. F., Armstrong, L. L., Goldman, M. P., & Lance, L. L. (2003). *Lexi-Comp's drug information handbook* (11th ed.). Hudson, OH: American Pharmaceutical Association.

Perry, J. C. (1998). Pharmacologic therapy of arrhythmias. In B. J. Deal, G. S. Wolff, & H. Gelband (Eds.), *Current concepts in diagnosis and management in infants and children* (pp. 267–305). Armonk, NY: Futura.

Porth, C. M. (Ed.). (2002). *Pathophysiology: Concepts of altered health states* (6th ed.). Philadelphia: Lippincott Williams & Wilkins.

# 41

# Antianginal Drugs

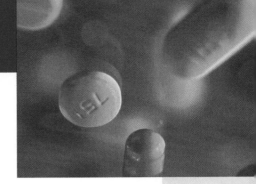

## OBJECTIVES

*After studying this chapter, the student will be able to:*

1 Describe general characteristics and types of antianginal drugs.

2 Discuss nitrate antianginal drugs in terms of indications for use, routes of administration, adverse effects, nursing process implications, and drug tolerance.

3 Differentiate between short-acting and long-acting dosage forms of nitrate antianginal drugs.

4 Discuss calcium channel blockers in terms of their effects on body tissues, clinical indications for use, common adverse effects, and nursing process implications.

5 Teach clients ways to prevent, minimize, or manage acute anginal attacks.

## CRITICAL THINKING SCENARIO

*M*rs. Hernandez, a 56-year-old housewife, experiences chest pressure after exercise. She is the mother of six children and works 30 hours a week word-processing documents for a law firm. When she is told that her chest discomfort is probably secondary to coronary artery disease, she cannot believe it. She states, "I'm just too young to have heart problems!" Mrs. Hernandez is referred to her health care provider and given sublingual nitroglycerin tablets to use as needed for chest pain.

✔ What assessment questions will you ask to determine Mrs. Hernandez's risk factors for heart disease?

✔ Evaluate Mrs. Hernandez's reaction to her new diagnosis and the client teaching implications.

✔ What lifestyle modifications would help minimize the progression of coronary artery disease?

## PROTOTYPE PROFILES

**nitroglycerin** (Nitro–Bid, others), p. 758

**propranolol** (Inderal), p. 759

# OVERVIEW

Angina pectoris is a clinical syndrome characterized by episodes of chest pain occurring from an imbalance in myocardial oxygen supply (myocardial ischemia) and demand. It is most often caused by atherosclerotic plaque in the coronary arteries but may also be caused by coronary vasospasm. The continuum of coronary artery disease (CAD) progresses from angina to myocardial infarction. The pathophysiology of the disease can be found in At the Foundation: Coronary Artery Disease. The degree and frequency of pain are dependent on multiple factors, including the type of angina. There are three main types of angina: classic angina, variant angina, and unstable angina (Box 41-1). The Canadian Cardiovascular Society classifies clients with angina into four classes according to the amount of physical activity they can tolerate before anginal pain occurs. The client's angina can be ranked from class I (occurring with strenuous or prolonged exertion) to class IV (inability to carry on any physical activity without discomfort or pain at rest). These categories can assist in clinical assessment and evaluation of therapy.

## Coronary Atherosclerosis

Classic anginal pain is usually described as substernal chest pain of a constricting, squeezing, or suffocating nature. It may radiate to the jaw, neck, or shoulder, down the left or both arms, or to the back. The discomfort is sometimes mistaken for arthritis, or for indigestion, and the pain may be associated with nausea, vomiting, dizziness, diaphoresis, shortness of breath, or fear of impending doom. The discomfort is usually brief, typically lasting 5 minutes or less until the balance of oxygen supply and demand is restored.

Current research indicates that gender differences exist in the type and quality of cardiac symptoms, with women reporting epigastric or back discomfort. Additionally, older adults may have atypical symptoms of CAD and may experience "silent" ischemia that may delay them from seeking professional help. Individuals with diabetes mellitus may present without classic angina, although they may experience related symptoms. The American Heart Association has released guidelines for the management of angina.

## Goals of Therapy

The goals of drug therapy are to relieve acute anginal pain; reduce the number and severity of acute anginal attacks; improve exercise tolerance and quality of life; delay progression of CAD; prevent myocardial infarction; and prevent sudden cardiac death. Both nonpharmacologic and pharmacologic management strategies are employed.

## Nonpharmacologic Management of Angina

For clients at any stage of CAD development, irrespective of anginal symptoms, optimal management involves lifestyle changes and medications to control or reverse risk factors for disease progression. Risk factors are frequently additive in nature and are classified as nonmodifiable and modifiable. Nonmodifiable risk factors include age, race, gender, and family history. The risk factors that can be altered include smoking, hypertension, hyperlipidemia, obesity, sedentary lifestyle, stress, and the use of drugs that increase cardiac workload (eg, adrenergics, corticosteroids). Thus, efforts are needed to assist clients in reducing blood pressure, weight, and serum cholesterol levels, when indicated, and developing an exercise program. For clients with diabetes mellitus, glucose and blood pressure control can reduce the microvascular changes associated with the condition. In addition, clients should

---

**AT THE FOUNDATION: *Coronary Artery Disease***

The development and progression of atherosclerotic plaque in the coronary arteries is called coronary artery disease (CAD). Factors contributing to plaque development and growth include endothelial injury, lipid infiltration (ie, cholesterol), recruitment of inflammatory cells (mainly monocytes and T lymphocytes), and smooth muscle cell proliferation. Atherosclerotic plaque narrows the lumen, decreases elasticity, and impairs dilation of coronary arteries. The result is impaired blood flow to the myocardium, especially with exercise or other factors that increase the cardiac workload and need for oxygen. Myocardial ischemia occurs when the coronary arteries are unable to provide sufficient blood and oxygen for normal cardiac functions. Also known as ischemic heart disease, CAD, and coronary heart disease, myocardial ischemia may present as an acute coronary syndrome with three main consequences. One consequence is unstable angina, with the occurrence of pain (symptomatic myocardial ischemia). A second is myocardial infarction (MI) that is silent or asymptomatic and diagnosed by biochemical markers only. A third is MI, with or without ST-segment elevation, which occurs when the ischemia is persistent or severe.

**BOX
41-1   Types of Angina Pectoris**

**Classic**

Classic angina (also called stable, typical, or exertional angina) occurs when atherosclerotic plaque obstructs coronary arteries and the heart requires more oxygenated blood than the blocked arteries can deliver. Chest pain is usually precipitated by situations that increase the workload of the heart, such as physical exertion, exposure to cold, and emotional upset. Recurrent episodes of classic angina usually have the same pattern of onset, duration, and intensity of symptoms. Pain is usually relieved by rest, a fast-acting preparation of nitroglycerin, or both.

**Variant**

Variant angina (also called atypical, Prinzmetal's, or vasospastic angina) is caused by spasms of the coronary artery that decrease blood flow to the myocardium. The spasms occur most often in coronary arteries that are already partly blocked by atherosclerotic plaque. Variant angina usually occurs during rest or with minimal exercise and often occurs at night. It often occurs at the same time each day. Pain is usually relieved by nitroglycerin. Long-term management includes avoidance of conditions that precipitate vasospasm, when possible (eg, exposure to cold, smoking, and emotional stress), as well as antianginal drugs.

**Unstable**

Unstable angina (also called rest, preinfarction, and crescendo angina) is a type of myocardial ischemia that falls between classic angina and myocardial infarction. It usually occurs in clients with advanced coronary atherosclerosis and produces increased frequency, intensity, and duration of symptoms. It often leads to myocardial infarction.

Unstable angina usually develops when a minor injury ruptures atherosclerotic plaque. The resulting injury to the endothelium causes platelets to aggregate at the site of injury, form a thrombus, and release chemical mediators that cause vasoconstriction (eg, thromboxane, serotonin, platelet-derived growth factor). The disrupted plaque, thrombus, and vasoconstriction combine to obstruct blood flow further in the affected coronary artery. When the plaque injury is mild, blockage of the coronary artery may be intermittent and cause silent myocardial ischemia or episodes of anginal pain at rest. Thrombus formation and vasoconstriction may progress until the coronary artery is completely occluded, producing myocardial infarction. Endothelial injury, with subsequent thrombus formation and vasoconstriction, may also result from therapeutic procedures (eg, angioplasty, atherectomy).

The Agency for Healthcare Research and Quality, in its clinical practice guidelines for the management of angina, defines unstable angina as meeting one or more of the following criteria:

- Anginal pain at rest that usually lasts longer than 20 minutes
- Recent onset (<2 months) of exertional angina of at least Canadian Cardiovascular Society Classification (CCSC) class III severity
- Recent (<2 months) increase in severity as indicated by progression to at least CCSC class III.

However, myocardial ischemia may also be painless or silent in a substantial number of clients. Overall, the diagnosis is usually based on chest pain history, electrocardiographic evidence of ischemia, and other signs of impaired cardiac function (eg, heart failure).

Because unstable angina often occurs hours or days before acute myocardial infarction, early recognition and effective management are extremely important in preventing progression to infarction, heart failure, or sudden cardiac death.

---

avoid circumstances known to precipitate acute attacks, and those who smoke should stop.

Additional nonpharmacologic management strategies include surgical revascularization (eg, coronary artery bypass graft) and interventional procedures that reduce blockages (eg, percutaneous transluminal coronary angioplasty [PTCA], intracoronary stents, laser therapy, and rotoblators). However, most clients still require a combination of measures to manage their disease effectively.

## ■ ANTIANGINAL DRUGS

Drugs used for myocardial ischemia are the organic nitrates, the beta-adrenergic blocking agents, and the calcium channel blocking agents. For relief of acute angina and prophylaxis before events that cause acute angina, nitroglycerin (sublingual tablets or translingual spray) is usually the primary drug of choice. For long-

term prevention or management of recurrent angina, a combination of oral or topical nitrates, beta-adrenergic blocking agents, or calcium channel blocking agents is common and effective. These drugs relieve anginal pain by reducing myocardial oxygen demand or increasing blood supply to the myocardium. Nitrates and beta blockers are described in the following sections, and dosage ranges are listed in Drugs at a Glance 40-1: Nitrate and Beta-Blocker Antianginal Drugs. Calcium channel blockers are described in a following section; indications for use and dosage ranges are listed in Drugs at a Glance 41-2: Calcium Channel Blockers. Age-related Considerations and Home Care Considerations are discussed in the accompanying boxes.

## Organic Nitrates

Organic nitrates relax smooth muscle in blood vessel walls. This action produces vasodilation, which relieves angi-

## DRUG TABLE 41-1

### *Drugs at a Glance*
### Nitrate and Beta-Blocker Antianginal Drugs

| Generic/Trade Name | Routes and Dosage Ranges | Comments |
|---|---|---|
| **Nitrates (Pregnancy Category C)** | | |
| *Short Acting* | | |
| **Nitroglycerin** (Nitro-Bid, Nitrostat, others) | See Prototype Profile 41-1: Nitroglycerin | See Prototype Profile 41-1: Nitroglycerin |
| *Long Acting* | | |
| **Isosorbide dinitrate** (Isordil, Sorbitrate) | SL, 2.5–10 mg PRN or q2–4h<br>PO, regular tablets, 10–60 mg q4–6h<br>PO, chewable tablets, 5–10 mg q2–3h<br>PO, sustained-release capsules, 40 mg q6–12h | Clients taking one or more long-acting antianginal drugs should carry a short-acting drug as well, to be used for acute attacks |
| **Isosorbide mononitrate** (ISMO, Monoket, Imdur) | PO, 20 mg twice daily, with first dose on arising and the second dose 7 h later<br>PO, extended-release tablets (Imdur), 30–60 mg once daily in the morning, increased after several days to 120 mg once daily if necessary | Seven-hour interval thought to delay development of nitrate tolerance<br>Produces a more constant therapeutic response than isosorbide dinitrate because it has no active metabolites |
| **Beta Blockers (Pregnancy Category C)** | | |
| **Propranolol** (Inderal) | See Prototype Profile 41-2: Propranolol | See Prototype Profile 41-2: Propranolol |
| **Atenolol** (Tenormin) | PO, 50 mg once daily, initially, increased to 100 mg/d after 1 wk if necessary | Use with caution in individuals with chronic lung disease (can cause bronchoconstriction with non-cardioselective agents) and type 1 diabetes mellitus (masks sympathetic nervous system signs of hypoglycemic reaction) |
| **Metoprolol** (Lopressor) | PO, 50 mg twice daily initially, increased up to 400 mg daily if necessary | |
| **Nadolol** (Corgard) | PO, 40–240 mg/d in a single dose | Taper dosage to discontinue after prolonged use or rebound angina can occur |

nal pain by several mechanisms. First, dilation of veins reduces venous pressure and venous return to the heart. This decreases blood volume and pressure within the heart (preload), which in turn decreases cardiac workload and oxygen demand. Second, nitrates dilate coronary arteries at higher doses and can increase blood flow to ischemic areas of the myocardium. Third, nitrates dilate arterioles, which lowers peripheral vascular resistance (afterload). This results in lower systolic blood pressure and, consequently, reduced cardiac workload. The prototype and most widely used nitrate is **P nitroglycerin**. Key information about this prototype can be found in Prototype Profile 41-1: Nitroglycerin.

Clinical indications for nitroglycerin and other nitrates are management and prevention of acute chest pain caused by myocardial ischemia. For acute angina and prophylaxis before a situation thought to trigger acute angina, fast-acting preparations (sublingual or chewable tablets, transmucosal spray or tablet) are used. For man-

agement of recurrent angina, long-acting preparations (oral and sustained-release tablets or transdermal ointment and discs) are used. However, they may not be effective in the long term because clients develop tolerance to the vasodilating (antianginal) effects of the drug, particularly those on high-dose, uninterrupted therapy. Although tolerance decreases the adverse effects of hypotension, dizziness, and headache, therapeutic effects also may be decreased. As a result, episodes of chest pain may occur more often or be more severe than expected. In addition, short-acting nitrates may be less effective in relieving acute pain. Intravenous (IV) nitroglycerin is used to manage angina that is unresponsive to organic nitrates by other routes or beta-adrenergic blocking agents. It also may be used to control blood pressure in perioperative or emergency situations and to reduce preload and afterload in severe heart failure.

Contraindications include hypersensitivity reactions, severe anemia, hypotension, and hypovolemia. The drugs

**DRUG TABLE 41-2**

*Drugs at a Glance*

## Calcium Channel Blockers

| Generic/Trade Name | Routes and Dosage Ranges | Comments |
|---|---|---|
| ***Pregnancy Category C*** | | |
| **Amlodipine** (Norvasc) | Angina or hypertension: PO, 5–10 mg once daily | |
| **Bepridil** (Vascor) | Angina: PO, 200 mg/d initially, increased to 300 mg daily after 10 d if necessary; maximum dose, 400 mg daily | Bepridil should be used with caution because its metabolites are excreted mainly in urine |
| **Diltiazem** (Cardizem, Dilacor) | Angina or hypertension: immediate-release, PO, 60–90 mg four times daily before meals and at bedtime<br>Hypertension: sustained-release only, PO, 120–180 mg twice daily<br>Arrhythmias (Cardizem IV only): IV injection, 0.25 mg/kg (average dose, 20 mg) over 2 min with a second dose of 0.35 mg/kg (average dose, 25 mg) in 15 min if necessary, followed by IV infusion of 5–15 mg/h up to 24 h | Individuals opportunely require reduced doses of cyclosporine while taking diltiazem, as diltiazem interferes with its metabolism and elimination |
| **Felodipine** (Plendil) | Hypertension: PO, 5–10 mg once daily | Plasma concentrations are higher in clients with renal impairment, and dosage should be reduced |
| **Isradipine** (DynaCirc) | Hypertension: PO, 2.5–5 mg twice daily | |
| **Nicardipine** (Cardene) | Angina: immediate-release only, PO, 20–40 mg three times daily<br>Hypertension: immediate-release, same as for angina, above; sustained-release, PO, 30–60 mg twice daily | |
| **Nifedipine** (Adalat, Procardia) | Angina: immediate-release, PO, 10–30 mg three times daily; sustained-release, PO, 30–60 mg once daily<br>Hypertension: sustained-release only, 30–60 mg once daily | Research has indicated an increased mortality exists in individuals who have the liquid contents of the capsule squeezed under the tongue, so the practice should be discontinued |
| **Nimodipine** (Nimotop) | Subarachnoid hemorrhage: PO, 60 mg q4h for 21 consecutive days. If patient unable to swallow, aspirate contents of capsule into a syringe with an 18-gauge needle, administer by nasogastric tube, and follow with 30 mL normal saline | Avoid concurrent use with grapefruit juice |
| **Nisoldipine** (Sular) | Hypertension: PO, initially 20 mg once daily, increased by 10 mg/wk or longer intervals to a maximum of 60 mg daily. Average maintenance dose, 20–40 mg daily. Adults with liver impairment or >65 y, PO, initially 10 mg once daily | Structurally similar to nifedipine but is 5 to 10 times more potent a vasodilator |
| **Verapamil** (Calan, Isoptin) | Angina: PO, 80–120 mg three times daily<br>Arrhythmias: PO, 80–120 mg three to four times daily; IV injection, 5–10 mg over 2 min or longer, with continuous monitoring of electrocardiogram and blood pressure<br>Hypertension: PO, 80 mg three times daily or 240 mg (sustained release) once daily | Do not crush sustained-release product |

## Age-related Considerations: Use of Antianginal Drugs

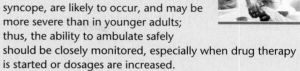

### USE IN CHILDREN

Safety and effectiveness of antianginal drugs have not been established for children. Nitroglycerin given intravenously for heart failure and intraoperative control of blood pressure, with the initial dose adjusted for weight and later doses titrated to response.

### USE IN OLDER ADULTS

Antianginal drugs are often used because cardiovascular disease and myocardial ischemia are common problems in older adults. Adverse drug effects, such as hypotension and

syncope, are likely to occur, and may be more severe than in younger adults; thus, the ability to ambulate safely should be closely monitored, especially when drug therapy is started or dosages are increased.

With calcium channel blockers, older adults may have higher plasma concentrations of verapamil, diltiazem, nifedipine, and amlodipine. This is attributed to decreased hepatic metabolism of the drugs. In addition, older adults may experience more hypotension with verapamil, nifedipine, and felodipine than younger clients. Blood pressure should be monitored with these drugs.

---

should be used cautiously in the presence of head injury or cerebral hemorrhage because they may increase intracranial pressure. Additionally, males taking nitroglycerin or any other nitrate should not take sildenafil (Viagra) for erectile dysfunction. Nitrates and sildenafil both decrease blood pressure, and the combined effect can produce profound, life-threatening hypotension.

### Individual Nitrates

**Nitroglycerin** (Nitro-Bid, others), the prototype drug, is used to relieve acute angina pectoris, prevent exercise-induced angina, and decrease the frequency and severity of acute anginal episodes. Oral dosage forms are rapidly metabolized in the liver, and relatively small proportions of doses reach the systemic circulation. In addition, oral doses act slowly and do not help relieve acute chest pain. Sublingual or chewable tablets of isosorbide dinitrate also may be used. Because nitrates are metabolized in the liver, they should be used with caution in clients with sig-

## Home Care Considerations: Use of Antianginal Drugs

***ASSESS:*** the frequency and severity of anginal attacks, how the attacks are managed, and lifestyle and environmental factors that may precipitate myocardial ischemia.

***MONITOR:*** the response to antianginal medications, modification of risk factors, and quality of life.

***EDUCATE:*** how to use, store, and replace medications to ensure a constant supply; about circumstances for which the client should seek emergency care. When anginal causative factors are identified, develop plan to avoid or minimize them. Significant others should be encouraged to receive bystander cardiopulmonary resuscitation training to expedite resuscitation measures in the event of sudden cardiac death.

nificant impairment of hepatic function. For these reasons, several alternative dosage forms have been developed, including transmucosal tablets and sprays administered sublingually or buccally, transdermal ointments and adhesive discs applied to the skin, and an IV preparation. Absorption of oral drugs or topical forms of nitroglycerin may be impaired in clients with extensive edema, heart failure, hypotension, or other conditions that impair blood flow to the gastrointestinal tract or skin. An IV form of nitroglycerin is used to relieve acute anginal pain that does not respond to other agents. Regardless of the route, nitroglycerin has a half-life of 1 to 5 minutes, supporting the beneficial use of transdermal patches and sustained-release tablets.

**Isosorbide dinitrate** (Isordil, Sorbitrate) is used to reduce the frequency and severity of acute anginal episodes. When given sublingually or in chewable tablets, it acts in about 2 minutes, and its effects last 2 to 3 hours. When higher doses are given orally, more drug escapes metabolism in the liver and produces systemic effects in approximately 30 minutes. Therapeutic effects last about 4 hours after oral administration. The effective oral dose is usually determined by increasing the dose until headache occurs, indicating the maximum tolerable dose. Sustained-release capsules also are available.

**Isosorbide mononitrate** (ISMO, Monoket, Imdur) is the metabolite and active component of isosorbide dinitrate. It is well absorbed after oral administration and is almost 100% bioavailable. Unlike other oral nitrates, this drug is not subject to first-pass hepatic metabolism. Onset of action occurs within 1 hour, peak effects occur between 1 and 4 hours, and the elimination half-life is approximately 5 hours. It is used only for prophylaxis of angina; it does not act rapidly enough to relieve acute attacks.

## Beta-Adrenergic Blocking Agents

Beta-adrenergic blocking agents are often prescribed in a variety of clinical conditions. Their actions, uses, and

## PROTOTYPE PROFILE 41-1

### P Nitroglycerin (nye troe GLI ser in)

**Drug Class**
*Chemical:* Nitrate
*Functional:* Antianginal agent; coronary vasodilator

**Trade Name**
Nitro-Bid

**Therapeutic Indications**
Relieve acute angina pectoris, prevent exercise-induced angina, and decrease the frequency and severity of acute anginal episodes by decreasing cardiac oxygen demand (decreasing preload and afterload and at higher doses, dilating coronary arteries)

**Pharmacokinetics**
*Absorption*
Absorbed directly into the systemic circulation

*Distribution*
Plasma protein binding: 60%

*Metabolism*
Oral dosage forms are rapidly metabolized in the liver, and relatively small proportions of doses reach the systemic circulation (extensive first-pass effect)

*Excretion*
Urine, as inactive metabolites

**Pharmacodynamics**
*Onset of Action*
Sublingual tablet: 1–3 min
Translingual spray: 2 min
Buccal tablet: 2–5 min
Sustained release: 20–45 min
Topical: 15–60 min
Transdermal: 40–60 min
Intravenous (as drip): immediate

*Duration*
Sublingual tablet: 30–60 min
Translingual spray: 30–60 min
Buccal tablet: 2 h
Sustained release: 4–8 h
Topical: 2–12 h

Transdermal: 18–24 h
Intravenous (as drip): 3–5 min

**Pregnancy Considerations**
Category C; excretion in breast milk is unknown

**Dosage**
*Short-acting:*
SL, 0.15–0.6 mg PRN for chest pain
Translingual spray, one or two metered doses (0.4 mg/dose) sprayed onto oral mucosa at onset of anginal pain, to a maximum of three doses in 15 min
IV, 5–10 mcg/min initially, increased in 10- to 20-mcg/min increments up to 100 mcg/min or more if necessary to relieve pain; use glass or special container because drug absorption occurs with soft plastic
*Long-acting:* Oral doses act slowly and do not help relieve acute chest pain.
PO, immediate-release tablets, 2.5–9 mg two or three times per day
PO, sustained-release tablets or capsules, 2.5 mg three or four times per day
Buccal tablet, 1 mg q3–5h while awake, placed between upper lip and gum or cheek and gum
Topical ointment, 1/2–2 inches q4–8h; do not rub in
Topical transdermal disc, applied once daily

**Side Effects/Adverse Reactions**
Headache
Hypotension
Nitrate tolerance minimized with a 8–12 h nitrate-free interval (administer 3 times a day rather than every 8 hours)

**Drug Interactions**
Males taking nitroglycerin or any other nitrate should not take sildenafil (Viagra) for erectile dysfunction because the combination can cause life-threatening hypotension
Hypotension may result if alcohol is ingested if nitrates are taken within 1 h or longer

### ? How Can You Avoid This Medication Error?

Mr. Ely has Nitropaste (nitroglycerin ointment), 1 inch, ordered every 6 hours to decrease blood pressure and control angina. The nurse carefully measures out 1 inch of ointment on the measuring paper and spreads the ointment with her finger. Before she is able to administer the medication, she feels dizzy and unwell. She hands the medication to another nurse and asks her to give it. Identify the error and how it could be prevented.

adverse effects are discussed in Chapter 16. In this chapter, the drugs are discussed only in relation to their use in angina pectoris.

Sympathetic stimulation of beta$_1$ receptors in the heart increases heart rate and force of myocardial contraction, both of which increase myocardial oxygen demand and may precipitate acute anginal attacks. Beta-blocking drugs prevent or inhibit sympathetic stimulation. Thus, the drugs reduce heart rate and myocardial contractility, particularly when sympathetic output is increased during exercise. A slower heart rate may improve coronary blood flow to the ischemic area. Beta blockers also reduce blood pressure, which in turn decreases myocardial workload and oxygen demand. In angina pectoris, beta-adrenergic blocking agents are used in long-term management to decrease the frequency and severity of anginal attacks, decrease the need for sublingual nitroglycerin, and increase exercise tolerance. When a beta blocker is being discontinued after prolonged use, it should be tapered in dosage and gradually discontinued, or rebound angina can occur.

These drugs should not be given to clients with known or suspected coronary artery spasms because they may intensify the frequency and severity of vasospasm. This probably results from unopposed stimulation of alpha-adrenergic receptors, which causes vasoconstriction, when beta-adrenergic receptors are blocked by the drugs. Clients who continue to smoke may have reduced efficacy with the use of beta blockers. Clients with asthma should be observed for bronchospasm from blockage of beta$_2$ receptors in the lung. Beta blockers should be used with caution in clients with diabetes mellitus because they can conceal signs of hypoglycemia (except for sweating and confusion).

**Propranolol,** the prototype beta blocker, is used to reduce the frequency and severity of acute attacks of angina. Studies indicate that beta blockers are more effective than nitrates or calcium channel blockers in decreas-ing the likelihood of silent ischemia and improving the mortality rate after transmural myocardial infarction. Key information about this prototype can be found in Prototype Profile 41-2: Propranolol.

**Atenolol, metoprolol,** and **nadolol** have the same actions, uses, and adverse effects as propranolol, but they have long half-lives and can be given once daily. Because they are excreted by the kidneys, the dosage must be reduced in clients with renal impairment.

## Calcium Channel Blocking Agents

Calcium channel blockers act on contractile and conductive tissues of the heart and on vascular smooth muscle. For these cells to function normally, the concentration of intracellular calcium must be increased. This is accomplished by movement of extracellular calcium ions into the cell (through calcium channels in the cell membrane) and release of bound calcium from the sarcoplasmic reticulum in the cell. Thus, calcium plays an important role in maintaining vasomotor tone, myocardial contractility, and conduction. Calcium channel blocking agents prevent the movement of extracellular calcium into the cell. As a result, coronary and peripheral arteries are dilated, myocardial contractility is decreased, and the conduction system is

---

**PROTOTYPE PROFILE 41-2**

*P* **Propranolol** (proe PRAN oh lole)

**Drug Class**
*Chemical:* Beta-adrenergic blocking agent
*Functional:* Antianginal; antihypertensive

**Trade Name**
Inderal

**Therapeutic Indications**
Reduce the frequency and severity of acute attacks of angina. Usually added to the antianginal drug regimen when nitrates do not prevent anginal episodes. Useful in preventing exercise-induced tachycardia, which can precipitate anginal attacks

**Dietary Considerations**
Administer with food

**Pharmacokinetics**
*Absorption*
Well absorbed after oral administration
*Distribution*
Plasma protein binding: Adults—93%; newborns—68%
*Metabolism*
Metabolized extensively in the liver; a relatively small proportion of an oral dose (approximately 30%)

reaches the systemic circulation (extensive first-pass effect). For this reason, oral doses of propranolol are much higher than IV doses

*Excretion*
Urine

**Pharmacodynamics**
*Onset of Action*
Onset of action is 30 minutes after oral administration and 1–2 min after IV injection
*Duration*
Approximately 6 h

**Pregnancy Considerations**
Category C; Category D second and third trimester; crosses placenta; small amounts found in breast milk

**Dosage**
PO, 10–80 mg two to four times a day
IV, 0.5–3 mg injected at a rate of 1 mg/min every 4 h until desired response is obtained
Because of variations in the degree of hepatic metabolism, clients vary widely in the dosages required to maintain a therapeutic response

*(continued)*

**PROTOTYPE PROFILE 41-2**

*P* **Propranolol (Continued)**

**Side Effects/Adverse Reactions**

Bronchospasm, laryngospasm
Congestive heart failure
Bradycardia
Agranulocytosis, thrombocytopenia

**Drug Interactions**

AV block with digitalis, calcium channel blockers
Increased inotropic effect with disopyramide and
verapamil

Increased beta-blocking effect with cimetidine
Decreased beta-blocking effect with smoking, norepinephrine, isoproterenol, barbiturates, dopamine,
dobutamine, rifampin
Increased effects of reserpine, digitalis, and neuromuscular blocking agents

---

depressed in relation to impulse formation (automaticity) and conduction velocity (Fig. 41-1).

In angina pectoris, the drugs improve the blood supply to the myocardium by dilating coronary arteries, and
they decrease the workload of the heart by dilating peripheral arteries. In variant angina, calcium channel blockers
reduce coronary artery vasospasm. In atrial fibrillation or
flutter and other supraventricular tachyarrhythmias, diltiazem and verapamil slow the rate of ventricular response.
In hypertension, the drugs lower blood pressure primarily by dilating peripheral arteries.

Calcium channel blockers are well absorbed after oral
administration but undergo extensive first-pass metabolism in the liver. Most of the drugs are more than 90%
protein bound and reach peak plasma levels within 1 to
2 hours (6 hours or longer for sustained-release forms).
Most also have short elimination half-lives (<5 hours);
hence, doses must be given three or four times daily
unless sustained-release formulations are used. Amlodipine (30 to 50 hours), bepridil (24 hours), and felodipine (11 to 16 hours) have long elimination half-lives and
therefore can be given once daily. An impaired liver produces fewer drug-binding plasma proteins such as albumin. This means that a greater proportion of a given dose
is unbound and therefore active.

In clients with cirrhosis, bioavailability of oral drugs
is greatly increased, and metabolism (of both oral and
parenteral drugs) is greatly decreased. Both of these effects
increase plasma levels of drug from a given dose (essentially an overdose). The effects result from shunting of
blood around the liver so that drug molecules circulating
in the bloodstream do not come in contact with drug-
metabolizing enzymes and therefore are not metabolized.
For example, the bioavailability of verapamil, nifedipine,
felodipine, and nisoldipine is approximately double and
the clearance of these drugs is approximately one third that
of clients without cirrhosis. Thus, the drugs should be used
with caution, dosages should be substantially reduced,
and clients should be closely monitored for drug effects

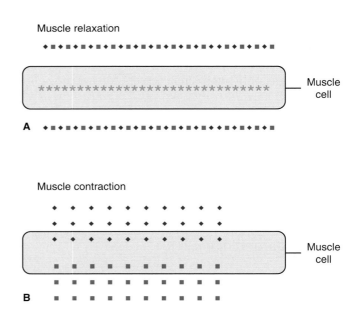

Muscle relaxation

A

Muscle contraction

B

Calcium-blocking drugs

C

FIGURE 41-1 Calcium channel blockers: mechanism of action.
(A) During muscle relaxation, potassium ions are inside the muscle
cell and calcium and sodium ions are outside the muscle cell. (B) For
muscle contraction to occur, potassium ions leave the cell and
sodium and calcium ions enter the cell through open channels in the
cell membrane. (C) When calcium channels are blocked by drug molecules, muscle contraction is decreased because calcium ions cannot move through the cell membrane into the muscle cell. (Calcium
ions = ◆; sodium ions = ■; potassium ions = ✱; calcium channel
blocking drugs = ▲.)

(including periodic measurements of liver enzymes). Dosage reductions are not necessary with renal disease except for bepridil and felodipine. Additionally, clients taking calcium channel blockers should avoid taking over-the-counter medications containing calcium because they reduce the therapeutic response.

The calcium channel blockers approved for use in the United States vary in their chemical structures and effects on body tissues. Seven of these are chemically dihydropyridines, of which nifedipine was the first available. Bepridil, diltiazem, and verapamil differ chemically from the dihydropyridines and each other. Nifedipine and related drugs act mainly on vascular smooth muscle to produce vasodilation, whereas verapamil and diltiazem have greater effects on the cardiac conduction system. Given the variations of drugs within the class, no prototype is identified here.

The drugs also vary in clinical indications for use; most are used for angina or hypertension, and only diltiazem and verapamil are used to manage supraventricular tachyarrhythmias. In clients with CAD, the drugs are effective as monotherapy but are commonly prescribed in combination with beta blockers. In addition, nimodipine is approved for use only in subarachnoid hemorrhage, in which it decreases spasm in cerebral blood vessels and limits the extent of brain damage. In animal studies, nimodipine exerted greater effects on cerebral arteries than on other arteries, probably because it is highly lipid soluble and penetrates the blood–brain barrier.

Contraindications include second- or third-degree heart block, cardiogenic shock, and severe bradycardia, heart failure, or hypotension. The drugs should be used cautiously with milder bradycardia, heart failure, or hypotension and with renal or hepatic impairment.

## Adjunctive Antianginal Drugs

In addition to antianginal drugs, several other drugs may be used to control risk factors and prevent progression of myocardial ischemia to myocardial infarction and sudden cardiac death. These may include the following:

- **Aspirin.** This drug has become the standard of care because of its antiplatelet (ie, antithrombotic) effects. Recommended doses vary from 81 mg daily to 325 mg daily or every other day; apparently all doses are beneficial in reducing the possibility of myocardial reinfarction, stroke, and death. Clopidogrel (see Chap. 45), 75 mg daily, is an acceptable alternative for individuals with aspirin allergy.
- **Antilipemics.** Clients who are unable to lower serum cholesterol levels sufficiently with a low-fat diet may require antilipemics (see Chap. 46). Lovastatin or a related "statin" is often used. The goal is usually to reduce the serum cholesterol level below 200 mg/dL and low-density lipoprotein cholesterol to below 130 mg/dL.
- **Antihypertensives.** These drugs (see Chap. 43) may be needed for clients with hypertension. Because beta blockers and calcium channel blockers are used to manage hypertension as well as angina, these drugs may be effective for both disorders.

*(text continues on page 766)*

---

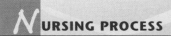

## NURSING PROCESS

### Assessment

Assess the client's condition in relation to angina pectoris. Specific assessment data vary with each client but usually should include the following:

- During the initial nursing history interview, try to answer the following questions:
  - How long has the client been taking antianginal drugs? For what purpose are they being taken (prophylaxis, treatment of acute attacks, or both)?
  - What is the frequency and duration of acute anginal attacks? Has either increased recently? (An increase could indicate worsening coronary atherosclerosis and increased risk of myocardial infarction.)
  - Do symptoms other than chest pain occur during acute attacks (eg, sweating, nausea)?
  - Are there particular activities or circumstances that provoke acute attacks? Do attacks ever occur when the client is at rest? Where does the client fit in the Canadian Cardiovascular Society classification system?
  - What measures relieve symptoms of acute angina?

- If the client takes nitroglycerin, ask how often it is required, how many tablets are needed for relief of pain, how often the supply is replaced, and where the client stores or carries the drug.
- Assess blood pressure and pulse, electrocardiogram (ECG) reports, serum cholesterol, and cardiac enzyme reports. Elevated cholesterol is a significant risk factor for coronary atherosclerosis and angina and the risk is directly related to the degree of elevation. Cardiac enzyme levels, such as troponin, creatine kinase (CK), lactate dehydrogenase (LDH), and aspartate aminotransferase (AST), should all be normal in clients with angina.
- During an acute attack, assess the following:
  - Location and quality of the pain. Chest pain is non-specific. It may be a symptom of numerous disorders, such as pulmonary embolism, esophageal spasm or inflammation (heartburn), costochondritis, or anxiety. Chest pain of cardiac origin is caused by myocardial ischemia and may indicate angina pectoris or myocardial infarction.

*(continued)*

## $N$URSING PROCESS (Continued)

- Precipitating factors. For example, what was the client doing, thinking, or feeling just before the onset of chest pain?
- Has the client had invasive procedures to diagnose or treat his or her coronary artery disease (CAD) (eg, cardiac catheterization, angioplasty, revascularization surgery)?

### Nursing Diagnoses

- Decreased Cardiac Output related to altered stroke volume or drug therapy
- Acute pain in chest related to inadequate perfusion of the myocardium
- Activity Intolerance related to chest pain
- Noncompliance related to drug therapy and lifestyle changes
- Deficient Knowledge related to management of disease process and drug therapy
- Ineffective Individual Coping related to chronic disease process
- Sexual Dysfunction related to fear of precipitating chest pain

### Planning/Goals

*The client will:*

- Receive or take antianginal drugs accurately
- Experience relief of acute chest pain
- Have fewer episodes of acute chest pain
- Have increased activity tolerance
- Identify and manage situations that precipitate anginal attacks
- Be closely monitored for therapeutic and adverse effects, especially when drug therapy is started
- Avoid preventable adverse effects
- Verbalize essential information about the disease process, needed dietary and lifestyle changes to improve health status, and drug therapy
- Recognize signs and symptoms that necessitate professional intervention
- Keep appointments for follow-up care and monitoring

### Interventions

Use the following measures to prevent acute anginal attacks:

- Assist in preventing, recognizing, and managing contributory disorders, such as atherosclerosis, hypertension, hyperthyroidism, hypoxia, and anemia. For example, hypertension is a common risk factor for CAD and morbidity and mortality increase progressively with the degree of either systolic or diastolic elevation. Management of hyper-

tension reduces morbidity and mortality rates. However, most studies indicate that the reductions stem more from fewer strokes, less renal failure, and less heart failure, than from less CAD.

- Help the client recognize and avoid precipitating factors (eg, heavy meals, strenuous exercise) when possible. If anxiety is a factor, relaxation techniques or psychological counseling may be helpful.
- Help the client to develop a more healthful lifestyle in terms of diet and weight control, adequate rest and sleep, regular exercise, and not smoking. Ideally, these self-help interventions are practiced before illness occurs and they can help prevent or delay illness. However, most individuals are unmotivated until illness develops, and perhaps after it develops as well. These interventions are beneficial at any stage of CAD. For example, for a client who already has angina, a supervised exercise program helps to develop collateral circulation. Smoking has numerous ill effects on the client with angina and decreases effectiveness of antianginal drugs.

During an acute anginal attack in a client known to have angina or CAD:

- Assume that any chest pain may be of cardiac origin.
- Have the client lie down or sit down to reduce cardiac workload and provide rest.
- Check vital signs and compare them with baseline values.
- Record the characteristics of chest pain and the presence of other signs and symptoms.
- Have the client take a fast-acting nitroglycerin preparation (previously prescribed), up to three sublingual tablets or three oral sprays, each 5 minutes apart, as necessary.
- If chest pain is not relieved with rest and nitroglycerin, assume that a myocardial infarction has occurred until proven otherwise. In a health care setting, keep the client at rest and notify the client's physician immediately. Outside of a health care setting, call 911 for immediate assistance.
- Leave sublingual nitroglycerin at the bedside of hospitalized clients (per hospital policy). The tablets or spray should be within reach so they can be used immediately. Record the number of tablets used daily, and ensure an adequate supply is available.

### Evaluation

- Observe and interview for relief of acute chest pain.
- Observe and interview regarding the number of episodes of acute chest pain.

## CLIENT TEACHING GUIDELINES
## Antianginal Drugs

### General Considerations

✔ Angina is chest pain that occurs because your heart is not getting enough blood and oxygen. The most common causes are hypertension and atherosclerosis of the coronary arteries. The chest pain usually lasts less than 5 minutes and episodes can be managed for years without causing permanent heart damage. However, if the pain is severe or prolonged, a heart attack and heart damage may develop. You need to seek information about your heart condition to prevent or decrease episodes of angina and prevent a heart attack.

✔ Several types of drugs are used in angina, and you may need a combination of drugs for the best effects. Most clients take one or more long-acting drugs to prevent anginal attacks and a fast, short-acting drug (usually nitroglycerin tablets that you dissolve under your tongue, or a nitroglycerin solution that you spray into your mouth) to relieve acute attacks. You should seek emergency care immediately if rest and three sublingual tablets or oral sprays 5 minutes apart do not relieve your chest pain. The long-acting medications are not effective in relieving sudden anginal pain.

✔ As with any medications for serious or potentially serious conditions, it is extremely important to take antianginal medications as prescribed. Do not increase dosage or discontinue the drugs without specific instructions from your health care provider.

✔ With sublingual nitroglycerin tablets, keep them in the original container, carry them so that they are always within reach but not where they are exposed to body heat, and replace them approximately every 6 months because they become ineffective.

✔ It may be helpful to record the number and severity of anginal episodes, the number of nitroglycerin tablets required to relieve the attack, and the total number of tablets taken daily. Such a record can help your health care provider know when to change your medications or your dosages.

✔ Headache and dizziness may occur with nitrate antianginal drugs, especially sublingual nitroglycerin. These effects are usually temporary and dissipate with continued therapy. If dizziness occurs, avoid strenuous activity and stand up slowly for approximately an hour after taking the drugs. If headache is severe, you may take aspirin or acetaminophen with the nitrate drug. Do not reduce drug dosage or take the drug less often to avoid headache. Loss of effectiveness may occur.

✔ Keep family members or support individuals informed about the location and use of antianginal medications in case help is needed.

✔ Avoid over-the-counter decongestants, cold remedies, and diet pills, which stimulate the heart and constrict blood vessels and thus may cause angina.

✔ With nitrate antianginal drugs, avoid alcohol. Both the drugs and alcohol dilate blood vessels and an excessive reduction in blood pressure (with dizziness and fainting) may occur with the combination.

✔ Several calcium channel blockers are available in both immediate-acting and long-acting (sustained-release) forms. The brand names often differ very little (eg, Procardia is a brand name of immediate-release nifedipine; Procardia XL is a long-acting formulation). It is extremely important that the correct formulation is used consistently.

### Self-administration
### or Caregiver Administration

✔ Take or give as instructed; specific instructions differ with the type of antianginal drug being taken.

✔ Take or give antianginal drugs on a regular schedule, at evenly spaced intervals. This increases drug effectiveness in preventing acute attacks of angina.

✔ With nitroglycerin and other nitrate preparations:

✔ Use according to instructions for the particular dosage form. The dosage forms were developed for specific routes of administration and are not interchangeable.

✔ For sublingual nitroglycerin tablets, place them under the tongue until they dissolve. Take at the first sign of an anginal attack, before severe pain develops. If chest pain is not relieved in 5 minutes, dissolve a second tablet under the tongue. If pain is not relieved within another 5 minutes, dissolve a third tablet. If pain continues or becomes more severe, notify your health care provider immediately or report to the nearest hospital emergency room. Sit down when you take the medications. This may help to relieve your pain and prevent dizziness from the drug.

✔ For the translingual solution of nitroglycerin, spray onto or under the tongue; do not inhale the spray.

✔ For transmucosal tablets of nitroglycerin, place them under the upper lip or between the cheek and gum and allow them to dissolve slowly over 3 to 5 hours. Do not chew or swallow the tablets.

✔ Take oral nitrates on an empty stomach with a glass of water. Oral isosorbide dinitrate is available in regular and chewable tablets; be sure each type is taken appropriately. Do not crush or chew sustained-release nitroglycerin tablets.

✔ For sublingual isosorbide dinitrate tablets, place them under the tongue until they dissolve.

✔ If an oral nitrate and topical nitroglycerin are being used concurrently, stagger the times of administration. This minimizes dizziness from low blood pressure and headache, which are common adverse effects of nitrate drugs.

✔ For nitroglycerin ointment, use the special paper to measure the dose. Place the ointment on a nonhairy part of the upper body and apply with the applicator

*(continued)*

CLIENT TEACHING GUIDELINES
## Antianginal Drugs (Continued)

paper. Cover the area with plastic wrap or tape. Rotate application sites (because the ointment can irritate the skin) and wipe off the previous dose before applying a new dose. Wash hands after applying the ointment.

The measured paper must be used for accurate dosage. The paper is used to apply the ointment because the drug is readily absorbed through the skin. Skin contact should be avoided except on the designated area of the body. Plastic wrap or tape aids absorption and prevents removal of the drug. It also prevents soiling of clothes and linens.

✔ For nitroglycerin patches, apply at the same time each day to clean, dry, hairless areas on the upper body or arms. Rotate sites. Avoid applying below the knee or elbow or in areas of skin irritation or scar tissue. Correct application is necessary to promote effective and consistent drug absorption. The drug is not as well absorbed from distal portions of the extremities because of decreased blood flow. Rotation of sites decreases skin irritation. Also, used patches must be disposed of properly because there is enough residual nitroglycerin to be harmful, especially to children and pets.

✔ With sustained-release forms of calcium channel blockers, which are usually taken once daily, do not take more often than prescribed and do not crush or chew.

## Nursing Actions
## Antianginal Drugs

| Nursing Actions | Rationale/Explanation |
|---|---|
| 1. Administer accurately. | |
| a. Check blood pressure and heart rate before each dose of an antianginal drug. Withhold the drug if systolic blood pressure is below 90 mm Hg. If the dose is omitted, record and report to the health care provider. | Hypotension is an adverse effect of antianginal drugs. Bradycardia is an adverse effect of propranolol and nadolol. Dosage adjustments may be necessary if these effects occur. |
| b. Give antianginal drugs on a regular schedule, at evenly spaced intervals. | To increase effectiveness in preventing acute attacks of angina |
| c. If oral nitrates and topical nitroglycerin are being used concurrently, stagger times of administration. | To minimize risks of additive hypotension and headache |
| d. For sublingual nitroglycerin and isosorbide dinitrate, instruct the client to place the tablets under the tongue until they dissolve. | |
| e. For oral isosorbide dinitrate, regular and chewable tablets are available. Be sure each type of tablet is taken appropriately. | |
| f. For sublingual nitroglycerin, check the expiration date on the container. | Sublingual tablets of nitroglycerin are volatile. Once the bottle has been opened, they become ineffective after approximately 6 mo and should be replaced. |
| g. To apply nitroglycerin ointment, use the special paper to measure the dose. Place the ointment on a non-hairy part of the body, and apply with the applicator paper. Cover the area with plastic wrap or tape. Rotate application sites and wipe off previous ointment before applying a new dose. | The measured paper must be used for accurate dosage. The paper is used to apply the ointment because the drug is readily absorbed through the skin. Skin contact should be avoided except on the designated area of the body. Plastic wrap or tape aids absorption and prevents removal of the drug. It also prevents soiling of clothes and linens. Application sites should be rotated because the ointment can irritate the skin. |
| h. For nitroglycerin patches, apply at the same time each day to clean, dry, hairless areas on the upper body or arms. Rotate sites. Avoid applying below the knee or elbow or in areas of skin irritation or scar tissue. | To promote effective and consistent drug absorption. The drug is not as well absorbed from distal portions of the extremities because of decreased blood flow. Rotation of sites decreases skin irritation. |
| i. For intravenous (IV) nitroglycerin, dilute the drug and give by continuous infusion, with frequent monitoring of blood pressure and heart rate. Use only with the special administration set supplied by the manufacturer to avoid drug adsorption onto tubing. | The drug should not be given by direct IV injection. The drug is potent and may cause hypotension. Dosage (flow rate) is adjusted according to response (pain relief or drop in systolic blood pressure of 20 mm Hg). |
| j. With IV verapamil, inject slowly, over 2–3 min. | To decrease hypotension and other adverse effects |

*(continued)*

## Nursing Actions
## Antianginal Drugs (Continued)

| Nursing Actions | Rationale/Explanation |
|---|---|
| 2. Observe for therapeutic effects. | |
| a. Relief of chest pain with acute attacks | Sublingual nitroglycerin usually relieves pain within 5 min. If pain is not relieved, two additional tablets may be given, 5 min apart. If pain is not relieved after three tablets, report to the health care provider or seek emergency care. |
| b. Reduced incidence and severity of acute attacks with prophylactic antianginal drugs | |
| c. Increased exercise tolerance | |
| 3. Observe for adverse effects. | |
| a. With nitrates, observe for hypotension, dizziness, lightheadedness, tachycardia, palpitations, and headache. | Adverse effects are extensions of pharmacologic action. Vasodilation causes hypotension, which in turn causes dizziness from cerebral hypoxia and tachycardia from compensatory sympathetic nervous system stimulation. Hypotension can decrease blood flow to coronary arteries and precipitate angina pectoris or myocardial infarction. Hypotension is most likely to occur within an hour after drug administration. Vasodilation also causes headache, the most common adverse effect of nitrates. |
| b. With beta-adrenergic blocking agents, observe for hypotension, bradycardia, bronchospasm, and heart failure. | Beta blockers lower blood pressure by decreasing myocardial contractility and cardiac output. Excessive bradycardia may contribute to hypotension and cardiac dysrhythmias. Bronchospasm is more likely to occur in clients with asthma or other chronic respiratory problems. |
| c. With calcium channel blockers, observe for hypotension, dizziness, lightheadedness, weakness, peripheral edema, headache, heart failure, pulmonary edema, nausea, and constipation. Bradycardia may occur with verapamil and diltiazem; tachycardia may occur with nifedipine and nicardipine. | Adverse effects result primarily from reduced smooth muscle contractility. These effects, except constipation, are much more likely to occur with nifedipine and other dihydropyridines. Nifedipine may cause profound hypotension, which activates the compensatory mechanisms of the sympathetic nervous system and the renin–angiotensin–aldosterone system. Peripheral edema may require the administration of a diuretic. Constipation is more likely to occur with verapamil. Diltiazem reportedly causes few adverse effects. |
| 4. Observe for drug interactions. | |
| a. Drugs that *increase* effects of antianginal drugs: | |
| (1) Antidysrhythmics, antihypertensive drugs, diuretics, phenothiazine antipsychotic agents | Additive hypotension |
| (2) Cimetidine | May increase beta-blocking effects of propranolol by slowing its hepatic clearance and elimination. Increases effects of all calcium channel blockers by inhibiting hepatic metabolism and increasing serum drug levels. |
| (3) Digoxin | Additive bradycardia when given with beta-blocking agents |
| b. Drugs that *decrease* effects of antianginal drugs: | |
| (1) Adrenergic drugs (eg, epinephrine, isoproterenol) | Adrenergic drugs, which stimulate beta receptors, can reverse bradycardia induced by beta blockers. |
| (2) Anticholinergic drugs | Drugs with anticholinergic effects can increase heart rate, offsetting slower heart rates produced by beta blockers. |
| (3) Calcium salts | May decrease therapeutic effectiveness of calcium channel blockers |
| (4) Carbamazepine, phenytoin, rifampin | May decrease effects of calcium channel blockers by inducing hepatic enzymes and thereby increasing their rate of metabolism |

## ? How Can You Avoid This Medication Error?

**Answer:** Actually, there are two errors in this situation. A nurse can only safely administer medication that she has prepared. In this situation, after the medication has been spread on the paper, the dosage will be unclear. Also, a nurse or a family member should never touch Nitropaste without wearing gloves. Hands should be washed after administration. This potent vasodilator is absorbed through the skin, causing systemic effects such as dizziness and headache.

## Critical Thinking Exercises

1. The nurse removes a client's transdermal nitroglycerin disc at bedtime as ordered to minimize nitrate tolerance. The client awakens during the night and complains of anginal symptoms. The nurse's first action is to:
   a. Notify the health care provider
   b. Apply a new transdermal disc
   c. Obtain further history of complaints
   d. Administer a short-acting nitrate as ordered

2. The health care provider prescribes nitroglycerin 2% ointment, 1.5-inch dose every 4 hours. To apply the ointment accurately, the client should be instructed to:
   a. Rub the ointment into the skin to enhance absorption
   b. Leave previous ointment on for 4 hours after applying a new dose
   c. Rotate application sites to decrease skin irritation
   d. Place the ointment on a distal part of the lower body to increase absorption

3. A client is receiving propranolol (Inderal) to manage her chronic angina pectoris. Because this drug is not cardioselective, the nurse should monitor the client for which adverse reaction?
   a. Seizures
   b. Confusion
   c. Bronchospasm
   d. Hypertensive crisis

4. A client, who is taking atenolol (Tenormin), is seen in the cardiac clinic following a myocardial infarction and reports that he continues to smoke. The nurse recognizes that smoking may contribute to what effect on beta-blocking activity?
   a. Reduce the efficacy
   b. Potentiate an increase in intracranial pressure
   c. Precipitate ventricular fibrillation
   d. Increase the incidence of side effects

5. A client with angina pectoris, being discontinued from beta blockers, asks the nurse, "Why can't I just stop taking the drug today if it's not working anyway?" The nurse instructs the client that failure to taper the drug slowly may lead to:
   a. Worsening of his angina symptoms
   b. Significant bronchoconstriction
   c. Development of congestive heart failure
   d. Drug fever

## SELECTED REFERENCES

Brater, D. C. (2000). Clinical pharmacology of cardiovascular drugs. In H. D. Humes (Ed.), *Kelley's textbook of internal medicine* (4th ed., pp. 651–672). Philadelphia: Lippincott Williams & Wilkins.

*Drug facts and comparisons.* (Updated monthly). St. Louis: Facts and Comparisons.

Jones, S. (2001). Oral or intravenous beta blockers in acute myocardial infarction. *Emergency Medicine Journal, 18*(4), 270–271.

Porth, C. M. (2002). *Pathophysiology: Concepts of altered health states* (6th ed., pp. 487–530). Philadelphia: Lippincott Williams & Wilkins.

Smith, S. C., & Goldberg, A. C. (2001). Ischemic heart disease. In S. N. Ahya, K. Flood, & S. Paranjothi (Eds.), *The Washington manual of medical therapeutics* (30th ed., pp. 96–130). Philadelphia: Lippincott Williams & Wilkins.

Talbert, R. L. (2002). Ischemic heart disease. In J. T. DiPiro, R. L. Talbert, G. C. Yee, G. R. Matzke, B. G. Wells, & L. M. Posey (Eds.), *Pharmacotherapy: A pathophysiologic approach* (5th ed., pp. 219–250). New York: McGraw-Hill.

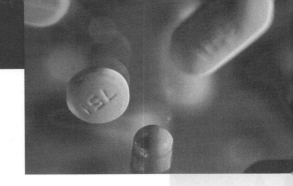

# 42

# Drugs Used in Hypotension and Shock

**OBJECTIVES**

*After studying this chapter, the student will be able to:*

1 Describe factors that control blood pressure.

2 Identify clients at risk for development of hypovolemia and shock.

3 List common causes of hypotension and shock.

4 Discuss assessment of a client in shock.

5 Describe therapeutic and adverse effects of vasopressor drugs used in the management of hypotension and shock.

**CRITICAL THINKING SCENARIO**

*B*etty Armstrong is in the cardiac care unit being managed for cardiogenic shock following an acute anterior myocardial infarction. She is currently on the following IV infusion: dobutamine (Dobutrex), 5 mcg/kg per minute, and dopamine hydrochloride (Inotropin), 5 mcg/kg per minute.

✔ Define shock. How does cardiogenic shock differ from hypovolemic shock, and how will this affect management?

✔ What symptoms would likely occur in a client experiencing cardiogenic shock?

✔ Review the autonomic nervous system (ANS). Describe the ANS effects of Mrs. Armstrong's medications and how they will be used to manage shock.

✔ Dopamine's effects differ depending on dosage. What effects will you most likely see in Mrs. Armstrong?

**PROTOTYPE PROFILE**

dopamine (Inotropin), p. 773

# OVERVIEW

Shock is a clinical syndrome characterized by decreased blood supply to body tissues. Clinical symptoms depend on the degree of impaired perfusion of vital organs (eg, brain, heart, and kidneys). To understand drug therapy used in the treatment of shock, it is necessary to understand the physiologic mechanisms that normally control blood pressure and the body's response to hypotension (see At the Foundation: Shock). Overall, regulation of blood pressure involves a complex, interacting, overlapping network of hormonal, neural, and vascular mechanisms, and any condition that affects heart rate, stroke volume, or peripheral vascular resistance affects arterial blood pressure. Many of these mechanisms are compensatory effects that try to restore balance when hypotension or hypertension occurs and are further described in Box 42-1.

Common signs and symptoms of shock include oliguria, heart failure, mental confusion, cool extremities, and coma. Most people in shock are hypotensive. In a previously hypertensive person, shock may be present if a drop in blood pressure of greater than 50 mm Hg has occurred, even if current blood pressure readings are "normal."

It is important to know the etiology of shock because management varies among the types. The types of shock, with their causes and symptoms, are summarized in Table 42-1.

# ANTISHOCK DRUGS

The goal of drug therapy in hypotension and shock is to restore and maintain adequate tissue perfusion, especially to vital organs. Drugs used in the management of shock are primarily the adrenergic drugs, which are discussed more extensively in Chapter 16. In this chapter, the drugs are discussed only in relation to their use in hypotension and shock. In these conditions, drugs with alpha-adrenergic activity (eg, norepinephrine, phenylephrine) are used to increase peripheral vascular resistance and raise blood pressure. Drugs with beta-adrenergic activity (eg, dobutamine, isoproterenol) are used to increase myocardial contractility and heart rate, which in turn raises blood pressure. Some drugs have both alpha- and beta-adrenergic activity (eg, dopamine, epinephrine). In many cases, a combination of drugs is used, depending on the type of shock and the client's response to treatment. In an emergency, the drugs may be used to maintain adequate perfusion of vital organs until sufficient fluid volume is replaced and circulation is restored.

The choice of drug depends primarily on the pathophysiology involved. Adrenergic drugs with beta activity

---

## AT THE FOUNDATION: *shock*

Shock is a clinical syndrome characterized by decreased blood supply to body tissues with resultant hypoxia at the cellular level. When decreased tissue perfusion occurs, the sympathetic nervous system (SNS) is stimulated, the hormones epinephrine and norepinephrine are secreted by the adrenal medulla, angiotensin II and aldosterone are formed, and the kidneys retain fluid. These compensatory mechanisms raise the blood pressure. Specific effects include (1) constriction of arterioles, which increases peripheral vascular resistance; (2) constriction of veins and increased venous tone; (3) stimulation of cardiac beta-adrenergic receptors, which increases heart rate and force of myocardial contraction; and (4) activation of the renin-angiotensin-aldosterone mechanism.

A consequence of inadequate blood flow to tissues is that cells change from aerobic (oxygen-based) to anaerobic metabolism. Lactic acid produced by anaerobic metabolism leads to generalized metabolic acidosis and eventually to organ failure and death if blood flow is not promptly restored.

There are three general categories of shock that are based on the circulatory mechanisms involved. These mechanisms are intravascular volume, the ability of the heart to pump, and vascular tone.

- *Hypovolemic shock* involves a loss of intravascular fluid volume that may be due to actual blood loss or relative loss from fluid shifts within the body.
- *Cardiogenic shock,* also called *pump failure,* occurs when the myocardium has lost its ability to contract efficiently and maintain an adequate cardiac output.
- *Distributive* or *vasogenic shock* is characterized by severe, generalized vasodilation, which results in severe hypotension and impairment of blood flow. Distributive shock is further divided into anaphylactic, neurogenic, and septic shock.
  - *Anaphylactic shock* results from a hypersensitivity (allergic) reaction to drugs or other substances (see Chap. 16).
  - *Neurogenic shock* results from inadequate SNS stimulation. The SNS normally maintains sufficient vascular tone (ie, a small amount of vasoconstriction) to support adequate blood circulation. Neurogenic shock may occur with depression of the vasomotor center in the brain or decreased sympathetic outflow to blood vessels.
  - *Septic shock* can result from almost any organism that gains access to the bloodstream but is most often associated with gram-negative and gram-positive bacterial infections and fungi.

## BOX 42-1 Mechanisms that Regulate Blood Pressure

### Neural

Neural regulation of blood pressure mainly involves the sympathetic nervous system (SNS). In the heart, SNS neurons control heart rate and force of contraction. In blood vessels, SNS neurons control muscle tone by maintaining a state of partial contraction, with additional constriction or dilation accomplished by altering this basal state. When hypotension and inadequate tissue perfusion occur, the SNS is activated and produces secretion of epinephrine and norepinephrine by the adrenal medulla, constriction of blood vessels in the skin, gastrointestinal tract, and kidneys, and stimulation of beta-adrenergic receptors in the heart, which increases heart rate and force of myocardial contraction. All of these mechanisms act to increase blood pressure and tissue perfusion, especially of the brain and heart.

The SNS is activated by the vasomotor center in the brain, which constantly receives messages from baroreceptors and chemoreceptors located in the circulatory system. Adequate function of these receptors is essential for rapid and short-term regulation of blood pressure. The vasomotor center interprets the messages from these receptors and modifies cardiovascular functions to maintain adequate blood flow.

More specifically, baroreceptors detect changes in pressure or stretch. For example, when a person moves from a lying to a standing position, blood pressure falls and decreases stretch in the aorta and arteries. This elicits increased heart rate and vasoconstriction to restore adequate circulation. The increased heart rate occurs rapidly and blood pressure is adjusted within 1 to 2 minutes. This quick response prevents orthostatic hypotension with dizziness and possible syncope. (Antihypertensive medications may blunt this response and cause orthostatic hypotension.)

Chemoreceptors, which are located in the aorta and carotid arteries, are in close contact with arterial blood and respond to changes in the oxygen, carbon dioxide, and hydrogen ion content of blood. Although their main function is to regulate ventilation, they also communicate with the vasomotor center and can induce vasoconstriction. Chemoreceptors are stimulated when blood pressure drops to a certain point because oxygen is decreased and carbon dioxide and hydrogen ions are increased in arterial blood.

The central nervous system (CNS) also regulates vasomotor tone and blood pressure. Inadequate blood flow to the brain results in ischemia of the vasomotor center. When this occurs, neurons in the vasomotor center stimulate widespread vasoconstriction in an attempt to raise blood pressure and restore blood flow. This reaction is called the CNS ischemic response, an emergency measure to preserve blood flow to vital brain centers. If blood flow is not restored within 3 to 10 minutes, the neurons of the vasomotor center are unable to function, the impulses that maintain vascular muscle tone stop, and blood pressure drops to a fatal level.

### Hormonal

The renin-angiotensin-aldosterone (RAA) system and vasopressin are important hormonal mechanisms in blood pressure regulation.

The *RAA system* is activated in response to hypotension and acts as a compensatory mechanism to restore adequate blood flow to body tissues. Renin is an enzyme that is synthesized, stored, and released from the kidneys in response to decreased blood pressure, SNS stimulation, or decreased sodium concentration in extracellular fluid. When released into the bloodstream, where its action lasts 30 to 60 minutes, renin converts angiotensinogen (a plasma protein) to angiotensin I. Angiotensin-converting enzyme (ACE) in the endothelium of pulmonary blood vessels then acts on angiotensin I to produce angiotensin II. Angiotensin II strongly constricts arterioles (and weakly constricts veins), increases peripheral resistance, and increases blood pressure by direct vasoconstriction, stimulation of the SNS, and stimulation of catecholamine release from the adrenal medulla. It also stimulates secretion of aldosterone from the adrenal cortex, which then causes the kidneys to retain sodium and water. Retention of sodium and water increases blood volume, cardiac output, and blood pressure.

*Vasopressin,* also called antidiuretic hormone or ADH, is a hormone secreted by the posterior pituitary gland that regulates reabsorption of water by the kidneys. It is released in response to decreased blood volume and decreased blood pressure. It causes retention of body fluids and vasoconstriction, both of which act to raise blood pressure.

### Vascular

The endothelial cells that line blood vessels synthesize and secrete several substances that play important roles in regulating cardiovascular functions, including blood pressure. These substances normally maintain a balance between vasoconstriction and vasodilation. When the endothelium is damaged (eg, by trauma, hypertension, hypercholesterolemia, or atherosclerosis), the resulting imbalance promotes production of vasoconstricting substances and also causes blood vessels to lose their ability to relax in response to dilator substances. In addition, changes in structure of endothelial and vascular smooth muscle cells (vascular remodeling) further impair vascular functions.

*Vasoconstrictors* increase vascular tone (ie, constrict or narrow blood vessels so that higher blood pressure is required to pump blood to body tissues). Vasoconstricting substances produced by the endothelium include angiotensin II, endothelin-1, platelet-derived growth factor (PDGF), and thromboxane $A_2$. Endothelin-1 is the strongest endogenous vasoconstrictor known. Angiotensin II and thromboxane $A_2$ can also be produced by other types of cells, but endothelial cells can produce both. Thromboxane $A_2$, a product of arachidonic acid metabolism, also promotes platelet aggregation and thrombosis.

*Vasodilators* decrease vascular tone and blood pressure. Major vasodilating substances produced by the endothelium include nitric oxide and prostacyclin (prostaglandin $I_2$)

*Nitric oxide (NO)* is a gas that can diffuse through cell membranes, trigger biochemical reactions, and then dissipate rapidly. It is formed by the action of the enzyme NO synthase on the amino acid L-arginine and continually

*(continued)*

BOX
42-1   **Mechanisms that Regulate Blood Pressure** (Continued)

released by normal endothelium. Its production is tightly regulated and depends on the amount of ionized calcium in the fluid portion of endothelial cells. Several substances (eg, acetylcholine, bradykinin, catecholamines, substance P, and products of aggregating platelets such as adenosine diphosphate and serotonin) act on receptors in endothelial cell membranes to increase the cytosolic concentration of ionized calcium, activate NO synthase, and increase NO production. In addition, increased blood flow or blood pressure increases shear stress at the endothelial surface and stimulates production of NO.

Once produced, endothelium-derived NO produces vasodilation primarily by activating guanylyl cyclase in vascular smooth muscle cells and increasing intracellular cyclic 3,5'-guanosine monophosphate as a second messenger. NO also inhibits platelet aggregation and production of platelet-derived vasoconstricting substances. Because NO is released into the vessel wall (to relax smooth muscle) and into the vessel lumen (to inactivate platelets), it is thought to have protective effects against vasoconstriction and thrombosis.

NO is also produced in leukocytes, fibroblasts, and vascular smooth muscle cells and may have pathologic effects when large amounts are produced. In these tissues, NO seems to have other functions, such as modifying nerve activity in the nervous system.

*Prostacyclin* is synthesized and released from endothelium in response to stimulation by several factors (eg, bradykinin, interleukin-1, serotonin, thrombin, PDGF). It produces vasodilation by activating adenylyl cyclase and increasing levels of cyclic adenosine monophosphate in smooth muscle cells. In addition, like NO, prostacyclin also inhibits platelet aggregation and production of platelet-derived vasoconstricting substances. The vasodilating effects of prostacyclin may occur independently or in conjunction with NO.

Overall, excessive vasoconstrictors or deficient vasodilators may contribute to the development of atherosclerosis, hypertension, and other diseases. Injury to the endothelial lining of blood vessels (eg, by the shear force of blood flow with hypertension or by rupture of atherosclerotic plaque) decreases vasodilators and leads to vasoconstriction, vasospasm, thrombus formation, and thickening of the blood vessel wall. All of these factors require the blood to flow through a narrowed lumen and increase blood pressure.

## Vascular Remodeling

Vascular remodeling is similar to the left ventricular remodeling that occurs in heart failure (see Chap. 38). It results from endothelial dysfunction and produces a thickening of the blood vessel wall and a narrowing of the blood vessel lumen. Thickening of the wall makes blood vessels less flexible and less able to respond to vasodilating substances. There are also changes in endothelial cell structure (ie, the connections between endothelial cells become looser) that lead to increased permeability. The mechanisms of these vascular changes, which promote and aggravate hypertension, are described below.

Normal endothelium helps maintain a balance between vasoconstriction and vasodilation, procoagulation and anticoagulation, proinflammation and antiinflammation, and progrowth and antigrowth. In the inflammatory process, normal endothelium acts as a physical barrier against the movement of leukocytes into the subendothelial space. Endothelial products such as nitric oxide may also inhibit leukocyte activity. However, inflammatory cytokines such as tumor necrosis factor–alpha and interleukin-1 activate endothelial cells to produce adhesion molecules (which allow leukocytes to adhere to the endothelium), interleukin-8 (which attracts leukocytes to the endothelium and allows them to accumulate in subendothelial cells), and foam cells (lipid-filled monocyte/macrophages that form fatty streaks, the beginning lesions of atherosclerotic plaque). Although activation of endothelial cells may be a helpful component of the normal immune response, the resulting inflammation may contribute to disease development.

In terms of cell growth, normal endothelium limits the growth of vascular smooth muscle that underlies the endothelium and forms the vessel wall. Growth-inhibiting products of the endothelium include nitric oxide, which also inhibits platelet activation and production of growth-promoting substances. When the endothelium is damaged, endothelial cells become activated and also produce growth-promoting products. Other endothelial products (eg, angiotensin II and endothelin-1) may also stimulate growth of vascular smooth muscle cells. Thus, damage or loss of endothelial cells stimulates growth of smooth muscle cells in the intimal layer of the blood vessel wall.

---

may be relatively contraindicated in shock states precipitated or complicated by cardiac dysrhythmias. Beta-stimulating drugs also should be used cautiously in cardiogenic shock after myocardial infarction because increased contractility and heart rate will increase myocardial oxygen consumption and extend the area of infarction.

For cardiogenic shock and decreased cardiac output, dopamine or dobutamine is given. With severe heart failure characterized by decreased cardiac output and high peripheral vascular resistance, vasodilator drugs (eg, nitroprusside, nitroglycerin) may be given along with the cardiotonic drug. The combination increases cardiac output

and decreases cardiac workload by decreasing preload and afterload. However, vasodilators should not be used alone because of the risk for severe hypotension and further compromise of tissue perfusion. Milrinone may be given when other drugs fail.

For distributive shock characterized by severe vasodilation and decreased peripheral vascular resistance, a vasoconstrictor or vasopressor drug, such as norepinephrine, is the drug of first choice. Drug dosage must be carefully titrated to avoid excessive vasoconstriction and hypertension, which cause impairment rather than improvement in tissue perfusion. Discussion of management

## TABLE 42-1  Types of Shock

| Types of Shock | Possible Causes | Clinical Manifestations |
|---|---|---|
| Hypovolemic | Trauma<br>Gastrointestinal bleed<br>Ruptured aneurysms<br>Third spacing<br>Dehydration | Hypotension<br>Tachycardia<br>Cool, clammy skin<br>Diaphoresis<br>Pallor<br>Oliguria |
| Cardiogenic | Acute myocardial infarction<br>Cardiac surgery<br>Dysrhythmias<br>Cardiomyopathy | Signs and symptoms of heart failure<br>Signs and symptoms of decreased cardiac output |
| Distributive<br>Neurogenic | Spinal cord damage<br>Spinal anesthesia<br>Severe pain<br>Drugs | Hypotension<br>Bradycardia<br>Warm, dry skin |
| Septic | Infection (eg, urinary tract, upper respiratory infections)<br>Invasive procedures | Hypotension<br>Cool or warm, dry skin<br>Hypothermia or hyperthermia |
| Anaphylactic | Contrast dyes<br>Drugs<br>Insect bites<br>Foods | Hypotension<br>Hives<br>Bronchospasm |

considerations in children and older adults is found in Age-related Considerations.

Individual drugs are described in the following section; indications for use and dosage ranges are listed in Drugs at a Glance 42-1: Drugs Used for Hypotension and Shock.

## INDIVIDUAL DRUGS

**Dopamine** is a naturally occurring catecholamine that functions as a neurotransmitter. Dopamine exerts its actions by stimulating alpha, beta, or dopaminergic receptors, depending on the dose being used. In addition, dopamine acts indirectly by releasing norepinephrine from sympathetic nerve endings and the adrenal glands. Peripheral dopamine receptors are located in splanchnic and renal vascular beds. At low doses (0.5 to 10 mcg/kg/min), dopamine selectively stimulates dopaminergic receptors that may increase renal blood flow and glomerular filtration rate (GFR). It has long been accepted that stimulation of dopamine receptors by low doses of exogenous dopamine produces vasodilation in the renal circulation and increases urine output. More recent studies indicate that low-dose dopamine enhances renal function only when cardiac function is improved. At doses greater than 3 mcg/kg per minute, dopamine binds to beta and alpha receptors, and the selectivity of dopaminergic receptors is lost beyond 10 mcg/kg per minute. At doses that stimulate beta receptors (3 to 20 mcg/kg/minute), there is an increase in heart rate, myocardial contractility, and blood pressure. At the highest doses (20 to 50 mcg/kg per minute), beta activity remains, but increasing alpha stimulation (vasoconstriction) may overcome its actions.

Dopamine, the prototype of the group, is useful in hypovolemic and cardiogenic shock and is described in detail in Prototype Profile 42-1: Dopamine. Adequate fluid therapy is necessary for the maximal pressor effect of dopamine. Acidosis decreases the effectiveness of dopamine.

**Dobutamine** is a synthetic catecholamine developed to provide less vascular activity than dopamine. It acts mainly on $beta_1$ receptors in the heart to increase the force of myocardial contraction with a minimal increase in heart rate. Dobutamine also may increase blood pressure with large doses. It is less likely to cause tachycardia, dysrhythmias, and increased myocardial oxygen demand than dopamine and isoproterenol. It is most useful in cases of shock that require increased cardiac output without the need for blood pressure support. It is recommended

(text continues on page 774)

## Age-related Considerations: Drugs Used in Hypotension and Shock

### USE IN CHILDREN

Little information is available about adrenergic drugs for the management of hypotension and shock in children. Children who lose up to one fourth of their circulating blood volume may experience minimal changes in arterial blood pressure and a relatively low heart rate. In general, management is the same as for adults, with drug dosages adjusted for weight.

### USE IN OLDER ADULTS

Older adults often have disorders such as atherosclerosis, peripheral vascular disease, and diabetes mellitus and may not demonstrate common symptoms of volume depletion (eg, thirst, skin turgor changes). Also, when adrenergic drugs are given, their vasoconstricting effects may decrease blood flow and increase risks for tissue ischemia and thrombosis. Careful monitoring of vital signs, skin color and temperature, urine output, and mental status is essential.

**DRUG TABLE 42-1** *Drugs at a Glance*

## Drugs Used for Hypotension and Shock

| Generic/Trade Name | Routes and Dosage Ranges | Comments/Uses |
|---|---|---|
| **Dopamine** (Intropin) | See Prototype Profile: Dopamine | |
| **Dobutamine** (Dobutrex) Pregnancy Category B | *Adults:* IV, 2.5–15 mcg/kg/min, increased to 40 mcg/kg/min if necessary. Reconstitute the 250-mg vial with 10 mL of sterile water or 5% dextrose injection. The resulting solution should be diluted to at least 50 mL with IV solution before administering (5000 mcg/mL). Add 250 mg of drug to 500 mL of diluent for a concentration of 500 mcg/mL. | Compatible IV with dopamine, epinephrine, isoproterenol, and lidocaine Administer with an infusion pump. |
| **Epinephrine** (Adrenalin) Pregnancy Category C | *Adults:* IV, 1–4 mcg/min. Prepare the solution by adding 2 mg (2 mL) of epinephrine injection 1:1000 to 250 or 500 mL of IV fluid. The final concentration is 8 or 4 mcg/mL, respectively. IV, direct injection, 100–1000 mcg of 1:10,000 injection, every 5–15 min, injected slowly. Prepare the solution by adding 1 mL epinephrine 1:1000 to 9 mL sodium chloride injection. The final concentration is 100 mcg/mL. Cardiac arrest, IV injection, 0.5–1.0 mg of 1:10,000 solution, repeated every 5 min as needed *Children:* IV infusion, 0.025 to 0.3 mcg/kg/min IV direct injection, 5 to 10 mcg/kg, slowly; Sub-Q, 0.01 mg/kg of 1:1000 solution | Treatment of anaphylactic shock Reversal of bronchoconstriction Treatment of cardiac arrest Compatible IV with dopamine, dobutamine, and diltiazem Incompatible IV with sodium bicarbonate and aminophylline |
| **Isoproterenol** (Isuprel) Pregnancy Category C | *Adults:* IV infusion, 0.5–10 mcg/min. Prepare solution by adding 2 mg to 250 mL of IV fluid. Final concentration is 8 mcg/mL. *Children:* IV infusion, 0.05–0.3 mcg/kg/min | Treatment of atropine-refractory bradycardias |
| **Metaraminol** (Aramine) Pregnancy Category C | *Adults:* IM, 2–10 mg IV injection, 0.5–5 mg IV infusion, add 15–500 mg of metaraminol to 250 or 500 mL of IV fluid. Adjust flow rate (dosage) to maintain the desired blood pressure. *Children:* IM, 0.1 mg/kg IV injection, 0.01 mg/kg IV infusion, 1 mg/25 mL of diluent. Adjust flow rate to maintain the desired blood pressure. | Treatment of hypotension due to spinal anesthesia |

*(continued)*

**DRUG TABLE 42-1**

*Drugs at a Glance*

## Drugs Used for Hypotension and Shock (Continued)

| Generic/Trade Name | Routes and Dosage Ranges | Comments/Uses |
|---|---|---|
| **Milrinone** (Primacor) Pregnancy Category C | *Adults:* IV injection (loading dose), 50 mcg/kg over 10 min. IV infusion (maintenance dose), 0.375–0.75 mcg/kg/min diluted in 0.9% or 0.45% sodium chloride or 5% dextrose solution. Maximum dose, 1.13 mg/kg/d. | Administer with an infusion pump Incompatible IV with furosemide and procainamide Compatible IV with atropine, epinephrine, digoxin, lidocaine, morphine, and sodium bicarbonate |
| **Norepinephrine** (Levophed) Pregnancy Category C | *Adults:* IV infusion, 2–4 mcg/min, to a maximum of 20 mcg/min. Prepare solution by adding 2 mg to 500 mL of IV fluid. Final concentration is 4 mcg/mL. *Children:* IV infusion, 0.03–0.1 mcg/kg/min | Central line administration required Potential for extravasation |
| **Phenylephrine** (Neo-Synephrine) Pregnancy Category C | *Adults:* IV infusion, 100–180 mcg/min initially, then 40–60 mcg/min Prepare solution by adding 10 mg of phenylephrine to 250 or 500 mL of IV fluid. Final concentration is 20 or 40 mcg/mL, respectively. IV injection, 0.1–0.5 mg every 10–15 min *Children:* SC, IM, 0.5–1 mg/25 lb | Potential for extravasation Allows for close titration of blood pressure due to short half-life |

---

## PROTOTYPE PROFILE 42-1

### 🅟 Dopamine (DOE pa meen)

**Drug Class**

*Chemical:* Catecholamine
*Functional:* Sympathomimetic agent; adrenergic agonist agent

**Trade Name**

Inotropin

**Therapeutic Indications**

Adjunct in treatment of shock persisting after adequate fluid volume replacement

**Pharmacokinetics**

*Absorption*
Immediate

*Distribution*
Widely distributed; does not cross blood–brain barrier

*Metabolism*
Half-life elimination 2 min

*Excretion*
Urine
Nonlinear pharmacokinetics in children; steady state may not be achieved for about 1 h instead of 20 min

**Pharmacodynamics**

*Onset of Action*
Adults: 5 min

*Duration*
Adults: <10 min

**Contraindications/Precautions**

Use with caution in clients with cardiovascular disease, especially post-MI, dysrhythmias, occlusive vascular disease; pheochromocytoma
Extravasation can cause tissue necrosis

**Pregnancy Considerations**

Category C
Excretion in breast milk is unknown

**Dosage**

*Requires use of infusion pump*
Renal perfusion: IV infusion, initial rate of ≤ 3 mcg/kg/min (no clear evidence that dopamine provides beneficial effect on renal function unless cardiac function is improved)

*(continued)*

## PROTOTYPE PROFILE 42-1
### P Dopamine (Continued)

Hypotension:

*Adults:* IV infusion, initial rate of 3–5 mcg/kg/min gradually titrated to desired response to a maximum of 20–50 mcg/kg/min

*Children:* IV infusion, 1–20 mcg/kg/min gradually titrated to desired response to a maximum of 50 mcg/kg/min

*Neonates:* IV infusion, 1–20 mcg/kg/min gradually titrated to desired response

### Side Effects/Adverse Reactions

Tachycardia, dysrhythmias, anginal pain, hypotension, palpitations, headache, nausea, vomiting

### Drug Interactions

*Increased Effects*

Effects of dopamine are prolonged and intensified by monoamine oxidase inhibitors, alpha- and beta-adrenergic blockers, cocaine, methyldopa, phenytoin, tricyclic antidepressants, reserpine, and general anesthesia

*Decreased Effects*

Effect of tricyclic antidepressants when used concomitantly

### Herbal and Dietary Supplements

None reported

---

for short-term use only. It may be used with dopamine to augment the $beta_1$ activity that is sometimes overridden by alpha effects when dopamine is used alone at doses greater than 10 mcg/kg per minute.

Dobutamine has a short plasma half-life and therefore must be administered by continuous intravenous (IV) infusion. A loading dose is not required because the drug has a rapid onset of action and reaches steady state within approximately 10 minutes after the infusion is begun. It is rapidly metabolized to inactive metabolites.

**Epinephrine** is a naturally occurring catecholamine produced by the adrenal glands. At low doses, epinephrine stimulates beta receptors, which increases cardiac output by increasing the rate and force of myocardial contractility. It also causes bronchodilation. Larger doses act on alpha receptors to increase blood pressure.

Epinephrine is the drug of choice for management of anaphylactic shock because of its rapid onset of action and antiallergic effects. It prevents the release of histamine and other mediators that cause symptoms of anaphylaxis, thereby reversing vasodilation and bronchoconstriction. In early management of anaphylaxis, it may be given subcutaneously to produce therapeutic effects within 5 to 10 minutes, with peak activity in approximately 20 minutes.

### ? How Can You Avoid This Medication Error?

Your postoperative patient is hypotensive and has low urine output. When a fluid bolus does not produce a significant increase in urine output, the physician orders low-dose IV dopamine. After the dopamine has infused for 2 hours, the patient complains of burning at the infusion site. When you assess the site, you do not detect swelling or warmth. You decide to continue to monitor the IV site rather than change it because you know starting another IV will be very difficult.

Epinephrine is also used to manage other kinds of shock and is usually given by continuous IV infusion. However, bolus doses may be given in emergencies, such as cardiac arrest. It may produce excessive cardiac stimulation, ventricular dysrhythmias, and reduced renal blood flow.

Epinephrine has an elimination half-life of about 2 minutes and is rapidly inactivated to metabolites, which are then excreted by the kidneys.

**Isoproterenol** is a synthetic catecholamine that acts exclusively on beta receptors to increase heart rate, myocardial contractility, and systolic blood pressure. However, it also stimulates vascular $beta_2$ receptors, which causes vasodilation, and may decrease diastolic blood pressure. For this reason, isoproterenol has limited usefulness as a pressor agent. It also may increase myocardial oxygen consumption and decrease coronary artery blood flow, which in turn causes myocardial ischemia. Cardiac dysrhythmias may result from excessive beta stimulation. Because of these limitations, use of isoproterenol is limited to shock associated with slow heart rates and myocardial depression.

**Metaraminol** is used mainly for hypotension associated with spinal anesthesia. It acts indirectly by releasing norepinephrine from sympathetic nerve endings. Thus, its vasoconstrictive actions are similar to those of norepinephrine, except that metaraminol is less potent and has a longer duration of action.

**Milrinone** is discussed in Chapter 39 as a treatment for heart failure. It is also used to manage cardiogenic shock in combination with other inotropic agents or vasopressors. It increases cardiac output and decreases systemic vascular resistance without significantly increasing heart rate or myocardial oxygen consumption. The increased cardiac output improves renal blood flow, which then leads to increased urine output, decreased circulating blood volume, and decreased cardiac workload.

**Norepinephrine** (Levophed) is a pharmaceutical preparation of the naturally occurring catecholamine norepinephrine. It stimulates alpha-adrenergic receptors and thus increases blood pressure primarily by vasoconstriction. It also stimulates beta$_1$ receptors and therefore increases heart rate, force of myocardial contraction, and coronary artery blood flow. It is useful in cardiogenic and septic shock, but reduced renal blood flow limits its prolonged use. Norepinephrine is used mainly in clients who are unresponsive to dopamine or dobutamine. As with all drugs used to manage shock, blood pressure should be monitored frequently during infusion.

**Phenylephrine** (Neo-Synephrine) is an adrenergic drug that stimulates alpha-adrenergic receptors. As a result, it constricts arterioles and raises systolic and diastolic blood pressures. Phenylephrine resembles epinephrine but has fewer cardiac effects and a longer duration of action. Reduction of renal and mesenteric blood flow limit prolonged use.

## GUIDELINES FOR MANAGEMENT OF HYPOTENSION AND SHOCK

■ Vasopressor drugs are less effective in the presence of inadequate blood volume, electrolyte abnormalities, and acidosis. These conditions also must be treated if present. In addition, normalizing the blood pH and body temperature facilitates the release of oxygen from hemoglobin to the cells.

## Nursing Process

### Assessment

Assess the client's condition in relation to hypotension and shock.

- Check blood pressure; heart rate; urine output; skin temperature and color of extremities; level of consciousness; orientation to person, place, and time; and adequacy of respiration. Abnormal values are not specific indicators of hypotension and shock, but they may indicate a need for further evaluation. In general, report blood pressure below 90/60, heart rate above 100, and urine output below 30 mL/hour.
- Assess electrocardiogram (ECG) and cardiac and hemodynamic status for indications of impaired cardiac function.
- Monitor available laboratory reports for abnormal values (eg, decreased oxygen saturation levels indicate decreased oxygenation of tissues; abnormal arterial blood gases may indicate metabolic acidosis; an increased hematocrit may indicate hypovolemia; an increased eosinophil count may indicate anaphylaxis; the presence of bacteria in blood cultures may indicate sepsis; an increased serum creatinine and blood urea nitrogen may indicate impending renal failure).

### Nursing Diagnoses

- Decreased Cardiac Output related to altered stroke volume
- Ineffective Tissue Perfusion: Decreased related to compromised cardiac output
- Deficient Fluid Volume related to fluid loss or vasodilation
- Anxiety related to potentially life-threatening illness
- Risk for Injury: Myocardial infarction, stroke, or renal damage related to decreased blood flow to vital organs

### Planning/Goals

*The client will:*

- Have improved tissue perfusion and relief of symptoms
- Have improved vital signs
- Be guarded against recurrence of hypotension and shock if possible
- Be assessed for therapeutic and adverse effects of adrenergic drugs
- Avoid preventable adverse effects of adrenergic drugs

### Interventions

Use measures to prevent or minimize hypotension and shock.

- General measures include those to maintain the airway, maintain fluid balance, control hemorrhage, manage infections, prevent hypoxia, and control other causative factors.
- Learn to recognize impending shock so management can be initiated early. Do not wait until symptoms are severe. The earlier the management, the greater the likelihood of reversing shock and preventing end-organ damage.
- Assist in recognizing and managing the underlying cause of shock in a particular client (eg, replacing fluids; preventing further loss of blood or other body fluids).

Monitor clients during shock and vasopressor drug therapy.

- Titrate adrenergic drug infusions to maintain blood pressure and tissue perfusion without causing hypertension.
- Check blood pressure and pulse constantly or at least every 5 to 15 minutes during acute shock and vasopressor drug therapy. Intra-arterial monitoring may be more reliable than cuff blood pressures in shock conditions.
- Monitor mental status, distal pulses, urine output, and skin temperature and color closely to assess tissue perfusion.
- Assess venipuncture sites frequently for signs of infiltration or extravasation. Have phentolamine (Regitine), an alpha-adrenergic blocking agent that reverses vasoconstriction, readily available in any setting where IV adrenergic drugs are used. If infiltration occurs, instill phentolamine through the IV catheter prior to removal.
- Keep family members informed about client status, management measures, including drug therapy, monitoring equipment, and the need for close observation of vital signs, IV infusion site, urine output, and so forth.

### Evaluation

Observe for improved vital signs, color and temperature of skin, urine output, and mental responsiveness.

■ Minimal effective doses of adrenergic drugs are recommended because of their extreme vasoconstrictive effects that can produce lactic acidosis at the cell level and create metabolic acidosis. Because catecholamine drugs have short half-lives, varying the flow rate of IV infusions can easily control dosage. Dosage and flow rate usually are titrated to maintain a low-normal blood pressure. Such titration depends on frequent and accurate blood pressure measurements.

■ Septic shock due to bacterial infection requires appropriate antibiotic therapy in addition to other management measures. If an abscess is the source of infection, it must be surgically drained.

■ Hypovolemic shock is most effectively managed by IV fluids that replace the type of fluid lost; that is, blood loss should be replaced with whole blood; gastrointestinal losses should be replaced with solutions containing electrolytes (eg, Ringer's lactate or sodium chloride solutions with added potassium chloride).

■ Cardiogenic shock may be complicated by pulmonary congestion, for which diuretic drugs are indicated and IV fluids are contraindicated (except to maintain a patent IV line).

■ Anaphylactic shock is often managed by nonadrenergic drugs as well as epinephrine. For example, the histamine-induced cardiovascular symptoms (eg, vasodilation and increased capillary permeability) are thought to be mediated through both types of histamine receptors. Thus, management may include a histamine-1 receptor blocker (eg, diphenhydramine, 1 mg/kg IV) and a histamine-2 receptor blocker (eg, cimetidine, 4 mg/kg IV), given over at least 5 minutes. In addition, IV corticosteroids are often given, such as methylprednisolone (20 to 100 mg) or hydrocortisone (100 to 500 mg). Doses may need to be repeated every 2 to 4 hours. Corticosteroids increase tissue responsiveness to adrenergic drugs in approximately 2 hours but do not produce anti-inflammatory effects for several hours.

## Nursing Actions
## Drugs Used in Hypotension and Shock

| Nursing Actions | Rationale/Explanation |
|---|---|
| 1. Administer accurately. | |
| a. Use a large vein for the venipuncture site. | To decrease risks of extravasation |
| b. Dilute drugs for continuous infusion in 250 or 500 mL of intravenous (IV) fluid. A 5% dextrose injection is compatible with all of the drugs and is most often used. For use of other IV fluids, consult drug manufacturers' literature. Dilute drugs for bolus injections to at least 10 mL with sodium chloride or water for injection. | To avoid adverse effects, which are more likely to occur with concentrated drug solutions |
| c. Use a separate IV line or a "piggyback" IV setup. | This allows the adrenergic drug solution to be regulated or discontinued without disruption of other IV lines. |
| d. Use an infusion pump | To administer the drug at a consistent rate and prevent wide fluctuations in blood pressure and other cardiovascular functions |
| e. Discard any solution with a brownish color or precipitate. | Most of the solutions are stable for 24–48 h. Epinephrine and isoproterenol decompose on exposure to light, producing a brownish discoloration. |
| f. Start the adrenergic drug slowly, and increase as necessary to obtain desired responses in blood pressure and other parameters of cardiovascular function. | Flow rate (dosage) is titrated according to client response. |
| g. Stop the drug gradually. | Abrupt discontinuance of pressor drugs may cause rebound hypotension. |
| h. Manage the client, not the monitor. | Abnormal monitor readings (ie, blood pressure monitors) should be confirmed with a manual reading before adjusting medication dosage. |
| 2. Observe for therapeutic effects. | |
| a. Systolic blood pressure of 80–100 mm Hg | These levels are adequate for tissue perfusion. Higher levels may increase cardiac workload, resulting in reflex bradycardia and decreased cardiac output. However, higher levels may be necessary to maintain cerebral blood flow in older adults. |

(continued)

## Nursing Actions

### Drugs Used in Hypotension and Shock (Continued)

| Nursing Actions | Rationale/Explanation |
|---|---|
| b. Heart rate of 60–100, improved quality of peripheral pulses | These indicate improved tissue perfusion and cardiovascular function. |
| c. Improved urine output | Increased urine output indicates improved blood flow to the kidneys. |
| d. Improved skin color and temperature | These indicate improved peripheral tissue perfusion. |
| e. Pulmonary capillary wedge pressure between 15 and 20 mm Hg in cardiogenic shock | Normal pulmonary capillary wedge pressure is 6–12 mm Hg. Higher levels are required to maintain cardiac output in cardiogenic shock. |

**3. Observe for adverse effects.**

| Nursing Actions | Rationale/Explanation |
|---|---|
| a. Bradycardia | Reflex bradycardia may occur with norepinephrine, metaraminol, and phenylephrine. |
| b. Tachycardia | This is most likely to occur with isoproterenol, but may occur with dopamine and epinephrine. |
| c. Dysrhythmias | Serious dysrhythmias may occur with any of the agents used in hypotension and shock. Causes may include high doses that result in excessive adrenergic stimulation of the heart, low doses that result in inadequate perfusion of the myocardium, or the production of lactic acid by ischemic tissue. |
| d. Hypertension | This is most likely to occur with high doses of norepinephrine, metaraminol, and phenylephrine. |
| e. Hypotension | This is most likely to occur with low doses of dopamine and isoproterenol, owing to vasodilation. |
| f. Angina pectoris—chest pain, dyspnea, palpitations | All pressor agents may increase myocardial oxygen consumption and induce myocardial ischemia. |
| g. Tissue necrosis if extravasation occurs | This may occur with solutions containing dopamine, norepinephrine, metaraminol, and phenylephrine, owing to local vasoconstriction and impaired blood supply. Tissue necrosis may be prevented by injecting 5–10 mg of phentolamine (Regitine) through the catheter or subcutaneously, around the area of extravasation. Phentolamine is most effective if injected within 12 h after extravasation. |

**4. Observe for drug interactions.**

a. Drugs that *increase* effects of pressor agents:

| Nursing Actions | Rationale/Explanation |
|---|---|
| (1) General anesthetics (eg, halothane) | Halothane and other halogenated anesthetics increase cardiac sensitivity to sympathomimetic drugs and increase the risks of cardiac dysrhythmias. |
| (2) Anticholinergic drugs (eg, atropine) | Atropine and other drugs with anticholinergic activity may potentiate the tachycardia that often occurs with pressor agents, especially isoproterenol. |
| (3) Monoamine oxidase (MAO) inhibitors (eg, tranylcypromine) | All effects of exogenously administered adrenergic drugs are magnified in clients taking MAO inhibitors because MAO is the circulating enzyme responsible for metabolism of adrenergic agents. |
| (4) Oxytocics (eg, oxytocin) | The risk of severe hypertension is increased. |

b. Drugs that *decrease* effects of pressor agents:

| Nursing Actions | Rationale/Explanation |
|---|---|
| (1) Beta-blocking agents (eg, propranolol) | Beta-blocking agents antagonize the cardiac stimulation of some pressor agents (eg, dobutamine, isoproterenol). Decreased heart rate, myocardial contractility, and blood pressure may result. |

## ? How Can You Avoid This Medication Error?

**Answer:** Considering that extravasation of this medication can cause very significant tissue damage, this was a very poor decision. IV medications sometimes infuse at very slow rates, so that swelling is not present when the IV solution has infiltrated. It is the responsibility of the nurse to be knowledgeable regarding which drugs are vesicants and to take special precautions. Vasopressor agents significantly constrict the vessels of the surrounding tissue, thus impeding blood flow and causing necrosis. Whenever possible, infuse these medications into central lines. When extravasation occurs, phentolamine (Regitine), an alpha-adrenergic blocker, can be injected into the tissue to reverse vasoconstriction and restore blood flow.

## Critical Thinking Exercises

1. During administration of dopamine, a client complains of pain at the infusion site. The nurse should recognize that the:
   a. Client is hypersensitive to the drug
   b. Infusion rate is too fast
   c. Infusion site should be immediately changed
   d. Medication is not effective

2. A client in cardiogenic shock is started on dobutamine (Dobutrex). The health care provider's order reads: dobutamine, 10 mcg/kg per minute IV. What effect should the nurse expect after beginning drug therapy?
   a. Enhanced cardiac contraction and contractility through stimulation of alpha$_1$, beta$_1$, and beta$_2$ receptors
   b. Dilated blood vessels through stimulation of dopamine receptors
   c. Increased cardiac output through stimulation of beta$_1$ receptors
   d. Constricted blood vessels and increased cardiac output through stimulation of alpha$_1$ receptors

3. A client receiving norepinephrine (Levophed) for shock has an arterial line in place. The client's blood pressure has been near 90/42 mm Hg for most of the morning. The blood pressure reading on the monitor suddenly shows a blood pressure of 130/80 mm Hg. The nurse should:
   a. Decrease the rate of the norepinephrine
   b. Call the health care provider
   c. Stop the norepinephrine infusion
   d. Confirm the blood pressure with a manual reading

4. A client with anaphylactic shock presents to the emergency department. The nurse should anticipate that the drug of choice for this type of shock would be:
   a. Dobutamine
   b. Dopamine
   c. Isoproterenol
   d. Epinephrine

## SELECTED REFERENCES

Dax, J. M., & Hermey, C. L. (2000). Shock and multiple organ dysfunction syndrome. In S. M. Lewis, M. M. Heitkemper, & S. R. Dirksen (Eds.), *Medical-surgical nursing: Assessment and management of clinical problems* (5th ed., pp. 1865–1894). St. Louis: Mosby.

Erstad, B. L. (2002). Hypovolemic shock. In J. T. DiPiro, R. L. Talbert, G. C. Yee, G. R. Matzke, B. G. Wells, & L. M. Posey (Eds.), *Pharmacotherapy: A pathophysiologic approach* (5th ed., pp. 453–466). New York: McGraw-Hill.

Hennessy, C. L., & Porth, C. M. (2002). Heart failure and circulatory shock. In C. M. Porth (Ed.), *Pathophysiology: Concepts of altered health states* (6th ed., pp. 547–574). Philadelphia: Lippincott Williams & Wilkins.

Karch, A. M. (2003). *Lippincott's 2003 nursing drug guide.* Philadelphia: Lippincott Williams & Wilkins.

Lacy, C. F., Armstrong, L. L., Goldman, M. P., & Lance, L. L. (2003). *Lexi-Comp's drug information handbook* (11th ed.). Hudson, OH: American Pharmaceutical Association.

Rudis, M. I., & Dasta, J. F. (2002). Vasopressors and inotropes in shock. In J. T. DiPiro, R. L. Talbert, G. C. Yee, G. R. Matzke, B. G. Wells, & L. M. Posey (Eds.), *Pharmacotherapy: A pathophysiologic approach* (5th ed., pp. 435–451). New York: McGraw-Hill.

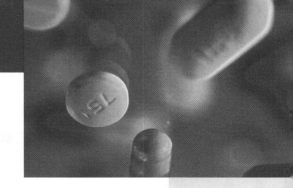

# 43

# Antihypertensive Drugs

## OBJECTIVES

*After studying this chapter, the student will be able to:*

1 Identify nonpharmacologic measures to control hypertension.

2 Review the effects of alpha-adrenergic blockers, beta-adrenergic blockers, calcium channel blockers, and diuretics in hypertension.

3 Discuss angiotensin-converting enzyme inhibitors and angiotensin II receptor antagonists in terms of mechanisms of action, indications for use, adverse effects, and nursing process implications.

4 Describe the rationale for using combination drugs in the management of hypertension.

5 Give interventions to increase therapeutic effects and minimize adverse effects of antihypertensive drugs.

6 Discuss the use of antihypertensive drugs in special populations.

## CRITICAL THINKING SCENARIO

*W*ally Ramos, a 36-year-old man, returns to the clinic for his third blood pressure check. Because his blood pressure is still elevated (178/96 mm Hg), the health care provider decides to start him on an angiotensin-converting enzyme inhibitor, captopril. He states, "I just can't believe I have high blood pressure. I feel just fine. I have heard stories that these medications have lots of undesirable side effects."

✔ Describe an appropriate teaching plan discussing hypertension and its effects.

✔ Describe an appropriate teaching plan discussing nonpharmacologic strategies to decrease blood pressure.

✔ How will you address Mr. Ramos' concerns about potential side effects?

✔ What factors could affect compliance with antihypertensive therapy?

## PROTOTYPE PROFILES

captopril (Capoten), p. 783

losartan (Cozaar), p. 785

prazosin (Minipress), p. 786

# OVERVIEW

Antihypertensive drugs are used to treat hypertension, a common, chronic disorder affecting an estimated 50 to 60 million adults and an unknown number of children and adolescents in the United States. Hypertension increases risks for myocardial infarction, heart failure, cerebral infarction and hemorrhage, and renal disease. To understand antihypertensive drug therapy, it is necessary to understand the physiologic mechanisms that normally control blood pressure and the body's response to hypertension. A description of these can be found in At the Foundation: Regulation of Blood Pressure and Hypertension.

Once the diagnosis of hypertension is established, a therapeutic regimen must be designed and implemented. The goal of management for most clients is to achieve and maintain normal blood pressure range (below 140/90 mm Hg in adults). If this goal cannot be achieved, lowering blood pressure to any extent is still considered beneficial in decreasing the incidence of coronary artery disease and stroke.

Hypertensive emergencies are episodes of severely elevated blood pressure that may be an extension of malignant (rapidly progressive) hypertension or caused by cerebral hemorrhage, dissecting aortic aneurysm, renal disease, pheochromocytoma, or eclampsia. These require immediate management, usually intravenous (IV) antihypertensive drugs, to lower blood pressure. Symptoms include severe headache, nausea, vomiting, visual disturbances, neurologic disturbances, disorientation, and decreased level of consciousness (drowsiness, stupor, coma). Hypertensive urgencies are episodes of less severe hypertension and are often managed with oral drugs. The goal of management is to lower blood pressure within 24 hours. In most instances, it is better to lower blood pressure gradually and to avoid wide fluctuations in blood pressure. Discussion of management considerations in children and older adults is found in Age-related Considerations. Guidelines for ongoing evaluation and intervention in the home are addressed in Home Care Considerations.

# NONPHARMACOLOGIC MANAGEMENT OF HYPERTENSION

Several nonpharmacologic measures are useful in reducing blood pressure. These measures include (1) weight reduction; (2) exercise; (3) salt restriction in diet; (4) stress reduction; (5) DASH eating plan (diet rich in fruits and vegetables and low in saturated and total fats); and (6) moderation in alcohol intake. If the systolic blood pressure cannot be maintained below 140 mm Hg through nonpharmacologic means, antihypertensive drugs are usually added to the treatment plan.

## AT THE FOUNDATION: *Regulation of Blood Pressure and Hypertension*

Arterial blood pressure reflects the force exerted on arterial walls by blood flow. Blood pressure normally stays relatively constant because of homeostatic mechanisms that adjust blood flow to meet tissue needs. The two major determinants of arterial blood pressure are cardiac output (systolic pressure) and peripheral vascular resistance (diastolic pressure).

Autoregulation is the ability of body tissues to regulate their own blood flow. Local blood flow is regulated mainly by nutritional needs of the tissue, such as lack of oxygen or accumulation of products of cellular metabolism (eg, carbon dioxide, lactic acid). Local tissues can form vasodilating and vasoconstricting substances to regulate local blood flow. Important tissue factors include histamine, bradykinin, serotonin, and prostaglandins.

Overall, regulation of blood pressure involves a complex, interacting, overlapping network of hormonal, neural, and vascular mechanisms. Any condition that affects heart rate, stroke volume, or peripheral vascular resistance affects arterial blood pressure. Many of these mechanisms are compensatory effects that try to restore balance when hypotension or hypertension occurs. The mechanisms are further described in Box 41-1 and referred to in the following discussion of antihypertensive drugs and their actions in lowering high blood pressure.

Hypertension profoundly alters cardiovascular function by increasing the workload of the heart and causing thickening and sclerosis of arterial walls. As a result of increased cardiac workload, the myocardium hypertrophies as a compensatory mechanism, and heart failure eventually occurs. As a result of endothelial dysfunction and arterial changes (vascular remodeling), the arterial lumen is narrowed, blood supply to tissues is decreased, and risks for thrombosis are increased. In addition, necrotic areas may develop in arteries, and these may rupture with sustained high blood pressure. The areas of most serious damage are the heart, brain, kidneys, and eyes. These are often called *target organs*.

When arterial blood pressure is elevated, the following sequence of events occurs: (1) kidneys excrete more fluid (increase urine output); (2) fluid loss reduces both extracellular fluid volume and blood volume; (3) decreased blood volume reduces venous blood flow to the heart and therefore decreases cardiac output; (4) decreased cardiac output reduces arterial blood pressure, and (5) the vascular endothelium produces vasodilating substances (eg, nitric oxide, prostacyclin), which reduce blood pressure.

# Age-related Considerations: Use of Antihypertensive Drugs

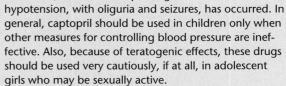

## USE IN CHILDREN

Most principles of managing adult hypertension apply to managing childhood and adolescent hypertension; some additional elements include the following:

- Children may have primary or secondary hypertension, but the incidence is unknown, and treatment is not well defined. In recent years, increased blood pressure measurements during routine pediatric examinations have led to the discovery of significant asymptomatic hypertension and the realization that mild elevations in blood pressure are more common during childhood, especially in adolescents, than previously thought. Hypertension in children and adolescents may indicate underlying disease processes (eg, cardiac, endocrine, renovascular, or renal parenchymal disorders) or the early onset of primary hypertension. Routine blood pressure measurement is especially important for children who are overweight or who have a hypertensive parent. Increased blood pressure in children often correlates with hypertension in young adults.
- National norms have been established for blood pressure in children and adolescents of comparable age, body size (height and weight), and sex. Normal blood pressure is defined as systolic and diastolic values less than the 90th percentile; hypertension is defined as an average of systolic or diastolic pressures that equals or exceeds the 95th percentile on three or more occasions. Blood pressure values obtained with a child or adolescent should be compared with the norms and recorded in permanent health care records. Multiple accurate measurements are especially important in diagnosing hypertension because blood pressure may be more labile in children and adolescents.
- The goals of management are to reduce blood pressure to below the 95th percentile and prevent the long-term effects of persistent hypertension. As in adults, prevention of obesity, avoiding excessive sodium intake, and exercise are important nonpharmacologic measures. Obese adolescents who lose weight may lower their blood pressure, especially when they also increase physical activity.
- Drug therapy should be cautious and conservative because few studies have been done in children, and long-term effects are unknown. The fewest drugs and the lowest doses should be used. Thus, if an initial drug is ineffective, it may be better to give a different single drug than to add a second drug to the regimen.
- Some guidelines for choosing drugs include the following:
  - Beta blockers are used in children of all ages; they should probably be avoided in children with resting pulse rates under 60 beats/minute.
  - Thiazide diuretics may be used, and they do not commonly produce hyperglycemia, hyperuricemia, or hypercalcemia in children as they do in adults.
  - Angiotensin II receptor blockers have not been established as safe and effective for use in children younger than 18 years of age.
  - Although ACE inhibitors have been used to treat hypertension in children, their safety and efficacy have not been established. Most clinical experience has been with captopril, with which hemodynamic effects are

stronger and last longer in newborns and young infants than in older children. Also, excessive and prolonged hypotension, with oliguria and seizures, has occurred. In general, captopril should be used in children only when other measures for controlling blood pressure are ineffective. Also, because of teratogenic effects, these drugs should be used very cautiously, if at all, in adolescent girls who may be sexually active.
  - Calcium channel blockers are used in treating acute and chronic childhood hypertension. With chronic hypertension, immediate-release forms have a short duration of action and require frequent administration, and long-acting forms contain dosages that are not suitable for young children.
  - Hydralazine seems to be less effective in childhood and adolescent hypertension than in adult disease.
- Although all clients with primary hypertension need regular supervision and assessment of blood pressure, this is especially important with young children and adolescents because of growth and developmental changes.

## USE IN OLDER ADULTS

- Most principles of managing hypertension in other populations apply to older adults (>65 years). In addition, the following factors require consideration:
- There are basically two types of hypertension in older adults. One is systolic hypertension, in which systolic blood pressure is above 160 mm Hg, but diastolic pressure is below 95 mm Hg or normal. The other type, systolic-diastolic hypertension, involves elevations of both systolic and diastolic pressures.
- Both types increase cardiovascular morbidity and mortality, especially heart failure and stroke, and should be treated.
- Nonpharmacologic management should be tried alone or with drug therapy. For example, weight reduction and moderate sodium restriction may be the initial management of choice if the client is hypertensive and overweight.
- If antihypertensive drug therapy is required, drugs used for younger adults may be used alone or in combination. A diuretic is usually the drug of first choice in older adults and may be effective alone. ACE inhibitors and calcium channel blocking agents may also be effective as monotherapy; beta blockers are usually less effective as monotherapy. Some ACE inhibitors (eg, lisinopril, ramipril, quinapril, moexipril) or their active metabolites produce higher plasma concentrations in older adults than in younger ones. This is attributed to decreased renal function rather than age itself. Additional guidelines include the following:
  - The goal of drug therapy for systolic-diastolic hypertension is usually a systolic pressure below 140 mm Hg and a diastolic below 90 mm Hg in clients with no other complications. For those with diabetes or renal failure, the goal is a systolic pressure below 130 mm Hg and a diastolic below 80 mm Hg. However, both goals may be difficult for most clients to meet because they require

*(continued)*

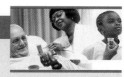

## Age-related Considerations: Use of Antihypertensive Drugs (Continued)

rather stringent lifestyle restrictions and may require two or more antihypertensive drugs.

• Older adults may be especially susceptible to the adverse effects of antihypertensive drugs because their homeostatic mechanisms are less efficient. For example, if hypotension occurs, the mechanisms that raise blood pressure are less efficient and syncope may occur. In addition, renal and liver function may be reduced, making accumulation of drugs more likely.

• Initial drug doses should be approximately half of the recommended doses for younger adults, and increases should be smaller and spaced at longer intervals. Lower drug doses (eg, hydrochlorothiazide, 12.5 mg daily) are

often effective and reduce risks for adverse effects.

• Blood pressure should be reduced slowly to facilitate adequate blood flow through arteriosclerotic vessels. Rapid lowering of blood pressure may produce cerebral insufficiency (syncope, transient ischemic attacks, stroke).

• A further incentive for successful management of hypertension in older clients is the benefit of reducing the incidence of dementia with antihypertensives.

• If blood pressure control is achieved and maintained for approximately 6 to 12 months, drug dosage should be gradually reduced, if possible.

---

## ANTIHYPERTENSIVE DRUGS

Drugs used in the management of primary hypertension belong to several different groups, including angiotensin-converting enzyme (ACE) inhibitors, angiotensin II receptor blockers (ARBs), also called angiotensin II receptor antagonists (AIIRAs), antiadrenergics, calcium channel blockers, diuretics, and direct vasodilators. In general, these drugs act to decrease blood pressure by decreasing cardiac output or peripheral vascular resistance.

## Angiotensin–converting Enzyme Inhibitors

ACE (also called *kininase*) is mainly located in the endothelial lining of blood vessels, which is the site of production of most angiotensin II. This same enzyme also metabolizes bradykinin, an endogenous substance with strong vasodilating properties.

ACE inhibitors block the enzyme that normally converts angiotensin I to the potent vasoconstrictor angi-

otensin II. By blocking production of angiotensin II, the drugs decrease vasoconstriction (having a vasodilating effect) and decrease aldosterone production (reducing retention of sodium and water). In addition to inhibiting formation of angiotensin II, the drugs also inhibit the breakdown of bradykinin, prolonging its vasodilating effects. These effects and possibly others help to prevent or reverse the remodeling of heart muscle and blood vessel walls that impairs cardiovascular function and exacerbates cardiovascular disease processes. Because of their effectiveness in hypertension and beneficial effects on the heart, blood vessels, and kidneys, these drugs are increasing in importance, number, and use. Widely used to treat heart failure and hypertension, the drugs may also decrease morbidity and mortality in other cardiovascular disorders. They improve postmyocardial infarction survival when added to standard therapy of aspirin, a beta blocker, and a thrombolytic.

ACE inhibitors may be used alone or in combination with other antihypertensive agents, such as thiazide diuretics. They may be effective alone in white hypertensive clients or in combination with a diuretic in African-American hypertensive clients. ACE inhibitors are also recommended for hypertensive adults with diabetes mellitus and kidney damage. Although the drugs can cause or aggravate proteinuria and renal damage in non-diabetic people, they decrease proteinuria and slow the development of nephropathy in diabetic clients. Based on research studies that indicate reduced morbidity and mortality from cardiovascular diseases, these drugs are increasingly being prescribed as a component of a multi-drug regimen.

Most ACE inhibitors (captopril, enalapril, fosinopril, lisinopril, ramipril, and quinapril) also are used in the management of heart failure because they decrease peripheral vascular resistance, cardiac workload, and ventricular remodeling. ℗ **Captopril,** the prototype of the group, is highlighted in Prototype Profile 43-1: Captopril. This drug and other ACE inhibitors are recommended as

## Home Care Considerations: Use of Antihypertensive Drugs

***ASSESS:*** blood pressure and signs of therapeutic and adverse response; for actual or potential barriers to compliance. For example, several antihypertensive medications are quite expensive, and clients may not take the drugs at all, or they may take fewer than the prescribed number of doses.

***MONITOR:*** drug effect and compliance with prescribed regimen (pharmacologic and lifestyle modifications).

***EDUCATE:*** about potential side effects that necessitate seeking professional help. Reinforce additional teaching points (see Client Teaching Guidelines: Antihypertensive Medications).

## PROTOTYPE PROFILE 43-1

### P Captopril (KAP toe pril)

**Drug Class**

*Chemical:* Angiotensin-converting enzyme (ACE) inhibitor
*Functional:* Antihypertensive agent

**Trade Name**

Capoten

**Therapeutic Indications**

Management of hypertension; treatment of heart failure, post–myocardial infarction left ventricular failure, diabetic nephropathy

**Pharmacokinetics**

*Absorption*

60%–75%; food reduces absorption 30%–40%

*Distribution*

Plasma protein binding: 25%–30%

*Metabolism*

50%

*Excretion*

Urine

**Pharmacodynamics**

*Onset of Action*

15 min; peak blood pressure reduction 1–1.5 h after administration

*Duration*

6–12 h; dose related; may require several weeks for full antihypertensive effect

**Contraindications/Precautions**

Hypersensitivity to captopril; heart failure; primary hyperaldosteronism; bilateral renal artery stenosis; pregnancy, particularly second and third trimesters

**Pregnancy Considerations**

Category: C/D (second and third trimester); reported to cause birth defects
Enters breast milk (compatible)

**Dosage**

*Adults:* PO, 25 mg, 2–3 times daily initially, gradually increased to 50, 100, or 150 mg 2–3 times daily, if necessary. Maximum dose, 450 mg/d
*Children:* PO, 1.5 mg/kg/d in divided doses, q8h; maximum dose, 6 mg/kg/d
*Neonates:* PO, 0.03–0.15 mg/kg/d, q8–24h maximum dose, 2 mg/kg/d

**Side Effects/Adverse Reactions**

Cough, hyperkalemia, nocturia, dizziness, taste disturbance, impotence, rash, angioedema, fetal injury

**Drug Interactions**

*Increased Effects*

Hypotensive effect with diuretics, nitrates, vasodilators, adrenergic blockers or other antihypertensive drugs
Risk for hyperkalemia with use with potassium supplements, angiotensin II receptor antagonists, or potassium-sparing diuretics

*Decreased Effects*

Effect of ACE inhibitors with high-dose aspirin therapy

**Herbal Supplements and Dietary Considerations**

Long-term use can result in a zinc deficiency that may decrease taste perception
Should be taken 1 h before or 2 h after eating

---

first-line agents for treating hypertension in diabetic clients, particularly those with type 1 diabetes mellitus or diabetic nephropathy, because they reduce proteinuria and slow the progression of renal impairment.

ACE inhibitors are well absorbed with oral administration, produce effects within 1 hour that last approximately 24 hours, have prolonged serum half-lives with impaired renal function, and most are metabolized to active metabolites that are excreted in urine and feces. These drugs are well tolerated, with a low incidence of serious adverse effects (eg, neutropenia, agranulocytosis, proteinuria, glomerulonephritis, and angioedema). However, a persistent cough develops in approximately 10% to 20% of clients and may lead to stopping the drug. Also, acute hypotension may occur when an ACE inhibitor is started, especially in clients with fluid volume deficit. Starting with a low dose, taken at bedtime, or stopping diuretics and reducing dosage of other antihypertensive drugs temporarily may prevent this reac-

tion. Hyperkalemia may develop in clients who have diabetes mellitus or renal impairment or who are taking nonsteroidal anti-inflammatory drugs, potassium supplements, or potassium-sparing diuretics. These drugs are contraindicated during pregnancy because serious illnesses, including renal failure, have occurred in neonates whose mothers took an ACE inhibitor during the second and third trimesters.

## Angiotensin II Receptor Blockers

ARBs were developed to block the strong blood pressure–raising effects of angiotensin II. Instead of decreasing production of angiotensin II, as the ACE inhibitors do, these drugs compete with angiotensin II for tissue binding sites and prevent angiotensin II from combining with its receptors in body tissues. Although multiple types of receptors have been identified, the AT1 receptors located in brain, renal, myocardial, vascular, and adrenal tissue determine most of the effects of angiotensin II on cardiovascular and renal functions. ARBs block the angiotensin II AT1 receptors and decrease arterial blood pressure by decreasing systemic vascular resistance (Fig. 43-1).

These drugs are similar to ACE inhibitors in their effects on blood pressure and hemodynamics and are as effective as ACE inhibitors in the management of hypertension and probably heart failure. They are less likely to cause hyperkalemia than ACE inhibitors, and the occurrence of a persistent cough is rare. Overall, the drugs are well tolerated, and the incidence of most adverse effects is similar to that of placebo.

ⓟ **Losartan,** the first ARB, is considered the prototype and is discussed in Prototype Profile 43-2: Losartan. The drug is readily absorbed and rapidly metabolized by the cytochrome P450 liver enzymes to an active metabolite. Both losartan and the metabolite are highly bound to plasma albumin, and losartan has a shorter duration of action than its metabolite. When losartan therapy is started, maximal effects on blood pressure usually occur within 3 to 6 weeks. If losartan alone does not control blood pressure, a low dose of a diuretic may be added. A combination product of losartan and hydrochlorothiazide is available.

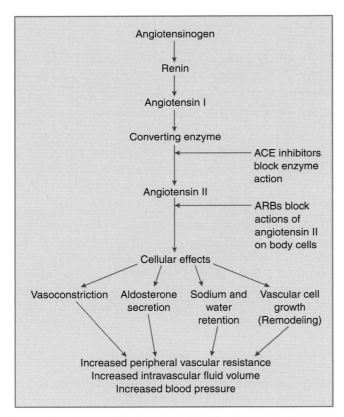

**FIGURE 43–1** Angiotensin-converting (ACE) enzyme inhibitors inhibit angiotensin-converting enzyme and thereby prevent formation of angiotensin II; angiotensin II receptor blockers (ARBs) prevent angiotensin II from connecting with its receptors and thereby prevent it from acting on body tissues containing those receptors (eg, blood vessels, adrenal cortex).

Dosage reductions of ARBs usually are not required for clients with renal impairment. However, fluid volume deficits (eg, from diuretic therapy) should be corrected before starting the drug, and blood pressure should be monitored closely during drug therapy. Clients on hemodialysis may have orthostatic hypotension with telmisartan and possibly other drugs of this group.

## Antiadrenergics

Antiadrenergic (sympatholytic) drugs inhibit activity of the sympathetic nervous system (SNS). When the SNS is stimulated, the nerve impulse travels from the brain and spinal cord to the ganglia. From the ganglia, the impulse travels along postganglionic fibers to effector organs (eg, heart, blood vessels). Although SNS stimulation produces widespread effects in the body, the effects relevant to this discussion are the increases in heart rate, force of myocardial contraction, cardiac output, and blood pressure that occur. When the nerve impulse is inhibited or blocked at any location along its pathway, the result is decreased blood pressure (see Chap. 17).

Alpha$_1$-adrenergic receptor blocking agents, such as ⓟ **prazosin** (see Prototype Profile 43-3: Prazosin), dilate blood vessels and decrease peripheral vascular resistance. These drugs can be used alone or in multidrug regimens. One adverse effect, called the *first-dose phenomenon,* results in orthostatic hypotension with palpitations, dizziness, and perhaps syncope 1 to 3 hours after the first dose or an increased dose. To prevent this effect, first doses and first increased doses are taken at bedtime. Another effect, associated with long-term use or higher doses, leads to sodium and fluid retention and a need for concurrent diuretic therapy. Centrally acting sympatholytics (eg, clonidine) stimulate presynaptic alpha$_2$ receptors in the brain and are classified as alpha$_2$ receptor agonists. When these drugs are taken, less norepinephrine is released, and sympathetic outflow from the vasomotor center is reduced. Stimulation of presynaptic alpha$_2$ receptors peripherally may also contribute to the decreased sympathetic activity. Reduced sympathetic activity leads to decreased cardiac output, heart rate, peripheral vascular resistance, and blood pressure. Chronic use of clonidine and related drugs may result in sodium and fluid retention, especially with higher doses. Clonidine is available in a skin patch that is applied once a week and reportedly reduces adverse effects and increases compliance. An additional advantage of transdermal clonidine is that clients who cannot take oral medications can use it. A disadvantage of this system is a delayed onset of effect (2 to 3 days); hence, other antihypertensive medications must also be given during the first 2 to 3 days of clonidine transdermal therapy. Other disadvantages include cost, a 20% incidence of local skin rash or irritation, and a 2- to 3-day delay in "offset" of action when transdermal therapy is discontinued.

Beta-adrenergic blocking agents (eg, propranolol) decrease heart rate, force of myocardial contraction, car-

## PROTOTYPE PROFILE 43-2

### Ⓟ Losartan (loe SAR tan)

**Drug Class**
*Chemical:* Angiotensin II receptor antagonist (ARB)
*Functional:* Antihypertensive agent

**Trade Name**
Cozaar

**Therapeutic Indications**
Treatment of hypertension, as single agent or in combination; nephropathy in type 2 diabetes mellitus with hypertension

**Pharmacokinetics**
*Absorption*
Well absorbed orally

*Distribution*
High level of plasma protein binding; does not cross blood–brain barrier

*Metabolism*
Liver, with extensive first-pass effect; active metabolite, carboxylic acid, responsible for most of the angiotensin receptor blockade (metabolite 40 times more potent that losartan)

*Excretion*
Feces (60%), urine (35%), remainder as unchanged drug

**Pharmacodynamics**
*Onset of Action*
6 h

*Duration*
Half-life elimination of losartan 1.5–2 h; metabolite 6–9 h

**Contraindications/Precautions**
Hypersensitivity, primary hyperaldosteronism, bilateral renal artery stenosis, pregnancy in second or third trimester; with caution, in clients with preexisting renal insufficiency, or significant mitral or aortic valvular disease, unilateral renal artery stenosis, volume depletion

**Pregnancy Considerations**
Category C; D in second and third trimesters
Excretion in breast milk unknown; not recommended

**Dosage**
*Adults:* Hypertension
Initial dose: PO, 50 mg daily (25 mg for those who have hepatic impairment or are taking a diuretic)
Maintenance dose: PO, 35–100 mg daily, in 1 or 2 doses, adjusted according to blood pressure control
Nephropathy:
Initial dose: PO, 50 mg once daily
Maintenance dose: PO, 50–100 mg once daily, adjusted according to blood pressure control
*Children:* Safety and efficacy not established

**Adverse Effects**
Chest pain, ventricular dysrhythmias, fatigue, cough, anemia

**Drug Interactions**
*Increased Effects*
Absorption of losartan with cimetidine
Increased blood levels of losartan with amiodarone, isoniazid, sulfonamides, fluoxetine, ritonavir, diltiazem, verapamil, erythromycin, itraconazole, ketoconazole
Increased risk for hyperkalemia with ACE inhibitors, potassium-sparing diuretics, potassium supplements

*Decreased Effects*
Decreased hypertensive effect with indomethacin and rifampin
Decreased efficacy of losartan with concomitant use with NSAIDs
Decreased losartan level with concomitant use of phenobarbital

**Herbal Supplements and Dietary Considerations**
St. John's wort may decrease levels
Dong quai has estrogenic effect so avoid if using for antihypertensive effect
Ginseng, ephedra, and yohimbe may worsen hypertension
Garlic may increase antihypertensive effect
May be taken with or without food
Grapefruit juice may decrease metabolism of losartan to its active form

---

diac output, and renin release from the kidneys. They are the drugs of first choice for clients younger than 50 years of age with high-renin hypertension, tachycardia, angina pectoris, myocardial infarction, or left ventricular hypertrophy. Most beta blockers are approved for use in hypertension and are probably equally effective. However, the cardioselective drugs (see Chap. 17) are preferred for hypertensive clients who also have asthma, peripheral vascular disease, or diabetes mellitus. Other antiadrenergic drugs include guanethidine and related drugs, which act at postganglionic nerve endings, and two other alpha

blockers (phentolamine and phenoxybenzamine), which occasionally are used in hypertension resulting from catecholamine excess. Individual antiadrenergic drugs are discussed in Chapter 17.

## Calcium Channel Blocking Agents

Calcium channel blockers (eg, verapamil) are used for several cardiovascular disorders. The mechanism of action and use in the management of tachydysrhythmias and angina pectoris are discussed in Chapters 40 and 41. In

## PROTOTYPE PROFILE 43-3

### *P* Prazosin (PRA zoe sin)

**Drug Class**
*Chemical:* Alpha-adrenergic blocking agent
*Functional:* Antihypertensive agent

**Trade Name**
Minipress

**Therapeutic Indications**
Treatment of hypertension

**Pharmacokinetics**
*Absorption*
GI: 60% (5% to circulation)

*Distribution*
Plasma protein binding: 92%–97%

*Metabolism*
Extensive hepatic metabolism

*Excretion*
Urine

**Pharmacodynamics**
*Onset of Action*
Less than 2 h

*Duration*
10–24 h

**Contraindications/Precautions**
Hypersensitivity to drug; "first-dose phenomenon" (orthostatic hypotension, syncope, loss of consciousness) may occur

**Pregnancy Considerations**
Category C
Excretion in breast milk unknown, so use with caution

**Dosage**
*Adults:* PO, 1 mg 2 to 3 times daily initially, increased if necessary to 20 mg in divided doses. Average maintenance dose, 6–15 mg daily
*Children:* initially 5 mcg/kg/min every 6 h, gradually increased to maximum of 25 mcg/kg/min

**Side Effects/Adverse Reactions**
Dizziness, orthostatic hypotension, headache, drowsiness, decreased energy, constipation

**Drug Interactions**
*Increased Effects*
Hypotensive effect with beta blockers, diuretics, ACE inhibitors, calcium channel blockers, and other antihypertensive medications
Risk for orthostasis with tricyclic antidepressants and low-potency antipsychotics

*Decreased Effects*
Antihypertensive effect with NSAIDs

**Herbal Supplements and Dietary Considerations**
Dong quai has estrogenic effect, so avoid if using for antihypertensive effect; also increases photosensitivity effect
Ginseng, ephedra, and yohimbe may worsen hypertension
Garlic may increase antihypertensive effect
Avoid ethanol as it may increase vasodilation
Food has a variable effect on absorption

---

hypertension, the drugs mainly dilate peripheral arteries and decrease peripheral vascular resistance by relaxing vascular smooth muscle.

Most of the available drugs are approved for use in hypertension. Nifedipine, a short-acting calcium channel blocker, has been used to treat hypertensive emergencies or urgencies, often by puncturing the capsule and squeezing the contents under the tongue or having the client bite and swallow the capsule. Such use is no longer recommended because this practice is associated with an increased risk of adverse cardiovascular events precipitated by rapid and severe decrease in blood pressure.

As a group, the calcium channel blockers are well absorbed from the gastrointestinal tract following oral administration and are highly bound to protein. The drugs are metabolized in the liver and excreted in urine. Calcium channel blockers may be used for monotherapy or in combination with other drugs. They may be especially useful for hypertensive clients who also have angina pectoris or other cardiovascular disorders. Note that sustained-release forms of nifedipine, diltiazem, and ver-

apamil, and other long-acting drugs (eg, amlodipine, felodipine) are recommended.

Calcium channel blockers are often used in clients with renal impairment because, in general, they are effective and well tolerated; they maintain renal blood flow even during blood pressure reduction in most clients; and they are mainly eliminated by hepatic metabolism. However, cautious use is still recommended because several agents produce active metabolites that are excreted by the kidneys.

## Diuretics

Antihypertensive effects of diuretics are usually attributed to sodium and water depletion. In fact, diuretics usually produce the same effects as severe dietary sodium restriction. In many cases of hypertension, diuretic therapy alone may lower blood pressure. When diuretic therapy is begun, blood volume and cardiac output decrease. With long-term administration of a diuretic, cardiac output returns to normal, but there is a persistent decrease in peripheral vascular resistance. This has been attributed to a persistent small reduction in extracellular water and plasma volume, decreased receptor sensitivity to vasopressor substances such as angiotensin, direct arteriolar vasodilation, and arteriolar vasodilation secondary to electrolyte depletion in the vessel wall.

Diuretics are preferred for initial therapy in older clients and African-American hypertensive clients. They should be included in any multidrug regimen for these and other populations. Thiazide-type diuretics should be used for most clients with uncomplicated hypertension. In moderate or severe hypertension that does not respond to a diuretic alone, the diuretic may be continued and another antihypertensive drug added, or monotherapy with a different type of antihypertensive drug may be tried.

The thiazide diuretic, hydrochlorothiazide, is most commonly used in the management of hypertension. Loop diuretics (eg, furosemide) or potassium-sparing diuretics (eg, spironolactone) may be useful in some circumstances; see Chapter 44 for discussion of diuretic drugs.

## Vasodilators (Direct Acting)

Vasodilator antihypertensive drugs directly relax smooth muscle in blood vessels, resulting in dilation and decreased peripheral vascular resistance. They also reduce afterload and may be used in management of heart failure. Hydralazine and minoxidil act mainly on arterioles; nitroprusside acts on arterioles and venules. These drugs have a limited effect on hypertension when used alone because the vasodilating action that lowers blood pressure also stimulates the SNS and triggers reflexive compensatory mechanisms (vasoconstriction, tachycardia, and increased cardiac output), which raise blood pressure. This effect can be prevented during long-term therapy by also giving a drug that prevents excessive sympathetic stimulation (eg, propranolol, an adrenergic blocker). These drugs also cause sodium and water retention, which may be minimized by concomitant diuretic therapy.

## ■ INDIVIDUAL DRUGS

Diuretics are discussed in Chapter 44 and listed in Table 44-1. Antiadrenergic drugs are discussed in Chapter 17 and listed in Tables 17-1 and 17-2. Antihypertensive agents are shown in the Drugs at a Glance 43-1: Antihypertensive Drugs, and combination products are listed in Drugs at a Glance 43-2: Oral Antihypertensive Combination Products.

## ■ MANAGEMENT ALGORITHM

The Seventh Report of the Joint National Committee on Prevention, Detection, Evaluation, and Treatment of High Blood Pressure (JNC 7) released a new management algorithm in May 2003. The updated report provides a new prehypertension classification of blood pressure, new treatment recommendations, and new recommendations on improving current hypertension control rates.

Initial interventions continue as lifestyle modifications (ie, reduction of weight, exercise, adoption of the DASH [Dietary Approaches to Stop Hypertension] eating plan, salt reduction, moderate alcohol intake, and no smoking). The JNC 7 management algorithm considers three groups of clients with hypertension: (1) those with stage 1 hypertension without associated conditions; (2) those with more severe, or stage 2, hypertension without associated conditions; and (3) those with associated conditions that require use of specific classes of blood pressure–lowering medication. For patients with stage 1 or stage 2 uncomplicated hypertension, the goal blood pressure is less than 140/90. In some patients in the third group (those with diabetes or chronic kidney disease), a goal blood pressure of less than 130/80 may be desirable.

Five classes of antihypertensive agents have been shown to reduce complications of hypertension: diuretics, ACE inhibitors, ARBs, beta blockers, and calcium channel blockers. Thiazide diuretics should be used as initial therapy for most patients with hypertension, either alone or in combination with an agent from one of the other four classes. Addition of a second drug from a different class should be initiated when use of a single drug in adequate doses fails to achieve the blood pressure goal. Two-thirds or more of patients require two or more drugs to control hypertension. The selection of the initial medication is probably less important than the need to achieve blood pressure control. Nevertheless, most clinical trials that have shown positive results in lowering blood pressure have included thiazide-type diuretics. Clinical trials have supported the benefits of each of these drug classes in reducing cardiovascular complications, and the most important benefits are related to lowering blood pressure. Overall, antihypertensive therapy has been associated with a more than 50% average reduction in the incidence of heart failure, a 35% to 40% reduction in strokes, and a 20% to 25% decrease in heart attacks. A reduction in the risk of dementia in the elderly also appears to occur through lowering of blood pressure.

Clients who have hypertension associated with specific conditions have been shown by clinical trials to benefit from particular drug tailoring. For example, for individuals who have had a heart attack, beta blockers and ACE inhibitors are preferred; for those at high risk for coronary heart disease, ACE inhibitors, beta blockers, and calcium channel blockers, along with diuretics, are recommended; and for chronic kidney disease, ACE inhibitors and angiotensin receptor blockers are drugs of first choice.

## ■ GENETIC AND ETHNIC CONSIDERATIONS

For most antihypertensive drugs, there have been few research studies comparing their effects in different genetic or ethnic groups. However, several studies indi-

(text continues on page 793)

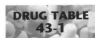

**DRUG TABLE 43-1**

## Drugs at a Glance
## Antihypertensive Drugs

| Generic/Trade Name | Routes and Dosage Ranges | Comments |
|---|---|---|
| **Angiotensin-converting Enzyme (ACE) Inhibitors** | | |
| **Benazepril** (Lotensin) Pregnancy Category C; D (second and third trimesters) | *Adults:* PO, 10 mg once daily initially, increased to 40 mg daily if necessary, in 1 or 2 doses | Observe for hypotensive effects within 1 to 3 h of first dose or increasing new dose as with all ACE Inhibitors |
| **Captopril** (Capoten) Pregnancy Category C; D (second and third trimesters) | See Prototype Profile 43-1: Captopril | |
| **Enalapril** (Vasotec) Pregnancy Category C; D (second and third trimesters) | *Adults:* PO, 5 mg once daily, increased to 10–40 mg daily, in 1 or 2 doses, if necessary *Children:* PO, 0.15 mg q12–24h | May cause depression |
| **Fosinopril** (Monopril) Pregnancy Category C; D (second and third trimesters) | *Adults:* PO, 10 mg once daily initially, increased to 40 mg daily if necessary, in 1 or 2 doses | |
| **Lisinopril** (Prinivil, Zestril) Pregnancy Category C; D (second and third trimesters) | *Adults:* PO, 10 mg once daily, increased to 40 mg if necessary | Angioedema may occur, particularly after first dose as with all ACE Inhibitors |
| **Moexipril** (Univasc) Pregnancy Category C; D (second and third trimesters) | *Adults:* PO, initial dose 7.5 mg (3.75 mg for those who have renal impairment or are taking a diuretic). Maintenance dose 7.5–30 mg daily, in 1 or 2 doses, adjusted according to blood pressure control. | ACE Inhibitors should not be taken during pregnancy |
| **Perindopril** (Aceon) Pregnancy Category C; D (second and third trimesters) | *Adults:* PO, 4–16 mg daily, in 1 or 2 doses | |
| **Quinapril** (Accupril) Pregnancy Category C; D (second and third trimesters) | *Adults:* PO, 10 mg once daily initially, increased to 20, 40, or 80 mg daily if necessary, in 1 or 2 doses | Wait at least 2 wk between dose increments |
| **Ramipril** (Altace) Pregnancy Category C; D (second and third trimesters) | *Adults:* PO, 2.5 mg once daily, increased to 20 mg daily if necessary, in 1 or 2 doses | |
| **Trandolapril** (Mavik) Pregnancy Category C; D (second and third trimesters) | *Adults:* PO, initial dose 1 mg once daily (0.5 mg for those who have hepatic or renal impairment or are taking a diuretic; 2 mg for African Americans). Maintenance dose 2–4 mg daily, in a single dose, adjusted according to blood pressure control | African Americans may require higher dosing |
| **Angiotensin II Receptor Blockers** | | |
| **Candesartan** (Atacand) Pregnancy Category C; D (second and third trimesters) | *Adults:* PO, 16 mg once daily initially, increased if necessary to a maximum of 32 mg daily, in 1 or 2 doses | Risk for lithium toxicity increased with simultaneous administration; avoid during pregnancy as with all drugs in class |
| **Eprosartan** (Teveten) Pregnancy Category C; D (second and third trimesters) | *Adults:* PO, 600 mg daily initially; may be increased to 800 mg daily, in 1 or 2 doses | No initial dosage adjustment is required for elderly or individuals with renal or hepatic impairment |
| **Irbesartan** (Avapro) Pregnancy Category C; D (second and third trimesters) | *Adults:* PO, 150 mg once daily initially, increased up to 300 mg once daily, if necessary | Dosage may need to be adjusted in volume-depleted clients |

*(continued)*

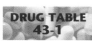

**DRUG TABLE 43-1**

*Drugs at a Glance*

## Antihypertensive Drugs (Continued)

| Generic/Trade Name | Routes and Dosage Ranges | Comments |
|---|---|---|
| **Losartan** (Cozaar)<br>Pregnancy Category C; D (second and third trimesters) | See Prototype Profile 43-2: Losartan | |
| **Olmesartan** (Benicar)<br>Pregnancy Category C; D (second and third trimesters) | *Adults:* PO, 20 mg daily initially, increased to 40 mg after 2 weeks | |
| **Telmisartan** (Micardis)<br>Pregnancy Category C (first trimester); D (second and third trimesters) | *Adults:* PO, 40 mg daily initially, increased to a maximum of 80 mg daily if necessary | May increase serum digoxin levels; decreases trough concentration of warfarin without change in INR |
| **Valsartan** (Diovan)<br>Pregnancy Category C; D (second and third trimesters) | *Adults:* PO, 80 mg daily initially, when used as monotherapy in clients who are not volume depleted. Maintenance dose may be increased. However, adding a diuretic is more effective than increasing dose beyond 80 mg. | Do not use with ACE inhibitors and beta blockers |
| *Antiadrenergic Agents*<br>*Alpha₁-blocking Agents* | | |
| **Doxazosin** (Cardura)<br>Pregnancy Category B | *Adults:* PO, 1 mg once daily initially, increased to 2 mg, then to 4, 8, and 16 mg daily if necessary | |
| **Prazosin** (Minipress)<br>Pregnancy Category C | See Prototype Profile 43-3: Prazosin | |
| **Terazosin** (Hytrin)<br>Pregnancy Category C | *Adults:* PO, 1 mg at bedtime initially, may be increased gradually. Usual maintenance dose, 1–5 mg once daily | |
| *Alpha₂ Agonists* | | |
| **Clonidine** (Catapres)<br>Pregnancy Category C | *Adults:* PO, 0.1 mg two times daily initially, gradually increased up to 2.4 mg daily, if necessary. Average maintenance dose, 0.2–0.8 mg daily<br>*Children:* PO, 5–25 mcg/kg/d, in divided doses, q6h; increase at 5- to 7-day intervals, if needed | |
| **Guanabenz** (Wytensin)<br>Pregnancy Category C | *Adults:* PO, 4 mg twice daily, increased by 4–8 mg daily every 1–2 wk if necessary to a maximum of 32 mg twice daily | Dosage adjustment in liver failure is probably necessary |
| **Guanfacine** (Tenex)<br>Pregnancy Category B | *Adults:* PO, 1 mg daily at bedtime, increased to 2 mg after 3–4 wk, then to 3 mg if necessary | |
| **Methyldopa** (Aldomet)<br>Pregnancy Category B | *Adults:* PO, 250 mg 2 or 3 times daily initially, increased gradually until blood pressure is controlled or a daily dose of 3 g is reached<br>*Children:* PO, 10 mg/kg/d in 2 to 4 divided doses initially, increased or decreased according to response. Maximum dose, 65 mg/kg/d or 3 g daily, whichever is less | |

*(continued)*

**DRUG TABLE 43-1**

## _Drugs at a Glance_

## Antihypertensive Drugs (Continued)

| Generic/Trade Name | Routes and Dosage Ranges | Comments |
|---|---|---|
| _Postganglionic-active Drugs_ | | |
| **Guanadrel** (Hylorel)<br>Pregnancy Category B | _Adults:_ PO, 10 mg daily initially. Usual dosage range, 20–75 mg daily in divided doses | Considered a second-line agent, usually with a diuretic; requires dosing adjustment in renal failure |
| **Guanethidine sulfate** (Ismelin)<br>Pregnancy Category C | _Adults:_ PO, 10 mg daily initially, increased every 5–7 days to a maximum daily dose of 300 mg if necessary. Usual daily dose, 25–50 mg<br>_Children:_ PO, 0.2 mg/kg/d initially, increased by the same amount every 7–10 d if necessary to a maximum dose of 3 mg/kg/d | |
| _Beta-adrenergic Blocking Agents_ | | |
| **Acebutolol** (Sectral)<br>Pregnancy Category B (manufacturer); D (second and third trimesters, by expert analysis) | _Adults:_ PO, 400 mg once daily initially, increased to 800 mg daily if necessary | Abrupt withdrawal should be avoided |
| **Atenolol** (Tenormin)<br>Pregnancy Category D | _Adults:_ PO, 50 mg once daily initially, increased in 1–2 wk to 100 mg once daily, if necessary | May cause fetal harm when administered during pregnancy |
| **Betaxolol** (Kerlone)<br>Pregnancy Category C (manufacturer); D (second and third trimesters, by expert analysis) | _Adults:_ PO, 10–20 mg daily | Used in the treatment of chronic open-angle glaucoma and ocular and malignant hypertension |
| **Bisoprolol** (Zebeta)<br>Pregnancy Category C (manufacturer); D (second and third trimesters, by expert analysis) | _Adults:_ PO, 5 mg once daily, increased to a maximum of 20 mg daily if necessary | Dosage adjustment necessary in renal insufficiency |
| **Carteolol** (Cartrol)<br>Pregnancy Category C (manufacturer); D (second and third trimesters, by expert analysis) | _Adults:_ PO, 2.5 mg once daily initially, gradually increased to a maximum of 10 mg daily if necessary. Usual maintenance dose, 2.5–5 mg once daily. Extend dosage interval to 48 h for a creatinine clearance of 20 to 60 mL/min and to 72 h for a creatinine clearance below 20 mL/min | Avoid abrupt withdrawal; monitor for orthostatic hypotension, depression, and confusion |
| **Metoprolol** (Lopressor)<br>Pregnancy Category C | _Adults:_ PO, 50 mg twice daily, gradually increased weekly or at longer intervals if necessary. Maximum dose, 450 mg daily | |
| **Nadolol** (Corgard)<br>Pregnancy Category C | _Adults:_ PO, 40 mg daily initially, gradually increased if necessary. Average dose, 80–320 mg daily | Dosage adjustment in hepatic failure probably necessary |
| **Penbutolol** (Levatol)<br>Pregnancy Category C | _Adults:_ PO, 20 mg once daily | |
| **Pindolol** (Visken)<br>Pregnancy Category B | _Adults:_ PO, 5 mg 2 or 3 times daily initially, increased by 10 mg/d at 3- to 4-wk intervals to a maximum of 60 mg daily | |

_(continued)_

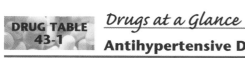

## DRUG TABLE 43-1 — *Drugs at a Glance*

## Antihypertensive Drugs (Continued)

| Generic/Trade Name | Routes and Dosage Ranges | Comments |
|---|---|---|
| **Propranolol** (Inderal)<br>Pregnancy Category C (manufacturer); D (second and third trimesters, by expert analysis) | *Adults:* PO, 40 mg twice daily initially, gradually increased to 160–640 mg daily<br>*Children:* PO, 1 mg/kg/d initially, gradually increased to a maximum of 10 mg/kg/d | Do not crush long-acting forms |
| **Timolol** (Blocadren)<br>Pregnancy Category C | *Adults:* PO, 10 mg twice daily initially, increased gradually if necessary. Average daily dose, 20–40 mg; maximal daily dose, 60 mg | Ophthalmic dosage form used for treatment of elevated intraocular pressure |
| *Alpha-beta-blocking Agents* | | |
| **Carvedilol** (Coreg)<br>Pregnancy Category C | *Adults:* PO, 6.25 mg twice daily for 7–14 d, then increase to 12.5 mg twice daily for 7–14 d, then increase to a maximal dose of 25 mg twice daily if tolerated and needed | |
| **Labetalol** (Trandate, Normodyne)<br>Pregnancy Category C (manufacturer); D (second and third trimesters, by expert analysis) | *Adults:* PO, 100 mg twice daily, increased by 100 mg twice daily every 2–3 d if necessary. Usual maintenance dose, 200–400 mg twice daily. Severe hypertension may require 1200–2400 mg daily<br>IV injection, 20 mg slowly over 2 min, followed by 40–80 mg every 10 min until the desired blood pressure is achieved or 300 mg has been given<br>IV infusion, add 200 mg to 250 mL of 5% dextrose or 0.9% sodium chloride solution (concentration 2 mg/3 mL) and infuse at a rate of 3 mL/min. Adjust flow rate according to blood pressure, and substitute oral labetalol when blood pressure is controlled | Take with food to reduce risk for hypotension |
| *Calcium Channel Blocking Agents* | | |
| **Amlodipine** (Norvasc)<br>Pregnancy Category C | *Adults:* PO, 5–10 mg once daily | Ingesting calcium salts while taking calcium channel blockers will reduce the therapeutic response |
| **Diltiazem** (sustained release) (Cardizem SR)<br>Pregnancy Category C | *Adults:* PO, 60–120 mg twice daily Extended-release tablets | Swallow whole, do not crush or chew |
| **Felodipine** (Plendil)<br>Pregnancy Category C | *Adults:* PO, 5–10 mg once daily Extended-release tablets | Swallow whole, do not crush or chew |
| **Isradipine** (DynaCirc)<br>Pregnancy Category C | *Adults:* PO, 2.5–5 mg twice daily | |
| **Nicardipine** (Cardene, Cardene SR, Cardene IV)<br>Pregnancy Category C | *Adults:* PO, 20–40 mg three times daily; sustained-release, PO, 30–60 mg twice daily; IV infusion, 5–15 mg/h | Alcohol may increase CNS depression |
| **Nifedipine** (Adalat, Procardia, Procardia XL)<br>Pregnancy Category C | *Adults:* Sustained-release only, PO, 30–60 mg once daily, increased over 1–2 wk if necessary | Puncturing short-acting capsules and administering sublingually is neither safe nor effective in hypertensive emergencies |

*(continued)*

**DRUG TABLE
43-1**

*Drugs at a Glance*

## Antihypertensive Drugs (Continued)

| Generic/Trade Name | Routes and Dosage Ranges | Comments |
|---|---|---|
| **Nisoldipine** (Sular)<br>Pregnancy Category C | *Adults:* PO, 20 mg once daily initially, increased by 10 mg/wk or longer intervals to a maximum of 60 mg daily. Average maintenance dose, 20–40 mg daily. Adults with liver impairment or >65 y, PO, 10 mg once daily initially | Avoid high-fat diet<br>Administer daily at the same time to minimize fluctuation of serum levels |
| **Verapamil** (Calan, Calan SR, Isoptin SR)<br>Pregnancy Category C | *Adults:* Immediate-release, PO, 80 mg 3 times daily; sustained-release, PO, 240 mg once daily; IV, see manufacturer's instructions<br>*Children:* IV, see manufacturer's instructions | May cause gingival hyperplasia |
| ***Other Vasodilators*** | | |
| **Diazoxide** (Hyperstat)<br>Pregnancy Category C | *Adults:* Rapid IV injection of 1–3 mg/kg up to a maximum of 150 mg in a single injection; dose may be repeated at 5- to 15-min intervals until desired response obtained | Use in hypertensive emergencies<br>Mini-bolus injections preferred over bolus administration of 300 mg |
| **Fenoldopam** (Corlopam)<br>Pregnancy Category B | *Adults:* IV infusion, initial dose based on body weight, then flow rate titrated to achieve desired response. Mix with 0.9% sodium chloride or 5% dextrose to a concentration of 40 mcg/mL (eg, 40 mg of drug [4 mL of concentrate] in 1000 mL of IV fluid) | Use in hypertensive emergencies<br>Contains sodium metabisulfite, so avoid in clients with hypersensitivity to sulfites |
| **Hydralazine** (Apresoline)<br>Pregnancy Category C | *Adults:* Chronic hypertension, PO, 10 mg four times daily for 2–4 d, gradually increased up to 300 mg/d, if necessary<br>*Children:* Chronic hypertension, 0.75 mg/kg/d initially in four divided doses<br>Gradually increased over 3–4 wk to a maximal dose of 7.5 mg/kg/d if necessary<br>*Adults:* Hypertensive crisis, IM, IV, 10–20 mg, increased to 40 mg if necessary<br>Repeat dose as needed<br>*Children:* Hypertensive crisis, IM, IV, 0.1–0.2 mg/kg every 4–6 h as needed | Assist client with rising; may cause orthostasis |
| **Minoxidil** (Loniten, Rogaine)<br>Pregnancy Category C | *Adults:* PO, 5 mg once daily initially, increased gradually until blood pressure is controlled. Average daily dose, 10–40 mg; maximal daily dose, 100 mg in single or divided doses<br>*Children <12 y:* PO, 0.2 mg/kg/d initially as a single dose, increased gradually until blood pressure is controlled. Average daily dose, 0.25–1.0 mg/kg; maximal dose, 50 mg/d | Also used as a topical application for alopecia |

*(continued)*

DRUG TABLE 43-1

## Drugs at a Glance
## Antihypertensive Drugs (Continued)

| Generic/Trade Name | Routes and Dosage Ranges | Comments |
|---|---|---|
| **Sodium nitroprusside** (Nipride) Pregnancy Category C | *Adults and Children:* IV infusion, 0.5–10 mcg/kg/min; average dose, 3 mcg/kg/min. Prepare solution by adding 50 mg of sodium nitroprusside to 250–1000 mL of 5% dextrose in water, and cover promptly to protect from light. | Drug is photosensitive so should be protected from light; do not use discolored solution. Drug is converted to cyanide ions in the bloodstream that may lead to acidosis, coma, convulsions, and almond smell on breath |

*Children's dosages from *Drug Facts and Comparisons* (2003).

cate that beta blockers have greater effects in people of Asian heritage compared with their effects in whites. For hypertension, Asians in general need much smaller doses because they metabolize and excrete beta blockers slowly. Other populations known to metabolize beta blockers slowly include Arab and Egyptian Americans and possibly German Americans. In African Americans, diuretics are effective and recommended as initial drug therapy; calcium channel blockers, alpha$_1$-receptor blockers, and the alpha–beta blocker labetalol are reportedly equally effective in African Americans and whites. ACE inhibitors, some ARBs (eg, losartan, telmisartan), and beta blockers are less effective as monotherapy in African Americans. When beta blockers are used, they are usually one component of a multidrug regimen, and higher doses may be required. Overall, African Americans are more likely to have severe hypertension and require multiple drugs.

## ◼ USE IN SURGICAL CLIENTS

The Joint National Committee on Detection, Evaluation, and Treatment of High Blood Pressure recommends that drug therapy be continued until surgery and restarted as soon as possible after surgery. If clients cannot take drugs orally, parenteral diuretics, antiadrenergic agents, ACE inhibitors, calcium blockers, or vasodilators may be given to avoid the rebound hypertension associated with abrupt discontinuance of some antiadrenergic antihypertensive agents. Transdermal clonidine also may be used. The anesthesiologist and surgeon must be informed about the client's hypertension and medication status.

## ◼ HYPERTENSIVE EMERGENCIES

Antihypertensive drugs are also used to treat hypertensive urgencies and emergencies, which involve dangerously high blood pressures and actual or potential damage to target organs. Although there are risks with severe hypertension, there are also risks associated with lowering blood pressure excessively or too rapidly, including stroke, myocardial infarction, and acute renal failure. Thus, the goal of management is usually to lower blood pressure over several minutes to several hours, with careful titration of drug dosage to avoid precipitous drops.

Urgencies can be treated with oral antihypertensive agents such as **captopril,** 25 to 50 mg every 1 to 2 hours, or **clonidine,** 0.2 mg initially, then 0.1 mg hourly until diastolic blood pressure falls below 110 mm Hg or 0.7 mg has been given.

A hypertensive emergency, defined as a diastolic pressure of 120 mm Hg or higher and target organ damage, requires an IV drug. The goal of management is usually to lower diastolic pressure to 100 to 110 mm Hg and maintain it there for several days to allow adjustment of the physiologic mechanisms that normally regulate blood pressure. Then, the blood pressure can be lowered to normotensive levels.

Several drugs can be given to treat a hypertensive emergency. **Diazoxide** is a fast-acting drug given undiluted and rapidly by IV injection. The drug was originally recommended for use by bolus administration. Recent studies have shown that mini-bolus injections are preferred over large bolus administration. **Fenoldopam** is a fast-acting drug indicated only for short-term use (<48 hours) in hospitalized clients. Dosage is calculated according to body weight and desired effects on blood pressure. Administration is by an infusion pump, with frequent monitoring of blood pressure. **Nitroglycerin** is especially beneficial in clients with both severe hypertension and myocardial ischemia. The dose is titrated according to blood pressure response and may range from 5 to 100 mcg/minute. Tolerance develops to IV nitroglycerin over 24 to 48 hours. **Nitroprusside,** which has a rapid onset and short duration of action, is given as a continuous infusion at a rate of 0.5 to 8 mcg/kg per minute. Intraarterial blood pressure should be monitored during the infusion. Nitroprusside is metabolized to thiocyanate, and serum

*(text continues on page 797)*

*Drugs at a Glance*

## Oral Antihypertensive Combination Products*

| | Components | | | | | | |
|---|---|---|---|---|---|---|---|
| Trade Name | Angiotensin II Receptor Antagonist | Angiotensin-Converting Enzyme Inhibitor | Beta Blocker | Calcium Channel Blocker | Diuretic | Non–Beta-Blocker Antiadrenergic | Dosage Ranges |
| Aldoril | | | | | HCTZ 15, 25, 30, or 50 mg | Methyldopa 250 or 500 mg | 1 tablet 2 to 3 times daily for 48 h, then adjusted according to response |
| Capozide | | Captopril 25 or 50 mg | | | HCTZ 15 or 25 mg | | 1 tablet 2 to 3 times daily |
| Combipres | | | | | Chlorthalidone 15 mg | Clonidine 0.1, 0.2, or 0.3 mg | 1 tablet twice daily |
| Corzide | | | Nadolol 40 or 80 mg | | Bendroflumethiazide 5 mg | | 1 tablet daily |
| Diovan HCT | Valsartan 80 or 160 mg | | | | HCTZ 12.5 mg | | 1 tablet daily |
| Hyzaar | Losartan 50 mg | | | | HCTZ 12.5 mg | | 1 tablet once daily |
| Inderide | | | Propranolol 40 or 80 mg | | HCTZ 25 mg | | 1–2 tablets twice daily |
| Inderide LA | | | Propranolol 80, 120, or 160 mg | | HCTZ 50 mg | | 1 capsule once daily |
| Lopressor HCT | | | Metoprolol 50 or 100 mg | | HCTZ 25 or 50 mg | | 1–2 tablets daily |
| Lotensin HCT | | Benazepril 5, 10, or 20 mg | | | HCTZ 12.5 or 25 mg | | 1 tablet daily |
| Lotrel | | Benazepril 10 or 20 mg | | Amlodipine 2.5 or 5 mg | | | 1 capsule daily |
| Minizide | | | | | Polythiazide 0.5 mg | Prazosin 1, 2, or 5 mg | 1 capsule 2 to 3 times daily |
| Prinzide | | Lisinopril 20 mg | | | HCTZ 12.5 or 25 mg | | 1 tablet daily |
| Tarka | | Trandolapril 1, 2, or 4 mg | | Verapamil 180 or 240 mg | | | 1 tablet daily |
| Tenoretic | | | Atenolol 50 or 100 mg | | Chlorthalidone 25 mg | | 1 tablet daily |
| Timolide | | | Timolol 10 mg | | HCTZ 25 mg | | 1–2 tablets 1 or 2 times daily |
| Vaseretic | | Enalapril | | | HCTZ 25 mg | | 1–2 tablets daily |
| Zestoretic | | Lisinopril 10 or 20 mg | | | HCTZ 12.5 or 25 mg | | 1 tablet daily |
| Ziac | | Bisoprolol 2.5, 5, or 10 mg | | | HCTZ 6.25 mg | | 1 tablet daily |

HCTZ, hydrochlorothiazide.
*Note that one trade name product may be available in multiple formulations, with variable amounts of antihypertensive, diuretic, or both components.

# NURSING PROCESS

## Assessment

Assess the client's condition in relation to hypertension.

- Identify conditions and risk factors that may lead to hypertension. These include:
  - Obesity
  - Elevated serum cholesterol (total and low-density lipoprotein) and triglycerides
  - Cigarette smoking
  - Sedentary lifestyle
  - Family history of hypertension or other cardiovascular disease
  - African-American race
  - Renal disease (eg, renal artery stenosis)
  - Adrenal disease (eg, hypersecretion of aldosterone, pheochromocytoma)
  - Other cardiovascular disorders (eg, atherosclerosis, left ventricular hypertrophy)
  - Diabetes mellitus
  - Oral contraceptives, corticosteroids, appetite suppressants, nasal decongestants, non-steroidal anti-inflammatory agents
  - Neurologic disorders (eg, brain damage)
- Observe for signs and symptoms of hypertension.
  - Check blood pressure accurately and repeatedly. As a rule, multiple measurements in which systolic pressure is above 140 mm Hg and/or diastolic pressure is above 90 mm Hg, are necessary to establish a diagnosis of hypertension.

    The importance of accurate blood pressure measurements cannot be overemphasized because there are many possibilities for errors. Some ways to improve accuracy and validity include using correct equipment (eg, proper cuff size), having the client rested and in the same position each time blood pressure is measured (eg, sitting or supine with arm at heart level), and using the same arm for repeated measurements.
  - In most cases of early hypertension, elevated blood pressure is the only clinical manifestation. If symptoms do occur, they are usually nonspecific (eg, headache, weakness, fatigue, tachycardia, dizziness, palpitations, epistaxis).
  - Eventually, signs and symptoms occur as target organs are damaged. Heart damage is often reflected as angina pectoris, myocardial infarction, or heart failure. Chest pain, tachycardia, dyspnea, fatigue, and edema may occur. Brain damage may be indicated by transient ischemic attacks or strokes of varying severity with symptoms ranging from syncope to hemiparesis. Renal damage may be reflected by proteinuria, increased blood urea nitrogen (BUN), and increased serum creatinine. Ophthalmoscopic examination may reveal hemorrhages, sclerosis of arterioles, and inflammation of the optic nerve (papilledema). Because arterioles can be visualized in the retina of the eye, damage to retinal vessels may indicate damage to arterioles in the heart, brain, and kidneys.

## Nursing Diagnoses

- Decreased Cardiac Output related to disease process or drug therapy
- Ineffective Coping related to long-term lifestyle changes and drug therapy
- Noncompliance related to lack of knowledge about hypertension and its management, costs and adverse effects of drug therapy, and psychosocial factors
- Disturbed Body Image related to the need for long-term management and medical supervision
- Fatigue related to antihypertensive drug therapy
- Deficient Knowledge related to hypertension, antihypertensive drug therapy, and nondrug lifestyle changes
- Sexual Dysfunction related to adverse drug effects

## Planning/Goals

*The client will:*

- Receive or take antihypertensive drugs correctly
- Be monitored closely for therapeutic and adverse drug effects, especially when drug therapy is started, when changes are made in drugs, and when dosages are increased or decreased
- Use nondrug measures to assist in blood pressure control
- Avoid, manage, or report adverse drug reactions
- Verbalize or demonstrate knowledge of prescribed drugs and recommended lifestyle changes
- Keep follow-up appointments

## Interventions

Implement measures to prevent or minimize hypertension. Preventive measures are mainly lifestyle changes to reduce risk factors. These measures should be started in childhood and continued throughout life. Once hypertension is diagnosed, lifetime adherence to a therapeutic regimen may be necessary to control the disease and prevent complications. The nurse's role is important in the prevention, early detection, and management of hypertension. Some guidelines for intervention at community, family, and personal levels include the following:

- Participate in programs to promote healthful lifestyles (eg, improving eating habits, increasing exercise, managing stress more effectively, and avoiding cigarette smoking).
- Participate in community screening programs, and make appropriate referrals when abnormal blood pressures are detected. If hypertension develops in women taking oral contraceptives, the drug should be discontinued for 3 to 6 months to see whether blood pressure decreases without antihypertensive drugs.
- Help the hypertensive client comply with prescribed therapy. Noncompliance is high among clients with hypertension. Reasons given for noncompliance include lack of symptoms, lack of motivation and self-discipline to make needed lifestyle changes (eg, lose weight, stop smoking, restrict salt intake), perhaps experiencing more symptoms from medications than from hypertension, the cost of

*(continued)*

## NURSING PROCESS (Continued)

therapy, and the client's failure to realize the importance of effective management, especially as related to prevention of major cardiovascular diseases (myocardial infarction, stroke, and death). In addition, several studies have shown that compliance decreases as the number of drugs and number of doses increase.

The nurse can help increase compliance by teaching the client about hypertension, helping the client make necessary lifestyle changes, and maintaining supportive interpersonal relationships. Losing weight, stopping smoking, and other changes are most likely to be effective if attempted one at a time.

- Use recommended techniques for measuring blood pressure. Poor techniques are too often used (eg, the client's

arm up or down rather than at heart level; cuff applied over clothing, too loosely, deflated too rapidly, or reinflated before completely deflated; a regular-sized cuff used on large arms that need a large cuff; using the stethoscope diaphragm rather than the bell). It is disturbing to think that antihypertensive drugs may be prescribed and dosages changed on the basis of inaccurate blood pressures.

### Evaluation

- Observe for blood pressure measurements within goal or more nearly normal ranges.
- Observe and interview regarding compliance with instructions about drug therapy and lifestyle changes.
- Observe and interview regarding adverse drug effects.

---

## CLIENT TEACHING GUIDELINES
## Antihypertensive Medications

### General Considerations

✔ Hypertension is a major risk factor for heart attack, stroke (sometimes called brain attack), and kidney failure. Although it rarely causes symptoms unless complications occur, it can be controlled by appropriate management. Consequently, you need to learn all you can about the disease process, the factors that cause or aggravate it, and its management. In few other conditions is your knowledge and understanding about your condition as important as with hypertension.

✔ For many people, lifestyle changes (ie, a diet to avoid excessive salt and control weight and fat intake, regular exercise, and avoiding smoking) may be sufficient to control blood pressure. If drug therapy is prescribed, these measures should be continued.

✔ When drug therapy is needed, your physician will try to choose a drug and develop a regimen that works for you. There are numerous antihypertensive drugs and many can be taken once a day, which makes their use more convenient and less disruptive of your usual activities of daily living. You may need several office visits to find the right drug or combination of drugs and the right dosage. Changes in drugs or dosages may also be needed later, especially if you develop other conditions or take other drugs that alter your response to the antihypertensive drugs.

✔ Antihypertensive drug therapy is usually long term, may require more than one drug, and may produce side effects. You need to know the brand and generic names of any prescribed drugs and how to take each drug for optimal benefit and minimal adverse effects.

✔ Antihypertensive drugs must be taken as prescribed for optimal benefits, even if you do not feel well when a medication is started or when dosage is increased. *No antihypertensive drug should be stopped abruptly.* If problems develop, they should be discussed with the health care provider who is treating the hypertension. If treatment is

stopped, blood pressure usually increases gradually as the medication(s) are eliminated from the body. Sometimes, however, blood pressure rapidly increases to pretreatment levels or even higher. With any of these situations, you are at risk of a heart attack or stroke. In addition, stopping one drug of a multidrug regimen may lead to increased adverse effects as well as decreased antihypertensive effectiveness. To avoid these problems, antihypertensive drugs should be tapered in dosage and discontinued gradually, as directed by your health care provider.

✔ Blood pressure measurements are the only way you can tell if your medication is working. Thus, you may want to monitor your blood pressure at home, especially when starting drug therapy, changing medications, or changing dosages. If so, a blood pressure machine may be purchased at a medical supply store. Follow instructions regarding use, take your blood pressure approximately the same time(s) each day (eg, before morning and evening meals), and keep a record to show to your health care provider.

✔ People sometimes feel dizzy or faint while taking antihypertensive medications. This usually means your blood pressure drops momentarily and is most likely to occur when you start a medication, increase dosage, or stand up suddenly from a sitting or lying position. This can be prevented or decreased by moving to a standing position slowly, sleeping with the head of the bed elevated, wearing elastic stockings, exercising legs, avoiding prolonged standing, and avoiding hot baths. If episodes still occur, you should sit or lie down to avoid a fall and possible injury.

✔ It is very important to keep appointments for follow-up care.

### Self-administration or Caregiver Administration

✔ Take or give antihypertensive drugs at prescribed time intervals, about the same time each day. For exam-

*(continued)*

## CLIENT TEACHING GUIDELINES
### Antihypertensive Medications (Continued)

ple, take once-daily drugs as close to every 24 hours as you can manage; twice-a-day drugs should be taken every 12 hours. If ordered four times daily, take approximately every 6 hours. Taking doses too close together can increase dizziness, weakness, and other adverse effects. Taking doses too far apart may not control blood pressure adequately and may increase risks of heart attack or stroke.

✔ Take oral captopril on an empty stomach. Food decreases drug absorption.

✔ Take most oral antihypertensive agents with or after food intake to decrease gastric irritation. Candesartan (Atacand), irbesartan (Avapro), losartan (Cozaar), telmisartan (Micardis), and valsartan (Diovan) may be taken with or without food.

✔ With prazosin, doxazosin, or terazosin, take the first dose and the first increased dose at bedtime to prevent dizziness and possible fainting.

✔ With the clonidine skin patch, apply to a hairless area on the upper arm or torso once every 7 days. Rotate sites.

---

### ? How Can You Avoid This Medication Error?

Fred Simosa, a nursing home resident, is having increasing difficulty with swallowing. You decide to crush his medications (Cardizem SR, Lasix, and Slow-K) and mix them with applesauce. What error, if any, has occurred? Reflect on potential effects of crushing these medications for this patient.

thiocyanate levels should be measured if the drug is given longer than 72 hours. The infusion should be stopped after 72 hours if the serum thiocyanate level is more than 12 mg/dL; it should be stopped at 48 hours in clients with renal impairment. Symptoms of thiocyanate toxicity (eg, nausea, vomiting, muscle twitching or spasm, and seizures) can be reversed with hemodialysis. Other drugs that may be used include IV **hydralazine, labetalol,** and **nicardipine;** see Drugs at a Glance 43-1 and 43-2.

## Herbal and Dietary Supplements

Use of nonprescription herbal and dietary supplements is frequently not reported by the client even though one third of the adults in the United States use these agents. Significant interactions can occur between herbs and dietary supplements when taken with prescribed drugs. Many nonprescription medications such as antihistamines, cold and cough preparations, and weight loss products can decrease the effectiveness of antihypertensive drugs or worsen hypertension. Caffeine, by its stimulating effects, may increase blood pressure. Ephedra (ma huang), used to suppress appetite; treat colds, nasal congestion, and asthma; and increase energy, increases blood pressure and increases risks for stroke. This product should be avoided by anyone with hypertension; it is not recommended for therapeutic use by anyone. Yohimbe, used to treat erectile dysfunction, is a central nervous system stimulant and can affect blood pressure. Additionally, ginseng may worsen hypertension; garlic may increase the antihypertensive effect of medications used for blood pressure control.

---

## *Nursing Actions*
## Antihypertensive Drugs

| Nursing Actions | Rationale/Explanation |
|---|---|
| **1. Administer accurately.** | |
| a. Give oral captopril and moexipril on an empty stomach, 1 h before meals. | Food decreases drug absorption. |
| b. Give most other oral antihypertensives with or after food intake. | To decrease gastric irritation |
| c. Give angiotensin II receptor blockers with or without food. | Food does not impair drug absorption. |
| d. For intravenous injection of propranolol or labetalol, the client should be attached to a cardiac monitor. In addition, parenteral atropine and isoproterenol (Isuprel) must be readily available. | For early detection and management of excessive myocardial depression and dysrhythmias. Atropine may be used to treat excessive bradycardia. Isoproterenol may be used to stimulate myocardial contractility and increase cardiac output. |

*(continued)*

## Nursing Actions

### Antihypertensive Drugs (Continued)

| Nursing Actions | Rationale/Explanation |
|---|---|
| e. Give the first dose and the first increased dose of prazosin, doxazosin, and terazosin at bedtime. | To prevent orthostatic hypotension and syncope |
| f. For administration of fenoldopam and nitroprusside, use the manufacturers' instructions to develop a unit protocol for preparation of infusion solutions, dosages, flow rates, durations of use, and monitoring of blood pressure during infusion. | These drugs are used to lower blood pressure rapidly in hypertensive emergencies, usually in an emergency department or critical care unit. They also have specific requirements for preparation and administration. A protocol established beforehand can save valuable time in an emergency situation. |
| **2. Observe for therapeutic effects.** | The choice of drugs and drug dosages often requires adjustment to maximize beneficial effects and minimize adverse effects. Thus, optimal therapeutic effects may not occur immediately after drug therapy is begun. |
| a. Decreased blood pressure. The usual goal is a normal blood pressure (ie, below 140/90). | |
| **3. Observe for adverse effects.** | Adverse effects are most likely to occur in clients who are elderly, have impaired renal function, and are receiving multiple antihypertensive drugs or large doses of antihypertensive drugs. |
| a. Orthostatic hypotension, dizziness, weakness | This is an extension of the expected pharmacologic action. Orthostatic hypotension results from drug blockage of compensatory reflexes (vasoconstriction, decreased venous pooling in extremities and increased venous return to the heart) that normally maintain blood pressure in the upright position. This adverse reaction may be aggravated by other conditions that cause vasodilation (eg, exercise, heat or hot weather, and alcohol consumption). Orthostatic hypotension is more likely to occur with guanethidine and methyldopa. |
| b. Sodium and water retention, increased plasma volume, perhaps edema and weight gain | These effects result from decreased renal perfusion. This reaction can be prevented or minimized by concurrent administration of a diuretic. |
| c. Prolonged atrioventricular conduction, bradycardia | Due to increased vagal tone and stimulation |
| d. Gastrointestinal disturbances, including nausea, vomiting, and diarrhea | These effects are more likely to occur with hydralazine, methyldopa, propranolol, and captopril. |
| e. Bronchospasm (with nonselective beta blockers) | The drugs may cause bronchoconstriction and are contraindicated in patients with asthma and other bronchoconstrictive lung disorders. |
| f. Hypertensive crisis (with abrupt withdrawal of clonidine or guanabenz). | This may be prevented by tapering dosage over several days before stopping the drug. |
| g. Cough and hyperkalemia with angiotensin-converting enzyme (ACE) inhibitors | A chronic, nonproductive cough is a relatively common adverse effect; hyperkalemia occurs in 1%–4% of clients. |
| **4. Observe for drug interactions.** | |
| a. Drugs that *increase* effects of antihypertensives: | |
| (1) Other antihypertensive agents | Combinations of two or three drugs with different mechanisms of action are often given for their additive effects and efficacy in controlling blood pressure when a single drug is ineffective. |
| (2) Alcohol, other central nervous system depressants (eg, opioid analgesics, phenothiazine antipsychotics) | These drugs have hypotensive effects when used alone and increased hypotension occurs when they are combined with antihypertensive drugs. |
| (3) Digoxin | Additive bradycardia with beta blockers |
| b. Drugs that *decrease* effects of antihypertensives: | |
| (1) Adrenergics | These drugs stimulate the sympathetic nervous system and raise blood pressure. They include over-the-counter nasal decongestants, cold remedies, bronchodilators, and appetite suppressants. |

(continued)

## Nursing Actions

### Antihypertensive Drugs (Continued)

| Nursing Actions | Rationale/Explanation |
|---|---|
| (2) Antacids | May decrease bioavailability of ACE inhibitors, especially captopril. Give antacids 2 h before or after ACE inhibitors. These drugs tend to increase blood pressure by causing retention of sodium and water. |
| (3) Nonsteroidal anti-inflammatory drugs, oral contraceptives | |

### ? How Can You Avoid This Medication Error?

**Answer:** If Mr. Simosa is having trouble swallowing, oral medications may not be safely taken at this time. Crushing the medications is also not indicated because Cardizem SR and Slow-K are sustained-release products. If Cardizem SR is crushed, the sustained-release properties will be lost. Immediately after administration, you will see a significant hypotensive effect because all the medication will be absorbed. Because none of the medication's absorption will be delayed, you may see a rebound hypertension at a later time. Slow-K will also lose the ability to absorb slowly, which might cause it to be excreted by the diuretic effects of the Lasix, which is not affected by crushing. The nurse should also assess the reason for Mr. Simosa's swallowing difficulty, if unknown, before administering his medications.

### Critical Thinking Exercises

1. A client is receiving propranolol (Inderal) to manage her chronic angina pectoris. Because this drug is not cardioselective, the nurse should monitor the client for which adverse reaction?
   a. Seizures
   b. Confusion
   c. Bronchospasm
   d. Hypertensive crisis

2. Which over-the-counter preparations should the nurse instruct Ms. Ellis to avoid now that she's taking diltiazem?
   a. Aspirin products
   b. Acetaminophen preparations
   c. Calcium tablets
   d. Antihistamines

3. Which disorder in a client's history would contraindicate propranolol therapy?
   a. Bronchial asthma
   b. Peptic ulcer disease
   c. Atrial tachycardia
   d. Migraine headaches

4. Which adverse reaction can occur during the first week of therapy with an ACE inhibitor?
   a. Tinnitus
   b. Dry, nonproductive, persistent cough
   c. Muscle weakness
   d. Constipation

### SELECTED REFERENCES

Applegate, W. B. (2002). Approach to the elderly patient with hypertension. In H. D. Humes (Ed.), *Kelley's textbook of internal medicine* (4th ed., pp. 3020–3026). Philadelphia: Lippincott Williams & Wilkins.

Carter, B. L., & Saseen, J. L. (2002). Hypertension. In J. T. DiPiro, R. L. Talbert, G. C. Yee, G. R. Matzke, B. G. Wells, & L. M. Posey (Eds.), *Pharmacotherapy: A pathophysiologic approach* (5th ed., pp. 157–183). New York: McGraw-Hill.

Chobanian, A. V., Bakris, G. L., Black, H. R., Cushman, W. C., Green, L. A., Izzo, J. L., et al. (2003). Seventh report of the joint national committee on prevention, detection, evaluation, and treatment of high blood pressure. *Hypertension, 42,* 1206–1252.

*Drug facts and comparisons.* (Updated monthly). St. Louis: Facts and Comparisons.

Franco, V., Oparil, S., & Carretero, O. A. (2004). Hypertensive therapy: Part I. *Circulation, 109*(24), 2953–2958.

Franco, V., Oparil, S., & Carretero, O. A. (2004). Hypertensive therapy: Part II. *Circulation, 109*(25), 3081–3088.

Grim, E., & Grim C. M. (2002). Alterations in blood pressure: Hypertension and orthostatic hypotension. In C. M. Porth, *Pathophysiology: Concepts of altered health states* (6th ed., pp. 459–485). Philadelphia: Lippincott Williams & Wilkins.

Huffstutler, S. Y. (2002). Managing hypertension in African American men. *Advance for Nurse Practitioners, 8*(4), 28–33, 92.

Karch, A. M. (2003). *Lippincott's nursing drug guide.* Philadelphia: Lippincott Williams & Wilkins.

Lacy, C. F., Armstrong, L. L., Goldman, M. P., & Lance, L. L. (2003). *Lexi-Comp's drug information handbook* (11th ed.). Hudson, OH: American Pharmaceutical Association.

Skidmore-Roth, L. (2001). *Mosby's handbook of herbs and natural supplements.* St. Louis: Mosby.

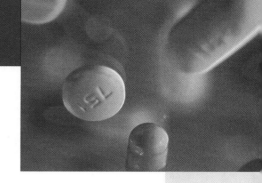

# 44

# Diuretics

## OBJECTIVES

*After studying this chapter, the student will be able to:*

1 List characteristics of diuretics in terms of mechanism of action, indications for use, principles of therapy, and nursing process implications.

2 Discuss major adverse effects of thiazide, loop, and potassium-sparing diuretics.

3 Identify clients at risk for developing adverse reactions to diuretic administration.

4 Differentiate between commonly used potassium-losing and potassium-sparing diuretics.

5 Discuss the rationale for using combination products containing a potassium-losing and a potassium-sparing diuretic.

6 Discuss the rationale for concomitant use of a loop diuretic and a thiazide or related diuretic.

7 Teach clients to manage diuretic therapy effectively.

## CRITICAL THINKING SCENARIO

*K*athleen White, an 82-year-old widow, is started on a thiazide diuretic to control her hypertension. She also has a history of osteoarthritis. She lives alone with her two cats and manages independently with only a little help from her neighbors. Her children live out-of-state, but she talks with them on the phone weekly.

✔ How do diuretics work to decrease blood pressure?

✔ How might a diuretic affect activities and normal daily functions?

✔ What are some key factors, particularly associated with diuretic therapy, that might pose safety risks for this widow? How might you minimize these risks?

✔ Develop an appropriate teaching plan for Mrs. White regarding her diuretic therapy.

## PROTOTYPE PROFILES

**furosemide** (Lasix), p. 807

**hydrochlorothiazide** (HydroDIURIL), p. 805

**spironolactone** (Aldactone), p. 808

# OVERVIEW

Diuretics are drugs that increase renal excretion of water, sodium, and other electrolytes, thereby increasing urine formation and output. They are important therapeutic agents widely used in the management of both edematous (eg, heart failure, renal and hepatic disease) and nonedematous (eg, hypertension, ophthalmic surgery) conditions. Diuretics are also useful in preventing renal failure by their ability to sustain urine flow. To aid understanding of diuretic drug therapy, renal physiology related to drug action is reviewed in the At the Foundation: Renal Physiology. Additionally, many clinical conditions alter renal function and produce edema and electrolyte imbalance requiring diuretic agents for management. Types of diuretics are described and individual drugs are listed in Drugs at a Glance 44-1: Diuretic Agents.

## Alterations in Renal Function

Many clinical conditions alter renal function. In some conditions, excessive amounts of substances (eg, sodium and water) are retained; in others, needed substances (eg, potassium, proteins) are eliminated. These conditions include cardiovascular, renal, hepatic, and other disorders that may be managed with diuretic drugs.

## Edema

*Edema* is the excessive accumulation of fluid in body tissues. It is a symptom of many disease processes and may occur in any part of the body. Additional characteristics include the following:

1. Edema formation results from one or more of the following mechanisms that allow fluid to leave the bloodstream (intravascular compartment) and enter interstitial (third) spaces.
   a. Increased capillary permeability occurs as part of the response to tissue injury. Thus, edema may occur with burns and trauma or allergic and inflammatory reactions.
   b. Increased capillary hydrostatic pressure results from a sequence of events in which increased blood volume (from fluid overload or sodium and water retention) or obstruction of venous blood flow causes a high venous pressure and a high capillary pressure. This is the primary mechanism for edema formation in heart failure, pulmonary edema, and renal failure.
   c. Decreased plasma oncotic pressure may occur with decreased synthesis of plasma proteins (caused by liver disease or malnutrition) or increased loss of plasma proteins (caused by burn injuries or the nephrotic syndrome). Plasma proteins are important in keeping fluids within the bloodstream. When plasma proteins are lacking, fluid seeps through the capillaries and accumulates in tissues.
2. Edema interferes with blood flow to tissues. Thus, it interferes with delivery of oxygen and nutrients and removal of metabolic waste products. If severe, edema may distort body features, impair movement, and interfere with activities of daily living.
3. Specific manifestations of edema are determined by its location and extent. A common type of localized edema occurs in the feet and ankles (dependent edema), especially with prolonged sitting or standing. A less common but more severe type of localized edema is pulmonary edema, a life-threatening condition that occurs with circulatory overload (eg, of intravenous [IV] fluids or blood transfusions) or acute heart failure. Generalized massive edema (anasarca) interferes with the functions of many body organs and tissues.

# DIURETIC DRUGS

Diuretic drugs act on the kidneys to decrease reabsorption of sodium, chloride, water, and other substances. Major subclasses are the thiazides and related diuretics,

## AT THE FOUNDATION: *Renal Physiology*

The primary function of the kidneys is to regulate the volume, composition, and pH of body fluids. The kidneys receive approximately 25% of the cardiac output. From this large amount of blood flow, the normally functioning kidney is efficient in retaining substances needed by the body and eliminating those not needed.

The nephron is the functional unit of the kidney; each kidney contains approximately 1 million nephrons. Each nephron is composed of a glomerulus and a tubule (Fig. 44-1). The nephron functions by three processes: glomerular filtration, tubular reabsorption, and tubular secretion. These processes normally maintain the fluid volume, electrolyte concentration, and pH of body fluids within a relatively narrow range. They also remove waste products of cellular metabolism. A minimum daily urine output of approximately 400 mL is required to remove normal amounts of metabolic end products.

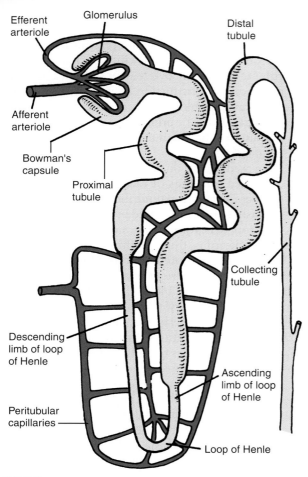

Efferent arteriole
Glomerulus
Distal tubule
Afferent arteriole
Bowman's capsule
Proximal tubule
Descending limb of loop of Henle
Ascending limb of loop of Henle
Peritubular capillaries
Collecting tubule
Loop of Henle

**FIGURE 44–1** The nephron is the functional unit of the kidney.

loop diuretics, and potassium-sparing diuretics, which act at different sites in the nephron (Fig. 44-2).

Major clinical indications for diuretics are edema, heart failure, and hypertension. In edematous states, diuretics mobilize tissue fluids by decreasing plasma volume. In hypertension, the exact mechanism by which diuretics lower blood pressure is unknown, but antihypertensive action is usually attributed to sodium depletion. Initially, diuretics decrease blood volume and cardiac output. With chronic use, cardiac output returns to normal, but there is a persistent decrease in plasma volume and peripheral vascular resistance. Sodium depletion may have a vasodilating effect on arterioles.

Diuretics are often used to manage edema and ascites in clients with hepatic impairment. They must be used with caution because diuretic-induced fluid and electrolyte imbalances may precipitate or worsen hepatic encephalopathy and coma. In clients with cirrhosis, diuretic therapy should be initiated in a hospital setting, with small doses and careful monitoring. To prevent hypokalemia and metabolic alkalosis, supplemental potassium or spironolactone may be needed.

The use of diuretic agents in the management of heart failure and hypertension is discussed further in Chapters 38 and 42, respectively. Discussion of management considerations in children and older adults is found in Age-related Considerations. Additionally, home care is an essential component in the management of clients requiring diuretic therapy. Guidelines for strategies for ongoing evaluation and intervention are addressed in Home Care Considerations.

**DRUG TABLE 44-1**

## Drugs at a Glance

### Diuretic Agents

| Generic/Trade Name | Routes and Dosage Ranges | Comments |
|---|---|---|
| **Thiazide and Related Diuretics** | | |
| **Chlorothiazide** (Diuril) Pregnancy Category C (by manufacturer); D (by expert analysis) | *Adults:* PO, 500–1000 mg 1 or 2 times daily; IV, 500 mg twice daily *Children:* PO, 22 mg/kg/d in 2 divided doses *Infants <6 mo:* PO, up to 33 mg/kg/d in 2 divided doses; IV, not recommended | |
| **Chlorthalidone** (Hygroton) Pregnancy Category B (by manufacturer); D (by expert analysis) | *Adults:* PO, 25–100 mg daily *Children:* PO, 3 mg/kg 3 times weekly, adjusted according to response | Requires dosage adjustment in renal failure |
| **Hydrochlorothiazide** (HydroDIURIL, Esidrix, Oretic) | See Prototype Profile 44-1: Hydrochlorothiazide | |
| **Loop Diuretics** | | |
| **Bumetanide** (Bumex) Pregnancy Category C (by manufacturer); D (by expert analysis) | *Adults:* PO, 0.5–2 mg daily as a single dose. May be repeated q4–6h to a maximum dose of 10 mg, if necessary. Giving on alternate days or for 3 to 4 d with rest | Be alert about complaints of hearing difficulties with IV injection; increased risk for hearing loss with rapid administration |

*(continued)*

## Drugs at a Glance

**DRUG TABLE 44-1**

### Diuretic Agents (Continued)

| Generic/Trade Name | Routes and Dosage Ranges | Comments |
|---|---|---|
| | periods of 1–2 d is recommended for long-term control of edema<br>IV, IM, 0.5–1 mg, repeated in 2–3 h if necessary, to a maximum daily dose of 10 mg; give injections over 1–2 min<br>*Children:* Not recommended for children <18 y | |
| **Ethacrynic acid**<br>Pregnancy Category B | *Adults:* Edema: PO, 50–100 mg daily, adjusted according to severity of condition and response, to maximum daily dose of 400 mg<br>Rapid mobilization of edema: IV, 50 mg or 0.5–1 mg/kg injected slowly to a maximum of 100 mg/dose<br>*Children:* PO, 25 mg daily<br>Dosage for infants has not been established<br>IV, no recommended parenteral dose in children | Not removed by hemodialysis or peritoneal dialysis |
| **Furosemide** (Lasix)<br>Pregnancy Category C | See Prototype Profile 44-2: Furosemide | |
| **Torsemide** (Demadex)<br>Pregnancy Category B | *Adults:* PO, IV, 5–20 mg once daily | Observe for orthostatic hypotension<br>Special adjustment in elderly is not necessary |
| ***Potassium-Sparing Diuretics*** | | All potassium-sparing diuretics may cause hyperkalemia |
| **Amiloride** (Midamor)<br>Pregnancy Category B | *Adults:* PO, 5–20 mg daily<br>*Children:* dosage not established | Administer with food or meals to avoid GI upset |
| **Spironolactone** (Aldactone)<br>Pregnancy Category D | See Prototype Profile 44-3: Spironolactone | |
| **Triamterene** (Dyrenium)<br>Pregnancy Category B (by manufacturer); D (by expert analysis) | *Adults:* PO, 100–300 mg daily in divided doses<br>*Children:* PO, 2–4 mg/kg/d in divided doses | Dosage adjustment recommended with cirrhosis<br>Will interfere with fluorescent measurement of quinidine levels |
| ***Osmotic Agents*** | | |
| **Glycerin** (Osmoglyn)<br>Pregnancy Category C | *Adults:* PO, 1–1.5 g/kg of body weight, usually given as a 50–75% solution, 1–2 h before ocular surgery<br>*Children:* Same as adults | Use may interrupt acute attacks of glaucoma |
| **Isosorbide** (Ismotic)<br>Pregnancy Category B | *Adults:* PO, 1.5–3 g/kg up to 4 times daily if necessary for glaucoma or ocular surgery | Less risk for nausea and vomiting than with other drugs in class |
| **Mannitol** (Osmitrol)<br>Pregnancy Category C | *Adults:* Diuresis: IV infusion, 50–200 g over 24 h, flow rate adjusted to maintain a urine output of 30–50 mL/h<br>Oliguria and prevention of acute renal failure: IV, 50–100 g<br>Reduction of intracranial or intraocular pressure: IV, 1.5–2 g/kg, given as a 20% solution, over 30–60 min<br>*Children:* Same as adults | May also be used as irrigation in transurethral surgical procedures |

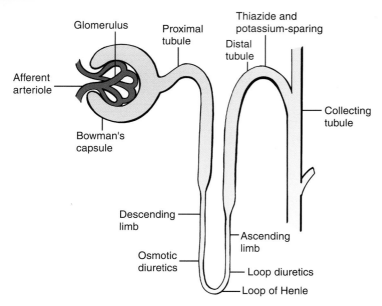

FIGURE 44-2 Diuretic sites of action in the nephron. Diuretics act at different sites in the nephron to decrease reabsorption of sodium and water and increase urine output.

## Thiazide and Related Diuretics

Thiazide diuretics are synthetic drugs that are chemically related to the sulfonamides and differ mainly in their duration of action. **ⓟ Hydrochlorothiazide** is the most commonly used and is considered the prototype (see Prototype Profile 44-1: Hydrochlorothiazide). Chlorothiazide is the only thiazide diuretic that can be given intravenously. Related diuretics are nonthiazides whose

pharmacologic actions are essentially the same as those of the thiazides; they include chlorthalidone, metolazone, and quinethazone.

Thiazides and related diuretics are frequently prescribed in the long-term management of heart failure and hypertension. They act to decrease reabsorption of sodium, water, chloride, and bicarbonate in the distal convoluted tubule. Most sodium is reabsorbed before it reaches the distal convoluted tubule, and only a small amount is reab-

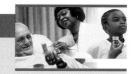

## Age-related Considerations: Use of Diuretics

### USE IN CHILDREN

Although they have not been extensively studied in children, diuretics are commonly used to manage heart failure, which often results from congenital heart disease; hypertension, which is usually related to cardiac or renal dysfunction; bronchopulmonary dysplasia and respiratory distress syndrome, which are often associated with pulmonary edema; and edema, which may occur with cardiac or renal disorders such as the nephrotic syndrome. Furosemide is the loop diuretic used most often in children. In preterm infants, furosemide stimulates production of prostaglandin $E_2$ in the kidneys and may increase the incidence of patent ductus arteriosus and neonatal respiratory distress syndrome. In neonates, furosemide may be given with indomethacin to prevent nonsteroidal anti-inflammatory drug–induced nephrotoxicity during therapeutic closure of a patent ductus arteriosus. In both preterm and full-term infants, furosemide half-life is prolonged but becomes shorter as renal and hepatic functions develop. Safety and effectiveness of bumetanide, ethacrynic acid, and torsemide have not been established. Spironolactone is the most widely used potassium-sparing diuretic in children. It is used with other diuretics to decrease potassium loss and hypokalemia. Spironolactone

accumulates in renal failure, and dosage should be reduced. It usually should not be used in severe renal failure.

### USE IN OLDER ADULTS

Thiazide diuretics are often prescribed for the management of hypertension and heart failure, which are common in older adults. Older adults are especially sensitive to adverse drug effects, such as hypotension and electrolyte imbalance. Thiazides may aggravate renal or hepatic impairment. With rapid or excessive diuresis, myocardial infarction, renal impairment, or cerebral thrombosis may occur from fluid volume depletion and hypotension. The smallest effective dose is recommended, usually a daily dose of 12.5 to 25 mg of hydrochlorothiazide or equivalent doses of other thiazides and related drugs. Risks for adverse effects may exceed benefits at doses of hydrochlorothiazide greater than 25 mg.

With loop diuretics, older adults are at greater risk for excessive diuresis, hypotension, fluid volume deficit, and possibly thrombosis or embolism. Rapid diuresis may cause urinary incontinence. With potassium-sparing diuretics, hyperkalemia is more likely to occur in older adults because of the renal impairment that occurs with aging.

## Home Care Considerations: Use of Diuretics

**ASSESS:** safe and effective use of medications, nutritional status and compliance with diet therapy, orthostatic blood pressures, weight, and use of over-the-counter medications that may aggravate edema or hypertension with each home visit.

**MONITOR:** client responses to therapy and provide teaching information as indicated. In some cases, the home care nurse may need to assist the client in obtaining medications or blood tests (eg, serum potassium levels).

**EDUCATE:** on how to take a blood pressure reading, recognizing signs and symptoms that necessitate professional follow up. Reinforce additional teaching points (see Client Teaching Guidelines: Diuretics).

These drugs are well absorbed, widely distributed in body fluids, and highly bound to plasma proteins. They accumulate only in the kidneys. Diuretic effects usually occur within 2 hours, peak at 4 to 6 hours, and last 6 to 24 hours. Antihypertensive effects usually last long enough to allow use of a single daily dose. Most of the drugs are excreted unchanged by the kidneys within 3 to 6 hours; some (eg, chlorthalidone) have longer durations of action (48 to 72 hours), attributed to slower excretion.

Thiazides and related drugs are contraindicated in clients allergic to sulfonamide drugs. They must be used cautiously during pregnancy because they cross the placenta and may have adverse effects on the fetus by compromising placental perfusion.

The effectiveness of thiazides decreases as the GFR decreases, and the drugs become ineffective when the GFR is less than 30 mL/minute. The drugs may accumulate and increase adverse effects in clients with impaired renal function. Thus, renal function tests should be performed periodically. If progressive renal impairment becomes evident (eg, a rising serum creatinine or blood urea nitrogen [BUN]), a thiazide usually should be discontinued, and metolazone, indapamide, or a loop diuretic may be given.

sorbed at this site. Thus, these drugs are not strong diuretics. In addition, they are ineffective when immediate diuresis is required (because of their slow onset of action) and relatively ineffective with decreased renal function. They work efficiently only when urine flow is adequate.

---

## PROTOTYPE PROFILE 44-1

### P Hydrochlorothiazide (hye droe klor oh THYE a zide)

**Drug Class**
*Chemical:* Thiazide diuretic
*Functional:* Diuretic; antihypertensive agent

**Trade Names**
HydroDIURIL, HCTZ, Oretic, Esidrix

**Therapeutic Indications**
Improvement of urine output; treatment of edema in heart failure, renal dysfunction, or hepatic cirrhosis; management of hypertension; investigational use for treatment of lithium-induced diabetes insipidus

**Pharmacokinetics**
*Absorption*
Readily absorbed (50%–80%) from GI tract

*Distribution*
Plasma protein binding: 65%

*Metabolism*
Not metabolized

*Excretion*
Urine (unchanged)

**Pharmacodynamics**
*Onset of Action*
2 h

*Duration*
6–12 h

**Contraindications/Precautions**
Hypersensitivity to thiazides or sulfonamide-derived drugs; pregnancy; severe electrolyte imbalance, hypovolemia, anuria, or renal decompensation

**Side Effects/Adverse Reactions**
Orthostatic hypotension, hypokalemia, dizziness, hyperglycemia, photosensitivity, anorexia or GI distress

**Pregnancy Considerations**
Category B (by manufacturer); D (by expert analysis). Enters breast milk; use with caution

**Dosage**
*Adults:* Edema: 25–100 mg/d in 1 to 2 doses; maximum of 200 mg/d
Hypertension: 25–50 mg/d
*Elderly:* 12.5–25 mg once daily
*Children:*
< 6 mo: 2–3 mg/kg/d in two doses
> 6 mo: 2 mg/kg/d in two doses

**Drug Interactions**
*Increased Effects*
Diuresis with Lasix and other loop diuretics
Hypotension with angiotensin-converting enzyme inhibitors

*(continued)*

**PROTOTYPE PROFILE 44-1**

**P Hydrochlorothiazide (Continued)**

Hyperglycemic effects in type 2 diabetes mellitus with beta blockers

Lithium toxicity due to reduced renal excretion of lithium

Potassium loss with steroids

Duration of neuromuscular blocking agents

*Decreased Effects*

Effects of oral hypoglycemics

Thiazide effect with colestipol and cholestyramine

Efficacy of thiazides with nonsteroidal anti-inflammatory drugs reducing the diuretic and antihypertensive effects

**Herbal Supplements and Dietary Considerations**

Dong quai has estrogenic effect, so avoid if using for antihypertensive effect; also increases photosensitivity effect

Ginseng, ephedra, and yohimbe may worsen hypertension

Garlic may increase antihypertensive effect

Peak serum hydrochlorothiazide levels may be decreased with ingestion with food

Produces a potassium loss

## Loop Diuretics

Loop diuretics inhibit sodium and chloride reabsorption in the ascending limb of the loop of Henle, where reabsorption of most filtered sodium occurs. Thus, these potent drugs produce significant diuresis, with their sodium-losing effect up to 10 times greater than that of thiazide diuretics. Dosage can be titrated upward as needed to produce greater diuretic effects. Overall, loop diuretics are the most effective and versatile diuretics available for clinical use.

Loop diuretics produce extensive diuresis for short periods, after which the kidney tubules regain their ability to reabsorb sodium. Actually, the kidneys reabsorb more sodium than usual during this postdiuretic phase; therefore, a high dietary intake of sodium can cause sodium retention and reduce or cancel the diuretic-induced sodium loss. Thus, dietary sodium restriction is required to achieve optimum therapeutic benefits.

Loop diuretics are the diuretics of choice when rapid effects are required (eg, in pulmonary edema) and when renal function is impaired (creatinine clearance <30 mL/minute). The drugs are contraindicated during pregnancy unless absolutely necessary.

Furosemide is the most commonly used loop diuretic and serves as the prototype for the group. Key considerations regarding furosemide are outlined in Prototype Profile 44-2: Furosemide. Bumetanide may be used to produce diuresis in some clients who are allergic to or no longer respond to furosemide. It is more potent than furosemide on a weight basis, and large doses can be given in small volumes. These drugs differ mainly in potency and produce similar effects at equivalent doses (eg, furosemide, 40 mg = bumetanide, 1 mg).

Loop diuretics are effective in clients with renal impairment. However, in chronic renal failure, they have lower peak concentrations at their site of action, which decreases diuresis. Renal elimination of the drugs is also prolonged. If renal dysfunction becomes more severe during treatment (eg, oliguria, increases in BUN

or creatinine), the diuretic may need to be discontinued. If high doses of furosemide are used, a volume-controlled IV infusion at a rate of 4 mg/minute or less may be used. If IV bumetanide is given to clients with chronic renal impairment, a continuous infusion (eg, 12 mg over 12 hours) produces more diuresis than equivalent-dose intermittent injections. Continuous infusion also produces lower serum drug levels and therefore may decrease adverse effects.

## Potassium–sparing Diuretics

Sodium is normally reabsorbed in the distal tubule in exchange for potassium and hydrogen ions. Potassium-sparing diuretics act at the distal tubule to decrease sodium reabsorption and potassium excretion. This group includes three drugs. One is spironolactone, an aldosterone antagonist. Aldosterone is a hormone secreted by the adrenal cortex that promotes retention of sodium and water and excretion of potassium by stimulating the sodium–potassium exchange mechanism in the distal tubule. Spironolactone blocks the sodium-retaining effects of aldosterone, and aldosterone must be present for spironolactone to be effective. This drug is the prototype of the class and is detailed in Prototype Profile 44-3: Spironolactone. The other two drugs, amiloride and triamterene, act directly on the distal tubule to decrease the exchange of sodium for potassium and have similar diuretic activity.

Potassium-sparing diuretics are weak diuretics when used alone. Thus, they are usually given in combination with potassium-losing diuretics to increase diuretic activity and decrease potassium loss. They are contraindicated in the presence of renal insufficiency because their use may cause hyperkalemia through the inhibition of aldosterone and subsequent retention of potassium. Hyperkalemia is the major adverse effect of these drugs; clients receiving potassium-sparing diuretics *should not* be given potassium supplements and *should not* be encouraged to eat foods high in potassium, or allowed to use salt substi-

## PROTOTYPE PROFILE 44-2

### *P* Furosemide (fyoor OH se mide)

**Drug Class**
*Chemical:* Loop diuretic
*Functional:* Antihypertensive agent; diuretic

**Trade Name**
Lasix

**Therapeutic Indications**
Management of edema associated with heart failure and renal and hepatic disease; treatment of hypertension

**Pharmacokinetics**
*Absorption*
60%–67% orally

*Distribution*
Plasma protein binding > 98%

*Metabolism*
Minimal hepatic metabolism

*Excretion*
Urine PO 50%; IV 80%; feces as unchanged drug

**Pharmacodynamics**
*Onset of Action*
Diuresis: PO in 30–60 min; IM in 30 min; IV in < 5 min

*Duration*
PO, 6–8 h; IV, 2 h

**Contraindications/Precautions**
Hypersensitivity to furosemide or sulfonylureas; anuria, severe electrolyte imbalance, hypovolemia, or hepatic coma

**Side Effects/Adverse Reactions**
Orthostatic hypotension, dehydration, dizziness, photosensitivity, hearing impairment (reversible or permanent with rapid IV or IM administration), electrolyte imbalances, ECG changes, or weakness

**Pregnancy Considerations**
Category C; diuretics usually avoided in pregnancy due to potential for decreased placental perfusion; crosses the placenta, increasing fetal urine production and electrolyte disturbances
Enters breast milk, so use with caution

**Dosage**
*Adults:* PO, 20–80 mg initially, increased in increments of 20–40 mg in intervals of 6–12 h to maximum of 600 mg/d

IV bolus or IM, 20–40 mg; may be repeated in 1–2 h and increased by 20 mg/dose until the desired response is obtained
IV continuous infusion, initial dose of 0.1 mg/kg bolus followed by infusion of 0.1 mg/kg/h; doubled every 2 h, not to exceed 4 mg/kg/h
*Children:* PO, 1–2 mg/kg/dose initially increased in increments of 1 mg/kg/dose in intervals of 6 h to maximum of 6 mg/kg/dose
IV or IM, 1 mg/kg/dose, increasing by 1 mg/kg/dose with each subsequent dose up to 6 mg/kg/dose until desired response obtained

**Drug Interactions**
*Increased Effects*
Drug-induced hypokalemia may increase risk of digoxin toxicity or dysrhythmias
Risk for toxicity with lithium or high-dose salicylates
Hypotension with angiotensin-converting enzyme inhibitors and nonsteroidal anti-inflammatory drugs (NSAIDs) potentiated by furosemide-induced hypovolemia
Risk for ototoxicity with other ototoxic agents (aminoglycosides or cisplatin)
Effects of peripheral adrenergic-blocking agents or ganglionic blockers

*Decreased Effects*
Effects of oral hypoglycemics
Furosemide effect with colestipol, cholestyramine, and sucralfate
Decreased furosemide concentration with metformin use
Hypotensive effect with aspirin, indomethacin, NSAIDs, phenobarbital, and phenytoin

**Herbal Supplements and Dietary Considerations**
Dong quai has estrogenic effect, so avoid if using furosemide for antihypertensive effect; also increases photosensitivity effect
Ginseng, ephedra, ginkgo, and yohimbe may worsen hypertension
Garlic may increase antihypertensive effect
Serum levels may be decreased if taken with food but may be administered with food in clients with GI distress

---

tutes. Salt substitutes contain potassium chloride rather than sodium chloride.

## Osmotic Diuretics

Osmotic agents produce rapid diuresis by increasing the solute load (osmotic pressure) of the glomerular filtrate. The increased osmotic pressure causes water to be pulled from extravascular sites into the bloodstream, thereby increasing blood volume and decreasing reabsorption of water and electrolytes in the renal tubules. Mannitol is useful in managing oliguria or anuria, and it may prevent acute renal failure during prolonged surgery, trauma, or infusion of cisplatin, an antineo-

You are working on a cardiac unit, caring for clients after bypass surgery. Mr. Vallera has Lasix 80 mg PO ordered bid to pull off extra fluid that is retained from the surgery. After administering the medication, you look through the chart as you document the medication you gave. You note that the nursing assistant has charted the following:

Vital signs: B/P 142/88 (lying), P 96 and regular; B/P
    108/60, P 128 and regular, R 18
Daily weight—164 lb (a 9-lb. drop from yesterday)
Yesterday's intake 1565 mL, output 3590 mL
Serum K+, 2.8 mEq/L
Were you wrong to administer the Lasix, and if so, why?

plastic agent. Mannitol is effective even when renal circulation and GFR are reduced (eg, in hypovolemic shock, trauma, or dehydration). Other important clinical uses of hyperosmolar agents include reduction of intracranial pressure before or after neurosurgery, reduction of intraocular pressure before certain types of ophthalmic surgery, and urinary excretion of toxic substances. Other osmotic agents are listed in Drugs at a Glance 44-1: Diuretic Agents.

## Combination Products

Thiazide and related diuretics are available in numerous fixed-dose combinations with nondiuretic antihypertensive agents (see Chap. 42) and with potassium-

---

**PROTOTYPE PROFILE 44-3**
**ⓟ Spironolactone**

**Drug Class**
*Chemical:* Potassium-sparing diuretic
*Functional:* Antihypertensive agent; diuretic

**Trade Name**
Aldactone

**Therapeutic Indications**
Management of hypertension; reduction of edema in heart failure, cirrhosis, and nephrotic syndrome; treatment of primary hyperaldosteronism

**Pharmacokinetics**
Well absorbed after oral administration

*Distribution*
Plasma protein binding: Adults—91%–96%

*Metabolism*
Hepatic; half-life 1.5–2 h

*Excretion*
Urine and feces

**Pharmacodynamics**
*Onset of Action*
24–48 h

*Duration*
48–72 h

**Contraindications/Precautions**
Anuria, acute renal insufficiency, hyperkalemia, clients receiving triamterene or amiloride

**Pregnancy Considerations**
Category C/D in pregnancy-induced hypertension
Enters breast milk

**Dosage**
Hypertension:
*Adults:* PO, 50–100 mg/d in 1 or 2 divided doses
*Children:* PO, 1–2 mg/kg/d in divided doses has been recommended
Edema:
*Adults:* PO, 25–200 mg/d in divided doses
*Children:* PO, 1.5–3.5 mg/kg/d in divided doses

**Side Effects/Adverse Reactions**
Drowsiness, lack of coordination, decreased mental alertness, GI cramping, diarrhea, thirst, impotence, breast enlargement in men

**Drug Interactions**
*Increased Effects*
Risk for hyperkalemia, especially in clients with renal impairment, with potassium supplements, angiotensin-converting enzyme inhibitors, angiotensin-receptor antagonists, other potassium-sparing diuretics, and co-trimoxazole
Risk for hyperchloremic acidosis with cholestyramine in clients with cirrhosis

*Decreased Effects*
Effects of digoxin and mitotane; may interfere with radioimmunoassay (RIA) tests to measure digoxin, producing falsely elevated serum digoxin values

**Herbal Supplements and Dietary Considerations**
Natural licorice increases mineralocorticoid activity and should be avoided
Food increases absorption
Avoid excessive ingestion of foods high in potassium (bananas, nuts) and salt substitutes

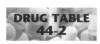

**Drugs at a Glance**
## Combination Diuretic Products

| Trade Name | Thiazide (Potassium-losing) Diuretic | Potassium-sparing Diuretic | Adult Dosage |
|---|---|---|---|
| **Aldactazide** 25/25 | HCTZ 25 mg | Spironolactone 25 mg | PO, 1–8 tablets daily |
| **Aldactazide** 50/50 | HCTZ 50 mg | Spironolactone 50 mg | PO, 1–4 tablets daily |
| **Dyazide, Maxzide** 25 mg | HCTZ 25 mg | Triamterene 37.5 mg | Hypertension: PO, 1 capsule bid initially, then adjusted according to response. Edema, PO, 1–2 capsules bid |
| **Maxzide** | HCTZ 50 mg | Triamterene 75 mg | PO, 1 tablet daily |
| **Moduretic** | HCTZ 50 mg | Amiloride 5 mg | PO, 1–2 tablets daily with meals |

HCTZ, hydrochlorothiazide.

sparing diuretics (Drugs at a Glance 44-2: Combination Diuretic Products). A major purpose of the antihypertensive combinations is to increase client convenience and compliance with drug therapy regimens. A major purpose of the diuretic combinations is to prevent potassium imbalances. Despite the convenience of a combination product, it may be better to give the drugs separately so that dosage can be titrated to the client's needs.

*(text continues on page 814)*

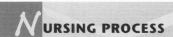

## NURSING PROCESS

### Assessment
Assess the client's status in relation to baseline data and conditions in which diuretic drugs are used.

- Useful baseline data include serum electrolytes, creatinine, glucose, blood urea nitrogen (BUN), and uric acid, because diuretics may alter these values. Other data are blood pressure readings, weight, amount and appearance of urine output, and measurement of edematous areas, such as ankles or abdomen.
- Observe for edema. Visible edema often occurs in the feet and legs of ambulatory clients. Rapid weight gain may indicate fluid retention.
  - With heart failure, numerous signs and symptoms result from edema of various organs and tissues. For example, congestion in the GI tract may cause nausea and vomiting, liver congestion may cause abdominal pain and tenderness, and congestion in the lungs (pulmonary edema) causes rapid, labored breathing, hypoxemia, frothy sputum, and other manifestations of severe respiratory distress.
  - Cerebral edema may be manifested by confusion, headache, dizziness, convulsions, unconsciousness, bradycardia, or failure of the pupils to react to light.
  - Ascites, which occurs with hepatic cirrhosis, is an accumulation of fluid in the abdominal cavity. The abdomen appears much enlarged.
- With heart failure, fatigue and dyspnea, in addition to edema, are common symptoms.

- Hypertension (blood pressure above 140/90 mm Hg on several measurements) may be the only clinical manifestation present.

### Nursing Diagnoses
- Excess Fluid Volume in edematous clients, related to retention of sodium and water
- Deficient Fluid Volume related to increased diuresis during diuretic drug therapy
- Imbalanced Nutrition: Less Than Body Requirements related to excessive loss of potassium with thiazide and loop diuretics
- Risk for Injury: Hypotension and dizziness as adverse drug effects
- Deficient Knowledge related to the need for and correct use of diuretics
- Sexual Dysfunction related to adverse drug effects

### Planning/Goals
*The client will:*
- Take or receive diuretic drugs as prescribed
- Experience reduced edema and improved control of blood pressure
- Reduce dietary intake of sodium and increase dietary intake of potassium
- Avoid preventable adverse drug effects
- Keep appointments for follow-up monitoring of blood pressure, edema, and serum electrolytes

*(continued)*

## *N*URSING PROCESS (Continued)

### Interventions

Promote measures to prevent or minimize conditions for which diuretic drugs are used.

- With edema, helpful measures include the following:
  - Decreasing dietary sodium intake
  - Losing weight, if obese
  - Elevating legs when sitting
  - Avoiding prolonged standing or sitting
  - Wearing support hose or elastic stockings
  - Treating the condition causing edema
- With heart failure and in older adults, administer IV fluids or blood transfusions carefully to avoid fluid overload and pulmonary edema. Fluid overload may occur with rapid administration or excessive amounts of IV fluids.
- With hypertension, helpful measures include decreasing dietary sodium intake, exercising regularly, and losing weight, if obese.
- With edematous clients, interventions to monitor fluid losses include weighing under standardized conditions, measuring urine output, and measuring edematous sites such as the ankles or the abdomen. Once the client reaches "dry weight," these measurements stabilize and can be done less often.
- With clients who are taking digoxin, a potassium-losing diuretic, and a potassium supplement, assist them to understand that the drugs act together to increase therapeutic effectiveness and avoid adverse effects (eg, hypokalemia and digoxin toxicity). Thus, stopping or changing dosage of one of these drugs can lead to serious illness.

### Evaluation

- Observe for reduced edema and body weight.
- Observe for reduced blood pressure.
- Observe for increased urine output.
- Monitor serum electrolytes for normal values.
- Interview regarding compliance with instructions for diet and drug therapy.
- Monitor compliance with follow-up appointments in outpatients.

## CLIENT TEACHING GUIDELINES
## Diuretics

### General Considerations

✔ Diuretics increase urine output and are commonly used to manage hypertension, heart failure, and edema (swelling) from heart, kidney, liver, and other disorders.

✔ While taking a diuretic drug, you need to maintain regular medical supervision so drug effects can be monitored and dosages adjusted when indicated.

✔ Reducing sodium intake in your diet helps diuretic drugs be more effective and allows smaller doses to be taken. Smaller doses are less likely to cause adverse effects. Thus, you need to avoid excessive table salt and obviously salty foods (eg, ham, packaged sandwich meats, potato chips, dill pickles, most canned soups). These foods may aggravate edema or hypertension by causing sodium and water retention.

✔ Diuretics may cause blood potassium imbalances, and either too little or too much damages heart function. Periodic measurements of blood potassium and other substances is one of the major reasons for regular visits to a health care provider.

Too little potassium (hypokalemia) may result from the use of potassium-losing diuretics such as hydrochlorothiazide, Lasix, and several others. To prevent or treat hypokalemia, your doctor may prescribe a potassium chloride supplement or a combination of a potassium-losing and a potassium-saving diuretic (either separately or as a combined product such as Dyazide, Maxzide, or Aldactazide). He or she may also recommend increased dietary intake of potassium-containing foods (eg, bananas, orange juice).

Too much potassium (hyperkalemia) can result from the use of potassium-saving diuretics, the overuse of potassium supplements, or from the use of salt substitutes. Potassium-saving diuretics are not a major cause of hyperkalemia because they are usually given along with a potassium-losing diuretic. If potassium supplements are prescribed, they should be taken as directed. You should not use salt substitutes without consulting your primary health care provider because they contain potassium chloride instead of sodium chloride. Hyperkalemia is most likely to occur in people with decreased kidney function, which often occurs in older adults and people with diabetes.

✔ With diuretic therapy, you will have increased urination, which usually lasts only a few days or weeks if you do not have edema. If you do have edema (eg, in your ankles), you can expect weight loss and decreased swelling as well as increased urination. It is a good idea to check and record your weight 2–3 times per week. Rapid changes in weight often indicate gain or loss of fluid.

✔ Some commonly used diuretics may increase blood sugar levels and cause or aggravate diabetes. If you have diabetes, you may need larger doses of your antidiabetic medications.

✔ Diuretics may cause sensitivity to sunlight. Thus, you need to avoid prolonged exposure to sunlight, use sunscreens, and wear protective clothing.

✔ Do not drink alcoholic beverages or take other medications without the approval of your health care provider.

*(continued)*

### CLIENT TEACHING GUIDELINES
**Diuretics** (Continued)

✔ If you are taking a diuretic to lower your blood pressure, especially with other antihypertensive drugs, you may feel dizzy or faint when you stand up suddenly. This can be prevented or decreased by changing positions slowly. If dizziness is severe, notify your health care provider.

**Self-administration or Caregiver Administration**

✔ Take or give a diuretic early in the day, if ordered daily, to decrease nighttime trips to the bathroom. Fewer bathroom trips means less interference with sleep and less risk of falls. Ask someone to help you to the bathroom if you are elderly, weak, dizzy, or unsteady in walking (or use a bedside commode).

✔ Take or give most diuretics with or after food to decrease stomach upset. Torsemide (Demadex) may be taken without regard to meals.

✔ If you are taking digoxin, a potassium-losing diuretic, and a potassium supplement, it is very important that you take these drugs as prescribed. This is a common combination of drugs for clients with heart failure and the drugs work together to increase beneficial effects and avoid adverse effects. Stopping or changing the dose of one of these medications while continuing the others can lead to serious illness.

## Nursing Actions
### Diuretics

| Nursing Actions | Rationale/Explanation |
|---|---|
| **1. Administer accurately.** | |
| a. Give in the early morning if ordered daily. | So that peak action will occur during waking hours and not interfere with sleep |
| b. Take safety precautions. Keep a bedpan or urinal within reach. Keep the call light within reach, and be sure the client knows how to use it. Assist to the bathroom anyone who is elderly, weak, dizzy, or unsteady in walking. | Mainly to avoid falls |
| c. Give amiloride and triamterene with or after food | To decrease gastrointestinal (GI) upset |
| d. Give intravenous (IV) injections of furosemide and bumetanide over 1–2 min; give torsemide over 2 min. | To decrease or avoid high peak serum levels, which increase risks of adverse effects, including ototoxicity |
| e. Give high-dose furosemide continuous IV infusions at a rate of 4 mg/min or less | |
| **2. Observe for therapeutic effects.** | |
| a. Decrease or absence of edema, increased urine output, decreased blood pressure | Most oral diuretics act within 2 h; IV diuretics act within minutes. Optimal antihypertensive effects occur in approximately 2–4 wk. |
| (1) Weigh the client daily while edema is present and two to three times weekly thereafter. Weigh under standard conditions: early morning before eating or drinking, after urination, with the same amount of clothing, and using the same scales. | Body weight is a very good indicator of fluid gain or loss. A weight change of 2.2 lb (1 kg) may indicate a gain or loss of 1000 mL of fluid. Also, weighing assists in dosage regulation to maintain therapeutic benefit without excessive or too rapid fluid loss. |
| (2) Record fluid intake and output every shift for hospitalized clients. | Normally, oral fluid intake approximates urinary output (1500 mL/24 h). With diuretic therapy, urinary output may exceed intake, depending on the amount of edema or fluid retention, renal function, and diuretic dosage. All sources of fluid gain, including IV fluids, must be included; all sources of fluid loss (perspiration, fever, wound drainage, GI tract drainage) are important. Clients with abnormal fluid losses have less urine output with diuretic therapy. Oliguria (decreased excretion of urine) may require stopping the drug. Output greater than 100 mL/h may indicate that side effects are more likely to occur. |

*(continued)*

## Nursing Actions

### Diuretics (Continued)

| Nursing Actions | Rationale/Explanation |
|---|---|
| (3) Observe and record characteristics of urine. | Dilute urine may indicate excessive fluid intake or greater likelihood of fluid and electrolyte imbalance due to rapid diuresis. Concentrated urine may mean oliguria or decreased fluid intake. |
| (4) Assess for edema daily or with each client contact: ankles for the ambulatory client, sacral area and posterior thighs for clients at bed rest. Also, it is often helpful to measure abdominal girth, ankles, and calves to monitor gain or loss of fluid. | Expect a decrease in visible edema and size of measured areas. If edema reappears or worsens, a thorough reassessment of the client is in order. Questions to be answered include:<br>(1) Is the prescribed diuretic being taken correctly?<br>(2) What type of diuretic and what dosage is ordered?<br>(3) Is there worsening of the underlying condition(s) that led to edema formation?<br>(4) Has other disease developed? |
| (5) In clients with heart failure or acute pulmonary edema, observe for decreased dyspnea, crackles, cyanosis, and cough. | Decreased fluid in the lungs leads to improved respirations as more carbon dioxide and oxygen gas exchange takes place and greater tissue oxygenation occur. |
| (6) Record blood pressure 2 to 4 times daily when diuretic therapy is initiated. | Although thiazide diuretics do not lower normal blood pressure, other diuretics may, especially with excessive or rapid diuresis. |
| 3. **Observe for adverse effects.** | Major adverse effects are fluid and electrolyte imbalances. |
| a. With potassium-losing diuretics (thiazides, bumetanide, furosemide, ethacrynic acid), observe for: | |
| (1) Hypokalemia<br>  (a) Serum potassium levels below 3.5 mEq/L<br>  (b) Electrocardiographic (ECG) changes (eg, low voltage, flattened T wave, depressed ST segment)<br>  (c) Cardiac dysrhythmias; weak, irregular pulse<br>  (d) Hypotension<br>  (e) Weak, shallow respirations<br>  (f) Anorexia, nausea, vomiting<br>  (g) Decreased peristalsis or paralytic ileus<br>  (h) Skeletal muscle weakness<br>  (i) Confusion, disorientation | Potassium is required for normal muscle function. Thus, potassium depletion causes weakness of cardiovascular, respiratory, digestive, and skeletal muscles. Clients most likely to have hypokalemia are those who are taking large doses of diuretics, potent diuretics (eg, furosemide), or adrenal corticosteroids; those who have decreased food and fluid intake; or those who have increased potassium losses through vomiting, diarrhea, chronic laxative or enema use, or GI suction. Clinically significant symptoms are most likely to occur with a serum potassium level below 3 mEq/L. |
| (2) Hyponatremia, hypomagnesemia, hypochloremic alkalosis, changes in serum and urinary calcium levels | In addition to potassium, sodium chloride, magnesium, and bicarbonate also are lost with diuresis. Thiazides and related diuretics cause hypercalcemia and hypocalciuria. They have been used to prevent calcium nephrolithiasis (kidney stones). Furosemide and other loop diuretics tend to cause hypocalcemia and hypercalciuria. |
| (3) Dehydration<br>  (a) Poor skin turgor, dry mucous membranes<br>  (b) Oliguria, urine of high specific gravity<br>  (c) Thirst<br>  (d) Tachycardia; hypotension<br>  (e) Decreased level of consciousness<br>  (f) Elevated hematocrit (above 45%) | Fluid volume depletion occurs with excessive or rapid diuresis. If it is prolonged or severe, hypovolemic shock may occur. |
| (4) Hyperglycemia—blood glucose above 120 mg/100 mL, polyuria, polydipsia, polyphagia, glycosuria | Hyperglycemia is more likely to occur in clients with known or latent diabetes mellitus. Larger doses of hypoglycemic agents may be required. The hyperglycemic effect may be reversible when diuretic therapy is discontinued. |

*(continued)*

## Nursing Actions
## Diuretics (Continued)

| Nursing Actions | Rationale/Explanation |
|---|---|
| | Long-term use of a thiazide or loop diuretic may alter glucose metabolism. One mechanism is thought to involve diuretic-induced hypokalemia and hypomagnesemia, which then leads to decreased postprandial insulin release. Another mechanism may be development or worsening of insulin resistance. |
| | Because glucose intolerance is an important risk factor for coronary artery disease, diuretics should be used with caution in prediabetic or diabetic hypertensive clients. |
| (5) Hyperuricemia—serum uric acid above 7.0 mg/ 100 mL | Hyperuricemia is usually asymptomatic except for clients with gout, a predisposition toward gout, or chronic renal failure. Apparently, decreased renal excretion of uric acid allows its accumulation in the blood. |
| (6) Pulmonary edema (with osmotic diuretics) | Pulmonary edema is most likely to occur in clients with heart failure who cannot tolerate the increased blood volume produced by the drugs. |
| (7) Ototoxicity (with furosemide and ethacrynic acid) | Reversible or transient hearing impairment, tinnitus, and dizziness are more common, although irreversible deafness may occur. Ototoxicity is more likely to occur with high serum drug levels (eg, high doses or use in clients with severe renal impairment) or when other ototoxic drugs (eg, aminoglycoside antibiotics) are being taken concurrently. |
| b. With potassium-sparing diuretics (spironolactone, triamterene, amiloride), observe for: | |
| (1) Hyperkalemia | Hyperkalemia is most likely to occur in clients with impaired renal function or those who are ingesting additional potassium (eg, salt substitutes) |
| (a) Serum potassium levels above 5 mEq/L | |
| (b) ECG changes (ie, prolonged P-R interval; wide QRS complex; tall, peaked T wave; depressed ST segment) | |
| (c) Cardiac dysrhythmias, which may progress to ventricular fibrillation and asystole | |
| 4. Observe for drug interactions. | |
| a. Drugs that *increase* effects of diuretics: | |
| (1) Aminoglycoside antibiotics | Additive ototoxicity with ethacrynic acid |
| (2) Antihypertensive agents | Additive hypotensive effects. In addition, angiotensin-converting enzyme inhibitor therapy significantly increases risks of hyperkalemia with spironolactone. |
| (3) Corticosteroids | Additive hypokalemia |
| b. Drugs that *decrease* effects of diuretics: | |
| (1) Nonsteroidal anti-inflammatory drugs (eg, aspirin, ibuprofen, others) | These drugs cause retention of sodium and water. |
| (2) Oral contraceptives | Retention of sodium and water |
| (3) Vasopressors (eg, epinephrine, norepinephrine) | These drugs may antagonize hypotensive effects of diuretics by decreasing responsiveness of arterioles. |

## ? How Can You Avoid This Medication Error?

**Answer:** The purpose of the diuretic therapy is to pull off excessive fluid, but the assessment data gathered from Mr. Vallera (significant weight loss—almost 10 lb in 1 day; orthostatic blood pressure with elevated pulse, which indicates volume depletion; and hypokalemia) indicate that diuresis is occurring too rapidly. It is always important to evaluate assessment data before giving a medication, so that a medication can be held if the client's condition warrants it.

## Critical Thinking Exercises

1. Mr. Smith has recently been started on hydrochlorothiazide, 25 mg PO daily, for heart failure. He also has a history of type 2 diabetes mellitus and takes an oral hypoglycemic agent. Which assessment finding should the nurse instruct Mr. Smith to observe for with long-term thiazide diuretic therapy?

   a. Hyponatremia
   b. Increased diuresis
   c. Hyperglycemia
   d. Increased hypotension

2. Like other potassium-sparing diuretics, spironolactone acts in the:

   a. Distal renal tubules
   b. Proximal renal tubules
   c. Ascending loop of Henle
   d. Glomerulus

3. Jason, 21 years of age, is brought to the emergency department with head trauma after a motorcycle accident. Shortly after admission, he becomes unresponsive. The health care provider prescribes mannitol (Osmitrol), 1.5 g/kg IV of 20% solution STAT. The nurse understands that mannitol will reduce Jason's intracranial pressure by:

   a. Increasing the osmotic pressure of plasma, glomerular filtrate, and tubular fluid
   b. Acting as an anti-inflammatory agent
   c. Blocking the action of the enzyme carbonic anhydrase
   d. Acting on the distal tubules, increasing water and sodium excretion

4. Mr. James is started on high dose aspirin therapy for rheumatoid arthritis. What effect will the addition of aspirin have on the effect of the diuretic Mr. James takes for his heart failure?

   a. No effect
   b. Increased effect
   c. Decreased effect
   d. Synergistic effect

5. Mr. Jones, 53 years of age, has had hypertension for 10 years and admits that he does not comply with his prescribed antihypertensive therapy. Recently, he has begun to experience shortness of breath and ankle swelling. The physician diagnoses renal insufficiency. What classification of diuretic is the drug choice for Mr. Jones?

   a. Thiazide
   b. Loop
   c. Osmotic
   d. Potassium sparing

## SELECTED REFERENCES

Applegate, W. B. (2000). Approach to the elderly client with hypertension. In H. D. Humes (Ed.), *Kelley's textbook of internal medicine* (4th ed., pp. 3026–3031). Philadelphia: Lippincott Williams & Wilkins.

Brater, D. C. (2000). Clinical pharmacology of cardiovascular drugs. In H. D. Humes (Ed.), *Kelley's textbook of internal medicine* (4th ed., pp. 651–672). Philadelphia: Lippincott Williams & Wilkins.

Carter, B. L., & Saseen, J. J. (2002). Hypertension. In J. T. DiPiro, R. L. Talbert, G. C. Yee, G. R. Matzke, B. G. Wells, & L. M. Posey (Eds.), *Pharmacotherapy: A pathophysiologic approach* (5th ed., pp. 157–183). New York: McGraw-Hill.

*Drug facts and comparisons.* (Updated monthly). St. Louis: Facts and Comparisons.

Guyton, A. C., & Hall, J. E. (2000). *Textbook of medical physiology* (10th ed.). Philadelphia: W. B. Saunders.

Johnson, J. A., Parker, R. B., & Patterson, J. H. (2002). Heart failure. In J. T. DiPiro, R. L. Talbert, G. C. Yee, G. R. Matzke, B. G. Wells, & L. M. Posey (Eds.), *Pharmacotherapy: A pathophysiologic approach* (5th ed., pp. 185–218). New York: McGraw-Hill.

Lacy, C. F., Armstrong, L. L., Goldman, M. P., & Lance, L. L. (2003). *Lexi-Comp's drug information handbook* (11th ed.). Hudson, OH: American Pharmaceutical Association.

Porth, C. M. (2002). *Pathophysiology: Concepts of altered health states* (6th ed.). Philadelphia: Lippincott Williams & Wilkins.

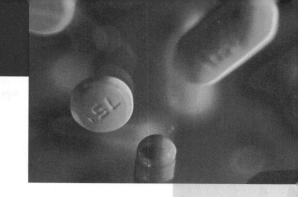

# 45

# Drugs That Affect Blood Coagulation

## OBJECTIVES

*After studying this chapter, the student will be able to:*

1 Describe important elements in the physiology of hemostasis and thrombosis.

2 Discuss potential consequences of blood clotting disorders.

3 Give characteristics and uses of anticoagulant, antiplatelet, and thrombolytic agents.

4 Compare and contrast heparin and warfarin in terms of indications for use, onset and duration of action, route of administration, blood tests used to monitor effects, and nursing process implications.

5 Teach clients on long-term warfarin therapy protective measures to prevent abnormal bleeding.

6 Discuss antiplatelet agents in terms of indications for use and effects on blood coagulation.

7 Describe thrombolytic agents in terms of indications and contraindications for use, routes of administration, and major adverse effects.

8 Describe systemic hemostatic agents for treating overdoses of anticoagulant and thrombolytic drugs.

## CRITICAL THINKING SCENARIO

*J*uan Sanchez, a 56-year-old migrant farmer without health insurance, is admitted to the hospital after an episode of syncope. He is diagnosed with atrial fibrillation and is started on a calcium channel blocker and warfarin (Coumadin). Before his discharge, you are responsible for patient teaching.

✔ What assessment data would be helpful to individualize your teaching plan?

✔ Discuss the rationale for use of warfarin in clients with atrial fibrillation.

✔ Identify side effects of warfarin therapy.

✔ Consider strategies that might help Mr. Sanchez comply with therapy and experience limited side effects.

## PROTOTYPE PROFILES

heparin (Hep–Lock), p. 823

warfarin (Coumadin), p. 825

# OVERVIEW

Anticoagulant, antiplatelet, and thrombolytic drugs are used in the prevention and management of thrombotic and thromboembolic disorders. Thrombosis involves the formation (thrombogenesis) or presence of a blood clot (thrombus) in the vascular system. Blood clotting is a normal body defense mechanism to prevent blood loss. Thus, thrombogenesis may be life saving when it occurs as a response to hemorrhage; however, it may be life threatening when it occurs at other times because the thrombus can obstruct a blood vessel and block blood flow to tissues beyond the clot. When part of a thrombus breaks off and travels to another part of the body, it is called an *embolus*.

Atherosclerosis is the basic disease process that often leads to pathologic thrombosis. Over time, plaque lesions become larger and extend farther into the lumen of the artery. Eventually, a thrombus may develop at plaque sites and partially or completely occlude an artery. In coronary arteries, a thrombus may precipitate myocardial ischemia (angina or infarction) (see Chap. 41); in carotid or cerebral arteries, a thrombus may precipitate a stroke; in peripheral arteries, a thrombus may cause intermittent claudication (pain in the legs with exercise) or acute occlusion. Thus, serious impairment of blood flow may occur with a large atherosclerotic plaque or a relatively small plaque with superimposed vasospasm and thrombosis.

Normally, thrombi are constantly being formed and dissolved (thrombolysis), but the blood stays fluid, and flow is not significantly obstructed. If the balance between thrombogenesis and thrombolysis is upset, thrombotic or bleeding disorders result. Thrombotic disorders occur much more often than bleeding disorders and are emphasized in this chapter; bleeding disorders may result from excessive amounts of drugs that inhibit clotting. Discussion of management considerations in children and older adults is found in Age-related Considerations.

To aid understanding of drug therapy for thrombotic disorders, normal hemostasis, endothelial functions in relation to blood clotting, platelet functions, blood coagulation, and characteristics of arterial and venous thrombosis are described in At the Foundation: Hemostasis and Clot Lysis.

# THROMBOTIC AND THROMBOEMBOLIC DISORDERS

Thrombosis may occur in both arteries and veins. Arterial thrombosis is usually associated with atherosclerotic plaque, hypertension, and turbulent blood flow. These conditions damage arterial endothelium and activate platelets to initiate the coagulation process. Arterial thrombi cause disease by obstructing blood flow. If the obstruction is incomplete or temporary, local tissue

---

## Age-related Considerations: Use of Anticoagulant Drugs

### USE IN CHILDREN

Little information is available about the use of anticoagulants in children. Heparin solutions containing benzyl alcohol as a preservative should not be given to premature infants because fatal reactions have been reported. When given for systemic anticoagulation, heparin dosage should be based on the child's weight (approximately 50 units/kg). Safety and effectiveness of low-molecular-weight heparin (LMWH) (eg, enoxaparin) have not been established in children.

Warfarin is given to children after cardiac surgery to prevent thromboembolism, but doses and guidelines for safe, effective use have not been developed. Accurate drug administration, close monitoring of blood coagulation tests, safety measures to prevent trauma and bleeding, avoidance of interacting drugs, and education of others in the child's environment (eg, teachers, babysitters, health care providers) are necessary.

Antiplatelet and thrombolytic drugs have no established indications for use in children.

### USE IN OLDER ADULTS

Older adults often have atherosclerosis and thrombotic disorders, including myocardial infarction, thrombotic stroke, and peripheral arterial insufficiency, for which they receive an anticoagulant or an antiplatelet drug. They are more likely than younger adults to experience bleeding and other complications of anticoagulant and antiplatelet drugs. For example, aspirin or clopidogrel is commonly used to prevent thrombotic stroke, but both drugs increase risk for hemorrhagic stroke.

With standard heparin, general principles for safe and effective use apply. With LMWH, elimination may be delayed in older adults with renal impairment, and the drugs should be used cautiously. They should also be used with caution in clients taking a platelet inhibitor (eg, aspirin, clopidogrel) to prevent myocardial infarction or thrombotic stroke, or an NSAID for arthritis pain. NSAIDs, which are commonly used by older adults, also have antiplatelet effects. Clients who take an NSAID daily may not need low-dose aspirin for antithrombotic effects.

With warfarin, dosage should be reduced because impaired liver function and decreased plasma proteins increase the risk for bleeding. Also, many drugs interact with warfarin to increase or decrease its effect, and older adults often take multiple drugs. Starting or stopping any drug may require that warfarin dosage be adjusted.

## AT THE FOUNDATION: *Hemostasis and Clot Lysis*

### Hemostasis

*Hemostasis* is prevention or stoppage of blood loss from an injured blood vessel and is the process that maintains the integrity of the vascular compartment. It involves activation of several mechanisms, including vasoconstriction, formation of a platelet plug (a cluster of aggregated platelets), sequential activation of clotting factors in the blood (Table 45-1), and growth of fibrous tissue (fibrin) into the blood clot to make it more stable and to repair the tear (opening) in the damaged blood vessel. Overall, normal hemostasis is a complex process involving numerous interacting activators and inhibitors, including endothelial factors, platelets, and blood coagulation factors (Box 45-1).

### Clot Lysis

When a blood clot is being formed, plasminogen (an inactive protein found in many body tissues and fluids) is bound to fibrin and becomes a component of the clot. After the outward blood flow is stopped and the tear in the blood vessel repaired, plasminogen is activated by plasminogen activator (produced by endothelial cells or the coagulation cascade) to produce plasmin. Plasmin is an enzyme that breaks down the fibrin meshwork that stabilizes the clot; this fibrinolytic or thrombolytic action dissolves the clot.

ischemia (deficient blood supply) occurs. If the obstruction is complete or prolonged, local tissue death or infarction occurs.

Venous thrombosis is usually associated with venous stasis. When blood flows slowly, thrombin and other procoagulant substances present in the blood become concentrated in local areas and initiate the clotting process. With a normal rate of blood flow, these substances are rapidly removed from the blood, primarily by Kupffer cells in the liver. A venous thrombus is less cohesive than an arterial thrombus, and an embolus can easily become detached and travel to other parts of the body.

Venous thrombi cause disease by two mechanisms. First, thrombosis causes local congestion, edema, and perhaps inflammation by impairing normal outflow of venous blood (eg, thrombophlebitis, deep vein thrombosis [DVT]). Second, embolization obstructs the blood supply when the embolus becomes lodged. The pulmonary arteries are common sites of embolization.

## DRUGS USED IN THROMBOTIC AND THROMBOEMBOLIC DISORDERS

Drugs given to prevent or treat thrombosis alter some aspect of the blood coagulation process. Anticoagulants are widely used in thrombotic disorders. They are more effective in preventing venous thrombosis than arterial

### TABLE 45-1 Blood Coagulation Factors

| Number | Name | Functions |
| --- | --- | --- |
| I | Fibrinogen | Forms fibrin, the insoluble protein strands that compose the supporting framework of a blood clot. Thrombin and calcium are required for the conversion. |
| II | Prothrombin | Forms thrombin, which catalyzes the conversion of fibrinogen to fibrin |
| III | Thromboplastin | Converts prothrombin to thrombin |
| IV | Calcium | Catalyzes the conversion of prothrombin to thrombin |
| V | Labile factor | Required for formation of active thromboplastin |
| VII | Proconvertin or stable factor | Accelerates action of tissue thromboplastin |
| VIII | Antihemophilic factor | Promotes breakdown of platelets and formation of active platelet thromboplastin |
| IX | Christmas factor | Similar to factor VIII |
| X | Stuart factor | Promotes action of thromboplastin |
| XI | Plasma thromboplastin antecedent | Promotes platelet aggregation and breakdown, with subsequent release of platelet thromboplastin |
| XII | Hageman factor | Similar to factor XI |
| XIII | Fibrin-stabilizing factor | Converts fibrin meshwork to the dense, tight mass of the completely formed clot |

### BOX 45-1    Hemostasis and Thrombosis

The blood vessels and blood normally maintain a balance between procoagulant and anticoagulant factors that favors anticoagulation and keeps the blood fluid. Injury to blood vessels and tissues causes complex reactions and interactions among vascular endothelial cells, platelets, and blood coagulation factors that shift the balance toward procoagulation and thrombosis.

#### Endothelial Cells

Endothelial cells play a role in all aspects of hemostasis and thrombosis. Normal endothelium helps to prevent thrombosis by producing anticoagulant factors, inhibiting platelet reactivity, and inhibiting activation of the coagulation cascade. However, endothelium promotes thrombosis when its continuity is lost (eg, the blood vessel wall is torn by rupture of atherosclerotic plaque, hypertension, trauma), its function is altered, or when blood flow is altered or becomes static. After a blood clot is formed, the endothelium also induces its dissolution and restoration of blood flow.

*Antithrombotic Functions*

- Synthesizes and releases prostacyclin (prostaglandin $I_2$), which inhibits platelet aggregation
- Releases endothelium-derived relaxing factor (nitric oxide), which inhibits platelet adhesion and aggregation
- Blocks platelet exposure to subendothelial collagen and other stimuli for platelet aggregation
- May inhibit platelet reactivity by inactivating adenosine diphosphate (ADP), a platelet product that promotes platelet aggregation
- Produces plasminogen activators (eg, tissue-type or tPA) in response to shear stress and such agonists as histamine and thrombin. These activators convert inactive plasminogen to plasmin, which then breaks down fibrin and dissolves blood clots (fibrinolytic effects).
- Produces thrombomodulin, a protein that helps prevent formation of intravascular thrombi by inhibiting thrombin-mediated platelet aggregation. Thrombomodulin also reacts with thrombin to activate proteins C and S, which inhibit the plasma cascade of clotting factors.

*Prothrombotic Functions*

- Produces antifibrinolytic factors. Normally, the balance between profibrinolysis and antifibrinolysis favors fibrinolysis (clot dissolution). In pathologic conditions, including atherosclerosis, fibrinolysis may be limited and thrombosis enhanced.
- In pathologic conditions, may induce synthesis of prothrombotic factors such as von Willebrand factor. Von Willebrand factor serves as a site for subendothelial platelet adhesion and as a carrier for blood coagulation factor VIII in plasma. Several disease states are associated with increased or altered production of von Willebrand factor, including atherosclerosis.
- Produces tissue factor, which activates the extrinsic coagulation pathway after exposure to oxidized low-density lipoprotein cholesterol, homocysteine, and cytokines (eg, interleukin-1, tumor necrosis factor–alpha)

#### Platelets

Platelets (also called *thrombocytes*) are fragments of large cells called *megakaryocytes.* They are produced in the bone marrow and released into the bloodstream, where they circulate for approximately 7 to 10 days before they are removed by the spleen. They contain no nuclei and therefore cannot repair or replicate themselves.

The cell membrane of a platelet contains a coat of glycoproteins that prevents the platelet from adhering to normal endothelium but allows it to adhere to damaged areas of endothelium and subendothelial collagen in the blood vessel wall. It also contains receptors for ADP, collagen, blood coagulation factors such as fibrinogen, and other substances. Breakdown of the cell membrane releases arachidonic acid (which can be metabolized to produce thromboxane $A_2$) and allows leakage of platelet contents (eg, thromboplastin and other clotting factors), which function to stop bleeding.

The cytoplasm of a platelet contains storage granules with ADP, fibrinogen, histamine, platelet-derived growth factor, serotonin, von Willebrand factor, enzymes that produce thromboxane $A_2$, and other substances. The cytoplasm also contains contractile proteins that contract storage granules so they empty their contents and help a platelet plug to retract and plug a hole in a torn blood vessel.

The only known function of platelets is hemostasis. When platelets come in contact with a damaged vascular surface, they become activated and undergo changes in structure and function. They enlarge, express receptors on their surfaces, release mediators from their storage granules, become sticky so that they adhere to endothelial and collagen cells, and form a platelet thrombus (ie, a cluster or aggregate of activated platelets) within seconds. The thrombus blocks the tear in the blood vessel and prevents further leakage of blood. Platelets usually disappear from a blood clot within 24 hours and are replaced by fibrin.

Formation of a platelet thrombus proceeds through the phases of activation, adhesion, aggregation, and procoagulation.

*Activation*

Platelet activation occurs when agonists such as thrombin, collagen, ADP, or epinephrine bind to their specific receptors on the platelet cell membrane surface. Activated platelets release von Willebrand factor, which aids platelet adhesion to blood vessel walls. They also secrete ADP and thromboxane $A_2$ into the blood. The ADP and thromboxane $A_2$ activate and recruit nearby platelets.

*Adhesion*

Platelet adhesion involves changes in platelets that allow them to adhere to endothelial cells and subendothelial collagen exposed by damaged endothelium. Adhesion is mediated by interactions between platelets and substances in the subendothelial tissues. Platelets contain binding sites for several subendothelial tissue proteins, including collagen and von Willebrand factor. In capillaries, where blood shear rates are high, platelets also can bind indirectly to collagen through von Willebrand factor. Von Willebrand factor is synthesized by

*(continued)*

**BOX 45-1** **Hemostasis and Thrombosis** (Continued)

endothelial cells and megakaryocytes. Although it contains binding sites for platelets and collagen, it does not normally bind with platelets until they are activated.

*Aggregation*

Aggregation involves the accumulation of platelets at a site of injury to a blood vessel wall and is stimulated by ADP, collagen, thromboxane $A_2$, thrombin, and other factors. It requires the binding of extracellular fibrinogen to platelet fibrinogen receptors. The fibrinogen receptor is located on a complex of two glycoproteins (GPIIb and IIIa) in the platelet cell membrane. Although many GP IIb/IIIa complexes are on the surface of each platelet, they do not function as fibrinogen receptors until the platelet is activated by an agonist. Each activated GP IIb/IIIa complex is capable of binding a single fibrinogen molecule. However, a fibrinogen molecule may bind to receptors on adjacent activated platelets, thus acting as a bridge to connect the platelets. Activated GP IIb/IIIa complexes can also bind von Willebrand factor and promote platelet aggregation when fibrinogen is lacking.

Aggregated platelets produce and release thromboxane $A_2$, which acts with ADP from platelet storage granules to promote additional GP IIb/IIIa activation, platelet secretion, and aggregate formation. The exposure of functional GP IIb/IIIa complexes is also stimulated by thrombin, which can directly stimulate thromboxane $A_2$ synthesis and granule secretion without initial aggregation. Collagen stimulates additional aggregation by increasing the production of thromboxane $A_2$ and storage granule secretion.

Overall, aggregated platelets release substances that recruit new platelets and stimulate additional aggregation. This activity helps the platelet plug become large enough to block blood flow out of a damaged blood vessel. If the opening is small, the platelet plug can stop blood loss. If the opening is large, a platelet plug and a blood clot are both required to stop the bleeding.

*Procoagulant Activity*

In addition to forming a platelet thrombus, platelets also activate and interact with circulating blood coagulation factors to form a larger and more stable blood clot. Activation of the previously inactive blood coagulation factors leads to formation of fibrin threads that attach to the platelets and form a tight meshwork of a fully developed blood clot.

More specifically, the platelet plug provides a surface on which coagulation enzymes, substrates, and cofactors interact at high local concentrations. These interactions lead to activation of coagulation factor X and the conversion of prothrombin to thrombin.

**Blood Coagulation**

The blood coagulation process causes hemostasis within 1 to 2 minutes. It involves sequential activation of clotting factors that are normally present in blood and tissues as inactive precursors and formation of a meshwork of fibrin strands that cements blood components together to form a stable, dense clot. Major phases include release of thromboplastin by disintegrating platelets and damaged tissue; conversion of prothrombin to thrombin, which requires thromboplastin and calcium ions; and conversion of fibrinogen to fibrin by thrombin.

Blood coagulation results from activation of the intrinsic or extrinsic coagulation pathway. Both pathways, which are activated when blood passes out of a blood vessel, are needed for normal hemostasis. The intrinsic pathway occurs in the vascular system; the extrinsic pathway occurs in the tissues. Although the pathways are initially separate, the terminal steps (ie, activation of factor X and thrombin-induced formation of fibrin) are the same.

The intrinsic pathway is activated when blood comes in contact with collagen in the injured vessel wall and coagulation factor XII interacts with biologic surfaces. The normal endothelium prevents factor XII from interacting with such surfaces. The activated form of factor XII is a protease that starts the interactions among factors involved in the intrinsic pathway (eg, prekallikrein, factor IX, factor VIII).

The extrinsic pathway is activated when blood is exposed to tissue extracts and tissue factor interacts with circulating coagulation factor VII. Activated factors VII and IX both act on factor X to produce activated factor X, which then interacts with factor V, calcium, and platelet factor 3. Platelet factor 3, a component of the platelet cell membrane, becomes available on the platelet surface only during platelet activation. The interactions among these substances lead to formation of thrombin, which then activates fibrinogen to form fibrin, and the clot is complete.

---

thrombosis. Home care is an essential component in the management of individuals on anticoagulants. Guidelines for strategies for ongoing evaluation and intervention are addressed in Home Care Considerations. Antiplatelet drugs are used to prevent arterial thrombosis. Thrombolytic agents are used to dissolve thrombi and limit tissue damage in selected thromboembolic disorders. These drugs are described in the following sections and in Drugs at a Glance 45-1: Anticoagulant, Antiplatelet, and Thrombolytic Agents. Discussion of specific manage-

ment considerations in children and older adults is found in Age-related Considerations.

## Anticoagulants

Anticoagulant drugs are given to prevent formation of new clots and extension of clots already present. They do not dissolve formed clots, improve blood flow in tissues around the clot, or prevent ischemic damage to tissues beyond the clot. Heparins and warfarin are commonly

## Home Care Considerations: Use of Anticoagulant Drugs

**ASSESS:** knowledge about prescribed drugs and ability and willingness to comply with instructions for taking the drugs, obtaining blood tests when indicated, and taking safety precautions. In addition, assess the environment for risk factors for injury.

**MONITOR:** for safe use of the drugs, for therapeutic response to treatment, including laboratory tests and signs and symptoms of bleeding. Also monitor for ability to obtain laboratory tests and other follow-up care.

**EDUCATE:** about the disorder (usually DVT), including the potential consequences of either overcoagulation or undercoagulation, precautions needed to decrease risks for bleeding, and the need for blood tests. Also teach to observe for signs that necessitate professional attention. Reinforce additional teaching points (see Client Teaching Guidelines: Drugs to Prevent or Treat Blood Clots).

used anticoagulants; danaparoid and lepirudin are newer agents. Clinical indications include prevention or management of thromboembolic disorders, such as thrombophlebitis, DVT, and pulmonary embolism. The main adverse effect is bleeding.

### Heparin

**Heparin** is a pharmaceutical preparation of the natural anticoagulant produced primarily by mast cells in pericapillary connective tissue. It is considered a prototype and is detailed in Prototype Profile 45-1: Heparin. Heparin is the anticoagulant of choice in acute venous thromboembolic disorders because the anticoagulant effect begins immediately with intravenous (IV) administration. When anticoagulation is required during pregnancy, heparin is used because it does not cross the placenta. Endogenous heparin is found in various body tissues, most abundantly in the liver and lungs. Exogenous heparin is obtained from bovine lung or porcine intestinal mucosa and standardized in units of biologic activity.

*(text continues on page 824)*

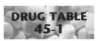

## DRUG TABLE 45-1 — Drugs at a Glance
### Anticoagulant, Antiplatelet, and Thrombolytic Agents

| Generic/Trade Name | Routes and Dosage Ranges (Adults) | Comments/Uses |
|---|---|---|
| **Anticoagulants** | | |
| **Heparin** | See Prototype Profile 45-1: Heparin | |
| **Argatroban** (Argatroban) Pregnancy Category B | IV continuous infusion, 2 mcg/kg/min | Thrombosis prophylaxis or management in heparin-induced thrombocytopenia |
| **Bivalirudin** (Angiomax) Pregnancy Category B | IV bolus dose of 1 mg/kg followed by 4 h infusion at rate of 2.5 mg/kg/min | Clients with unstable angina undergoing PTCA in conjunction with aspirin |
| **Dalteparin** (Fragmin) Pregnancy Category B | Abdominal surgery, Sub-Q 2500 IU 1–2 h before surgery and then once daily for 5–10 days after surgery<br>Hip replacement surgery, Sub-Q 2500 IU 1–2 h before surgery and the evening of surgery (at least 6 h after first dose) and then 5000 IU once daily for 5 days | Prophylaxis of DVT in clients having hip replacement surgery; also clients at high risk for thromboembolic disorders who are having abdominal surgery |
| **Danaparoid** (Orgaran) Pregnancy Category B | Sub-Q, 750 IU twice daily, with first dose 1–24 h before surgery, then daily for 7–14 days after surgery | Prophylaxis of DVT in clients having hip replacement surgery |
| **Enoxaparin** (Lovenox) Pregnancy Category B | DVT prophylaxis in clients having hip or knee replacement surgery, Sub-Q, 30 mg twice daily, with first dose within 12–24 h after surgery and continued for 7–10 days<br>Abdominal surgery, Sub-Q, 40 mg once daily with first dose given 2 h before surgery, for 7–10 days<br>DVT/pulmonary embolism management, outpatients, Sub-Q, 1 mg/kg q12h; inpatients, 1 mg/kg q12h or 1.5 mg/kg q24h | Prevention and management of DVT and pulmonary embolism<br>Management of unstable angina, to prevent myocardial infarction |

*(continued)*

**DRUG TABLE 45-1**

## *Drugs at a Glance*
### Anticoagulant, Antiplatelet, and Thrombolytic Agents (Continued)

| Generic/Trade Name | Routes and Dosage Ranges (Adults) | Comments/Uses |
|---|---|---|
| | Unstable angina: 1 mg/kg q12h in conjunction with oral aspirin (100–325 mg once daily) | |
| **Fondaparinux** (Arixtra) Pregnancy Category B | Sub-Q, 2.5 mg daily, with first dose 6–8 h after surgery and continuing for a maximum of 11 days | Prevention of DVT following hip fracture surgery or knee or hip replacement |
| **Lepirudin** (Refludan) Pregnancy Category B | IV injection, 0.4 mg/kg over 15–20 sec, followed by continuous IV infusion of 0.15 mg/kg for 2–10 days or longer if needed | Heparin alternative for anticoagulation of clients with heparin-induced thrombocytopenia and associated thromboembolic disorders |
| **Tinzaparin** (Innohep) Pregnancy Category B | Sub-Q, 175 anti-Xa IU/kg daily for at least 6 days and until adequately anticoagulated with warfarin | Management of DVT, with or without PE; may be given in conjunction with warfarin |
| **Warfarin** (Coumadin) | See Prototype Profile 45-2: Warfarin | |
| ***Antiplatelet Agents*** | | |
| **Aspirin** Pregnancy Category D | PO, 81–325 mg daily | Prevention of myocardial infarction Prevention of thromboembolic disorders in clients with prosthetic heart valves or transient ischemic attacks |
| **Abciximab** (ReoPro) Pregnancy Category C | IV bolus injection, 0.25 mg/kg 10–60 min before starting PTCA, then a continuous IV infusion of 10 mcg/min for 12 h | Used with PTCA to prevent rethrombosis of treated arteries Intended for use with aspirin and heparin |
| **Anagrelide** (Agrylin) Pregnancy Category C | PO, 0.5 mg four times daily or 1 mg twice daily initially, then titrate to lowest dose effective in maintaining platelet count <600,000/mm³ | Essential thrombocythemia, to reduce the elevated platelet count, the risk for thrombosis, and associated symptoms |
| **Cilostazol** (Pletal) Pregnancy Category C | PO, 100 mg twice daily, 30 min before or 2 h after breakfast and dinner; reduce to 50 mg twice daily with concurrent use of fluconazole, itraconazole, erythromycin, or diltiazem | Treatment of intermittent claudication, to increase walking distance (before leg pain occurs) |
| **Clopidogrel** (Plavix) Pregnancy Category B | PO, 75 mg once daily with or without food | May reduce atherosclerotic events (myocardial infarction, stroke, vascular death) in clients with atherosclerosis documented by recent stroke, recent myocardial infarction, or established peripheral artery disease |
| **Dipyridamole** (Persantine) Pregnancy Category B | PO, 25–75 mg three times per day, 1 h before meals | Prevention of thromboembolism after cardiac valve replacement, given with warfarin |
| **Dipyridamole and Aspirin** (Aggrenox) Pregnancy Category B (dipyridamole), D (aspirin) | PO, 1 capsule (200 mg extended-release dipyridamole/25 mg aspirin) twice daily | Same as above |
| **Eptifibatide** (Integrilin) Pregnancy Category B | IV bolus injection, 180 mcg/kg, followed by continuous infusion of 2 mcg/kg/min See manufacturer's instructions for preparation and administration | Used in clients with acute coronary syndromes, including clients who are to be managed medically and those undergoing PTCA |

*(continued)*

**DRUG TABLE 45-1**

*Drugs at a Glance*

## Anticoagulant, Antiplatelet, and Thrombolytic Agents (Continued)

| Generic/Trade Name | Routes and Dosage Ranges (Adults) | Comments/Uses |
|---|---|---|
| **Ticlopidine** (Ticlid) Pregnancy Category B | PO, 250 mg twice daily with food | May prevent thrombosis in clients with coronary artery or cerebral vascular disease (eg, clients who have had stroke precursors or a completed thrombotic stroke) |
| **Tirofiban** (Aggrastat) Pregnancy Category B | IV infusion, 0.4 mcg/kg/min for 30 min, then 0.1 mcg/kg/min. Patients with severe renal impairment (creatinine clearance <30 mL/min) should receive half the usual rate of infusion. See manufacturer's instructions for preparation and administration | Management of acute coronary syndromes, with heparin, for clients who are to be managed medically or those undergoing PTCA; also acute myocardial infarction and pulmonary embolism |
| **Treprostinil** (Remodulin) Pregnancy Category B | Continuous infusion by Sub-Q catheter and infusion pump at initial dose of 1.25 mg/kg/min, increasing by no more than 1.25 mg/kg/min per week for first 4 wk, and then by no more than 2.5 mg/kg/min per week for remaining duration of infusion | Treatment of pulmonary arterial hypertension |
| ***Thrombolytic Agents*** | | |
| **Alteplase** (Activase) Pregnancy Category C | IV infusion, 100 mg over 3 h (first hour, 60 mg with a bolus of 6–10 mg over 1–2 min initially; second hour, 20 mg; third hour, 20 mg) | Synonymous with tissue-type plasminogen activator (t-PA); alteplase and anistreplase may act more specifically on the fibrin in a clot and cause less systemic depletion of fibrinogen, but these agents are very expensive Management of acute ischemic stroke, acute myocardial infarction, and pulmonary emboli |
| **Anistreplase, recombinant** (Eminase) Pregnancy Category C | IV injection, 30 units over 2–5 min | Decreases infarct size in acute myocardial infarction |
| **Drotrecogin alfa, activated** (Xigris) Pregnancy Category C | IV infusion of 24 mcg/kg/h for 96 h | Reduction of mortality in severe sepsis |
| **Reteplase, recombinant** (Retavase) Pregnancy Category C | IV injection, 10 units over 2 min, repeated in 30 min. Inject into a flowing IV infusion line that contains no other medications | Acute myocardial infarction; a derivative of t-PA with less risk of hemorrhage |
| **Streptokinase** (Streptase) Pregnancy Category C | IV 250,000 units over 30 min, then 100,000 units/h for 24–72 h | Management of acute, severe pulmonary emboli or iliofemoral thrombophlebitis Used to dissolve clots in arterial or venous cannulas or catheters May be injected into a coronary artery to dissolve a thrombus if done within 6 h of onset of symptoms The least expensive agent of the class, but may cause allergic reactions because it is a foreign protein. Combination therapy (eg, with alteplase and streptokinase) may also be used |

*(continued)*

## DRUG TABLE 45-1

## *Drugs at a Glance*

## Anticoagulant, Antiplatelet, and Thrombolytic Agents (Continued)

| Generic/Trade Name | Routes and Dosage Ranges (Adults) | Comments/Uses |
|---|---|---|
| **Tenecteplase** (TNKase) Pregnancy Category C | IV bolus dose based on weight, 30 mg (for <60 kg) not to exceed 50 mg (>90 kg) | For use with acute myocardial infarction; administered rapidly in one dose |
| **Urokinase** (Abbokinase) Pregnancy Category B | IV 4400 units/kg over 10 min, followed by continuous infusion of 4400 units/kg/h for 12 h For clearing IV catheters, see manufacturer's instructions | Used for coronary artery thrombi and pulmonary emboli; causes less allergic reaction as it is not susceptible to antistreptokinase antibodies Clearance of clogged IV catheters |

DVT, deep vein thrombosis; PE, pulmonary embolism; PTCA, percutaneous transluminal coronary angioplasty or atherectomy.

## PROTOTYPE PROFILE 45-1

### *P* Heparin (HEP a rin)

**Drug Class**

*Chemical:* Anticoagulant
*Functional:* Anticoagulant

**Trade Name**

Hep-Lock

**Therapeutic Indications**

Prevention and management of thromboembolic disorders (eg, DVT, pulmonary embolism, atrial fibrillation with embolization); treatment of disseminated intravascular coagulation (DIC); prevention of clotting during cardiac and vascular surgery, extracorporeal circulation, hemodialysis, blood transfusions, and in blood samples to be used in laboratory tests

**Pharmacokinetics**

*Absorption*
Well absorbed

*Distribution*
Plasma protein binding: >80%

*Metabolism*
Hepatic

*Excretion*
Urine

**Pharmacodynamics**

*Onset of Action*
Anticoagulation: IV, immediately; Sub-Q, 20 to 30 min

*Duration*
IV, 2–6 h; Sub-Q, 8–12 h

**Contraindications/Precautions**

Contraindications include GI ulcerations (eg, peptic ulcer disease, ulcerative colitis), blood dyscrasias, severe kidney or liver disease, severe hypertension, polycythemia vera, and recent surgery of the eye,

spinal cord, or brain. It should be used with caution in clients with hypertension, renal or hepatic disease, alcoholism, history of GI ulcerations, drainage tubes (eg, nasogastric tubes, indwelling urinary catheters), and any occupation with high risk for traumatic injury Low-dose heparin prophylaxis is either ineffective or contraindicated in major orthopedic surgery, abdominal prostatectomy, and brain surgery Do not administer IM owing to local tissue reactions (pain, irritation, and/or hematoma formation)

**Pregnancy Considerations**

Category C
Does not enter breast milk
Is anticoagulant of choice for use during pregnancy and lactation

**Dosage**

Weight-based dosing per institutional nomogram recommended
*Adults:* IV injection, 5000 units initially, followed by 5000–10,000 units q4–6h, to a maximum dose of 25,000 units/d
IV infusion, 5000 units (loading dose), then 15–25 units/kg/h
DIC: IV injection, 50–100 units/kg q4h; IV infusion, 20,000–40,000 units/d at initial rate of 0.25 units/kg/min, then adjusted according to aPTT
Sub-Q, 10,000–12,000 units q8h, or 14,000–20,000 units q12h
Low-dose prophylaxis: Sub-Q, 5000 units 2 h before surgery, then q12h until discharged from hospital or fully ambulatory
*Children:* DIC: IV injection, 25–50 units/kg q4h
IV infusion, 50 units/kg initially, followed by 100 units/kg q4h or 20,000 units/m² over 24 h

*(continued)*

## PROTOTYPE PROFILE 45-1
### Ⓟ Heparin (Continued)

**Side Effects/Adverse Reactions**
Hemorrhage, itching, burning, ecchymosis

**Drug Interactions**
*Increased Effects*
Anticoagulant effect with aspirin, NSAIDs, warfarin, dextran, thrombolytics, probenecid, dipyridamole, ticlopidine

*Decreased Effects*
Anticoagulant effect with protamine sulfate (antidote), nitroglycerin

**Herbal Supplements and Dietary Considerations**
Avoid dong quai, evening primrose, cat's claw, feverfew, red clover, horse chestnut, garlic, green tea, ginseng, and ginkgo due to their additional antiplatelet activity
**When taken for more than 6 mo, may interfere with calcium absorption**

---

Heparin combines with antithrombin III (a natural anticoagulant in the blood) to inactivate clotting factors IX, X, XI, and XII, inhibit the conversion of prothrombin to thrombin, and prevent thrombus formation. After thrombosis has developed, heparin can inhibit additional coagulation by inactivating thrombin, preventing the conversion of fibrinogen to fibrin, and inhibiting factor XIII (the fibrin-stabilizing factor). Other effects include inhibiting factors V and VIII and platelet aggregation.

### Low–Molecular-Weight Heparins
Standard heparin is a mixture of high– and low–molecular-weight fractions, but most anticoagulant activity is attributed to the low–molecular-weight portion. **Low-molecular-weight heparins** (LMWHs) contain the low–molecular-weight fraction and are as effective as IV heparin in treating thrombotic disorders. Indications for use include prevention or management of thromboembolic complications associated with surgery or ischemic complications of unstable angina and myocardial infarction. Currently available LMWHs (dalteparin, enoxaparin, tinzaparin) differ from standard heparin and each other; they cannot be used interchangeably (ie, unit for unit).

LMWHs are given subcutaneously and do not require close monitoring of blood coagulation tests. These characteristics allow outpatient anticoagulant therapy, an increasing trend. The drugs are also associated with less thrombocytopenia than standard heparin. However, platelet counts should be monitored during therapy.

### Regulation of Heparin Dosage
**Heparin** dosage is regulated by the activated partial thromboplastin time (aPTT), which is sensitive to changes in blood clotting factors, except factor VII. Thus, normal or control values indicate normal blood coagulation; therapeutic values indicate low levels of clotting factors and delayed blood coagulation. During heparin therapy, the aPTT should be maintained at approximately 1.5 to 2.5 times the control or baseline value. The normal control value is 25 to 35 seconds; therefore, therapeutic values are 45 to 70 seconds, approximately. With continuous IV infusion, blood for the aPTT may be drawn at any time; with intermittent administration, blood for the aPTT should be drawn approximately 1 hour before a dose of heparin is scheduled. Monitoring of aPTT is not necessary with low-dose standard heparin given subcutaneously for prophylaxis of thromboembolism or with LMWH (eg, enoxaparin).

### Warfarin
**Warfarin** is the most commonly used oral anticoagulant. It is considered a prototype and is described in Prototype Profile 45-2: Warfarin. The drug acts in the liver to prevent synthesis of vitamin K–dependent clotting factors (ie, factors II, VII, IX, and X). Warfarin is similar to vitamin K in structure and therefore acts as a competitive antagonist to hepatic use of vitamin K.

Warfarin is the anticoagulant of choice for long-term maintenance therapy (ie, several weeks or months) because it can be given orally. Anticoagulant effects do not occur for 3 to 5 days after warfarin is started because clotting factors already in the blood follow their normal pathway of elimination. Warfarin has no effect on circulating clotting factors or on platelet function. Smaller doses are being used now than formerly, with similar antithrombotic effects and decreased risks for bleeding.

### Regulation of Warfarin Dosage
Warfarin dosage is regulated according to the international normalized ratio (INR), for which therapeutic values are 2.0 to 3.0 in most conditions. An average daily dose of 4 to 5 mg maintains a therapeutic INR; stopping warfarin returns an elevated INR to normal in approximately 4 days in most clients.

The INR is based on prothrombin time (PT). PT is sensitive to changes in three of the four vitamin K–dependent coagulation factors. Thus, normal or control values indicate normal levels of these factors; therapeutic values indicate low levels of the factors and delayed blood coagulation. A normal baseline or control PT is approximately 12 seconds; a therapeutic value is approximately 1.5 times the control, or 18 seconds.

## PROTOTYPE PROFILE 45-2

### P Warfarin (WAR far in)

**Drug Class**
*Chemical:* Anticoagulant
*Functional:* Anticoagulant

**Trade Name**
Coumadin

**Therapeutic Indications**
Long-term prevention or management of venous thromboembolic disorders, including DVT, pulmonary embolism, and embolization associated with atrial fibrillation and prosthetic heart valves. In addition, warfarin therapy after myocardial infarction may decrease re-infarction, stroke, venous thromboembolism, and death

**Pharmacokinetics**
*Absorption*
Well absorbed

*Distribution*
Plasma protein binding: >98%

*Metabolism*
Hepatic; half-life variable among individuals

*Excretion*
Urine and bile

**Pharmacodynamics**
*Onset of Action*
36–72 h

*Duration*
2–5 d

**Contraindications/Precautions**
Contraindicated in clients with GI ulcerations, blood disorders associated with bleeding, severe kidney or liver disease, severe hypertension, and recent surgery of the eye, spinal cord, or brain
Use cautiously with mild hypertension, renal or hepatic disease, alcoholism, history of GI ulcerations, drainage tubes (eg, nasogastric tubes, indwelling urinary catheters), and occupations with high risk for traumatic injury. In addition, warfarin is contraindicated during pregnancy

**Pregnancy Considerations**
Category D; crosses placenta and produces fetal abnormalities
Does not cross breast milk, only metabolites are excreted

**Dosage**
PO, 2–5 mg/d for 2–3 days, then adjusted according to the INR; average maintenance daily dose, 2–5 mg

**Side Effects/Adverse Reactions**
Bleeding, anorexia, diarrhea, abdominal cramps, nausea, vomiting, taste disturbance

**Drug Interactions**
*Increased Effects*
Bleeding tendency with cephalosporins, dipyridamole, indomethacin, salicylates, phenylbutazone, quinidine, quinine
Anticoagulant effect with oral antibiotics, chloral hydrate, clofibrate, ethacrynic acid, sulfonamides, sulfonylureas, allopurinol, ethanol, omeprazole, statins, acetaminophen, gemfibrozil

*Decreased Effects*
Anticoagulant effect with barbiturates, nafcillin, carbamazepine, phenytoin, estrogens, aluminum hydroxide, cholestyramine, colestipol, spironolactone, and vitamin K (antidote)

**Herbal Supplements and Dietary Considerations**
Multivitamin supplements may contain 25–28 mcg of vitamin K and should be taken consistently to avoid fluctuating vitamin K levels. St. John's wort may reduce warfarin levels. Avoid dong quai, evening primrose, cat's claw, feverfew, red clover, horse chestnut, garlic, green tea, ginseng, and ginkgo owing to their additional antiplatelet activity. Many enteral products contain vitamin K
A consistent intake of vitamin K in diet (green leafy vegetables and alfalfa contain large amounts of vitamin K)

---

When warfarin is started, PT and INR should be assessed daily until a stable daily dose is reached (the dose that maintains PT and INR within therapeutic ranges and does not cause bleeding). Thereafter, PT and INR are determined every 2 to 4 weeks for the duration of oral anticoagulant drug therapy. If the warfarin dose is changed, PT and INR are needed more often until a stable daily dose is again established.

For many years, the PT was used to regulate warfarin dosage. PT is determined by adding a mixture of thromboplastin and calcium to citrated plasma and measuring the time (in seconds) it takes for the blood to clot. However, values vary among laboratories according to the type of thromboplastin and the instrument used to measure PT. The INR system standardizes the PT by comparing a particular thromboplastin with a standard thromboplastin designated by the World Health Organization. Advantages of the INR include consistent values among laboratories, more consistent warfarin dosage with less risk for bleeding or thrombosis, and more consistent reports of clinical trials and other research studies. Some laboratories report both PT and INR.

Warfarin dosage may need to be reduced in clients with biliary tract disorders (eg, obstructive jaundice), liver disease (eg, hepatitis, cirrhosis), malabsorption syndromes (eg, steatorrhea), and hyperthyroidism or fever. These conditions increase anticoagulant drug effects by reducing absorption of vitamin K, decreasing hepatic synthesis of blood clotting factors, or increasing the breakdown of clotting factors. Despite these influencing factors, however, the primary determinant of dosage is the PT and INR.

Warfarin interacts with many other drugs to cause increased, decreased, or unpredictable anticoagulant effects (see Nursing Actions: Drugs That Affect Blood Coagulation, later in the chapter). Thus, warfarin dosage may need to be increased or decreased when other drugs are given concomitantly. Most drugs can be given if warfarin dosage is titrated according to the PT or INR and altered appropriately when an interacting drug is added or stopped. INR or PT measurements and vigilant observation are needed whenever a drug is added to or removed from a drug therapy regimen containing warfarin.

### Other Anticoagulant Drugs

**Danaparoid**, a heparinoid, is a low–molecular weight, heparin-like drug derived from porcine mucosa. It has antithrombotic effects and is given subcutaneously to prevent postoperative thromboembolism in clients having hip replacement surgery, in the management of ischemic stroke, and as an alternative anticoagulant in clients who cannot tolerate heparin. Although related to heparin and LMWH, it does not contain heparin and cannot be used interchangeably with standard heparin or LMWH.

**Fondaparinux** produces anticoagulant effects by directly binding to circulating and clot-bound factor Xa, accelerating the activity of antithrombin and inhibiting thrombin production. It is used in the prevention of DVT in clients having surgery for hip fracture or joint replacement surgery of the knee or hip.

**Lepirudin, bivalirudin,** and **argatroban** are direct thrombin inhibitors that prevent blood coagulation by inactivating thrombin. They are used as a heparin substitute for clients who need anticoagulation but have thrombocytopenia with heparin.

## Antiplatelet Drugs

Antiplatelet drugs prevent one or more steps in the prothrombotic activity of platelets. As described previously, platelet activity is very important in both physiologic hemostasis and pathologic thrombosis. Arterial thrombi, which are composed primarily of platelets, may form on top of atherosclerotic plaque and block blood flow in the artery. They may also form on heart walls and valves and embolize to other parts of the body.

Drugs used clinically for antiplatelet effects act by a variety of mechanisms to inhibit platelet activation, adhesion, aggregation, or procoagulant activity. These include drugs that block platelet receptors for thromboxane $A_2$, adenosine diphosphate (ADP), glycoprotein (GP) IIb/IIIa, and phosphodiesterase.

### Thromboxane $A_2$ Inhibitors

**Aspirin** is a commonly used analgesic–antipyretic–anti-inflammatory drug (see Chap. 7) with potent antiplatelet effects. Aspirin exerts pharmacologic actions by inhibiting synthesis of prostaglandins. In this instance, aspirin acetylates cyclooxygenase, the enzyme in platelets that normally synthesizes thromboxane $A_2$, a prostaglandin product that causes platelet aggregation. Thus, aspirin prevents formation of thromboxane $A_2$ and thromboxane $A_2$–induced platelet aggregation and thrombus formation. A single dose of 300 to 600 mg or multiple doses of 30 mg (eg, daily for several days) inhibit the cyclooxygenase in circulating platelets almost completely. These antithrombotic effects persist for the life of the platelet (7 to 10 days). Aspirin may be used long term for prevention of myocardial infarction or stroke, and in clients with prosthetic heart valves. It is also used for the immediate treatment of suspected or actual acute myocardial infarction, for transient ischemic attacks (TIAs), and for evolving thrombotic strokes. Adverse effects are uncommon with the small doses used for antiplatelet effects. However, there is an increased risk for bleeding, including hemorrhagic stroke. Because approximately 85% of strokes are thrombotic, the benefits of aspirin or other antiplatelet agents are thought to outweigh the risk for hemorrhagic stroke (approximately 15%).

**Nonsteroidal anti-inflammatory drugs** (NSAIDs), including ibuprofen and many other aspirin-related drugs, inhibit cyclooxygenase reversibly. Their antiplatelet effects subside when the drugs are eliminated from the circulation, and the drugs usually are not used for antiplatelet effects. However, clients who take an NSAID daily (eg, for arthritis pain) may not need to take additional aspirin for antiplatelet effects. Acetaminophen does not affect platelets in usual doses.

### Adenosine Diphosphate Receptor Antagonists

**Ticlopidine** inhibits platelet aggregation by preventing ADP-induced binding between platelets and fibrinogen. This reaction inhibits platelet aggregation irreversibly, and effects persist for the lifespan of the platelet. The drug is indicated for prevention of thrombotic stroke in people who have had stroke precursor events (eg, TIAs) or a completed thrombotic stroke. Ticlopidine is considered a second-line drug for clients who cannot take aspirin. The adverse effects (eg, neutropenia, diarrhea, skin rashes) and greater cost make it prohibitive for use by many clients. Contraindications include active bleeding disorders (eg, GI bleeding from peptic ulcer or intracranial bleeding), neutropenia, thrombocytopenia, severe liver disease, and hypersensitivity to the drug.

**Clopidogrel** is chemically related to ticlopidine and causes similar effects. It is indicated for reduction of myocardial infarction, stroke, and vascular death in clients with atherosclerosis and reportedly causes fewer or less severe adverse effects than ticlopidine. Aspirin has long been the most widely used antiplatelet drug for prevention of myocardial reinfarction and arterial thrombosis in clients with TIAs and prosthetic heart valves. However, clopidogrel may be more effective than aspirin. Clopidogrel does not need dosage reduction in clients with renal impairment.

### Glycoprotein IIb/IIIa Receptor Antagonists

**Abciximab** is a monoclonal antibody that prevents the binding of fibrinogen, von Willebrand factor, and other molecules to GP IIb/IIIa receptors on activated platelets. This action inhibits platelet aggregation.

Abciximab is used with percutaneous transluminal coronary angioplasty or removal of atherosclerotic plaque to prevent rethrombosis of treated arteries. It is used with aspirin and heparin and is contraindicated in clients who have recently received an oral anticoagulant or IV dextran. Other contraindications include active bleeding, thrombocytopenia, history of a serious stroke, surgery or major trauma within the previous 6 weeks, uncontrolled hypertension, or hypersensitivity to drug components.

**Eptifibatide** and **tirofiban** inhibit platelet aggregation by preventing activation of GP IIb/IIIa receptors on the platelet surface and the subsequent binding of fibrinogen and von Willebrand factor to platelets. Antiplatelet effects occur during drug infusion and stop when the drug is stopped. The drugs are indicated for acute coronary syndrome (eg, unstable angina, myocardial infarction) in clients who are to be managed medically or by angioplasty or atherectomy.

Drug half-life is approximately 2.5 hours for eptifibatide and 2 hours for tirofiban; the drugs are cleared mainly by renal excretion. With tirofiban, plasma clearance is approximately 25% lower in older adults and approximately 50% lower in clients with severe renal impairment (creatinine clearance <30 mL/minute).

The drugs are contraindicated in clients with hypersensitivity to any component of the products; current or previous bleeding (within the previous 30 days); a history of thrombocytopenia after previous exposure to tirofiban; a history of stroke within 30 days or any history of hemorrhagic stroke; major surgery or severe physical trauma within the previous month; severe hypertension (systolic blood pressure >180 mm Hg with tirofiban or >200 mm Hg with eptifibatide, or diastolic blood pressure >110 mm Hg with either drug); a history of intracranial hemorrhage, neoplasm, arteriovenous malformation, or aneurysm; a platelet count less than 100,000 mm³; serum creatinine 2 mg/dL or above (for the 180-mcg/kg bolus and the 2-mcg/kg per minute infusion) or 4 mg/dL or above (for the 135-mcg/kg bolus

and the 0.5-mcg/kg per minute infusion); or dependency on dialysis (eptifibatide).

Bleeding is the most common adverse effect, with most major bleeding occurring at the arterial access site for cardiac catheterization. If bleeding occurs and cannot be controlled with pressure, the drug infusion and heparin should be discontinued.

These drugs should be used cautiously if given with other drugs that affect hemostasis (eg, warfarin, thrombolytics, other antiplatelet drugs).

### Phosphodiesterase Inhibitor

**Cilostazol** inhibits phosphodiesterase, an enzyme that metabolizes cyclic adenosine monophosphate (cAMP). The inhibition increases intracellular cAMP, which then inhibits platelet aggregation and produces vasodilation. The drug reversibly inhibits platelet aggregation induced by various stimuli (eg, thrombin, ADP, collagen, arachidonic acid, epinephrine, and shear stress). It is indicated for management of intermittent claudication. Symptoms usually improve within 2 to 4 weeks, but may take as long as 12 weeks. The drug is contraindicated in clients with heart failure.

Cilostazol is highly protein bound (95% to 98%), mainly to albumin, extensively metabolized by hepatic cytochrome P450 enzymes, and excreted in urine (74%) and feces. The drug and two active metabolites accumulate with chronic administration and reach steady state within a few days. The most common adverse effects are diarrhea and headache.

### Miscellaneous Agents

**Anagrelide** inhibits platelet aggregation induced by cAMP phosphodiesterase, ADP, and collagen. However, it is indicated only to reduce platelet counts in clients with essential thrombocythemia (a disorder characterized by excessive numbers of platelets). Doses to reduce platelet production are smaller than those required to inhibit platelet aggregation. Anagrelide may be given to clients with renal impairment (eg, serum creatinine <2 mg/dL) if potential benefits outweigh risks.

**Dipyridamole** inhibits platelet adhesion, but its mechanism of action is unclear. It is used for prevention of thromboembolism after cardiac valve replacement and is given with warfarin.

## Thrombolytic Agents

Thrombolytic agents are given to dissolve thrombi. They stimulate conversion of plasminogen to plasmin (also called fibrinolysin), a proteolytic enzyme that breaks down fibrin, the framework of a thrombus. The main use of thrombolytic agents is for management of acute, severe thromboembolic disease, such as myocardial infarction, pulmonary embolism, and iliofemoral thrombosis.

The goal of thrombolytic therapy is to reestablish blood flow and prevent or limit tissue damage. Heparin and warfarin are given after completion of thrombolytic therapy to manage further clot formation. Thrombolytic drugs are also used to dissolve clots in arterial or venous cannulas or catheters. Before a thrombolytic agent is begun, INR, aPTT, platelet count, and fibrinogen should be checked to establish baseline values and to determine whether a blood coagulation disorder is present. Two or 3 hours after thrombolytic therapy is started, the fibrinogen level can be measured to determine whether fibrinolysis is occurring. Alternatively, INR or aPTT can be checked for increased values because the breakdown products of fibrin exert anticoagulant effects.

**Alteplase, reteplase,** and **tenecteplase** are tissue plasminogen activators used mainly in acute myocardial infarction to dissolve clots obstructing coronary arteries and reestablish perfusion of tissues beyond the thrombotic area. The drugs bind to fibrin in a clot and act locally to dissolve the clot. The most common adverse effect is bleeding, which may be internal (eg, intracranial, gastrointestinal [GI], genitourinary) or external (eg, venous or arterial puncture sites, surgical incisions). The drugs are contraindicated in the presence of bleeding, a history of stroke, central nervous system surgery or trauma within the previous 2 months, and severe hypertension.

**Anistreplase, streptokinase,** and **urokinase** are enzymes that break down fibrin. They are used mainly to lyse coronary artery clots in acute myocardial infarction. Streptokinase may also be used to dissolve clots in vascular catheters and to treat acute, severe pulmonary emboli or iliofemoral thrombophlebitis. It works indirectly by binding to plasminogen to form an active complex; the complex catalyzes the conversion of other plasminogen molecules into plasmin, an enzyme that digests the fibrin meshwork. An advantage of anistreplase is that it can be given in a single IV injection. Urokinase is recommended for use in clients allergic to streptokinase. As with other anticoagulants and thrombolytic agents, bleeding is the main adverse effect.

**Drotrecogin alfa** (Xigris) is a recombinant version of human activated protein C that is approved for use in severe sepsis or septic shock. Severe sepsis is characterized by an excessive inflammatory reaction to infection, inappropriate blood clot formation, and impaired breakdown of clots. Drotrecogin alfa is given for its thrombolytic effects, along with other therapies for inflammation and infection. The major adverse effect is bleeding.

## Drugs Used to Control Bleeding

Anticoagulant, antiplatelet, and thrombolytic drugs profoundly affect hemostasis, and their major adverse effect is bleeding. As a result, systemic hemostatic agents (antidotes) may be needed to prevent or treat bleeding episodes. Antidotes should be used cautiously because overuse can increase the risk for recurrent thrombotic disorders. The drugs are described in this section and in Drugs at a Glance 45-2: Systemic Hemostatic Drugs.

**DRUG TABLE 45-2**

*Drugs at a Glance*

## Systemic Hemostatic Drugs

| Generic/Trade Name | Routes and Dosage Ranges | Comments |
|---|---|---|
| **Aminocaproic acid** (Amicar) Pregnancy Category C | PO, IV infusion, 5 g initially, followed by 1.0 to 1.25 g/h for 8 h or until bleeding is controlled; maximum dose, 30 g/24 h | Control bleeding caused by overdoses of thrombolytic agents or bleeding disorders caused by hyperfibrinolysis (eg, cardiac surgery, blood disorders, hepatic cirrhosis, prostatectomy, neoplastic disorders) |
| **Aprotinin** (Trasylol) Pregnancy Category B | See manufacturer's literature | Used in selected clients undergoing coronary artery bypass graft surgery to decrease blood loss and blood transfusions |
| **Protamine sulfate** Pregnancy Category C | Depends on the amount of heparin given within the previous 4 h | Treatment of heparin overdosage |
| **Tranexamic acid** (Cyklokapron) Pregnancy Category B | PO, 25 mg/kg 3 to 4 times daily, starting 1 d before surgery, or IV 10 mg/kg immediately before surgery, followed by 25 mg/kg PO 3 to 4 times daily for 2–8 d | Control bleeding caused by overdoses of thrombolytic agents Prevent or decrease bleeding from tooth extraction in clients with hemophilia |
| **Phytonadione/Vitamin K** (Mephyton) Pregnancy Category C | PO, 10–20 mg in a single dose | Antidote for warfarin overdosage |

**Aminocaproic acid** and **tranexamic acid** are used to stop bleeding caused by overdoses of thrombolytic agents. Aminocaproic acid also may be used in other bleeding disorders caused by hyperfibrinolysis (eg, cardiac surgery, blood disorders, hepatic cirrhosis, prostatectomy, neoplastic disorders). Tranexamic acid also is used for short periods (2 to 8 days) in clients with hemophilia to prevent or decrease bleeding from tooth extraction. Dosage of tranexamic acid should be reduced in the presence of moderate or severe renal impairment.

**Aprotinin** is a natural protease inhibitor obtained from bovine lung that has a variety of effects on blood coagulation. It inhibits plasmin and kallikrein, thus inhibiting fibrinolysis, and inhibits breakdown of blood clotting factors. It is used to decrease bleeding in selected clients undergoing coronary artery bypass surgery.

**Protamine sulfate** is an antidote for standard heparin and LMWH. Because heparin is an acid and protamine sulfate is a base, protamine neutralizes heparin activity. Protamine dosage depends on the amount of heparin administered during the previous 4 hours. Each milligram of protamine neutralizes approximately 100 units of heparin or dalteparin and 1 mg of enoxaparin. A single dose should not exceed 50 mg.

The drug is given by slow IV infusion over at least 10 minutes (to prevent or minimize adverse effects of hypotension, bradycardia, and dyspnea). Protamine effects occur immediately and last for approximately 2 hours. A second dose may be required because heparin activity lasts approximately 4 hours.

Protamine sulfate can cause severe hypotensive and anaphylactoid reactions. Thus, it should be given in settings with equipment and personnel for resuscitation and management of anaphylactic shock.

**Vitamin K** is the antidote for warfarin overdosage. An oral dose of 10 to 20 mg usually stops minor bleeding and returns the INR to a normal range within 24 hours.

## Herbal and Dietary Supplements

Many commonly used herbs and supplements have a profound effect on drugs used for anticoagulation. Multivitamin supplements may contain 25 to 28 mcg of vitamin K and should be taken consistently to avoid fluctuating vitamin K levels. Doses of vitamin C in excess of 500 mg/day may lower INR, and vitamin E in excess of 400 IU/day may increase warfarin effects. Herbs commonly used that may increase the effects of warfarin include alfalfa, celery, clove, feverfew, garlic, ginger, ginkgo, ginseng, and licorice. Clients taking warfarin should be questioned carefully about their use of herbs as well as vitamin or mineral supplements.

*(text continues on page 835)*

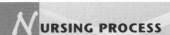

## URSING PROCESS

### Assessment

Assess the client's status in relation to thrombotic and thromboembolic disorders.

- Risk factors for thromboembolism include:
  - Immobility (eg, limited activity or bed rest for more than 5 days)
  - Obesity
  - Cigarette smoking
  - History of thrombophlebitis, deep vein thrombosis (DVT), or pulmonary emboli
  - Congestive heart failure
  - Pedal edema
  - Lower limb trauma
  - Myocardial infarction
  - Atrial fibrillation
  - Mitral or aortic stenosis
  - Prosthetic heart valves
  - Abdominal, thoracic, pelvic, or major orthopedic surgery
  - Atherosclerotic heart disease or peripheral vascular disease
  - Use of oral contraceptives
- Signs and symptoms of thrombotic and thromboembolic disorders depend on the location and size of the thrombus.
  - DVT and thrombophlebitis usually occur in the legs. The conditions may be manifested by edema (the affected leg is often measurably larger than the other) and pain,

especially in the calf when the foot is dorsiflexed (Homans' sign). If thrombophlebitis is superficial, it may be visible as a red, warm, tender area following the path of a vein.
  - Pulmonary embolism, if severe enough to produce symptoms, is manifested by chest pain, cough, hemoptysis, tachypnea, and tachycardia. Massive emboli cause hypotension, shock, cyanosis, and death.
  - Disseminated intravascular coagulation (DIC) is usually manifested by bleeding, which may range from petechiae or oozing from a venipuncture site to massive internal bleeding or bleeding from all body orifices.

### Nursing Diagnoses

- Ineffective Tissue Perfusion related to thrombus or embolus or drug-induced bleeding
- Acute Pain related to tissue ischemia
- Impaired Physical Mobility related to bed rest and pain
- Ineffective Coping related to the need for long-term prophylaxis of thromboembolic disorders or fear of excessive bleeding
- Anxiety related to fear of myocardial infarction or stroke
- Deficient Knowledge related to anticoagulant or antiplatelet drug therapy
- Risk for Injury related to drug-induced impairment of blood coagulation

*(continued)*

## N URSING PROCESS (Continued)

### Planning/Goals

*The client will:*

- Receive or take anticoagulant and antiplatelet drugs correctly
- Be monitored closely for therapeutic and adverse drug effects, especially when drug therapy is started and when changes are made in drugs or dosages
- Use nondrug measures to decrease venous stasis and prevent thromboembolic disorders
- Act to prevent trauma from falls and other injuries
- Inform any health care provider when taking an anti-coagulant or antiplatelet drug
- Avoid or report adverse drug reactions
- Verbalize or demonstrate knowledge of safe management of anticoagulant drug therapy
- Keep follow-up appointments for tests of blood coagulation and drug dosage regulation
- Avoid preventable bleeding episodes

### Interventions

Use measures to prevent thrombotic and thromboembolic disorders.

- Have the client ambulate and exercise legs regularly, especially after surgery.
- For clients who cannot ambulate or do leg exercises, do passive range-of-motion and other leg exercises several times daily when changing the client's position or performing other care.
- Have the client wear elastic stockings. Elastic stockings should be removed every 8 hours and replaced after inspecting the skin. Improperly applied elastic stockings can impair circulation rather than aid it. For clients on bed rest, intermittent pneumatic compression devices can also be used.
- Avoid trauma to lower extremities.
- Maintain adequate fluid intake (1500–3000 mL/day) to avoid dehydration and hemoconcentration.
- Assist clients to promote good blood circulation (eg, exercise) and avoid situations that impair circulation (eg, wearing tight clothing, crossing the legs at the knees, prolonged sitting or standing, bed rest, and placing pillows under the knees when in bed).

For the client receiving anticoagulant therapy, implement safety measures to prevent trauma and bleeding.

- For clients who cannot ambulate safely because of weakness, sedation, or other conditions, keep the call light within reach, keep bedrails elevated, and assist in ambulation.
- Provide an electric razor for shaving.

- Avoid intramuscular injections, venipunctures, and arterial punctures when possible.
- Avoid intubations when possible (eg, nasogastric tubes, indwelling urinary catheters).

For the client receiving tirofiban or eptifibatide:

- Monitor the femoral artery access site closely. This is the most common site of bleeding.
- Avoid invasive procedures as much as possible (eg, arterial and venous punctures, intramuscular injections, urinary catheters, nasotracheal suction, nasogastric tubes). If venipuncture must be done, avoid sites where pressure cannot be applied (eg, subclavian or jugular veins).
- While the vascular sheath is in place, keep clients on complete bed rest with the head of the bed elevated 30 degrees and the affected limb restrained in a straight position.
- Discontinue heparin for 3 to 4 hours and be sure the activated clotting time is less than 180 seconds or the activated partial thromboplastin time (aPTT) is below 45 seconds before removing the vascular sheath.
- After the vascular sheath is removed, apply pressure to the site and observe closely. For outpatients, be sure there is no bleeding for at least 4 hours before hospital discharge.

For the client receiving a thrombolytic drug or a revascularization procedure for acute myocardial infarction:

- Monitor closely for bleeding.
- Assist the client and family to understand the importance of diligent efforts to reverse risk factors contributing to coronary artery disease (eg, diet and perhaps medication to lower serum cholesterol to below 200 mg/dL and low-density lipoprotein cholesterol to below 130 mg/dL, weight reduction if overweight, control of blood pressure if hypertensive, avoidance of smoking, stress reduction techniques, exercise program designed and supervised by a health care provider).
- Assist the client and family to understand the importance of complying with medication orders to prevent re-infarction and other complications, and continued medical supervision.

### Evaluation

- Observe for signs and symptoms of thromboembolic disorders or bleeding.
- Check blood coagulation tests for therapeutic ranges.
- Observe and interview regarding compliance with instructions about drug therapy.
- Observe and interview regarding adverse drug effects.

## CLIENT TEACHING GUIDELINES
## Drugs to Prevent or Treat Blood Clots

### General Considerations

✔ Antiplatelet and anticoagulant drugs are given to people who have had, or who are at risk of having, a heart attack, stroke, or other problems from blood clots. For prevention of a heart attack or stroke, you are most likely to be given an antiplatelet drug (eg, aspirin, clopidogrel) or warfarin (Coumadin). For home management of deep vein thrombosis, which usually occurs in the legs, you are likely to be given heparin injections for a few days, followed by warfarin for long-term therapy. These medications help to prevent the blood clot from getting larger, traveling to your lungs, or recurring later.

✔ All of these drugs can increase your risk of bleeding, so you need to take safety precautions to prevent injury.

✔ To help prevent blood clots from forming and decreasing blood flow through your arteries, you need to reduce risk factors that contribute to cardiovascular disease. This can be done by a low-fat, low-cholesterol diet (and medication if needed) to lower total cholesterol to below 200 mg/dL and low-density lipoprotein cholesterol to below 130 mg/dL; weight reduction if overweight; control of blood pressure if hypertensive; avoidance of smoking; stress reduction techniques; and regular exercise.

✔ To help prevent blood clots from forming in your leg veins, avoid or minimize situations that slow blood circulation, such as wearing tight clothing; crossing the legs at the knees; prolonged sitting or standing; and bed rest. For example, on automobile trips, stop and walk around every 1 to 2 hours; on long plane trips, exercise your feet and legs at your seat and walk around when you can.

✔ Following instructions regarding these medications is extremely important. Too little medication increases your risk of problems from blood clot formation; too much medication can cause bleeding.

✔ While taking any of these medications, you need regular medical supervision and periodic blood tests. The blood tests can help your health care provider regulate drug dosage and maintain your safety.

✔ You need to take the drugs as directed; avoid taking other drugs without the health care provider's knowledge and consent; inform any health care provider (including dentists) that you are taking an antiplatelet or anticoagulant drug before any invasive diagnostic tests or treatments are begun; and keep all appointments for continuing care.

✔ With warfarin therapy, you need to avoid walking barefoot; avoid contact sports; use an electric razor; avoid injections when possible; and carry an identification card, necklace, or bracelet (eg, MedicAlert) stating the name of the drug and the health care provider's name and telephone number. Also, avoid large amounts of certain vegetables (eg, broccoli, brussels sprouts, cabbage, cauliflower, chives, collard greens, kale, lettuce, mustard greens, peppers, spinach, turnips, and watercress), tomatoes, bananas, or fish; these foods contain vitamin K and may decrease anticoagulant effects.

✔ For home management of deep vein thrombosis, both warfarin and enoxaparin (Lovenox) are given for 3 months or longer. With Lovenox, you need an injection, usually every 12 hours. You or someone close to you may be instructed in injecting the medication, or a visiting nurse may do the injections, if necessary.

Even if a nurse is not needed to give the injections, one will usually visit your home each day to perform a finger stick blood test. The results of this test determine your daily dose of warfarin. Once the blood test and the warfarin dose stabilize, the blood tests are done less often (eg, every 2 weeks).

✔ Report any sign of bleeding (eg, excessive bruising of the skin, blood in urine or stool). If superficial bleeding occurs, apply direct pressure to the site for 3 to 5 minutes or longer if necessary.

### Self-administration

✔ Take aspirin with food or after meals, with 8 oz of water, to decrease stomach irritation. However, stomach upset is uncommon with the small doses used for antiplatelet effects. Do not crush or chew coated tablets (long-acting preparations).

✔ Take cilostazol (Pletal) 30 minutes before or 2 hours after morning and evening meals for better absorption and effectiveness.

✔ Take ticlopidine (Ticlid) with food or after meals to decrease GI upset. Clopidogrel (Plavix) may be taken with or without food.

✔ With Lovenox, wash hands and cleanse skin to prevent infection; inject deep under the skin, around the navel, upper thigh, or buttocks; and change the injection site daily. If excessive bruising occurs at the injection site, rubbing an ice cube over an area before the injection may be helpful.

**? How Can You Avoid This Medication Error?**

Helen Innes is admitted to your medical unit for management of bacterial pneumonia. She has been on oral antibiotics for 7 days but her respiratory condition has not improved. In addition to her intravenous antibiotics, you administer her usual dose of Coumadin that she takes for a history of pulmonary emboli. When you document the medications given, you notice that her international normalized ratio (INR) is 6.

## Nursing Actions

## Drugs That Affect Blood Coagulation

| Nursing Actions | Rationale/Explanation |
|---|---|
| 1. Administer accurately. | |
| a. With standard heparin: | |
| (1) When handwriting a heparin dose, write out "units" rather than using the abbreviation "U." | This is a safety precaution to avoid erroneous dosage. For example, 1000 U (1000 units) may be misread as 10,000 units. Underdosage may cause thromboembolism, and overdosage may cause bleeding. In addition, heparin is available in several concentrations (1000, 2500, 5000, 10,000, 15,000, 20,000, and 40,000 units/mL). |
| (2) Check dosage and vial label carefully. | |
| (3) For Sub-Q heparin: | |
| (a) Use a 26-gauge, ½-inch needle. | To minimize trauma and risk of bleeding |
| (b) Leave a small air bubble in the syringe to follow dose | Locks drug into subcutaneous space and minimizes trauma |
| (c) Grasp a skinfold and inject the heparin into it, at a 90-degree angle, without aspirating. | To give the drug in a deep subcutaneous or fat layer, with minimal trauma |
| (d) Do not massage site after injection | |
| (4) For intermittent IV administration: | |
| (a) Give by direct injection into a heparin lock or tubing injection site. | These methods prevent repeated venipunctures. |
| (b) Dilute the dose in 50 to 100 mL of any IV fluid (usually 5% dextrose in water). | |
| (5) For continuous IV administration: | This is usually the preferred method because it maintains consistent serum drug levels and decreases risks of bleeding. |
| (a) Use a volume-control device and an infusion-control device. | To regulate dosage and flow rate accurately |
| (b) Add only enough heparin for a few hours. One effective method is to fill the volume-control set (eg, Volutrol) with 100 mL of 5% dextrose in water and add 5000 units of heparin to yield a concentration of 50 units/mL. Dosage is regulated by varying the flow rate. For example, administration of 1000 units/h requires a flow rate of 20 mL/h.<br>    Another method is to add 25,000 units of heparin to 500 mL of IV solution. | To avoid inadvertent administration of large amounts. Whatever method is used, it is desirable to standardize concentration of heparin solutions within an institution. Standardization is safer, because it reduces risks of errors in dosage. |
| b. With low–molecular-weight heparins: | |
| (1) Give by deep Sub-Q injection, into an abdominal skin fold, with the patient lying down, using the same technique as standard heparin. Do not rub the injection site. | To decrease bruising |
| (2) Rotate sites. | |

*(continued)*

## *Nursing Actions*

## Drugs That Affect Blood Coagulation (Continued)

| Nursing Actions | Rationale/Explanation |
|---|---|
| c. After the initial dose of warfarin, check the international normalized ratio (INR) before giving a subsequent dose. Do not give the dose if the INR is above 3.0. Notify the health care provider. | The INR is measured daily until a maintenance dose is established, then periodically throughout warfarin therapy. An elevated INR indicates a high risk of bleeding. |
| d. Give ticlopidine with food or after meals; give cilostazol 30 min before or 2 h after morning and evening meals; give clopidogrel with or without food. | |
| e. With eptifibatide, tirofiban, and thrombolytic agents, follow manufacturers' instructions for reconstitution and administration. | These drugs require special preparation and administration techniques. |
| 2. **Observe for therapeutic effects.** | |
| a. With prophylactic heparins and warfarin, observe for the absence of signs and symptoms of thrombotic disorders. | |
| b. With therapeutic heparins and warfarin, observe for decrease or improvement in signs and symptoms (eg, less edema and pain with deep vein thrombosis, less chest pain and respiratory difficulty with pulmonary embolism). | |
| c. With prophylactic or therapeutic warfarin, observe for an INR between 2.0 and 3.0. | Frequency of INR determinations varies, but the test should be done periodically in all clients taking warfarin. |
| d. With therapeutic heparin, observe for an activated partial thromboplastin time of 1.5 to 2 times the control value. | |
| e. With anagrelide, observe for a decrease in platelet count. | Platelet counts should be done every 2 days during the first week of management and weekly until a maintenance dose is reached. Counts usually begin to decrease within the first 2 wk of therapy. |
| f. With aspirin, clopidogrel, and other antiplatelet drugs, observe for the absence of thrombotic disorders (eg, myocardial infarction, stroke) | |
| g. With cilostazol, observe for ability to walk farther without leg pain (intermittent claudication). | Improvement may occur within 2 to 4 wk or take as long as 12 wk. |
| 3. **Observe for adverse effects.** | |
| a. Bleeding: | Bleeding is the major adverse effect of anticoagulant drugs. It may occur anywhere in the body, spontaneously or in response to minor trauma. With eptifibatide and tirofiban, most major bleeding occurs at the arterial access site for cardiac catheterization. Hypotension and tachycardia may indicate internal bleeding. |
| (1) Record vital signs regularly. | Gastrointestinal (GI) bleeding is fairly common; risks are increased with intubation. Blood in stools may be bright |
| (2) Check stools for blood (melena). | red, tarry (blood that has been digested by GI secretions), or occult (hidden to the naked eye but present with a guaiac test). Hematemesis also may occur. |
| (3) Check urine for blood (hematuria). | Genitourinary bleeding also is fairly common; risks are increased with catheterization or instrumentation. Urine may be red (indicating fresh bleeding) or brownish or smoky gray (indicating old blood). Or bleeding may be microscopic (red blood cells are visible only on microscopic examination during urinalysis). |
| (4) Inspect the skin and mucous membranes daily. | Bleeding may occur in the skin as petechiae, purpura, or ecchymoses. Surgical wounds, skin lesions, parenteral injection sites, the nose, and gums may be bleeding sites. |
| (5) Assess for excessive menstrual flow. | *(continued)* |

## *Nursing Actions*

## Drugs That Affect Blood Coagulation (Continued)

| Nursing Actions | Rationale/Explanation |
|---|---|
| b. Other adverse effects:<br>  (1) With heparin, tissue irritation at injection sites, transient alopecia, reversible thrombocytopenia, paresthesias, and hypersensitivity | These effects are uncommon. They are more likely to occur with large doses or prolonged administration. |
|   (2) With warfarin, dermatitis, diarrhea, and alopecia | These effects occur only occasionally. Warfarin has been given for prolonged periods without toxicity. |
|   (3) With anagrelide, adverse cardiovascular effects (eg, tachycardia, vasodilation, heart failure) | These effects are most likely to occur in clients with known heart disease. |
|   (4) With clopidogrel and ticlopidine, GI upset, skin rash, neutropenia, and thrombocytopenia | Neutropenia and thrombocytopenia are more likely to occur with ticlopidine than clopidogrel. |
| c. With thrombolytic drugs, observe for bleeding with all uses and reperfusion dysrhythmias when used for acute myocardial infarction. | Bleeding is most likely to occur at sites of venipuncture or other invasive procedures. Reperfusion dysrhythmias may occur when blood supply is restored to previously ischemic myocardium. |
| 4. Observe for drug interactions.<br>  a. Drugs that *increase* risks of bleeding with anticoagulant, antiplatelet, and thrombolytic agents:<br>    (1) Any one of these drugs in combination with any other drug that affects hemostasis<br>    (2) A combination of these drugs | These drugs are often used concurrently or sequentially to decrease risks of myocardial infarction or stroke. |
|   b. Drugs that *increase* effects of heparins:<br>    (1) Antiplatelet drugs (eg, aspirin, clopidogrel, others)<br>    (2) Warfarin<br>    (3) Parenteral penicillins and cephalosporins | Additive anticoagulant effects and increased risks of bleeding<br>Some may affect blood coagulation and increase risks of bleeding |
|   c. Drugs that *decrease* effects of heparins:<br>    (1) Antihistamines, digoxin, tetracyclines<br><br>    (2) Protamine sulfate | These drugs antagonize the anticoagulant effects of heparin. Mechanisms are not clear.<br>The antidote for heparin overdose |
|   d. Drugs that *increase* effects of warfarin:<br>    (1) Analgesics (eg, acetaminophen, aspirin and other nonsteroidal anti-inflammatory drugs)<br>    (2) Androgens and anabolic steroids<br>    (3) Antibacterial drugs (eg, aminoglycosides, erythromycin, fluoroquinolones, isoniazid, metronidazole, penicillins, cephalosporins, trimethoprim-sulfamethoxazole, tetracyclines)<br>    (4) Antifungal drugs (eg, fluconazole, ketoconazole, miconazole), including intravaginal use<br>    (5) Antiseizure drugs (eg, phenytoin)<br>    (6) Cardiovascular drugs (eg, amiodarone, beta blockers, loop diuretics, gemfibrozil, lovastatin, propafenone, quinidine)<br>    (7) Gastrointestinal drugs (eg, cimetidine, omeprazole)<br>    (8) Thyroid preparations (eg, levothyroxine) | Mechanisms by which drugs may increase effects of warfarin include inhibiting warfarin metabolism, displacing warfarin from binding sites on serum albumin, causing antiplatelet effects, inhibiting bacterial synthesis of vitamin K in the intestinal tract, and others. |
|   e. Drugs that *decrease* effects of warfarin:<br>    (1) Antacids and griseofulvin<br>    (2) Carbamazepine, disulfiram, rifampin<br><br>    (3) Cholestyramine<br>    (4) Diuretics<br>    (5) Estrogens, including oral contraceptives | May decrease GI absorption<br>These drugs activate liver metabolizing enzymes, which accelerate the rate of metabolism of warfarin.<br>Decreases absorption<br>Increase synthesis and concentration of blood clotting factors<br>Increase synthesis of clotting factors and have thromboembolic effect |

*(continued)*

## Nursing Actions

### Drugs That Affect Blood Coagulation (Continued)

| Nursing Actions | Rationale/Explanation |
|---|---|
| (6) Vitamin K | Restores prothrombin and other vitamin K–dependent clotting factors in the blood. Antidote for overdose of warfarin. |
| f. Drug that may *increase* or *decrease* effects of warfarin:<br>(1) Alcohol | Alcohol may induce liver enzymes, which *decrease* effects by accelerating the rate of metabolism of the anticoagulant drug. However, with alcohol-induced liver disease (ie, cirrhosis), effects may be *increased* owing to impaired metabolism of warfarin. |
| g. Drugs that *increase* effects of cilostazol:<br>(1) Diltiazem<br>(2) Erythromycin<br>(3) Itraconazole, ketoconazole | These drugs inhibit the main cytochrome P450 enzyme (CYP3A4) that metabolizes cilostazol. Grapefruit juice also inhibits drug metabolism and should be avoided. |

## ? How Can You Avoid This Medication Error?

**Answer:** Ms. Innes' INR is too high, which could significantly increase her risk for bleeding. Therapeutic INR levels are usually between 2 and 3. Before giving anticoagulants, it is important to check lab work (activated partial thromboplastin time for heparin, prothrombin time or INR for Coumadin) to determine whether the dose should be administered. For Ms. Innes, antibiotic therapy may have interfered with the synthesis of vitamin K in the intestine, thus increasing the risk of bleeding. Notify Ms. Innes' physician. Because no signs of bleeding have been noted, he or she may decrease the Coumadin dosage.

## Critical Thinking Exercises

**1.** How soon after oral anticoagulation therapy with warfarin begins will the maximum anticoagulation and antithrombotic effects be achieved?
   a. 24 hours
   b. 1 to 3 days
   c. 3 to 5 days
   d. 5 to 10 days

**2.** The major adverse reaction associated with heparin is bleeding. Which drug will the physician probably prescribe if a client on heparin develops a significant bleeding problem?
   a. Phytonadione
   b. Protamine sulfate
   c. Streptokinase
   d. Dicumarol

**3.** Mr. Samuels, age 43 years, has a prosthetic aortic heart valve. He is taking prophylactic warfarin sodium (Coumadin), 7.5 mg PO daily. Which laboratory test measures the peak concentration levels of warfarin?
   a. Prothrombin time (PT)
   b. Bleeding time
   c. Partial thromboplastin time (PTT)
   d. Activated partial thromboplastin time (aPTT)

**4.** Mr. Green, age 54 years, comes to the emergency department complaining of chest pain unrelieved by nitroglycerin. The physician makes a diagnosis of acute evolving transmural myocardial infarction and prescribes an initial loading dose of streptokinase (Streptase), 20,000 IU by intracoronary infusion, followed by 2,000 IU/minute for 60 minutes. What is streptokinase's mechanism of action?
   a. It prevents further thrombus formation at the infarction site.
   b. It lyses the clot by activating plasminogen.
   c. It decreases the size of the thrombus by decreasing platelet aggregation.
   d. It blocks the synthesis of vitamin K–dependent clotting factors.

**5.** Which adverse reaction should the nurse monitor for that is commonly associated with streptokinase use?

a. Hypotension
b. Seizures
c. Heart failure
d. Allergic reaction

## SELECTED REFERENCES

Activated protein C (Xigris) for severe sepsis (2002). *The Medical Letter on Drugs and Therapeutics, 44*(1124), 17–18.

Deblinger, L. (2000). The challenges of oral anticoagulation. *Patient Care for the Nurse Practitioner, 3*(12), 12–25.

*Drug facts and comparisons.* (Updated monthly). St. Louis: Facts and Comparisons.

Duplaga, B. A., Rivers, C. W., & Nutescu, E. (2001). Dosing and monitoring of low-molecular-weight heparins in special populations. *Pharmacotherapy, 21*(2), 218–234.

Ezekowitz, M. D. (2000). Use of anticoagulant drugs. In H. D. Humes (Ed.), *Kelley's textbook of internal medicine* (4th ed., pp. 673–684). Philadelphia: Lippincott Williams & Wilkins.

Gaspard, K. J. (2002). Alterations in hemostasis. In C. M. Porth (Ed.), *Pathophysiology: Concepts of altered health states* (6th ed., pp. 259–269). Philadelphia: Lippincott Williams & Wilkins.

Haines, S. T, Racine, E., & Zeolla, M. (2002). Venous thromboembolism. In J. T. DiPiro, R. L. Talbert, G. C. Yee, G. R. Matzke, B. G. Wells, & L. M. Posey (Eds.), *Pharmacotherapy: A pathophysiologic approach* (5th ed., pp. 337–373). New York: McGraw-Hill.

Karch, A. M. (2003). *Lippincott's nursing drug guide.* Philadelphia: Lippincott Williams & Wilkins.

Lacy, C. F., Armstrong, L. L., Goldman, M. P., & Lance, L. L. (2003). *Lexi-Comp's drug information handbook* (11th ed.). Hudson, OH: American Pharmaceutical Association.

North American Nursing Diagnosis Association. (2001). *Nursing diagnoses: Definitions and classification, 2001–2002.* Philadelphia: Author.

Sachdev, G. P., Ohlrogge, K. D., & Johnson, C. L. (1999). Review of the Fifth American College of Chest Physicians consensus conference on antithrombotic therapy: Outpatient management for adults. *American Journal of Health-System Pharmacy, 56*, 1505–1514.

Skidmore-Roth, L. (2001). *Mosby's handbook of herbs and natural supplements.* St. Louis: Mosby.

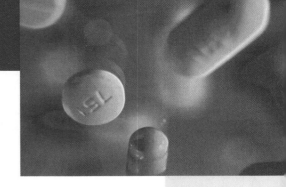

# 46

# Drugs for Dyslipidemia

## OBJECTIVES

*After studying this chapter, the student will be able to:*

1 Identify sources and functions of cholesterol and triglycerides.

2 Describe dyslipidemic drugs in terms of mechanism of action, indications for use, major adverse effects, and nursing process implications.

3 Teach clients pharmacologic and nonpharmacologic measures to prevent or reduce dyslipidemia.

## CRITICAL THINKING SCENARIO

*D*uring a routine physical examination, 26-year-old William Hall is diagnosed with dyslipidemia. His father died at 46 years of age of a massive myocardial infarction (MI). Mr. Hall jogs 3 miles three to four times a week. He eats out, mostly at fast-food places. He is very serious when he listens to the doctor explain his diagnosis. He responds by asking, "Does this mean I am going to die young like my dad?"

✔ What might be the emotional impact of this diagnosis for Mr. Hall, in light of his family history?

✔ What is the underlying pathophysiology of atherosclerosis? What are possible consequences of atherosclerosis other than MI?

✔ What are some ways to explain the significance of laboratory values (cholesterol, low-density lipoproteins, high-density lipoproteins, triglycerides)?

✔ Develop a plan for teaching and follow-up regarding lifestyle modification.

## PROTOTYPE PROFILE

lovastatin (Mevacor, Altocor), p. 844

# OVERVIEW

Dyslipidemic drugs are used in the management of clients with elevated blood lipids, a major risk factor for atherosclerosis and vascular disorders such as coronary artery disease, stroke, and peripheral arterial insufficiency. These drugs have proven efficacy and are being used increasingly to reduce morbidity and mortality from coronary heart disease and other atherosclerosis-related cardiovascular disorders. To understand clinical use of these drugs, it is necessary to understand atherosclerosis, characteristics of blood lipids, and types of blood lipid disorders (see At the Foundation: Blood Lipids).

The Third Report of The National Cholesterol Education Program Expert Panel on Detection, Evaluation and Treatment of High Blood Cholesterol in Adults classifies blood lipid levels as follows:

*Total Serum Cholesterol (mg/dL)*

Normal or desirable = less than 200
Borderline high = 200 to 239
High = 240 or above

*Low-Density Lipoprotein (LDL) Cholesterol (mg/dL)*

Optimal = less than 100
Near or above optimal = 100 to 129
Borderline high = 130 to 159
High = 160 to 189
Very high = 190 or above

*High-Density Lipoprotein (HDL) Cholesterol (mg/dL)*

High = more than 60
Low = less than 40

*Triglycerides (mg/dL)*

Normal or desirable = less than 150
Borderline high = 150 to 199
High = 200 to 499
Very high = 500 or above

Overall, the most effective blood lipid profile for prevention or management of atherosclerosis and its sequelae is high HDL cholesterol, low LDL cholesterol, and low total cholesterol. A low triglyceride level is also desirable. For accurate interpretation of a client's lipid profile, blood samples for laboratory testing of triglycerides should be drawn after the client has fasted for 12 hours. Fasting is not required for cholesterol testing.

# DYSLIPIDEMIA

Dyslipidemia (also called hyperlipidemia) is associated with atherosclerosis and its many pathophysiologic effects (eg, myocardial ischemia and infarction, stroke, peripheral arterial occlusive disease). Ischemic heart disease has a high rate of morbidity and mortality. Elevated total cholesterol and LDL cholesterol and reduced HDL cholesterol are the abnormalities that are major risk factors for coronary artery disease. Elevated triglycerides also play a role in cardiovascular disease. For example, high blood levels reflect excessive caloric intake (excessive dietary fats are stored in adipose tissue; excessive proteins and carbohydrates are converted to triglycerides and also stored in adipose tissue) and obesity. High caloric intake also increases the conversion of very-low-density lipoprotein (VLDL) to LDL cholesterol, and high dietary intake

## AT THE FOUNDATION: *Blood Lipids*

Blood lipids, which include cholesterol, phospholipids, and triglycerides, are derived from the diet or synthesized by the liver and intestine. Most cholesterol is found in body cells, where it is a component of cell membranes and performs other essential functions. In cells of the adrenal glands, ovaries, and testes, cholesterol is required for the synthesis of steroid hormones (eg, cortisol, estrogen, progesterone, and testosterone). In liver cells, cholesterol is used to form cholic acid. The cholic acid is then conjugated with other substances to form bile salts, which promote absorption and digestion of fats. In addition, a small amount is found in blood serum. Serum cholesterol is the portion of total body cholesterol involved in formation of atherosclerotic plaques. Unless a person has a genetic disorder of lipid metabolism, the amount of cholesterol in the blood is strongly related to dietary intake of saturated

fat. Phospholipids are essential components of cell membranes, and triglycerides provide energy for cellular metabolism.

Blood lipids are transported in plasma by specific proteins called *lipoproteins*. Each lipoprotein contains cholesterol, phospholipid, and triglyceride bound to protein. The lipoproteins vary in density and amounts of lipid and protein. Density is determined mainly by the amount of protein, which is more dense than fat. Thus, density increases as the proportion of protein increases. The lipoproteins are differentiated according to these properties, which can be measured in the laboratory. For example, HDL cholesterol contains larger amounts of protein and smaller amounts of lipid; LDL cholesterol contains less protein and larger amounts of lipid. Other plasma lipoproteins are chylomicrons and VLDL. Additional characteristics of lipoproteins are described in Box 46-1.

BOX
46-1 **Types of Lipoproteins**

**Chylomicrons,** the largest lipoprotein molecules, are synthesized in the wall of the small intestine. They carry recently ingested dietary cholesterol and triglycerides that have been absorbed from the gastrointestinal tract. Hyperchylomicronemia normally occurs after a fatty meal, reaches peak levels in 3 to 4 hours, and subsides within 12 to 14 hours. Chylomicrons carry triglycerides to fat and muscle cells, where the enzyme lipoprotein lipase breaks down the molecule and releases fatty acids to be used for energy or stored as fat. This process leaves a remnant containing cholesterol, which is then transported to the liver. Thus, chylomicrons transport triglycerides to peripheral tissues and cholesterol to the liver.

**Low-density lipoprotein (LDL) cholesterol,** sometimes called "bad cholesterol," transports approximately 75% of serum cholesterol and carries it to peripheral tissues and the liver. LDL cholesterol is removed from the circulation by receptor and nonreceptor mechanisms. The receptor mechanism involves the binding of LDL cholesterol to receptors on cell surface membranes. The bound LDL molecule is then engulfed into the cell, where it is broken down by enzymes and releases free cholesterol into the cytoplasm.

Most LDL cholesterol receptors are located in the liver. However, nonhepatic tissues (eg, adrenal glands, smooth muscle cells, endothelial cells, and lymphoid cells) also have receptors by which they obtain the cholesterol needed for building cell membranes and synthesizing hormones. These cells can regulate their cholesterol intake by adding or removing LDL receptors.

Approximately two thirds of the LDL cholesterol is removed from the bloodstream by the receptor-dependent mechanism. The number of LDL receptors on cell membranes determines the amount of LDL degradation (ie, the more receptors on cells, the more LDL is broken down). Conditions that decrease the number or function of receptors (eg, high dietary intake of cholesterol, saturated fat, or calories), increase blood levels of LDL.

The remaining one third is removed by mechanisms that do not involve receptors. Nonreceptor uptake occurs in various cells, especially when levels of circulating LDL cholesterol are high. For example, macrophage cells in arterial walls can attach LDL, thereby promoting accumulation of cholesterol and the development of atherosclerosis. The amount of LDL cholesterol removed by nonreceptor mechanisms is increased with inadequate numbers of receptors or excessive amounts of LDL cholesterol.

A high serum level of LDL cholesterol is atherogenic and a strong risk factor for coronary heart disease. The body normally attempts to compensate for high serum levels by inhibiting hepatic synthesis of cholesterol and cellular synthesis of new LDL receptors.

**Very-low-density lipoprotein (VLDL)** contains approximately 75% triglycerides and 25% cholesterol. It transports endogenous triglycerides (those synthesized in the liver and intestine, not those derived exogenously, from food) to fat and muscle cells. There, as with chylomicrons, lipoprotein lipase breaks down the molecule and releases fatty acids to be used for energy or stored as fat. The removal of triglycerides from VLDL leaves a cholesterol-rich remnant, which returns to the liver. Then the cholesterol is secreted into the intestine, mostly as bile acids, or it is used to form more VLDL and recirculated.

**High-density lipoprotein (HDL) cholesterol,** often referred to as "good cholesterol," is a small but very important lipoprotein. It is synthesized in the liver and intestine and some is derived from the enzymatic breakdown of chylomicrons and VLDL. It contains moderate amounts of cholesterol. However, this cholesterol is transported from blood vessel walls to the liver for catabolism and excretion. This reverse transport of cholesterol has protective effects against coronary heart disease.

The mechanisms by which HDL cholesterol exerts protective effects are unknown. Possible mechanisms include clearing cholesterol from atheromatous plaque; increasing excretion of cholesterol so less is available for reuse in the formation of LDL cholesterol; and inhibiting cellular uptake of LDL cholesterol. Regular exercise and moderate alcohol consumption are associated with increased levels of HDL cholesterol; obesity, diabetes mellitus, genetic factors, smoking, and some medications (eg, steroids and beta blockers) are associated with decreased levels. HDL cholesterol levels are not directly affected by diet.

of triglycerides and saturated fat decreases the activity of LDL receptors and increases synthesis of cholesterol. Very high triglyceride levels are associated with acute pancreatitis.

Dyslipidemia may be primary (ie, genetic or familial) or secondary to dietary habits, other diseases (eg, diabetes mellitus, alcoholism, hypothyroidism, obesity, obstructive liver disease), and medications (eg, beta blockers, cyclosporine, oral estrogens, glucocorticoids, sertraline, thiazide diuretics, anti–human immunodeficiency virus protease inhibitors). Types of dyslipidemia (also called *hyperlipoproteinemia* because increased blood levels of lipoproteins accompany increased blood lipid levels) are described in Box 46-2. Although hypercholesterolemia is usually emphasized, hypertriglyceridemia is also associated with most types of hyperlipoproteinemia.

##  INITIAL MANAGEMENT OF DYSLIPIDEMIA

The National Cholesterol Education Program recommends management of clients according to their blood levels of total and LDL cholesterol and their risk factors

| BOX 46-2 | **Types of Dyslipidemia** |
| --- | --- |

**Type I** is characterized by elevated or normal serum cholesterol, elevated triglycerides, and chylomicronemia. This rare condition may occur in infancy and childhood.

**Type IIa** (familial hypercholesterolemia) is characterized by a high level of low-density lipoprotein (LDL) cholesterol, a normal level of very–low-density lipoprotein (VLDL), and a normal or slightly increased level of triglycerides. It occurs in children and is a definite risk factor for development of atherosclerosis and coronary artery disease.

**Type IIb** (combined familial hyperlipoproteinemia) is characterized by increased levels of LDL, VLDL, cholesterol, and triglycerides and lipid deposits (xanthomas) in the feet, knees, and elbows. It occurs in adults.

**Type III** is characterized by elevations of cholesterol and triglycerides plus abnormal levels of LDL and VLDL. This type usually occurs in middle-aged adults (40 to 60 years) and is associated with accelerated coronary and peripheral vascular disease.

**Type IV** is characterized by normal or elevated cholesterol levels, elevated triglycerides, and increased levels of VLDL. This type usually occurs in adults and may be the most common form of hyperlipoproteinemia. Type IV is often secondary to obesity, excessive intake of alcohol, or other diseases. Ischemic heart disease may occur at 40 to 50 years of age.

**Type V** is characterized by elevated cholesterol and triglyceride levels with an increased level of VLDL and chylomicronemia. This uncommon type usually occurs in adults. Type V is not associated with ischemic heart disease. Instead, it is associated with fat and carbohydrate intolerance, abdominal pain, and pancreatitis, which are relieved by lowering triglyceride levels.

for cardiovascular disease (Table 46-1). Note that both dietary and drug therapy are recommended at lower serum cholesterol levels in clients who already have cardiovascular disease or diabetes mellitus. Also, the target LDL serum level is lower in these clients. Guidelines include the following:

■ Assess for and treat, if present, conditions known to increase blood lipids (eg, diabetes mellitus, hypothyroidism).
■ Stop medications known to increase blood lipids, if possible.
■ Start a low-fat diet. A Step I diet contains no more than 30% of calories from fat, less than 10% of calories from saturated fats (eg, meat, dairy products), and less than 300 mg of cholesterol per day. A Step II diet contains no more than 30% of calories from fat, less than 7% of calories from saturated fat, and less than 200 mg of cholesterol per day. The Step II diet is more stringent and may be used initially in clients with more severe dyslipidemia, cardiovascular disease, or diabetes mellitus. It can decrease LDL cholesterol levels by 8% to 15%. Diets with more stringent fat restrictions than the Step II diet are not recommended because they produce little additional reduction in LDL cholesterol, they raise serum triglyceride levels, and they lower HDL cholesterol concentrations.

■ Use the "Mediterranean diet," which includes moderate amounts of monounsaturated fats (eg, canola and olive oils) and polyunsaturated fats (eg, safflower, corn, cottonseed, sesame, soybean, sunflower oils), to also decrease risk for cardiovascular disease.
■ Increase dietary intake of soluble fiber (eg, psyllium preparations, oat bran, pectin, fruits and vegetables). This diet lowers serum LDL cholesterol by 5% to 10%.
■ Dietary supplements (eg, Cholestin) and cholesterol-lowering margarines (eg, Benecol and Take Control) can help reduce cholesterol levels. These products are considered to be foods, not drugs, and are costly.
■ Start a weight reduction diet if the client is overweight or obese. Weight loss can increase HDL and decrease LDL.
■ Emphasize regular aerobic exercise (usually 30 minutes at least three times weekly). This increases blood levels of HDL.
■ If the client smokes, assist to develop a cessation plan. In addition to numerous other benefits, HDL levels are higher in nonsmokers.

### TABLE 46-1 National Cholesterol Education Program Recommendations for Treatment of Dyslipidemia

| Patient's Cardiovascular Disease Status | Diet Therapy | | Drug Therapy | | Goal of Therapy (mg/dL) |
| --- | --- | --- | --- | --- | --- |
| | Total Cholesterol (mg/dL) | LDL Cholesterol (mg/dL) | Total Cholesterol (mg/dL) | LDL Cholesterol (mg/dL) | |
| No or one risk factor | 240 | 160 | 275 | 190 | LDL <160 |
| More than two risk factors | 200 | 130 | 240 | 160 | LDL <130 |
| Has cardiovascular disease | 160 | 100 | 200 | 130 | LDL <100 |

LDL, low-density lipoprotein.

- If the client is postmenopausal, hormone replacement therapy can raise HDL and lower LDL.
- If the client has elevated serum triglycerides, initial management includes efforts to achieve desirable body weight, ingest low amounts of saturated fat and cholesterol, exercise regularly, stop smoking, and reduce alcohol intake, if indicated. The goal is to reduce serum triglyceride levels to 200 mg/dL or less.
- Unless lipid levels are severely elevated, a minimum of 6 months of intensive diet therapy and lifestyle modification should be undertaken before drug therapy is considered. It is essential that diet therapy continue because the benefits of diet and drug therapy are additive.

## Genetic and Ethnic Considerations

Little information has been reported on racial or ethnic differences for lipid-lowering drugs. Members of minority populations (eg, African Americans, Mexican Americans) are less likely to be treated than white Americans. Despite an increased prevalence of diabetes and obesity, American Indians appear to have lower cholesterol levels than the United States population as a whole. This suggests that diet and exercise may be more useful than lipid-lowering drugs for this group.

## Herbal and Dietary Supplements

Use of nonprescription herbal and dietary supplements is frequently not reported by the client even though one third of the adults in the United States use these agents. Significant interactions can occur between herbs and dietary supplements when taken with prescribed drugs. Flax or flax seed is used internally as a laxative and a dyslipidemic agent. Absorption of all medications may be decreased when taken with flax, resulting in less than a therapeutic effect. Garlic is reportedly used as a dyslipidemic agent and a possible antihypertensive, but there is little scientific support for such use. Bleeding may be increased when garlic is used with anticoagulants, and insulin doses may need to be decreased as a result of the hypoglycemic effect of garlic. Green tea is commonly used for its dyslipidemic effect, and the caffeinated product can be a central nervous system stimulant. Soy is used as a food source and has been researched extensively. Use of soy to lower cholesterol (LDL and total cholesterol) has been documented. Significant interactions with other herbs or drugs have not been reported.

## ▨ DRUG THERAPY OF DYSLIPIDEMIA

Dyslipidemic drugs are used to decrease blood lipids, to prevent or delay the development of atherosclerotic plaque, to promote the regression of existing atherosclerotic plaque, and to reduce morbidity and mortality from cardiovascular disease. Clinical data suggest that drug therapy may be efficacious even for those with mild to moderate elevations of LDL cholesterol. The drugs act by altering the production, metabolism, or removal of lipids and lipoproteins. Drug therapy is recommended when approximately 6 months of dietary and other lifestyle changes fail to decrease dyslipidemia to an acceptable level. It is also recommended for clients with signs and symptoms of coronary heart disease, a strong family history of coronary heart disease or dyslipidemia, or other risk factors for atherosclerotic vascular disease (eg, hypertension, diabetes mellitus, cigarette smoking). Considerations for use of dyslipidemic drugs to treat children and older adults are given in Age-related Considerations. The nurse also must adjust treatment for home care (see Home Care Considerations). Although several dyslipidemic drugs are available, none is effective in all types of dyslipidemia. Categories of drugs are described in this section; individual drugs are listed in Drugs at a Glance 46-1: Dyslipidemic Agents.

Drug selection is based on the type of dyslipidemia and its severity. For single-drug therapy to lower cholesterol, a statin is preferred. To lower both cholesterol and triglycerides, a statin, gemfibrozil, or niacin may be used. To lower triglycerides, gemfibrozil or niacin may be used. Gemfibrozil is usually preferred for people with diabetes because niacin increases blood sugar.

When monotherapy is not effective, combination therapy is rational because the drugs act by different mechanisms. In general, a statin and a bile acid sequestrant or niacin and a bile acid sequestrant are the most effective combinations in reducing total and LDL cholesterol. A fibrate or niacin may be included when a goal of therapy is to increase levels of HDL cholesterol. However, a fibrate-statin combination should be avoided because of increased risk for severe myopathy, and a niacin-statin combination increases the risk for hepatotoxicity.

The **HMG-CoA reductase inhibitors** or statins (eg, ℗ lovastatin) inhibit an enzyme (hydroxymethylglutaryl–coenzyme A reductase) required for hepatic synthesis of cholesterol. By decreasing production of cholesterol, these drugs decrease total serum cholesterol, LDL cholesterol, VLDL cholesterol, and triglycerides. They reduce LDL cholesterol within 2 weeks and reach maximal effects in approximately 4 to 6 weeks. HDL cholesterol levels remain unchanged or may increase.

Overall, these drugs are useful in treating most of the major types of dyslipidemia and are the most widely used dyslipidemics. In this drug class, lovastatin is the prototype and is outlined in Prototype Profile 46-1: Lovastatin. Studies indicate that these drugs can reduce the blood levels of C-reactive protein (CRP), which is associated with severe arterial inflammation that leads to heart attacks and strokes. The incidence of coronary artery disease is reduced by 25% to 60% and the risk for death from any cause by approximately 30%. They also reduce the risk for angina pectoris and peripheral arterial disease as well as the need

## Age-related Considerations: Use of Drugs for Dyslipidemia

### USE IN CHILDREN

As with adults, initial management consists of diet therapy (for 6 to 12 months) and management of any secondary causes, especially with younger children. With additional risk factors or primary familial hypercholesterolemia (type IIa), however, these measures are not likely to be effective without drug therapy.

Dyslipidemic drugs are not recommended for children younger than 10 years of age. Lovastatin recently received U.S. Food and Drug Administration (FDA) approval for use in children 10 to 17 years old. Oral dosing recommendations are 10 to 20 mg daily with a meal, initially, and increasing up to 40 mg daily as necessary, with increases made at least 4 weeks apart. Other statin drugs are not recommended in children younger than 18 years of age, and the safety and effectiveness of the fibrates have not been established. Bile acid sequestrants are considered the drugs of choice, and niacin also may be used. Despite considerable use of bile acid sequestrants, children's dosages have only been established for cholestyramine. Recommendations for oral dosing of cholestyramine are 240 mg/kg per day to be given in three divided doses. Niacin dosage is 55 to 87 mg/kg per day to be given orally three to four times a day with or just after meals. The long-term consequences of dyslipidemic drug therapy in children are unknown.

### USE IN OLDER ADULTS

As with younger adults, diet, exercise, and weight control should be tried first. When drug therapy is required, statins are effective for lowering LDL cholesterol and usually are well tolerated by older adults. However, they are expensive. Niacin and bile acid sequestrants are effective, but older adults do not tolerate their adverse effects very well. In postmenopausal women, estrogen replacement therapy increases HDL cholesterol.

Older adults often have diabetes, impaired liver function, or other conditions that raise blood lipid levels. Thus, management of secondary causes is especially important. They are also likely to have cardiovascular and other disorders that increase the adverse effects of dyslipidemic drugs. Overall, use of dyslipidemic drugs should be cautious, with close monitoring for therapeutic and adverse effects. Lower starting dosages are recommended for fenofibrate (67 mg/day), pravastatin (10 mg/day), and simvastatin (5 mg/day).

---

for angioplasty and coronary artery grafting to increase or restore blood flow to the myocardium.

Absorption following oral administration varies by drug. Lovastatin and pravastatin are poorly absorbed; fluvastatin has the highest rate of absorption. Most of the statins undergo extensive first-past metabolism by the liver, which results in low levels of drug available for general circulation. Metabolism occurs in the liver, with 80% to 85% of drug metabolites excreted in feces and the remaining excreted in urine.

## Home Care Considerations: Use of Drugs for Dyslipidemia

**ASSESS:** knowledge about prescribed drugs, diet therapy, and ability and willingness to comply with instructions for taking the drugs and obtaining blood tests when indicated.

**MONITOR:** compliance with medication regime and diet therapy. Also monitor for ability to obtain laboratory tests and other follow-up care.

**EDUCATE:** about the role of blood lipids in causing myocardial infarction, stroke, and peripheral arterial insufficiency; the prescribed management regimen and its goals; and the importance of improving dyslipidemia in preventing or improving cardiovascular disorders. Reinforce additional teaching points (see Client Teaching Guidelines: Dyslipidemic Drugs).

Statins are usually well tolerated; the most common adverse effects (nausea, constipation, diarrhea, abdominal cramps or pain, headache, skin rash) are usually mild and transient. More serious reactions include rare occurrences of hepatotoxicity and myopathy. The drugs are contraindicated in women who are or who may become pregnant because studies have demonstrated fetal abnormalities or fetal risk. Because the drug enters breast milk, women who are breast-feeding should not use the drug.

Statins are metabolized by the liver and excreted partly through the kidneys (their main route of excretion is through bile). Liver function tests are recommended before starting a statin, at 6 and 12 weeks after starting the drug or increasing the dose, then every 6 months. Monitor clients who have increased serum aminotransferases until the abnormal values resolve. If the increases are more than three times the upper limit of normal levels and persist, the dose should be reduced or the drug discontinued. Drug plasma concentrations may be increased in clients with renal impairment, and they should be used cautiously; some need reduced dosage.

**Bile acid sequestrants** (eg, cholestyramine) bind bile acids in the intestinal lumen. This causes the bile acids to be excreted in feces and prevents their being recirculated to the liver. Loss of bile acids stimulates hepatic synthesis of more bile acids from cholesterol. As more hepatic cholesterol is used to produce bile acids, more serum cholesterol moves into the liver to replenish the supply, thereby lowering serum cholesterol (especially LDL). LDL

(text continues on page 845)

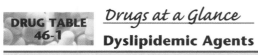

**DRUG TABLE 46-1**

*Drugs at a Glance*

## Dyslipidemic Agents

| Generic/Trade Name | Routes and Dosage Ranges | Comments |
|---|---|---|
| **HMG-CoA Reductase Inhibitors (Statins)** | | |
| **Atorvastatin** (Lipitor) Pregnancy Category X | For types IIa and IIb dyslipidemia *Adults:* PO, 10–80 mg daily in a single dose | May take without regard to food |
| **Fluvastatin** (Lescol, Lescol XL) Pregnancy Category X | For types IIa and IIb dyslipidemia *Adults:* PO, 40–80 mg daily in one or two doses | Administer at least 2 h after niacin or bile acid–binding resins if used together for lipid-lowering effect; may take without regard to food |
| **Lovastatin** (Mevacor, Altocor) Pregnancy Category X | See Prototype Profile 46-1: Lovastatin | |
| **Pravastatin** (Pravachol) Pregnancy Category X | For types IIa and IIb dyslipidemia *Adults:* PO, 40–80 mg once daily *Elderly:* PO, 10 mg once daily | As with all statins, observe for liver enzyme elevations during therapy; may take without regard to food |
| **Simvastatin** (Zocor) Pregnancy Category X | For types IV and V (hypertriglyceridemia) *Adults:* PO, 5–80 mg once daily in the evening *Elderly:* PO, 5–20 mg once daily in the evening | Take with food; 6–8 wk of therapy is necessary to determine efficacy |
| **Fibrates** | | |
| **Fenofibrate** (Tricor) Pregnancy Category C | For types IV, V (hypertriglyceridemia) *Adults:* PO, 67 mg daily, increased if necessary to a maximum dose of 201 mg daily | May potentiate the effect of warfarin and sulfonylureas Cyclosporine blood levels may be reduced with concurrent therapy |
| **Gemfibrozil** (Lopid) Pregnancy Category C | For types IV, V (hypertriglyceridemia) *Adults:* PO, 900–1500 mg daily, usually 1200 mg in two divided doses, 30 min before morning and evening meals | May decrease absorption of folic acid, iron, and calcium, especially with long-term use or high doses May also decrease absorption of PO digoxin, warfarin, thiazide diuretics, propranolol, phenobarbital, thyroid hormone, amiodarone, NSAIDs, and other drugs |
| **Bile Acid Sequestrants** | | |
| **Cholestyramine** (Questran, LoCholest) Pregnancy Category C | For type IIa dyslipidemia *Adults:* PO tablets, 4 g once or twice daily initially, gradually increased at monthly intervals to 8–16 g daily in two divided doses. Maximum daily dose, 24 g PO powder, 4 g one to six times daily *Children:* 240 mg/kg/d in three divided doses | Use with caution in clients with constipation No significant effect on absorption of digoxin, lovastatin, metoprolol, quinidine, valproic acid, or warfarin reported |
| **Colesevelam** (Welchol) Pregnancy Category B | For type IIa dyslipidemia *Adults:* 3.75 g daily in one or two doses. Maximum daily dose, 4.375 g | |

*(continued)*

**DRUG TABLE 46-1**

*Drugs at a Glance*

**Dyslipidemic Agents** (Continued)

| Generic/Trade Name | Routes and Dosage Ranges | Comments |
|---|---|---|
| **Colestipol**<br>Pregnancy Category C | For type IIa dyslipidemia<br>*Adults:* PO tablets, 2 g once or twice daily initially, gradually increased at 1- to 2-mo intervals, up to 16 g daily<br>PO granules, 5 g daily initially, gradually increased at 1- to 2-mo intervals, up to 30 g daily in single or divided doses | The absorption of numerous medications affected with concurrent use. Give other medications 1 h before or 4 h after administering colestipol |
| *Miscellaneous* | | |
| **Nicotinic acid (niacin)**<br>Pregnancy Category A/C (with dose exceeding RDA recommendations) | For types II, III, IV, V dyslipidemia<br>*Adults:* PO, 2–6 g daily, in three or four divided doses, with or just after meals<br>*Children:* PO, 55–87 mg/kg/d, in three or four divided doses, with or just after meals | Instruct to avoid sudden changes in posture; observe closely for signs of hepatotoxicity and myositis |
| **Niacin (extended release)**<br>Pregnancy Category A/C (with dose exceeding RDA recommendations) | For types IIa, IIb dyslipidemia<br>*Adults:* PO, 500–2000 mg daily | Do not crush timed release forms |

---

## PROTOTYPE PROFILE 46-1

### *P* Lovastatin (LOE va sta tin)

**Drug Class**
*Chemical:* HMG-CoA reductase inhibitors, statin
*Functional:* Antilipemic

**Trade Names**
Mevacor, Altocor

**Therapeutic Indications**
To decreased elevated serum total and LDL cholesterol concentrations in primary hypercholesterolemia

**Pharmacokinetics**
*Absorption*
30%; Increased with extended release tablets

*Distribution*
Plasma protein binding: 95%

*Metabolism*
Extensively in the liver; a relatively small proportion of an oral dose reaches the systemic circulation (extensive first-pass effect)

*Excretion*
Predominately feces

**Pharmacodynamics**
*Onset of Action*
LDL cholesterol reduction—3 d

*Duration*
Unknown

**Contraindications/Precautions**
Hypersensitivity to lovastatin, active liver disease, pregnancy, or breast-feeding

**Pregnancy Considerations**
Category X; safety and efficacy have not been established; the medication should be discontinued if pregnancy occurs
Enters breast milk, contraindicated

**Dosage**
*Adults:* PO, 10–80 mg/d in 1 to 2 divided doses with meals
*Children:* <10 y: not recommended
10–17 y: PO, usual range 10 to 40 mg/d with evening meal, adjusted at 4-wk intervals

**Side Effects/Adverse Reactions**
Nausea, abdominal pain or cramps, flatulence, constipation, myalgia
May elevate aminotransferases, so liver function tests should be routinely performed

*(continued)*

## PROTOTYPE PROFILE 46-1
### P Lovastatin (Continued)

**Drug Interactions**

*Increased Effects*

Effect of warfarin

Effect with other antilipemics

*Decreased Effects*

Cholestyramine may reduce lovastatin absorption and effect

**Herbal Supplements and Dietary Considerations**

St. John's wort may decrease lovastatin levels

Quantities of grapefruit juice exceeding 1 quart/d may increase serum concentration of lovastatin

Use cautiously and in reduced dosages, in clients who ingest substantial amounts of alcohol

---

cholesterol levels decrease within a week of starting these drugs and reach maximal reductions within a month. When the drugs are stopped, pretreatment LDL cholesterol levels return within a month.

These drugs are used mainly to reduce LDL cholesterol further in clients who are already receiving a statin drug. The inhibition of cholesterol synthesis by a statin makes bile acid–binding drugs more effective. In addition, the combination increases HDL cholesterol and can further reduce the risk for cardiovascular disorders. With long-term use, bile acid sequestrants may also reduce absorption of folic acid and the fat-soluble vitamins: A, D, E, and K. Poor absorption of vitamin K can significantly affect prothrombin times.

These drugs are not absorbed systemically, and their main adverse effects are abdominal fullness, flatulence, and constipation. They may decrease absorption of many oral medications (eg, digoxin, folic acid, glipizide, propranolol, tetracyclines, thiazide diuretics, thyroid hormones, fat-soluble vitamins, and warfarin). Other drugs should be taken at least 1 hour before or 4 hours after cholestyramine or colestipol. In addition, dosage of the interactive drug may need to be changed when a bile acid sequestrant is added or withdrawn.

**Fibrates** are derivatives of fibric acid (eg, gemfibrozil, fenofibrate) and are similar to endogenous fatty acids. The drugs increase the oxidation of fatty acids in liver and muscle tissue and thereby decrease hepatic production of triglycerides, decrease VLDL cholesterol, and increase

HDL cholesterol. These are the most effective drugs for reducing serum triglyceride levels, and their main indication for use is high serum triglyceride levels (>500 mg/dL). They are also useful in clients with low HDL cholesterol levels. In clients with coronary artery disease, management with gemfibrozil is associated with regression of atherosclerotic lesions on angiography.

These drugs are well absorbed following oral administration. Metabolism occurs in the liver, and excretion is mainly by the kidneys. **Fibrates** may cause hepatotoxicity. Abnormal elevations of serum aminotransferases have occurred with both gemfibrozil and fenofibrate, but they usually subside when the drug is discontinued. Fenofibrate is contraindicated in clients with severe hepatic impairment, including clients with primary biliary cirrhosis, pre-existing gallbladder disease, and persistent elevations in liver function test results. In addition, hepatitis (hepatocellular, chronic active, and cholestatic) has been reported after use of fenofibrate from a few weeks to several years. Liver function tests should be monitored during the first year of drug administration. The drug should be discontinued if elevated enzyme levels persist at more than three times the normal limit. With excretion mainly by the kidneys, there is an accumulation in the serum of clients with renal impairment. Drug and dose effects on renal function and triglyceride levels should be evaluated before dosage is increased. The main adverse effects are gastrointestinal discomfort and diarrhea, which may occur less often with fenofibrate than with gemfibrozil. The drugs may also increase cholesterol concentration in the biliary tract and cause gallstones. For clients receiving warfarin, warfarin dosage should be substantially decreased because fibrates displace warfarin from binding sites on serum albumin.

**Niacin** (nicotinic acid) decreases both cholesterol and triglycerides. It inhibits mobilization of free fatty acids from peripheral tissues, thereby reducing hepatic synthesis of triglycerides and secretion of VLDL, which leads to decreased production of LDL cholesterol. Niacin is the most effective drug for increasing the concentration of HDL cholesterol. Disadvantages of niacin are the high doses required for dyslipidemic effects and the subsequent adverse effects. Niacin commonly causes skin flushing, pruritus, and gastric irritation and may cause

**?** **How Can You Avoid This Medication Error?**

Mrs. Gribble, a 79-year-old nursing home resident, likes to take all of her medications together. You mix up her cholestyramine (Questran) in a large glass of orange juice and give it to her with her digoxin, Lasix, captopril, and Slow-K. You monitor her pulse and blood pressure before administration and they are within normal limits. What, if any, additional precautions should be used when Questran is administered?

hyperglycemia, hyperuricemia, elevated hepatic aminotransferase enzymes, and hepatitis. Flushing can be reduced by starting with small doses, gradually increasing doses, taking doses with meals, and taking aspirin, 325 mg, about 30 minutes before niacin doses.

Niacin is rapidly absorbed from the gastrointestinal tract. Minimal metabolism occurs by the liver, and most of the drug is excreted unchanged in the urine. Niacin may cause hepatotoxicity, especially with doses above 2 g daily, with timed-release preparations, and if given in combination with a statin or fibrate.

Niacin is most effective in preventing heart disease when used in combination with another dyslipidemic drug such as a bile acid sequestrant or a fibrate. Its use with a statin lowers serum LDL cholesterol more than either drug alone, but the combination has not been studied in relation to preventing cardiovascular disease.

*(text continues on page 850)*

# NURSING PROCESS

## Assessment

Assess the client's status in relation to atherosclerotic vascular disease.

- Identify risk factors:
  - Hypertension
  - Diabetes mellitus
  - High intake of dietary fat and refined sugars
  - Obesity
  - Inadequate exercise
  - Cigarette smoking
  - Family history of atherosclerotic disorders
  - Dyslipidemia
- Signs and symptoms depend on the specific problem:
  - **Dyslipidemia** is manifested by elevated serum cholesterol (>240 mg/100 mL) or triglycerides (>200 mg/100 mL), or both.
  - **Coronary artery atherosclerosis** is manifested by myocardial ischemia (angina pectoris, myocardial infarction).
  - **Cerebrovascular insufficiency** may be manifested by syncope, memory loss, transient ischemic attacks (TIAs), or strokes. Impairment of blood flow to the brain is caused primarily by atherosclerosis in the carotid, vertebral, or cerebral arteries.
  - **Peripheral arterial insufficiency** is manifested by impaired blood flow in the legs (weak or absent pulses; cool, pale extremities; intermittent claudication; leg pain at rest; and development of gangrene, usually in the toes because they are most distal to blood supply). This condition results from atherosclerosis in the distal abdominal aorta, the iliac arteries, and the femoral and smaller arteries in the legs.

## Nursing Diagnoses

- Ineffective Tissue Perfusion: related to interruption of arterial blood flow
- Imbalanced Nutrition: More Than Body Requirements of fats and calories
- Anxiety related to risks of atherosclerotic cardiovascular disease
- Disturbed Body Image related to the need for lifestyle changes
- Noncompliance related to dietary restrictions and adverse drug reactions
- Deficient Knowledge related to drug and diet therapy of dyslipidemia

## Planning/Goals

*The client will:*

- Take lipid-lowering drugs as prescribed
- Decrease dietary intake of saturated fats and cholesterol
- Lose weight if obese and maintain the lower weight
- Have periodic measurements of blood lipids
- Avoid preventable adverse drug effects
- Receive positive reinforcement for efforts to lower blood lipid levels
- Report feeling less anxious and more in control as risks of atherosclerotic cardiovascular disease are decreased

## Interventions

Use measures to prevent, delay, or minimize atherosclerosis.

- Help clients to control risk factors. Ideally, primary prevention begins in childhood with healthful eating habits (ie, avoiding excessive fats, meat, and dairy products; obtaining adequate amounts of all nutrients, including dietary fiber; avoiding obesity), exercise, and avoiding cigarette smoking. However, changing habits to a more healthful lifestyle is helpful at any time, before or after disease manifestations appear. Weight loss often reduces blood lipids and lipoproteins to a normal range. Changing habits is difficult for most people, even those with severe symptoms.
- Use measures to increase blood flow to tissues:
  - Exercise is helpful in developing collateral circulation in the heart and legs. Collateral circulation involves use of secondary vessels in response to tissue ischemia related to obstruction of the principal vessels. Clients with angina pectoris or previous myocardial infarction require a carefully planned and supervised program of progressive exercise. Those with peripheral arterial insufficiency usually can increase exercise tolerance by walking regularly. Distances should be determined by occurrence of pain and must be individualized.
  - Posture and position may be altered to increase blood flow to the legs in peripheral arterial insufficiency. Elevating the head of the bed and having the legs horizontal or dependent may help. Elevating the feet is usually contraindicated unless edema is present or likely to develop.
- Although drug therapy is being increasingly used to prevent or manage atherosclerotic disorders, a major thera-

*(continued)*

## N URSING PROCESS (Continued)

peutic option for management of occlusive vascular disease is surgical removal of atherosclerotic plaque or revascularization procedures. Thus, severe angina pectoris may be relieved by a coronary artery bypass procedure that detours blood flow around occluded vessels. This procedure also may be done after a myocardial infarction. The goal is to prevent infarction or reinfarction. TIAs may be relieved by carotid endarterectomy; the goal is to prevent a stroke. Peripheral arterial insufficiency may be relieved by aortofemoral, femoropopliteal, or other bypass grafts that detour around occluded vessels. Although these procedures increase blood flow to ischemic tissues, they do not halt progression of atherosclerosis.

The nursing role in relation to these procedures is to provide excellent preoperative and postoperative nursing care to promote healing, prevent infection, maintain patency of grafts, and help the client to achieve optimum function.

- Any dyslipidemic drug therapy must be accompanied by an appropriate diet; refer clients to a nutritionist. Overeating or gaining weight may decrease or cancel the lipid-lowering effects of the drugs.

- Encourage adult clients to have their serum cholesterol measured at least once every 5 years. Adults and children with a personal or family history of dyslipidemia or other risk factors should be tested more often.
- The most effective measures for preventing dyslipidemia and atherosclerosis are those related to a healthful lifestyle (diet low in cholesterol and saturated fats, weight control, exercise).
- Assist clients and family members to understand the desirability of lowering high blood lipid levels before serious cardiovascular diseases develop.

### Evaluation

- Observe for decreased blood levels of total and low-density lipoprotein (LDL) cholesterol and triglycerides; observe for increased levels of high-density lipoprotein (HDL) cholesterol.
- Observe and interview regarding compliance with instructions for drug, diet, and other therapeutic measures.
- Observe and interview regarding adverse drug effects.
- Validate the client's ability to identify foods high and low in cholesterol and saturated fats.

---

## CLIENT TEACHING GUIDELINES
## Dyslipidemic Drugs

### General Considerations

✔ Heart and blood vessel disease causes a great deal of illness and many deaths. The basic problem is usually atherosclerosis, in which the arteries are partly blocked by cholesterol deposits. Cholesterol, a waxy substance made in the liver, is necessary for normal body functioning. However, excessive amounts in the blood increase the likelihood of having a heart attack, stroke, or leg pain from inadequate blood flow. One type of cholesterol (low-density lipoprotein [LDL] or "bad") attaches to artery walls, where it can enlarge over time and block blood flow. The other type (high-density lipoprotein [HDL] or "good") carries cholesterol away from the artery and back to the liver, where it can be broken down. Thus, the healthiest blood cholesterol levels are low total cholesterol (<200 mg/dL), low LDL (<130 mg/dL), and high HDL (>35 mg/dL). High levels of blood triglycerides, another type of fat, are also unhealthy.

✔ Dyslipidemic drugs are given to lower high concentrations of fats (total cholesterol, LDL cholesterol, and triglycerides) in your blood. The goal of management is to prevent heart attack, stroke, and peripheral arterial disease. If you already have heart and blood vessel disease, the drugs can improve your symptoms, activity level, and quality of life.

✔ A low-fat diet is needed. This is often the first step in treating high cholesterol or triglyceride levels, and may be prescribed for 6 months or longer before drug

therapy is begun. When drug therapy is prescribed, the diet should be continued. An important part is reducing the amount of saturated fat (from meats, dairy products). In addition, eating a bowl of oat cereal daily can help lower cholesterol by 5% to 10%. Diet counseling by a dietitian or nutritionist can be helpful in developing guidelines that fit your needs and lifestyle. Overeating or gaining weight may decrease or cancel the lipid-lowering effects of the drugs.

✔ Other lifestyle changes that can help improve cholesterol levels include regular aerobic exercise (raises HDL); losing weight (raises HDL, lowers LDL, lowers triglycerides); and not smoking (HDL levels are higher in nonsmokers).

✔ Adults should have measurements of total cholesterol and HDL cholesterol at least once every 5 years. People with a personal or family history of dyslipidemia or other risk factors for cardiovascular disease should be tested more often.

✔ Atorvastatin and other statin-type dyslipidemic drugs may increase sensitivity to sunlight. Avoid prolonged exposure to the sun, use sunscreens, and wear protective clothing.

✔ Gemfibrozil may cause dizziness or blurred vision and should be used cautiously while driving or performing other tasks that require alertness, coordination, or

*(continued)*

## CLIENT TEACHING GUIDELINES
### Dyslipidemic Drugs (Continued)

physical dexterity. It also may cause abdominal pain, diarrhea, nausea, or vomiting. Notify a health care provider if these symptoms become severe.

✔ Skin flushing may occur with niacin. If it is distressing, taking one regular aspirin tablet (325 mg) 30 to 60 minutes before the niacin dose may decrease this reaction. Flushing usually decreases in a few days, but may recur when niacin dosage is increased. Ask your health care provider if there is any reason you should not take aspirin.

✔ Cholestyramine and colestipol can cause constipation. Increasing intake of dietary fiber can help prevent this adverse effect.

### Self-administration

✔ Take lovastatin with food; take atorvastatin, fluvastatin, pravastatin, or simvastatin in the evening, with or without food. Food decreases stomach upset associated with lovastatin. All of these drugs may be more effective if taken in the evening or at bedtime, probably because

more cholesterol is produced at nighttime and the drugs block cholesterol production.

✔ Take fenofibrate with food; food increases drug absorption.

✔ Take gemfibrozil on an empty stomach, 30 minutes before morning and evening meals.

✔ Take immediate-release niacin with meals to decrease stomach upset; take timed-release niacin without regard to meals.

✔ Mix cholestyramine powder and colestipol granules with water or other fluids, soups, cereals, or fruits such as applesauce and follow with more fluid. These drug forms should not be taken dry.

✔ Do not take cholestyramine or colestipol with other drugs because they may prevent absorption of the other drugs. If taking other drugs, take them 1 hour before or 4 to 6 hours after cholestyramine or colestipol.

✔ Swallow colestipol tablets whole; do not cut, crush, or chew.

## *Nursing Actions*
## Drugs for Dyslipidemia

| *Nursing Actions* | *Rationale/Explanation* |
| --- | --- |
| 1. **Administer accurately.** | |
| a. Give lovastatin with food; give fluvastatin on an empty stomach or at bedtime. Atorvastatin, pravastatin, or simvastatin may be given with or without food in the evening. Avoid giving with grapefruit juice. | Food decreases gastrointestinal (GI) upset associated with lovastatin. These drugs are more effective if taken in the evening or at bedtime, because more cholesterol is produced by the liver at night and the drugs block cholesterol production. Grapefruit juice increases serum drug levels. Food increases drug absorption. |
| b. Give fenofibrate with food. | |
| c. Give gemfibrozil on an empty stomach, about 30 min before morning and evening meals. | |
| d. Give immediate-release niacin with meals; give timed-release niacin without regard to meals. | The immediate-release formulation may cause gastric irritation. |
| e. Mix cholestyramine powder and colestipol granules with water or other fluids, soups, cereals, or fruits such as applesauce and follow with more fluid. | These drug forms should not be taken dry. |
| f. Do not give cholestyramine or colestipol with other drugs; give them 1 h before or 4–6 h after cholestyramine or colestipol. | Cholestyramine and colestipol prevent absorption of many drugs. |
| g. Instruct clients to swallow colestipol tablets whole; do not cut, crush, or chew. | |
| 2. **Observe for therapeutic effects.** | |
| a. Decreased levels of total serum cholesterol, low-density lipoprotein cholesterol, and triglycerides, and increased levels of high-density lipoprotein cholesterol. | With statins, effects occur in 1–2 wk, with maximum effects in 4–6 wk. With fibrates and niacin, effects occur in approximately 1 mo. With cholestyramine and colestipol, maximum effects occur in approximately 1 mo. |

*(continued)*

## Nursing Actions

### Drugs for Dyslipidemia (Continued)

| Nursing Actions | Rationale/Explanation |
|---|---|
| 3. Observe for adverse effects. | |
| a. GI problems—nausea, vomiting, flatulence, constipation or diarrhea, abdominal discomfort | GI symptoms are the most common adverse effects of dyslipidemic drugs. Constipation is especially common with cholestyramine and colestipol. |
| b. With lovastatin and related drugs, observe for GI upset (see 3a), skin rash, pruritus, and myopathy | Adverse effects are usually mild and of short duration. A less common but potentially serious effect is liver dysfunction, usually manifested by increased levels of serum aminotransferases. Serum aminotransferases (aspartate and alanine aminotransferase) should be measured before starting the drug, every 4–6 wk during the first 3 mo, then every 6–12 wk or after dosage increases for 1 y, then every 6 mo. |
| c. With nicotinic acid, flushing of the face and neck, pruritus, and skin rash may occur, as well as tachycardia, hypotension, and dizziness. | These symptoms may be prominent when nicotinic acid is used to lower blood lipids because relatively high doses are required. Aspirin 325 mg, 30 min before nicotinic acid, decreases the flushing reaction. |
| 4. Observe for drug interactions. | |
| a. Drugs that *increase* effects of lovastatin and related drugs: | |
| (1) Azole antifungals (eg, fluconazole, itraconazole) | Risk of myopathy is increased. It is recommended that statin therapy be interrupted temporarily if systemic azole antifungals are needed. |
| (2) Cyclosporine | Risk of severe myopathy or rhabdomyolysis is increased. |
| (3) Erythromycin | Risk of severe myopathy or rhabdomyolysis is increased. |
| (4) Fibrate dyslipidemics (eg, fenofibrate, gemfibrozil) | Risk of severe myopathy or rhabdomyolysis is increased. These drugs should not be given concurrently with statin dyslipidemic drugs. |
| (5) Niacin | Risk of severe myopathy or rhabdomyolysis is increased. |
| (6) Drugs that increase effects of fluvastatin: | |
| (a) Alcohol, cimetidine, ranitidine, omeprazole | Increased blood levels |
| b. Drugs that *decrease* effects of lovastatin and related drugs: | |
| (1) Bile acid sequestrant dyslipidemics | Decreased blood levels unless the drugs are taken 1–4 h apart |
| (2) Antacids | Decrease absorption of atorvastatin |
| (3) Isradipine | This calcium channel blocker may decrease blood levels of lovastatin and its metabolites by increasing their hepatic metabolism. |
| (4) Rifampin | Decreases blood levels of fluvastatin |
| c. Drugs that *decrease* effects of fibrate dyslipidemic drugs: | |
| (1) Bile acid sequestrant dyslipidemic drugs | Decrease absorption unless the fibrate is taken about 1 h before or 4–6 h after the bile acid sequestrant |

### ? How Can You Avoid This Medication Error?

**Answer:** Questran should not be administered at the same time as other oral medications because it interferes with the absorption of many other drugs, including digoxin. Give other drugs 1 hour before or 4 to 6 hours after Questran is administered.

## Critical Thinking Exercises

1. It is important for a nurse to teach a client on long-term cholestyramine therapy that she may experience a deficiency in vitamin:

   a. $B_1$
   b. $B_6$
   c. C
   d. K

2. Ms. Adams, age 40 years, has type III hyperlipoproteinemia. When she fails to respond to nonpharmacologic therapy, the physician prescribes gemfibrozil (Lopid). This drug is most effective when the patient has:

   a. Coronary artery disease
   b. Angina
   c. Peripheral vascular disease
   d. No previous history of coronary artery disease

3. A 46-year-old man visits the health care provider for his annual check-up. Assessment findings reveal a slight increase in blood pressure and a serum cholesterol level of 340 mg/dL. What can the nurse anticipate as the preferred treatment for this client?

   a. A low-lipid diet and exercise program
   b. A low-lipid diet and a cholesterol synthesis inhibitor
   c. An exercise program and a fibric acid derivative
   d. A low-lipid diet, an exercise program, and niacin

4. A 32 year-old female client has been taking lovastatin, 40 mg PO daily, for 18 months for type IIb dyslipidemia. At a clinic appointment, she tells the nurse she is 2 months pregnant. The nurse understands that her pregnancy will require:

   a. Supplementation of additional prenatal vitamins
   b. Cessation of the drug immediately
   c. Reduction of dosage to 20 mg PO daily
   d. Increase of the dosage to 40 mg PO twice daily

5. A client on gemfibrozil (Lopid) develops right upper quadrant pain and steatorrhea. The nurse should suspect which of the following disorders?

   a. Peptic ulcer
   b. Stomach cancer
   c. Mononucleosis
   d. Cholelithiasis

## SELECTED REFERENCES

Braun, L. T., & Rosenson, R. S. (2001). Assessing coronary heart disease risk and managing lipids. *Nurse Practitioner, 26*(12), 30–41.

*Drug facts and comparisons.* (Updated monthly). St. Louis: Facts and Comparisons.

Hatcher, T. (2001). The proverbial herb. *American Journal of Nursing, 101*(2), 36–43.

Karch, A. M. (2003). *Lippincott's nursing drug guide.* Philadelphia: Lippincott Williams & Wilkins.

Lacy, C. F., Armstrong, L. L., Goldman, M. P., & Lance, L. L. (2003). *Lexi-Comp's drug information handbook* (11th ed.). Hudson, OH: American Pharmaceutical Association.

McCormick, J. J., & Deeg, M. A. (2000). Pharmacologic treatment of dyslipidemia. *American Journal of Nursing, 100*(2), 55–60.

National Institute of Health Expert Panel (2001). *Third report of the national cholesterol education program (NCEP) expert panel on detection, evaluation, and treatment of high blood cholesterol in adults (Adult Treatment Panel III).* (NIH Publication No. 01-3670). Bethesda, MD: National Institutes of Health.

North American Nursing Diagnosis Association. (2001). *Nursing diagnoses: Definitions and classification, 2001–2002.* Philadelphia: Author.

Pennachio, D. L. (2000). Drug-herb interactions: How vigilant should you be? *Patient Care for the Nurse Practitioner, 3*(10), 17–45.

Porth, C. M., & Hennessy, C. L. (2002). Alterations in cardiac function. In C. M. Porth (Ed.), *Pathophysiology: Concepts of altered health states* (6th ed., pp. 487–530). Philadelphia: Lippincott Williams & Wilkins.

Skidmore-Roth, L. (2001). *Mosby's handbook of herbs and natural supplements.* St. Louis: Mosby.

Talbert, R. L. (2002). Hyperlipidemia. In J. T. DiPiro, R. L. Talbert, G. C. Yee, G. R. Matzke, B. G. Wells, & L. M. Posey (Eds.), *Pharmacotherapy: A pathophysiologic approach* (5th ed., pp. 395–418). New York: McGraw-Hill.

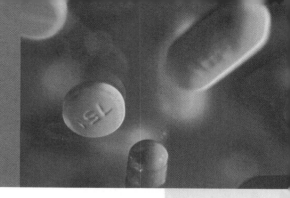

# Section 11
# Drugs Affecting the Digestive System

# 47

# Drugs Used for Peptic Ulcer and Acid Reflux Disorders

## OBJECTIVES

*After studying this chapter, the student will be able to:*

1 Describe the main elements of peptic ulcer disease and gastroesophageal reflux disease.

2 Differentiate the types of drugs used to treat peptic ulcers and acid reflux disorders.

3 Discuss the advantages and disadvantages of proton pump inhibitors.

4 Differentiate between prescription and over-the-counter uses of histamine-2 receptor blocking agents.

5 Discuss significant drug–drug interactions with cimetidine.

6 Describe characteristics, uses, and effects of selected antacids.

7 Discuss the rationale for using combination antacid products.

8 Teach clients nonpharmacologic measures to manage peptic ulcers and gastroesophageal reflux disease.

## CRITICAL THINKING SCENARIO

Annette Greenspan, a 46-year-old homemaker, has rheumatoid arthritis that has been treated with aspirin, nonsteroidal anti-inflammatory drugs (NSAIDs), and prednisone for the last 10 years. During the past week, Mrs. Greenspan has been feeling increasingly weak. She is dizzy when getting up and has had one episode of syncope (fainting). A workup indicates that she has a peptic ulcer. Omeprazole, a proton pump inhibitor, is ordered.

✔ What are Mrs. Greenspan's risk factors that contributed to the development of her ulcer?

✔ Consider how symptoms of weakness, dizziness, and syncope are associated with a peptic ulcer.

✔ How do proton pump inhibitors work to heal ulcers?

✔ What therapies (drugs and nondrugs) can be used to prevent a recurrence of her ulcer?

## PROTOTYPE PROFILES

cimetidine (Tagamet), p. 859

omeprazole (Prilosec), p. 861

# ◻ OVERVIEW

Drugs to prevent or treat peptic ulcer and acid reflux disorders are composed of several groups of drugs, most of which alter gastric acid and its effects on the mucosa of the upper gastrointestinal (UGI) tract. To aid understanding of drug effects, peptic ulcer disease is described in At the Foundation: Peptic Ulcer Disease; related UGI disorders are described in Box 47-1.

# Gastroesophageal Reflux Disease

Gastroesophageal reflux disease (GERD), the most common disorder of the esophagus, is characterized by regurgitation of gastric contents into the esophagus and exposure of esophageal mucosa to gastric acid and pepsin. The same amount of acid-pepsin exposure may lead to different amounts of mucosal damage, possibly related to individual variations in esophageal mucosal resistance.

## AT THE FOUNDATION: *Peptic Ulcer Disease*

Peptic ulcer disease is characterized by ulcer formation in the esophagus, stomach, or duodenum, areas of the GI mucosa that are exposed to gastric acid and pepsin. Gastric and duodenal ulcers are more common than esophageal ulcers.

Peptic ulcers are attributed to an imbalance between cell-destructive and cell-protective effects (ie, increased destructive mechanisms or decreased protective mechanisms). *Cell-destructive effects* include those of gastric acid (hydrochloric acid), pepsin, *Helicobacter pylori* infection, and ingestion of nonsteroidal anti-inflammatory drugs (NSAIDs). Gastric acid, a strong acid that can digest the stomach wall, is secreted by the parietal cells in the mucosa of the stomach antrum, near the pylorus. The parietal cells contain receptors for acetylcholine, gastrin, and histamine, substances that stimulate gastric acid production. Acetylcholine is released by vagus nerve endings in response to stimuli, such as thinking about or ingesting food. Gastrin is a hormone released by cells in the stomach and duodenum in response to food ingestion and stretching of the stomach wall. It is secreted into the bloodstream and eventually circulated to the parietal cells. Histamine is released from cells in the gastric mucosa and diffuses into nearby parietal cells. An enzyme system (H+-K+-ATPase) catalyzes the production of gastric acid and acts as a gastric acid (proton) pump to move gastric acid from parietal cells in the mucosal lining of the stomach into the stomach lumen.

Pepsin is a proteolytic enzyme that helps digest protein foods and also can digest the stomach wall. Pepsin is derived from a precursor called *pepsinogen,* which is secreted by chief cells in the gastric mucosa. Pepsinogen is converted to pepsin only in a highly acidic environment (ie, when the pH of gastric juices is 3 or less).

*H. pylori* is a gram-negative bacterium found in the gastric mucosa of most clients with chronic gastritis, about 75% of clients with gastric ulcers, and more than 90% of clients with duodenal ulcers. It is spread mainly by the fecal-oral route. However, iatrogenic spread by contaminated endoscopes, biopsy forceps, and nasogastric tubes has also occurred. Once in the body, the organism colonizes the mucus-secreting epithelial cells

of the stomach mucosa and is thought to produce gastritis and ulceration by impairing mucosal function. Eradication of the organism accelerates ulcer healing and significantly decreases the rate of ulcer recurrence.

*Cell-protective effects* (eg, secretion of mucus and bicarbonate, dilution of gastric acid by food and secretions, prevention of diffusion of hydrochloric acid from the stomach lumen back into the gastric mucosal lining, the presence of prostaglandin E, alkalinization of gastric secretions by pancreatic juices and bile, and perhaps other mechanisms) normally prevent autodigestion of stomach and duodenal tissues and ulcer formation.

A gastric or duodenal ulcer may penetrate only the mucosal surface, or it may extend into the smooth muscle layers. When superficial lesions heal, no defects remain. When smooth muscle heals, however, scar tissue remains, and the mucosa that regenerates to cover the scarred muscle tissue may be defective. These defects contribute to repeated episodes of ulceration.

Although there is considerable overlap in etiology, clinical manifestations, and treatment of gastric and duodenal ulcers, there are differences as well. **Gastric ulcers** (which may be preceded by less severe mucosal defects such as erosions or gastritis) are often associated with stress (eg, major trauma or severe medical illness), NSAID ingestion, or *H. pylori* infection of the stomach. They are often manifested by painless bleeding and take longer to heal than duodenal ulcers. Gastric ulcers associated with stress may occur in any age group and are usually acute in nature; those associated with *H. pylori* infection or NSAID ingestion are more likely to occur in older adults, especially in the sixth and seventh decades, and to be chronic in nature. **Duodenal ulcers** are strongly associated with *H. pylori* infection and NSAID ingestion, may occur at any age, occur about equally in men and women, are often manifested by abdominal pain, and are usually chronic in nature. They are also associated with cigarette smoking. Compared with nonsmokers, smokers are more likely to develop duodenal ulcers, their ulcers heal more slowly with treatment, and the ulcers recur more rapidly.

BOX
47-1    **Selected Upper Gastrointestinal Disorders**

### Gastritis

Gastritis, a common disorder, is an acute or chronic inflammatory reaction of gastric mucosa. Patients with gastric or duodenal ulcers usually also have gastritis. *Acute gastritis* (also called gastropathy) usually results from irritation of the gastric mucosa by such substances as alcohol, aspirin or other nonsteroidal anti-inflammatory drugs (NSAIDs), and others. *Chronic gastritis* is usually caused by *H. pylori* infection and it persists unless the infection is treated effectively. *H. pylori* organisms may cause gastritis and ulceration by producing enzymes (eg, urease, others) that break down mucosa; they also alter secretion of gastric acid.

### Nonsteroidal Anti-inflammatory Drug Gastropathy

NSAID gastropathy indicates damage to gastroduodenal mucosa by aspirin and other NSAIDs. The damage may range from minor superficial erosions to ulceration and bleeding. NSAID gastropathy is one of the most common causes of gastric ulcers, and it may cause duodenal ulcers as well. Many people take NSAIDs daily for pain, arthritis, and other conditions. Chronic ingestion of NSAIDs causes local irritation of gastroduodenal mucosa, inhibits the synthesis of prostaglandins (which normally protect gastric mucosa by inhibiting acid secretion, stimulating secretion of bicarbonate and mucus, and maintaining mucosal blood flow), and increases the synthesis of leukotrienes and possibly other inflammatory substances that may contribute to mucosal injury.

### Stress Ulcers

Stress ulcers indicate gastric mucosal lesions that develop in patients who are critically ill from trauma, shock, hemorrhage, sepsis, burns, acute respiratory distress syndrome, major surgical procedures, or other severe illnesses. The lesions may be single or multiple ulcers or erosions. Stress ulcers are usually manifested by painless upper gastrointestinal (GI) bleeding. The frequency of occurrence has decreased, possibly because of prophylactic use of antacids and antisecretory drugs and improved management of sepsis, hypovolemia, and other disorders associated with critical illness.

Although the exact mechanisms of stress ulcer formation are unknown, several factors are thought to play a role, including mucosal ischemia, reflux of bile salts into the stomach, reduced GI tract motility, and systemic acidosis. Acidosis increases severity of lesions, and correction of acidosis decreases their formation. In addition, lesions do not form if the pH of gastric fluids is kept about 3.5 or above and lesions apparently form only when mucosal blood flow is diminished.

### Zollinger-Ellison Syndrome

Zollinger-Ellison syndrome is a rare condition characterized by excessive secretion of gastric acid and a high incidence of ulcers. It is caused by gastrin-secreting tumors in the pancreas, stomach, or duodenum. Approximately two thirds of the gastrinomas are malignant. Symptoms are those of peptic ulcer disease, and diagnosis is based on high levels of serum gastrin and gastric acid. Treatment may involve long-term use of a proton pump inhibitor to diminish gastric acid, or surgical excision.

---

Acid reflux often occurs after the evening meal and decreases during sleep. The main symptom is heartburn (pyrosis), which increases with a recumbent position or bending over. Effortless regurgitation of acidic fluid into the mouth, especially after a meal and at night, is often indicative of GERD. Depending on the frequency and extent of acid-pepsin reflux, GERD may result in mild to severe esophagitis or esophageal ulceration. Pain on swallowing usually means erosive or ulcerative esophagitis.

The main cause of GERD is thought to be an incompetent lower esophageal sphincter (LES). Normally, the LES is contracted or closed and prevents the reflux of gastric contents. It opens or relaxes on swallowing, to allow passage of food or fluid, then contracts again. Several circumstances contribute to impaired contraction of the LES and the resulting reflux, including foods (eg, fats, chocolate), fluids (alcohol, caffeinated beverages), medications (eg, beta-adrenergic agents, calcium channel blockers, nitrates), gastric distention, cigarette smoking, and recumbent posture.

GERD occurs in men, women, and children but is especially common during pregnancy and after 40 years of age.

## TYPES OF DRUGS

Drugs used in the treatment of acid-peptic disorders promote healing of lesions and prevent recurrence of lesions by decreasing cell-destructive effects or increasing cell-protective effects. Several types of drugs are used, alone and in various combinations. Antacids neutralize gastric acid and decrease pepsin production; antimicrobials and bismuth can eliminate *Helicobacter pylori* infection; histamine-2 receptor antagonists ($H_2RAs$) and proton pump inhibitors (PPIs) decrease gastric acid secretion; sucralfate provides a barrier between mucosal erosions or ulcers and gastric secretions; and misoprostol restores prostaglandin activity. All of these drugs are commonly taken in the home setting, usually by self-administration. Guidelines for strategies for ongoing evaluation and intervention in the home are addressed in Home Care Considerations. In addition, age-specific considerations are also important in the treatment of these conditions. Discussion of specific management factors in children and older adults is found in Age-related Considerations. Types of

## Home Care Considerations: Use of Drugs for Peptic Ulcer and Acid Reflux Disorders

**ASSESS:** the client and family's knowledge of condition and medication regimen and for compliance with the prescribed regimen. If cimetidine is being taken, assess for potential drug–drug interactions.

**MONITOR:** for compliance with the prescribed regimen, therapeutic and adverse drug effects, especially with changes in drugs or dosages; for excessive or prolonged use of antacids or OTC H₂RAs and refer for evaluation of peptic ulcer disease or GERD and that client is keeping appointments for observation and follow-up care.

**EDUCATE:** on safe use of the drugs, on ways to minimize adverse effects, and on efforts to minimize acid reflux. With OTC H₂RAs, clients should be instructed to avoid daily use of maximum doses for longer than 2 weeks. With misoprostol, report possibility of pregnancy or plans to become pregnant. Women should not take the first dose of misoprostol until the second or third day of their menstrual period (to be sure that they are not pregnant). Reinforce additional teaching points (see Client Teaching Guidelines: Antiulcer and Anti-Heartburn Drugs).

drugs and individual agents are described in the following sections; dosages are listed in Drugs at a Glance 47-1: Representative Antacid Products, and Drugs at a Glance 47-2: Drugs for Acid-Peptic Disorders.

## Antacids

Antacids are alkaline substances that neutralize acids. They react with hydrochloric acid in the stomach to produce neutral, less acidic, or poorly absorbed salts and to raise the pH (alkalinity) of gastric secretions. Raising the pH to approximately 3.5 neutralizes more than 90% of gastric acid and inhibits conversion of pepsinogen to pepsin. Commonly used antacids are aluminum, magnesium, and calcium compounds.

Antacids differ in the amounts needed to neutralize gastric acid (50 to 80 mEq of acid is produced hourly), in onset of action, and in adverse effects. *Aluminum compounds* have a low neutralizing capacity (ie, relatively large doses are required) and a slow onset of action. They can cause constipation. In people who ingest large amounts of aluminum-based antacids over a long period, hypophosphatemia and osteomalacia may develop because aluminum combines with phosphates in the gastrointestinal (GI) tract and prevents phosphate absorption. Aluminum compounds are rarely used alone for acid-peptic disorders. *Magnesium-based antacids* have a high neutralizing capacity and a rapid onset of action. They may cause diarrhea and hypermagnesemia. *Calcium compounds* have a rapid onset of action but may cause hypercalcemia and hypersecretion of gastric acid ("acid rebound"), owing to stimulation of gastrin release, if large doses are used. Consequently, calcium compounds are rarely used in peptic ulcer disease.

Commonly used antacids are mixtures of aluminum hydroxide and magnesium hydroxide (eg, Gelusil, Mylanta,

## Age-related Considerations: Use of Drugs for Peptic Ulcer and Acid Reflux Disorders

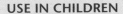

### USE IN CHILDREN

Antacids may be given to ambulatory children in doses of 5 to 15 mL every 3 to 6 hours or after meals and at bedtime, as for adults with acid-peptic disorders. For prevention of GI bleeding in critically ill children, 2 to 5 mL may be given to infants, and 5 to 15 mL to children every 1 to 2 hours. Safety and effectiveness of other antiulcer drugs have not been established for children.

Although PPIs are not approved by the U.S. Food and Drug Administration (FDA) for use in children and are not available in pediatric dosage formulations, they are widely used in the treatment of peptic ulcer and gastroesophageal disease. They are also used to eradicate *H. pylori* organisms. Most published reports involve adult doses for children older than 3 years of age. Some clinicians titrate dosage by a child's weight, such as an initial dose of 0.7 mg/kg/day.

### USE IN OLDER ADULTS

All of the antiulcer, antiheartburn drugs may be used in older adults. With antacids, smaller doses may be effective because older adults usually secrete less gastric acid than younger

adults. Further, with decreased renal function, older adults are more likely to experience adverse effects, such as neuromuscular effects with magnesium-containing antacids. Many health care providers recommend calcium carbonate antacids (eg, Tums) as a calcium supplement to prevent or treat osteoporosis in older women.

With H₂RAs, older adults are more likely to experience adverse effects, especially confusion, agitation, and disorientation with cimetidine. In addition, older adults often have decreased renal function, and doses need to be reduced.

Older adults often take large doses of NSAIDs for arthritis and therefore are at risk for development of acute gastric ulcers and GI bleeding. Thus, they may be candidates for treatment with misoprostol. Dosage of misoprostol may need to be reduced to prevent severe diarrhea and abdominal cramping.

PPIs and sucralfate are well tolerated by older adults. A PPI is probably the drug of choice for treating symptomatic GERD because evidence suggests that clients 60 years of age and older require stronger antisecretory effects than younger adults. No dosage reduction is recommended for older adults.

## Drugs at a Glance

## DRUG TABLE 47-1 Representative Antacid Products

| Trade Name | Magnesium Oxide or Hydroxide | Aluminum Hydroxide | Calcium Carbonate | Other | Route and Dosage Ranges (Adults) | Comments |
|---|---|---|---|---|---|---|
| **Aludrox** Pregnancy Category C | 103 mg/5 mL | 307 mg/5 mL | | | PO, 10 mL q4h, or as needed | Overall indications for use of drug class: temporary relief of symptoms associated with gastric acidity including heartburn, sour stomach, or acid indigestion |
| **Amphojel** Pregnancy Category C | | 300 or 600 mg/tab, 320 mg/5 mL | | | PO, 10 mL or 600 mg 5 or 6 times daily | |
| **Di-Gel** Pregnancy Category C | | 200 mg/5 mL | | Simethicone 20 mg/5 mL | PO, 2 tsp liquid q2h, after meals or between meals, and at bedtime. Maximal dose, 20 tsp/24 h. Do not use maximal dose longer than 2 wk | |
| **Gelusil** Pregnancy Category C | 200 mg/tab | 200 mg/tab | | Simethicone 25 mg/tab | PO, 10 or more mL or 2 or more tablets after meals and at bedtime or as directed by physician to a maximum of 12 tablets or tsp/24 h | |
| **Maalox** suspension Pregnancy Category C | 200 mg/5 mL | 225 mg/5 mL | | | PO, 30 mL 4 times daily, after meals and at bedtime or as directed by physician; maximal dose, 16 tsp/24 h | |
| **Mylanta** Pregnancy Category C | 200 mg/tab, 200 mg/5 mL | 200 mg/tab, 200 mg/5 mL | | Simethicone 25 mg/tab, 20 mg/5 mL | PO, 5–10 mL or 1–2 tablets q2–4h, between meals and at bedtime or as directed by physician | |
| **Mylanta Double-strength** Pregnancy Category C | 400 mg/tab, 400 mg/5 mL | 400 mg/tab, 400 mg/5 mL | | Simethicone 30 mg/tab, 30 mg/5 mL | Same as Mylanta | |
| **Titralac** Pregnancy Category C | | | 420 mg/tab, 1 g/5 mL | Glycine 180 mg/tab, 300 mg/5 mL | PO, 1 tsp or 2 tablets, after meals or as directed by prescriber, to maximal dose of 19 tablets or 8 tsp/24 h | |

**DRUG TABLE 47-2**

*Drugs at a Glance*

## Drugs for Acid-Peptic Disorders

| Generic/Trade Name | Routes and Dosage Ranges | Comments |
|---|---|---|
| *Histamine-2 Receptor Antagonists* | | **Overall indications for use of drug class:** Treatment of peptic ulcers and GERD, to promote healing, then maintenance to prevent recurrence<br>Prevention of stress ulcers, GI bleeding, and aspiration pneumonitis<br>Treatment of Zollinger-Ellison syndrome<br>Treatment of heartburn |
| **Cimetidine** (Tagamet)<br>Pregnancy Category B | See Prototype Profile 47-1: Cimetidine | |
| **Famotidine** (Pepcid)<br>Pregnancy Category B<br>Famotidine 10 mg, calcium carbonate 800 mg, & magnesium hydroxide 165 mg (Pepcid Complete)<br>Pregnancy Category B | Duodenal or gastric ulcer: PO, 40 mg once daily at bedtime or 20 mg twice daily for 4–8 wk; maintenance, PO, 20 mg once daily at bedtime<br>Zollinger-Ellison syndrome: PO, 20 mg q6h, increased if necessary<br>IV injection, 20 mg q12h, diluted to 5 or 10 mL with 5% dextrose or 0.9% sodium chloride<br>IV infusion, 20 mg q12h, diluted with 100 mL of 5% dextrose or 0.9% sodium chloride<br>Impaired renal function (creatinine clearance <50 mL/min): PO, IV 20 mg q24–48h<br>GERD: PO, 20 mg twice daily for 6–12 wk<br>Heartburn (Pepcid Complete): PO, 1–2 tablets, chewed, daily as needed | Administer IV infusion over 15–30 min<br>PO bioavailability may be increased with food |
| **Nizatidine** (Axid)<br>Pregnancy Category B | Duodenal or gastric ulcer: PO, 300 mg once daily at bedtime or 150 mg twice daily; maintenance, PO, 150 mg once daily at bedtime<br>GERD: PO, 150 mg twice daily<br>Heartburn: PO, 75–150 mg twice daily as needed<br>Impaired renal function (creatinine clearance [CrCl] 20–50 mL/min): PO, 150 mg daily; (CrCl <20 mL/min): PO, 150 mg q48h | Giving nocturnal dose at 6 PM rather than at 10 PM; may better suppress nighttime acid secretion<br>May take several days before medication relieves stomach discomfort; if client instructed to also take antacids, wait 30–60 min between medications |
| **Ranitidine** (Zantac)<br>Pregnancy Category B | Duodenal ulcer, PO 300 mg once daily at bedtime or 150 mg twice daily<br>IM, 50 mg q6–8h<br>IV injection, 50 mg diluted in 20 mL of 5% dextrose or 0.9% sodium chloride solution q6–8h<br>IV intermittent infusion, 50 mg diluted in 100 mL of 5% dextrose or 0.9% sodium chloride solution<br>Gastric ulcer or GERD PO 150 mg twice daily<br>Impaired renal function (CrCl <50 mL/min), PO 150 mg q24h; IV, IM 50 mg q18–24h | May take several days before medication relieves stomach discomfort; if client instructed also to take antacids, wait 30–60 min between medications |

*(continued)*

**DRUG TABLE 47-2**

*Drugs at a Glance*

## Drugs for Acid-Peptic Disorders (Continued)

| Generic/Trade Name | Routes and Dosage Ranges | Comments |
|---|---|---|
| **Proton Pump Inhibitors** | | **Overall indications for use of drug class:** Treatment of gastric and duodenal ulcers, for 4–8 wk<br>Treatment of GERD with erosive esophagitis for 4–8 wk to promote healing, then maintenance to prevent recurrence<br>Treatment of Zollinger-Ellison syndrome |
| **Esomeprazole** (Nexium)<br>Pregnancy Category B | GERD with erosive esophagitis: PO, 20–40 mg once daily for 4–8 wk; maintenance, 20 mg once daily | Tablets should be swallowed whole and not chewed or crushed<br>Take at least one hour before meals |
| **Lansoprazole** (Prevacid)<br>Pregnancy Category B | Duodenal ulcer: PO, 15 mg daily for healing and maintenance<br>Gastric ulcer: PO, 30 mg once daily, up to 8 wk<br>Erosive esophagitis: PO, 30 mg daily up to 8 wk; maintenance, 15 mg daily<br>*H. pylori* infection: PO, 30 mg (with amoxicillin and clarithromycin) twice daily for 14 d<br>Hypersecretory conditions: PO, 60–90 mg daily | Tablets should be swallowed whole and not chewed or crushed<br>Take before meals<br>Serum levels may be decreased if taken with food |
| **Omeprazole** (Prilosec)<br>Pregnancy Category C | See Prototype Profile 47-2: Omeprazole | |
| **Pantoprazole** (Protonix, Protonix IV)<br>Pregnancy Category B | GERD with erosive esophagitis: PO, IV, 40 mg once daily<br>Zollinger-Ellison syndrome: PO, IV, 40–80 mg q12h | Tablets should be swallowed whole and not chewed or crushed<br>May be taken with or without food |
| **Rabeprazole** (Aciphex)<br>Pregnancy Category B | Duodenal ulcer: PO, 20 mg once daily up to 4 wk<br>GERD: PO, 20 mg once daily for healing and maintenance<br>Zollinger-Ellison syndrome: PO, 60 mg once or twice daily | May be taken with or without food, but high-fat meals may delay absorption |

Maalox). Some antacid mixtures contain other ingredients, such as simethicone or alginic acid. Simethicone is an antiflatulent drug available alone as Mylicon. When added to antacids, simethicone does not affect gastric acidity. It reportedly decreases gas bubbles, thereby reducing GI distention and abdominal discomfort. Alginic acid (eg, in Gaviscon) produces a foamy, viscous layer on top of gastric acid and thereby decreases backflow of gastric acid onto esophageal mucosa while the person is in an upright position.

Antacids act primarily in the stomach and are used to prevent or treat peptic ulcer disease, GERD, esophagitis, heartburn, gastritis, GI bleeding, and stress ulcers. Aluminum-based antacids also are given to clients with chronic renal failure and hyperphosphatemia to decrease absorption of phosphates in food. Magnesium-based antacids are contraindicated in clients with renal failure.

*Antacids* are often used as needed to relieve heartburn and abdominal discomfort. If used to treat acid-peptic disorders, they are more often used with other agents than alone and require a regular dosing schedule. The choice of antacid should be individualized to find a preparation that is acceptable to the client in terms of taste, dosage, and convenience of administration. Some guidelines include the following:

**1.** Most commonly used antacids combine aluminum hydroxide and magnesium hydroxide. The combination decreases the adverse effects of diarrhea (with magnesium products) and constipation (with aluminum products). Calcium carbonate is effective in relieving heartburn, but it is infrequently used to treat peptic ulcers or GERD.

2. Antacids may be used more often now that low doses (eg, 2 antacid tablets 4 times a day) have been shown to be effective in healing gastric and duodenal ulcers. All of the low-dose regimens contained aluminum, and the aluminum rather than acid neutralization may be the important therapeutic factor. Compared with other drugs for acid-peptic disorders, low-dose antacids are inexpensive and cause few adverse effects. In addition, tablets are as effective as liquids and are usually more convenient to use.

3. Antacids with magnesium are contraindicated in renal disease because hypermagnesemia may result; those with high sugar content are contraindicated in diabetes mellitus.

4. Additional ingredients may be helpful to some clients. Simethicone has no effect on intragastric pH but may be useful in relieving flatulence or gastroesophageal reflux. Alginic acid may be useful in clients with daytime acid reflux and heartburn. *Sucralfate* must be taken before meals, and this is inconvenient for some clients.

## Guidelines for Therapy With Antacids

1. To prevent stress ulcers in critically ill clients and to treat acute GI bleeding, nearly continuous neutralization of gastric acid is desirable. Dose and frequency of administration must be sufficient to neutralize approximately 50 to 80 mEq of gastric acid each hour. This can be accomplished by a continuous intragastric drip through a nasogastric tube or by hourly administration.

2. When a client has a nasogastric tube in place, antacid dosage may be titrated by aspirating stomach contents, determining pH, and then basing the dose on the pH. (Most gastric acid is neutralized and most pepsin activity is eliminated at a pH above 3.5.)

3. When prescribing antacids to treat active ulcers, it has long been recommended to take them 1 hour and 3 hours after meals and at bedtime for greater acid neutralization. This schedule is effective but inconvenient for many clients. More recently, lower doses taken less often have been found effective in healing duodenal or gastric ulcers even though less acid neutralization occurs.

4. It was formerly thought that liquid antacid preparations were more effective. Now, tablets are considered as effective as liquids.

5. When antacids are used to relieve pain, they usually may be taken as needed. However, they should not be taken in high doses or for prolonged periods because of potential adverse effects.

## *Helicobacter pylori* Agents

Multiple drugs are required to eradicate *H. pylori* organisms and heal related ulcers. Effective combinations include two antimicrobials and a PPI or an H$_2$RA. For the antimicrobial component, two of the following drugs—**amoxicillin, clarithromycin, metronidazole,** or **tetracycline**—are used. A single antimicrobial agent is not used because of concern about emergence of drug-resistant *H. pylori* organisms. For clients with an active ulcer, adding an antisecretory drug (ie, H$_2$RA or PPI) to an antimicrobial regimen accelerates symptom relief and ulcer healing. In addition, antimicrobial-antisecretory combinations are associated with low ulcer recurrence rates.

A bismuth preparation is added to some regimens. Bismuth exerts antibacterial effects against *H. pylori* by disrupting bacterial cell walls, preventing the organism from adhering to gastric epithelium, and inhibiting bacterial enzymatic and proteolytic activity. It also increases secretion of mucus and bicarbonate, inhibits pepsin activity, and accumulates in ulcer craters.

Although several regimens are effective in *H. pylori* infection, three-drug regimens with a PPI and two antibacterial drugs may be preferred. The regimen using metronidazole, a bismuth compound, tetracycline, and an antisecretory drug is very effective in healing ulcers. However, this regimen is not well tolerated, partly because of the multiple daily doses required. In addition, metronidazole inhibits alcohol's typical metabolism and may precipitate a disulfiram-like reaction (flushing, tachycardia, diaphoresis, nausea, vomiting, or headache) if alcohol ingestion occurs with use.

Because client compliance is a difficulty with all the *H. pylori* eradication regimens, some drug combinations are packaged as individual doses to increase convenience. For example, Helidac contains bismuth, metronidazole, and tetracycline (taken with an H$_2$RA); Prevpac contains amoxicillin, clarithromycin, and lansoprazole.

## Histamine–2 Receptor Antagonists

Histamine is a substance found in almost every body tissue and released in response to certain stimuli (eg, allergic reactions, tissue injury). Once released, histamine causes contraction of smooth muscle in the bronchi, GI tract, and uterus; dilation and increased permeability of capillaries; dilation of cerebral blood vessels; and stimulation of sensory nerve endings to produce pain and itching.

Histamine also causes strong stimulation of gastric acid secretion. Vagal stimulation causes release of histamine from cells in the gastric mucosa. The histamine then acts on receptors located on the parietal cells to increase production of hydrochloric acid. These receptors are called the H$_2$ receptors.

Traditional antihistamines, or H$_1$-receptor antagonists, prevent or reduce other effects of histamine but do not block histamine effects on gastric acid production. The H$_2$RAs inhibit both basal secretion of gastric acid and the secretion stimulated by histamine, acetylcholine, and gastrin. They decrease the amount, acidity, and pepsin content of gastric juices. A single dose of an H$_2$RA can inhibit acid secretion for 6 to 12 hours, and a continuous intravenous (IV) infusion can inhibit secretion for prolonged periods.

$H_2RAs$ have been replaced as first-choice drugs by the PPIs for most indications, but are still widely used. Clinical indications for use include prevention and treatment of peptic ulcer disease, GERD, esophagitis, GI bleeding due to acute stress ulcers, and Zollinger-Ellison syndrome. With gastric or duodenal ulcers, healing occurs within 6 to 8 weeks; with esophagitis, healing occurs in about 12 weeks. Over-the-counter oral preparations, at lower dosage strengths, are approved for the treatment of heartburn.

There are no known contraindications, but the drugs should be used with caution in children, pregnant women, older adults, and clients with impaired renal or hepatic function. Dosage should be reduced in the presence of impaired renal function.

Adverse effects occur infrequently with usual doses and duration of treatment. They are more likely to occur with prolonged use of high doses and in older adults or those with impaired renal or hepatic function.

**Cimetidine, ranitidine, famotidine,** and **nizatidine** are the four available $H_2RAs$. *P* **Cimetidine** serves as the prototype, and it is still widely used (see Prototype Profile 47-1: Cimetidine). It is well absorbed after oral administration. For acutely ill clients, cimetidine is given intravenously. A major disadvantage of cimetidine is that it affects the cytochrome P450 drug-metabolizing system in the liver, inhibiting hepatic metabolism of numerous

---

## PROTOTYPE PROFILE 47-1

### *P* Cimetidine (sye MET I deen)

**Drug Class**
*Chemical:* Histamine-2 ($H_2$) antagonist
*Functional:* Antihistamine; $H_2$ blocker

**Trade Name**
Tagamet

**Therapeutic Indications**
Treatment of duodenal or gastric ulcers; GERD; prevention of UGI bleeding; heartburn

**Pharmacokinetics**
*Absorption*
Immediate

*Distribution*
Plasma protein binding: 20%–40%

*Metabolism*
Partially hepatic

*Excretion*
Predominately urine; some excretion in bile and eliminated in feces

**Pharmacodynamics**
*Onset of Action*
1 h

*Duration*
72 h

**Contraindications/Precautions**
Hypersensitivity; with caution with renal or hepatic impairment or with drugs metabolized through the cytochrome P450 system

**Pregnancy Considerations**
Category B
Crosses the placenta
Excreted in breast milk, compatible

**Dosage**
Duodenal or gastric ulcer: PO, 800 mg once daily at bedtime or 300 mg four times daily or 400 mg twice daily

Maintenance: PO, 400 mg at bedtime
IV injection, 300 mg, diluted in 20 mL of 0.9% NaCl solution q6–8h
IV intermittent infusion, 300 mg diluted in 50 mL of dextrose or saline solution q6h
IM, 300 mg q6–8h
GERD: PO, 800 mg twice daily or 400 mg four times daily
Prevention of UGI bleeding: IV continuous infusion, 50 mg/h
Heartburn: PO, 200 mg once or twice daily as needed
Impaired renal function: PO, IV, 300 mg q8–12h

**Adverse Effects**
Headache, agitation, dizziness, diarrhea, nausea, vomiting, agranulocytosis, thrombocytopenia

**Drug Interactions**
*Increased Effects*
Increased warfarin effect
Serum concentration of multiple drugs metabolized through the cytochrome P450 system, including calcium channel blockers, phenytoin, quinidine, carbamazepine, procainamide, triamterene, quinolone antibiotics, theophylline, citalopram, flecainide, amiodarone, tacrine, tricyclic antidepressants (TCAs), and some benzodiazepines, and beta blockers.

*Decreased Effects*
Decreased serum concentration with ketoconazole, itraconazole, fluconazole
Decreased delavirdine absorption with concurrent use
Avoid concurrent use with other $H_2$ antagonists

**Herbal Supplements and Dietary Considerations**
St. John's wort decreases cimetidine levels

other drugs, thereby increasing blood levels and risk for toxicity with the inhibited drug.

Ranitidine is more potent than cimetidine on a weight basis, and smaller doses can be given less frequently. In addition, ranitidine causes fewer drug interactions than cimetidine. Oral ranitidine reaches peak blood levels 1 to 3 hours after administration and is metabolized in the liver; approximately 30% is excreted unchanged in the urine. Parenteral ranitidine reaches peak blood levels in about 15 minutes; 65% to 80% is excreted unchanged in the urine. Famotidine and nizatidine are similar to cimetidine and ranitidine.

Compared with cimetidine, the other drugs cause similar effects, except they are less likely to cause mental confusion and gynecomastia (antiandrogenic effects). In addition, they do not interfere with the metabolism of other drugs.

Cimetidine may be less expensive, but it may cause confusion and antiandrogenic effects. It also increases the risk for toxicity with several commonly used drugs. Compared with cimetidine, other $H_2$RAs are more potent on a weight basis and have a longer duration of action, so they can be given in smaller, less frequent doses. In addition, they do not alter the hepatic metabolism of other drugs.

Over-the-counter $H_2$RAs are indicated for the treatment of heartburn. In some cases, clients may depend on self-medication with over-the-counter (OTC) drugs and delay seeking treatment for peptic ulcer disease or GERD. For prescription or nonprescription uses, cimetidine is preferably taken by clients who are taking no other medications.

### Guidelines for Therapy With Histamine-2 Receptor Antagonists

1. For an acute ulcer, full dosage may be given for up to 8 weeks. When the ulcer heals, dosage may be reduced by 50% for maintenance therapy to prevent recurrence.

2. For duodenal ulcers, a single evening or bedtime dose produces the same healing effects as multiple doses. Commonly used nocturnal doses are cimetidine, 800 mg; ranitidine, 300 mg; nizatidine, 300 mg; or famotidine, 40 mg.

3. For gastric ulcers, the optimal $H_2$RA dosage schedule has not been established. Gastric ulcers heal more slowly than duodenal ulcers, and most authorities prescribe 6 to 8 weeks of drug therapy.

4. To maintain ulcer healing and prevent recurrence, long-term $H_2$RA therapy is often used. The drug is usually given as a single bedtime dose, but the amount is reduced by 50% (ie, cimetidine, 400 mg; ranitidine, 150 mg; nizatidine, 150 mg; or famotidine, 20 mg).

5. For Zollinger-Ellison syndrome, high doses given as often as every 4 hours may be required.

6. For severe reflux esophagitis, multiple daily doses may be required for adequate symptom control.

7. Dosage of all these drugs should be reduced in the presence of impaired renal function.

8. Antacids are often given concurrently with $H_2$RAs to relieve pain. They should not be given at the same time (except for Pepcid Complete) because the antacid reduces absorption of the other drug. $H_2$RAs usually relieve pain after 1 week of administration.

9. These drugs are available in a wide array of products, and precautions must be taken to ensure the correct formulation, dosage strength, and method of administration for the intended use. For example, cimetidine is available in tablets of 100, 200, 300, 400, and 800 mg, an oral liquid with 300 mg/5 mL, and injectable solutions. Ranitidine is available in tablets of 75, 150, and 300 mg, effervescent tablets of 150 mg, capsules (Zantac GELdose) of 150 and 300 mg, a liquid syrup with 15 mg/mL, effervescent granules of 150 mg, and injectable solutions of 1 mg/mL and 25 mg/mL. Nizatidine is available in tablets of 75 mg and capsules of 150 and 300 mg, and famotidine in tablets of 10, 20, and 40 mg, chewable tablets of 10 mg, orally disintegrating tablets (Pepcid RPD) of 20 and 40 mg, a powder for oral suspension that contains 40 mg/5mL when reconstituted, and injection solutions of 10 mg/mL and 20 mg/50 mL.

10. All of the drugs are available by prescription and OTC. When prescriptions are given, clients should be advised to avoid concomitant use of OTC versions of the same or similar drugs.

## Proton Pump Inhibitors

Proton pump inhibitors are strong inhibitors of gastric acid secretion. These drugs bind irreversibly to the gastric proton pump (ie, the enzyme $H^+$-$K^+$-ATPase) to prevent the "pumping" or release of gastric acid from parietal cells into the stomach lumen, therefore blocking the final step of acid production. Inhibition of the proton pump suppresses gastric acid secretion in response to all primary stimuli, histamine, gastrin, and acetylcholine. Thus, the drugs inhibit both daytime (including meal-stimulated) and nocturnal (unstimulated) acid secretion.

PPIs are the drugs of first choice in most situations. They heal gastric and duodenal ulcers more rapidly and may be more effective in erosive esophagitis, erosive gastritis, and Zollinger-Ellison syndrome than $H_2$RAs. They are also effective in eradicating *H. pylori* infection when combined with two antibacterial drugs. Most PPIs are given orally only; pantoprazole (Protonix IV) is a parenteral formulation. PPIs are more expensive than $H_2$RAs. Compared with $H_2$RAs, PPIs suppress gastric acid more strongly and for a longer time. This effect provides faster symptom relief and faster healing in acid-related diseases. The drugs are also effective in maintenance therapy to prevent recurrence of esophagitis. In clients with *H. pylori*–associated ulcers, eradication of the organism with antimicrobial drugs is preferable to long-term maintenance therapy with antisecretory drugs.

The drugs usually are well tolerated; adverse effects are minimal with both short- and long-term use. Nausea, diarrhea, and headache are the most frequently reported adverse effects. However, long-term consequences of profound gastric acid suppression are unknown.

**Omeprazole, esomeprazole, lansoprazole, pantoprazole,** and **rabeprazole** are available PPIs. *P* **Omeprazole** was the first, is still widely used, and serves as the prototype (see Prototype Profile 47-2: Omeprazole).

It is well absorbed after oral administration, highly bound to plasma proteins (about 95%), metabolized in the liver, and excreted in the urine (about 75%) and bile or feces. Acid-inhibiting effects occur within 2 hours and last 72 hours or longer. When the drug is discontinued, effects persist for 48 to 72 hours or longer, until the gastric parietal cells can synthesize additional $H^+$-$K^+$-ATPase. The other drugs are very similar to omeprazole. Omepra-

zole (Prilosec) has been approved for OTC sales for treating heartburn. If heartburn is not improved within 14 days of treatment, clients should be evaluated by their health care provider. Prescription omeprazole has been very expensive; with nonprescription use, the cost should be much less.

## Guidelines for Therapy With Proton Pump Inhibitors

1. Recommended doses of PPIs heal most gastric and duodenal ulcers in about 4 weeks. Large gastric ulcers may require 8 weeks.
2. The drugs may be used to maintain healing of gastric and duodenal ulcers and decrease the risk for ulcer recurrence.
3. A PPI and two antimicrobial drugs are the most effective regimens for eradication of *H. pylori* organisms.
4. With GERD, higher doses or longer therapy may be needed for severe disease and esophagitis. Lower doses can maintain symptom relief and esophageal healing.

---

## PROTOTYPE PROFILE 47-2
### *P* Omeprazole (oh ME pray zol)

**Drug Class**
*Chemical:* Proton pump inhibitor
*Functional:* Gastric acid secretion inhibitor

**Trade Name**
Prilosec

**Therapeutic Indications**
Short-term treatment of duodenal or gastric ulcer disease; GERD; Zollinger-Ellison syndrome; and part of drug regimen for *H. pylori* eradication

**Pharmacokinetics**
*Absorption*
Well absorbed

*Distribution*
Plasma protein binding: 95%

*Metabolism*
Hepatic

*Excretion*
Urine

**Pharmacodynamics**
*Onset of Action*
Antisecretory: approximately 1 h; peak effect 2 h

*Duration*
72 h

**Contraindications/Precautions**
Hypersensitivity; use with caution in elderly

**Pregnancy Considerations**
Category C
Crosses the placenta
Excreted in breast milk; use with caution

**Dosage**
*Adults:* gastric ulcer: PO, 40 mg once daily for 4–8 wk
Duodenal ulcer: PO, 20 mg once daily for 4–8 wk
GERD: PO, 20 mg once daily
Zollinger-Ellison syndrome: PO, 60 mg once daily
*H. pylori* eradication: dose varies with regimen; 20 mg once daily or 40 mg as single dose or in two divided doses in conjunction with antibiotic
*Children:* Safety and efficacy in children <2 y have not been established

**Adverse Effects**
Headache, dizziness, GI distress, cough, back pain, diarrhea

**Drug Interactions**
*Increased Effects*
Increased half-life of digoxin, phenytoin, diazepam, warfarin, and other drugs metabolized in the liver
Increased serum levels of omeprazole with voriconazole

*Decreased Effects*
Decreased clinical effects of itraconazole, ketoconazole, and drugs dependent on acid for absorption
Theophylline clearance increased slightly

**Herbal Supplements and Dietary Considerations**
St. John's wort may decrease omeprazole levels
Should be taken on an empty stomach

## Prostaglandin

Naturally occurring prostaglandin E, which is produced in mucosal cells of the stomach and duodenum, inhibits gastric acid secretion and increases mucus and bicarbonate secretion, mucosal blood flow, and perhaps mucosal repair. It also inhibits the mucosal damage produced by gastric acid, aspirin, and NSAIDs. When synthesis of prostaglandin E is inhibited, erosion and ulceration of gastric mucosa may occur. This is the mechanism by which aspirin and other NSAIDs are thought to cause gastric and duodenal ulcers (see Chap. 7).

**Misoprostol** is a synthetic form of prostaglandin E approved for concurrent use with NSAIDs to protect gastric mucosa from NSAID-induced erosion and ulceration. It is indicated for clients at high risk for GI ulceration and bleeding, such as those taking high doses of NSAIDs for arthritis and older adults. It is contraindicated in women of childbearing potential, unless effective contraceptive methods are being used, and during pregnancy, because it may induce abortion. The most common adverse effects are diarrhea (occurs in 10% to 40% of recipients) and abdominal cramping. Older adults may be unable to tolerate misoprostol-induced diarrhea and abdominal discomfort.

## Sucralfate

**Sucralfate** is a preparation of sulfated sucrose and aluminum hydroxide that binds to normal and ulcerated mucosa. It is used to prevent and treat peptic ulcer disease. It is effective even though it does not inhibit secretion of gastric acid or pepsin, and it has little neutralizing effect on gastric acid. Its mechanism of action is unclear, but it is thought to act locally on the gastric and duodenal mucosa. Possible mechanisms include binding to the ulcer and forming a protective barrier between the mucosa and gastric acid, pepsin, and bile salts; neutralizing pepsin; stimulating prostaglandin synthesis in the mucosa; and exerting healing effects through the aluminum component. Sucralfate is effective in healing duodenal ulcers and in maintenance therapy to prevent ulcer recurrence. In general, the rates of ulcer healing with sucralfate are similar to the rates with H₂RAs.

Adverse effects are low in incidence and severity because sucralfate is not absorbed systemically. Constipation and dry mouth are most often reported. The main disadvantages of using sucralfate are that the tablet is large; it must be given at least twice daily; it requires an acid pH for activation and should not be given with an antacid, H₂RA, or PPI; and it may bind other drugs and prevent their absorption. In general, sucralfate should be given 2 hours before or after other drugs.

### Guidelines for Therapy With Sucralfate

**1.** When sucralfate is used to treat an ulcer, it should be administered for 4 to 8 weeks unless healing is confirmed by radiologic or endoscopic examination.

**2.** When used long term to prevent ulcer recurrence, dosage should be reduced.

## Dietary and Herbal Supplements

Several herbal supplements are promoted as aiding heartburn, gastritis, and peptic ulcer disease. Most have not been studied in humans, and there is little, if any, evidence that they are either safe or effective for the proposed uses. Given the known safety and effectiveness of available drugs and the possible consequences of delaying effective treatment, the use of herbal supplements for any acid-peptic disorder should be discouraged.

## ■ DRUG USE IN SPECIFIC SITUATIONS

## Effects of Acid–Suppressant Drugs on Other Drugs

**Antacids** may prevent absorption of most drugs taken at the same time, including benzodiazepine antianxiety drugs, corticosteroids, digoxin, H₂RAs (eg, cimetidine), iron supplements, phenothiazine antipsychotic drugs, phenytoin, fluoroquinolone antibacterials, and tetracyclines. Antacids increase absorption of a few drugs, including levodopa, quinidine, and valproic acid. These interactions can be avoided or minimized by separating administration times by 1 to 2 hours.

**H₂RAs** may alter the effects of several drugs. Most significant effects occur with cimetidine, which interferes with the metabolism of many commonly used drugs. Consequently, the affected drugs are eliminated more slowly, their serum levels are increased, and they are more likely to cause adverse effects and toxicity unless dosage is reduced.

Interacting drugs include antidysrhythmics (lidocaine, propafenone, quinidine), the anticoagulant warfarin, anticonvulsants (carbamazepine, phenytoin), benzodiazepine antianxiety or hypnotic agents (alprazolam, diazepam, flurazepam, triazolam), beta-adrenergic blocking agents (labetalol, metoprolol, propranolol), the bronchodilator theophylline, calcium channel blocking agents (eg, verap-

> **? How Can You Avoid This Medication Error?**
>
> You are passing medications in a skilled nursing facility. Mrs. Fallot has difficulty swallowing. She has lansoprazole (Prevacid) ordered for gastroesophageal reflux disease (GERD). You are planning to open the capsule and mix it with applesauce and her blenderized meal. Another nurse approaches you stating that you should never open capsules because they are time-released and this will impact the onset and duration of the drug. She suggests you see if she can take the capsule with water. How can this drug be safely given to Mrs. Fallot?

# NURSING PROCESS

## Assessment

Assess the client's status in relation to peptic ulcer disease, GERD, and other conditions in which antiulcer drugs are used.

- Identify risk factors for peptic ulcer disease:
  - Cigarette smoking. Effects are thought to include stimulation of gastric acid secretion and decreased blood supply to gastric mucosa. (Nicotine constricts blood vessels.) Moreover, clients with peptic ulcers who continue to smoke heal more slowly and have more recurrent ulcers, despite usually adequate treatment, than those who stop smoking.
  - Stress, including physiologic stress (eg, shock, sepsis, burns, surgery, head injury, severe trauma, or medical illness) and psychological stress. One mechanism may be that stress activates the sympathetic nervous system, which then causes vasoconstriction in organs not needed for "fight or flight." Thus, stress may lead to ischemia in gastric mucosa, with ulceration if ischemia is severe or prolonged.
  - Drug therapy with aspirin and other NSAIDs, corticosteroids, and antineoplastics.
- Signs and symptoms depend on the type and location of the ulcer:
  - Periodic epigastric pain, which occurs 1 to 4 hours after eating or during the night and is often described as burning or gnawing, is a symptom of chronic duodenal ulcer.
  - Gastrointestinal (GI) bleeding occurs with acute or chronic ulcers when the ulcer erodes into a blood vessel. Clinical manifestations may range from mild (eg, occult blood in feces and eventual anemia) to severe (eg, hematemesis, melena, hypotension, and shock).
- GERD produces heartburn (a substernal burning sensation).

## Nursing Diagnoses

- Pain related to effects of gastric acid on peptic ulcers or inflamed esophageal tissues
- Imbalanced Nutrition: Less Than Body Requirements related to anorexia and abdominal discomfort
- Constipation related to aluminum- or calcium-containing antacids and sucralfate
- Diarrhea related to magnesium-containing antacids and misoprostol
- Deficient Knowledge related to drug therapy and non-pharmacologic management of GERD and peptic ulcer disease

## Planning/Goals

**The client will:**

- Take or receive antiulcer, anti-heartburn drugs accurately
- Experience relief of symptoms
- Avoid situations that cause or exacerbate symptoms, when possible
- Be observed for GI bleeding and other complications of peptic ulcer disease and GERD
- Maintain normal patterns of bowel function
- Avoid preventable adverse effects of drug therapy

## Interventions

Use measures to prevent or minimize peptic ulcer disease and gastric acid–induced esophageal disorders.

- With peptic ulcer disease, helpful interventions may include the following:
  - General health measures such as a well-balanced diet, adequate rest, and regular exercise
  - Avoiding cigarette smoking and gastric irritants (eg, alcohol, aspirin and NSAIDs, caffeine)
  - Reducing psychological stress (eg, by changing environments) or learning healthful strategies of stress management (eg, relaxation techniques, physical exercise). There is no practical way to avoid psychological stress because it is part of everyday life.
  - Long-term drug therapy with small doses of $H_2RAs$, antacids, or sucralfate. With "active" peptic ulcer disease, helping the client follow the prescribed therapeutic regimen helps to promote healing and prevent complications.
  - Diet therapy is of minor importance in prevention or treatment of peptic ulcer disease. Some physicians prescribe no dietary restrictions, whereas others suggest avoiding or minimizing highly spiced foods, gas-forming foods, and caffeine-containing beverages.
- With heartburn and esophagitis, helpful measures are those that prevent or decrease gastroesophageal reflux of gastric contents (eg, avoiding irritant, highly spiced, or fatty foods; eating small meals; not lying down for 1 to 2 hours after eating; elevating the head of the bed; and avoiding obesity, constipation, or other conditions that increase intra-abdominal pressure).

## Evaluation

- Observe and interview regarding drug use.
- Observe and interview regarding relief of symptoms.
- Observe for signs and symptoms of complications.
- Observe and interview regarding adverse drug effects.

---

amil), tricyclic antidepressants (eg, amitriptyline), and sulfonylurea antidiabetic drugs. In addition, cimetidine may increase serum levels (eg, fluorouracil, procainamide, and its active metabolite) and pharmacologic effects of other drugs (eg, respiratory depression with opioid analgesics) by unidentified mechanisms. Cimetidine also may decrease effects of several drugs, including drugs that require an acidic environment for absorption (eg, iron salts, indomethacin, fluconazole, tetracyclines) and miscellaneous drugs (eg, digoxin, tocainide) by unknown mechanisms.

Ranitidine, famotidine, and nizatidine do not inhibit the cytochrome P450–metabolizing enzymes. Ranitidine decreases absorption of diazepam if given at the

## CLIENT TEACHING GUIDELINES
## Antiulcer and Anti-Heartburn Drugs

### General Considerations

✔ These drugs are commonly used to prevent and treat peptic ulcers and heartburn. Peptic ulcers usually form in the stomach or first part of the small bowel (duodenum), where tissues are exposed to stomach acid. Two common causes of peptic ulcer disease are stomach infection with a bacterium called *Helicobacter pylori* and taking non-steroidal anti-inflammatory drugs (NSAIDs) such as ibuprofen and many others. Heartburn (also called gastroesophageal reflux disease) is caused by stomach acid splashing back onto the esophagus.

Peptic ulcer disease and heartburn are chronic conditions that are usually managed on an outpatient basis. Complications such as bleeding require hospitalization. Overall, these conditions can range from mild to serious, and it is important to seek information about the disease process, ways to prevent or minimize symptoms, and drug therapy.

✔ With heartburn, try to minimize acid reflux by elevating the head of the bed; avoiding stomach distention by eating small meals; not lying down for 1 to 2 hours after eating; minimizing intake of fats, chocolate, citric juices, coffee, and alcohol; avoiding smoking (stimulates gastric acid production); and avoiding obesity, constipation, or other conditions that increase intra-abdominal pressure. In addition, take tablets and capsules with 8 oz of water and do not take medications at bedtime unless instructed to do so. Some medications (eg, tetracycline, potassium chloride tablets, iron supplements, nonsteroidal anti-inflammatory drugs [NSAIDs]) may cause "pill-induced" irritation of the esophagus (esophagitis) if not taken with enough liquid.

✔ Most medications for peptic ulcer disease and heartburn decrease stomach acid. An exception is the antibiotics used to treat ulcers caused by *H. pylori* infection. The strongest acid reducers are omeprazole (Prilosec), esomeprazole (Nexium), lansoprazole (Prevacid), pantoprazole (Protonix), and rabeprazole (Aciphex). These are prescription drugs. (Omeprazole is approved for nonprescription use.) Histamine-blocking drugs such as cimetidine (Tagamet), famotidine (Pepcid), and others are available as both prescription and over-the-counter (OTC) preparations. OTC products are indicated for heartburn, and smaller doses are taken than for peptic ulcer disease. These drugs usually should not be taken longer than 2 weeks without the advice of a health care provider. The concern is that OTC drugs may delay diagnosis and treatment of potentially serious illness. In addition, cimetidine can increase toxic effects of numerous drugs and should be avoided if you are taking other medications.

Misoprostol (Cytotec) is given to prevent ulcers from NSAIDs, which are commonly used to relieve pain and inflammation with arthritis and other conditions. This drug should be taken only while taking a traditional NSAID such as ibuprofen. Related drugs such as celecoxib (Celebrex), rofecoxib (Vioxx), and valdecoxib (Bextra) are less likely to cause peptic ulcer disease. Do not take misoprostol if pregnant and do not become pregnant while taking the drug. If pregnancy occurs during misoprostol therapy, stop the drug and notify your health care provider immediately. Misoprostol can cause abdominal cramps and miscarriage.

Numerous antacid preparations are available, but they are not equally safe in all people and should be selected carefully. For example, products that contain magnesium have a laxative effect and may cause diarrhea; those that contain aluminum or calcium may cause constipation. Some commonly used antacids (eg, Maalox, Mylanta) are a mixture of magnesium and aluminum preparations, an attempt to avoid both constipation and diarrhea. People with kidney disease should not take products that contain magnesium because magnesium can accumulate in the body and cause serious adverse effects. Thus, it is important to read product labels and, if you have a chronic illness or take other medications, ask your physician or pharmacist to help you select an antacid and an appropriate dose.

### Self-administration or Caregiver Administration

✔ Take antiulcer drugs as directed. Underuse decreases therapeutic effectiveness; overuse increases adverse effects. For acute peptic ulcer disease or esophagitis, drugs are given in relatively high doses for 4 to 8 weeks to promote healing. For long-term maintenance therapy, dosage is reduced.

✔ With Prilosec, Aciphex, Nexium, and Protonix, swallow the capsule whole; do not open, chew, or crush. With Prevacid, the capsule can be opened and the granules sprinkled on applesauce for patients who are unable to swallow capsules. Also, the granules are available in a packet for preparing a liquid suspension. Follow instructions for mixing the granules exactly. The granules should not be crushed or chewed.

✔ Take cimetidine with meals or at bedtime. Take famotidine, nizatidine, and ranitidine with or without food. Do not take an antacid for 1 hour before or after taking one of these drugs.

✔ Take sucralfate on an empty stomach at least 1 hour before meals and at bedtime. Also, do not take an antacid for 1 hour before or after taking sucralfate.

✔ Take misoprostol with food.

✔ For treatment of peptic ulcer disease, take antacids 1 and 3 hours after meals and at bedtime (4 to 7 doses daily), 1 to 2 hours before or after other medications. Antacids decrease absorption of many medications if taken at the same time. Also, chew chewable tablets thoroughly before swallowing, then drink a glass of water; allow effervescent tablets to dissolve completely and almost stop bubbling before drinking; and shake liquids well before measuring the dose.

same time and increases hypoglycemic effects of glipizide. Nizatidine increases serum salicylate levels in people taking high doses of aspirin.

**PPIs** have relatively few effects on other drugs. Omeprazole increases blood levels of some benzodiazepines (diazepam, flurazepam, triazolam), phenytoin, and warfarin, probably by inhibiting hepatic metabolism. These interactions have not been reported with the other PPIs.

**Sucralfate** decreases absorption of ciprofloxacin and other fluoroquinolones, digoxin, phenytoin, and warfarin. Sucralfate binds to these drugs when both are present in the GI tract. This interaction can be avoided or minimized by giving the interacting drug 2 hours before giving sucralfate.

## Effects of Acid Suppressant Drugs on Nutrients

Dietary folate, iron, and vitamin $B_{12}$ are better absorbed from an acidic environment. When gastric fluids are made less acidic by antacids, $H_2$RAs, or PPIs, deficiencies of these nutrients may occur. In addition, sucralfate interferes with absorption of fat-soluble vitamins, and magnesium-containing antacids interfere with absorption of vitamin A.

## *Nursing Actions*
## Antiulcer Drugs

| *Nursing Actions* | *Rationale/Explanation* |
|---|---|
| 1. Administer accurately. | |
|   a. With proton pump inhibitors: | |
|     (1) Give most of the drugs before food intake; give oral pantoprazole with or without food. | Manufacturer's recommendations |
|     (2) Ask clients to swallow the tablets or capsules whole, without crushing or chewing. | Drug formulations are delayed-release and long-acting. Opening, crushing or chewing destroys these effects. |
|     (3) For clients who are unable to swallow capsules, the lansoprazole capsule can be opened and the granules mixed with 60 mL of orange or tomato juice or sprinkled on 1 tablespoon of applesauce, Ensure pudding, cottage cheese, or yogurt, and swallowed immediately, without chewing. | Manufacturer's recommendations. Enteric-coated, delayed-release granules are in oral capsules or separate packets. Chewing or crushing destroys the coating; mixing the granules with applesauce or other acidic substances preserves the coating of the granules, allowing them to remain intact until they reach the small intestine. |
|     (4) To give lansoprazole granules as a liquid suspension, mix 1 packet with 30 mL of water (use no other liquids), stir well, and ask the client to swallow immediately, without chewing the granules. | |
|     (5) Give IV pantoprazole over 15 min, injected into a dedicated line or the Y-site of an IV infusion. Use the in-line filter provided; if injecting in a Y-site, the filter should be placed below the Y-site closest to the patient. Flush the IV line with 5% dextrose, 0.9% NaCl, or lactated Ringer's before and after pantoprazole administration. | |
|   b. With histamine ($H_2$) blockers: | |
|     (1) Give single oral doses at bedtime; give multiple oral doses of cimetidine with meals and at bedtime and other drugs without regard to food intake. | The drugs are effective and convenient in a single oral dose at bedtime. |
|     (2) To give cimetidine or ranitidine IV, dilute in 20 mL of 5% dextrose or normal saline solution, and inject over at least 2 min. For intermittent infusion, dilute in at least 50 mL of 5% dextrose or 0.9% sodium chloride solution, and infuse over 15–20 min. | |
|     (3) To give famotidine IV, dilute with 5–10 mL of 0.9% sodium chloride injection, and inject over at least 2 min. For intermittent infusion, dilute in 100 mL of 5% dextrose or 0.9% sodium chloride, and infuse over 15–30 min. | |

*(continued)*

## Nursing Actions

### Antiulcer Drugs (Continued)

| Nursing Actions | Rationale/Explanation |
|---|---|
| c. With antacids:<br>  (1) Do not give doses within approximately 1 h of oral H$_2$ antagonists or sucralfate.<br>  (2) Shake liquids well before measuring the dose.<br><br>  (3) Instruct clients to chew antacid tablets thoroughly and follow with a glass of water.<br>d. Give sucralfate 1 h before meals and at bedtime.<br><br><br><br>e. Give misoprostol with food.<br>f. Follow package instructions for administering combination drug regimens for *H. pylori* infection (eg, Prevpac, Helidac). | Antacids decrease absorption and therapeutic effectiveness of the other drugs.<br>These preparations are suspensions and must be mixed thoroughly to give the correct dose.<br>To increase the surface area of drug available to neutralize gastric acid<br>To allow the drug to form its protective coating over the ulcer before high levels of gastric acidity. Sucralfate requires an acidic environment. After it has adhered to the ulcer, antacids and food do not affect drug action. |
| 2. **Observe for therapeutic effects.**<br>  a. Decreased epigastric pain with gastric and duodenal ulcers; decreased heartburn with gastroesophageal reflux disorders<br>  b. Decreased gastrointestinal (GI) bleeding (eg, absence of visible or occult blood in vomitus, gastric secretions, or feces)<br>  c. Higher pH of gastric contents<br>  d. Radiologic or endoscopic reports of ulcer healing | Therapeutic effects depend on the reason for use.<br>Antacids should relieve pain within a few minutes. Proton pump inhibitors and H$_2$ antagonists relieve pain in 7–10 days by healing effects on peptic ulcers or esophagitis.<br><br><br>The minimum acceptable pH with antacid therapy is 3.5. Healing usually occurs within 4 to 8 weeks. |
| 3. **Observe for adverse effects.**<br>  a. With proton pump inhibitors, observe for headache, diarrhea, abdominal pain, nausea, and vomiting.<br>  b. With H$_2$ antagonists, observe for diarrhea or constipation, headache, dizziness, muscle aches, fatigue, skin rashes, mental confusion, delirium, coma, depression, fever.<br><br><br><br><br><br>  c. With antacids containing magnesium, observe for diarrhea and hypermagnesemia.<br><br><br><br><br>  d. With antacids containing aluminum or calcium, observe for constipation.<br><br><br><br>  e. With sucralfate, observe for constipation.<br><br>  f. With misoprostol, observe for diarrhea, abdominal pain, nausea, and vomiting, headache, uterine cramping, vaginal bleeding.<br>  g. With bismuth, observe for black stools. | These effects occur infrequently and are usually well tolerated.<br><br>Adverse effects are uncommon and usually mild with recommended doses. Central nervous system effects have been associated with high doses in elderly clients or those with impaired renal function. With long-term administration of cimetidine, other adverse effects have been observed. These include decreased sperm count and gynecomastia in men and galactorrhea in women.<br>Diarrhea may be prevented by combining these antacids with other antacids containing aluminum or calcium. Hypermagnesemia may occur in clients with impaired renal function. These antacids should not be given to clients with renal failure.<br>Constipation may be prevented by combining these antacids with other antacids containing magnesium. A high-fiber diet, adequate fluid intake (2000–3000 mL daily), and exercise also help prevent constipation.<br>The drug is not absorbed systemically and constipation is the most commonly reported adverse effect.<br>Diarrhea commonly occurs and may be severe enough to indicate dosage reduction or stopping the drug.<br><br>This is a harmless discoloration of feces; it does not indicate GI bleeding. |

*(continued)*

## Nursing Actions

## Antiulcer Drugs (Continued)

| Nursing Actions | Rationale/Explanation |
|---|---|
| 4. Observe for drug interactions. | Most significant drug interactions alter the effect of the other drug rather than that of the antiulcer or anti–gastroesophageal reflux disease (GERD) drug. |
| a. Drugs that alter effects of proton pump inhibitors: | |
| (1) Clarithromycin *increases* effects of omeprazole. | May increase blood levels |
| (2) Sucralfate *decreases* effects of lansoprazole. | Decreases absorption of lansoprazole, which should be given about 30 min before sucralfate if both are used. |
| b. Drugs that *decrease* effects of H₂ antagonists: | |
| (1) Antacids | Antacids decrease absorption of cimetidine and probably ranitidine. The drugs should not be given at the same time. |
| c. Drugs that alter effects of antacids: | |
| (1) Anticholinergic drugs (eg, atropine) *increase* effects | May increase effects by delaying gastric emptying and by decreasing acid secretion themselves |
| (2) Cholinergic drugs (eg, dexpanthenol [Ilopan]) *decrease* effects | May decrease effects by increasing GI motility and rate of gastric emptying |
| d. Drugs that *decrease* effects of sucralfate: | |
| (1) Antacids | Antacids should not be given within 30 min before or after administration of sucralfate. |

## ? How Can You Avoid This Medication Error?

**Answer:** Mrs. Fallot should not be given this drug with water because she has difficulty swallowing and is at risk for aspiration. Many capsules are time-released and should not be emptied prior to administration. This is not the case with lansoprazole, because the protective granules within the capsule can be preserved if given with acidic foods such as applesauce or yogurt. The granules should not be chewed. When a dispute regarding medications arises, it is wise to consult a drug resource or a pharmacist.

## Critical Thinking Exercises

1. A client asks the nurse what factors contributed to the development of his duodenal ulcer. The nurse explains that the factor most closely associated with ulcer formation is:
   a. Secretion of mucus and bicarbonate
   b. A diet high in spices
   c. The presence of *Helicobacter pylori*
   d. The presence of prostaglandin E

2. When taking a client's history, the nurse notes that the client is taking warfarin and cimetidine concurrently. The nurse should anticipate that the:
   a. Warfarin effects would be increased
   b. Cimetidine effects would be increased
   c. Warfarin effects would be decreased
   d. Cimetidine effects would be decreased

3. One of the most common adverse effects of misoprostol that makes the drug difficult to tolerate in older adults is:
   a. Diarrhea
   b. Headache
   c. Constipation
   d. Hyperphosphatemia

4. A client is started on sucralfate. The nurse, during discharge instructions, explains to the client that the medication should be administered:
   a. At the same time as an antacid
   b. After meals
   c. With meals
   d. 2 hours before other drugs

**5.** A client with *H. pylori* develops a related ulcer. He is placed on ranitidine and Helidac, a drug combination that contains bismuth, metronidazole, and tetracycline. The client is instructed not to consume alcohol, ignores the teaching, and drinks a six-pack of beer. The client presents to the emergency department with tachycardia, headache, diaphoresis, and nausea and vomiting. This disulfiram-like reaction likely occurred because of the interaction between the alcohol and which drug in the combination?

a. Ranitidine
b. Bismuth
c. Metronidazole
d. Tetracycline

## SELECTED REFERENCES

*Drug facts and comparisons.* (Updated monthly). St. Louis: Facts and Comparisons.

Guyton, A. C., & Hall, J. E. (2000). *Textbook of medical physiology* (10th ed.). Philadelphia: W. B. Saunders.

Henderson, R. P., & Lander, R. D. (2000). Peptic ulcer disease. In E. T. Herfindal & D. R. Gourley (Eds.), *Textbook of therapeutics: Drugs and disease management* (7th ed., pp. 515–531). Philadelphia: Lippincott Williams & Wilkins.

Hale-Pradhan, P. B., Landry, H. K., & Sypula, W. T. (2002). Esomeprazole for acid peptic disorders. *Annals of Pharmacotherapy, 36*(4), 655–663.

Lacy, C. F., Armstrong, L. L., Goldman, M. P., & Lance, L. L. (2003). *Lexi-Comp's drug information handbook* (11th ed.). Hudson, OH: American Pharmaceutical Association.

Meurer, L. N., & Bower, D. J. (2002). Management of *Helicobacter pylori* infection. *American Family Physician, 65*(7), 1327–1336.

Metz, D. C., & Walsh, J. H. (2000). Gastroduodenal ulcer disease and gastritis. In H. D. Humes (Ed.), *Kelley's textbook of internal medicine* (4th ed., pp. 824–844). Philadelphia: Lippincott Williams & Wilkins.

Porth, C. M. (Ed.). (2002). *Pathophysiology: Concepts of altered health states* (6th ed., pp. 831–858). Philadelphia: Lippincott Williams & Wilkins.

Richter, J. E. (2000). Diseases of the esophagus. In H. D. Humes (Ed.), *Kelley's textbook of internal medicine* (4th ed., pp. 813–824). Philadelphia: Lippincott Williams & Wilkins.

Vanderhoff, B. T., & Tahboub, R. M. (2002). Proton pump inhibitors: An update. *American Family Physician, 66*(2), 273–280.

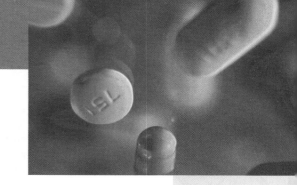

# 48

# Antiemetics

## OBJECTIVES

*After studying this chapter, the student will be able to:*

1 Identify clients at risk for developing nausea and vomiting.

2 Give guidelines for preventing, minimizing, or treating nausea and vomiting.

3 Differentiate the major types of antiemetic drugs.

4 Discuss characteristics, effects, and nursing process implications of selected antiemetic drugs.

## CRITICAL THINKING SCENARIO

*K*elly Morgan, a 44-year-old woman, is having elective abdominal surgery. In the past, she has experienced significant postoperative nausea. Her health care provider orders lorazepam (Ativan), prochlorperazine (Compazine), and metoclopramide (Reglan) on an as needed basis to treat postoperative nausea and vomiting.

✔ What factors contribute to nausea and vomiting in the postoperative client?

✔ How does each ordered antiemetic work to decrease nausea and vomiting?

✔ Why is more than one antiemetic ordered?

✔ How will you make decisions regarding which antiemetic medications to give Ms. Morgan?

## PROTOTYPE PROFILE

ondansetron (Zofran), p. 873

## OVERVIEW

Antiemetic drugs are used to prevent or treat nausea and vomiting. *Nausea* is an unpleasant sensation of abdominal discomfort accompanied by a desire to vomit. *Vomiting* is the expulsion of stomach contents through the mouth. Nausea may occur without vomiting, and vomiting may occur without prior nausea, but the two symptoms often occur together.

Nausea and vomiting are common symptoms experienced by virtually everyone. These symptoms may accompany almost any illness or stress situation. Causes of nausea and vomiting include the following:

- Gastrointestinal (GI) disorders, including infection or inflammation in the GI tract, liver, gallbladder, or pancreas; impaired GI motility and muscle tone (eg, gastroparesis); and overeating or ingestion of foods or fluids that irritate the GI mucosa
- Cardiovascular, infectious, neurologic, or metabolic disorders
- Drug therapy. Nausea and vomiting are the most common adverse effects of drug therapy. Although the symptoms may occur with most drugs, they are especially associated with alcohol, aspirin, digoxin, anticancer drugs, antimicrobials, estrogen preparations, and opioid analgesics.
- Pain and other noxious stimuli, such as unpleasant sights and odors
- Emotional disturbances, physical or mental stress
- Radiation therapy
- Motion sickness
- Postoperative status, which may include pain, impaired GI motility, and receiving various medications

## ANTIEMETIC DRUGS

Drugs used to prevent or treat nausea and vomiting belong to several different therapeutic classifications, and most have anticholinergic, antidopaminergic, antihistaminic, or antiserotonergic effects. In general, the drugs are more effective in prophylaxis than treatment. Most antiemetics prevent or relieve nausea and vomiting by acting on the vomiting center, chemoreceptor trigger zone (CTZ), cerebral cortex, vestibular apparatus, or a combination of these. This mechanism is described in At the Foundation: Triggering the Vomiting Center. Major drugs are described in the following sections and in Drugs at a Glance 48-1: Antiemetic Drugs.

## Phenothiazines

Phenothiazines are central nervous system depressants used in the treatment of psychosis and psychotic symptoms in other disorders (see Chap. 9). These drugs have widespread effects on the body. Their therapeutic effects in nausea and vomiting (as in psychosis) are attributed to their ability to block dopamine from receptor sites in the brain and CTZ (antidopaminergic effects). When used as antiemetics, phenothiazines act on the CTZ and the vomiting center. Not all phenothiazines are effective antiemetics.

Phenothiazines are usually effective in preventing or treating nausea and vomiting induced by drugs, radiation therapy, surgery, and most other stimuli, but they are usually ineffective in motion sickness. These drugs cause sedation; prochlorperazine (Compazine) and promethazine (Phenergan) are commonly used.

## Antihistamines

Antihistamines are used primarily to prevent histamine from exerting its widespread effects on body tissues (see Chap. 38). Antihistamines used as antiemetic agents are the "classic" antihistamines or $H_1$-receptor blocking agents (as differentiated from cimetidine and related drugs, which are $H_2$-receptor blocking agents). The drugs are thought to relieve nausea and vomiting by blocking the action of acetylcholine in the brain (anticholinergic effects). Antihistamines may be effective in preventing

---

**AT THE FOUNDATION:** *Triggering the Vomiting Center*

Vomiting occurs when the vomiting center (a nucleus of cells in the medulla oblongata) is stimulated. Stimuli are relayed to the vomiting center from peripheral (eg, gastric mucosa, peritoneum, intestines, joints) and central (eg, cerebral cortex, vestibular apparatus of the ear, and neurons in the fourth ventricle, called the *chemoreceptor trigger zone* [CTZ]) sites. The vomiting center, CTZ, and GI tract contain benzodiazepine, cholinergic, dopamine, histamine, opiate, and serotonin receptors, which are stimulated by emetogenic drugs and toxins circulating in blood and cerebrospinal fluid. For example, in cancer chemotherapy, emetogenic drugs stimu-

late the CTZ, which then transmits signals to the vomiting center. In motion sickness, rapid changes in body motion stimulate receptors in the inner ear (vestibular branch of the auditory nerve, which is concerned with equilibrium), and nerve impulses are transmitted to the CTZ and the vomiting center.

When stimulated, the vomiting center initiates efferent impulses that cause closure of the glottis, contraction of abdominal muscles and the diaphragm, relaxation of the gastroesophageal sphincter, and reverse peristalsis, which moves stomach contents toward the mouth for ejection.

**DRUG TABLE 48-1**

*Drugs at a Glance*

## Antiemetic Drugs

| Generic/Trade Name | Routes and Dosage Ranges | Comments |
|---|---|---|
| **Phenothiazines** | | |
| **Prochlorperazine** (Compazine)<br>Pregnancy Category C | *Adults:* PO, 5–10 mg 3 or 4 times daily (sustained-release capsule, 10 mg twice daily)<br>IM, 5–10 mg q3–4h to a maximum of 40 mg daily<br>Rectal suppository 25 mg twice daily<br>*Children:* >10 kg: PO, 0.4 mg/kg/d, in 3 or 4 divided doses<br>IM, 0.2 mg/kg as a single dose<br>Rectal suppository 0.4 mg/kg/d, in 3 or 4 divided doses | May cause drowsiness<br>Injection formulation may contain sulfites that may cause allergic reactions |
| **Promethazine** (Phenergan)<br>Pregnancy Category C | *Adults:* PO, IM, rectal suppository 12.5–25 mg q4–6h<br>*Children:* >3 mo: PO, IM, rectal suppository 0.25–0.5 mg/kg q4–6h | May cause drowsiness<br>Injection formulation may contain sulfites that may cause allergic reactions |
| **Antihistamines** | | |
| **Cyclizine** (Marezine)<br>Pregnancy Category B | *Adults:* Motion sickness, PO 50 mg 30 min before departure, then q4–6h as needed, to a maximal daily dose of 200 mg<br>IM, 50 mg q4–6h as needed<br>*Children:* 6–12 y: Motion sickness, PO, 25 mg up to three times daily (maximal daily dose 75 mg) | OTC preparation<br>Drowsiness common; avoid alcohol |
| **Dimenhydrinate** (Dramamine)<br>Pregnancy Category B | *Adults:* PO, 50–100 mg q4–6h as needed (maximal dose, 400 mg in 24 h)<br>IM, 50 mg as needed<br>IV, 50 mg in 10 mL of sodium chloride injection, over 2 min<br>*Children:* 6–12 y: PO, 25–50 mg q6–8h (maximal dose, 150 mg in 24 h)<br>IM, 1.25 mg/kg 4 times daily (maximal dose, 300 mg in 24 h) | Possesses anticholinergic activity |
| **Hydroxyzine** (Vistaril)<br>Pregnancy Category C | *Adults:* IM, 25–100 mg q4–6h as needed<br>*Children:* IM, 0.5–1.1 mg/kg/dose q4–6h as needed | IM administration in children should be given into the midlateral muscles of thigh |
| **Meclizine** (Antivert, Bonine)<br>Pregnancy Category B | *Adults:* Motion sickness, PO, 25–50 mg 1 h before travel<br>Vertigo, PO, 25–100 mg daily in divided doses<br>*Children:* Dosage not established | May cause drowsiness; CNS depression increased with alcohol ingestion |
| **Prokinetic Agent** | | |
| **Metoclopramide** (Reglan)<br>Pregnancy Category B | *Adults:* PO, 10 mg 30 min before meals and at bedtime for 2–8 wk<br>IV, 2 mg/kg 30 min before injection of cisplatin and 2 h after injection of cisplatin, then 1–2 mg/kg q2–3h if needed, up to 4 doses<br>*Children:* Dosage not established | Give IV dose over 1–2 min; rapid bolus causes transient restlessness and anxiety followed by drowsiness |

*(continued)*

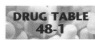

*Drugs at a Glance*

**Antiemetic Drugs** (Continued)

| Generic/Trade Name | Routes and Dosage Ranges | Comments |
|---|---|---|
| **5-HT₃ (Serotonin) Receptor Antagonists** | | |
| **Dolasetron** (Anzemet)<br>Pregnancy Category B | *Adults:* Prevention of postoperative nausea and vomiting (PONV), PO, 100 mg 2 h before surgery<br>Prevention or treatment of PONV, IV, 12.5 mg as a single dose, 15 min before cessation of anesthesia or as soon as nausea or vomiting develops<br>Prevention of chemotherapy-induced nausea and vomiting, PO, 100 mg within 1 h before chemotherapy; IV, 1.8 mg/kg as a single dose approximately 30 min before chemotherapy<br>*Children:* 2–16 y: Prevention of PONV, PO, 1.2 mg/kg within 2 h before surgery. Maximum dose, 100 mg<br>Prevention or treatment of PONV, IV, 0.35 mg/kg as a single dose, 15 min before cessation of anesthesia or as soon as nausea or vomiting develops. Maximum dose, 12.5 mg<br>Prevention of chemotherapy-induced nausea and vomiting, PO, 1.8 mg/kg within 1 h before chemotherapy, maximum dose, 100 mg; IV 1.8 mg/kg as a single dose approximately 30 min before chemotherapy, maximum dose 100 mg | Administer cautiously in clients with cardiac conduction prolongation, especially prolonged QT intervals; electrocardiogram changes directly related to hydrodolasetron concentration, the drug's active metabolite |
| **Granisetron** (Kytril)<br>Pregnancy Category B | *Adults:* Cancer chemotherapy, PO, 1 mg twice daily, first dose approximately 1 h before emetogenic drug, second dose 12 h later, only on days receiving chemotherapy; IV, 10 mcg/kg infused over 5 min, 30 min before emetogenic drug, only on days receiving chemotherapy<br>*Children:* 2–16 y: IV 10 mcg/kg | Drug should be administered on a scheduled basis, not on a PRN basis because drug prevents nausea and vomiting; is not successful in the treatment of nausea and vomiting |
| **Ondansetron** (Zofran)<br>Pregnancy Category B | See Prototype Profile 48-1: Ondansetron | |

and treating motion sickness. Not all antihistamines are effective as antiemetic agents.

## Corticosteroids

Although corticosteroids are used mainly as antiallergic, anti-inflammatory, and antistress agents (see Chap. 36), they have antiemetic effects as well. The mechanism by which the drugs exert antiemetic effects is unknown; they may block prostaglandin activity in the cerebral cortex. Dexamethasone and methylprednisolone are commonly used in the management of chemotherapy-induced emesis, usually in combination with one or more other

antiemetic agents. Regimens vary from a single dose before chemotherapy to doses every 4 to 6 hours for 24 to 48 hours. With this short-term use, adverse effects are mild (eg, euphoria, insomnia, mild fluid retention).

## Benzodiazepine Antianxiety Drugs

Benzodiazepine antianxiety drugs (see Chap. 8) are not antiemetics, but they are often used in multidrug regimens to prevent nausea and vomiting associated with cancer chemotherapy. They produce relaxation and inhibit cerebral cortex input to the vomiting center. They are often prescribed for clients who experience anticipatory nausea and vomiting before administration of anticancer drugs. Lorazepam (Ativan) is commonly used.

## 5-Hydroxytryptamine₃ (5-HT₃ or Serotonin) Receptor Antagonists

**P** **Ondansetron (Zofran), granisetron** (Kytril), and **dolasetron** (Anzemet) are used to prevent or treat moderate to severe nausea and vomiting associated with cancer chemotherapy, radiation therapy, and postoperative status. Some anticancer drugs apparently cause nausea and vomiting by combining with a subset of 5-HT₃ receptors located in the CTZ and GI tract. These drugs antagonize receptors peripherally on vagal nerve terminals and centrally in the CTZ and prevent their activation by emetogenic anticancer drugs.

These three drugs may be given intravenously or orally and are metabolized in the liver. Adverse effects are usually mild to moderate, and common ones include diarrhea, headache, dizziness, constipation, muscle aches, and transient elevation of liver enzymes.

Ondansetron was the first drug of this group and serves as the prototype (see Prototype Profile 48-1: Ondansetron). Its half-life is 3 to 5.5 hours in most clients and 9 to 20 hours in clients with moderate or severe liver impairment. With oral drug, action begins in 30 to 60 minutes and peaks in about 2 hours. With intravenous (IV) drug, onset and peak of drug action are immediate.

Granisetron has a half-life 6 hours with oral drug and 5 to 9 hours with IV drug; its half-life in clients with liver impairment is unknown. Action begins rapidly with IV injection and peaks in 30 to 45 minutes; action begins more slowly with oral drug and peaks in 60 to 90 minutes.

Dolasetron has a half-life of about 7 hours with both IV and oral drug, which is extended to 11 hours in clients with severe liver impairment. Action onset and peak occur rapidly with IV administration; onset is rapid, and peak occurs in 1 to 2 hours with oral drug.

---

### PROTOTYPE PROFILE 48-1

**P** **Ondansetron** (on DAN se tron)

**Drug Class**
*Chemical:* Serotonin antagonists; 5-HT₃ receptor antagonist
*Functional:* Antiemetic

**Trade Name**
Zofran

**Therapeutic Indications**
Prevention of nausea and vomiting associated with emetogenic cancer chemotherapy; postoperatively when nausea and vomiting should be avoided

**Pharmacokinetics**
*Absorption*
Bioavailability: PO, 56%

*Distribution*
Plasma protein binding: 70 to 76%

*Metabolism*
Hepatic

*Excretion*
Urine, feces

**Pharmacodynamics**
*Onset of Action*
Approximately 30 min; peak PO approximately 2 h

*Duration*

**Contraindications/Precautions**
Contraindicated with hypersensitivity, with caution in clients with progressive ileus or gastric distention

**Pregnancy Considerations**
Category B
Excretion in breast milk unknown

**Dosage**
*Cancer chemotherapy:*
*Adults:* PO, 8 mg 30 min before emetogenic drug, repeat in 8 h, then 8 mg q12h for 1–2 d
IV, 0.15 mg/kg for 3 doses (first 30 min before emetogenic drug, then at 4 and 8 h after the first dose) or a single dose of 32 mg 30 min before emetogenic drug
*Children:* 4–11 y: PO, 4 mg 30 min before emetogenic drug, repeat in 4 and in 8 h, then q8h for 1–2 d
4–18 y: IV, 0.15 mg/kg for 3 doses as for adults
2–12 y: ≤ 40 kg: IV, 0.1 mg/kg; > 40 kg: IV, 4 mg as a single dose
*Postoperative nausea and vomiting:*
*Adults:* PO, 16 mg 1 h before anesthesia or IV 4 mg just before anesthesia or postoperatively

**Adverse Effects**
Malaise, drowsiness, fatigue, headache, constipation, diarrhea, anxiety, cold sensation

**Drug Interactions**
*Increased Effects*
Altered clearance of ondansetron with cimetidine, allopurinol, disulfiram

*Decreased Effects*
Altered clearance of ondansetron with phenytoin, phenylbutazone, rifampin, allopurinol, barbiturates, carbamazepine

**Herbal Supplements and Dietary Considerations**
St. John's wort may decrease ondansetron levels
Orally disintegrating tablets contain phenylalanine
Food increases the extent of absorption

## Miscellaneous Antiemetics

**Dronabinol** (Marinol) is a cannabinoid (derivative of marijuana) used in the management of nausea and vomiting associated with anticancer drugs and unrelieved by other drugs. Dronabinol causes the same adverse effects as marijuana, including psychiatric symptoms, has a high potential for abuse, and may cause a withdrawal syndrome when abruptly discontinued. As a result, it is a Schedule III drug under federal narcotic laws.

Withdrawal symptoms (eg, insomnia, irritability, restlessness, others) may occur if dronabinol is abruptly stopped. Onset occurs within 12 hours, with peak intensity within 24 hours and dissipation within 96 hours. These symptoms are most likely to occur with high doses or prolonged use. Sleep disturbances may persist for several weeks.

**Metoclopramide** (Reglan) is a prokinetic agent that increases GI motility and the rate of gastric emptying by increasing the release of acetylcholine from nerve endings in the GI tract (peripheral cholinergic effects). As a result, it can decrease nausea and vomiting associated with gastroparesis and other nonobstructive disorders characterized by gastric retention of food and fluids. Metoclopramide also has central antiemetic effects; it antagonizes the action of dopamine, a catecholamine neurotransmitter. Metoclopramide is given orally in diabetic gastroparesis and esophageal reflux. Large doses of the drug are given intravenously during chemotherapy with cisplatin (Platinol) and other emetogenic antineoplastic drugs.

With oral administration, action begins in 30 to 60 minutes and peaks in 60 to 90 minutes. With intramuscular (IM) use, action onset occurs in 10 to 15 minutes and peaks in 60 to 90 minutes. With IV use, action onset occurs in 1 to 3 minutes and peaks in 60 to 90 minutes. Adverse effects include sedation, restlessness, and extrapyramidal reactions (eg, akathisia, dystonia, symptoms of Parkinson's disease).

Metoclopramide may increase the effects of alcohol and cyclosporine (by increasing their absorption) and decrease the effects of cimetidine and digoxin (by accelerating passage through the GI tract and decreasing time for absorption).

**Phosphorated carbohydrate solution** (Emetrol) is a hyperosmolar solution with phosphoric acid. It is thought to reduce smooth muscle contraction in the GI tract and is available over-the-counter.

**Scopolamine,** an anticholinergic drug (see Chap. 19), is effective in relieving nausea and vomiting associated with motion sickness. A transdermal patch is often used to prevent seasickness.

## Indications for Use

Antiemetic drugs are indicated to prevent and treat nausea and vomiting associated with surgery, pain, motion sickness, cancer chemotherapy, radiation therapy, and other causes. Because of their adverse effects (eg, sedation, cognitive impairment), phenothiazines are mainly indicated when other antiemetic drugs are ineffective or only a few doses are needed.

## Contraindications to Use

Antiemetic drugs are usually contraindicated when their use may prevent or delay diagnosis, when signs and symptoms of drug toxicity may be masked, and for routine use to prevent postoperative vomiting. Metoclopramide is relatively contraindicated in Parkinson's disease because it further depletes dopamine and reduces the effectiveness of levodopa, a major antiparkinson drug.

## Management Considerations

### Drug Selection

Choice of an antiemetic drug depends largely on the cause of nausea and vomiting and the client's condition.

1. The 5-HT$_3$ receptor antagonists (ondansetron, granisetron, and dolasetron) are usually the drugs of first choice for clients with chemotherapy-induced or postoperative nausea and vomiting. In chemotherapy, studies indicate greater effectiveness when combined with a corticosteroid (eg, dexamethasone).
2. Drugs with anticholinergic and antihistaminic properties are preferred for motion sickness. Antihistamines such as meclizine and dimenhydrate are also useful for vomiting caused by labyrinthitis, uremia, or postoperative status.
3. For ambulatory clients, drugs causing minimal sedation are preferred. However, most antiemetic drugs cause some sedation in usual therapeutic doses.
4. Promethazine (Phenergan), a phenothiazine, is often used clinically for its antihistaminic, antiemetic, and sedative effects.
5. Although phenothiazines are effective antiemetic agents, they may cause serious adverse effects (eg, hypotension, sedation, anticholinergic effects, extrapyramidal reactions that simulate signs and symptoms of Parkinson's disease). Consequently, phenothiazines other than promethazine usually should not be used, especially in pregnant, young, elderly, and postoperative clients, unless vomiting is severe and cannot be controlled by other measures.
6. Metoclopramide (Reglan) may be preferred when nausea and vomiting are associated with nonobstructive gastric retention.

### Dosage and Administration Factors

Dosage and route of administration depend primarily on the reason for use.

1. Doses of phenothiazines are much smaller for antiemetic effects than for antipsychotic effects.
2. Most antiemetic agents are available in oral, parenteral, and rectal dosage forms. As a general rule, oral dosage

## Home Care Considerations: Use of Antiemetics

**ASSESS:** the client and family's knowledge of condition and medication regimen and for compliance with the prescribed regimen.

**MONITOR:** for therapeutic and adverse drug effects, for circumstances that aggravate nausea and vomiting, and that client is keeping appointments for follow-up care.

**EDUCATE:** regarding importance of reading and following medication instructions, not exceeding recommended dosages without consulting a health care provider, and interventions to minimize adverse effects of these drugs and decrease risks for injury from sedating drugs. Reinforce additional teaching points regarding specific drug preparations (see Client Teaching Guidelines: Antiemetic Drugs).

forms are preferred for prophylactic use, and rectal or parenteral forms are preferred for therapeutic use.

3. Antiemetic drugs are often ordered as needed (PRN). As for any PRN drug, the client's condition should be assessed before drug administration.

4. The use of antiemetic drugs is usually short term, from a single dose to a few days.

5. The home care nurse may need to assess clients for possible causes of nausea and vomiting and assist clients and caregivers with appropriate use of the drugs and other interventions to prevent fluid and electrolyte depletion. Guidelines for ongoing evaluation and intervention in the home are addressed in Home Care Considerations. In addition, age-specific considerations are also important in the treatment of these conditions. Discussion of specific management factors in children and older adults is found in Age-related Considerations.

### Timing of Drug Administration

When nausea and vomiting are likely to occur because of travel, administration of emetogenic anticancer drugs, diagnostic tests, or therapeutic procedures, an antiemetic drug should be given before the emetogenic event. Pretreatment usually increases client comfort and allows use of lower drug doses. It also may prevent aspiration and other potentially serious complications of vomiting.

## Herbal and Dietary Supplements

**Ginger,** commonly used in cooking, is promoted for use in preventing nausea and vomiting associated with motion sickness, pregnancy, postoperative status, and other conditions. A few studies have investigated its antiemetic activity in humans. The results in one randomized, double-blind study indicated that ginger was comparable to metoclopramide, and that both treatments were more effective than a placebo in preventing

## Age-related Considerations: Use of Antiemetics

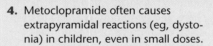
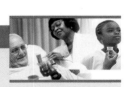

### USE IN CHILDREN

Few studies of antiemetics have been done in children, and their use is not clearly defined. Thus, antiemetic drug therapy should be cautious and limited to prolonged vomiting of known etiology.

1. With the 5-HT$_3$ receptor antagonists, safety and efficacy of granisetron and dolasetron have not been established for children younger than 2 years of age, and there is little information available about the use of ondansetron in children 3 years of age and younger.

2. Phenothiazines are more likely to cause dystonias and other neuromuscular reactions in children than in adults. Promethazine is preferred because its action is more like that of the antihistamines than the phenothiazines. However, promethazine should not be used in children with hepatic disease, Reye's syndrome, a history of sleep apnea, or a family history of sudden infant death syndrome. Excessive doses may cause hallucinations, convulsions, and sudden death.

3. Several antiemetics are not recommended for use in children younger than 12 years of age (eg, buclizine, cyclizine, scopolamine).

4. Metoclopramide often causes extrapyramidal reactions (eg, dystonia) in children, even in small doses.

5. Dronabinol may be used to prevent or treat chemotherapy-induced nausea and vomiting in children who do not respond to other antiemetic drugs. However, the drug should be used cautiously in children because of its psychoactive effects.

### USE IN OLDER ADULTS

Most antiemetic drugs cause drowsiness, especially in older adults, and therefore should be used cautiously. Efforts should be made to prevent nausea and vomiting when possible. Older adults are at risk for fluid volume depletion and electrolyte imbalances with vomiting.

Dronabinol should be used cautiously because older adults are usually more sensitive to the drug's psychoactive effects than young or middle-aged adults.

postoperative nausea and vomiting. Similar results were obtained in another study using oral metoclopramide in gynecologic surgery clients. Other studies have not supported the use of ginger. The general consensus seems to be that it is premature to recommend ginger for any therapeutic use until long-term, controlled studies are done.

## DRUG USE IN SPECIFIC SITUATIONS

### Chemotherapy-induced Nausea and Vomiting

Several anticancer drugs may cause severe nausea and vomiting and much discomfort for clients. Cisplatin is one of the most emetogenic drugs. For this reason, new antiemetics are usually compared with older drugs in the treatment of cisplatin-induced nausea and vomiting. Some general management guidelines include the following:

1. Chemotherapy may be given during sleeping hours.

2. Some clients may experience less nausea and vomiting if they avoid or decrease food intake for a few hours before scheduled chemotherapy.

3. Antiemetic drugs should be given before the emetogenic drug to prevent nausea and vomiting when possible. Most often, they are given intravenously for rapid effects and continued for 2 to 3 days. Continuous intravenous infusion may be more effective than intermittent bolus injections.

4. The 5-HT$_3$ receptor antagonists (eg, ondansetron) are usually considered the most effective antiemetics. They may be given in a single daily dose.

5. Metoclopramide, given intravenously in high doses, may be used alone or in combination with various other drugs. Diphenhydramine (Benadryl) may be given at the same time or PRN because high doses of metoclopramide often cause extrapyramidal effects (see Chap. 9).

6. Various combinations of antiemetic and sedative-type drugs are used, and research continues in this area. A commonly used regimen for prophylaxis is a corticosteroid (eg, dexamethasone, 8 to 10 mg) and a 5-HT$_3$ receptor antagonist (eg, dolasetron, 1.8 mg/kg; granisetron, 10 mcg/kg; or ondansetron, 16 to 32 mg).

## NURSING PROCESS

### Assessment

Assess for nausea and vomiting.

- Identify risk factors (eg, digestive or other disorders in which nausea and vomiting are symptoms; drugs associated with nausea and vomiting).
- Interview regarding frequency, duration, and precipitating causes of nausea and vomiting. Also, question the client about accompanying signs and symptoms, characteristics of vomitus (amount, color, odor, presence of abnormal components, such as blood), and any measures that relieve nausea and vomiting. When possible, observe and measure the vomitus.

### Nursing Diagnoses

- Deficient Fluid Volume related to uncontrolled vomiting
- Imbalanced Nutrition: Less Than Body Requirements related to impaired ability to ingest and digest food
- Altered Tissue Perfusion: Hypotension related to fluid volume depletion or antiemetic drug effect
- Risk for Injury related to adverse drug effects
- Deficient Knowledge related to nondrug measures to reduce nausea and vomiting and appropriate use of antiemetic drugs

### Planning/Goals

*The client will:*

- Receive antiemetic drugs at appropriate times, by indicated routes
- Take antiemetic drugs as prescribed for outpatient use
- Obtain relief of nausea and vomiting

- Eat and retain food and fluids
- Have increased comfort
- Maintain body weight
- Maintain normal bowel elimination patterns
- Have fewer vomiting episodes and less discomfort with cancer chemotherapy or surgical procedures

### Interventions

Use measures to prevent or minimize nausea and vomiting:

- Assist clients to identify situations that cause or aggravate nausea and vomiting.
- Avoid exposure to stimuli when feasible (eg, unpleasant sights and odors; excessive ingestion of food, alcohol, or nonsteroidal anti-inflammatory drugs).
- Because pain may cause nausea and vomiting, administration of analgesics before painful diagnostic tests and dressing changes or other therapeutic measures may be helpful.
- Administer antiemetic drugs 30 to 60 minutes before a nausea-producing event (eg, radiation therapy, cancer chemotherapy, or travel), when possible.
- Many oral drugs cause less gastric irritation, nausea, and vomiting if taken with or just after food. For any drug likely to cause nausea and vomiting, check reference sources to determine whether it can be given with food without altering beneficial effects.
- When nausea and vomiting occur, assess the client's condition and report to the physician. In some instances, a drug (eg, digoxin, an antibiotic) may need to be discontin-

*(continued)*

## Nursing Process (Continued)

ued or reduced in dosage. In other instances (eg, paralytic ileus, GI obstruction), preferred treatment is restriction of oral intake and nasogastric intubation.

- Eating dry crackers before rising in the morning may help prevent nausea and vomiting associated with pregnancy.
- Avoid oral intake of food, fluids, and drugs during acute episodes of nausea and vomiting. Oral intake may increase vomiting and risks of fluid and electrolyte imbalances.
- Minimize activity during acute episodes of nausea and vomiting. Lying down and resting quietly are often helpful.

Give supportive care during vomiting episodes:

- Give replacement fluids and electrolytes. Offer small amounts of food and fluids orally when tolerated and according to client preference.
- Record vital signs, intake and output, and body weight at regular intervals if nausea or vomiting occurs frequently.

- Decrease environmental stimuli when possible (eg, noise, odors). Allow the client to lie quietly in bed when nauseated. Decreasing motion may decrease stimulation of the vomiting center in the brain.
- Help the client rinse his or her mouth after vomiting. This decreases the bad taste and corrosion of tooth enamel by gastric acid.
- Provide requested home remedies when possible (eg, a cool, wet washcloth to the face and neck).

### Evaluation

- Observe and interview for decreased nausea and vomiting.
- Observe and interview regarding ability to maintain adequate intake of food and fluids.
- Compare current weight with baseline weight.
- Observe and interview regarding appropriate use of antiemetic drugs.

---

## CLIENT TEACHING GUIDELINES
### Antiemetic Drugs

#### General Considerations

✔ Try to identify the circumstances that cause or aggravate nausea and vomiting and avoid them when possible.

✔ Drugs are more effective in preventing nausea and vomiting than in stopping them. Thus, they should be taken before the causative event when possible.

✔ Do not eat, drink, or take oral medications during acute vomiting episodes, to avoid aggravating the stomach upset.

✔ Lying down may help nausea and vomiting to subside; activity tends to increase stomach upset.

✔ Once your stomach has settled down, try to take enough fluids to prevent dehydration and potentially serious problems. Tea, broth, and gelatins are usually tolerated.

✔ Do not drive an automobile or operate dangerous machinery if drowsy from antiemetic drugs to avoid injury.

✔ If taking antiemetic drugs regularly, do not drink alcohol or take other drugs without consulting a health care provider. Several drugs interact with antiemetic agents, to increase adverse effects.

✔ Dronabinol, which is derived from marijuana and recommended only for nausea and vomiting associated with cancer chemotherapy, can cause dizziness, drowsiness, mood changes, and other mind-altering effects. You should avoid alcohol and other drugs that cause drowsiness. Also, do not drive or perform hazardous tasks requiring alertness, coordination, or physical dexterity, to decrease risks of injury.

#### Self-administration or Caregiver Administration

✔ Take the drugs as prescribed: Do not increase dosage, take more often, or take when drowsy, dizzy, or unsteady on your feet. Several of the drugs cause sedation and other adverse effects, which are more severe if too much is taken.

✔ To prevent motion sickness, take medication 30 minutes before travel and then every 4 to 6 hours, if necessary, to avoid or minimize adverse effects.

✔ Take or give antiemetic drugs 30 to 60 minutes before a nausea-producing event, when possible. This includes cancer chemotherapy, radiation therapy, painful dressings, or other treatments.

✔ Take dronabinol only when you can be supervised by a responsible adult because of its sedative and mind-altering effects.

## Nursing Actions

## Antiemetics

| Nursing Actions | Rationale/Explanation |
|---|---|
| **1. Administer accurately.** | |
| a. For prevention of motion sickness, give antiemetics 30 min before travel and q4–6h, if necessary. | To allow time for drug dissolution and absorption |
| b. For prevention of vomiting with cancer chemotherapy and radiation therapy, give antiemetic drugs 30–60 min before treatment. | Drugs are more effective in preventing than in stopping nausea and vomiting. |
| c. Inject intramuscular antiemetics deeply into a large muscle mass (eg, gluteal area). | To decrease tissue irritation |
| d. In general, do not mix parenteral antiemetics in a syringe with other drugs. | To avoid physical incompatibilities |
| e. Omit antiemetic agents and report to the physician if the client appears excessively drowsy or is hypotensive. | To avoid potentiating adverse effects and central nervous system (CNS) depression |
| f. Mix intravenous (IV) ondansetron in 50 mL of 5% dextrose or 0.9% sodium chloride injection and infuse over 15 min. | |
| g. Mix granisetron in 20–50 mL of 5% dextrose or 0.9% sodium chloride injection and infuse over 5 min. | |
| h. With dolasetron: | |
| (1) Give oral drug 1–2 h before chemotherapy; give IV drug about 30 min before chemotherapy. | For oral administration to clients who cannot swallow tablets, dolasetron injection can be mixed in apple or apple–grape juice. Specific instructions should be obtained from a pharmacy. When kept at room temperature, the diluted oral solution should be used within 2 h. |
| (2) Give IV drug (up to 100-mg dose) by direct injection over 30 sec or longer or dilute up to 50 mL with 0.9% sodium chloride, 5% dextrose, or 5% dextrose and 0.45% sodium chloride and infuse over 15 min. | |
| **2. Observe for therapeutic effects.** | |
| a. Verbal reports of decreased nausea | |
| b. Decreased frequency or absence of vomiting | |
| **3. Observe for adverse effects.** | |
| a. Excessive sedation and drowsiness | Excessive sedation may occur with usual doses of antiemetics and is more likely to occur with high doses. This may be minimized by avoiding high doses and assessing the client's level of consciousness before each dose. |
| b. Anticholinergic effects—dry mouth, urinary retention | These effects are common to many antiemetic agents and are more likely to occur with large doses. |
| c. Hypotension, including orthostatic hypotension | Most likely to occur with phenothiazines; may also occur with 5-HT₃ antagonists |
| d. Extrapyramidal reactions—dyskinesia, dystonia, akathisia, parkinsonism | These disorders may occur with phenothiazines and metoclopramide. |
| e. With ondansetron and related drugs, observe for headache, diarrhea or constipation, dizziness, fatigue, and muscle aches. Bradycardia and hypotension may also occur. | These drugs are usually well tolerated, with mild to moderate adverse effects. |
| f. With dronabinol, observe for alterations in mood, cognition, and perception of reality, dysphoria, drowsiness, dizziness, anxiety, tachycardia, and conjunctivitis. | Tachycardia may be prevented with a beta-adrenergic blocking drug, such as propranolol (Inderal). |
| **4. Observe for drug interactions.** | |
| a. Drugs that *increase* effects of antiemetic agents: | |
| (1) CNS depressants (alcohol, sedative-hypnotics, antianxiety agents, other antihistamines or antipsychotic agents) | Additive CNS depression |

*(continued)*

## Nursing Actions
## Antiemetics (Continued)

| Nursing Actions | Rationale/Explanation |
|---|---|
| (2) Anticholinergics (eg, atropine) | Additive anticholinergic effects. Some phenothiazines and antiemetic antihistamines have strong anticholinergic properties. |
| (3) Antihypertensive agents | Additive hypotension |
| b. Drugs that alter effects of 5-HT$_3$ receptor antagonists: | |
| (1) Atenolol and cimetidine *increase* effects of dolasetron | The drugs decrease dolasetron metabolism and clearance. |
| (2) Rifampin (and presumably other enzyme inducers) *decreases* effects of dolasetron and granisetron | Enzyme inducers accelerate metabolism of affected drugs. |

## Critical Thinking Exercises

1. Ondansetron suppresses nausea and vomiting by:
   a. Reducing smooth muscle contraction in the GI tract
   b. Blocking dopamine receptors in the CTZ
   c. Increasing the release of acetylcholine from nerve endings in the GI tract
   d. Blocking serotonin receptors in the CTZ and on vagal nerve terminals

2. A diabetic client is given metoclopramide (Reglan) orally for diabetic gastroparesis. The drug produces a central antiemetic effect by:
   a. Antagonizing the action of dopamine, a catecholamine neurotransmitter
   b. Reducing smooth muscle contraction in the GI tract
   c. Increasing the release of acetylcholine from nerve endings in the GI tract
   d. Blocking serotonin receptors in the CTZ and on vagal nerve terminals

3. The use of promethazine can be considered in a child with which of the following conditions?
   a. Hepatic disease
   b. Reye's syndrome
   c. A history of sleep apnea
   d. Chemotherapy-induced nausea and vomiting

4. A client with cancer finds dronabinol, a cannabinoid, successful in managing nausea and vomiting associated with anticancer drugs. The nurse should observe for:
   a. Bradycardia
   b. Altered perception of reality
   c. Hypotension
   d. Nausea and vomiting

5. Metoclopramide is given to a client intravenously in high doses for chemotherapy-induced nausea and vomiting. Diphenhydramine (Benadryl) may be given at the same time or PRN because high doses of metoclopramide often cause:
   a. Dehydration
   b. Constipation
   c. Extrapyramidal effects
   d. Bradycardia

## SELECTED REFERENCES

Clayton, B. D., & Frye, C. B. (2000). Nausea and vomiting. In E. T. Herfindal & D. R. Gourley (Eds.), *Textbook of therapeutics: Drug and disease management* (7th ed., pp. 553–570). Philadelphia: Lippincott Williams & Wilkins.

*Drug facts and comparisons.* (Updated monthly). St. Louis: Facts and Comparisons.

Fetrow, C. W., & Avila, J. R. (1999). *Professional's handbook of complementary and alternative medicines.* Springhouse, PA: Springhouse Corporation.

Hasler, W. L. (2000). Approach to the patient with nausea and vomiting. In H. D. Humes (Ed.), *Kelley's textbook of internal medicine* (4th ed., pp. 729–738). Philadelphia: Lippincott Williams & Wilkins.

Lacy, C. F., Armstrong, L. L., Goldman, M. P., & Lance, L. L. (2003). *Lexi-Comp's drug information handbook* (11th ed.). Hudson, OH: American Pharmaceutical Association.

Miguel, R. (1999). Supportive care: Controlling chemotherapy-induced and postoperative nausea and vomiting. *Journal of the Moffitt Cancer Center, 6,* 393–397.

Porth, C. M. (2002). Alterations in gastrointestinal function. In C. M. Porth (Ed.), *Pathophysiology: Concepts of altered health states* (6th ed., pp. 831–858). Philadelphia: Lippincott Williams & Wilkins.

Rosen, R. H. (2002). Management of chemotherapy-induced nausea and vomiting. *Journal of Pharmacy Practice, 15*(1), 32–41.

Taylor, A. T. (2002). Nausea and vomiting. In J. T. DiPiro, R. L. Talbert, G. C. Yee, G. R. Matzke, B. G. Wells, & L. M. Posey (Eds.), *Pharmacotherapy: A pathophysiologic approach* (5th ed., pp. 641–653). New York: McGraw-Hill.

# Recently Approved and Miscellaneous Drugs

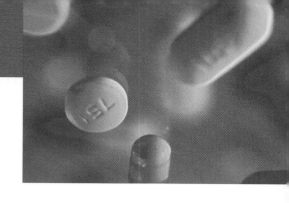

| Generic/Trade Name | Routes and Doses | Classification/Characteristics |
|---|---|---|
| **Alfuzosin** (UroXatral)<br>Pregnancy Category B | PO, 10 mg once daily, reduced with renal impairment | Alpha$_1$ blocker for treatment of benign prostatic hyperplasia |
| **Antithrombin III Human** (Thrombate III)<br>Pregnancy Category B | Dosage individualized | Replaces a substance normally found in plasma in individuals with thrombotic disorders |
| **Atomoxetine** (Strattera)<br>Pregnancy Category C | PO, 40–100 mg daily, in 1 to 2 doses | A selective norepinephrine reuptake inhibitor used in attention deficit-hyperactivity disorder (ADHD); nonstimulant with low risk for abuse (not a controlled substance) |
| **Balsalazide** (Colazal)<br>Pregnancy Category B | PO, 2.25 g 3 times daily for 8–12 wk | Anti-inflammatory agent used in treatment of ulcerative colitis |
| **Dutasteride** (Avodart)<br>Pregnancy Category X | PO, 0.5 mg daily | A 5 alpha-reductase inhibitor that produces antiandrogen effects for clients with benign prostatic hypertrophy |
| **Eplerenone** (Inspira)<br>Pregnancy Category B | PO, 50 mg once daily | An aldosterone receptor antagonist used in the treatment of hypertension alone or in combination with other agents |
| **Epoprostenol** (Flolan)<br>Pregnancy Category B | IV infusion via central venous catheter; see manufacturer's instructions for dosage | Prostaglandin used in treatment of pulmonary hypertension; use restricted |
| **Escitalopram** (Lexapro)<br>Pregnancy Category C | Adults: PO, 10 mg daily; may be increased to 20 mg daily after at least one wk | Similar to other selective serotonin reuptake inhibitors (SSRIs) for treatment of depression |
| **Glipizide/metformin** (Metaglip)<br>Pregnancy Category C | PO, 2.5/250 mg once daily, increased if necessary | Combination oral agent for type 2 diabetes mellitus; each tablet contains metformin 250 or 500 mg and glipizide 2.5 or 5 mg |
| **Ibandronate** (Boniva)<br>Pregnancy Category C | PO, 2.5 mg once daily | Bisphosphonate used for the prevention and treatment of postmenopausal osteoporosis |
| **Mesalamine** (Asacol, Pentasa, Rowasa)<br>Pregnancy Category B | Tablets: PO, 800 mg 3 times daily<br>Capsules: PO, 1 g 4 times daily for up to 8 wk<br>Rectally: 500 mg suppository twice daily or enema 60 mL once daily | Anti-inflammatory agent for treatment of ulcerative colitis and proctitis |
| **Midodrine** (ProAmatine)<br>Pregnancy Category C | PO, 10 mg 3 times daily | Alpha$_1$ agonist used for treatment of severe symptoms associated with orthostatic hypotension |
| **Olsalazine** (Dipentum)<br>Pregnancy Category C | PO, 500 mg twice daily | Anti-inflammatory agent used in the treatment of ulcerative colitis |
| **Omalizumab** (Xolair)<br>Pregnancy Category B | IV or Sub-Q dose based on pretreatment IgE serum levels and body weight | Anti-IgE monoclonal antibody agent for treatment of asthma in individuals with documented reactivity to a perennial aeroallergen uncontrolled with inhaled corticosteroids; not used to manage acute asthma symptoms |
| **Palonosetron** (Aloxi)<br>Pregnancy Category B | IV, 0.25 mg 30 min before chemotherapy on day one of therapy (not more than once weekly) | A selective 5-HT$_3$ receptor antagonist used to prevent or treat chemotherapy-induced nausea and vomiting |

*(continued)*

| Generic/Trade Name | Routes and Doses | Classification/Characteristics |
|---|---|---|
| **Pentosan polysulfate sodium** (Elmiron) Pregnancy Category B | PO, 100 mg 3 times daily | Urinary analgesic used to prevent mucosal irritation and bladder pain associated with interstitial cystitis |
| **Rasburicase** (Elitek) Pregnancy Category C | IV infusion, 0.15–0.2 mg/kg once daily for 5 d, begin chemotherapy 4–24 h after the first dose | Urate-oxidase enzyme used to manage serum uric acid levels in children with malignancies; may cause anaphylaxis |
| **Rifaximin** (Xifaxan) Pregnancy Category C | PO, 200 mg 3 times daily for 3 days | Nonsystemic antibiotic, a derivative of rifampin, for treatment of travelers' diarrhea |
| **Riluzole** (Rilutek) Pregnancy Category C | PO, 50 mg q12h; no increased benefit expected from higher doses | Glutamate inhibitor used in the treatment of amyotrophic lateral sclerosis (can extend survival or time to tracheostomy) |
| **Rosuvastatin** (Crestor) Pregnancy Category X | Adults: PO, 10 mg once daily to maximum dose of 40 mg/d | For treatment of type IIa, IIb, IV dyslipidemia |
| **Sevelamer** (Renagel) Pregnancy Category C | PO, 2–4 capsules 3 times daily | Phosphate binder used to reduce serum phosphorus levels |
| **Sulfasalazine** (Azulfidine) Pregnancy Category B; D at term | PO, 2–4 g daily in divided doses | Anti-inflammatory agent used to treat ulcerative colitis and rheumatoid arthritis |
| **Tegaserod** (Zelnorm) Pregnancy Category B | PO, 6 mg twice daily for 6 wk | Serotonin 5-HT$_4$ receptor agonist used to manage constipation-dominant irritable bowel syndrome (IBS) |
| **Tiotropium** (Spiriva) Pregnancy Category C | Inhalation capsule, once daily | Long-acting anticholinergic medication given for once-daily maintenance treatment of COPD; used to prevent bronchospastic attacks |
| **Trospium** (Sanctura) Pregnancy Category C | PO, 20 mg twice daily | Antimuscarinic/antispasmodic agent for treatment of overactive bladder |

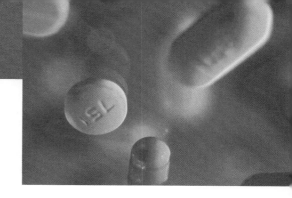

# Fluids and Electrolytes

Water is required for cellular metabolism and excretion of metabolic waste products; 2000 to 3000 mL is needed daily. Treatment of fluid deficiency is aimed toward increasing intake or decreasing loss, depending on causative factors. The safest and most effective way of replacing body fluids is to give oral fluids when possible. To meet fluid needs over a longer period, a nasogastric or other gastrointestinal tube may be used to administer fluids when clients can't take fluids orally. Clients may also receive fluids by the IV route. Treatment of fluid excess is aimed toward decreasing intake and increasing loss. In acute circulatory overload or pulmonary edema, the usual treatment is to stop fluid intake (if the client is receiving IV fluids, slow the rate but keep the vein open for medication) and administer an IV diuretic. Because fluid excess may be a life-threatening emergency, prevention is better than treatment.

Minerals occur in the body and foods mainly in ionic form. Ions are electrically charged particles. Metals (eg, sodium, potassium, calcium, magnesium) form positive ions or cations; nonmetals (eg, chlorine, phosphorus, sulfur) form negative ions or anions. These cations and anions combine to form compounds that are physiologically inactive and electrically neutral. When placed in solution, such as a body fluid, the components separate into electrically charged particles called *electrolytes*. For example, sodium and chlorine combine to form sodium chloride (NaCl or table salt). In a solution, NaCl separates into $Na^+$ and $Cl^-$ ions. (The plus sign after Na means that Na is a cation; the minus sign after Cl means that

Cl is an anion.) At any given time, the body must maintain an equal number of positive and negative charges. Therefore, the ions are constantly combining and separating to maintain electrical neutrality or electrolyte balance.

Electrolytes also maintain the acid–base balance of body fluids, which is necessary for normal body functioning. When foods are digested in the body, they produce mineral residues that react chemically as acids or bases. Acids are usually anions, such as chloride, bicarbonate, sulfate, and phosphate. Bases are usually cations, such as sodium, potassium, calcium, and magnesium. If approximately equal amounts of cations and anions are present in the mineral residue, the residue is essentially neutral, and the pH of body fluids does not require adjustment. If there is an excess of cations (base), the body must draw on its anions (acid) to combine with the cations, render them physiologically inactive, and restore the normal pH of the blood. Excess cations are excreted in the urine, mainly in combination with the anion phosphate. If there is an excess of anions (acid), usually sulfate or phosphate, they combine with hydrogen ions or other cations and are excreted in the urine.

Some minerals (calcium, phosphorus, sodium, potassium, magnesium, chlorine) are required in relatively large amounts (>100 mg) and thus are sometimes called *macronutrients*. Imbalances of macronutrients are classified as deficiency states and excess states. Selected individual drugs used to manage these states are described in the following tables.

| | Type/Characteristics | Uses | Comments |
|---|---|---|---|
| **Dextrose Injection** | | | |
| | Available in preparations containing 2.5%, 5%, 10%, 20%, 25%, 30%, 40%, 50%, 60%, and 70% dextrose | To provide water and calories Treat hypoglycemia (eg, insulin overdose) | The dextrose in $D_5W$ is rapidly used, leaving "free" water for excreting waste products, maintaining renal function, and maintaining urine output. |
| | The most frequently used concentration is 5% dextrose in water ($D_5W$) or sodium chloride injection. | As a component of parenteral nutritional mixtures | |
| | 5% dextrose in water is isotonic with blood. It provides water and 170 kcal/L. | | |
| | 10% dextrose solution provides twice the calories in the same volume of fluid but is hypertonic and therefore may cause phlebitis. | | Coinfusion of 10% dextrose solutions with lipid emulsions in peripheral parenteral nutrition may prevent or decrease phlebitis. |
| | Except for 25% or 50% solutions sometimes used to treat hypoglycemia, the higher concentrations are used in parenteral nutrition. They are hypertonic and must be given through a central or subclavian catheter. | | |
| **Dextrose and Sodium Chloride Injection** | | | |
| | Available in several concentrations | Maintenance fluids, usually with added potassium chloride, in clients who cannot eat or drink | |
| | Frequently used are 5% dextrose in 0.225% (also called $D_5$1/4 normal saline) and 5% dextrose in 0.45% sodium chloride ($D_5$1/2 normal saline) | Replacement fluids when large amounts are lost | |
| | These provide approximately 170 kcal/L, water, sodium, and chloride. | To keep IV lines open Administration of IV medications | |
| **Crystalline Amino Acid Solutions (Aminosyn, Freamine)** | | | |
| | Contain essential and nonessential amino acids | As a component of peripheral or central IV parenteral nutrition, with concentrated dextrose solutions | Special formulations are available for use in patients with renal or hepatic failure. |
| **Fat Emulsions (Intralipid, Liposyn)** | | | |
| | Provide concentrated calories and essential fatty acids | As a component of peripheral or central total parenteral nutrition | More calories can be supplied with a fat emulsion than with dextrose-protein solutions alone. |
| | Available in 10% and 20% emulsions | | |
| | 500 mL of 10% emulsion provides 550 calories. | | |

## Agents Used in Mineral–Electrolyte and Acid–Base Imbalances

| Drug | Routes and Dosage Ranges | Overall Indications for Use of Drug Class |
|---|---|---|
| **Alkalinizing Agent** | | |
| **Sodium bicarbonate** Pregnancy Category C | *Adults:* PO, 325 mg to 2 g, up to 4 times daily; maximum daily dose, 16 g for adults <60 y, 8 g for adults >60 y <br> IV dosage individualized according to arterial blood gases <br> *Children:* IV dosage individualized according to arterial blood gases | Treatment of metabolic acidosis; urine alkalinization |
| **Sodium Preparations** | | |
| **Sodium chloride (NaCl) injection** Pregnancy Category C | *Adults:* IV, 1500–3000 mL of 0.22% or 0.45% solution/24 h depending on the client's fluid needs; approximately 50 mL/h to keep IV lines open | Treatment of hyponatremia |
| **Magnesium Preparations** | | |
| **Magnesium oxide** Pregnancy Category B <br> **Magnesium hydroxide** Pregnancy Category B <br> **Magnesium sulfate** Pregnancy Category B | *Adults:* Hypomagnesemia, PO, magnesium oxide 250–500 mg 3–4 times daily, milk of magnesia 5 mL 4 times daily, or a magnesium-containing antacid 15 mL 3 times daily; IM (magnesium sulfate), 1–2 g (2–4 mL of 50% solution) 1–2 times daily based on serum magnesium levels <br> Eclampsia, IM, 1–2 g (2–4 mL of 50% solution) initially, then 1 g every 30 min until seizures stop <br> Convulsive seizures, IM, 1 g (2 mL of 50% solution) repeated PRN <br> IV, do not exceed 150 mg/min (1.5 mL/min of a 10% solution, 3 mL/min of a 5% solution) <br> *Children:* Convulsions: IM, 20–40 mg/kg in a 20% solution; repeat as necessary | To prevent or treat hypomagnesemia <br> To treat hypertension or convulsions associated with toxemia of pregnancy or acute nephritis in children |
| **Potassium Preparations** | | |
| **Potassium chloride (KCl)** Pregnancy Category A | *Adults:* PO, 15–20 mEq 2–4 times daily <br> IV, 40–100 mEq/24 h, depending on serum potassium levels. <br> KCl **must** be diluted in dextrose or NaCl IV solution for IV use. <br> **Maximum** *for serum K$^+$ >2.5 mEq:* diluted 40 mEq/L, infused 10 mEq/h to maximum dose of 200 mEq in 24 h <br> **Maximum** *for serum K$^+$ <2.5 mEq:* diluted 80 mEq/L, infused 40 mEq/h to maximum dose of 400 mEq in 24 h <br> *Children:* IV infusion, up to 3 mEq/kg or 40 mEq/m$^2$ daily. <br> Adjust amount of fluids to body size. | Prevention or treatment of hypokalemia |
| **Cation Exchange Resin** | | |
| **Sodium polystyrene sulfonate** (Kayexalate) Pregnancy Category C | *Adults:* PO, 15 g in 100–200 mL of water and 70% sorbitol, 1–4 times daily <br> *Rectally* (retention enema): 30–50 g in 100–200 mL of water and 70% sorbitol q6h | Treatment of hyperkalemia |

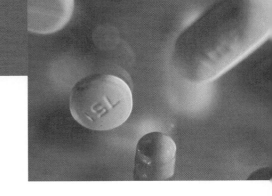

# Therapeutic Serum Drug Concentrations for Selected Drugs

Listed below are generally accepted therapeutic serum drug concentrations, in conventional and SI units, for several commonly used drugs. In addition, toxic concen-trations are listed for selected drugs. SI units have not been established for some drugs.

| Drug | Conventional Units | SI Units |
|------|-------------------|----------|
| Acetaminophen | 0.2–0.6 mg/dL | 13–40 µmol/L |
| | Toxic >5 mg/dL | >300 µmol/L |
| Amikacin | (peak) 16–32 mcg/mL | 20–30 mg/L |
| | (trough) ≤8 mcg/mL | |
| Amitriptyline | 110–250 ng/mL | 375–900 nmol/L |
| Carbamazepine | 4–12 mcg/mL | 17–50 µmol/L |
| Desipramine | 125–300 ng/mL | 470–825 nmol/L |
| Digoxin | 0.5–2.2 ng/mL | 1–2.6 nmol/L |
| Disopyramide | 2–8 mcg/mL | 6–18 µmol/L |
| Ethosuximide | 40–110 mcg/mL | 280–780 µmol/L |
| Gentamicin | (peak) 4–8 mcg/mL | 5–10 mg/L |
| | (trough) ≤2 mcg/mL | |
| Imipramine | 200–350 ng/mL | 530–950 nmol/L |
| Lidocaine | 1.5–6 mcg/mL | 6–21 µmol/L |
| Lithium | 0.5–1.5 mEq/L | 0.5–1.5 µmol/L |
| Maprotiline | 50–200 ng/mL | 180–270 nmol/L |
| Netilmicin | (peak) 6–10 mcg/mL | 5–10 mg/L |
| | (trough) ≤2 mcg/mL | |
| Nortriptyline | 50–150 ng/mL | 190–570 nmol/L |
| Phenobarbital | 15–50 mcg/mL | 65–170 µmol/L |
| Phenytoin | 10–20 mcg/mL | 40–80 µmol/L |
| Primidone | 5–12 mcg/mL | 25–45 µmol/L |
| Procainamide | 4–8 mcg/mL | 17–40 µmol/L |
| Propranolol | 50–200 ng/mL | 190–770 nmol/L |
| Protriptyline | 100–300 ng/mL | 380–1140 nmol/L |
| Quinidine | 2–6 mcg/mL | 4.6–9.2 µmol/L |
| Salicylate | 100–200 mg/L | 724–1448 µmol/L |
| | Toxic >200 mg/L | >1450 µmol/L |
| Theophylline | 10–20 mcg/mL | 55–110 µmol/L |
| Tobramycin | (peak) 4–8 mcg/mL | 5–10 mg/L |
| | (trough) ≤2 mcg/mL | |
| Valproic acid | 50–100 mcg/mL | 350–700 µmol/L |
| Vancomycin | (peak) 30–40 mg/mL | (peak) 20–40 mg/L |
| | (trough) 5–10 mg/mL | (trough) 5–10 mg/L |

mcg, microgram; ng, nanogram; µmol, micromole.

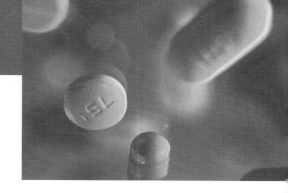

# Anesthetic Agents

Anesthesia means loss of sensation with or without loss of consciousness. Anesthetic drugs are given to prevent pain and promote relaxation during surgery, childbirth, some diagnostic tests, and some treatments. They interrupt the conduction of painful nerve impulses from a site of injury to the brain. The two basic types of anesthesia are general and regional.

*General anesthesia* is a state of profound central nervous system (CNS) depression, during which there is complete loss of sensation, consciousness, pain perception, and memory. It has three components: hypnosis, analgesia, and muscle relaxation. Several different drugs are usually combined to produce desired levels of these components without excessive CNS depression. This *balanced anesthesia* also allows lower dosages of potent general anesthetics.

*Regional anesthesia* involves loss of sensation and motor activity in localized areas of the body. It is induced by application or injection of local anesthetic drugs. The drugs act to decrease the permeability of nerve cell membranes to ions, especially sodium.

This action stabilizes and reduces excitability of cell membranes. When excitability falls low enough, nerve impulses cannot be initiated or conducted by the anesthetized nerves. As a result, the drugs prevent the cells from responding to pain impulses and other sensory stimuli.

Major classes of agents used in anesthesia are included in the following tables.

## General Anesthetics

| Generic/Trade Name | Characteristics | Comments |
|---|---|---|
| ***General Inhalation Anesthetics*** | | |
| **Desflurane** (Suprane)<br>Pregnancy Category B | Similar to isoflurane | Used for induction and maintenance of general anesthesia |
| **Enflurane** (Ethrane)<br>Pregnancy Category B | Nonexplosive, nonflammable volatile liquid; similar to halothane but may produce better analgesia and muscle relaxation; sensitizes heart to catecholamines—increases risk of cardiac dysrhythmias; renal or hepatic toxicity not reported | A frequently used agent |
| **Halothane** (Fluothane)<br>Pregnancy Category C | Nonexplosive, nonflammable volatile liquid<br>Advantages:<br>1. Produces rapid induction with little or no excitement; rapid recovery with little excitement or nausea and vomiting<br>2. Does not irritate respiratory tract mucosa; therefore does not increase saliva and tracheobronchial secretions<br>3. Depresses pharyngeal and laryngeal reflexes, which decreases risk of laryngospasm and bronchospasm<br>Disadvantages:<br>1. Depresses contractility of the heart and vascular smooth muscle, which causes decreased cardiac output, hypotension, and bradycardia<br>2. Circulatory failure may occur with high doses. | Halothane has largely been replaced by newer agents with increased efficacy, decreased adverse effects, or both.<br>It may be used in balanced anesthesia with other agents. Although quite potent, it may not produce adequate analgesia and muscle relaxation at a dosage that is not likely to produce significant adverse effects. Therefore, nitrous oxide is given to increase analgesic effects; a neuromuscular blocking agent is given to increase muscle relaxation; and an IV barbiturate is used to produce rapid, smooth induction, after which halothane is given to maintain anesthesia. |

*(continued)*

| Generic/Trade Name | Characteristics | Comments |
|---|---|---|
| | 3. Causes cardiac dysrhythmias. Bradycardia is common; ventricular dysrhythmias are uncommon unless ventilation is inadequate.<br>4. Sensitizes heart to catecholamines; increases risk of cardiac dysrhythmias<br>5. Depresses respiration and may produce hypoxemia and respiratory acidosis (hypercarbia)<br>6. Depresses functions of the kidneys, liver, and immune system<br>7. May cause jaundice and hepatitis<br>8. May cause malignant hyperthermia | |
| **Isoflurane** (Forane)<br>Pregnancy Category C | Similar to halothane but less likely to cause cardiovascular depression and ventricular dysrhythmias. Isoflurane may cause malignant hyperthermia but apparently does not cause hepatotoxicity. | Used for induction and maintenance of general anesthesia |
| **Nitrous oxide**<br>Pregnancy Category C | Nonexplosive gas; good analgesic, weak anesthetic; one of oldest and safest anesthetics; causes no appreciable damage to vital organs unless hypoxia is allowed to develop and persist; administered with oxygen to prevent hypoxia; rapid induction and recovery. Note: Nitrous oxide is an incomplete anesthetic; that is, by itself, it cannot produce surgical anesthesia. | Used in balanced anesthesia with IV barbiturates, neuromuscular blocking agents, opioid analgesics, and more potent inhalation anesthetics. It is safer for prolonged surgical procedures (see "Characteristics"). It is used alone for analgesia in dentistry, obstetrics, and brief surgical procedures. |
| **Sevoflurane** (Ultane)<br>Pregnancy Category B | Similar to isoflurane | Used for induction and maintenance of general anesthesia |
| *General Intravenous Anesthetics* | | |
| **Alfentanil** (Alfenta)<br>Pregnancy Category C | Opioid analgesic–anesthetic related to fentanyl and sufentanil. Rapid acting. | May be used as a primary anesthetic or an analgesic adjunct in balanced anesthesia |
| **Etomidate** (Amidate)<br>Pregnancy Category C | A nonanalgesic hypnotic used for induction and maintenance of general anesthesia | May be used with nitrous oxide and oxygen in maintenance of general anesthesia for short operative procedures such as uterine dilation and curettage |
| **Fentanyl and droperidol combination** (Innovar)<br>Pregnancy Category C; high dose at term | Droperidol (Inapsine) is related to the antipsychotic agent haloperidol. It produces sedative and antiemetic effects. Fentanyl citrate (Sublimaze) is a very potent opioid analgesic whose actions are similar to those of morphine but of shorter duration. Innovar is a fixed-dose combination of the two drugs. Additional doses of fentanyl are often needed because its analgesic effect lasts approximately 30 minutes, whereas droperidol's effects last 3–6 hours. The Food and Drug Administration recently issued a warning about serious cardiac dysrhythmias, including torsades de pointes, associated with the use of droperidol. | Either drug may be used alone, but they are often used together for neuroleptanalgesia and combined with nitrous oxide for neuroleptanesthesia.<br>Neuroleptanalgesia is a state of reduced awareness and reduced sensory perception during which a variety of diagnostic tests or minor surgical procedures can be done, such as bronchoscopy and burn dressings.<br>Neuroleptanesthesia can be used for major surgical procedures. Consciousness returns rapidly, but respiratory depression may last 3–4 hours into the postoperative recovery period. |

*(continued)*

| Generic/Trade Name | Characteristics | Comments |
|---|---|---|
| **Ketamine** (Ketalar)<br>Pregnancy Category D | Rapid-acting nonbarbiturate anesthetic; produces marked analgesia, sedation, immobility, amnesia, and a lack of awareness of surroundings (called dissociative anesthesia); may be given IV or IM; awakening may require several hours; during recovery, unpleasant psychic symptoms may occur, including dreams and hallucinations; vomiting, hypersalivation, and transient skin rashes also may occur during recovery. | Used most often for brief surgical, diagnostic, or therapeutic procedures. It also may be used to induce anesthesia. If used for major surgery, it must be supplemented by other general anesthetics. It is generally contraindicated in clients with increased intracranial pressure, severe coronary artery disease, hypertension, or psychiatric disorders. Hyperactivity and unpleasant dreams occur less often with children than adults. |
| **Methohexital sodium** (Brevital)<br>Pregnancy Category C | An ultrashort-acting barbiturate similar to thiopental | See thiopental, below. |
| **Midazolam** (Versed)<br>Pregnancy Category D | Short-acting benzodiazepine. May cause respiratory depression, apnea, death with IV administration. Smaller doses are needed if other CNS depressants (eg, opioid analgesics, general anesthetics) are given concurrently. | Given IM for preoperative sedation. Given IV for conscious sedation during short endoscopic or other diagnostic procedures; induction of general anesthesia; and maintenance of general anesthesia with nitrous oxide and oxygen for short surgical procedures |
| **Propofol** (Diprivan)<br>Pregnancy Category B | A rapid-acting hypnotic used with other agents in balanced anesthesia. May cause hypotension, apnea, and other signs of CNS depression. Recovery is rapid, occurring within minutes after the drug is stopped. | Given by IV bolus or infusion for induction or maintenance of general anesthesia or sedation in intensive care |
| **Remifentanil** (Ultiva)<br>Pregnancy Category C | An opioid analgesic–anesthetic with a rapid onset and short duration of action | Used for induction and maintenance of general anesthesia |
| **Sufentanil** (Sufenta)<br>Pregnancy Category C | A synthetic opioid analgesic-anesthetic related to fentanyl. Compared with fentanyl, it is more potent and faster acting and may allow a more rapid recovery. | May be used as a primary anesthetic or an analgesic adjunct in balanced anesthesia |
| **Thiopental sodium**<br>  (Pentothal)<br>Pregnancy Category C | Ultrashort-acting barbiturate, used almost exclusively in general anesthesia; excellent hypnotic but does not produce significant analgesia or muscle relaxation; given IV by intermittent injection or by continuous infusion of a dilute solution. | Thiopental is commonly used. A single dose produces unconsciousness in less than 30 seconds and lasts 20–30 minutes. Usually given to induce anesthesia. It is used alone only for brief procedures. For major surgery, it is usually supplemented by inhalation anesthetics and muscle relaxants. |

## Neuromuscular Blocking Agents (Skeletal Muscle Relaxants)

| Generic/Trade Name | Characteristics | Clinical Uses |
|---|---|---|
| **Depolarizing Type** | | |
| **Succinylcholine** (Anectine) Pregnancy Category C | Short acting after single dose; action can be prolonged by repeated injections or continuous intravenous infusion. Malignant hyperthermia may occur | All types of surgery and brief procedures, such as endoscopy and endotracheal intubation |
| **Nondepolarizing Type** | | |
| **Atracurium** (Tracrium) Pregnancy Category C | Intermediate acting* | Adjunct to general anesthesia |
| **Cisatracurium** (Nimbex) Pregnancy Category C | Intermediate acting* | Same as rocuronium, below |
| **Doxacurium** (Nuromax) Pregnancy Category C | Long acting* | Adjunct to general anesthesia |
| **Metocurine** (Metubine) Pregnancy Category C | Long acting; more potent than tubocurarine* | Adjunct to general anesthesia; to facilitate endotracheal intubation and mechanical ventilation |
| **Mivacurium** (Mivacron) Pregnancy Category C | Short acting* | Adjunct to general anesthesia |
| **Pancuronium** (Pavulon) Pregnancy Category C | Long acting* | Mainly during surgery after general anesthesia has been induced; occasionally to aid endotracheal intubation or mechanical ventilation |
| **Pipecuronium** (Arduan) Pregnancy Category C | Long acting* | Adjunct to general anesthesia; recommended only for procedures expected to last 90 minutes or longer |
| **Rocuronium** (Zemuron) Pregnancy Category C | Intermediate acting* | Adjunct to general anesthesia to aid endotracheal intubation and provide muscle relaxation during surgery or mechanical ventilation |
| **Tubocurarine** Pregnancy Category | Long acting; the prototype of nondepolarizing drugs* | Adjunct to general anesthesia; occasionally to facilitate mechanical ventilation |
| **Vecuronium** (Norcuron) Pregnancy Category C | Intermediate acting* | Adjunct to general anesthesia; to facilitate endotracheal intubation and mechanical ventilation |

*All the nondepolarizing agents may cause hypotension; effects of the drugs can be reversed by neostigmine (Prostigmin).

## Local Anesthetics

| Generic/Trade Name | Characteristics | Comments/Clinical Uses |
|---|---|---|
| **Articaine** (Septocaine, Septodont) Pregnancy Category C | Newer drug, formulated with epinephrine Effects occur in 1–6 min and last 1 h | Local infiltration and nerve block for dental and periodontal procedures or oral surgery |
| **Benzocaine** (Americaine) Pregnancy Category C | Poorly water soluble Minimal systemic absorption Available in numerous preparations, including aerosol sprays, throat lozenges, rectal suppositories, lotions, and ointments May cause allergic reactions Effects occur in 5 min or less and last 15–45 min | Topical anesthesia of skin and mucous membrane to relieve pain and itching of sunburn, other minor burns and wounds, skin abrasions, earache, hemorrhoids, sore throat, and other conditions |
| **Bupivacaine** (Marcaine) Pregnancy Category C | Given by injection May cause systemic toxicity Effects occur in 5 min and last 2–4 h with injection, 10–20 min and 3–5 h with epidural administration | Regional anesthesia by infiltration, nerve block, and epidural anesthesia during childbirth. Not used for spinal anesthesia |
| **Chloroprocaine** (Nesacaine) Pregnancy Category C | Related to procaine, but its potency is greater and duration of action is shorter Rapidly metabolized and less likely to cause systemic toxicity than other local anesthetics Given by injection Effects occur in 6–12 min and last 30 min | Regional anesthesia by infiltration, nerve block, and epidural anesthesia |
| **Cocaine** Pregnancy Category C; X with nonmedicinal use | A naturally occurring plant alkaloid Readily absorbed through mucous membranes A Schedule II controlled substance with high potential for abuse, largely because of euphoria and other CNS stimulatory effects; produces psychic dependence and tolerance with prolonged use Too toxic for systemic use Effects occur in 1–5 min and last 30–60 min | Topical anesthesia of ear, nose, and throat |
| **Dyclonine** (Dyclone) Pregnancy Category C | Absorbed through skin and mucous membranes Effects occur in <10 min and last <60 min | Topical anesthesia in otolaryngology |
| **Levobupivacaine** (Chirocaine) Pregnancy Category B | Newer drug May be given by local infiltration and epidurally When given epidurally, effects occur within 10 min and last about 8 h | Local or regional anesthesia for surgery and obstetrics and for postoperative pain management |
| **Lidocaine** (Xylocaine) Pregnancy Category B, manufacturer; C, expert analysis | Given topically and by injection One of the most widely used local anesthetic drugs Topical patches are available for the relief of painful conditions such as postherpetic neuralgia; the patches are to be applied for 12 h daily only Acts as an antidysrhythmic drug by decreasing myocardial irritability With injection, effects occur in <2 min and last 30–60 min With epidural use, effects occur in 5–15 min and last 1–3 h With topical use, effects occur in 2–5 min and last 15–45 min | Topical anesthesia and regional anesthesia by local infiltration, nerve block, spinal, and epidural anesthesia Intravenously to prevent or treat cardiac dysrhythmias (see Chap. 40). (**Warning:** Do not use preparations containing epinephrine for dysrhythmias.) |

*(continued)*

## Local Anesthetics (Continued)

| Generic/Trade Name | Characteristics | Comments/Clinical Uses |
|---|---|---|
| **Lidocaine 2.5% and prilocaine 2.5%** (EMLA) Pregnancy Category B | Formulated to be absorbed through intact skin; contraindicated for use on mucous membranes or abraded skin Must be applied at least 1 h before the planned procedure Effects occur in 1–2 h and last 1–2 h | Topical anesthesia for vaccinations or venipunctures in children |
| **Mepivacaine** (Carbocaine) Pregnancy Category C | Related to lidocaine; action slower in onset and longer in duration than lidocaine With injection, effects occur in 3–5 min and last 0.75–1.5 h Epidurally, effects occur in 5–15 min and last 1–3 h | Infiltration, nerve block, and epidural anesthesia |
| **Pramoxine** (Tronothane) Pregnancy Category C | Not injected or applied to nasal mucosa because it irritates tissues Effects occur in 3–5 min | Topical anesthesia for skin wounds, dermatoses, hemorrhoids, endotracheal intubation, sigmoidoscopy |
| **Prilocaine** (Citanest) Pregnancy Category B | Similar to lidocaine in effectiveness but has a slower onset, longer duration, and less toxicity because it is more rapidly metabolized and excreted With injection, effects occur in <2 min and last 60 min Epidurally, effects occur in 5–15 min and last 1–3 h | Regional anesthesia by infiltration, nerve block, and epidural infusion |
| **Procaine** (Novocain) Pregnancy Category C | Rarely used Rapidly metabolized With injection, effects occur in 2–5 min and last 15–60 min | Regional anesthesia by infiltration, nerve block, and spinal anesthesia. Not used topically |
| **Proparacaine** (Alcaine) Pregnancy Category C | Causes minimal irritation of the eye but may cause allergic contact dermatitis of the fingers | Topical anesthesia of the eye for tonometry and for removal of sutures, foreign bodies, and cataracts |
| **Ropivacaine** (Naropin) Pregnancy Category B | Given by injection or epidural infusion With epidural infusion, effects occur in 10–30 min and last up to 6 h | Obstetric or postoperative analgesia and local or regional surgical anesthesia |
| **Tetracaine** (Pontocaine) Pregnancy Category C | Applied topically Formerly injected for regional anesthesia but now rarely injected because of possible allergic reactions | Topical anesthesia |

# *E*

# Vitamins and Minerals

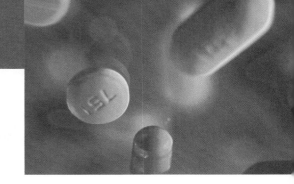

Vitamins and minerals are required for normal body metabolism, growth, and development. Vitamins are components of enzyme systems that release energy from proteins, fats, and carbohydrates. They also are required for formation of red blood cells, nerve cells, hormones, genetic materials, bones, and other tissues. Minerals occur in the body and foods mainly in ionic form. Minerals function to maintain fluid and electrolyte balance (see Appendix B) and acid–base balance. They also maintain osmotic pressure; maintain nerve and muscle function; assist in transfer of compounds across cell membranes; and influence the growth process.

Vitamins are typically classified as fat soluble (A, D, E, K) and water soluble (B complex, C). Fat-soluble vitamins are absorbed from the intestine with dietary fat, and absorption requires the presence of bile salts and pancre-

atic lipase. Water-soluble vitamins are readily absorbed. Vitamin drug preparations are described below.

Several minerals are considered necessary for human nutrition and are mainly obtained from foods or supplements. Some minerals (calcium, phosphorus, sodium, potassium, magnesium, chlorine) are required in relatively large amounts (>100 mg) and thus are sometimes referred to as *macronutrients*; sodium, potassium, magnesium, chlorine are discussed in Appendix B. Calcium and phosphorus are discussed in Chapter 20. Other minerals are required in small amounts (<100 mg); these are often called *micronutrients* or *trace elements*. Key trace elements (iodine, iron, and zinc), have relatively well-defined roles in human nutrition. Iron and zinc drug preparation are outlined in this section. Iodine is discussed in Chapter 21.

## Vitamin Drug Preparations

| Generic/Trade Name | Routes and Dosage Ranges | Comments |
| --- | --- | --- |
| ***Fat-soluble Vitamins*** | | |
| **Vitamin A** (also called retinol) Pregnancy Category A; X if dose exceeds RDA recommendations | *Adults:* Deficiency: PO, IM, 100,000 IU daily for 3 d, then 50,000 IU daily for 2 wk, then 10,000–20,000 IU daily for another 2 mo<br>*Children:* Kwashiorkor: Retinol, 30 mg IM, followed by intermittent oral therapy Xerophthalmia (>1 y old): Retinyl palmitate, 110 mg PO or 55 mg IM plus another 110 mg PO at 1 and 3 or 4 days later | IM administration indicated when oral not feasible, as in anorexia, nausea, vomiting, preoperative and postoperative conditions, or malabsorption syndromes<br>With xerophthalmia, vitamin E 40 IU should be co-administered to increase effectiveness of the retinol |
| **Vitamin D** Pregnancy Category C | See Chapter 20. | |
| **Vitamin E** Pregnancy Category A; C if dose exceeds RDA recommendations | *Adults:* PO, 100–400 IU daily<br>*Children:* PO, 15–30 IU daily | Should not be given IV because IV use has been associated with 38 infant deaths |
| **Vitamin K** **Phytonadione** (Mephyton, Aqua-Mephyton) Pregnancy Category C | *Adults:* Anticoagulant-induced prothrombin deficiency, PO, Sub-Q, IM, 2.5–10 mg initially, repeat after 6–8 h (injected dose) or 12–48 h (oral dose) if needed (ie, if prothrombin time still prolonged)<br>Hypoprothrombinemia due to other causes, PO, Sub-Q, IM, 2.5–25 mg<br>*Older children:* Same as adults | Do not give IV; serious, anaphylaxis-like reactions have occurred |

*(continued)*

| Generic/Trade Name | Routes and Dosage Ranges | Comments |
|---|---|---|
| | *Newborns:* Prevention of hemorrhagic disease, IM, 0.5–1 mg within 1 h after birth; may be repeated after 2–3 wk if mother received anticoagulant, anticonvulsant, antitubercular, or recent antibiotic drug therapy during pregnancy<br>Treatment of hemorrhagic disease: Sub-Q, IM, 1 mg | |
| *Water-soluble Vitamins*<br>**B-Complex Vitamins** | | |
| **Calcium pantothenate** ($B_5$)<br>Pregnancy Category C | *Adults:* Total parenteral nutrition, IV, 15 mg daily<br>*Children:* Total parenteral nutrition, >11 y, IV, 15 mg daily; 1–11 y, IV, 5 mg | Deficiency states seen only with severe, multiple B-complex deficiency states |
| **Cyanocobalamin** ($B_{12}$)<br>Pregnancy Category A; C if dose exceeds RDA<br>**Nasal** (Nascobal)<br>Pregnancy Category C | *Adults:* PO, 100–250 mcg daily<br>IM, 30 mcg daily for 5–10 d, then 100–200 mcg monthly<br>Intranasal gel, 1 spray (500 mcg) in one nostril, once per wk<br>*Children:* PO, IM, Sub-Q, 10–100 mcg daily for 5–15 d, then 100–200 mcg monthly | Oral drug, alone or in multivitamin preparations, is given for nutritional deficiencies. Parenteral $B_{12}$ should be given for pernicious anemia<br>Intranasal drug should not be used if rhinitis, nasal congestion, or upper respiratory infection is present |
| **Folic acid**<br>Pregnancy Category A; C if dose exceeds RDA | *Adults:* Deficiency, megaloblastic anemia PO, Sub-Q, IM, IV, up to 1 mg daily until symptoms decrease and blood tests are normal, then maintenance dose of 0.4 mg daily<br>*Children:* PO, Sub-Q, IM, IV, up to 1 mg daily until symptoms decrease and blood tests are normal, then a daily maintenance dose as follows: infants, 0.1 mg; <4 y, up to 0.3 mg; >4 y, 0.4 mg | Oral administration preferred unless severe intestinal malabsorption is present |
| **Niacin** (nicotinic acid), **niacinamide** (nicotinamide)<br>Pregnancy Category A; C if dose exceeds RDA | *Adults:* Deficiency: PO, 50–100 mg daily<br>Pellagra: PO, up to 500 mg daily<br>Hyperlipidemia: PO, 2–6 g daily (maximum dose, 6 g/d)<br>*Children:* Safety and effectiveness not established for amounts exceeding the RDA | To reduce flushing with larger doses, start with smaller doses and gradually increase them |
| **Pyridoxine** ($B_6$)<br>Pregnancy Category A; C if dose exceeds RDA | *Adults:* Deficiency: PO, IM, IV, 2–5 mg daily<br>Anemia, peripheral neuritis: 50–200 mg daily<br>*Children:* Safety and effectiveness not established for amounts exceeding the RDA | Usually given with isoniazid, an antitubercular drug, to prevent peripheral neuropathy |
| **Riboflavin**<br>Pregnancy Category A; C if dose exceeds RDA | *Adults:* Deficiency: PO, 5–10 mg daily<br>In total parenteral nutrition, 3.6 mg/d<br>*Children:* In total parenteral nutrition, IV, >11 y, 3.6 mg/d; 1–11 y, 1.4 mg/d | Deficiency rarely occurs alone; more likely with other vitamin deficiency states |
| **Thiamine** ($B_1$)<br>Pregnancy Category A; C if dose exceeds RDA | *Adults:* Deficiency: PO, 10–30 mg daily; IM, 10–20 mg three times daily for 2 wk, supplemented with 5–10 mg orally; IV, 50–100 mg/d<br>*Children:* Safety and effectiveness not established for amounts exceeding the RDA | Deficiency is common in individuals with alcoholism |
| **Vitamin C**<br>Vitamin C (ascorbic acid)<br>Pregnancy Category A; C if dose exceeds RDA | *Adults:* Deficiency, PO, IM, IV, 100–500 mg daily<br>Urinary acidification, 2 g daily in divided doses<br>Prophylaxis, 50–100 mg daily<br>*Children:* Infants receiving formula, 35–50 mg daily for first few weeks of life | Excessive doses (eg, 2000 mg or more daily) cause adverse effects and should be avoided |

## Individual Drugs Used in Trace Mineral Imbalances

| Drug | Routes and Dosage Ranges | Comments |
|---|---|---|
| *Iron Preparations* | | |
| **Ferrous gluconate** (Fergon) Pregnancy Category A | *Adults:* PO, 320–640 mg (40–80 mg elemental iron) 3 times daily *Children:* PO, 100–300 mg (12.5–37.5 mg elemental iron) 3 times daily *Infants:* PO, 100 mg or 30 drops of elixir initially, gradually increased to 300 mg or 5 mL of elixir daily (15–37.5 mg elemental iron), in divided doses | For treatment of iron deficiency anemia |
| **Ferrous sulfate** (Feosol) Pregnancy Category A | *Adults:* PO, 325 mg–1.2 g (60–240 mg elemental iron) daily in 3 or 4 divided doses *Children: 6–12 y:* PO 120–600 mg (24–120 mg elemental iron) daily, in divided doses *<6 y:* 300 mg (60 mg elemental iron) daily, in divided doses | |
| **Iron dextran injection** (InFeD) Pregnancy Category C | *Adults:* Dosage is calculated for individual clients according to hemoglobin and weight (see manufacturer's literature). A small test dose is required before therapeutic doses are given. *Children:* Dosage is calculated for individual clients according to hemoglobin and weight (see manufacturer's literature). A small test dose is required before therapeutic doses are given. | |
| *Zinc Preparation* | | |
| **Zinc sulfate** Pregnancy Category C | *Adults:* PO, 25–50 mg elemental zinc (eg, zinc sulfate 110–220 mg) daily | To prevent or treat zinc deficiency |

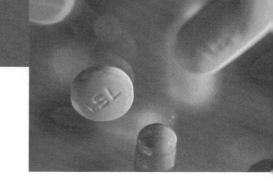

# Drugs Used in Dermatologic Conditions

Many different agents are used to prevent or treat dermatologic disorders. Most agents fit into one or more of the following categories:

- **Antimicrobials** are used to treat infections caused by bacteria, fungi, and viruses (see Chaps. 28 through 33). When used in dermatologic infections, antimicrobials may be administered locally (topically) or systemically (orally or parenterally).
- **Antiseptics** kill or inhibit the growth of bacteria, viruses, or fungi. They are used primarily to prevent infection. They are occasionally used to treat dermatologic infections. Skin surfaces should be clean before application of antiseptics.
- **Astringents** (eg, dilute solutions of aluminum salts) are used for their drying effects on exudative lesions.
- **Corticosteroids** (see Chap. 36) are used to treat the inflammation present in many dermatologic conditions. They are most often applied topically but also may be given orally or parenterally.
- **Emollients** or lubricants (eg, mineral oil, lanolin) are used to relieve pruritus and dryness of the skin.
- **Enzymes** are used to débride burn wounds, decubitus ulcers, and venous stasis ulcers. They promote healing by removing necrotic tissue.
- **Immunomodulators** are newer drugs with immunosuppressant and anti-inflammatory effects. They are not steroids, do not cause the adverse effects associated with corticosteroids, and may be used as corticosteroid substitutes. They are used to treat moderate to severe atopic dermatitis.
- **Keratolytic agents** (eg, salicylic acid) are used to remove warts, corns, calluses, and other keratin-containing skin lesions.
- **Retinoids** are vitamin A derivatives that are active in proliferation and differentiation of skin cells. These agents are commonly used to treat acne, psoriasis, aging and wrinkling of skin from sunlight exposure, and skin cancers. These drugs have been associated with severe fetal abnormalities.
- **Sunscreens** are used to protect the skin from the damaging effects of UV radiation, thereby decreasing skin cancer and signs of aging, including wrinkles.

Most dermatologic medications are applied topically. To be effective, topical agents must be in contact with the underlying skin or mucous membrane. Numerous dosage forms have been developed for topical application of drugs to various parts of the body and for various therapeutic purposes. Basic components of topical agents are one or more active ingredients and a usually inactive vehicle. Commonly used vehicles and dosage forms include ointments, creams, lotions, aerosols, gels, otic solutions, and vaginal and rectal suppositories. Many topical drug preparations are available in several dosage forms. Topical medications are used primarily for local effects; systemic effects are usually undesirable. Common topical antimicrobial agents, corticosteroids, and miscellaneous agents are described in the following tables.

## Topical Antimicrobial Agents

| Generic/Trade Name | Indications for Use | Application |
|---|---|---|
| *Antibacterial Agents* | | |
| **Azelaic acid** (Azelex) Pregnancy Category B | Acne | To lesions, twice daily |
| **Bacitracin** (Baciguent) Pregnancy Category C | Bacterial skin infections | To affected area, after cleansing, 1–3 times daily, small amount. Cover with a sterile dressing, if desired. Do not use longer than 1 wk. |
| **Benzoyl peroxide** Pregnancy Category C | Acne | To affected areas, after cleansing, 1–3 times daily |
| **Clindamycin** (Cleocin T) Pregnancy Category B | Acne vulgaris | To affected areas, twice daily |
| **Erythromycin** (Aknemycin) Pregnancy Category B | Acne vulgaris | To affected areas, after cleansing, twice daily, morning and evening |
| **Gentamicin** (Garamycin) Pregnancy Category C | Skin infections caused by susceptible strains of streptococci, staphylococci, and gram-negative organisms | To infected areas, 3–4 times daily. Cover with dressing if desired. |
| **Mafenide** (Sulfamylon) Pregnancy Category C | Treatment of burn wounds | To affected area, after cleansing, once or twice daily, using sterile technique |
| **Metronidazole** (MetroLotion) Pregnancy Category B | Rosacea | To affected areas, after cleansing, twice daily, morning and evening |
| **Mupirocin** (Bactroban) Pregnancy Category B | Impetigo caused by *Staphylococcus aureus,* beta-hemolytic streptococci, or *Streptococcus pyogenes* Eradication of nasal colonization with methicillin-resistant *S. aureus* | Impetigo: Ointment, to affected areas, 3 times daily. Cover with dressing, if desired. Other skin lesions: Cream, 3 times daily for 10 d. Cover with dressing, if desired. Eradication of nasal colonization: Ointment from single-use tube, one half in each nostril, morning and evening for 5 d |
| **Neomycin** (Myciguent) Pregnancy Category C | Bacterial skin infections | To affected area, after cleansing, 1–3 times daily, small, fingertip-size amount. Cover with a sterile dressing, if desired. Do not use longer than 1 wk. |
| **Silver sulfadiazine** (Silvadene) Pregnancy Category B | Prevent or treat infection in burn wounds caused by *Pseudomonas* and many other organisms | To affected area, after cleansing, once or twice daily, using sterile technique |
| **Sulfacetamide sodium** (Sebizon) Pregnancy Category C | Bacterial skin infections Seborrheic dermatitis | Skin infections: 2–4 times daily until infection clears Seborrhea: to scalp and adjacent skin areas, at bedtime |
| **Tetracycline** (Topicycline) Pregnancy Category D | Acne vulgaris | To affected areas, twice daily, morning and evening |
| *Combination Products* | | |
| **Bacitracin and polymyxin B** (Polysporin) Pregnancy Category C | Bacterial skin infections | To lesions, 2–3 times daily |
| **Erythromycin/benzoyl peroxide** (Benzamycin) Pregnancy Category C | Acne | To affected areas, after cleansing, twice daily, morning and evening |
| **Neomycin, polymyxin B and bacitracin** (Neosporin) Pregnancy Category C | Bacterial skin infections | To lesions, 2–3 times daily |

*(continued)*

## Topical Antimicrobial Agents (Continued)

| Generic/Trade Name | Indications for Use | Application |
|---|---|---|
| *Antifungal Agents* | | |
| **Amphotericin B** (Fungizone) Pregnancy Category B | Cutaneous candidiasis | To affected areas, 2–4 times daily |
| **Butenafine** (Mentax) Pregnancy Category B | Tinea pedis | To affected area, once daily for 4 wk |
| **Ciclopirox** (Loprox) Pregnancy Category B | Tinea infections Cutaneous candidiasis | To affected area, twice daily for 2–4 wk |
| **Clioquinol** (Vioform) Pregnancy Category C | Fungal skin infection and inflammation | To affected areas, 2–3 times daily. Do not use for >1 wk. |
| **Clotrimazole** (Lotrimin, Mycelex) Pregnancy Category B | Tinea infections Cutaneous candidiasis | To affected areas, twice daily, morning and evening |
| **Econazole** (Spectazole) Pregnancy Category C | Tinea infections Cutaneous candidiasis | Tinea infections: To affected areas, once daily Cutaneous candidiasis: To affected areas, twice daily |
| **Ketoconazole** (Nizoral) Pregnancy Category C | Tinea infections Cutaneous candidiasis Seborrheic dermatitis | Tinea infections and cutaneous candidiasis: To affected areas, once daily for 2–4 wk Seborrheic dermatitis: To affected areas twice daily for 4 wk or until clinical clearing |
| **Miconazole** (Micatin) Pregnancy Category C | Tinea infections Cutaneous candidiasis | To affected areas, twice daily for 2–4 wk |
| **Naftifine** (Naftin) Pregnancy Category B | Tinea infections | To affected areas, once daily with cream, twice daily with gel |
| **Nystatin** (Mycostatin) Pregnancy Category B | Candidiasis of skin and mucous membranes | To affected areas, after cleansing, 2–3 times daily until healing is complete |
| **Oxiconazole** (Oxistat) Pregnancy Category B | Tinea infections | To affected areas, once or twice daily for 2–4 wk |
| **Sulconazole** (Exelderm) Pregnancy Category C | Tinea infections | To affected areas, once or twice daily |
| **Terbinafine** (Lamisil) Pregnancy Category B | Tinea infections | To affected areas, twice daily for 1–4 wk |
| *Antiviral Agents* | | |
| **Acyclovir** (Zovirax) Pregnancy Category B | Herpes genitalis Herpes labialis in immunosuppressed clients | To lesions, q3h six times daily for 7 d |
| **Penciclovir** (Denavir) Pregnancy Category B | Herpes labialis | To lesions, q2h while awake for 4 d |

## Topical Corticosteroids

| Generic/Trade Name | Dosage Forms | Potency |
|---|---|---|
| **Alclometasone** (Aclovate) Pregnancy Category C | Cream, ointment | Low |
| **Amcinonide** (Cyclocort) Pregnancy Category C | Cream, lotion, ointment | High |
| **Augmented betamethasone dipropionate** (Diprolene) Pregnancy Category C | Cream, gel, lotion, ointment | Ointment very high; cream high |
| **Betamethasone dipropionate** (Alphatrex, others) Pregnancy Category C | Aerosol, cream, lotion, ointment | Cream and ointment high; lotion medium |
| **Betamethasone valerate** (Valisone, others) Pregnancy Category C | Cream, foam, lotion, ointment | Ointment high; cream medium |
| **Clobetasol** (Temovate) Pregnancy Category C | Cream, gel, ointment, scalp application | Very high |
| **Clocortolone** (Cloderm) Pregnancy Category C | Cream | Medium |
| **Desonide** (Tridesilon) Pregnancy Category C | Cream, lotion, ointment | Low |
| **Desoximetasone** (Topicort) Pregnancy Category C | Cream, gel, ointment | Medium |
| **Dexamethasone** (Decaderm, Decadron) Pregnancy Category C | Aerosol, cream | Low |
| **Diflorasone** (Florone, Maxiflor) Pregnancy Category C | Cream, ointment | Ointment, very high; cream, high |
| **Fluocinolone** (Synalar, others) Pregnancy Category C | Cream, oil, ointment, shampoo, solution | High |
| **Fluocinonide** (Lidex) Pregnancy Category C | Cream, gel, ointment, solution | High |
| **Flurandrenolide** (Cordran) Pregnancy Category C | Cream, lotion, ointment, tape | Medium |
| **Fluticasone** (Cutivate) Pregnancy Category C | Cream, ointment | Medium |
| **Halcinonide** (Halog) Pregnancy Category C | Cream, ointment, solution | High |
| **Halobetasol** (Ultravate) Pregnancy Category C | Cream, ointment | Very high |
| **Hydrocortisone** (Cortril, Hydrocortone, others) Pregnancy Category C | Cream, lotion, ointment, solution, spray, roll-on stick | Medium or low |
| **Mometasone** (Elocon) Pregnancy Category C | Cream, lotion, ointment | Medium |
| **Triamcinolone acetonide** (Aristocort, Kenalog, others) Pregnancy Category C | Aerosol, cream, lotion, ointment | 0.5% cream and ointment, high; lower concentrations, medium |

## Miscellaneous Dermatologic Agents

| Generic/Trade Name | Dermatologic Effects | Clinical Indications | Method of Administration |
|---|---|---|---|
| *Enzymes* | | | |
| **Collagenase** (Santyl) Pregnancy Category C | Débriding effects | Enzymatic débridement of infected wounds (eg, burn wounds, decubitus ulcers) | Topically once daily until the wound is cleansed of necrotic material |
| **Trypsin** (Granulex) Pregnancy Category unknown | Débriding effects | Débridement of infected wounds (eg, decubitus and varicose ulcers) | Topically by spray twice daily |
| *Immunomodulators* | | | |
| **Pimecrolimus** (Elidel) Pregnancy Category C | Anti-inflammatory | Atopic dermatitis | Topically to affected skin, once daily |
| **Tacrolimus** (Protopic) Pregnancy Category C | Anti-inflammatory | Atopic dermatitis | Topically to affected skin, twice daily |
| *Retinoids* | | | |
| **Acitretin** (Soriatane) Pregnancy Category X | A metabolite of etretinate | Severe psoriasis | PO, 25–50 mg/d |
| **Adapalene** (Differin) Pregnancy Category C | Reportedly causes less burning, itching, redness, and dryness than tretinoin | Acne vulgaris | Topically to skin lesions once daily |
| **Isotretinoin** (Accutane) Pregnancy Category X | Inhibits sebum production and keratinization | Severe cystic acne Disorders characterized by excessive keratinization (eg, pityriasis, ichthyosis) *Mycosis fungoides* | PO, 1–2 mg/kg/d, in 2 divided doses, for 15–20 wk |
| **Tazarotene** (Tazorac) Pregnancy Category X | A prodrug, mechanism of action is unknown | Acne Psoriasis | Topically to skin, after cleansing, once daily in the evening |
| **Tretinoin** (Retin-A) Pregnancy Category C | Irritant | Acne vulgaris | Topically to skin lesions once daily |
| *Other Agents* | | | |
| **Anthralin** (Anthra-Derm, others) Pregnancy Category C | Slows the rate of skin cell growth and replication | Psoriasis | Topically to lesions once daily or as directed |
| **Becaplermin** (Regranex) Pregnancy Category C | A recombinant human platelet-derived growth factor | Diabetic skin ulcers | Topically to ulcer, amount calculated according to size of the ulcer |
| **Calcipotriene** (Dovonex) Pregnancy Category C | Synthetic analog of vitamin D that helps to regulate skin cell production and development | Psoriasis | Topically to lesions twice daily |
| **Capsaicin** (Zostrix) Pregnancy Category C | Depletes substance P (which transmits pain impulses) in sensory nerves of the skin | Relief of pain associated with rheumatoid arthritis, osteo-arthritis, and neuralgias | Topically to affected area, up to 3–4 times daily |
| **Coal tar** (Balnetar, Zetar, others) Pregnancy Category C | Irritant | Psoriasis Dermatitis | Topically to skin, in various con-centrations and preparations (eg, creams, lotions, shampoos, bath emulsion). Also available in combination with hydrocortisone and other substances |
| **Colloidal oatmeal** (Aveeno) Pregnancy Category A | Antipruritic | Pruritus | Topically as a bath solution (1 cup in bathtub of water) |

*(continued)*

## Miscellaneous Dermatologic Agents (Continued)

| Generic/Trade Name | Dermatologic Effects | Clinical Indications | Method of Administration |
|---|---|---|---|
| **Dextranomer** (Debrisan) Pregnancy Category Unknown | Absorbs exudates from wound surfaces | Cleansing of ulcers (eg, venous stasis, decubitus) and wounds (eg, burn, surgical, traumatic) | Apply to a clean, moist wound surface q12h initially, then less often as exudate decreases |
| **Fluorouracil** (Efudex) Pregnancy Category X | Antineoplastic | Actinic keratoses Superficial basal cell carcinomas | Topically to skin lesions twice daily for 2–6 wk |
| **Masoprocol** (Actinex) Pregnancy Category B | Inhibits proliferation of keratin-containing cells | Actinic keratoses | Topically to skin lesions morning and evening for 28 d |
| **Salicylic acid** Pregnancy Category C; D third trimester | Keratolytic, antifungal | Removal of warts, corns, calluses Superficial fungal infections Seborrheic dermatitis Acne Psoriasis | Topically to lesions |
| **Selenium sulfide** (Selsun) Pregnancy Category C | Antifungal, antidandruff | Dandruff Tinea versicolor | Topically to scalp as shampoo once or twice weekly |

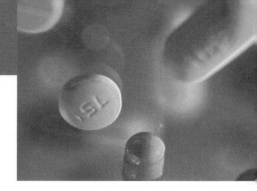

# G

# Ophthalmics and Otics

Drugs used to diagnose or treat ophthalmic and otic disorders represent a variety of therapeutic classifications, most of which are discussed in other chapters. Drug therapy of ophthalmic conditions is unique because of the location, structure, and function of the eye. Many systemic drugs are unable to cross the blood–eye barrier and achieve therapeutic concentrations in ocular structures. In general, penetration is greater if the drug achieves a high concentration in the blood, is fat soluble, and is poorly bound to serum proteins, and if inflam- mation is present. Because of the difficulties associated with systemic therapy, various methods of administering drugs locally have been developed. The most common and preferred method is topical application of oph- thalmic solutions (eyedrops) to the conjunctiva.

Drugs used to manage infective otic conditions are preparations that are used to treat similar infections aris- ing in other areas of the body. Major classes used in oph- thalmic and external otic preparations are included in the following tables.

## Ophthalmic Agents

| Generic/Trade Name | Routes and Dosage Ranges (Adults) | Overall Indications for Use of Drug Class |
|---|---|---|
| *Autonomic Drugs* | | |
| **ADRENERGICS** | | Decreases production of aqueous humor, produces mydriasis, decreases IOP, and reduces photophobia |
| **Dipivefrin** (0.1% solution) (Propine) Pregnancy Category B | 1 drop in affected eye(s) q12h | |
| **Epinephrine** (0.5%, 1%, and 2% solutions) (Epifrin, Glaucon) Pregnancy Category C | 1 drop in each eye once or twice daily *Children:* Same as adults | |
| **Phenylephrine** (2.5% and 10% solutions) (Neo-Synephrine) Pregnancy Category C | Before ophthalmoscopy or refraction, 1 drop of 2.5% or 10% solution Preoperatively, 1 drop of 2.5% or 10% solution 30–60 min before surgery Postoperatively, 1 drop of 10% solution once or twice daily *Children:* refraction, 1 drop of 2.5% solution | |
| **ALPHA$_2$-ADRENERGIC AGONISTS** | | Decreases IOP |
| **Apraclonidine** (Iopidine) Pregnancy Category C | 1–2 drops in affected eye(s) 3 times daily | |
| **Brimonidine** (Alphagan) Pregnancy Category B | 1 drop in affected eye(s) 3 times daily, q8h | |
| **BETA BLOCKERS** | | Decreases production of aqueous humor and reduces IOP |
| **Betaxolol** (Betoptic) Pregnancy Category C by manu- facturer; D, second and third trimesters by expert opinion | 1–2 drops in affected eye(s) twice daily | |
| **Carteolol** (Ocupress) Pregnancy Category C by manufac- turer; D, second and third trimesters by expert opinion | 1 drop in affected eye(s) twice daily | |

*(continued)*

| Generic/Trade Name | Routes and Dosage Ranges (Adults) | Overall Indications for Use of Drug Class |
|---|---|---|
| **Levobunolol** (Betagan) Pregnancy Category C | 1–2 drops in affected eye(s) once or twice daily | |
| **Metipranolol** (OptiPranolol) Pregnancy Category C | 1 drop in affected eye(s) twice daily | |
| **Timolol maleate** (Timoptic, Timoptic-XE) Pregnancy Category C by manufacturer; D, second and third trimesters by expert opinion | 1 drop in affected eye(s) twice daily; gel, 1 drop once daily | |
| **CHOLINERGICS** | | Increases outflow of aqueous humor; miosis |
| **Pilocarpine** (0.25%–10% solutions) (Isopto Carpine, Pilocar) Pregnancy Category C | Glaucoma, 1 drop of 1% or 2% solution in each eye 3–4 times daily | |
| **Pilocarpine ocular system** (Ocusert Pilo-20 or -40) Pregnancy Category C | One system in conjunctival sac per week | |
| **Carbachol** (Carboptic) Pregnancy Category C | 2 drops of 0.75%–3% solution into eye(s) up to 3 times daily | |
| **ANTICHOLINESTERASE AGENT** | | Treatment of glaucoma, through increased outflow of aqueous humor; miosis |
| **Demecarium bromide** (Humorsol) Pregnancy Category X | 1 drop of 0.125%–0.25% solution in each eye twice a day to twice a week | |
| **ANTICHOLINERGICS** | | For mydriasis, cycloplegia, and treatment of photophobia |
| **Atropine sulfate** (0.5%–3% solutions) Pregnancy Category C | Before intraocular surgery, 1 drop After intraocular surgery, 1 drop once daily | |
| **Cyclopentolate hydrochloride** (Cyclogyl) Pregnancy Category C | For refraction, 1 drop of 0.5% or 2% solution Before ophthalmoscopy, 1 drop of 0.5% solution *Children:* For refraction, 1 drop of 0.5%, 1%, or 2% solution, repeated in 10 min | |
| **Homatropine hydrobromide** (2% and 5% solutions) Pregnancy Category C | Refraction, 1 drop of 5% solution every 5 min for 2 or 3 doses or 1–2 drops of 2% solution every 10–15 min for 5 doses Uveitis, 1 drop of 2% or 5% solution 2–3 times daily | |
| **Tropicamide** (0.5% and 1% solutions) (Mydriacyl) Pregnancy Category C | Before refraction or ophthalmoscopy, 1 drop, repeated in 5 min, then every 20–30 min as needed to maintain mydriasis | |
| *Diuretics* | | |
| **CARBONIC ANHYDRASE INHIBITORS** | | Decrease production of aqueous humor; decrease IOP |
| **Acetazolamide** (Diamox, Diamox Sequels) Pregnancy Category C | PO, 250 mg q6h Sustained-release capsules: PO, 500 mg q12h IV, IM, 5–10 mg/kg/d in divided doses, q6h *Children:* PO, 10–15 mg/kg/d in divided doses, q6–8h IV, IM, 5–10 mg/kg q6h | |
| **Brinzolamide** (Azopt) Pregnancy Category C | 1 drop 3 times daily | |
| **Dorzolamide** (Trusopt) Pregnancy Category C | 1 drop 3 times daily | |

*(continued)*

| Generic/Trade Name | Routes and Dosage Ranges (Adults) | Overall Indications for Use of Drug Class |
|---|---|---|
| **OSMOTIC AGENTS** | | Reduces volume of vitreous humor; decreases IOP |
| **Glycerin** (Osmoglyn) Pregnancy Category C | PO, 1–1.5 g/kg, usually as a 50% or 75% solution 1–1½ h before surgery *Children:* Same as adults | |
| **Isosorbide** (Ismotic) Pregnancy Category C | Emergency reduction of IOP, PO, 1.5 g/kg up to 4 times daily | |
| **Mannitol** (Osmitrol) Pregnancy Category C | IV, 1.5–2 g/kg as a 20% solution over 30–60 min *Children:* Same as adults | |
| **PROSTAGLANDIN ANALOGS** | | Decreases IOP |
| **Bimatoprost** (Lumigan) Pregnancy Category C | 1 drop once daily in the evening | |
| **Latanoprost** (Xalatan) Pregnancy Category C | 1 drop once daily in the evening | |
| **Travoprost** (Travatan) Pregnancy Category C | 1 drop once daily in the evening | |
| **Unoprostone** (Rescula) Pregnancy Category C | 1 drop twice daily | |
| *Miscellaneous Agents* | | |
| **ANESTHETICS, LOCAL** | | Provides surface anesthesia of conjunctiva and cornea |
| **Proparacaine** (Alcaine, Ophthaine) Pregnancy Category C | Minor procedures, 1–2 drops of 0.5% solution | |
| **Tetracaine** (Pontocaine) Pregnancy Category C | Minor procedures, 1–2 drops of 0.5% solution | |
| **LUBRICANTS** | | Serves as "artificial tears" or to moisten contact lenses |
| **Methylcellulose** (Methulose) Pregnancy Category C | 1–2 drops as needed | |
| **Polyvinyl alcohol** (Liquifilm) Pregnancy Category C | 1–2 drops as needed | |
| *Antibacterial Agents* | | Treatment of bacterial infections of eye |
| **Ciprofloxacin 3.5 mg/mL solution** (Ciloxan) Pregnancy Category C | *Adults:* Corneal ulcer, day 1, 2 drops q15 min for 6 h, then q30min for rest of day; day 2, 2 drops q1h; days 3–14, 2 drops q4h *Children:* Conjunctivitis, 1–2 drops q2h while awake for 2 d, then 1–2 drops q4h while awake for 5 d Safety and efficacy not established in infants <1 y | |
| **Erythromycin 5% ointment** (Ilotycin) Pregnancy Category B | *Children:* Prevention of neonatal gonococcal or chlamydial conjunctivitis, 0.5–1 cm in each eye | |
| **Gentamicin 3 mg/mL solution or 3 mg/g ointment** (Garamycin) Pregnancy Category C | 1 drop q1–4h; ointment, instill 2–3 times daily | |
| **Levofloxacin 5 mg/mL solution** (Quixin) Pregnancy Category C | 1–2 drops q2h up to 8 doses/d for 1–2 d, then q4h up to 4 doses/d for 5 d Dosage not established | |
| **Norfloxacin 3 mg/mL solution** (Chibroxin) Pregnancy Category C | 1–2 drops, 4 times daily, up to 7 d Same as adults for children 1 y and older | |

| Generic/Trade Name | Routes and Dosage Ranges | Overall Indications for Use of Drug Class |
|---|---|---|
| **Ofloxacin 3 mg/mL solution** (Ocuflox) <br> Pregnancy Category C | Conjunctivitis, 1–2 drops q2–4h while awake for 2 d, then 4 times daily for 3–5 d <br> Same as adults for children 1 y and older <br> Corneal ulcer, 1–2 drops q30min while awake, q4–6h during sleep, for 1–2 d, then q1h while awake for 4–6 d, then q4h while awake until healed <br> Dosage not established | |
| **Sulfacetamide 10% solution or ointment** (Bleph-10 Liquifilm), **15% solution** (Isopto Cetamide), **10% and 30% solution, 10% ointment** (Sodium Sulamyd) <br> Pregnancy Category C | Conjunctivitis, corneal ulcers, or other superficial infections caused by susceptible organisms: 1–2 drops q4h or 0.5 inch ointment 3–4 times daily, for 7–10 days <br> Safety and efficacy not established. Contraindicated in infants <2 mo of age | |
| **Sulfisoxazole 4% solution** (Gantrisin) <br> Pregnancy Category B; D (near term) | *Adults:* 1–2 drops 3 or more times daily <br> *Children:* Safety and efficacy not established. Contraindicated in infants <2 mo of age | |
| **Tobramycin (0.3% solution and 3 mg/g ointment)** (Tobrex) <br> Pregnancy Category C | *Adults:* 1–2 drops 2–6 times daily or ointment 2–3 times daily <br> *Children:* See manufacturer's instructions | |
| *Antiviral Agent* | | Treatment of viral infections of eye |
| **Trifluridine 1% solution** (Viroptic) <br> Pregnancy Category C | *Adults:* Keratoconjunctivitis or corneal ulcers caused by herpes simplex virus: 1 drop q2h while awake (maximum, 9 drops/d) until corneal ulcer heals, then 1 drop q4h (minimum, 5 drops/d), for 7 d <br> *Children: >6 y:* Same as adults | |
| *Antifungal Agent* | | Treatment of fungal eye infections |
| **Natamycin 5% suspension** (Natacyn) <br> Pregnancy Category C | *Adults:* 1 drop q1–2h for 3–4 d, then q3–4h, for 14–21 d <br> *Children:* Safety and efficacy not established | |
| *Antiallergic Agents* | | Treatment of allergic conjunctivitis |
| **Azelastine** (Optivar) <br> Pregnancy Category C | *Adults:* 1 drop in affected eye(s) twice daily | Treatment of seasonal allergic conjunctivitis, keratitis, and keratoconjunctivitis |
| **Cromolyn** (Crolom, Opticrom) <br> Pregnancy Category B | *Adults:* 1–2 drops in each eye 4–6 times daily at regular intervals | |
| **Emedastine** (Emadine) <br> Pregnancy Category B | *Adults:* 1–2 drops twice daily | |
| **Ketotifen** (Zaditor) <br> Pregnancy Category C | *Adults:* 1 drop in affected eye(s) q8–12h | |
| **Levocabastine** (Livostin) <br> Pregnancy Category C | *Adults:* 1 drop in affected eyes 4 times daily, for up to 2 wk | |
| **Lodoxamide** (Alomide) <br> Pregnancy Category B | *Adults:* 1–2 drops in affected eye(s) 4 times daily, for up to 3 mo | |
| **Olopatadine** (Patanol) <br> Pregnancy Category C | *Adults:* 1–2 drops twice daily | |

*(continued)*

| Generic/Trade Name | Routes and Dosage Ranges | Overall Indications for Use of Drug Class |
|---|---|---|
| *Corticosteroids* | | Treatment of Inflammatory disorders of the conjunctiva, cornea, eyelid, and anterior eyeball (e.g. conjunctivitis, keratitis) |
| **Dexamethasone** (Decadron, Maxidex) <br> Pregnancy Category C | *Adult:* Solution or suspension 1–2 drops q1h daytime, q2h nighttime until response; then 1 drop q4h <br> Postoperative inflammation, 1–2 drops 4 times daily, starting 24 h after surgery, for 2 wk <br> Ointment thin strip 3–4 times daily until response, then once or twice daily | Treatment of corneal injury from chemical, radiation or thermal burns, or penetration of foreign bodies <br> Prevention of graft rejection after corneal transplant |
| **Fluorometholone** (FML) <br> Pregnancy Category C | *Adults:* Solution 1 drop q1–2h until response, then less often <br> Ointment thin strip 3–4 times daily until response, then once or twice daily | |
| **Loteprednol** (Lotemax, Alrex) <br> Pregnancy Category C | *Adults:* Allergic conjunctivitis, 0.2%, 1 drop in affected eye(s) 4 times daily <br> Keratitis, 0.5%, 1–2 drops in affected eye(s) 4 times daily <br> Postoperative inflammation, 0.5%, 1–2 drops in affected eye(s) 4 times daily starting 24 h after surgery and continuing for 2 wk | |
| **Medrysone** (HMS) <br> Pregnancy Category C | *Adults:* 1 drop q1–2h until response obtained, then less frequently | |
| **Prednisolone** (Econopred, others) <br> Pregnancy Category C | *Adults:* Solution or suspension 1–2 drops q1–2h until response, then 1 drop q4h, then less frequently <br> Ointment thin strip 3–4 times daily until response, then once or twice daily | |
| **Rimexolone** (Vexol) <br> Pregnancy Category C | *Adults:* Uveitis, 1–2 drops in affected eye q1h during waking hours for 1 wk, then 1 drop q2h for 1 wk, then taper until uveitis resolved <br> Postoperative inflammation, 1–2 drops in affected eye(s) 4 times daily starting 24 h after surgery and continuing for 2 wk | |
| *Nonsteroidal Anti-inflammatory Drugs* | | Multiple Indications highlighted below |
| **Diclofenac** (Voltaren) <br> Pregnancy Category B; D (third trimester) | *Adults:* 1 drop to affected eye 4 times daily, starting 24 h after surgery, for 2 wk | Treatment of inflammation after cataract surgery |
| **Flurbiprofen** (Ocufen) <br> Pregnancy Category C; D (third trimester) | *Adults:* 1 drop every 30 min for 4 doses, starting 2 h before surgery | Inhibition of pupil constriction during eye surgery |
| **Ketorolac** (Acular) <br> Pregnancy Category C | *Adults:* 1 drop 4 times daily for approximately 1 wk | Treatment of ocular itching due to seasonal allergic conjunctivitis |
| **Suprofen** (Profenal) <br> Pregnancy Category C | *Adults:* 2 drops at 3, 2, and 1 h before surgery or q4h while awake the day before surgery | Inhibition of pupil constriction during eye surgery |

IOP, intraocular pressure.

## Otic Preparations

| Generic/Trade Name | Routes and Dosage Ranges | Overall Indications for Use of Drug Class |
|---|---|---|
| *Cerumenolytics* | | Cerumenolytics soften and facilitate removal of impacted ear wax |
| **Antipyrine and benzocaine** (Auralgan) Pregnancy Category C | Ear pain: fill ear canal and place moistened cotton plug in external ear; may repeat every 1–2 h until pain and congestion is relieved Ear wax removal: instill drops 3–4 times daily for 2–3 d | Added analgesic relieves the pain associated with acute otitis media, otitis externa, and swimmer's ear |
| **Triethanolamine polypeptide oleate-condensate** (Cerumenex) Pregnancy Category C | Ear wax removal: fill ear canal and place cotton plug in external ear. After 15–30 min, flush ear with lukewarm water Repeat procedure for particularly hard impactions | |
| *Antibiotics* | | Treatment of bacterial infections of ear |
| **Acetic acid, propylene glycol diacetate, and hydrocortisone** (Acetasol) Pregnancy Category C | Instill 4 drops in ear(s) 3–4 times daily | Combination antibiotic and corticosteroid |
| **Chloramphenicol** (Chloromycetin Otic) Pregnancy Category C | Instill 4 drops in ear(s) 3–4 times daily | Antibiotic |
| **Polymyxin B** Pregnancy Category B by expert opinion | 1–2 drops 3–4 times daily | Antibiotic used in combinations with other drugs |

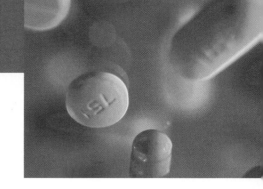

# Nasal Decongestants, Antitussives, and Expectorants

The drugs discussed here are used to treat upper respiratory disorders and symptoms such as the common cold, sinusitis, nasal congestion, cough, and excessive secretions.

Some of these diverse drugs are discussed more extensively in other chapters; they are discussed in the following table in relation to their use in upper respiratory conditions.

## Nasal Decongestants, Antitussives, and Expectorants

| Generic/Trade Name | Routes and Dosage Ranges | Overall Indications for Use of Drug Class |
|---|---|---|
| *Nasal Decongestants* | | Relieves nasal obstruction and discharge |
| **Ephedrine sulfate 0.25% solution**<br>Pregnancy Category C | *Adults:* Topically, 2–3 sprays in each nostril no more often than q4h. Maximum, 6 doses/24 h<br>*Children:* ≥12 y: Same as adults<br>6–11 y: 2–3 sprays in each nostril no more often than q4h<br>Maximum, 6 doses/24 h<br><6 y: Not recommended | |
| **Naphazoline** (Privine) 0.05% spray or drops<br>Pregnancy Category C | *Adults:* Topically, 1–2 sprays or drops no more often than q6h. Maximum, 4 doses/24 h<br>*Children:* ≥12 y: Same as adults<br><12 y: Not recommended | |
| **Oxymetazoline** (Afrin) **0.05% spray**<br>Pregnancy Category C | *Adults:* Topically, 2–3 sprays in each nostril, q10–12h<br>Maximum, 2 doses/24 h<br>*Children:* ≥6 y: Same as adults<br><6 y: Not recommended | |
| **Phenylephrine** (Neo-Synephrine)<br>Pregnancy Category C | *Adults:* PO, 10–20 mg q4h<br>Maximum, 120 mg/24 h<br>Topically, 2–3 sprays or drops of 0.25%, 0.5%, or 1% solution in each nostril no more often than q4h. Maximum, 6 doses/24 h<br>*Children:* ≥12 y: Same as adults<br>6–11 y: PO, 10 mg q4h<br>Maximum, 60 mg/24 h<br>Topically, 2–3 sprays of 0.25% solution in each nostril no more often than q4h<br>Maximum, 6 doses/24 h<br>2–5 y: topically, 2–3 drops of 0.125% solution no more often than q4h<br>Maximum, 6 doses/24 h | |

*(continued)*

| Generic/Trade Name | Routes and Dosage Ranges | Overall Indications for Use of Drug Class |
|---|---|---|
| **Pseudoephedrine** (Sudafed, Dimetapp)<br>Pregnancy Category C | *Adults:* Regular tablets, PO, 60 mg q4–6h<br>Extended-release tablets, PO, 120 mg q12h or 240 mg q24h<br>Maximum, 240 mg in 24 h<br>*Children:* ≥12 y: Same as adults for regular and extended release tablets<br>6–12 y: 30 mg q4–6h<br>Maximum, 120 mg/24 h<br>2–5 y: PO, 15 mg q4–6h<br>Maximum, 60 mg/24 h<br><2 y: Consult pediatrician | |
| **Tetrahydrozoline** (Tyzine)<br>0.1% solution<br>Pregnancy Category C | *Adults:* Topically, 2–4 drops or 3–4 sprays in each nostril, no more often than q3h<br>Maximum, 8 doses/24 h<br>*Children:* ≥6 y: Same as adults<br>2–5 y: Spray not recommended. 2–3 drops of 0.05% solution in each nostril no more often than q3h<br>Maximum, 8 doses/24 h | |
| **Xylometazoline** (Otrivin)<br>Pregnancy Category C | *Adults:* Topically, 0.1% solution, 1–3 sprays or 2–3 drops in each nostril q8–10h<br>Maximum, 3 doses/24 h<br>*Children:* ≥12 y: Same as adult<br>2–11 y: Topically, 0.05%, 1 spray, or 2–3 drops in each nostril q8–10h<br>Maximum, 3 doses/24 h | |
| *Narcotic Antitussive* | | Suppresses cough center in the medulla oblongata of the cough receptors in the throat, trachea, or lungs |
| **Codeine**<br>Pregnancy Category C; D with prolonged use or high doses at term | *Adults:* PO, 10–20 mg q4–6h<br>Maximum, 120 mg/24 h<br>*Children:* 6–12 y: PO, 5–10 mg q4–6h<br>Maximum, 60 mg/24 h<br>2–6 y: PO, 2.5–5 mg q4–6h<br>Maximum, 30 mg/24 h | |
| *Nonnarcotic Antitussive* | | |
| **Dextromethorphan** (Benylin DM, others)<br>Pregnancy Category C | *Adults:* Liquid, lozenges, and syrup, 10–30 mg q4–8h<br>Maximum, 120 mg/24 h<br>Sustained action liquid (Delsym), PO, 60 mg q12h<br>*Children:* >12 y: Same as adults<br>6–12 y: 5–10 mg q4h or 15 mg q6–8h<br>Maximum, 60 mg/24 h<br>2–6 y: 2.5–7.5 mg q4–8h<br>Maximum, 30 mg/24 h<br>6–12 y: PO, 5–10 mg q4h or 15 mg q6–8h<br>Maximum dose, 60 mg/24h<br>Sustained action liquid, 6–12 y: 30 mg q12h<br>2–5 y: 15 mg q12h | |

*(continued)*

## Nasal Decongestants, Antitussives, and Expectorants (Continued)

| Generic/Trade Name | Routes and Dosage Ranges | Overall Indications for Use of Drug Class |
|---|---|---|
| *Expectorant* | | Liquefies respiratory secretions and allows for easier removal |
| **Guaifenesin** (glyceryl guaiacolate) (Robitussin, others) Pregnancy Category C | PO, 100–400 mg q4h Maximum, 2400 mg/24 h *Children:* 12 y and older: Same as adults 6–12 y: PO, 100–200 mg q4h Maximum, 1200 mg/24 h 2–6 y: PO, 50–100 mg q4h Maximum, 600 mg/24 h | |
| *Mucolytic* | | Liquefies mucus in the respiratory tract |
| **Acetylcysteine** (Mucomyst) Pregnancy Category B | *Adults:* Nebulization, 1–10 mL of a 20% solution or 2–20 mL of a 10% solution q2–6h Instillation, 1–2 mL of a 10% or 20% solution q1–4h Acetaminophen overdosage: PO, 140 mg/kg initially, then 70 mg/kg q4h for 17 doses; dilute a 10% or 20% solution to a 5% solution with cola, fruit juice, or water *Children:* Acetaminophen overdosage; see literature | |

## Representative Multi-ingredient Nonprescription Cold, Cough, and Sinus Remedies

| Trade Name | Antihistamine | Ingredients | | | |
|---|---|---|---|---|---|
| | | Nasal Decongestant | Analgesic | Antitussive | Expectorant |
| Actifed Cold & Allergy | Triprolidine, 2.5 mg/tab | Pseudoephedrine, 60 mg/tab | | | |
| Advil Cold and Sinus Tablets | | Pseudoephedrine, 30 mg | Ibuprofen, 200 mg | | |
| Cheracol D Cough Liquid | | | | Dextromethorphan, 10 mg/5 mL | Guaifenesin, 100 mg/5 mL |
| Comtrex Cold & Sinus Tablets | Brompheniramine, 2 mg/tab | Pseudoephedrine, 30 mg/tab | Acetaminophen, 500 mg/tab | | |
| Contac Day & Night Cold & Flu Tablets | (Day) (Night) Diphenhydramine, 50 mg/tab | Pseudoephedrine, 60 mg/tab Pseudoephedrine, 60 mg/tab | Acetaminophen, 650 mg/tab Acetaminophen, 650 mg/tab | Dextromethorphan, 30 mg/tab | |
| Coricidin D Cold, Flu & Sinus Tablets | Chlorpheniramine, 2 mg/tab | Pseudoephedrine, 30 mg/tab | Acetaminophen, 325 mg/tab | | |
| Dimetapp Cold and Allergy Elixir | Brompheniramine, 1 mg/5 mL | Pseudoephedrine, 15 mg/5 mL | | | |
| Dristan Cold Formula | Chlorpheniramine, 2 mg/tab | Phenylephrine, 5 mg/tab | Acetaminophen, 325 mg/tab | | |

*(continued)*

| Trade Name | Antihistamine | Ingredients | | | |
| --- | --- | --- | --- | --- | --- |
| | | Nasal Decongestant | Analgesic | Antitussive | Expectorant |
| Motrin Sinus Tablets | | Pseudoephedrine, 30 mg/tab | Ibuprofen, 200 mg/tab | | |
| Robitussin Cold and Flu Tablets | | Pseudoephedrine, 10 mg/tab | Acetaminophen, 325 mg/tab | Dextromethorphan, 10 mg/tab | Guaifenesin, 200 mg/tab |
| Sinutab Sinus Allergy Maximum Strength Tablets | Chlorpheniramine, 2 mg/tab | Pseudoephedrine, 30 mg/tab | Acetaminophen, 500 mg/tab | | |
| TheraFlu Flu, Cold, and Cough Powder | Chlorpheniramine, 4 mg/pack | Pseudoephedrine, 60 mg/pack | Acetaminophen, 650 mg/pack | Dextromethorphan, 20 mg/pack | |
| Vicks NyQuil Cold & Flu Capsules | Doxylamine, 6.25 mg/capsule | Pseudoephedrine, 30 mg/capsule | Acetaminophen, 250 mg/capsule | Dextromethorphan, 10 mg/capsule | |

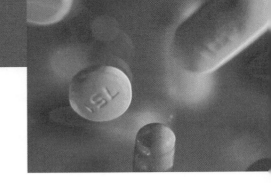

# Drugs That Modify Stool Consistency: Antidiarrheals, Laxatives, and Cathartics

Antidiarrheal drugs are used to treat diarrhea, defined as the frequent expulsion of liquid or semiliquid stools. Diarrhea is a symptom of numerous conditions that increase bowel motility, cause secretion or retention of fluids in the intestinal lumen, and cause inflammation or irritation of the gastrointestinal (GI) tract. As a result, bowel contents are rapidly propelled toward the rectum, and absorption of fluids and electrolytes is limited. Antidiarrheal drugs include a variety of agents, most of which are discussed in other chapters. When used for treatment of diarrhea, the drugs may be given to relieve the symptom (nonspecific therapy) or the underlying cause of the symptom (specific therapy).

Laxatives and cathartics are drugs used to promote bowel elimination (defecation). The term *laxative* implies mild effects and elimination of soft, formed stool. The term *cathartic* implies strong effects and elimination of liquid or semiliquid stool. Because the different effects depend more on the dose than on the particular drug used, the terms often are used interchangeably. Laxatives and cathartics are widely available on a nonprescription basis and are among the most frequently abused drugs. One reason for overuse is the common misconception that a daily bowel movement is necessary for health and well-being, even with little intake of food or fluids. This notion may lead to a vicious cycle of events in which a person fails to have a bowel movement, takes a strong laxative, again fails to have a bowel movement, and takes another laxative before the fecal column has had time to become reestablished (2 to 3 days with normal food intake). Thus, a pattern of laxative dependence and abuse is established. Individual drugs used to modify stool consistency are listed in the following tables.

## Antidiarrheal Drugs

| Generic/Trade Name | Routes and Dosage Ranges | Overall Indications for Use of Drug Class |
|---|---|---|
| *Opiate-related Drugs* | | |
| **Paregoric**<br>Pregnancy Category B; D with prolonged use or at high doses | *Adults:* PO, 5–10 mL one to four times daily (maximum of four doses) until diarrhea is controlled<br>*Children:* PO, 0.25–0.5 mL/kg one to four times daily (maximum of four doses) until diarrhea is controlled | Symptomatic treatment of acute diarrhea<br>Morphine is the active ingredient.<br>A Schedule III drug alone and a Schedule V in the small amounts combined with other drugs.<br>Recommended doses and short-term use do not produce euphoria, analgesia, or dependence. |
| **Difenoxin with atropine sulfate** (Motofen)<br>Pregnancy Category C | *Adults:* PO, 2 mg initially, then 1 mg after each loose stool or 1 mg q3–4h as needed; maximum dose, 8 mg (8 tablets)/24 h<br>*Children:* Safety and effectiveness not established for children <12 y | An active metabolite of diphenoxylate<br>Overdose may cause respiratory depression and coma.<br>Each tablet contains 1 mg of difenoxin and 0.025 mg of |

*(continued)*

| Generic/Trade Name | Routes and Dosage Ranges | Overall Indications for Use of Drug Class |
|---|---|---|
| | | atropine. The atropine is added to discourage overdose and abuse for opioid effects.<br>Contraindicated in children <2 y of age and clients who are allergic to the ingredients or have hepatic impairment.<br>A Schedule IV drug |
| **Diphenoxylate with atropine sulfate** (Lomotil)<br>Pregnancy Category C | *Adults:* PO, 5 mg (2 tablets or 10 mL of liquid) 3 or 4 times daily; maximal daily dose, 20 mg<br>*Children:* Liquid preparation (2.5 mg diphenoxylate and 0.025 mg atropine per 5 mL), PO, 4 times daily, as follows: 2 y, 11–14 kg: 1.5–3 mL; 3 y, 12–16 kg: 2–3 mL; 4 y, 14–20 kg: 2–4 mL; 5 y, 16–23 kg: 2.5–4.5 mL; 6–8 y, 17–32 kg: 2.5–5 mL; 9–12 y, 23–55 kg: 3.5–5 mL | A derivative of meperidine (Demerol).<br>Commonly prescribed; decreases intestinal motility<br>In recommended doses, does not produce euphoria, analgesia, or dependence. In high doses, produces morphine-like effects, including euphoria, dependence, and respiratory depression.<br>Naloxone (Narcan) is the antidote for overdose<br>Each tablet or 5 mL of liquid contains 2.5 mg of diphenoxylate and 0.025 mg of atropine<br>The atropine is added to discourage drug abuse<br>Contraindicated in severe liver disease, glaucoma, and children <2 y of age<br>A Schedule V drug |
| **Loperamide** (Imodium)<br>Pregnancy Category B | *Adults:* PO, 4 mg initially, then 2 mg after each loose stool to a maximum daily dose of 16 mg. For chronic diarrhea, dosage should be reduced to the lowest effective amount (average 4–8 mg daily)<br>*Children:* 2–5 y, 13–20 kg: PO, 1 mg three times daily; 6–8 y, 20–30 kg: PO, 2 mg twice daily; 8–12 y, >30 kg: PO, 2 mg 3 times daily | A derivative of meperidine; decreases intestinal motility<br>As effective as diphenoxylate, with fewer adverse effects in recommended doses. High doses may produce morphine-like effects<br>Safety not established for children <2 y of age<br>Naloxone (Narcan) is the antidote for overdose. |

### *Antibacterial Agents*

| Generic/Trade Name | Routes and Dosage Ranges | Overall Indications for Use of Drug Class |
|---|---|---|
| **Ciprofloxacin** (Cipro)<br>Pregnancy Category C | *Adults:* PO, 500 mg q12h for 5–7 days<br>*Children:* Not recommended for use | Diarrhea caused by susceptible strains of *Escherichia coli, Campylobacter jejuni,* and *Shigella* species<br>A fluoroquinolone (see Chap. 30) |
| **Erythromycin** (E-Mycin)<br>Pregnancy Category B | *Adults:* PO, 250 mg 4 times daily for 10–14 d<br>*Children:* PO, 30–50 mg/kg/d, in divided doses, for 10–14 d | Intestinal amebiasis caused by *Entamoeba histolytica*<br>A macrolide (see Chap. 30) |
| **Metronidazole** (Flagyl)<br>Pregnancy Category B; may be contraindicated in first trimester | *Adults: Clostridium difficile* infection: PO, 500 mg 3 times daily or 250 mg 4 times daily<br>Intestinal amebiasis: PO, 750 mg 3 times daily for 5–10 d<br>*Children:* Dosage not established for *C. difficile* infection<br>Intestinal amebiasis: PO, 35–50 mg/kg/24 h (maximum 750 mg/dose), in 3 divided doses for 10 d | Diarrhea and colitis caused by *C. difficile* organisms<br>Intestinal amebiasis (see Chap. 33) |

*(continued)*

| Generic/Trade Name | Routes and Dosage Ranges | Overall Indications for Use of Drug Class |
|---|---|---|
| **Trimethoprim-sulfamethoxazole** (TMP-SMX) (Bactrim, Septra) Pregnancy Category C | *Adults:* PO, 160 mg of TMP and 800 mg of SMX q12h for 5 d or longer *Children:* PO, 8 mg/kg of TMP and 40 mg/kg of SMX daily, in divided doses, q12h, for 5 d or longer | Diarrhea caused by susceptible strains of *E. coli* or *Shigella* organisms Traveler's diarrhea |
| ***Miscellaneous Drugs*** | | |
| **Bismuth subsalicylate** (Pepto-Bismol) Pregnancy Category C; D in third trimester | *Adults:* PO, 2 tablets or 30 mL every 30–60 min, if needed, up to 8 doses in 24 h *Children:* 9–12 y: PO, 1 tablet or 15 mL; 6–9 y: PO, 2/3 tablet or 10 mL; 3–6 y: PO, 1/3 tablet or 5 mL; under <3 y, consult pediatrician | Control of diarrhea, including traveler's diarrhea, and relief of abdominal cramping Has antimicrobial, antisecretory, and possibly anti-inflammatory effects |
| **Cholestyramine** (Questran) Pregnancy Category C | *Adults:* PO, 16–32 g/d in 120–180 mL of water, in two to four divided doses before or during meals and at bedtime | Diarrhea due to bile salts reaching the colon and causing a cathartic effect. "Bile salt diarrhea" is associated Crohn's disease or surgical excision of the ileum Binds and inactivates bile salts in the intestine |
| **Colestipol** (Colestid) Pregnancy Category C | *Adults:* PO, 15–30 g/d in 120–180 mL of water, in two to four divided doses before or during meals and at bedtime | Same as cholestyramine, above |
| **Octreotide** (Sandostatin) Pregnancy Category B | *Adults:* Sub-Q, IV, 50 mcg two to three times daily initially, then adjusted according to response *Children:* Dosage not established | Diarrhea associated with carcinoid tumors, HIV/AIDS, cancer chemotherapy or radiation, or diarrhea unresponsive to other drugs In GI tract, decreases secretions and motility |
| **Pancreatin or pancrelipase** (Viokase, Pancrease, Cotazym) Pregnancy Category C | *Adults:* PO, 1–3 tablets or capsules or 1–2 packets of powder with meals and snacks *Children:* PO, 1–3 tablets or capsules or 1–2 packets of powder with each meal | Diarrhea and malabsorption due to deficiency of pancreatic enzymes. Pancreatic enzymes used only for replacement Possibly effective for symptomatic treatment of diarrhea |
| **Psyllium preparations** (Metamucil) Pregnancy Category B | *Adults:* PO, 1–2 tsp, 2 or 3 times daily, in 8 oz of fluid | Absorbs water and decreases fluidity of stools |

## Laxatives and Cathartics

| Generic/Trade Name | Routes and Dosage Ranges | Overall Indications for Use of Drug Class |
|---|---|---|
| **Bulk-forming Laxatives** | | Swelling of substance adds bulk to fecal mass that stimulates peristalsis and defecation |
| **Methylcellulose** (Citrucel) <br> Pregnancy Category C | *Adults:* PO, 1 heaping tbsp 1–3 times daily with water (8 oz or more) <br> *Children:* PO, 1 level tbsp 1–3 times daily with water (4 oz) | |
| **Polycarbophil** (FiberCon, Mitrolan) <br> Pregnancy Category C | *Adults:* PO, 1 g 4 times daily or PRN with 8 oz of fluid; maximum dose, 6 g/24 h <br> *Children: 6–12 y:* PO, 500 mg 1–3 times daily or PRN; maximum dose, 3 g/24 h <br> *2–6 y:* PO, 500 mg 1 or 2 times daily or PRN; maximum dose, 1.5 g/24 h | |
| **Psyllium preparations** (Metamucil, Effersyllium, Serutan, Perdiem Plain) <br> Pregnancy Category B | *Adults:* PO, 4–10 g (1–2 tsp) 1–3 times daily, stirred in at least 8 oz of water or other liquid | |
| **Surfactant Laxatives (Stool Softeners)** | | To decrease surface tension of fecal mass to allow water to penetrate stool, act as a detergent to facilitate admixing of fat and water in stool |
| **Docusate sodium** (Colace, Doxinate) <br> Pregnancy Category C | *Adults:* PO, 50–200 mg daily <br> *Children: >12 y:* same dosage as adults <br> *3–12 y:* 20–120 mg daily <br> *<3 y:* 10–40 mg daily | |
| **Docusate calcium** (Surfak) <br> Pregnancy Category C | *Adults:* PO, 50–240 mg daily <br> *Children: >12 y:* same dosage as adults <br> *2–12 y:* 50–150 mg daily <br> *<2 y:* 25 mg daily | |
| **Docusate potassium** (Dialose) <br> Pregnancy Category C | *Adults:* PO, 100–300 mg daily <br> *Children: 6–12 y:* 100 mg at bedtime | |
| **Saline Cathartics** | | To increase osmotic pressure in the intestinal lumen and cause water to be retained when rapid bowel evacuation is needed |
| **Magnesium citrate solution** <br> Pregnancy Category B <br> **Magnesium hydroxide** (milk of magnesia, magnesia magma) <br> Pregnancy Category B | *Adults:* PO, 200 mL at bedtime <br> *Adults:* Regular liquid, PO, 15–60 mL at bedtime. Concentrated liquid, PO, 10–20 mL at bedtime <br> *Children:* Regular liquid, PO, 2.5–5 mL | |
| **Polyethylene glycol–electrolyte solution** (PEG 3350, sodium sulfate, sodium bicarbonate, sodium chloride, potassium chloride) (CoLyte, GoLYTELY) <br> Pregnancy Category C | *Adults:* For bowel cleansing before gastrointestinal examination: PO, 240 mL (8 oz) every 10 min until 4 L is consumed <br> *Children:* No recommended children's dose | |
| **Sodium phosphate and sodium biphosphate** (Fleet Phosphosoda, Fleet Enema) <br> Pregnancy Category C | *Adults:* PO, 20–40 mL in 8 oz of water <br> Rectal enema, 60–120 mL <br> *Children: ≥10 y:* PO, 10–20 mL in 8 oz of water <br> *5–10 y:* PO, 5–10 mL in 8 oz of water <br> Rectal enema, 60 mL | |
| **Stimulant Cathartics** | | To irritate the GI mucosa and pull water into bowel lumen. This moves feces to bowel rapidly to allow colonic absorption of fecal water, so that a watery stool is eliminated |
| **Bisacodyl** (Dulcolax) <br> Pregnancy Category C | *Adults:* PO, 10–15 mg <br> Rectal suppository, 10 mg <br> *Children: ≥6 y:* PO, 5–10 mg <br> *<2 y:* rectal suppository 5 mg | |
| **Cascara sagrada** <br> Pregnancy Category C | *Adults:* PO, tablets, 325 mg; fluid extract, 0.5–1.5 mL; aromatic fluid extract, 5 mL <br> *Children: ≥12 y:* Same as adults | |

*(continued)*

| Generic/Trade Name | Routes and Dosage Ranges | Overall Indications for Use of Drug Class |
|---|---|---|
| **Castor oil** (Neoloid)<br>Pregnancy Category C | *Adults:* PO, 15–60 mL<br>*Children:* 5–15 y: PO, 5–30 mL depending on strength of emulsion<br>*<2 y:* PO, 1.25–7.5 mL depending on strength of emulsion | |
| **Glycerin**<br>**Senna** preparations (Senokot, Black Draught)<br>Pregnancy Category C | *Adults:* Rectal suppository, 3 g<br>Granules, PO, 1 level tsp once or twice daily; geriatric, obstetric, gynecologic clients, PO 0.5 level tsp once or twice daily<br>Syrup, PO, 2–3 tsp once or twice daily; geriatric, obstetric, gynecologic clients, 1–1½ tsp once or twice daily<br>Tablets, PO, 2 tablets once or twice daily; geriatric, obstetric, gynecologic clients, 1 tablet once or twice daily<br>Suppositories, 1 suppository at bedtime<br>*Children <6 y:* rectal suppository 1–1.5 g<br>*Weight >27 kg:* granules, syrup, tablets, suppositories—½ adult dose | |
| *Lubricant Laxative*<br>**Mineral oil** (Agoral Plain, Milkinol, Fleet Mineral Oil Enema)<br>Pregnancy Category C | *Adults:* PO, 15–30 mL at bedtime<br>Rectal enema, 30–60 mL<br>*Children:* >6 y: PO, 5–15 mL at bedtime<br>Rectal enema, 30–60 mL | Lubricates fecal mass and slows colonic absorption of water from the fecal mass |
| *Miscellaneous Laxatives*<br>**Lactulose** (Chronulac, Cephulac)<br>Pregnancy Category B | *Adults:* PO, 15–30 mL daily; maximum dose 60 mL daily<br>Portal system encephalopathy, PO, 30–45 mL 3–4 times daily, adjusted to produce two or three soft stools daily<br>Rectally as retention enema, 300 mL with 700 mL water or normal saline, retained 30–60 min, q4–6h<br>*Infants:* PO, 2.5–10 mL daily in divided doses<br>*Older Children:* PO, 40–90 mL daily in divided doses | Pulls water into intestinal lumen, exerting a laxative effect |
| **Sorbitol**<br>Pregnancy Category C | *Adults:* PO, 30–50 g daily | |

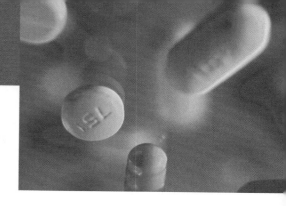

# Drugs Used in Oncologic Disorders

Drugs used in oncologic disorders include those used to kill, damage, or slow the growth of cancer cells and those used to prevent or treat adverse drug effects. Antineoplastic drug therapy, commonly called *chemotherapy*, is a major treatment modality for cancer, along with surgery and radiation therapy.

Some general characteristics of antineoplastic drugs include:

- Most drugs kill malignant cells by interfering with cell replication, with the supply and use of nutrients (eg, amino acids, purines, pyrimidines), or with the genetic materials in the cell nucleus (DNA or RNA).
- The drugs act during the cell's reproductive cycle. Some, called *cell cycle specific*, act mainly during specific phases such as DNA synthesis or formation of the mitotic spindle. Others act during any phase of the cell cycle and are called *cell cycle nonspecific*.
- Cytotoxic drugs are most active against rapidly dividing cells, both normal and malignant. Commonly damaged normal cells are those of the bone marrow, the lining of the gastrointestinal tract, and the hair follicles.
- Each drug dose kills a specific percentage of cells. To achieve a cure, all malignant cells must be killed or reduced to a small number that can be killed by the person's immune system.
- Antineoplastic drugs may induce drug-resistant malignant cells. Mechanisms may include inhibiting drug uptake or activation, increasing the rate of drug inactivation, pumping the drug out of the cell before it can act, increasing cellular repair of DNA damaged by the drugs,

or altering metabolic pathways and target enzymes of the drugs. Mutant cells also may emerge.

- Most cytotoxic antineoplastic drugs are potential teratogens.
- Most antineoplastic drugs are given orally or intravenously; some are given topically, intrathecally, or by instillation into a body cavity.
- A few drugs are available in liposomal preparations. These preparations increase drug concentration in malignant tissues and decrease concentration in normal tissues, thereby increasing effectiveness while decreasing toxicity. For example, liposomal doxorubicin and daunorubicin reduce the drugs' cardiotoxic effects.

Cytotoxic antineoplastic drugs are usually classified in terms of their mechanisms of action (alkylating agents and antimetabolites) or their sources (plant alkaloids, antibiotics). Other drugs used in chemotherapy are immunostimulants (see Chap. 36), hormones, hormone inhibitors, and cytoprotectants.

Current cancer treatment modalities are limited in their ability to distinguish between normal and malignant cells. Cytoprotective agents are used to preferentially protect normal cells, but not malignant cells, from cytotoxic agents. These agents allow for protection from side-effects or toxicities from the cytotoxic agents, allowing for alterations in protocols and improved quality of life for the client.

Commonly used drugs, dosages, and routes of administration for these medications are listed in the following tables.

## Cytotoxic Antineoplastic Drugs

| Generic/Trade Name | Routes and Dosage Ranges* | Clinical Uses | Adverse Effects |
|---|---|---|---|
| *Alkylating Drugs* | | | |
| **NITROGEN MUSTARD DERIVATIVES** | | | |
| **Chlorambucil** (Leukeran) <br> Pregnancy Category D | PO, 0.1–0.2 mg/kg/d for 3–6 wk. Maintenance therapy, 0.03–0.1 mg/kg/d | Chronic lymphocytic leukemia, Hodgkin's and non-Hodgkin's lymphomas | Bone marrow depression, hepatotoxicity, secondary leukemia |
| **Cyclophosphamide** (Cytoxan) <br> Pregnancy Category D | Induction therapy, PO, 1–5 mg/kg/d; IV, 20–40 mg/kg in divided doses over 2–5 days <br> Maintenance therapy, PO, 1–5 mg/kg daily | Hodgkin's disease, non-Hodgkin's lymphomas, leukemias, cancer of breast, lung or ovary, multiple myeloma, neuroblastoma | Bone marrow depression, nausea, vomiting, alopecia, hemorrhagic cystitis, hypersensitivity reactions, secondary leukemia or bladder cancer |
| **Ifosfamide** (Ifex) <br> Pregnancy Category D | IV, 1.2 g/m$^2$/d for 5 consecutive d. Repeat every 3 wk or after white blood cell and platelet counts return to normal after a dose | Germ cell testicular cancer | Bone marrow depression, hemorrhagic cystitis, nausea and vomiting, alopecia, CNS depression, seizures |
| **Melphalan** (Alkeran) <br> Pregnancy Category D | PO, 6 mg/d for 2–3 wk, then 28 drug-free days, then 2 mg daily <br> IV, 16 mg/m$^2$ every 2 wk for 4 doses, then every 4 wk | Multiple myeloma, ovarian cancer | Bone marrow depression, nausea and vomiting, hypersensitivity reactions |
| **NITROSOUREAS** | | | |
| **Carmustine** (BiCNU, Gliadel) <br> Pregnancy Category D | IV, 150–200 mg/m$^2$ every 6 wk <br> Wafer, implanted in brain after tumor resection | Hodgkin's disease, non-Hodgkin's lymphomas, multiple myeloma, brain tumors | Bone marrow depression, nausea, vomiting |
| **Lomustine** (CCNU) <br> Pregnancy Category D | PO, 130 mg/m$^2$ every 6 wk | Hodgkin's disease, brain tumors | Nausea and vomiting, bone marrow depression |
| **PLATINUM COMPOUNDS** | | | |
| **Carboplatin** (Paraplatin) <br> Pregnancy Category D | IV infusion, 360 mg/m$^2$ on day 1 every 4 wk | Palliation of ovarian cancer | Bone marrow depression, nausea and vomiting, nephrotoxicity |
| **Cisplatin** (Platinol) <br> Pregnancy Category D | IV, 100 mg/m$^2$ once every 4 wk | Advanced carcinomas of testes, bladder, ovary | Nausea, vomiting, anaphylaxis, nephrotoxicity, bone marrow depression, ototoxicity |
| **Oxaliplatin** (Eloxatin) <br> Pregnancy Category D | IV infusion, 85 mg/m$^2$ every 2 wk | Advanced colon cancer | Anaphylaxis, anemia, increased risk for bleeding or infection |
| *Antimetabolites* | | | |
| **Capecitabine** (Xeloda) <br> Pregnancy Category D | PO, 1250 mg/m$^2$ q12h for 2 wk, then a rest period of 1 wk, then repeat cycle | Metastatic breast cancer, colorectal cancer | Bone marrow depression, nausea, vomiting, diarrhea, mucositis |
| **Cladribine** (Leustatin) <br> Pregnancy Category D | IV infusion, 0.09 mg/kg/d for 7 consecutive d | Hairy cell leukemia | Bone marrow depression, nausea, vomiting |
| **Cytarabine** (Cytosar-U) <br> Pregnancy Category D | IV infusion, 100 mg/m$^2$/d for 7 d <br> IV, 100 mg/m$^2$ q12h for 7 d | Leukemias of adults and children | Bone marrow depression, nausea, vomiting, anaphylaxis, mucositis, diarrhea |
| **Fludarabine** (Fludara) <br> Pregnancy Category D | IV, 25 mg/m$^2$/d for 5 consecutive d; repeat every 28 d | Chronic lymphocytic leukemia | Bone marrow depression, nausea, vomiting, diarrhea |

*(continued)*

| Generic/Trade Name | Routes and Dosage Ranges* | Clinical Uses | Adverse Effects |
|---|---|---|---|
| **Fluorouracil (5-FU)** (Adrucil, Efudex, Fluoroplex) Pregnancy Category D; X topical | IV, 12 mg/kg/d for 4 d, then 6 mg/kg every other day for 4 doses Topical, apply to skin cancer lesion twice daily for several weeks | Carcinomas of the breast, colon, stomach, and pancreas Solar keratoses, basal cell carcinoma | Bone marrow depression, nausea, vomiting, mucositis Pain, pruritus, burning at site of application |
| **Gemcitabine** (Gemzar) Pregnancy Category D | IV, 1000 mg/m² once weekly up to 7 wk or toxicity, withhold for 1 wk, then once weekly for 3 wk and withhold for 1 wk | Lung and pancreatic cancer | Bone marrow depression, nausea, vomiting, flulike symptoms, skin rash |
| **Mercaptopurine** (Purinethol) Pregnancy Category D | PO, 2.5 mg/kg/d (100–200 mg for average adult) | Acute and chronic leukemias | Bone marrow depression, nausea, vomiting, mucositis |
| **Methotrexate** (MTX) (Rheumatrex) Pregnancy Category X | Acute leukemia in children, induction: PO, IV, 3 mg/m²/d; Maintenance: PO, 30 mg/m² twice weekly Choriocarcinoma: PO, IM, 15 mg/m² daily for 5 d | Leukemias, non-Hodgkin's lymphomas, osteosarcoma, choriocarcinoma of testes, cancers of breast, lung, head and neck | Bone marrow depression, nausea, vomiting, mucositis, diarrhea, fever, alopecia |
| *Antitumor Antibiotics* | | | |
| **Bleomycin** (Blenoxane) Pregnancy Category D | IV, IM, Sub-Q, 0.25–0.5 units/kg once or twice weekly | Squamous cell carcinoma, Hodgkin's and non-Hodgkin's lymphomas, testicular carcinoma | Pulmonary toxicity, mucositis, alopecia, nausea, vomiting, hypersensitivity reactions |
| **Dactinomycin** (Actinomycin D) (Cosmegen) Pregnancy Category C | IV, 15 mcg/kg/d for 5 d and repeated every 2–4 wk | Rhabdomyosarcoma, Wilms' tumor, choriocarcinoma, testicular carcinoma, Ewing's sarcoma | Bone marrow depression, nausea, vomiting Extravasation may lead to tissue necrosis |
| **Daunorubicin conventional** Pregnancy Category D | IV, 25–45 mg/m² daily for 3 d every 3–4 wk | Acute leukemias, lymphomas | Same as doxorubicin, below |
| **Daunorubicin liposomal** (DaunoXome) Pregnancy Category D | IV infusion, 40 mg/m² every 2 wk | AIDS-related Kaposi's sarcoma | Bone marrow depression, nausea, vomiting |
| **Doxorubicin conventional** (Adriamycin) Pregnancy Category D | *Adults:* IV, 60–75 mg/m² every 21 d *Children:* IV, 30 mg/m² daily for 3 d, repeated every 4 wk | Acute leukemias, lymphomas, carcinomas of breast, lung, and ovary | Bone marrow depression, alopecia, mucositis, GI upset, cardiomyopathy Extravasation may lead to tissue necrosis |
| **Doxorubicin liposomal** (Doxil) Pregnancy Category D | IV infusion, 20 mg/m², once every 3 wk | AIDS-related Kaposi's sarcoma | Bone marrow depression, nausea, vomiting, fever, alopecia |
| **Epirubicin** (Ellence) Pregnancy Category D | IV infusion, 120 mg/m² every 3–4 wk | Breast cancer | Cardiotoxicity |
| **Idarubicin** (Idamycin) Pregnancy Category D | IV injection, 12 mg/m²/d for 3 d, with cytarabine | Acute myeloid leukemia | Same as doxorubicin, above |
| **Mitomycin** (Mutamycin) Pregnancy Category D | IV, 20 mg/m² every 6–8 wk | Metastatic carcinomas of stomach and pancreas | Bone marrow depression, nausea, vomiting Extravasation may lead to tissue necrosis |
| **Mitoxantrone** (Novantrone) Pregnancy Category D | IV infusion, 12 mg/m² on days 1–3, for induction of remission in leukemia | Acute nonlymphocytic leukemia, prostate cancer | Bone marrow depression, congestive heart failure, nausea |

*(continued)*

| Generic/Trade Name | Routes and Dosage Ranges* | Clinical Uses | Adverse Effects |
|---|---|---|---|
| **Pentostatin** (Nipent) Pregnancy Category D | IV, 4 mg/m² every other week | Hairy cell leukemia unresponsive to interferon-alpha | Bone marrow depression, hepatotoxicity, nausea, vomiting |
| **Valrubicin** (Valstar) Pregnancy Category C | Intravesically, 800 mg once weekly for 6 wk | Bladder cancer | Dysuria, urgency, frequency, bladder spasms, hematuria |
| *Plant Alkaloids* | | | |
| CAMPTOTHECINS | | | |
| **Irinotecan** (Camptosar) Pregnancy Category D | IV infusion, 125 mg/m² once weekly for 4 wk, then a 2-wk rest period; repeat regimen | Metastatic cancer of colon or rectum | Bone marrow depression, diarrhea |
| **Topotecan** (Hycamtin) Pregnancy Category D | IV infusion, 1.5 mg/m² daily for 5 consecutive days every 21 d | Advanced ovarian cancer, small cell lung cancer | Bone marrow depression, nausea, vomiting, diarrhea |
| PODOPHYLLOTOXINS | | | |
| **Etoposide** (Toposar, VePesid) Pregnancy Category D | IV, 50–100 mg/m²/d on days 1–5, or 100 mg/m²/d on days 1, 3, and 5, every 3–4 wk PO, 2 times the IV dose | Testicular cancer, small cell lung cancer | Bone marrow depression, allergic reactions, nausea, vomiting, alopecia |
| **Teniposide** (Vumon) Pregnancy Category D | IV infusion, 165 mg/m² twice weekly for 8–9 doses | Acute lymphocytic leukemia in children | Same as etoposide, above |
| TAXANES | | | |
| **Docetaxel** (Taxotere) Pregnancy Category D | IV infusion, 60–100 mg/m², every 3 wk | Advanced breast cancer, non–small cell lung cancer | Bone marrow depression, nausea, vomiting, hypersensitivity reactions |
| **Paclitaxel** (Taxol) Pregnancy Category D | IV infusion, 135 mg/m² every 3 wk | Advanced ovarian cancer, advanced breast cancer, non–small cell lung cancer, AIDS-related Kaposi's sarcoma | Bone marrow depression, allergic reactions, hypotension, bradycardia, nausea, vomiting |
| VINCA ALKALOIDS | | | |
| **Vinblastine** (Velban) Pregnancy Category D | *Adults:* IV, 3.7–11.1 mg/m² (average, 5.5–7.4 mg/m²) weekly *Children:* IV, 2.5–7.5 mg/m² weekly | Metastatic testicular carcinoma, Hodgkin's disease | Bone marrow depression, nausea, vomiting Extravasation may lead to tissue necrosis |
| **Vincristine** (Oncovin) Pregnancy Category D | *Adults:* IV, 1.4 mg/m² weekly *Children:* IV, 2 mg/m² weekly | Hodgkin's and other lymphomas, acute leukemia, neuroblastoma, Wilms' tumor | Peripheral neuropathy Extravasation may lead to tissue necrosis |
| **Vinorelbine** (Navelbine) Pregnancy Category D | IV injection, 30 mg/m² once weekly | Non–small cell lung cancer | Bone marrow depression, peripheral neuropathy Extravasation may lead to tissue necrosis |
| *Monoclonal Antibodies* | | | |
| **Gemtuzumab** ozogamicin (Mylotarg) Pregnancy Category D | IV infusion, 9 mg/m², for 2 doses, 14 d apart | Acute myeloid leukemia | Chills, fever, nausea, vomiting, diarrhea |
| **Ibritumomab** tiuxetan (Zevalin) Pregnancy Category D | See literature | Non-Hodgkin's lymphoma, with rituximab | Severe or fatal infusion reaction, severe bone marrow depression |

*(continued)*

## Cytotoxic Antineoplastic Drugs (Continued)

| Generic/Trade Name | Routes and Dosage Ranges* | Clinical Uses | Adverse Effects |
|---|---|---|---|
| **Rituximab** (Rituxan) Pregnancy Category C | IV infusion, 375 mg/m² once weekly for 4 doses | Non-Hodgkin's lymphoma | Hypersensitivity reactions, cardiac dysrhythmias |
| **Trastuzumab** (Herceptin) Pregnancy Category B | IV infusion, 4 mg/kg, then 2 mg/kg once weekly | Metastatic breast cancer | Cardiotoxicity (dyspnea, edema, heart failure) |
| *Miscellaneous Agents* | | | |
| **Asparaginase** (Elspar) Pregnancy Category C | IV, 1000 IU/kg/d for 10 d | Acute lymphocytic leukemia | Hypersensitivity reactions, including anaphylaxis |
| **Hydroxyurea** (Droxia, Mylocel, Hydrea) Pregnancy Category D | PO, 80 mg/kg as a single dose every third day or 20–30 mg/kg as a single dose daily | Chronic myelocytic leukemia, melanoma, ovarian cancer, head and neck cancer | Bone marrow depression, nausea, vomiting, peripheral neuritis |
| **Levamisole** (Ergamisol) Pregnancy Category C | PO, 50 mg q8h for 3 d every 2 wk | Colon cancer, with fluorouracil | Nausea, vomiting, diarrhea |
| **Procarbazine** (Matulane) Pregnancy Category D | PO, 2–4 mg/kg/d for 1 wk, then 4–6 mg/kg/d | Hodgkin's disease | Bone marrow depression, mucositis, CNS depression |
| **Temozolomide** (Temodar) Pregnancy Category D | PO, 150 mg/m² once daily for 5 d, then 200 mg/m² every 28 d | Brain tumors | Bone marrow depression |

*Dosages may vary significantly or change often, according to use in different types of cancer and in different combinations.

## Antineoplastic Hormones and Hormone Inhibitors

| Generic/Trade Name | Routes and Dosage Ranges | Clinical Uses | Adverse Effects |
|---|---|---|---|
| *Antiestrogens* | | | |
| **Fulvestrant** (Faslodex) Pregnancy Category D | IM, 250 mg once monthly (one 5-mL or two 2.5-mL injections) | Advanced breast cancer in postmenopausal women | GI upset, hot flashes, injection site reactions |
| **Tamoxifen** (Nolvadex) Pregnancy Category D | PO, 20 mg once or twice daily | Breast cancer: after surgery or radiation; prophylaxis in high-risk women; and treatment of metastatic disease | Hot flashes, nausea, vomiting, vaginal discharge, risk for endometrial cancer in non-hysterectomized women |
| **Toremifene** (Fareston) Pregnancy Category D | PO, 60 mg once daily | Metastatic breast cancer in postmenopausal women | Hot flashes, nausea, hypercalcemia, tumor flare |
| *Aromatase Inhibitors* | | | |
| **Anastrazole** (Arimidex) Pregnancy Category D | PO, 1 mg once daily | Advanced breast cancer in postmenopausal women | Nausea, hot flashes, edema |
| **Exemestane** (Aromasin) Pregnancy Category D | PO, 25 mg once daily | Advanced breast cancer in postmenopausal women | Hot flashes, nausea, depression, insomnia, anxiety, dyspnea, pain |
| **Letrozole** (Femara) Pregnancy Category D | PO, 2.5 mg once daily | Advanced breast cancer | Nausea, hot flashes |
| **Goserelin** (Zoladex) Pregnancy Category X | Sub-Q implant, 3.6 mg every 28 d or 10.8 mg every 12 wk | Advanced prostatic or breast cancer, endometriosis | Hot flashes, transient increase in bone pain |

*(continued)*

| Generic/Trade Name | Routes and Dosage Ranges | Clinical Uses | Adverse Effects |
|---|---|---|---|
| **Leuprolide** (Eligard, Lupron, Viadur) Pregnancy Category X | Sub-Q, 7.5 mg/month IM, 7.5 mg/mo, 22.5 mg/ 3 mo, or 30 mg/4 mo IM implant, 65 mg/12 mo | Advanced prostatic cancer | Same as for goserelin, above |
| **Triptorelin** (Trelstar LA, Trelstar Depot) Pregnancy Category X | IM, 3.75 mg/28 d or 11.25 mg/ 3 mo | Advanced prostatic cancer | Same as for goserelin and leuprolide, above |

## Cytoprotective Agents

| Generic/Trade Name | Routes and Dosage Ranges | Clinical Uses |
|---|---|---|
| **Amifostine** (Ethyol) Pregnancy Category C | Reduction of cisplatin-induced renal toxicity | IV infusion 910 mg/m$^2$ once daily within 30 min of starting chemotherapy |
| **Dexrazoxane** (Zinecard) Pregnancy Category C | Reduction of doxorubicin-induced cardio-myopathy in women with metastatic breast cancer who have received a cumulative dose of 300 mg/m$^2$ and need additional doxorubicin | IV 10 times the amount of doxorubicin (eg, dexrazoxane 500 mg/m$^2$ per dox-orubicin 50 mg/m$^2$), then give doxoru-bicin within 30 min of completing dexrazoxane dose |
| **Erythropoietin** (Epogen, Procrit) Pregnancy Category C | Treatment of chemotherapy-induced anemia | SC 150–300 units/kg 3 times weekly, adjusted to maintain desired hematocrit |
| **Filgrastim** (Neupogen) Pregnancy Category C | Treatment of chemotherapy-induced neutropenia | SC, IV 5 mcg/kg/d, at least 24 h after cyto-toxic chemotherapy, up to 2 wk or an absolute neutrophil count of 10,000/mm$^3$ |
| **Leucovorin** (Wellcovorin) Pregnancy Category C | "Rescue" after high-dose methotrexate for osteosarcoma Advanced colorectal cancer, with 5-fluorouracil | "Rescue," PO, IV, IM 15 mg q6h for 10 doses, starting 24 h after methotrexate begun Colorectal cancer, IV 20 mg/m$^2$ or 200 mg/m$^2$, followed by 5-fluorouracil, daily for 5 d, repeated every 28 d |
| **Mesna** (Mesnex) Pregnancy Category B | Prevention of ifosfamide-induced hemor-rhagic cystitis | IV, 20% of ifosfamide dose for 3 doses (at time of ifosfamide dose, then 4 h and 8 h after ifosfamide dose) |
| **Oprelvekin** (Neumega) Pregnancy Category C | Prevention of thrombocytopenia | Sub-Q, 50 mcg/kg once daily, usually for 10–21 d |
| **Sargramostim** (Leukine) Pregnancy Category C | Myeloid reconstitution after bone marrow transplantation; to decrease chemotherapy-induced neutropenia | IV infusion, 250 mcg/m$^2$/d until absolute neutrophil count is >1500/mm$^3$ for 3 d, up to 42 d |

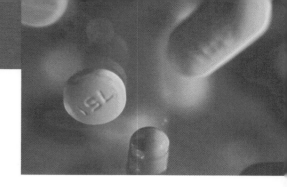

# Potential Drug Interactions With Grapefruit Juice

Grapefruit juice affects the metabolism of several drugs that undergo metabolism by the cytochrome P450 system (particularly at isoenzymes CYP1A2, and CYP3A4) in the intestinal wall or liver. Grapefruit and its juice contain various bioflavonoids that alters the metabolism of these drugs by binding to the isoenzyme and interfering with first-pass metabolism. Other mechanisms have also been suggested, including the potential that grapefruit juice may also inhibit P-glycoprotein, a drug transporter in intestinal mucosa. Additionally, Seville orange juice is now thought to have similar effects as grapefruit juice on medications. The research designs of studies that have demonstrated potential drug interactions with grapefruit juice are varied; findings and indications of the drugs are outlined in the following table.

| Drug | Findings | Consequences |
|---|---|---|
| Albendazole (Albenza) | Increased serum concentration | Potential for increased side effects |
| Amiodarone (Cordarone) | Increased bioavailability and serum concentration | Potential for dysrhythmias |
| Benzodiazepines, oral<br>**Diazepam** (Valium)<br>**Midazolam** (Versed)<br>**Triazolam** (Halcion) | Increased serum concentration | Potential for increased sedation |
| **Budesonide** (Encort EC) | Increased oral absorption | Potential for hypercorticism |
| **Buspirone** (BuSpar) | Increased absorption and serum concentration | Action of drug does not seem significantly affected, although ingestion of large amounts of grapefruit juice should be avoided |
| **Caffeine** | Decreased drug clearance | Potential for increased side effects, including insomnia and nervousness |
| Calcium Channel Blockers<br>**Amlodipine** (Norvasc)<br>**Diltiazem** (Cardizem)<br>**Felodipine** (Plendil, Renedil)<br>**Nicardipine** (Cardene)<br>**Nifedipine** (Adalat, Procardia)<br>**Nimodipine** (Nimotop)<br>**Nisoldipine** (Sular)<br>**Verapamil** (Calan) | Increased serum concentration | Varies with each individual; potential for signs of toxicity |
| **Carbamazepine** (Tegretol) | Increased peak and trough serum concentrations | Potential increased signs of toxicity |
| **Carvedilol** (Coreg) | Increased bioavailability | Significance unknown |
| **Clomipramine** (Anafranil) | Increased serum concentration | Potential for increased side effects |
| **Cyclosporine** (Sandimmune) | Increased serum concentrations | Potential for increased signs of toxicity |

*(continued)*

| Drug | Findings | Consequences |
|---|---|---|
| **Erythromycin** (E-Mycin, others) | Increased serum peak concentration | No significant unfavorable effects; increased antibiotic concentrations may be beneficial for treatment of susceptible infections |
| **Estrogens** | Increased absorption and serum concentrations of 17-beta-estradiol and ethinyl-estradiol | Significance unknown |
| **Fexofenadine** (Allegra) | Possible decreased oral absorption and reduced drug levels | Significance unknown |
| HMG-CoA Reductase Inhibitors (Statins): **Atorvastatin** (Lipitor) **Lovastatin** (Mevacor) **Simvastatin** (Zocor) | Increased absorption and serum concentration | Potential for increased toxicity |
| **Itraconazole** (Sporanox) | Impaired absorption | Significance unknown |
| **Methylprednisolone** (Medrol) | Increased serum concentration with oral administration | Significance small except in sensitive clients |
| **Quinidine** (Quinaglute, Quinidex) | Delayed absorption and increased time to peak concentration | Minor but possibly significant changes in the metabolism |
| **Sildenafil** (Viagra) | Altered metabolism | Increased time to effectiveness |

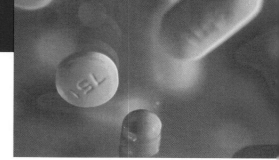

# Index

Note: Page numbers followed by f, t, and b indicate figures, tables, and boxed material, respectively.

## A

AACAP. *See* American Academy of Child and Adolescent Psychiatry
AACT. *See* American Academy of Clinical Toxicology
abacavir (Ziagen), 572t
  administration of, 578b
  adverse effects of, 580b
  in children, 564b
abacavir/lamivudine/zidovudine (Trizivir), 572t
Abbokinase. *See* urokinase
abbreviations, in medication orders, 39, 40t
abciximab (ReoPro), 821t, 827
abdominal fat, 463
Abelcet. *See* amphotericin B lipid complex
abortifacients, 403, 404t, 407b
absence seizures, 195
absolute refractory period, 730b
absorption, of drugs, 11
acarbose (Precose), 375t
  administration of, 382b, 386b
  adverse effects of, 387b
  drug interactions of, 389b
  in older adults, 368b
  in pregnancy, 398b
  sulfonylurea plus, 384
Accolate. *See* zafirlukast
AccuNeb. *See* albuterol
Accupril. *See* quinapril
Accutane. *See* isotretinoin
acebutolol (Sectral), 288t
  as antidysrhythmic drug, 739t, 745
  as antihypertensive drug, 790t
  duration of action of, 291
  intrinsic sympathomimetic activity of, 291
  receptor selectivity of, 291
ACE inhibitors. *See* angiotensin-converting enzyme inhibitors
Aceon. *See* perindopril
acetaminophen (Tylenol), 102, 107t, 114–115
  for cancer pain, 122
  in children, 112b
  client teaching guidelines for, 118b–119b
  in combination products, 85t, 910t, 911t

hepatotoxicity of, 23
indications for, 104–105
mechanism of action of, 102–103
for migraine, 119
for rheumatoid arthritis, 122
therapeutic serum drug concentrations of, 886t
therapy guidelines for, 114–115
toxicity of, 25t, 115
Acetasol. *See* acetic acid, propylene glycol diacetate, and hydrocortisone
acetazolamide (Diamox, Diamox Sequels), 903t
acetic acid derivatives, 111–112
acetic acid, propylene glycol diacetate, and hydrocortisone (Acetasol), 907t
acetylcholine, 299b
  and Alzheimer's disease, 299
  cholinergic drugs and, 299
  and myasthenia gravis, 299
acetylcysteine (Mucomyst), 910t
  for acetaminophen poisoning, 25t, 115
acetyltransferase, and drug actions, 19
Achromycin. *See* tetracycline
acid-base balance, 883t
acid-peptic disorders, 852–853
  drug therapy for, 853–862, 856t–857t (*See also* antacids)
    adverse effects of, 866b
    age-related considerations for, 854b
    client teaching guidelines for, 864b
    dietary and herbal supplements, 862
    drug interactions of, 867b
    *Helicobacter pylori* agents, 858
    histamine-2 receptor antagonists, 856t, 858–860
    in home care, 854b
    nursing actions for, 865b–867b
    nursing process for, 863b
    prostaglandin, 862
    proton pump inhibitors, 857t, 860–861
    sucralfate, 862
    therapeutic effects of, 866b
acid reflux, 853
Aciphex. *See* rabeprazole
acitretin (Soriatane), 900t
Aclovate. *See* alclometasone

acquired immunity, 610b
  active, 610b
    vaccines and toxoids for, 613t–619t
  passive, 610b
    immune serums for, 619t–621t
acquired immunodeficiency syndrome (AIDS). *See also* human immuno-deficiency virus infection
  corticosteroids for, 660
  drug therapy for, 428t, 572t–574t, 574–576
  in pregnancy, 401
ACTH. *See* corticotropin
Acthar Gel. *See* corticotropin
ActHIB. *See* *Haemophilus B* (Hib) conjugate vaccine
Actifed Cold & Allergy, 910t
Actinex. *See* masoprocol
Actinomycin D. *See* dactinomycin
Actiq. *See* fentanyl
Activase. *See* alteplase
activated charcoal, 27
activated partial thromboplastin time (aPTT), 824
active immunity
  acquired, 610b
    vaccines and toxoids for, 613t–619t
  agents for, 611–612
Activelle, 419t
active transport, of drugs, 10
Actonel. *See* risedronate
Actos. *See* pioglitazone
Acular. *See* ketorolac
acute gastritis, 853b
Acute Pain Management Guideline Panel, 84b
acute renal failure (ARF)
  and drug therapy, 71
  nutritional support products for, 456–457
  and pharmacokinetics, 21t–22t
  sulfonamides and, 542
acyclovir (Zovirax)
  adverse effects of, 580b
  for dermatologic conditions, 898t
  drug interactions of, 580b
  for herpesvirus infections, 569–574, 570t
Adalat. *See* nifedipine
adapalene (Differin), 900t

# Student Resource CD-ROM for Foundations of Clinical Drug Therapy

**This unique resource provides you with the tools needed to succeed!**

## Self-Study Dosage Calculation Questions and Dosage Calculator

Nearly 100 dosage calculation problems allow you to practice the techniques learned in Chapter 3: Dosage Calculations. The questions are organized by chapter, with questions included for all drug chapters. A handy dosage calculator provides an additional resource.

## NCLEX Review Questions

The CD-ROM includes 594 questions, giving you extensive opportunity to practice for the NCLEX. Each question provides a rationale, reinforcing key concepts and facilitating understanding. Additional NCLEX-style questions are found at the end of each chapter in the text.

## Animations

Clear animations help you understand underlying physiologic concepts behind pharmacology, including:
- The Cell Cycle
- Absorption
- Distribution
- Drug Binding
- Excretion
- Intramuscular Medication
- Intravenous Medication

## Preventing Medication Errors Video

This comprehensive video provides a tutorial, reviewing all aspects of medication error prevention. Topics include:
- Interpreting Medication Orders
- Transcribing Medication Orders
- Reviewing Medication Orders
- Preparing Medications
- Administering Medications
- Assessing Patient Response
- Procedural Safeguards
- Reporting Medication Errors

## Drug Monographs

The resource provides monographs for the top 100 most commonly prescribed drugs. Gain easy access to essential information, including indications, dosages, contraindications, pharmacokinetics, and nursing considerations.

## Patient Teaching Resource

Access and print out patient teaching guidelines for almost 800 drugs. The sheets allow you to customize the teaching handouts, filling in the patient's name and indication for use. Instructions for use teach safe self-administration.